Current Practice of Medicine

Volume 2

Current Practice of Medicine

Series Editor
ROGER C. BONE, MD
President
The Medical College of Ohio
Toledo, Ohio

V DERMATOLOGY

Jeffrey P. Callen, MD

Professor of Medicine and Chief, Division of Dermatology
Department of Medicine
University of Louisville School of Medicine
Louisville, Kentucky

VI RHEUMATOLOGY

Daniel J. McCarty, MD

Director, Arthritis Institute
Department of Medicine
Medical College of Wisconsin
Milwaukee, Wisconsin

VII ALLERGY AND IMMUNOLOGY

Phillip L. Lieberman, MD

Clinical Professor, Division of Allergy and Immunology
Department of Medicine and Pediatrics
University of Tennessee, Memphis, College of Medicine
Memphis, Tennessee

VIII INFECTIOUS DISEASES

Harold C. Neu, MD

Professor of Medicine and
  Pharmacology
Department of Medicine
Columbia University College of
  Physicians and Surgeons
New York, New York

Robert H. Rubin, MD

Associate Professor of Medicine
Harvard Medical School;
Director, Center for Experimental
  Pharmacology and Therapeutics
Harvard-MIT Division of Health Sciences
  and Technology;
Chief of Transplantation Infectious Diseases
Massachusetts General Hospital
Boston, Massachusetts

CHURCHILL LIVINGSTONE, INC. • CURRENT MEDICINE, INC.

Distributed Worldwide by
CHURCHILL LIVINGSTONE, INC.
650 Avenue of the Americas
New York, NY 10003

DEVELOPED BY CURRENT MEDICINE, INC.
PHILADELPHIA

MANAGING EDITOR: . . . . Lori J. Bainbridge
PROJECT EDITOR: . . . . Peter Stevenson
DEVELOPMENTAL EDITORS: . . . . Jim Slade, Karen Nevers, Barbara Cohen-Kligerman
EDITORIAL ASSISTANTS: . . . . Charlene French, Danielle Shaw
INDEXER . . . . Maria Coughlin
ART DIRECTOR: . . . . Paul Fennessy
LAYOUT: . . . . Jerilyn Bockorick, Lisa Caro, Robert LeBrun, Patrick Whelan
COVER DESIGN: . . . . Jerilyn Bockorick
ILLUSTRATION DIRECTOR: . . . . Ann Saydlowski
ILLUSTRATOR: . . . . Gary Welch
PRODUCTION MANAGER: . . . . David Myers
ASSISTANT PRODUCTION MANAGER: . . . . Lori Holland
TYPESETTING MANAGER: . . . . Colleen Ward

Printed in Hong Kong by Paramount Printing Group Limited.

ISBN: 0-443-07894-7 (*series*)
ISBN: 0-443-07891-2 (*volume*)
ISSN: 1079-980X
5 4 3 2 1

Although every effort has been made to ensure that drug doses and other information are presented accurately in this publication, the ultimate responsibility rests with the prescribing physician. Neither the publishers nor the authors can be held responsible for errors or for any consequences arising from the use of information contained herein. Products mentioned in this publication should be used in accordance with the prescribing information prepared by the manufacturers. No claims or endorsements are made for any drug or compound at present under clinical investigation.

Contributors

V. DERMATOLOGY

SECTION EDITOR

JEFFREY P. CALLEN, MD
Professor of Medicine;
Chief, Division of Dermatology
Department of Medicine
University of Louisville School of Medicine
Louisville, Kentucky

JAMIE A. ALPERT, MD
Assistant Professor
Division of Dermatology
Department of Medicine
University of Vermont College of Medicine
Burlington, Vermont

GRANT J. ANHALT, MD
Professor and Vice Chairman
Department of Dermatology and Pathology
Johns Hopkins University School of
 Medicine
Baltimore, Maryland

KENNETH A. ARNDT, MD
Professor of Dermatology
Harvard Medical School;
Dermatologist-in-Chief
Beth Israel Hospital
Boston, Massachusetts

RAYMOND L. BARNHILL, MD
Associate Professor of Pathology
Harvard Medical School;
Director, Dermatopathology Division
Brigham and Women's and Children's
 Hospital;
Attending Dermatologist
Brigham and Women's Hospital
Boston, Massachusetts

JEFFREY D. BERNHARD, MD
Professor of Medicine
Director, Dermatology Division
University of Massachusetts Medical Center
Worcester, Massachusetts

RICHARD A.F. CLARK, MD
Professor and Chairman
Department of Dermatology
State University of New York at Stony
 Brook Health Sciences Center
Stony Brook, New York

PHILIP P. COHEN, MD
Assistant Professor
Departments of Dermatology and
 Pathology
University of Texas Medical School at
 Houston;
Section of Dermatology
Department of Medical Specialties
University of Texas M.D. Anderson Cancer
 Center
Houston, Texas

BONI E. ELEWSKI, MD
Associate Professor
Department of Dermatology
Case Western Reserve University School of
 Medicine
Cleveland, Ohio

VINCENT FALANGA, MD, FACP
Associate Professor of Dermatology and
 Medicine
Department of Dermatology and
 Cutaneous Surgery
University of Miami School of Medicine
Miami, Florida

FRANKLIN P. FLOWERS, MD
Professor and Chairman
Division of Dermatology
Department of Medicine
University of Florida College of Medicine
Gainesville, Florida

STEVEN M. HACKER, MD
Assistant Clinical Professor
Division of Dermatology and Cutaneous
 Surgery
Department of Medicine
University of Florida College of Medicine
Gainesville, Florida

TISSA R. HATA, MD
Chief Resident
Department of Dermatology
Harvard Medical School
Boston, Massachusetts

TERRENCE HOPKINS, MD
Clinical Assistant Professor
Department of Dermatology
State University of New York at Stony Brook
 Health Sciences Center School of Medicine
Stony Brook, New York

JOSEPH L. JORIZZO, MD
Professor and Chairman
Department of Dermatology
Bowman Gray School of Medicine of Wake
 Forest University
Winston-Salem, North Carolina

SETH G. KATES, MD
Instructor, Division of Dermatology
University of Massachusetts Medical School;
Chairman, Department of Dermatology
Fallon Clinic
Worcester, Massachusetts

FRANCISCO A. KERDEL, BSc, MBBS
Associate Professor of Dermatology
Department of Dermatology and
 Cutaneous Surgery
University of Miami School of Medicine
Miami, Florida

PAUL A. KRUSINSKI, MD
Professor of Medicine;
Director, Division of Dermatology
University of Vermont School of Medicine
Burlington, Vermont

CAROL L. KULP-SHORTEN, MD
Assistant Clinical Professor of Medicine
University of Louisville School of Medicine
Louisville, Kentucky

GRACE S. LIANG-FEDERMAN, MD
Department of Dermatology and
 Cutaneous Surgery
University of Miami School of Medicine
Miami, Florida

HENRY W. LIM, MD
Professor of Dermatology
The Ronald O. Perelman Department of
 Dermatology
New York University School of Medicine;
Chief of Staff
Veterans Affairs Medical Center
New York, New York

DONALD P. LOOKINGBILL, MD
Professor of Medicine;
Chief, Division of Surgery
The Milton S. Hershey Medical Center
Pennsylvania State University College of
 Medicine
Hershey, Pennsylvania

NICHOLAS J. LOWE, MD
Clinical Professor of Dermatology
University of California, Los Angeles,
    School of Medicine
Los Angeles, California

LYNN MCKINLEY-GRANT, MD
Department of Dermatology
Washington Hospital Center;
Chief, Division of Dermatology
Veterans Affairs Medical Center
Washington, DC

RONALD L. MOY, MD
Assistant Clinical Professor
Division of Dermatology
University of California, Los Angeles,
    School of Medicine
Los Angeles, California

PAUL I. OH, MD, FRCPC
Lecturer
Sunnybrook Health Science Center
University of Toronto Faculty of Medicine
Toronto, Ontario, Canada

JEFFREY B. PARDES, MD
Wound Healing Fellow
Department of Dermatology and
    Cutaneous Surgery
University of Miami School of Medicine
Miami, Florida

DANIEL RIVLIN, MD
Director of Mohs Microsurgery Unit
Mount Sinai Medical Center
Miami Beach, Florida

LISA M. SEUNG, MD
Resident
Section of Dermatology
Department of Medicine
University of Chicago Pritzker School of
    Medicine
Chicago, Illinois

NEIL H. SHEAR, MD, FRCPC, FACP
Director, Clinical Pharmacology;
Deputy Director, Dermatology;
Director, Drug Safety Research Group;
University of Toronto Faculty of Medicine;
Associate Professor of Medicine,
    Pharmacology, Pediatrics and Pharmacy
Sunnybrook Health Science Centre
Toronto, Ontario, Canada

KAREN SIMPSON, MD
Research Fellow
Department of Dermatology
University of California, Irvine, College of
    Medicine
Irvine, California

ARTHUR J. SOBER, MD
Associate Professor of Dermatology
Harvard Medical School;
Associate Chief of Dermatology
Massachusetts General Hospital
Boston, Massachusetts

YARDY TSE, MD
Fellow, Dermatologic and Mohs
    Micrographic Surgery
The Ronald O. Perelman Department of
    Dermatology
New York University Medical Center
New York, New York

GUY F. WEBSTER, MD, PHD
Associate Professor
Department of Dermatology and Internal
    Medicine
Jefferson Medical College of Thomas
    Jefferson University
Philadelphia, Pennsylvania

VICTORIA P. WERTH, MD
Assistant Professor
Department of Dermatology
University of Pennsylvania School of
    Medicine;
Chief, Division of Dermatology
Veterans Affairs Hospital
Philadelphia, Pennsylvania

VI. RHEUMATOLOGY

SECTION EDITOR
DANIEL J. MCCARTY, MD
Director, Arthritis Institute
Department of Medicine
Medical College of Wisconsin
Milwaukee, Wisconsin

ALAN J. BRIDGES, MD
Associate Professor
Department of Medicine
University of Wisconsin Medical School;
Chief, Rheumatology
William S. Middleton Memorial Veterans
    Hospital
Madison, Wisconsin

**W. WATSON BUCHANAN, MD, FACP,
FACR (HON)**
Emeritus Professor
Department of Medicine
McMaster University School of Medicine
Hamilton, Ontario, Canada

JUAN J. CANOSO, MD
Adjunct Professor
Department of Medicine
Tufts University School of Medicine

Boston, Massachusetts;
American British Cowdray Hospital
Mexico City, Mexico

JAMES T. CASSIDY, MD
Professor of Medicine
Department of Child Health
University of Missouri Health Sciences
    Center
Columbia, Missouri

JAMES J. CASTLES, MD
Professor and Executive Associate Dean
Department of Internal Medicine
University of California, Davis, School of
    Medicine
Davis, California

CATHERINE CORMIER, MD
Assistant Professor of Medicine
Hopital Cochin
Department of Rheumatology
Paris, France

ROSE S. FIFE, MD
Professor of Medicine;
Assistant Dean for Research
Department of Medicine, Biochemistry,
    and Molecular Biology
Indiana University School of Medicine
Indianapolis, Indiana

ELLEN M. GINZLER, MD, MPH
Professor of Medicine
Department of Medicine
State University of New York Health
    Science Center at Brooklyn College of
    Medicine
Brooklyn, New York

DON L. GOLDENBERG, MD
Professor of Medicine
Department of Medicine
Tufts University School of Medicine
Boston, Massachusetts;
Newton-Wellesley Hospital
Newton, Massachusetts

NORTIN M. HADLER, MD
Professor of Medicine
Department of Medicine and Microbiology
University of North Carolina at Chapel Hill
    School of Medicine;
Attending Rheumatologist
University of North Carolina Hospital
Chapel Hill, North Carolina

BASHAR KAHALEH, MD
Professor of Medicine
Department of Medicine;
Medical Specialties Clinic
Medical College of Ohio
Toledo, Ohio

MUHAMMAD A. KHAN, MD, FRCP
Professor of Medicine
Case Western Reserve School of Medicine
Cleveland, Ohio

ROBERT W. LIGHTFOOT, JR., MD
Professor of Medicine
Department of Internal Medicine
University of Kentucky College of Medicine
Lexington, Kentucky

MONICA LUCHI, MD
Clinical Assistant in Medicine
Division of Rheumatology
Department of Medicine
University of Pennsylvania School of
  Medicine
Philadelphia, Pennsylvania

CHARLES J. MENKES, MD
Professor of Medicine
Department of Rheumatology
Universite Rene Descartes;
Hopital Cochin
Paris, France

DAVID W. PUETT, MD
Carolina Arthritis Associates
Wilmington, North Carolina

ANN K. ROSENTHAL, MD
Assistant Professor
Department of Medicine
Medical College of Wisconsin
Milwaukee, Wisconsin

LAWRENCE M. RYAN, MD
Professor of Medicine
Department of Medicine
Medical College of Wisconsin
Milwaukee, Wisconsin

H. RALPH SCHUMACHER, JR., MD
Professor of Medicine
Department of Medicine
University of Pennsylvania School of
  Medicine;
Veterans Affairs Medical Center
Philadelphia, Pennsylvania

FRANK R. SCHMID, MD
Professor of Medicine
Department of Medicine
Northwestern University Medical School;
Northwestern Medical Faculty Foundation
Chicago, Illinois

JOHN S. SERGENT, MD
Professor of Medicine
Department of Medicine
Vanderbilt University School of Medicine;

Chief, Medical Service
Department of Medicine
St. Thomas Hospital
Nashville, Tennessee

JEFFREY L. TANJI, MD
Associate Professor
Family Practice and Exercise Science
University of California, Davis, School of
  Medicine
Davis, California

DAVID E. TRENTHAM, MD
Associate Professor of Medicine
Department of Medicine
Harvard Medical School;
Physician and Chief
Division of Rheumatology
Beth Israel Hospital
Boston, Massachusetts

JENNIE H. UTSINGER
Research Assistant in Rheumatology
Chestnut Hill Hospital
Philadelphia, Pennsylvania

PETER D. UTSINGER, MD
Chief of Rheumatology
Chestnut Hill Hospital
Philadelphia, Pennsylvania

JOAN M. VON FELDT, MD
Assistant Professor of Medicine
Department of Medicine
University of Pennsylvania School of
  Medicine
Philadelphia, Pennsylvania

VICTORIA P. WERTH, MD
Assistant Professor
Department of Dermatology
University of Pennsylvania School of
  Medicine
Philadelphia, Pennsylvania

R. GEOFFREY WILBER, MD
Assistant Professor of Orthopedics
Case Western Reserve Hospital;
Chief, Spine Surgery
MetroHealth Medical Center;
The Cleveland Clinic Foundation
Cleveland, Ohio

ROBERT L. WORTMANN, MD
Professor and Chairman
Department of Medicine
East Carolina University School of
  Medicine;
Pitt County Hospital
Greenville, North Carolina

VII. ALLERGY AND IMMUNOLOGY

SECTION EDITOR
PHILLIP L. LIEBERMAN, MD
Clinical Professor
Division of Allergy and Immunology
Department of Medicine and Pediatrics
University of Tennessee, Memphis, College
  of Medicine
Memphis, Tennessee;

EMIL J. BARDANA, JR., MD
Professor of Medicine
Department of Medicine
Oregon Health Sciences University School
  of Medicine
Portland, Oregon

LEONARD BIELORY, MD
Associate Professor
Division of Pediatrics and Ophthalmology
Department of Medicine
New Jersey Medical School
Newark, New Jersey

MICHAEL S. BLAISS, MD
Associate Professor of Pediatrics;
Assistant Professor of Medicine
Department of Medicine
University of Tennessee, Memphis, College
  of Medicine;
Le Bonheur Children's Medical Center
Memphis, Tennessee

JOHN E. ERFFMEYER, MD
Section of Allergy and Clinical
  Immunology
Department of Medicine
Ochsner Clinic of Baton Rouge
Baton Rouge, Louisiana

JORDAN N. FINK, MD
Professor of Medicine
Department of Medicine
Medical College of Wisconsin
Milwaukee, Wisconsin

ROGER W. FOX, MD
Associate Professor
Department of Internal Medicine and
  Public Health
University of South Florida College of
  Medicine;
Asthma and Allergy Associates of Tampa
  Bay
Tampa, Florida

HENRY G. HERROD, MD
Le Bonheur Professor of Pediatrics;
Vice Chairman, Department of Pediatrics
University of Tennessee, Memphis, College
of Medicine;
Le Bonheur Children's Medical Center
Memphis, Tennessee

JAMES HOLBERT, MD, PhD, MBA
Clinical Associate Professor
Department of Medicine and Pediatrics
University of Tennessee, Memphis, College
of Medicine;
Hematology Consultants
Memphis, Tennessee

DENNIS K. LEDFORD, MD
Associate Professor
Department of Medicine
University of South Florida College of
Medicine;
Asthma and Allergy Associates of Tampa Bay
Tampa, Florida

RICHARD F. LOCKEY, MD
Professor of Medicine, Pediatrics, and
Public Health;
Director, Division of Allergy and
Immunology
University of South Florida College of
Medicine;
Chief, Allergy and Immunology Section
James A. Haley Veterans' Hospital
Tampa, Florida

GAILEN D. MARSHALL, JR., MD, PhD
Associate Professor of Medicine and
Pathology
Department of Internal Medicine
University of Texas Medical School at
Houston;
Service Chief, Division of Allergy and
Clinical Immunology
Hermann Hospital
Houston, Texas

DEAN D. METCALFE, MD
Section Head
Allergic Diseases Section
National Institutes of Health Clinical Center
Bethesda, Maryland

RAYMOND G. SLAVIN, MD
Professor of Medicine
Department of Internal Medicine
St. Louis University School of Medicine
St. Louis, Missouri

SHELDON L. SPECTOR, MD
Clinical Professor
Department of Medicine
University of California, Los Angeles,
School of Medicine;

Allergy Research Foundation, Inc.
Los Angeles, California

VIII. INFECTIOUS DISEASES

SECTION EDITORS
HAROLD C. NEU, MD,
Professor of Medicine and Pharmacology
Department of Medicine
Columbia University College of Physicians
and Surgeons
New York, New York

ROBERT H. RUBIN, MD
Associate Professor of Medicine
Harvard Medical School;
Director, Center for Experimental
Pharmacology and Therapeutics
Harvard-MIT Division of Health Sciences
and Technology;
Chief of Transplantation Infectious
Diseases
Massachusetts General Hospital
Boston, Massachusetts

JAMES S. BALDASSARRE, MD
Assistant Medical Director;
Director, Anti-infectives
Robert Wood Pharmaceutical Research
Institute
Spring House, Pennsylvania

NESLI BASGOZ, MD
Instructor in Medicine
Harvard Medical School;
Assistant Physician
Infectious Disease and Transplant Units
Massachusetts General Hospital
Boston, Massachusetts

BYRON E. BATTEIGER, MD
Associate Professor
Department of Medicine
Indiana University School of Medicine
Indianapolis, Indiana

STEVEN L. BERK, MD
Professor of Medicine
Department of Medicine
East Tennessee State University
James H. Quillen College of Medicine
Johnson City, Tennessee

GERALD P. BODEY, AB, MD
Professor of Medicine
Department of Medicine;
Chairman, Department of Medical
Specialties
University of Texas M.D. Anderson Cancer
Center
Houston, Texas

ROGER C. BONE, MD
President
Medical College of Ohio
Toledo, Ohio

ANTHONY W. CHOW, MD, FRCPC, FACP
Professor of Medicine
Division of Infectious Diseases
Department of Medicine
University of British Columbia Faculty of
Medicine;
Division of Infectious Diseases
Vancouver Hospital Health Sciences
Center
Vancouver, British Columbia, Canada

BRANDON CLINT, MD
Clinical Assistant Professor
Department of Internal Medicine
Baylor College of Medicine
Houston, Texas;
Sid Peterson Memorial Hospital
Kerrville, Texas

RAYMOND J. DATTWYLER, MD
Associate Professor of Medicine
Division of Allergy
Department of Medicine
State University of New York at Stony
Brook Health Sciences Center
Stony Brook, New York

JAY DOBKIN, MD
Associate Professor of Clinical Medicine
Department of Medicine
Columbia University College of Physicians
and Surgeons
New York, New York

MARY T. FLOOD, MD, PhD
Professor of Clinical Medicine
Division of Infectious Diseases
Department of Medicine
Columbia University College of Physicians
and Surgeons;
Presbyterian Hospital
New York, New York

PIERCE GARDNER, MD
Professor of Medicine
Department of Medicine;
Associate Dean for Academic Affairs
State University of New York at Stony
Brook Health Sciences Center
Stony Brook, New York

LAYNE O. GENTRY, MD
Infectious Disease Section
St. Luke's Episcopal Hospital
Houston, Texas

Larry J. Goodman, MD
Associate Professor
Department of Internal Medicine
Rush Medical College of Rush University
Chicago, Illinois

Marie R. Griffin, MD, MPH
Professor of Medicine
Department of Preventive Medicine
Vanderbilt University School of Medicine
Nashville, Tennessee

Douglas A. Holt, MD
Associate Professor of Medicine
Division of Infectious Diseases and Tropical
  Medicine
Department of Internal Medicine
University of South Florida College of
  Medicine;
Infectious Disease Center
Tampa General Hospital
Tampa, Florida

Richard Allen Johnson, MD
Clinical Instructor
Department of Dermatology
Harvard Medical School;
New England Deaconess Hospital
Boston, Massachusetts

Evelyn Kim, BA
University of South Florida College of
  Medicine;
Infectious Disease Center
Tampa General Hospital
Tampa, Florida

Matthew E. Levison, MD
Professor of Medicine
Department of Medicine
Medical College of Pennsylvania
Philadelphia, Pennsylvania

George M. Lordi, MD
Associate Professor
Department of Medicine
University of Medicine and Dentistry of
  New Jersey
Newark, New Jersey

Benjamin J. Luft, MD
Associate Professor of Medicine
Department of Medicine
State University of New York at Stony
  Brook Health Sciences Center
Stony Brook, New York

Wafeeq A. Mahmood, MD, FRCPC
Senior Fellow
Division of Infectious Diseases
Department of Medicine

University of British Columbia Faculty of
  Medicine;
Fellow
Division of Infectious Diseases
Vancouver Hospital Health Sciences
  Center
Vancouver, British Columbia, Canada

Harish Moorjani, MD
Clinical Instructor in Medicine
Department of Medicine
New York Medical College
Valhalla, New York

Michael H. Picard, MD
Assistant Professor
Department of Medicine
Harvard Medical School;
Associate Director, Cardiac Ultrasound
Massachusetts General Hospital
Boston, Massachusetts

Lee B. Reichman, MD, MPH
Professor of Medicine
Division of Preventive Medicine and
  Community Health
Department of Medicine
New Jersey Medical School
Newark, New Jersey

Kenneth V.I. Rolston, MD
Associate Professor
Department of Medical Specialties
University of Texas M.D. Anderson Cancer
  Center
Houston, Texas

Carole A. Sable, MD
Assistant Professor
Department of Internal Medicine
University of Virginia
Charlottesville, Virginia

Jay P. Sanford, MD
Professor of Internal Medicine
Department of Internal Medicine
University of Texas Southwestern Medical
  Center;
Dean Emeritus
Uniformed Services University of the
  Health Sciences
Dallas, Texas

George A. Sarosi, MD
Professor of Medicine
Department of Medicine
Stanford University School of Medicine
Stanford, California;
Department of Medicine
Santa Clara Valley Medical Center
San Jose, California

William Schaffner, MD
Professor of Medicine
Division of Infectious Diseases
Departments of Preventive Medicine and
  Medicine
Vanderbilt University School of Medicine
Nashville, Tennessee

Brian E. Scully, MD, BCH, MA
Associate Professor of Clinical Medicine
Department of Medicine
Columbia University College of Physicians
  and Surgeons;
Columbia Presbyterian Medical Center
New York, New York

John T. Sinnott IV, MA, MD
Professor of Medicine
Division of Infectious Diseases, Surgery,
  and Tropical Medicine
Department of Internal Medicine
University of South Florida College of
  Medicine;
Tampa General Hospital
Tampa, Florida

Jack D. Sobel, MD
Professor of Medicine
Department of Internal Medicine
Wayne State University School of
  Medicine;
The Detroit Medical Center
Detroit, Michigan

Kurt B. Stevenson, MD
(private practice)
Boise, Idaho

Gordon M. Trenholme, MD
James R. Lowenstine Professor of Medicine
Rush Medical College of Rush University;
Rush-Presbyterian-St. Luke's Medical
  Center
Chicago, Illinois

Brian Wispelwey, MS, MD
Asssociate Professor of Medicine
Division of Infectious Diseases
Department of Medicine;
Director, Infectious Diseases Clinic
University of Virginia School of Medicine
Charlottesville, Virginia

Foreword

During the past few decades, the practice of medicine has evolved from an "art form" applied at a leisurely pace to a "science" demanding rapid and accurate diagnosis with quick and effective therapies. This textbook, *Current Practice of Medicine*, is designed to offer the primary care physician a ready reference for the practice of such a science. Its chapters are condensed but comprehensive, and are greatly enhanced by the liberal application of figures and tables. Key concepts are presented in a form that can be assimilated and applied directly to the management of a patient. Perhaps the most remarkable advancement in clinical practice has been the ever-increasing armamentarium of methods for imaging the organs of pathology, either directly by endoscopy, or indirectly by computed tomography or magnetic resonance imaging. The images obtained from such tools are represented plentifully in this textbook. In this era of rapid scientific developments, it is essential for a textbook to be up to date. To circumvent the lead time required to produce a work of this magnitude, each of the four volumes of *Current Practice of Medicine* will be updated regularly. For ease of use, a companion CD-ROM version is planned, allowing the text to be linked to MEDLINE for extensive evaluation of cited references. *Current Practice of Medicine* is a modern textbook well suited for the practicing internist of today. No doubt it will serve its purpose well.

Tadataka Yamada, MD
Ann Arbor, Michigan

Series Preface

Medical knowledge is said to double approximately every five years. Complicated diagnostic tools, emerging pharmaceuticals, and innovative treatment protocols continually challenge today's physician. To provide the highest quality health care to patients, the general practitioner must keep pace with the burgeoning medical literature.

Today's physicians have access to many good sources of information, including continuing education courses, journals and textbooks, and interactive computer software. However, until now, a complete medical information source that is always within an arm's reach has been lacking. As Editor of the *Current Practice of Medicine* series, I am proud to introduce a comprehensive medical reference source that will satisfy the substantial informational needs of the general practitioner. The series is designed to provide the general practitioner with easily accessible, in-depth commentary on contemporary medicine.

Four bound volumes, each filled with hundreds of photographs, tables, and detailed medical illustrations, cover every aspect of internal medicine:

- Allergy and Immunology
- Cardiology
- Dermatology
- Endocrinology and Metabolic Disease
- Gastroenterology
- General Internal Medicine
- Hematology
- Hepatology
- Infectious Diseases
- Nephrology
- Neurology
- Oncology
- Psychiatry
- Pulmonary and Critical Care Medicine
- Rheumatology

The Section Editors have asked the premier specialists of their respective fields to contribute up-to-date and reliable chapters specifically intended for the general practitioner.

Current Practice of Medicine is an ambitious series. It is a valuable addition to the reference libraries of all physicians who deal with the complicated mysteries presented by patients. I am proud to oversee the important and essential information that these volumes contribute to medical knowledge.

I would like to thank all of the contributing authors and the Section Editors, whose efforts are central to the great success of this series. I also offer my sincere thanks to Abe Krieger, President of Current Medicine; Lori J. Bainbridge, Managing Editor; Pete Stevenson and Jim Slade, Developmental Editors; and everyone on the staff of Current Medicine who helped to make this project possible.

Roger C. Bone, MD
Toledo, Ohio

Series Contents

Volume Contents

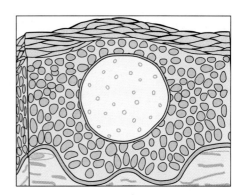

DERMATOLOGY

V

The Dermatology section of *Current Practice of Medicine* presents common and complex areas of the field in a format that makes diagnosis and treatment decisions easier for the general practitioner. Chapter topics ranging from common bacterial infections of the skin to life-threatening dermatoses are presented. Easy-to-follow algorithms and tables offer a practical approach to diagnostic evaluation and therapeutic interventions. Color photographs are an important part of any dermatologic text, and this section is liberally illustrated.

As Section Editor, I recruited recognized specialists in the field to write these chapters. Many of these authors have published extensively on their assigned topics, several have written texts, and many are department chairs or division heads at their respective medical schools and hospitals.

I believe that the practical approach of this text will increase the knowledge base of generalists and specialists alike, ultimately improving patient care.

Section Editor
Jeffrey P. Callen

Principles of Diagnosis
Donald P. Lookingbill

1

> ### *Key Points*
> - Dermatologic diagnosis is based upon the history of the patient, skin examination, and laboratory testing as necessary.
> - In new patients the complete skin surface should be examined.
> - Dermatologic disorders are divided into growths and rashes.
> - Growths are subdivided into epidermal, pigmented or dermal processes.
> - Rashes are first separated according to the presence or absence of epidermal involvement, and then further subdivided according to the nature of the epidermal change or the type of dermal inflammation.
> - The configuration and distribution of rashes may serve as secondary diagnostic considerations.
> - If a clinical diagnosis cannot be made, a dermatologist should be consulted.

To diagnose a skin disease, the physician must 1) take a history, 2) carefully examine the skin, and 3) occasionally perform laboratory testing. In the skin examination, particular attention is given to identifying the nature of the primary lesion. By correlating the clinical appearance of the primary lesion with the responsible pathologic change, an algorithmic approach to diagnosis can be developed. Two algorithms have been developed: one for growths (Fig. 1-1) and one for rashes (Fig. 1-2). In diagnosing rashes, it is sometimes also helpful to note the way in which the lesions are arranged and their distribution on the body surface. Laboratory tests are less often employed in dermatologic diagnosis than in many other fields of medicine, but a few simple skin tests are invaluable in diagnosing some skin conditions.

HISTORY

For many skin disorders, a brief history will suffice. For nearly every patient, the physician should obtain at least three pieces of historical information: 1) the duration and progression of the problem, 2) associated symptoms, and 3) prior treatment. For skin disorders, the most important symptom is itch. In regard to therapy, careful and often repeated inquiry is necessary to elicit all the topical and systemic medications that the patient may have used. This obviously includes over-the-counter as well as prescription products.

Following the brief preliminary history-taking, the physical examination should be performed. After this, additional history will sometimes be needed. For example, if during the physical examination the physician notes a butterfly rash suggestive of cutaneous lupus erythematosus, the patient should be asked about other signs or symptoms associated with systemic lupus erythematosus.

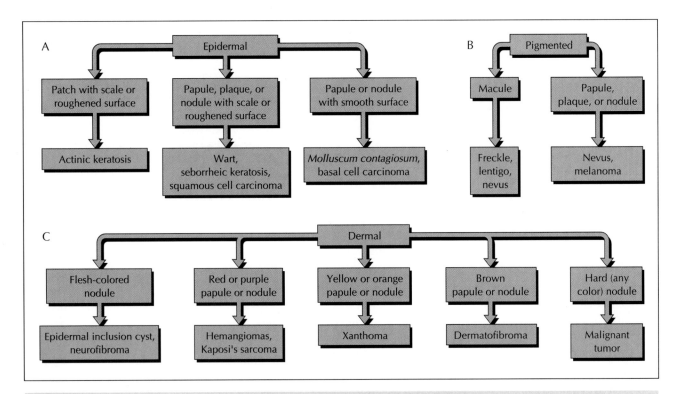

FIGURE 1-1 Algorithm of (*panel A*) epidermal, (*panel B*) pigmented and (*panel C*) dermal growths.

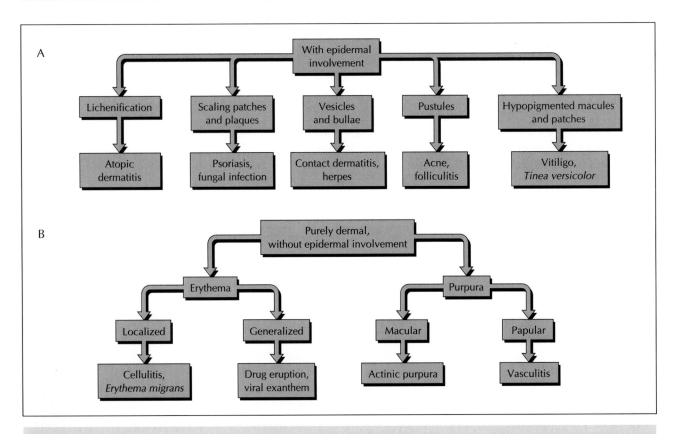

FIGURE 1-2 Algorithm of rashes (*panel A*) with epidermal, and (*panel B*) with purely dermal involvement.

If the physical examination suggests a diagnosis of contact dermatitis, the patient should be questioned regarding exposures to possible contact allergens. Because the nature of a responsible environmental allergen is not always obvious, this type of history-taking is often painstaking and can tax the skills of even the most seasoned dermatologic detective [1•].

PHYSICAL EXAMINATION

For new patients, a complete skin examination is strongly recommended. The reasons for this are twofold: 1) the physician may discover that a rash involves more areas than the patient realized (or admitted) and this can help in making the diagnosis; and 2) an incidental important growth might be found, for example, an early melanoma, detection of which could be lifesaving. In two studies that determined the frequency of finding an incidental skin cancer from a complete examination, the yield in the first was 1.9%, and in the second, 3.4% [2,3]. One of the cancers detected in the first study was Kaposi's sarcoma, and this represented the initial finding that led to a diagnosis of AIDS in that patient.

Environment

To properly examine a patient's skin, the patient should be disrobed, gowned, and examined under adequate light. Ideally, this should include bright overhead lighting, as well as a movable incandescent light for bright local illumination. A penlight is particularly helpful for "sidelighting" lesions in order to determine whether they are flat or elevated. A Wood's light is a black light that has been used in the past to diagnose *tinea capitis*. The Wood's light is not useful for diagnosing fungal infection in any other body location, and in recent years even most of the cases of *tinea capitis* are of the type that do not fluoresce with Wood's light. Wood's light can be helpful, however, in accentuating pigment changes in the skin (*eg*, hypopigmented spots in patients of light complexion).

Examination

Inspection of skin lesions can sometimes be enhanced with the use of a hand lens, but for the diagnosis of most skin lesions magnification is not required. *Palpation* of skin lesions, however, is almost always a useful maneuver. With palpation, the physician can determine the texture and consistency of the skin lesions. For example, if a nodule feels hard, the physician should suspect the possibility of malignancy. Even in these days of AIDS, gloves need not be worn for palpation of dry skin lesions. Gloves should be worn for examining exudative, mucosal, and genital lesions.

In addition to examining the skin, the physician should look at the nails and the mouth, where irregularities may be detected that will aid in the dermatologic diagnosis (*eg*, oral hairy leukoplakia on the sides of the tongue strongly suggests a diagnosis of AIDS).

TERMINOLOGY OF SKIN LESIONS

In determining a dermatologic diagnosis, the physician must first be prepared to describe what is seen. Dermatologic vocabulary terms are used to describe the morphology of the primary lesion (Table 1-1). Proceeding from description to diagnosis, the physician will find it helpful to employ clinical pathologic considerations. An algorithmic approach can then be used (*eg*, it is critical to distinguish a vesicle from a papule because the differential diagnosis for each of these is entirely different). Similarly, erythema must be distinguished from purpura; this distinction is made by determining whether or not the redness is blanchable. As a

TABLE 1-1 TERMINOLOGY OF SKIN LESIONS	
Lesion	**Appearance**
Macule	Flat with color (*eg*, red, brown)
Patch	Flat with color and surface change (*eg*, scale)
Papule	Elevated <0.5 cm in diameter
Plaque	Elevated >0.5 cm in diameter, but without depth
Nodule	Elevated *and* indurated, >0.5 cm in diameter and depth
Cyst	A nodule filled with fluid or semisolid content
Vesicle	A small blister, filled with visible clear fluid, <0.5 cm
Bullae	Same as vesicle but >0.5 cm
Pustule	Same as vesicle except fluid is yellow
Wheal	Edematuous plaque (hive)
Erosion	Shallow sore from partial denudation of the epidermis
Ulcer	Deeper wound with loss of all of the epidermis and part or all of dermis
Descriptive terms	
Colors	
Erythema	Blanchable redness from dilated blood vessels
Purpura	Nonblanchable, deep red or purple color from extravasated blood
Hyperpigmented	Increased brown pigment, usually melanin
Hypopigmented	Whiter than normal
Surface change	
Crust	Dried serum, pus or blood on surface of skin (scab)
Scale	White or whitish flakes on surface of skin from thickened stratum corneum
Lichenification	Thickened skin with accentuated surface markings

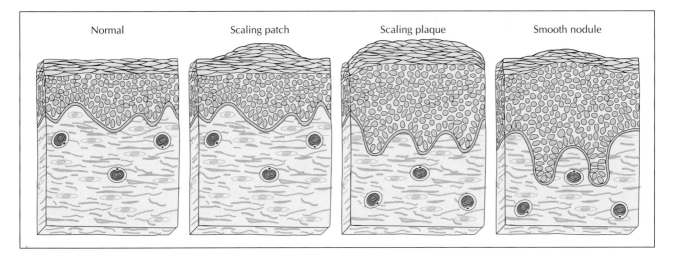

| Normal | Scaling patch | Scaling plaque | Smooth nodule |

FIGURE 1-3 Epidermal growths. These growths arise from thickening of the stratum corneum and/or the epidermis.

final example, crust and scale must be distinguished from each other. A crust represents dried blood or serum on the surface of the skin, and hence indicates the preexistence of a vesicle, bulla, or pustule. Scale, on the other hand, represents thickened stratum corneum and suggests an entirely different differential diagnosis.

ALGORITHMIC APPROACH TO DIAGNOSIS

It is useful to divide dermatologic disorders into growths and rashes [4•]. This is often the way patients describe their complaint (*eg*, "I'm concerned about this bump on my skin," or "I have developed this itchy rash").

Growths

Growths can be subdivided into those that arise from the epidermis, those that are pigmented, and those that are derived from processes confined to the dermis (Fig. 1-1).

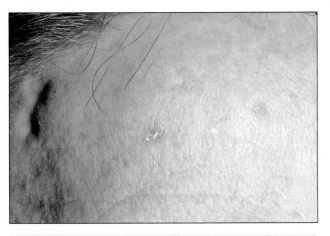

FIGURE 1-4 Actinic keratosis. Epidermal growth appearing as a (often subtle) scaling patch.

The clinicopathologic correlation for epidermal growths is demonstrated in Figure 1-3, and illustrated with the examples in Figures 1-4 through 1-6. The clinicopathologic correlation for pigmented growths is illustrated in Figure 1-7, and exemplified by Figures 1-8 and 1-9. Dermal growths represent proliferation of cellular elements in the dermis (Fig. 1-10), and examples of such growths are shown in Figures 1-11 through 1-15. Most dermal growths appear as nodules in the skin. If a nodule cannot be clinically diagnosed, a biopsy should be done to rule out malignancy.

Rashes

The algorithmic approach for the diagnosis of rashes is shown in Figure 1-2. Rashes are inflammatory processes, so by definition there is vascular involvement, and this therefore always involves the dermis, as there are no blood vessels in the epidermis. The physician must first decide whether there is also epidermal involvement. The possible types of epidermal involvement are depicted in Figure 1-16 with specific examples shown in Figures 1-17 through 1-21. Correctly identifying the type of epidermal involvement will lead to selection of the proper differential diagnosis and ultimately the correct final diagnosis of a rash. If, for example, the physician mistakes crust for scale, the chances of determining a correct final diagnosis are very remote.

If a rash has no surface change, then it is described as purely dermal (Fig. 1-22). For these rashes, the physician must determine whether the redness from the inflammation is blanchable. Erythema represents blanchable redness (Fig. 1-23). Common causes for these types of rashes are listed in Figure 1-2. Purpura represents extravasated blood in the dermis. (Figs. 1-24 and 1-25). If purpura is elevated, it is termed palpable purpura, an important finding that indicates necrotizing vasculitis in the skin.

The algorithmic approaches place emphasis on correctly describing and identifying the primary process affecting the skin in terms of its morphology.

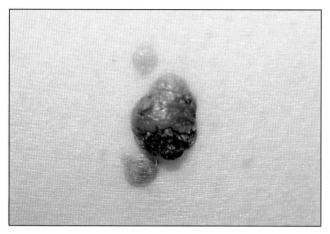

FIGURE 1-5 Seborrheic keratosis. Epidermal growth appearing as a plaque with scale, a rough surface, or both.

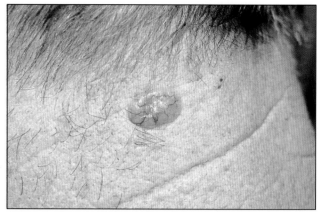

FIGURE 1-6 Basal cell carcinoma. Epidermal growth appearing as a smooth, "pearly" nodule. (*From* Lookingbill and Marks [4•]; with permission.)

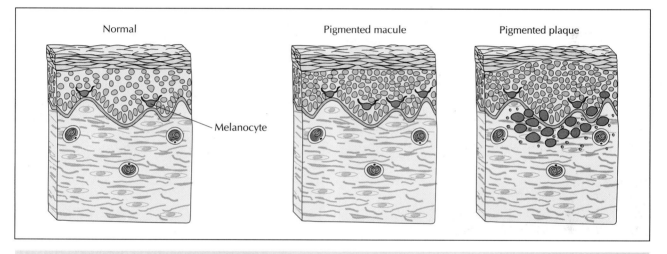

Normal | Pigmented macule | Pigmented plaque

Melanocyte

FIGURE 1-7 Pigmented growths. These growths are due to increased pigment with or without an increase in pigment-producing cells.

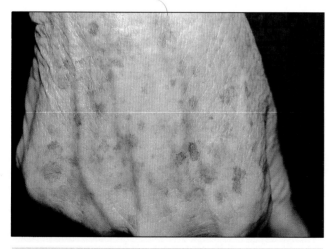

FIGURE 1-8 Lentigines (liver spots). Pigmented growths appearing as macules. (*From* Lookingbill and Marks [4•]; with permission.)

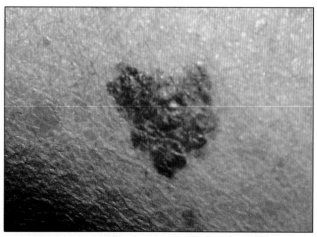

FIGURE 1-9 Melanoma. Pigmented growth appearing as plaque.

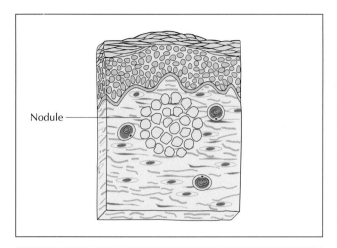

FIGURE 1-10 Dermal growths. These nodules result from proliferation of cells in the dermis.

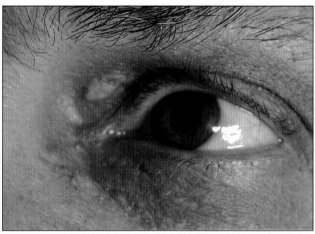

FIGURE 1-11 Epidermal inclusion cyst. Dermal growth appearing as a flesh-colored nodule resulting from an epidermal-lined, keratin-containing cyst in the dermis.

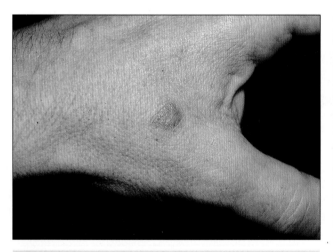

FIGURE 1-12 Kaposi's sarcoma. Dermal growth appearing as a purple nodule that results from a proliferation of vascular elements in the dermis.

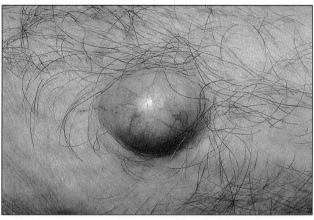

FIGURE 1-13 Xanthelasma. Dermal growth appearing as a yellow plaque derived from a collection of lipid-laden cells in the dermis.

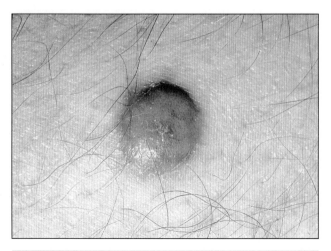

FIGURE 1-14 Dermatofibroma. Dermal growth due to increased number of fibroblasts in the dermis. The pigment, however, is epidermal.

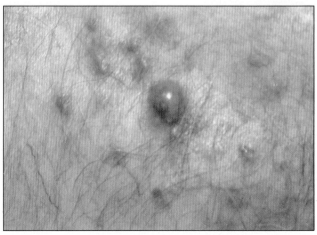

FIGURE 1-15 Metastatic adenocarcinoma. Dermal growth forming a hard nodule from malignant cells that have aggregated in the dermis.

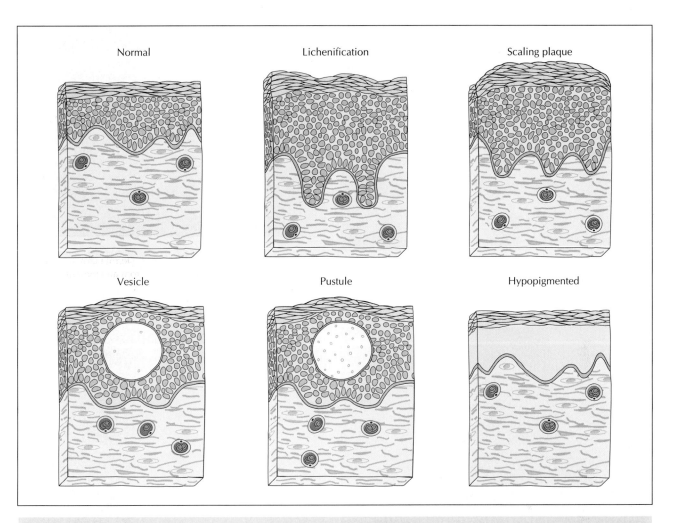

Normal

Lichenification

Scaling plaque

Vesicle

Pustule

Hypopigmented

FIGURE 1-16 Rashes with epidermal involvement. These rashes are characterized by epidermal thickening (lichenification), scaling, disruption (vesicles and pustules), or hypopigmentation.

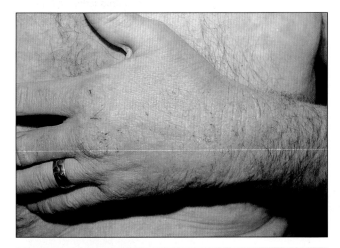

FIGURE 1-17 Atopic dermatis. Rash with epidermal involvement—lichenification.

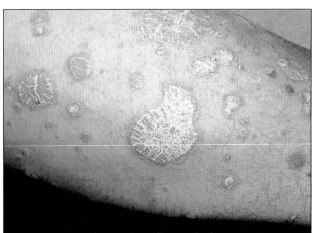

FIGURE 1-18 Psoriasis. Rash with epidermal involvement—scaling plaques.

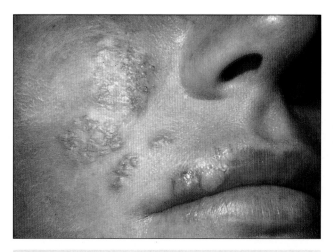

FIGURE 1-19 Herpes simplex. Rash with epidermal involvement—vesicles.

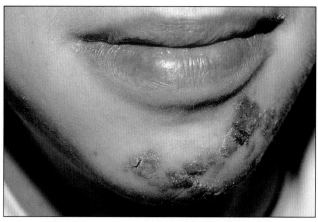

FIGURE 1-20 Impetigo. Rash with epidermal involvement—pustules. The pustules have ruptured and dried to form honey-colored crusts.

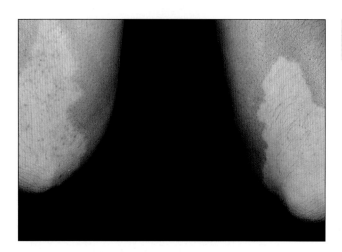

FIGURE 1-21 Vitiligo. Rash with epidermal involvement—hypopigmentation.

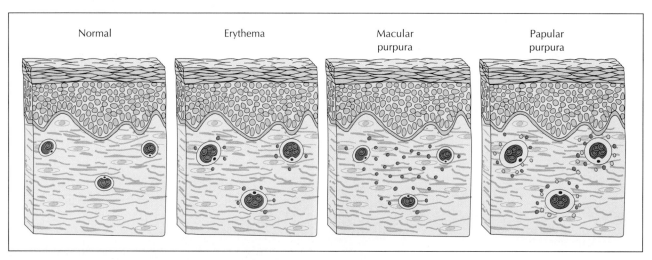

FIGURE 1-22 Rashes, purely dermal. These rashes have no epidermal involvement. They are characterized by dermal vascular changes resulting in erythema (blanchable redness) or purpura (purple that is not blanchable). Noninflammatory purpura is macular; inflammatory purpura is papular (palpable).

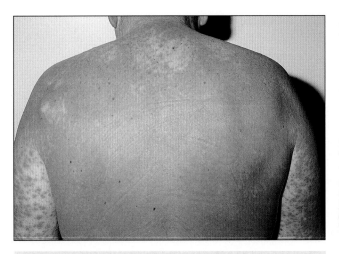

FIGURE 1-23 Drug eruption. Purely dermal rash character-ized by erythematous macules and papules, confluent and generalized.

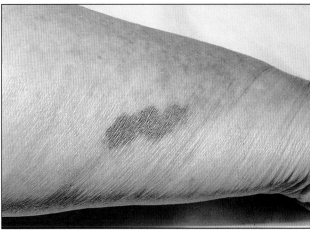

FIGURE 1-24 Actinic purpura. Purely dermal rash from non-inflammatory extravasation of blood from fragile blood vessels. (*From* Lookingbill and Marks [4•]; with permission.)

CONFIGURATION AND DISTRIBUTION OF RASHES

Occasionally, additional diagnostic information can be obtained for rashes if the lesions are arranged in a special way or distributed in particular locations (Table 1-2, Figs. 1-26 and 1-27). As is shown in these common configura-tions, when vesicles appear in streaks, a contact dermatitis is virtually always the cause. Streaks of papules can be seen in patients with psoriasis or lichen planus.

The distribution of a rash can sometimes help with the diagnosis (*eg*, scaling plaques in psoriasis commonly occur on the scalp, elbows, knees, and intergluteal cleft, and scabies frequently involves the finger webs and genital areas, but rarely involves the head).

LABORATORY TESTS

For the majority of patients with skin disease, laboratory tests are not needed. In some circumstances, however, dermatologic testing is invaluable [5]. The tests most frequently employed are office microscopic examinations and skin biopsies. Patch tests, which are also useful, are done by dermatologists (*see* When to Refer section).

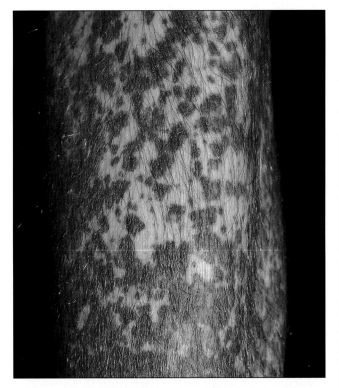

FIGURE 1-25 Necrotizing vasculitis. Purely dermal rash due to inflammatory necrosis of dermal blood vessels, resulting in palpable purpura.

TABLE 1-2 RASHES ASSOCIATED WITH SPECIFIC CONFIGURATIONS	
Configuration	**Disease**
Vesicles	
Linear	Contact dermatitis
Grouped	Herpes simplex
Grouped and dermatomal	Herpes zoster
Papules, scaling	
Linear	Psoriasis
	Lichen planus
Papules, nonscaling	
Grouped	Insect bites
Annular scaling patches and plaques	*Tinea corporis*

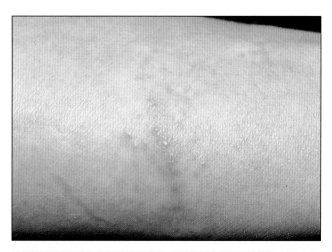

FIGURE 1-26 Vesicles in linear configuration. Streaks of vesicles signify a dermatitis to an external contactant, for example poison ivy.

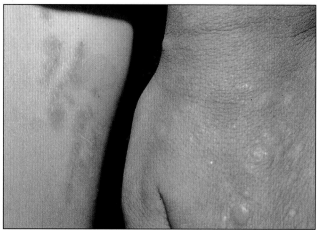

FIGURE 1-27 Koebner phenomenon. In psoriasis and lichen planus (*shown here*), external trauma such as scratching may precipitate streaks of papules.

Office Microscopic Examination

For dermatologic diagnosis, the microscope is most frequently used for examining potassium hydroxide preparations. For scaling rashes, if the diagnosis is uncertain, the physician should follow the admonition that "if it scales, scrape it." A #15 scalpel blade is used to scrape scale from the edge of a lesion onto a glass slide, to which one drop of 10% or 20% potassium hydroxide is applied, covered with a coverslip, gently heated, blotted, and microscopically examined under low power and low illumination. Suspicious elements are examined under high power to confirm whether or not they represent fungal hyphae. The finding of even one definite hypha is diagnostic for cutaneous fungal infection.

Other microscopic examinations sometimes employed for dermatologic diagnosis include the Gram stain, Tzanck preparation for diagnosis of herpes infections, and scabies scrapings. For a scabies scraping, a #15 scalpel blade is moistened with oil, and a suspicious lesion (preferably a burrow) is vigorously scraped at right angles to the skin. The material is transferred to a drop of oil on a glass slide, covered with the coverslip, and examined for presence of mites, eggs, or mite feces.

Skin Biopsy

Skin biopsies are sometimes necessary to determine the diagnosis of a growth or rash. Since the skin is an external organ, a biopsy is a simple procedure. Two common methods for performing a skin biopsy are with shave or punch. For either procedure, the skin is first prepped with an antiseptic and numbed with an injection of xylocaine. A shave biopsy can be used for diagnosing a superficial process, while a punch biopsy is needed to reach the depth of a nodular growth or deep inflammatory process. Biopsies of growths are usually diagnostic, while biopsy results from rashes may often be nonspecific. Accordingly, a physician performing a biopsy of a rash, should provide the pathologist with a meaningful differential diagnosis and also be prepared to place the pathology report into a clinicopathologic correlation context. If the clinician seeing the patient is unequipped to provide the forgoing, a random biopsy of an undiagnosed rash is unlikely to be helpful to that physician. A dermatologist should be consulted instead.

WHEN TO REFER

Referral to a dermatologist is recommended when the primary physician is unable to make a diagnosis, or not equipped for or not successful with therapy. A dermatologist will also be needed if patch testing is indicated.

Patch testing, an invaluable method for determining allergens that might be responsible for contact dermatitis, is done almost exclusively by dermatologists and requires the necessary materials and careful attention to detail. Because patch testing is used for the detection of delayed hypersensitivity to specific allergens, the method differs from that of scratch testing, which detects immediate hypersensitivity reactions to systemic (inhaled and ingested) allergens. In patch testing, the materials are placed on the skin under a patch for 48 hours, at which point the patches are removed and an initial reading is taken. A second reading is taken at 96 hours, and any positive results must be interpreted in light of the patient's history: that is, it must be determined whether a positive result is relevant to the patient's dermatitis [6].

REFERENCES AND RECOMMENDED READING

Recently published papers of particular interest have been highlighted as:

• Of interest

1.• Marks JG, DeLeo VA: *Contact and Occupational Dermatology.* St. Louis: Mosby Yearbook; 1992.

2. Lookingbill DP: Yield from a complete skin examination: findings in 1157 new dermatology patients. *J Am Acad Dermatol* 1988, 18:31–37.

3. Lee G, Massa MC, Welykyj S, *et al.*: Yield from total skin examination and effectiveness of skin cancer awareness program. Findings in 874 new dermatology patients. *Cancer* 1991, 67:202–205.

4.• Lookingbill DP, Marks JGM: *Principles of Dermatology*, edn 2. Philadelphia: WB Saunders; 1993.

5. McBurney EI: Diagnostic dermatologic methods. *Ped Clin North Am* 1983, 30:419–434.

6. Adams RM: Patch testing—a recapitulation. *J Am Acad Dermatol* 1981, 5:629–643.

Common Bacterial Infections of the Skin

Steven M. Hacker
Franklin P. Flowers

2

> ### Key Points
> - One of the most important mechanisms of prevention of cutaneous infection is an intact stratum corneum.
> - The most common cutaneous infections tend to be caused by gram-positive cocci such as *Staphylococcus aureus*.
> - Diagnosis of cutaneous infections is based on characteristic clinical presentation and history. It is confirmed by Gram stain and culture.
> - The therapeutic approach to cutaneous infection may involve local measures, systemic measures, or both.
> - Local therapy should always include good basic skin hygiene with antibacterial soaps and topical antibiotics.
> - Systemic therapy should be based on antibiotic sensitivity for the causative organisms.

Resident and transient flora harmlessly colonize the skin; their numbers and distribution varying with site, age, climate, underlying disease, and medication. By contrast, pathogenic organisms are normally prevented from invading and colonizing the skin by an intact stratum corneum, rapid cell turnover, skin surface lipids, and skin surface pH. Moreover, normal skin flora elaborate protein-complex antibiotics in the presence of potential pathogens [1].

Impetigo, folliculitis, furuncles, and other skin infections are almost all caused by β-hemolytic organisms—either group A streptococci or *Staphylococcus aureus*. Less common infections are caused by gram-negative microbes and by *Pseudomonas aeruginosa*.

IMPETIGO

Impetigo occurs in a vesiculo-pustular form with thick golden crusts and in a bullous form (Table 2-1). Although it is seen in all age groups, it is one of the most common skin infections in children. Impetigo may spread rapidly when left untreated, and it may take several weeks before spontaneous healing occurs.

Diagnosis

The diagnosis of impetigo is based on clinical presentation with laboratory confirmation. Nonbullous impetigo begins as superficial vesicles that may become pustular or develop a honey-colored crust (Fig. 2-1). These crusts can be easily removed, and doing so leaves a smooth, red, moist surface that may produce fresh exudate. At times, a halo of erythema surrounds the lesion. Typically, the lesions

TABLE 2-1 TYPES OF IMPETIGO

Type	Characteristic lesion	Most common site	Most common causative organism	Treatment
Nonbullous impetigo (*impetigo contagiosa*)	Honey-colored crusting at site of previous vesicle or pustule	Legs then arms, face, and trunk	*Staphylococcus aureus* group A β-hemolytic streptococcus	If mild, topical antibiotics and good hygiene; if severe, systemic antibiotics
Bullous impetigo	Bulla, and ruptured bulla that leave an inflamed red base with thin varnish-like crust	Face	Group II *S. aureus*, usually plaque type 71	Systemic antibiotics
Ecthyma	Thick crust that when removed reveals a superficial ulceration; scars may occur	Lower legs	Group A β-hemolytic streptococcus	If mild, removal of crust followed by topical antibiotic; if severe, systemic antibiotics

are not painful but on occasion may itch, especially those that are preceded by a bug bite. Nonbullous impetigo commonly occurs on such exposed surfaces as the extremities and the face where minor trauma, insect bites, contact dermatitis, or abrasions may occur.

Laboratory evaluation includes a Gram stain and culture of an early lesion or a base of a crust. A Gram stain reveals gram-positive cocci. A bacterial culture yields *S. aureus*, streptococci, or both.

A serious complication of nonbullous impetigo is acute glomerulonephritis (AGN). It is most often associated with the nephrotigenic strains of streptococci (types 49, 55, 57, 60 and strand M-type 2). The incidence of AGN with impetigo varies from 2% to 15% depending upon the strain of streptococcus. It is a complication most commonly seen in children under 6 years old. The prognosis is better for children than adults. Treatment of the impetigo does not alter the risk for the development of AGN. There is no evidence suggesting that bullous impetigo is associated with the development of AGN. Other disorders associated with

streptococcal skin infections include scarlet fever, lymphangitis, and transient postinflammatory pigmentary changes. Rheumatic fever has not been reported following nonbullous impetigo.

Bullous impetigo classically represents a toxin-induced lesion that remains nonpurulent. It is unusual to find bullous lesions that are secondarily infected by streptococci or other bacteria. This may be a result of the production of bacteriocins produced by group II *S. aureus*. Clinically, the lesions of bullous impetigo begin as small vesicles which quickly enlarge to form bullae (Fig. 2-2). The bullae will usually rupture within 24 to 48 hours and leave a thin varnish-like brown to black crust. Bullous impetigo frequently begins on nontraumatized skin of the buttocks, perineum, trunk, or face. However, these lesions may be found anywhere on the body. They are shallow lesions that are rarely associated with regional lymphadenopathy. The group II strains of *S. aureus* are also associated with neonatal bullous impetigo, staphylococcal scalded skin syndrome, and staphylococcal scarlet fever.

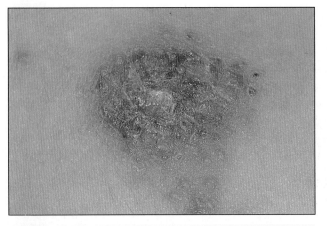

FIGURE 2-1 Nonbullous impetigo (note the honey-colored crusting).

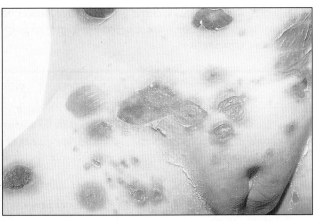

FIGURE 2-2 Bullous impetigo.

		TABLE 2-2 TOPICAL ANTIBIOTICS USED FOR SKIN INFECTIONS		
Agent	**Dose**	**Duration**		**Indication**
Bacitracin ointment	bid to tid	2–3 wk, or 1 wk after lesion has healed		Impetigo, ecthyma
Mupirocin ointment				
Neomycin-bacitracin-polymyxin B				
Erythromycin 2%	bid	2–3 wk or 1 wk after lesion has healed		Folliculitis

bid—twice daily; tid—three times daily.

Treatment

Topical therapy should be reserved for those cases where only a few lesions are present (Table 2-2). It would be impractical to treat dozens of lesions topically when systemic therapy would be equally efficacious and probably provide better compliance. Also, a patient using topical therapy should be able to demonstrate reasonably good hygiene and reliability in applying the medication. Some disadvantages of topical therapy are slower rates of healing, continued development of new lesions, inability to eradicate streptococci concomitantly present in the respiratory tract, and practical difficulties in applying medication for numerous lesions. Topical therapy is not effective in bullous impetigo.

Probably the two most effective topical therapies for nonbullous impetigo are mupirocin and neomycin-bacitracin-polymyxin B [2]. Mupirocin is highly effective against all species of staphylococci, including methicillin-resistant *S. aureus* and most species of *Streptococcus pyogenes* [3]. It is ineffective against most gram-positive bacilli, anaerobes, and aerobic gram-negative bacilli. It is as efficacious as oral erythromycin for the treatment of impetigo [4•].

Neomycin is active against staphylococci but less so against streptococci and gram-negative bacilli. It does, however, have activity against *P. aeruginosa* and obligate anaerobe bacteria. Bacitracin inhibits both staphylococci and streptococci as well as other gram-positive bacilli. Bacitracin ointment alone has been shown to be effective in the treatment of nonbullous impetigo [5]. Polymyxin B is active against aerobic gram-negative bacilli, including *P. aeruginosa*. Combining these medications into one topical medication thus provides a spectrum of activity that may be adequate for the treatment of pyoderma.

Systemic therapy combined with topical therapy is advised in more severe cases (Table 2-3). Treatment with dicloxacillin, erythromycin, or cephalexin rather than with penicillin has been suggested because of the recent emergence of *S. aureus* as the primary pathogen. However, because of an increase in the number of erythromycin-resistant strains of *S. aureus* [6,7], cephalexin or dicloxacillin should be the initial treatment. A comparison of twice daily cephalexin versus four times daily dicloxacillin revealed the cephalexin to be equally efficacious to dicloxacillin in the treatment of impetigo [8]. Recently, 5 days of azithromycin

		TABLE 2-3 SYSTEMIC ANTIBIOTICS USED FOR SKIN INFECTIONS	
Type	**Dose/frequency**	**Duration**	**Indication**
Penicillin-VK	50 mg/kg/d in four divided doses	7–10 d	Erysipelas
Erythromycin ethylsuccinate	30–40 mg/kg/d in three divided doses	7–10 d	Impetigo, folliculitis, ecthyma, paronychia, furuncles, cellulitis
Dicloxacillin	15 mg/kg/d in four divided doses	7–10 d	Impetigo, folliculitis, ecthyma, paronychia, furuncles, cellulitis
Cephalexin	50 mg/kg/d in two divided doses	7–10 d	Impetigo, folliculitis, ecthyma, paronychia, furuncles, cellulitis
Azithromycin	500 mg orally on d 1, then 250 mg oraly once daily x 4 d	5 d	Impetigo, folliculitis, ecthyma, paronychia, furuncles, cellulitis
Ciprofloxacin	500–750 mg orally twice daily	7–10 d	Impetigo, folliculitis, ecthyma, paronychia, furuncles, cellulitis
Amoxicillin clavulanate	500 mg orally three times daily	7–10 d	Impetigo, folliculitis, ecthyma, paronychia, furuncles, cellulitis, deep nodular gram-negative folliculitis

was shown to be as or more effective than 7 days of erythromycin or cloxacillin in the treatment of impetigo as well as carbuncles, furuncles, paronychia, folliculitis, and erysipelas [9•].

Prevention

Good hygiene and appropriate clothing that covers exposed skin in those patients susceptible to insect bites is recommended as a preventive measure. Topical antibiotics applied prophylactically to areas of minor skin trauma in children in a daycare center significantly reduced the development of cutaneous infections [3]. Additionally, eradication of nasal carriers of *S. aureus* by the administration of 5 days of topical mupirocin four times a day was shown to be effective [10].

ECTHYMA

Ecthyma is a form of impetigo that involves deeper layers of the skin. In this disorder the process erodes through the epidermis and results in a shallow ulcer. The lesions typically begin as vesiculopustules that quickly crust over (Fig. 2-3). The crust of ecthyma differs from the crust of impetigo because it is larger, heaped up, and harder. Upon removal, it reveals an ulcer. An individual lesion will usually heal within a few weeks and may or may not form a scar. The most common area of the body affected is the lower extremities. The most common organism is β-hemolytic streptococci.

The disease is more common in children, due to trauma that occurs during normal recreational activity. Other predisposing factors include insect bites, scratches, pediculosis, scabies, and eczema, especially in those patients with underlying poor hygiene in warm, humid environments.

Treatment

The treatment of ecthyma includes removal of the overlying crust and application of a topical antibiotic to the ulcer

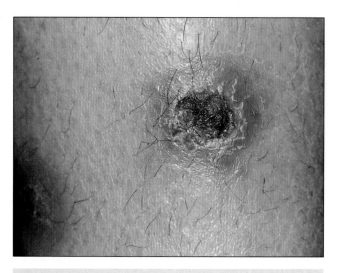

FIGURE 2-3 Ecthyma on the leg.

base (Table 2-2). The removal of the crust may be facilitated by prior softening with warm, gentle soap compresses. A topical antibiotic such as mupirocin may be used. In more severe cases oral antibiotics such as dicloxacillin, erythromycin, or azithromycin should be instituted (Table 2-3). Encouragement of proper skin hygiene is paramount.

FOLLICULITIS

Folliculitis is classified according to depth of involvement and etiology (Table 2-4). All types involve the hair follicle in some manner.

Superficial Folliculitis

Superficial folliculitis (Bockhart's impetigo, superficial pustular perifolliculitis, impetigo follicularis) is caused by coagulase-positive *S. aureus*. Predisposing conditions include poor hygiene, maceration, and occlusive therapies

TABLE 2-4 TYPES OF FOLLICULITIS				
Type	Characteristic lesion	Most common site	Most common organism	Treatment
Superficial folliculitis (Bockhart's impetigo)	Small dome-shaped pustule at the follicular orifice	In children, the scalp; adults—scalp, back, and extremities	*Staphylococcus aureus*	Topical erythromycin 2% solution
Gram-negative folliculitis				
Superficial variant	Superficial pustules	Centrofacial, perinasal area	Enterobacter, klebsiella	If mild, topical antibiotics
Deep variant	Fluctuant, deep-seated nodules	Centrofacial, perinasal area	Proteus	If severe, systemic antibiotics or isotretinoin
Hot tub folliculitis	Follicularly oriented erythematous papules topped by a small pustule	Buttocks, axilla, lateral aspects of trunk	*Pseudomonas aeruginosa* (serotype 0:11)	Discontinue use of hot tub

and dressings. Occupational exposures to cutting oils, solvents and tar preparations may also induce this disorder.

Superficial folliculitis is a clinical diagnosis supported by Gram stain and culture. Characteristically, the lesion is approximately a 1- to 4-mm dome-shaped yellow pustule located at the follicular orifice. There may be multiple or single lesions. The usual sites of involvement are the scalp, back, and extremities (Figs. 2-4 and 2-5). Any hair-bearing area, however, may be involved. In children, the most common site of involvement is the scalp. The course of individual lesions typically reveals a pustule that may rupture or become excoriated and leave a crust in its wake. A bacterial culture of the lesion will usually yield coagulase-positive staphylococci.

Treatment

Superficial folliculitis may spontaneously resolve without therapy. However, appropriate antibiotic therapy will accelerate the clearing process. Local care is usually both effective and sufficient for the treatment of superficial folliculitis. Soap and water cleansing should be performed routinely prior to the application of topical antibiotics (Table 2-2). Erythromycin 2% solution applied twice a day to affected areas can also be useful. This treatment is empiric, and culturing pustules to determine antibiotic sensitivities for the causative organism is usually unnecessary except in severe resistant cases.

Gram-Negative Folliculitis

Another variant, gram-negative folliculitis, presents in two forms: superficial pustules around the nose, and deep nodular or cystic lesions. It predominantly occurs as a superinfection in a patient who has received long-term antibiotics for acne vulgaris. The usual cause of the superficial variant is klebsiella or enterobacter. The deep nodular type is associated with proteus. Although Gram stain is usually nega-

tive, cultures will often be positive. The superficial variant may be treated with topical antibiotics while the deep nodular variant often requires oral antibiotics such as ampicillin-clavulanate, trimethoprim-sulfamethoxazole or ciprofloxacin (Table 2-3). In severe cases, the treatment of choice is isotretinoin [6].

Hot Tub Folliculitis

Hot tub folliculitis is a variant of folliculitis caused by *P. aeruginosa*. Although *Pseudomonas* has been associated with folliculitis after prolonged therapy of topical corticosteroids under occlusion, it is being increasingly recognized after the recreational use of whirlpools and hot tubs [11]. *Pseudomonas* species tend to flourish in pools that have low chloride levels, high pH, and high water temperatures.

Clinically, the skin lesions are erythematous papules topped by a pustule ranging from 2 to 10 mm in size that occurs in a follicular distribution. The lesions are often very pruritic and are characteristically found on the buttocks, hips, axilla, and lateral aspects of the trunk. Those areas that are not submerged in the hot tub are typically spared and include the head, neck, and mucous membranes. The eruption may begin anywhere from 6 hours to 5 days after the exposure; however, the incubation period is typically 2 days. The diagnosis is made clinically and supported by bacterial culture. The organism may be cultured from a pustule as well as the pool water. Serotype O:11 is most often affiliated with hot tub folliculitis.

Hot tub folliculitis is a self-limited disease and does not require therapy. However, hot tub use should be discontinued until the water source is appropriately adjusted. Topical corticosteroids should also be avoided. Serious infections have occurred in immunosuppressed patients infected with *P. aeruginosa* O–11 [12]. Thus, it may be prudent to advise immunosuppressed patients to avoid recreational hot tub use because of the theoretical possibility of serious infection.

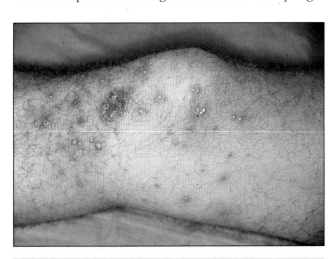

FIGURE 2-4 Superficial folliculitis on the leg.

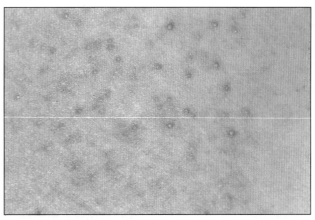

FIGURE 2-5 Folliculitis (note the dome-shaped pustules in a follicular distribution).

FURUNCLES AND CARBUNCLES

A furuncle or a boil is an acute perifollicular staphylococcal abscess of the skin and subcutaneous tissue. A carbuncle is an aggregation of interconnected furuncles that drain through a number of points in the skin surface. The lesions always begin near a hair follicle or a sebaceous gland. True furuncles are not thought to occur in hairless areas. Although the exact cause of furuncles is unknown, sebaceous gland obstruction or ingrown hairs probably play an important role.

Diagnosis

Predisposing factors to furunculosis or multiple recurrent furuncles include poor hygiene, occupational exposure to grease and oil, infection of preexisting dermatoses, malnutrition, alcoholism, and underlying hypogammoglobulonemia or leukopenia. Furuncles also tend to be more common in participants in contact sports. However, most cases do not have any predisposing local or systemic cause. Although furuncleosis tends to be more severe in diabetics, it is felt that diabetes alone does not predispose to furunculosis.

Clinically, furuncles prefer the following sites: nape, face, buttocks, thighs, perineum, breasts, and axillae (Fig. 2-6). Carbuncles occur in thick skin since these areas tend to favor lateral extension of subcutaneous abscesses (Fig. 2-7). These areas include the nape, shoulders, buttocks, outer thighs, and hips. Carbuncles develop more slowly than furuncles but attain larger sizes and are more painful. Because of the overlying thick skin, the drainage of the suppurative process is delayed and favors formation of necrosis within the abscess. This necrotic process extends laterally along the fibrous trabeculae to other follicles and produces more abscesses. The surface of the overlying skin often reveals a dull red color and indurated texture. It is tense with sieve-like changes that allow pus drainage from multiple follicular orifices. Furuncles are painful when they occur in skin that is tightly bound down, such as over the external auditory canal or nasal cartilage, while carbuncles are almost always painful, regardless of location.

Treatment

The initial treatment of furuncles and carbuncles should be warm compresses and good hygiene. Also, an oral semisynthetic penicillinase-resistant penicillin such as dicloxacillin, cephalosporin, or azithromycin [8,9•] should be prescribed, for at least a 2-week minimum (Table 2-3). In the event that furunculosis is severe and associated with systemic symptoms and lymphadenitis, intravenous antibiotics may be indicated. If drainage has already occurred and only a few lesions are present, local therapy is indicated. Surgical excision should be avoided in early lesions. Additionally, squeezing the lesion to extract hair or pus should not be performed. Both of these maneuvers may cause local or systemic extension.

When it begins to suppurate and become boggy, the lesion may be drained by "nicking" with a #11 blade. Draining lesions should be covered with topical antibiotics (Table 2-2) and loose dressings that are changed frequently to prevent autoinoculation. Medicated wicks or rubber drains should not be used as they prevent healing and may lead to scarring. Typically, after a lesion has been drained it will completely resolve after 2 weeks. However, the overlying violaceous color of the skin may not resolve for weeks to months.

Prevention

Prevention of recurrences may be difficult and unrewarding. Avoidance of skin irritants, good personal hygiene, and daily antibiotic washes may be attempted but are often ineffective. Topical washes that have shown some success in preventing furunculosis include chlorhexidine. Attempts to

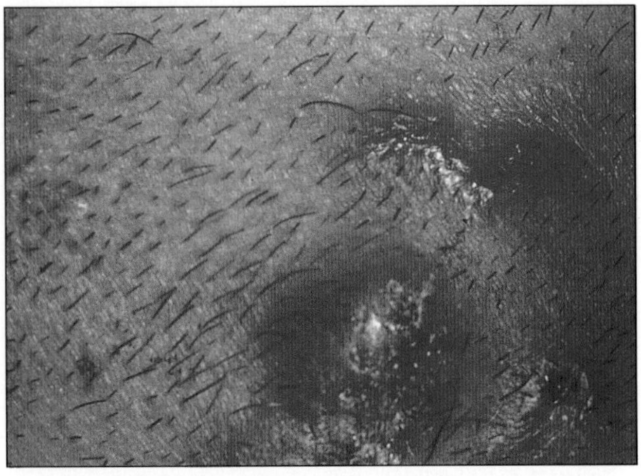

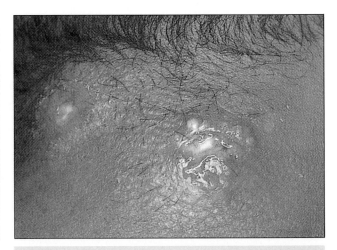

FIGURE 2-6 Furuncle (note the discrete hard subcutaneous nodule with an overlying erythematous hue).

FIGURE 2-7 Carbuncle on the nape (notice the multiple number of drainage points through the skin).

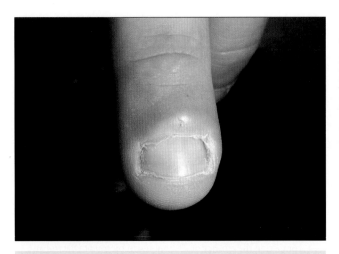

FIGURE 2-8 Acute staphylococcal paronychia (note the acute swollen, inflamed erythematous paronychial folds).

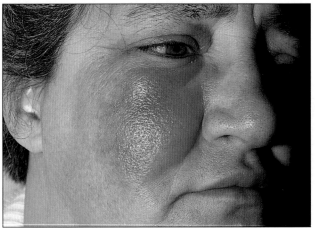

FIGURE 2-9 Erysipelas (note the erythematous and edematous skin with a sharply demarcated margin).

eliminate the *S. aureus* carrier state with nasal mupirocin have been effective [10].

PARONYCHIA

Paronychia is inflammation of the nail folds. The potential space surrounding the nail fold provides an excellent setting for infection. The infection begins in the paronychium at the site of the nail and usually manifests as swelling, local redness, and pain (Fig. 2-8). Pyonychia is a term that is used to refer to pyoderma involving the perionychium. In acute paronychia, the most common causative bacteria include staphylococci, beta-hemolytic streptococci, and gram-negative enteric bacteria. Chronic paronychia is usually caused by *Candida*.

Gentle pressure on the tender swollen paronychium will usually express a drop of pus. It is also not unusual to see pus through the nail or at the paronychial fold. As the syndrome progresses, the tender red swollen area extends around the nail fold and spares the distal edge. Resolution typically occurs within a few days. However, if it does not occur rapidly, the nail matrix may become disturbed and a permanent dystrophy of the nail plate may occur.

Common predisposing factors include minor trauma that results in a break of the skin, such as a hangnail, a splinter lodged under the distal edge of the nail, or a prick from a thorn. Paronychia may be secondary to hematoma.

Treatment

Medical treatment includes wet compresses (Burow's solution) or hot bland soaks combined with appropriate systemic antibiotic therapy. Topical antibiotics are of limited value because of poor penetration throughout the nail plate to the affected area. If medical treatment does not resolve these measures and a pocket of pus remains, then surgical drainage of the loculation is indicated.

ERYSIPELAS

Erysipelas or superficial cellulitis is characterized by an edematous, brawny, infiltrated, well-demarcated plaque that is bright red and warm (Fig. 2-9). It spreads peripherally without central clearing. Although the infection may occur anywhere, the most common sites are the face and scalp. The characteristic leading border is often palpable and distinct from the uninvolved skin. Clinically, the patient with erysipelas is febrile and appears ill.

The most common causative organism is group A β-hemolytic streptococci. Other less common causes include group B, group C, or group G streptococci. Predisposing factors include poor skin hygiene, prior wounds and injuries, and preexisting ulcers or suppurative cutaneous processes. Additionally, underlying conditions that lower the host's resistance and predispose to erysipelas include: cachexia, malnutrition, and underlying systemic disease.

The diagnosis is made clinically since diagnostic techniques such as culture and Gram stain are frequently unrewarding. The treatment of choice is penicillin either via oral, intramuscular, or intravenous routes continued for at least 10 days. It is very effective and rapid improvement may be seen within 24 to 48 hours. Local treatment should include elevation of the affected body part, rest, and cold compresses.

Complications of erysipelas include *elephantiasis verrucosa nostra* in those patients in whom recurrent erysipelas of the lower extremity occurs. Other complications include septicemia or deep cellulitis and these are more common in the elderly and newborn.

CELLULITIS

Cellulitis is a diffuse suppurative inflammation involving the subcutaneous tissue. Clinically there is local erythema and warmth. The cutaneous erythema is poorly demarcated

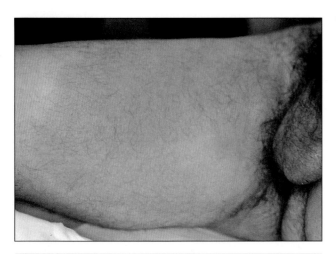

FIGURE 2-10 Cellulitis on the inner thigh (note the vague demarcation between normal and affected skin).

from uninvolved areas and thus presents a contrasting clinical picture to that of the distinct palpable margin of erysipelas (Fig. 2-10). Associated with cellulitis are systemic symptoms such as malaise, fever, and chills. The most common causes of cellulitis are beta-hemolytic streptococci and *S. aureus.*

Cellulitis is a clinical diagnosis since the causative organism is often very difficult to recover. Nonetheless, attempts to retrieve the causative organisms by skin biopsy, blood culture, or aspiration of the advancing edge have been positive on occasion.

Treatment should include bed rest, elevation of the affected parts, and systemic antibiotic therapy that will provide adequate coverage for either streptococci or staphylococci (Table 2-3). Complications of cellulitis include gangrene, metastatic abscess, and sepsis. These are more common in immunocompromized adults or very young children.

REFERENCES AND RECOMMENDED READING

Recently published papers of particular interest have been highlighted as:
• Of interest
•• Of outstanding interest

1. Roth R, James W: Microbiology of the skin: resident flora, ecology, infection. *J Am Acad Dermatol* 1989, 20:367–390.

2. Hirschmann JV: Topical antibiotics in dermatology. *Arch Dermatol* 1988, 124:1691–1700.

3. Leyden J: Mupirocin: A new topical antibiotic. *J Am Acad Dermatol* 1990, 22:879–883.

4.• McLin S: A bacteriologically controlled randomized study comparing the efficacy of 2% mupirocin ointment (Bactroban) with oral erythromycin in the treatment of patients with impetigo. *J Am Acad Dermatol* 1990, 22:883–885.

5. Dillon H: Topical and systemic therapy for pyodermas. *Int J Dermatol* 1980, 19:443–451.

6. James WD, Leyden JJ: Treatment of gram-negative folliculitis with isotretinoin: positive clinical and microbiologic response. *J Am Acad Dermatol* 1985, 12:319.

7. Grossman KL, Rasmussen JE: Recent advances in pediatric infectious disease and their impact on dermatology. *J Am Acad Dermatol* 1991, 24:379–389.

8. Dillon H: Treatment of staphylococcal skin infections: a comparison of cephalexin and dicloxacillin. *J Am Acad Dermatol* 1983, 8:177–181.

9.• Daniel R: Azithromycin, erythromycin and cloxacillin in the treatment of infections of skin and associated soft tissues. *J Int Med Res* 1991, 19:433–445.

10. Casewell MW, Hill LR: Elimination of nasal carriage of staphylococcus aureus with mupirocin "pseudomonic acid"—a control trial. *J Antimicrob Chemother* 1986, 17:365–372.

11. Fox A, Hambrick G: Recreationally associated pseudomonas aeruginosa folliculitis. *Arch Dermatol* 1984, 120:1304–1307.

12. Aze P, Thyss A, Caldani C, *et al.*: Pseudomonas aeruginosa O–11 folliculitis: development into ecthyma gangrenosum in immunosuppressed patients. *Arch Dermatol* 1985, 121:873–876.

Common Viral Infections of the Skin

Paul A. Krusinski

3

Key Points

- Genital molluscum contagiosum, in spite of its banal nature, implies unprotected sexual exposure, and testing for syphilis, hepatitis B, and HIV may be necessary.
- Recently published Centers for Disease Control and Prevention guidelines for the treatment of recurrent genital herpes simplex with acyclovir suggest a 5-day course of 200 mg five times daily, 400 mg three times daily, or 800 mg twice daily.
- Zoster therapy now includes a choice of either acyclovir or famciclovir. Additional agents will become available in the next few years.
- Post-herpetic neuralgia is no longer considered separately, but is a category of all "zoster-associated pain."
- The viral etiologies of erythema infectiosum (Fifth disease) and roseola (exantheum subitum) have now been elucidated. Exposure to these agents may have serious consequences for some patients.

Even though the primary emphasis of this chapter is on the manifestations, diagnosis, and treatment of cutaneous viral infections, these do not occur in a vacuum. Infected skin envelops a human being, and even the most banal cutaneous viral skin lesions have systemic implications. For example, some forms of papillomavirus that cause warts are associated with the development of carcinoma of the cervix and squamous cell carcinoma. Genital molluscum contagiosum implies unprotected sex, and questions about syphilis, hepatitis B, and HIV must be discussed. Herpes simplex and zoster infections may become life-threatening in the immunocompromised individual. This chapter discusses common viral infections of the skin and points out when the clinician must be on the lookout for more serious complications and systemic effects.

HUMAN PAPILLOMAVIRUS INFECTIONS

Warts are extremely common, usually banal, and characteristically fall into the category of a clinical nuisance. The various clinical types include: common warts (*verrucae vulgaris*), plantar warts (*verrucae plantaris*), flat warts (*verrucae plana*), and genital warts (*condyloma acuminata*). These types are described as separate clinical entities because their appearance and treatment sometimes vary considerably.

Common Warts

This condition can occur on almost any area of the body, most often in children but also in any age group, and many warts may persist for years. However, in children one half of all warts will spontaneously regress in 1 year and two thirds of all warts will clear in 2 years without therapy. The verrucous papules are so common that recognition and diagnosis are usually easy (Fig. 3-1). For treatment, one may use keratolytic acid paintings that are available over the counter

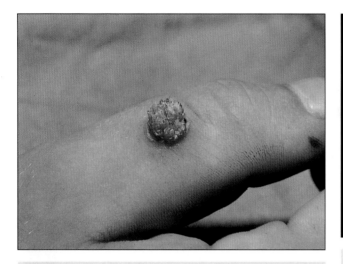

FIGURE 3-1 Verrucous papule of a common wart. (*From* Flowers and Krusinski [24]; with permission.)

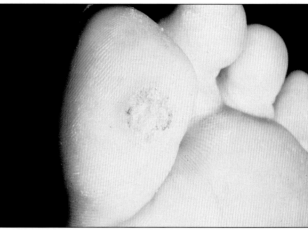

FIGURE 3-2 Planter warts interrupt the skin lines and have dark dots (thrombosed vessels) within them. (*From* Flowers and Krusinski [24]; with permission.)

under a variety of names. Each contains 17% salicylic acid, and should be applied twice daily (Table 3-1). For warts that are few in number or fail to be relieved by topical keratolytic acids, liquid nitrogen cryosurgery is successful 70% to 80% of the time. This procedure should be performed at monthly intervals and may take three or four applications to achieve clearing on areas of thicker skin.

Plantar Warts

Plantar warts, appearing on the soles of the feet, are particularly recalcitrant to therapy. They occur most frequently on weight-bearing prominences, and at times are extremely painful. They must be differentiated from calluses that have increased skin lines and also from hard corns. Dark dots that represent thrombosed blood vessels are usually present in plantar warts (Fig. 3-2). The differential diagnosis

includes verrucous carcinoma and amelanotic melanoma that can also occur on the sole. Plantar warts may be treated with the same modalities used for common warts (Table 3-1) [1•]. However, liquid nitrogen cryosurgery may be painful when used on the sole and is usually only effective for plantar warts of very small diameter and thickness. It can be combined with paring and topical chemodestruction to enhance its effectiveness. Topical formalin and glutaraldehyde represent alternatives to keratolytic acid paintings for persistent plantar warts. CO_2 laser vaporization has a 90% success rate and should be used in place of electrodesiccation and curettage because it usually causes less scarring.

Flat Warts

Flat warts are found most often on the face in children, the beard region in men, and on the legs in women where shaving causes inoculation along the minor nicks from a razor. They are asymptomatic flat papules and plaques that may be pink, flesh-colored, or slightly hyperpigmented (Fig. 3-3). They range in size from 1 mm to greater than

TABLE 3-1 TREATMENT OF COMMON AND PLANTAR WARTS
Keratolytic acid paintings
File with emery board after bath or shower
Apply 17% salicylic acid twice daily
If irritation develops, apply castor oil in place of acid twice daily
Resume acid paintings twice daily
Liquid nitrogen cryosurgery
Freeze 3–4 mm around wart
Curettage and electrodesiccation
May lead to substantial scarring
CO_2 laser vaporization
For periungual or recalcitrant warts

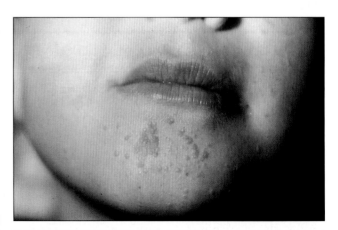

FIGURE 3-3 Flat warts.

1 cm and are often multiple. As with warts in general, they will spontaneously clear in many patients. When clearing occurs, it is frequently heralded by pruritus and erythema. The treatment of choice for verrucae plana is topical tretinoin cream, Retin-A (Ortho Pharmaceuticals, Raritan, NJ), applied twice daily, with application of 0.5% for facial and 0.1% for hands or legs. The condition may take several months to clear.

GENITAL WARTS

Genital warts are one of the most common sexually transmissible diseases. Most patients have asymptomatic flesh-colored or pink verrucous papules that are easily diagnosed (Fig. 3-4). However, in some patients they may be extensive, persistent, and resistant to treatment. In patients with condyloma acuminata, questions regarding unprotected sex and the possibility of other diseases (*eg*, syphilis, hepatitis B, and HIV) need to be discussed and ruled out. Some human papillomavirus types associated with condyloma acuminata have been shown to be oncogenic but the vast majority of venereal warts are caused by nononcogenic strains [2]. There is no question that carcinoma of the cervix, carcinoma of the head of the penis, and intraanal squamous cell carcinomas have been linked to oncogenic strains of papillomavirus [3]. This extremely common epidemiologic problem is compounded by the existence of subclinical human papillomavirus infection of the genitals in both men and women, which is very difficult to diagnose and treat.

Genital warts need to be differentiated from molluscum contagiosum, folliculitis, nevi, and skin tags. Sometimes this can be accomplished through the use of acetowhitening. Five percent acetic acid (white vinegar) is applied by compresses over the genital region for 3 to 5 minutes. The typical white appearance of condyloma acuminata aids in the diagnosis. One should realize that many false-positive and false-negative reactions occur with this method. Occasionally biopsies of genital warts may be helpful, but histo-

logically this may sometimes be confounding. The use of monoclonal antibody immunohistochemical stains to characterize the human papillomavirus type are not readily available in most clinical laboratories at the present time. Women who have external genital condylomata should have frequent pap smears and colposcopy examinations. Likewise, women who come in contact with men with genital warts should have frequent pap smears even if clinical examination is negative for warts. The frequency of sexual abuse as a cause of childhood genital or perianal warts is controversial, but issues relating to abuse need to be raised when the diagnosis is made [4].

There are many different treatments available for condyloma acuminata (Table 3-2). Careful follow-up is necessary as recurrences or newly developing warts will occur during the course of treatment.

HERPES SIMPLEX VIRUS INFECTIONS

Herpes simplex virus infections can occur anywhere on the body. Type I infections will occur above the waist 70% to 90% of the time, and type II below the waist 70% to 90% of the time. The primary infection of herpes simplex type 1 (HSV 1) manifests itself as a painful, erosive gingivostomatitis. The patient appears febrile and extremely toxic, but in the immunocompetent host it will resolve in 2 to 3 weeks. Primary HSV 1 gingivostomatitis is extremely rare, and most infected individuals have a subclinical infection that is never clinically diagnosed. The most frequently observed manifestation of HSV 1 infection is recurrent herpes labialis. It typically occurs at the mucocutaneous junction frequently in or around the same location after a 12 to 24 hour prodrome of itching and tingling (Fig. 3-5). Precipitating factors of a febrile illness or upper respiratory infections have led to the term cold sore or fever blister. Other precipitating events include exposure to ultraviolet

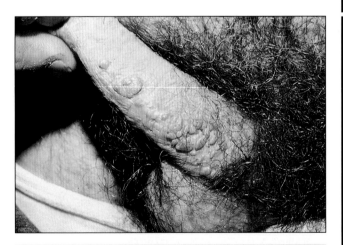

FIGURE 3-4 Condyloma acuminata. (*From* Flowers and Krusinski [24]; with permission.)

TABLE 3-2 TREATMENT OF GENITAL WARTS
Podophyllin 25% in tincture of benzoin
Apply once weekly (by physician)
Wash off as tolerated in 4–6 h
Podophyllotoxin (Condylox*) [5]
Apply twice daily 3 d/wk (by patient)
Use for 1 mo
Liquid nitrogen cryocautery
5-Fluorouracil cream, 5%
Apply daily or twice daily 4 d/wk
Use for 2 mo
CO₂ laser vaporization
*Oclassen Pharmaceuticals, San Rafael, CA.

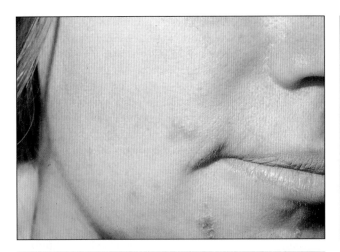

FIGURE 3-5 Grouped vesicles on an erythematous base that recur in the same location are characteristic of herpes simplex.

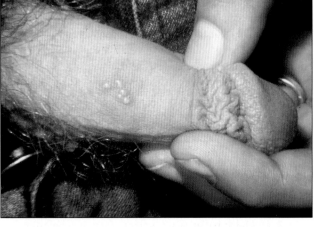

FIGURE 3-6 Recurrent genital herpes. (*From* Flowers and Krusinski [24]; with permission.)

light, trauma, and psychological stress. Recurrent cold sores typically last 7 to 10 days, and may cause considerable discomfort as well as cosmetic concern.

As in orolabial herpes simplex, primary genital infection may be subclinical. When infection does occur, multiple discreet bilateral vesicles and erosions may appear on the external genitalia. This may be associated with systemic symptoms of fever, malaise, and acute toxicity in both sexes, but healing will occur spontaneously in 2 to 3 weeks in the immunocompetent individual. In women with vaginal and cervical involvement, additional symptoms of vaginal discharge, dysuria, urinary retention, and lumbosacral reticulopathy may occur. Men may have bilateral inguinal lymphadenopathy. Primary genital herpes simplex may be due to HSV 1 or HSV 2. Genital herpes is almost always due to HSV 2. The typical morphology of recurrent genital herpes simplex consists of tightly clustered vesicles on an erythematous base, which occur in and around the same location before healing spontaneously in 7 to 10 days (Fig. 3-6). Fifty percent of patients will experience a prodrome of itching, burning, or tingling. This sexually transmitted disease is the source of potentially life-threatening neonatal herpes simplex infection. Maternal asymptomatic shedding may occur 1% of the time and accounts for most neonatal infections [6•]. Also, there is possible increased susceptibility to HIV infection if mucosal erosions are present during sexual intercourse.

Localized herpes simplex infection of the fingertip is called herpetic whitlow. In 10% of patients, usually children, it is caused by HSV 1 related to thumb and finger sucking. The remaining 90% of patients have HSV 2 obtained through sexual contact [7]. The usual herpes morphology of grouped vesicles on a red base helps distinguish herpetic whitlow from a felon or other digital inflammatory conditions (Fig. 3-7). Considerable edema is associated with the lesion and the pain is frequently quite severe.

Herpes gladiatorum is the term for herpes simplex lesions on the torso of competitive wrestlers, caused by HSV 1 infection [8]. Both herpes simplex and molluscum contagiosum skin infections may disqualify athletes from competitive wrestling.

Perianal erosions of herpetic proctitis may be present with or without the usual morphology of herpes simplex. It is often associated with pain, discharge, and tenesmus. It is most frequently seen in homosexual men and heterosexual women.

Diagnosis

The diagnosis of herpes simplex on the skin is usually easily made on clinical grounds. However, before using expensive antiviral chemotherapeutic agents one should obtain laboratory confirmation. A Tzanck smear is taken from scrapings from the floor of a herpetic vesicle. It may be stained with Wright stain in the examiner's office or sent to the laboratory for a Papanicolaou's stain. The results are positive approximately 50% of the time in active vesicular lesions.

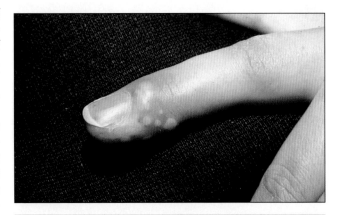

FIGURE 3-7 Herpetic whitlow. (*From* Flowers and Krusinski [24]; with permission.)

Viral culture early in the course of a recurrence will yield positive results 80% to 90% of the time. Current serologic assays are only helpful in identifying individuals at risk for reactivation who are about to undergo organ transplantation. However, they are otherwise of little clinical use.

Complications

A banal cold sore may represent a severe and possibly life-threatening problem in selected individuals. Specifically, patients undergoing organ transplantation and patients with AIDS may develop severe chronic herpetic infections that may lack the usual morphology (Fig. 3-8), and may lead to disseminated infection. Herpes simplex is also the most common infectious cause of erythema multiforme (*see* Kulp-Shorten, Urticaria and Reactive Dermatoses). Patients with severe atopic dermatitis, Darier's disease, and mycosis fungoides may get Kaposi's varicelliform eruption caused by herpes simplex (Fig. 3-9). Prompt diagnosis and early, aggressive treatment is necessary for these serious complications.

Treatment

Topical, oral, and intravenous acyclovir or Zovirax (Burroughs-Wellcome Laboratories, Research Triangle Park, NC) are effective against herpes simplex virus infections. However, topical acyclovir is only slightly more beneficial than placebo when evaluated in clinical trials. Its only clinical utility is in the treatment of cutaneous infections in immunocompromised individuals, where it has definitely been shown to shorten the clinical course of their disease. For primary and recurrent herpetic infections that are not very frequent, episodic treatment with oral acyclovir is indicated (Table 3-3). Those patients who have frequently recurring genital herpes simplex may wish to take a suppressive regimen of acyclovir 200 mg orally three times daily or 400 mg orally twice daily for 1 year prophylactically. Immunocompromised individuals, those with disseminated infection, or complications of herpes simplex infec-

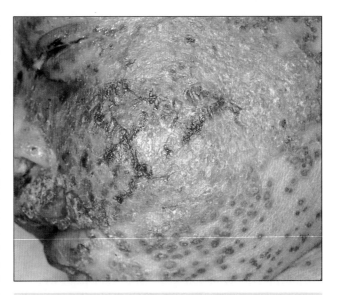

FIGURE 3-9 Kaposi's varicelliform eruption.

TABLE 3-3 TREATMENT OF HERPES SIMPLEX INFECTIONS

Orolabial

Primary

   Toxic patient: acyclovir 10 mg/kg i.v. every 8 h for 5 d

Recurrent

   Infrequent: topical antibiotic cream or ointment 3 times daily (placebo therapy)

   Frequent, severe, or immunocompromised: acyclovir 200 mg orally 5 times daily for 5 d

Herpes gladiatorum or herpetic whitlow

Acyclovir 200 mg orally 5 times daily for 5 d

Genital herpes

Primary: acyclovir 200 mg orally 5 times daily for 7–10 d

Recurrent

   Infrequent: acyclovir 200 mg orally 5 times daily for 5 d

   Or acyclovir 400 mg orally 3 times daily for 5 d

   Or acyclovir 800 mg orally 2 times daily for 5 d

   Acyclovir 200 mg orally 3 times daily for 1 y or

   Acyclovir 400 mg orally twice daily for 1 y

Complications of herpes simplex

Recurrent erythema multiforme and Stevens-Johnson syndrome

Suppressive regimen (*see above* Genital herpes)

Disseminated herpes simplex (immunocompromised or eczema herpeticum): acyclovir 200–400 mg orally 5 times daily for 10–14 d or longer, or in severe cases acyclovir i.v. (*see above* Primary)

Acyclovir 10 mg/kg i.v. every 8 h for 10 d

Foscarnet 60 mg/kg every 8 h i.v. (in patients with AIDS with acyclovir-resistant infection)

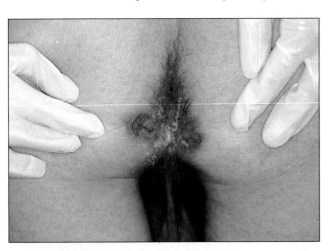

FIGURE 3-8 Chronic ulceration in an AIDS patient with herpes simplex virus.

tion may need intravenous therapy. Immunocompromised individuals may also need to be treated for much longer periods of time to achieve clinical clearing. Patients with AIDS may need to be treated frequently or continuously with oral acyclovir. Thymidine kinase-negative strains of herpes simplex resistant to acyclovir have been isolated from patients with AIDS after intravenous courses of acyclovir. These patients may be treated successfully with intravenous foscarnet therapy [9].

VARICELLA ZOSTER VIRUS INFECTIONS

Varicella

Varicella or chickenpox is usually a banal infection, most often occurring in children aged between 5 and 15 years old [10]. Mild symptoms consist of fever and a pruritic, polymorphic skin eruption that begins on the torso and spreads centrifugally (Fig. 3-10). Eruptions begin as macules and papules that develop into vesicles, pustules, and frequently, hemorrhagic erosions. Punched-out, pocklike scars may occur, especially after secondary bacterial infection. The eruption usually occurs 14 to 21 days after exposure to another individual who has chickenpox, and is spread in expired respiratory droplets [11].

Diagnosis

The Tzanck smear may be very helpful in the diagnosis of varicella zoster virus (VZV) infections. Results are positive 80% of the time when taken from a varicella or zoster vesicle. Viral culture for this virus takes at least 2 weeks, is expensive, and is only positive approximately 50% of the time. Serologic testing for VZV is only helpful in determining susceptibility to varicella.

Treatment

Acyclovir has been shown to be helpful for the treatment of varicella in healthy children [12•]. Its use decreases fever and duration of illness, and also decreases the number of cutaneous lesions. However, complications of chickenpox have not been reduced in these early studies. It is reported that perhaps 20% of all patients with chickenpox who have a more severe course might benefit substantially from this therapy. However, in most children it is a banal disease, and therapy may not be necessary. The Oka vaccine for varicella may soon be available in the United States [13]. It is to be given with the measles, mumps, and rubella immunizations at 18 months and 5 years of age. It has been shown to diminish life-threatening varicella infections in children with leukemia.

Zoster or Shingles

Reactivation of the varicella virus from its latent state in the dorsal root ganglia with migration along sensory nerves to the adjacent skin dermatome leads to the clinical development of zoster [14]. A prodrome of 5 to 7 days of hyperesthesia or radicular pain in the same dermatome is quite common. Clinically, one sees tightly grouped vesicles on an erythematous base in a dermatomal pattern (Fig. 3-11). However, occasionally two or three adjacent dermatomes may be involved. In otherwise healthy individuals zoster will resolve in 2 to 3 weeks. It is felt that zoster is more frequent in the elderly and in patients with decreasing cell-mediated immunity, Hodgkin's disease, and AIDS. Disseminated zoster may occur in severely immunosuppressed patients. It is diagnosed when the patient has ten or more extradermatomal vesicles. Pneumonitis, hepatitis, and meningoencephalitis represent life-threatening visceral complications.

Treatment

Oral or intravenous acyclovir decreases viral shedding and acute pain associated with zoster. Acyclovir should be used in patients with ophthalmic involvement to prevent the occurrence of blindness. Acute pain from zoster is usually well controlled with oral acyclovir, and some studies suggest a decrease in the incidence of postzoster neuralgia with the

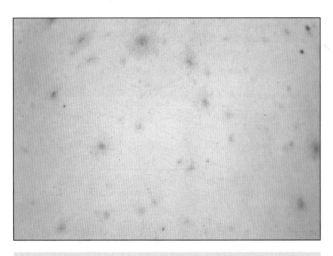

FIGURE 3-10 The lesions of chickenpox (varicella) are polymorphous and congregate on the torso.

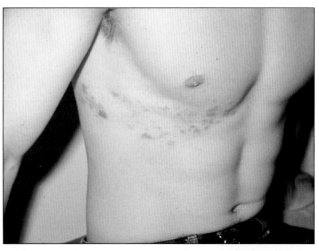

FIGURE 3-11 Zoster: vesicles in a dermatomal pattern.

TABLE 3-4 TREATMENT OF VARICELLA-ZOSTER INFECTION

Varicella

Children: acyclovir 20 mg/kg daily orally in 4 divided doses for 7 d

Adults: acyclovir 800 mg 5 times daily orally for 7–10 d

Zoster

Localized: acyclovir 800 mg orally 5 times daily for 7–10 d or, famciclover orally 500 mg 3 times daily

Burroughs solution compresses 3 to 4 times daily

Topical antibiotic ointment after compresses

Disseminated: acyclovir 10 mg/kg i.v. every 8h for 7 d

Post-zoster neuralgia

Topical capsaicin cream 0.075% 6 times daily

Amitriptyline 50 mg orally every h

Oral analgesics

Local nerve block by anesthesiologist

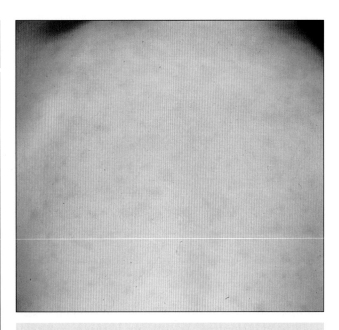

FIGURE 3-12 Roseola infantum. (*From* Flowers and Krusinski [24]; with permission.)

use of acyclovir [15]. Systemic corticosteroids have not been proven to be helpful in large, placebo-controlled studies [16].

Zoster requires larger doses of acyclovir than herpes simplex and acyclovir should be administered 800 mg orally five times per day for 7 to 10 days (Table 3-4). Severely immunocompromised patients who are at high risk for developing dissemination should be treated with intravenous acyclovir 10 mg per kg three times daily [17]. Institution of this therapy early in their disease decreases dissemination and visceral involvement.

Famciclovir is also available for the treatment of zoster in immunocompetent patients. Because of its greater bioavailability than acyclovir (77% absorption versus 20–30%) and its longer intracellular half-life, its recommended dosage is 500 mg orally three times daily. It has been shown to decrease viral shedding and shorten healing time in a similar manner to acyclovir. Some studies have shown that it may decrease zoster-associated pain perhaps even sooner than acyclovir. Famciclovir's safety profile appears to be similar to acyclovir. BVaraU (another nucleoside analogue) and valaciclovir are also being developed for their antizoster effect.

POST-HERPETIC NEURALGIA

Persistent pain greater than 3 to 6 months after resolution of the cutaneous symptoms of zoster is more frequently seen in elderly patients. At times, it is so severe as to be debilitating. Treatment with 0.075% capsaicin cream [18] topically four to six times daily or oral tricyclic antidepressants [19] has been shown to be helpful in 50% or more of patients. Many other therapies have also been suggested for postzoster neuralgia, but they have not been studied in a systematic

fashion. Use of nerve blocks performed by anesthesiologists may sometimes prove to be very helpful when all else fails.

The International Antiviral Consortium [20] has agreed that there is no universal definition for post-herpetic neuralgia. They suggest all pain during and after the eruption be called "zoster-associated pain." Studies of newer antivirals will use this terminology when assessing efficacy of zoster pain relief.

HERPESVIRUS TYPE 6

Exanthem subitum or roseola occurs in children between 6 months and 4 years of age and has been linked to human herpesvirus-6 (HH6) [21]. Characteristically, high fever remains constant for 3 to 5 days, developing with no other positive physical findings. Febrile seizures may occur in some of these patients. The rash appears at the time of defervescence and consists of discreet to confluent pink macules, primarily on the trunk (Fig. 3-12). Most infections due to HH6 in children present as a febrile illness with nonspecific findings, and therefore roseola is not diagnosed. Reactivation of HH6 later in life during periods of immunosuppression has recently been described.

HUMAN PARVOVIRUS

Erythema infectiosum or Fifth disease has now been linked to human parovirus B-19 [22]. Mild fever may accompany the distinctive eruption in this disease that consists of striking erythema of the cheeks with circumoral pallor or a slapped-cheek appearance (Fig. 3-13) and a reticulate erythematous, asymptomatic eruption on the extremities (Fig. 3-14). Some patients may have arthralgias associated

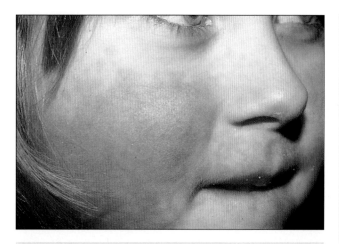

FIGURE 3-13 "Slapped cheek" facial erythema of Fifth disease. (*From* Flowers and Krusinski [24]; with permission.)

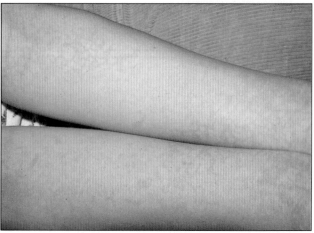

FIGURE 3-14 Reticulate eruption of Fifth disease.

with this distinctive eruption. Erythema infectiosum is self-limited and no treatment is necessary. However, epidemiologic studies have linked this virus to an increase in spontaneous abortion in women who are exposed early in pregnancy, and to aplastic crisis in patients with hemoglobinopathies and hematologic disorders [23]. Unfortunately, once the rash appears the patient is no longer infectious, and diagnosis is frequently made too late to prevent exposure to the above individuals, who are susceptible to serious complications.

MOLLUSCUM CONTAGIOSUM

Molluscum contagiosum are small, 2 to 6 mm flesh-colored or pink papules with a central umbilication. They are caused by a member of the poxvirus family and most frequently infect children, with lesions occurring on the trunk and face. In sexually active adults, the same clinical lesions will occur on the genitals and inner thighs as a sexually transmissible disease (Fig. 3-15). In patients with AIDS, molluscum contagiosum is quite common. These patients characteristically may develop hundreds of lesions which may grow to be quite large and become cosmetically disfiguring. The disease is self-limited and many children will observe spontaneous resolution within 6 to 18 months. However, patients with AIDS may have persistent lesions which require aggressive treatment. In adults, the papules may be curetted, nicked with a scalpel blade, or treated with liquid nitrogen cryocautery. The differential diagnosis in this group of patients includes condyloma acuminata and folliculitis. Sexual transmission of these lesions occurs during unprotected sexual exposure and questions regarding the symptoms and testing for syphilis, hepatitis B, and HIV must be raised in this group of patients.

HAND, FOOT, AND MOUTH DISEASE

A few strains of coxsackie virus (coxsackie A5,10,15, and 16) will cause this relatively mild disease. After a 7 to 10 day incubation period, patients develop a small number of 2 to 4 mm, flat-topped, gray pustules on their palms and soles with concomitant development of similar pustules involving the oral mucosa. These quickly rupture and may present as small, tender erosions. Only mild constitutional symptoms and low-grade fever accompany the cutaneous findings. The disease is self-limited and resolves spontaneously after 5 to 7 days. Infrequently, pneumonitis may complicate the illness. No treatment is available and usually none is necessary.

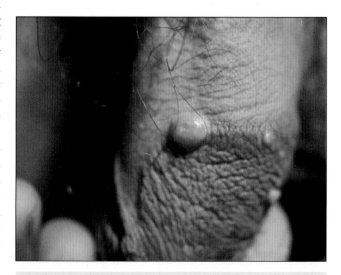

FIGURE 3-15 Molluscum contagiosum. (*From* Flowers and Krusinski [24]; with permission.)

REFERENCES AND RECOMMENDED READING

Recently published papers of particular interest have been highlighted as:
- • Of interest
- •• Of outstanding interest

1.• Ramsey ML: Plantar warts: choosing treatment for active patients. *Physician and Sportsmed* 1992, 20:69–88.

2. Koutsky LA, Holmes KK, Critchlow CW, *et al.*: A cohort study of the risk of cervical intraepithelial neoplasia grade 2 or 3 in relation to papillomavirus infection. *N Engl J Med* 1992, 326:1272–1278.

3. Franco EL: Human papillomavirus and the natural history of cervical cancer. *Infect Med* 1993, 10:57–64.

4. Raimer SS, Raimer BG: Family violence, child abuse, and anogenital warts. *Arch Dermatol* 1992, 128:842–843.

5. Beutner KR, Friedman-Kien AE, Artman NN, *et al.*: Patient-applied podofilox for treatment of genital warts. *Lancet* 1989, i:831–834.

6.• Prober CG, Corey L, Brown ZA, *et al.*: The management of pregnancies complicated by genital infections with herpes simplex virus. *Clin Infect Dis* 1992, 15:1031–1038.

7. Gill MJ, Arlette J, Buchan KA: Herpes simplex virus infection of the hand. *J Am Acad Dermatol* 1990, 22:111–116.

8. Belongia EA, Goodman JL, Holland EJ, *et al.*: An outbreak of herpes gladiatorum at a high-school wrestling camp. *N Engl J Med* 1991, 324:906–910.

9. DeTorres O: Focus on foscarnet: a pyrophosphate analog for use in CMV retinitis and other viral infections. *Hosp Formul* 1991, 26:929–947.

10. Krusinski PA: Varicella (chickenpox). In *Clinical Dermatology*. Edited by Demis DJ. Philadelphia: JB Lippincott; 1988:1–7.

11. Weller TH: Varicella and herpes zoster: changing concepts of the natural history, control, and importance of a not-so-benign virus. *N Engl J Med* 1983, 308:1362–1367; *continues* 1434–1440.

12.• Dunkle LM, Arvin AM, Whitley RJ, *et al.*: A controlled trial of acyclovir for chickenpox in normal children. *N Engl J Med* 1991, 325:1539–1544.

13. Weibel RE, Neff BJ, Kuter BJ, *et al.*: Live attenuated varicella virus vaccine. *N Engl J Med* 1984, 310:1409–1415.

14. Krusinski PA: Herpes zoster. In *Clinical Dermatology*. Edited by Demis DJ. Philadelphia: JB Lippincott; 1988: 1–7.

15. Huff JC, *et al.*: Therapy of herpes zoster with oral acyclovir. *Am J Med* 1988, 85(suppl 2A):84–89.

16. Esmann V, Kroon S, Peterslund NA, *et al.*: Prednisolone does not prevent post-herpetic neuralgia. *Lancet* 1987, ii:126–129.

17. Shepp DH: Treatment of varicella-zoster virus infections in severely immunocompromised patients. *N Engl J Med* 1986, 314:208–212.

18. Bernstein JE, Bickers DR, Dahl MV, *et al.*: Treatment of chronic postherpetic neuralgia with topical capsaicin. *J Am Acad Dermatol* 1987, 17:93–96.

19. Watson CT, Evans RJ, Reed K, *et al.*: Amitriptyline versus placebo in postherpetic neuralgia. *Neurology* 1982, 32:671–673.

20. Wood M: How can the burden of zoster-associated pain be reduced? *International Herpes Management Forum*, Worthing: PPS Europe; 1993.

21. Yamanishi K, Shiraki K, Kondo T, *et al.*: Identification of human herpesvirus-6 as a causal agent for exanthem subitum. *Lancet* 1988, i:1065–1067.

22. Bell LM, Naides SJ, Stoffman P, *et al.*: Human parvovirus B19 infection among hospital staff members after contact with infected patients. *N Engl J Med* 1989, 321:485–491.

23. Ware R: Human parvovirus infection. *J Pediatr* 1989, 114:343–348.

24. Flowers FP, Krusinski PA: Dermatology in ambulatory and emergency medicine: a clinical guide with algorithms. Chicago: Year Book Medical Publishers; 1984.

Common Fungal Infections of the Skin

Boni E. Elewski

Key Points

- The dermatophyte fungi are the largest group of mycotic pathogens causing cutaneous diseases.
- Predisposing factors for the dermatophytoses include contact with infected animals, crowded living conditions, participation in contact sports, and use of gymnasiums.
- Not all annular or ringlike dermatoses are caused by dermatophytes. Similarly, only approximately 50% of dystrophic nails are caused by fungal organisms.
- There is an epidemic of *Trichophyton tonsurans* in urban areas of the United States. Prominent cervical lymphadenopathy, scale, and patches of alopecia are typical of the clinical presentation.
- Newer topical and systemic antifungals have significantly improved therapy. Oral antifungals are generally required when treating tinea capitis, onychomycosis, and extensive disease, and in those patients immunocompromised by disease or by therapy.

Cutaneous infections by the dermatophytes *Candida* and *Malassezia furfur* (*Pityrosporum*) are discussed in this chapter. Diagnosis and therapeutic options as well as common presentations of clinical disease are reviewed.

DERMATOPHYTOSES

Dermatophytoses are caused by a closely related group of organisms that are similar in morphology, pathogenicity, and physiology and have a special affinity for the keratinized tissues of the hair, skin, and nails [1•,2]. The dermatophytes encompass only three genera—*Epidermophyton*, *Microsporum*, and *Trichophyton*—but are collectively the largest group of fungi causing cutaneous diseases [2]. They are also referred to as ringworms because of the characteristic ring that develops on the infected skin. Diseases produced by these organisms are prefaced by the adjective *tinea*, and are named according to the body part infected (*eg*, tinea capitis refers to dermatophytosis of scalp hair, and tinea pedis to dermatophytosis of the plantar surface; Table 4-1). Although the causative organisms are closely related, the various dermatophytoses produce protean manifestations and can resemble numerous cutaneous diseases (Table 4-2).

Clinical Manifestations

Dermatophytoses have various presentations dependent upon the body site infected and the infecting fungus. For example, in a hair-bearing area, follicular invasion can result in folliculitis or alopecia. Disease in the nail unit can result in dystrophy, onycholysis, or loss of nail. Infection on the palm and sole can be particularly chronic owing to the lack of sebaceous glands, which contain fungistatic material [1•]. In addition, disease produced by some organisms, especially that acquired from animal sources, can be quite inflammatory and may

TABLE 4-1 SPECIFIC DERMATOPHYTOSES AND AREAS OF INFECTION	
Disease	**Area**
Tinea barbae	Beard region
Tinea corporis	Glabrous skin
Tinea cruris	Groin
Tinea pedis	Plantar surface or toe webs
Tinea manuum	Palmar surface
Tinea capitis	Scalp hair
Tinea unguium	Nails

TABLE 4-2 DIFFERENTIAL DIAGNOSIS OF DERMATOPHYTOSIS
Tinea corporis, cruris, and pedis
Psoriasis, eczematous dermatitis, pityriasis rosea, granuloma annulare, bacterial pyoderma, subacute cutaneous lupus erythematosus
Tinea pedis
Psoriasis, eczema, candidiasis, eczematous dermatitis, erythrasma
Tinea cruris
Candidiasis, erythrasma, eczematous dermatitis, neurodermatitis
Tinea unguium or onychomycosis
Nail psoriasis, lichen planus
Tinea capitis
Inflammatory variety—bacterial pyoderma
Noninflammatory variety—alopecia areata trichotillomania, discoid lupus, seborrheic dermatitis, psoriasis

resemble bacterial pyoderma [2]. In this chapter, presentations of common tineas are discussed.

Tinea corporis

Tinea corporis is dermatophytosis of the glabrous skin of the trunk, extremities, and face and occurs in all ages, ethnic backgrounds, and nationalities. It is most common in warm, humid climates. Predisposing factors include contact with animals (especially kittens, cattle, and horses), crowded living conditions, participation in contact sports and use of gymnasiums, and a variety of systemic disorders including diabetes mellitus and HIV infection. Contact with infected animals is a common cause as certain animals can harbor the organisms, resulting in disease in exposed persons. Kittens are particularly a problem, and large epidemics have resulted from a single infected animal.

Typical lesions of tinea corporis are pruritic, oval, annular (ringlike), erythematous, scaly patches that may have a slightly elevated border (Fig. 4-1). However, the presentation of tinea corporis is quite variable and can mimic many other dermatoses. It should be stressed that not all annular or ringlike dermatoses are tinea corporis. The diagnosis is especially challenging if blistering or pustular lesions occur

(Fig. 4-2). The use of topical steroids may change the clinical appearance and produce tinea incognito (Fig. 4-3). Scratching may lead to lichenification and the appearance of a neurodermatitis or eczematous response. Occasionally, this lichenified presentation may mimic psoriasis. The diagnosis can be confirmed by potassium hydroxide preparation and by fungal culture.

Tinea pedis

Tinea pedis refers to dermatophytosis of the plantar surface or toe webs. There are three common recognized patterns: 1) moccasin or chronic hyperkeratotic; 2) interdigital; and 3)

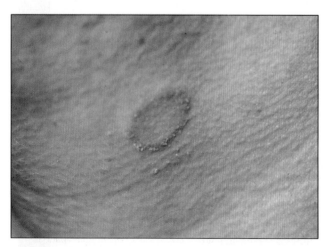

FIGURE 4-1 Tinea corporis. Annular scaly patch typical of dermatophytosis.

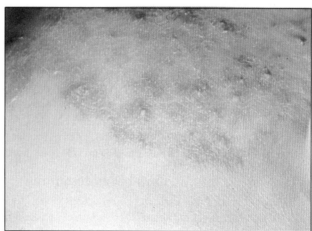

FIGURE 4-2 Tinea corporis with pustular lesions. This rash mimicked bacterial folliculitis.

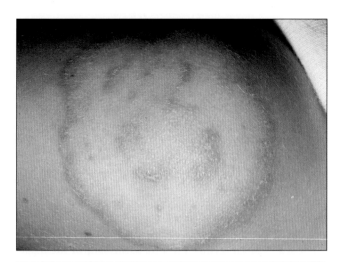

FIGURE 4-3 Tinea corporis. Use of topical steroids spread a small annular patch but reduced scale and itching. The rash progressed in size, but became less inflammatory.

inflammatory or vesicular [1•,2,3]. The interdigital variety is the most common, and the patient typically presents with macerated, fissured, scaling, interdigital lesions usually involving the web space of the fourth and fifth toes. Bacterial infections and cutaneous candidiasis can be differentiated by culture. Wood's light examination revealing bright coral red fluorescence is typical of infection by *Corynebacterium minutissimum* or erythrasma. In the vesicular variety of tinea pedis, the patient presents with painful pruritic vesicles or bullous lesions on the instep of one or both feet. Infection may be disabling, and this variety has historically been a particular problem in the military. The dermatophytid reaction can be associated with the vesicular variety. When this reaction occurs, the patient may have an eczematous-appearing rash on one or both hands that may resemble dishidrotic eczema on the palms or sides of

fingers. This rash is considered a hypersensitivity reaction to the fungal foot infection, and both cultures and potassium hydroxide (KOH) preparation taken from the hand produce negative results. The hyperkeratotic variety of tinea pedis or moccasin foot is characterized by dry, scaly, hyperkeratotic changes on the plantar surface of one or both feet (Fig. 4-4). Fungal nail disease is generally present, and the patient may also have palmar infection (tinea manuum). Chronic infections that are recalcitrant to therapy typically occur.

Tinea cruris

Tinea cruris refers to dermatophytosis of the inguinal region, including the gluteal folds, the crural folds, and proximal medial thighs. Intense pruritus is common and has led to the lay term "jock itch." Adult men are more commonly infected than women. Risk factors include maceration and occlusion. The scrotal skin appears immune to infection by dermatophytes, although candidiasis and erythrasma occur in this region (Fig. 4-5). Women are more likely to present with cutaneous candidiasis in the genital and inguinal areas than with dermatophytosis.

Tinea unguium

The terms *tinea unguium* and *onychomycosis* are often used interchangeably; however, the former specifies dermatophytic infection of the nail unit, whereas onychomycosis encompasses all forms of fungal infection causing nail disease. Onychomycosis is responsible for approximately 50% of dystrophic nails and occurs in an estimated 15% to 20% of people 40 to 60 years old [1•].

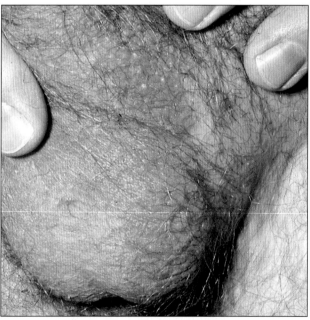

FIGURE 4-5 Tinea cruris. Note scrotal involvement—patient has cutaneous candidiasis, not dermatophytosis. The treatment would therefore be different than for dermatophytosis as griseofulvin would be ineffective.

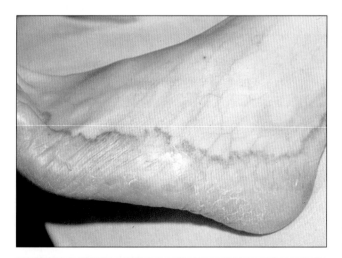

FIGURE 4-4 Moccasin tinea pedis. Entire plantar surface extending to lateral and medial borders of foot is red and scaly. (*From* Elewski [1•]; with permission.)

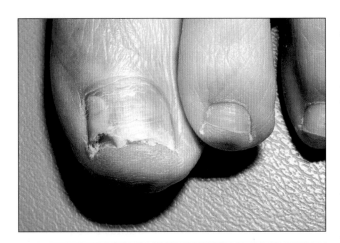

FIGURE 4-6 Tinea unguium or oncyomycosis. Note thickened nail bed with hyperkeratosis and onycholysis.

Toenails are more often involved than fingernails. The most common presentation is distal subungual variety manifested by subungual debris and thickening with associated onycholysis and thickening of the nail plate (Fig. 4-6) [4]. However, there are other presentations of fungal nail disease, including white superficial onychomycosis and candidiasis in nails [1•]. It is important to stress that not all patients with dystrophic nails have fungal disease. For example, psoriasis and lichen planus can mimic onychomycosis and can be differentiated by a culture.

Tinea capitis

Tinea capitis refers to dermatophytosis of the scalp hair follicle and occurs mostly in children [5]. Currently, there is an epidemic of *Trichophyton tonsurans* infection in urban areas of the United States [6–10]. Many infected children are black or Hispanic, and infection is often recalcitrant to griseofulvin therapy. The clinician must be suspicious of infection as this organism does not cause hair fluorescence [11], and therefore the diagnosis must made on clinical signs and by culture.

There are inflammatory and noninflammatory varieties of tinea capitis. With the inflammatory variety, the clinical picture varies from a few pustules in the scalp to widespread abscesses or kerions [5]. Alopecia and tender cervical lymphadenopathy are generally associated (Fig. 4-7). If untreated, a permanent scarring alopecia may result. The noninflammatory type may resemble alopecia areata and present with oval, generally scaly patches of alopecia. Prominent cervical adenopathy, presence of scale, and lack of exclamation point hairs in patches of alopecia point to a diagnosis of tinea capitis. As only a few species of dermatophytes are able to yield hair fluorescence under Wood's light examination, the diagnosis should be based upon culturing a dermatophyte, not on the presence or absence of scalp fluorescence [11]. It should be stressed that the presence of fluorescence is dependent upon the infecting dermatophyte rather than the clinical presentation.

Diagnosis

The clinical diagnosis of dermatophyte infection can be confirmed by direct microscopy of skin scrapings (KOH) and by fungal culture [2]. Methods of specimen collection vary depending on the body site infected. In nail disease, the specimen is best collected by cutting back diseased nails and curetting or scraping the hyperkeratotic and thickened nail bed in the area proximal to the cuticle area or proximal nail fold. With scalp infection, 10 to 12 hairs in the diseased area or at the border of alopecia should be epilated, and scale in the area can also be included in the specimen. With infections on the foot, hand, or elsewhere, the active raised border is the best site for collection of specimens. A glass slide or scalpel blade can be used to scrape off sufficient scale. In blistering conditions, the roof of the blister would be the best specimen. Once the specimen is obtained, a portion can be used for a KOH preparation and the remainder for culture. A KOH preparation is a simple, easy office procedure. Potassium hydroxide is a keratin-clearing agent and will dissolve the keratin in the specimen, permitting visualization of the fungal hyphae. As the KOH of all dermatophytes are indistinguishable, specific identification of the organism requires a culture (Fig. 4-8). Because dermatophytes can be acquired from animal, human, and soil sources, knowing the causative pathogen will help determine the pattern of spread [2]. Fungal cultures take considerable experience to correctly identify the genus and species. For this reason, many clinicians use a screening media, such as dermatophyte test media, that contains a phenol red indicator. With dermatophyte growth, the medium changes from yellow to red. Although a useful screen for dermatophytes, false-positive and false-negative results are common. In addition, *Candida albicans* will not change the color of the dermatophyte test media and therefore may lead to incorrect diagnoses [2]. Many reference laboratories are available for precise identification of fungal organisms.

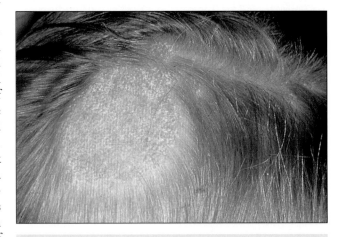

FIGURE 4-7 Tinea capitis. Patch of alopecia in a child's scalp. Note that not all patients with tinea capitis will fluoresce under Wood's light examination.

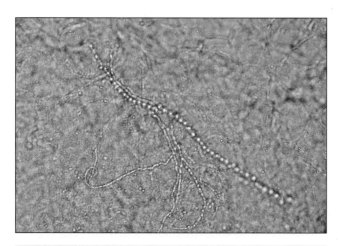

Figure 4-8 Positive potassium hydroxide preparation. Note branching hyphae typical of dermatophyte infection. The exact organism must be determined by culture.

TABLE 4-3 ACTIVITY SPECTRUM OF ORAL ANTIFUNGALS

	Dermatophytes	Candida	Malassezia furfur
Griseofulvin	+	−	−
Ketoconazole	+	+	+
Fluconazole	+	+	+
Itraconazole	+	+	+
Terbinafine	+	+/±	−

+, effective; −, ineffective; +/±. probably effective.

Therapy

Newer topical and systemic antifungals have significantly improved the therapy for dermatophyte infections [12•, 13–17]. Oral antifungals available for therapy include griseofulvin, ketoconazole, itraconazole, fluconazole, and terbinafine (Table 4-3) [18]. Topical agents include the imidazoles, allylamines, ciclopiroxolamine, and a variety of miscellaneous agents (Table 4-4).

An oral therapeutic agent is necessary when treating tinea capitis and onychomycosis. Tinea capitis is generally treated until the patient is culture-negative and new hair is regrowing, and with griseofulvin, the duration of therapy is generally 2 to 3 months. Patients and their families should

also use an antifungal shampoo—ketoconazole or selenium sulfide—on a daily basis [19]. In patients with *Microsporum canis* infections, the infected cat or dog should be appropriately treated. Onychomycosis has been historically treated with griseofulvin, which is administered until the new fungal-free nail has regrown [18]. Because of the slow growth of nails, this progress can take up to 2 years for toenails and 6 to 9 months for fingernails. Upon cessation of therapy, recurrence is common. However, newer agents appear promising using short-term or pulse courses (Table 4-5) and may prevent some relapses [14,17]. Further stud-

TABLE 4-4 ACTIVITY SPECTRUM OF TOPICAL ANTIFUNGALS

	Dermatophytes	Candida	Malassezia furfur
Imidazoles	+	+	+
Clotrimazole			
Ketoconazole			
Miconazole			
Oxiconazole			
Sulconazole			
Allylamines	+	+	+
Naftifine			
Terbinafine			
Ciclopiroxolamine	+	+	+
Miscellaneous			
Tolnaftate	+	−	+
Nystatin	−	+	+
Selenium sulfide, 2.5%	−	−	+

+, effective; −, ineffective.

TABLE 4-5 THERAPY FOR DERMATOPHYTOSIS

Tinea corporis, cruris, and pedis

Topical imidazole, allylamine, or other effective agent twice daily for 4 wk or until clinically and mycologically resolved

Tinea capitis

Griseofulvin 5–15 mg/kg until mycologic cure obtained and normal hair is regrowing

*Itraconazole 100 mg/d for 30 d (dosage may vary according to body weight; duration may vary according to severity and clinical response)

Tinea unguium (toenails)

Griseofulvin (ultramicrosize strength) until nail has regrown and is culture-negative (generally 1–2 y toenail, 6–9 mo fingernail)

*Itraconazole 200 mg qd for 12 wk toenail, for 6 wk fingernail

*Itraconazole 400 mg qd for 1 wk–1 wk/mo 3–4 mo, toenail; 2 mo, fingernail

*Terbinafine 250 mg qd for 12 wk, toenail; for 6 wk, fingernail

*Fluconazole 100 mg qd or pulse dose† 300 mg/wk until nail has regrown and is culture negative

*Currently investigational in United States; dosage and duration may vary according to response. †With pulse dosage, nail is often not clinically normal when drug is discontinued.

ies are necessary to prove their effectiveness and dosage schedules.

Topical agents will generally suffice for tinea pedis, cruris, and corporis. The patient should be instructed to apply the topical agent twice a day to the involved skin and approximately 2 cm around the diseased area for 4 to 8 weeks. However, topical terbinafine has been shown effective for interdigital tinea pedis after a single 1-week course [20•]. In patients with extensive disease and patients immunocompromised by disease or therapy, an oral agent is justified as adjuvant therapy [21•]. Two weeks of ketoconazole 200 mg every day, or griseofulvin 250 mg twice daily (ultramicrosize) or 1 week of itraconazole 200 mg to 400 mg every day can be used adjunctively with appropriate topical therapy [18].

CUTANEOUS CANDIDIASIS

Both cutaneous and oral candidiasis are commonly encountered fungal infections. *Candida albicans* is the most frequently isolated species of *Candida* and is part of the normal flora of the alimentary tract and mucocutaneous areas, but is not ordinarily found on normal intact skin. Predisposing factors for clinical disease include: 1) underlying systemic disease; 2) impaired host immunity; 3) treatment with systemic antibiotics (>7 d) or immunosuppressive agents; 4) extremes of age; and 5) disrupted epithelial barrier (moisture, occlusion) [1•].

Clinical Presentation

Candida produces protean manifestations of the skin and mucous membranes. In many instances, disease may resemble dermatophyte or bacterial infection. The presence of risk factors should alert the clinician to Candida infection.

Candida intertrigo
With maceration, heat, occlusion, and friction, Candida overgrowth can occur. Areas predisposed include the groin, axillary vault, gluteal region, and under the pannus or pendulous breasts. The typical presentation is a bright red, moist skin surface with scaling borders and satellite papules or pustules (Fig. 4-9).

Candida paronychia
With prolonged exposure to water or manipulation of the cuticle, *Candida* can infect the proximal nail fold, developing erythema and edema with a purulent discharge. In chronic disease, the nail becomes dystrophic.

Candida diaper dermatitis
The occlusive nature of diapers promotes Candida overgrowth. The diaper area, including the folds of the groin, becomes red with satellite pustules (Fig. 4-10) [22].

Acute pseudomembranous candidiasis or thrush
White-gray curdlike patches develop in the buccal mucosa, tongue, gingiva, and pharynx. Risk factors include use of dentures, diabetes mellitus, systemic antibiotics (>7 d), HIV infection, and other immunocompromised states.

Angular cheilitis or perleche
Infection of the oral commisures is commonly caused by *Candida*, resulting in maceration, erythema, and scaling (Fig. 4-11).

Diagnosis
The diagnosis of all forms of cutaneous and mucosal candidiasis can be made by the potassium hydroxide wet mount, which reveals yeast and pseudohyphae. A fungal culture confirms the diagnosis [1•,2].

Therapy
Most cutaneous and oral candidiasis can be treated by topical agents. Topical agents such as ketoconazole or econazole creams are generally used twice daily for 2 to 4 weeks. In oral candidiasis, clotrimazole troches are very effective. Whenever possible, risk factors such as dentures should also

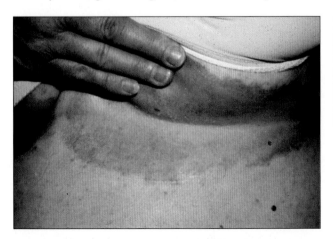

FIGURE 4-9 Red macerated rash under pendulous breasts is a common presentation of cutaneous candidiasis.

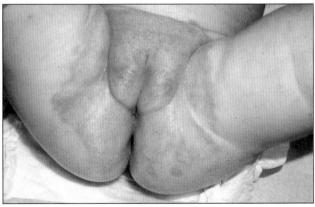

FIGURE 4-10 *Candida* diaper dermatitis. Note involvement of the folds of the groin that serve as a differentiating point from diaper dermatitis.

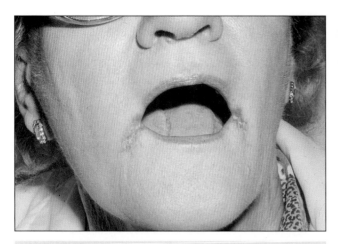

FIGURE 4-11 Perleche in an edentulous woman is a common presentation of cutaneous candidiasis.

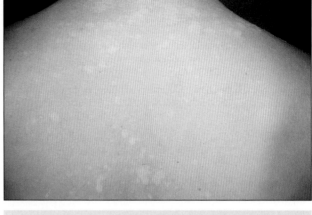

FIGURE 4-12 Pityriasis or tinea versicolor. Note hypopigmented and scaly patches on trunk and proximal extremities.

be removed. Oral agents can be used as adjunct to topical agents, and may be necessary in extensive infections, immunocompromised conditions, and diabetes mellitus. Systemic ketoconazole 200 to 400 mg every day for 5 to 7 days is a very effective systemic therapy. Fluconazole has been reported to be successful in vaginal candidiasis with a one-time dose of 150 mg [1•,12•].

TINEA VERSICOLOR OR PITYRIASIS VERSICOLOR

Pityriasis or tinea versicolor is caused by the yeast *M. furfur* [1•,2]. The typical presentation is asymptomatic, slightly scaly, hypopigmented or hyperpigmented, or even erythematous to salmon-colored patches on the trunk and upper arms (Fig. 4-12). Disease is most common during the summer months, and chronic infections are common.

The diagnosis is made by a KOH preparation showing short hyphae and yeast cells. Culture is not routinely done.

The treatment of pityriasis or tinea versicolor is topical application of an antifungal agent twice daily for up to 4 weeks (Table 4-4). Oral agents may occasionally be indicated (Table 4-3) [23,24,25•]. Ketoconazole 200 mg every day for 5 to 10 days is very effective, as is a single 400-mg dose of fluconazole. To avoid recurrence, prophylactic oral or topical treatment regimens may be important. Patients should also be instructed to avoid heavy oils on affected areas that may promote the growth of *M. furfur*.

REFERENCES AND RECOMMENDED READING

Recently published papers of particular interest have been highlighted as:
• Of interest
•• Of outstanding interest

1.•   Elewski BE, ed. *Cutaneous Fungal Infections.* New York: Igaku-Shoin Medical Publishers; 1992.

2.   Elewski BE, Hazen PG: The superficial mycoses and the dermatophytes. *J Am Acad Dermatol* 1989, 21:655–673.

3.   Kearse HL, Miller OF: Tinea pedis in prepubertal children: does it occur? *J Am Acad Dermatol* 1988, 19:619–622.

4.   Daniel CR III, Lawson LA: Tinea unguium. *Cutis* 1987, 40:326–327.

5.   Herbert A: Tinea capitis. *Arch Dermatol* 1988, 124:1554–1557.

6.   Bronson RM, Desai DR, Barsky S, *et al.*: An epidemic of infection with Trichophyton tonsurans revealed in a 20-year survey of fungal infections in Chicago. *J Am Acad Dermatol* 1983, 8:322–330.

7.   Rasmussen JE, Ahmed R: Trichophyton reactions in children with tinea capitis. *Arch Dermatol* 1978, 114:371–372.

8.   Babel DE, Baughman SA: Evaluation of the adult carrier state in juvenile tinea capitis caused by Trichophyton tonsurans. *J Am Acad Dermatol* 1989, 21:1209–1212.

9.   Sharma V, Hall JC, Knapp JF, *et al.*: Scalp colonization by Trichophyton tonsurans in an urban pediatric clinic. *Arch Dermatol* 1988, 124:1511–1513.

10.   Hebert AA, Head ES, MacDonald EM: Tinea capitis caused by Trichophyton tonsurans. *Pediatr Dermatol* 1985, 2:219–223.

11.   Prevost E: The rise and fall of fluorescent tinea capitis. *Pediatr Dermatol* 1983, 1:127–133.

12.• Elewski BE: Mechanisms of action of antifungal drugs. *J Am Acad Dermatol* 1993, 28:S28–S34.

13.   Lambert DR, Siegle RJ, Camisa C: Griseofulvin and ketoconazole in the treatment of dermatophyte infections. *Int J Dermatol* 1989, 28:300–304.

14.   Hay RJ, Clayton YM, Moore MK, *et al.*: An evaluation of itraconazole in the management of onychomycosis. *Br J Dermatol* 1988, 119:359–366.

15.   Lesher JL Jr, Smith JG Jr: Antifungal agents in dermatology. *J Am Acad Dermatol* 1987, 173:383–396.

16.   Zaias N, Serrano L: The successful treatment of fingernail Trichophyton rubrum onychomycosis with oral terbinafine. *Clin Exp Dermatol* 1989, 14:120–124.

17.   Goodfield MJD, Rowell NR, Forster RA, *et al.*: Treatment of dermatophyte infection of the finger and toenails with terbinafine (SF86-327, Lamisil), an orally active fungicidal agent. *Br J Dermatol* 1989, 12:1753–1757.

18.   Gupta AK, Sauder DN, Shear NH: Antifungal agents: an overview, part II. *J Am Acad Dermatol* 1994, 30:911–933.

19. Allen HB, Honig RJ, Leyden JJ, *et al.*: Selenium sulfide: adjunctive therapy for tinea capitis. *Pediatr* 1982, 69:81–83.

20.• Bergstresser P, Elewski B, Hanifin J, *et al.*: Comparison of cure and relapse rates with 1- and 4-week regimens of terbinafine and clotrimazole 1% cream in patients with interdigital tinea pedis: results of a double blind, multicenter study. *J Am Acad Dermatol* 1993, 28:648–651.

21.• Elewski BE, Sullivan J: Dermatophytes as opportunistic pathogens. *J Am Acad Dermatol* 1994, 30:1021–1022.

22. Honig P, Gribetz B, Leyden JJ, *et al.* Amoxicillin and diaper dermatitis. *J Am Acad Dermatol* 1988, 19:275–279.

23. Lopez-Lopez JR, Gonzalez-Benavides JD: Pityriasis versicolor in children. *Med Cutan Ibero Lat Am* 1985, 13:381–383.

24. Ford GP, Ive FA, Midgley G: Pityrosporum folliculitis and ketoconazole. *Br J Dermatol* 1982, 107:691–695.

25.• Delescluse RCJ: Itraconazole in tinea versicolor: a review. *J Am Acad Dermatol* 1990, 23:551–554.

Premalignant and Malignant Epithelial Tumors

5

5

Lisa M. Seung
Daniel Rivlin
Ronald L. Moy

Key Points

- Epithelial malignant neoplasms have many potential etiologies, but the most common one and the one that can be protected against easily is actinic damage from the sun.
- Actinic keratosis is the most common precancerous lesion, and can be treated effectively with a variety of methods.
- Basal cell carcinoma is the most common epithelial malignancy and rarely if ever metastasizes, but can cause local destruction.
- Squamous cell carcinoma is the second most common epithelial malignancy and can metastasize.
- There are many methods for treating basal cell carcinoma and squamous cell carcinoma effectively, but Mohs micrographic surgery has the highest cure rate.

Although not all skin tumors are sun-related, ultraviolet radiation is the single most important cause of both premalignant and malignant epithelial tumors. Prevention plays a pivotal role in reducing the incidence of skin cancer. Thus, the risks of sun exposure and benefits of high-potency sun screens, with a sun protection factor of greater than 15, should be made common knowledge to all patients. In addition, generalists should learn to recognize premalignant lesions as early diagnosis and treatment of such lesions will decrease the morbidity rate of patients as well as the cost of treatment. When in doubt, a suspicious lesion should be biopsied rather than observed and allowed to develop into a malignant tumor.

PREMALIGNANT LESIONS

Actinic Keratoses

Actinic keratoses, also known as solar keratoses, are scaly, red papules of about 3 to 6 mm in diameter that develop on sun-exposed skin surfaces [1]. They are usually rough, keratotic lesions that are best detected by palpation (Fig. 5-1).

Actinic keratoses are most often induced by ultraviolet radiation and are thus more likely to develop in individuals who have had extensive sun exposure and are fair in complexion. The elderly, who have experienced the most cumulative sun exposure, are at the highest risk for development of actinic keratoses. The lesions are often multiple and most commonly appear on the face, dorsal surfaces of the hands and forearms, and the bald scalp.

If left untreated actinic keratoses have the potential to transform into squamous cell carcinoma. It is estimated that 12% to 25% of patients with actinic keratoses will develop invasive squamous cell carcinoma [2]; however, metastasis

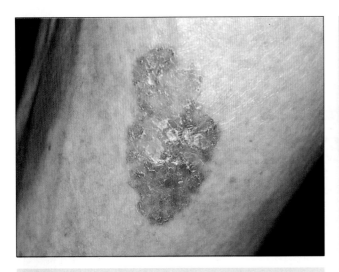

FIGURE 5-1 Red, scaly, erythematous plaque typical of both superficial basal cell carcinoma and Bowen's disease. This particular case represents superficial basal cell carcinoma.

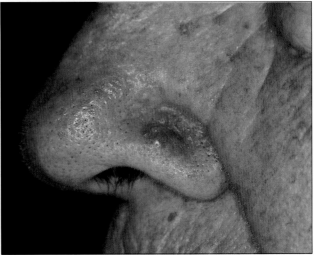

FIGURE 5-2 Typical nodular basal cell carcinoma with a pearly telangiectatic border and central erosion.

is rare in this type of squamous cell carcinoma [3•]. Although there have been controversies regarding whether treatment of actinic keratoses actually reduces morbidity in patients [4,5], it is generally accepted that the risks involved are too great to forgo therapy.

Treatment

Treatment of actinic keratoses in patients with a few lesions is best accomplished by cryosurgery or curettage. In cryosurgery, liquid nitrogen is sprayed onto the affected lesion or applied with a cotton-tipped swab. With curettage, an instrument (curette) is used to scrape out the lesions. A success rate of 99% has been shown for treatment with each of these procedures [1,3•]. In addition, both cryosurgery and curettage are quick procedures, and healing is usually prompt. However, with both procedures there may be some residual hypopigmentation.

In patients with numerous lesions, topical application of 5-fluorouracil (Efudex; Roche Dermatologics, Nutley, NJ, and Fluoroplex; Allergan Herbert, Irvine, CA) is extremely effective. One to five percent 5-fluorouracil is available in a cream or solution form and can be applied topically once or twice a day for about 4 to 6 weeks. A newer topical agent, masoprocol cream (Actinex; Reed & Carnrick, Jersey City, NJ), has also demonstrated effectiveness in treating multiple actinic keratoses. Masoprocol and 5-fluorouracil are especially useful, as they can destroy subclinical lesions as well as fully developed actinic keratoses. Unfortunately, they have uncomfortable side effects such as inflammation, erythema and irritation. In addition, patients should be warned that complications such as persistent redness may infrequently occur. Any lesion resistant to 5-fluorouracil or masoprocol can be further treated with cryosurgery or curettage.

Even after treatment, patients with actinic keratoses should be closely monitored at regular intervals for the development of further lesions. Also, proper precautions (*ie*, protection from the sun) should always be advised. The use of sunscreens and photoprotective clothing has been associated with spontaneous resolution of existing lesions, as well as reduction of new lesions.

Bowen's Disease

Bowen's disease is an in situ squamous cell carcinoma that has the potential to become invasive. It has been described as a well-demarcated, scaly, indurated red plaque that is often confused with benign dermatoses, such as chronic eczema or psoriasis (Fig. 5-2) [6••]. As a result of the confusion over its initial diagnosis, Bowen's disease is usually not properly diagnosed until a biopsy is performed. More often than not, the biopsy is taken after the presumed "dermatitis" has been present for several years and has been resistant to corticosteroid treatment.

Bowen's disease most frequently occurs in middle-aged to older white adults and can arise on both sun-exposed as well as nonexposed skin surfaces. A variety of agents have been implicated in the pathogenesis of Bowen's disease: 1) actinic damage (which accounts for the development of lesions on sun-exposed areas such as the face), 2) inorganic arsenic (a chemical formerly present in certain "bromide" medications and in fungicides and pesticides), 3) a viral factor (several human papillomavirus types have been linked to Bowen's disease), and 4) radiation exposure [7••]. In addition, a connection between Bowen's disease and internal cancer has been a topic of debate in the past. However, recent consensus is that there is no real increased risk of concurrent or subsequent visceral malignancy associated with Bowen's disease [8•].

Treatment options for Bowen's disease include surgical excision, curettage with electrodesiccation, topical 5-fluorouracil, cryosurgical destruction, radiation therapy, and laser surgery. For recurrent lesions Mohs micrographic surgery can be performed (*see* section on Squamous cell carcinoma).

MALIGNANT LESIONS

Squamous Cell Carcinoma

Squamous cell carcinoma is the second most frequent malignancy of the skin, second only to basal cell carcinoma. The lesions of squamous cell carcinoma arise from the keratin-producing squamous cells of the epithelium. Squamous cell carcinoma tends to occur on the sun-exposed skin regions of the elderly, such as the face, hands, and forearms. Also, it is often seen in conjunction with weathered and actinically damaged skin. In comparison with basal cell carcinoma, squamous cell carcinoma has the potential to metastasize and is able to develop from skin that has been chronically inflamed or irritated. In most instances, squamous cell carcinoma appears as a erythematous plaque, nodule, or ulceration (Table 5-1).

Etiology

The most common cause of squamous cell carcinoma is ultraviolet radiation and, in particular, ultraviolet-B exposure. Thus, fair-skinned individuals are the most likely victims of cutaneous squamous cell carcinoma. Other known causes of squamous cell carcinoma include certain chronic dermatoses, polycyclic aromatic hydrocarbons (seen in tars and petroleum), arsenic (which often causes lesions to appear on the palms and soles), human papillomavirus (especially types 16 and 18), genetic predisposition, and immunosuppression [9••]. Of special note is the well-documented incidence of squamous cell carcinoma arising in previously irradiated or burned skin, as well as its development from scars. Squamous cell carcinoma arising in such areas of skin injury is referred to as Marjolin's ulcer, and is usually located on the extremities [10]. Although Marjolin's ulcer is a rare entity, it is known to be an especially aggressive form of squamous cell carcinoma. Therefore, any chronic, intractable ulcer should be biopsied.

Keratoacanthoma, although originally believed to be a separate disorder, is now considered to be one form of squamous cell carcinoma. Keratoacanthomas tend to follow a course in which the lesions spontaneously involute. Nevertheless, they should be treated as other types of squamous cell carcinomas and excised or destroyed when discovered, as lesions have been known to metastasize.

Appearance

Squamous cell carcinoma may present with a variety of features. The lesions range in color from red to tan. In comparison with basal cell carcinoma, squamous cell carcinoma usually appears more scaly and may have some degree of ulceration, crusting, or erosion [11] (Fig. 5-3). In addition, the lesions usually lack the pearly hue and telangiec-

TABLE 5-1 METASTATIC RATES FOR SQUAMOUS CELL CARCINOMA	
Location of primary lesion	**Recurrence, %**
Sun-damaged skin	5.2
External ear	8.8
Lower lip	13.7
Osteomyelitic sinus	31.0
Scar	37.9

Data from Rowe and coworkers [18].

tasias commonly associated with basal cell carcinoma. Because the appearance of squamous cell carcinoma may be variable, a biopsy should always be performed to establish diagnosis.

Local invasion and metastasis

Squamous cell carcinoma is known to grow more rapidly than basal cell carcinoma. However, it can penetrate through the subcutaneous and muscle layers and travel along nerve routes or through the lymphatics or the bloodstream. If allowed to grow indefinitely, the lesions may result in pain, necrosis of involved tissues, and functional impairment, including the loss of vision.

In metastasis, the regional lymph nodes are the most frequent targets of regional invasion. Distant organs such as bone, lung, and brain may also become sites of metastasis, but this is unusual. Once metastasis has taken place, (usually within 2 years of diagnosis of squamous cell carcinoma), prognosis tends to be poor. Tumors associated with ulcers, chronic irritation, or radiation exposure are more likely to metastasize, as are higher grade tumors. In addition, tumors of greater depth and size and those located on mucosal regions are more likely to metastasize as well as

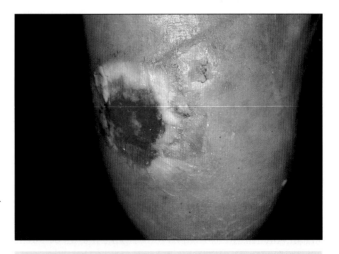

FIGURE 5-3 This ulcerated nodule with hyperkeratatic borders represents a deeply invasive squamous cell carcinoma.

recur. The incidence of metastasis is about 11% for patients with squamous cell carcinoma located on mucosal regions, 10% to 40% in patients with Marjolin's ulcer, and about 3% in patients with cutaneous squamous cell carcinoma [12].

Treatment

A number of different therapeutic options are available for squamous cell carcinoma, depending upon the location of the tumor, its size and depth of invasion, the age of the patient, and whether the tumor is a primary or recurrent lesion. Regardless of the choice of treatment, adequate follow-up is essential as recurrences tend to occur within the first 2 years after treatment of the primary lesion (Table 5-2).

Surgical excision

The conventional method for treating squamous cell carcinoma involves conservative surgical excision. This method achieves high success rates with rapid healing and good cosmetic results. After excision, margins should be examined histologically. The disadvantage of this form of treatment is that it may not be able to completely eradicate the tumor, especially if there is significant subclinical extension.

Cryosurgery and curettage

Options for small, primary lesions derived from sun damage (*ie*, actinically derived lesions) include destructive methods such as cryosurgery or curettage with electrodesiccation. These two modalities of treatment should only be performed on small lesions with distinct borders. In addition, they do not always achieve acceptable cosmetic results, and should be used with caution for lesions appearing on the face. When used for appropriate, small lesions, cryosurgery or curettage with electrodesiccation can achieve success rates equivalent to surgical excision. In addition, both are quick and economical modes of treatment.

Radiation treatment

Radiation treatment is especially useful for treating elderly or debilitated patients who are poor surgical candidates. Treatment requires multiple office visits and is costly. Other disadvantages to radiation therapy include lower success rates compared with other treatment modalities, and the often significant side effects with treatment.

Mohs micrographic surgery

To achieve the greatest amount of tissue preservation with the highest success rates, Mohs micrographic surgery is an important treatment. This procedure allows the physician to serially remove thin pieces of the specimen and microscopically examine 100% of the borders with frozen horizontal sections. Orientation is preserved and the edges of each slice are color-coded with dyes so that a map can be drawn, indicating any residual tumor [13]. The procedure is repeated but only in regions where, according to the map, the tumor is still remaining. Mohs surgery is the best treatment for large tumors, recurrent tumors, and for those

TABLE 5-2 RECURRENCE RATES IN PATIENTS TREATED FOR SQUAMOUS CELL CARCINOMA	
Therapeutic modality	**5-Year recurrence, %**
Cryotherapy	3.2
Curettage and electrodessication	3.7
Surgical excision	8.1
Radiation therapy	10.0
Mohs micrographic surgery	3.1

Data from Rowe and coworkers [18••].

regions where tissue preservation is deemed paramount (*ie*, for lesions on the face).

Metastatic disease

Treatment options for metastatic disease are limited. If there is invasion into regional lymph nodes, the options include lymph node dissection or radiation therapy [14••]. However, both lymph node dissection and radiation therapy can be used concomitantly. Once there are distant metastases (*eg*, metastases to the bones or lungs), prognosis is dismal. Combination chemotherapy for distant metastasis has been employed but has had limited effectiveness.

Basal Cell Carcinoma

Basal cell carcinoma is the most common cutaneous malignancy in the white population. Like squamous cell carcinoma, it has a tendency to occur in fair-skinned, elderly individuals who have been exposed to the harmful effects of the sun. Basal cell carcinoma appears most frequently on the face and neck as a small, pink, crusted, pearly lesion, often with rolled borders and telangiectasias. Of all the cutaneous malignancies, basal cell carcinoma is the slowest growing and is the least likely to metastasize. On initial presentation to a physician, patients often complain of a sore that tends to bleed or crust over, but which fails to heal.

Etiology

Many of the causes of basal cell carcinoma overlap with those of squamous cell carcinoma. For example, exposure to ultraviolet-B radiation, arsenic, and immunosuppressive states are known to predispose individuals to basal cell tumors. Occasionally, basal cell carcinoma may develop from trauma and scars including smallpox scars. However, unlike Marjolin's ulcers, they usually appear on the face and neck regions [15].

Appearance

Whenever basal cell carcinoma is suspected, the first step is to confirm the diagnosis with a biopsy. Nodular or nodular-ulcerative basal cell carcinoma is the most common basal cell carcinoma and presents as a small, pearly papule or nodule with a rolled border. Overlying telangiectasias are

TABLE 5-3 RECURRENCE RATES IN PATIENTS TREATED FOR BASAL CELL CARCINOMA

Therapeutic modality	5-Year recurrence, %
Surgical excision	10.1
Curettage and electrodessication	7.7
Radiation therapy	8.7
Cryotherapy	7.5
Mohs micrographic surgery	1.0

Data from Rowe and coworkers [19•].

frequently visible in these lesions. As they grow a central ulceration may develop along with crusting.

Superficial basal cell carcinoma is another common basal cell carcinoma that may present as multiple, red, scaly patches. The lesion commonly appears as a red plaque or patch with well-defined borders that may be pearly and scaly in appearance [16]. If allowed to develop for some time, these lesions tend to become nodular and may ulcerate.

Sclerosing or morpheaform basal cell carcinoma is a less common form of basal cell carcinoma that has the resemblance of a scar. It is yellowish-white in color and usually appears as a firm, indurated plaque with indistinct borders. Sclerosing basal cell carcinoma is a more aggressive form of basal cell carcinoma, as it often has subclinical extensions. These subclinical extensions make complete removal difficult and result in higher rates of recurrence.

Two other variants of basal cell carcinoma deserve mention. Pigmented basal cell carcinoma is a tumor that often resembles malignant melanoma but has the biologic behavior of common basal cell carcinoma. The other variant, infiltrating basal cell carcinoma, is a more aggressive tumor that, like sclerosing basal cell carcinoma, may have significant subclinical spread and high recurrence rates. The lesions of infiltrating basal cell carcinoma are ill-defined plaques that can resemble sclerosing basal cell carcinoma.

Local invasion and metastasis

Basal cell carcinoma tends to invade locally and rarely metastasizes. Like squamous cell carcinoma, local invasion can lead to infection, necrosis, and eventually pain and impairment of vital organs. The tumor can spread along nerves and bones. Basal cell carcinoma has an especially slow growth rate due to its dependence upon the stroma and an adequate blood supply for growth. Also, it may enter phases of regression alternating with periods of more aggressive growth.

Although recurrence rates for basal cell carcinoma vary greatly, two-thirds of recurrent lesions are known to develop within 3 years of diagnosis of the primary tumor [14••]. Tumors more likely to recur include those located on the nose, ear, or periorbital region (in descending order of

likelihood of recurrence). Also, tumors greater than 2 cm in diameter are more likely to recur [17] as are those with poor margins, such as sclerosing or infiltrating basal cell carcinoma. In general, any tumor with significant subclinical extension has a higher chance of recurring.

Treatment

As with squamous cell carcinoma, there are a number of methods to treat basal cell carcinoma. For small primary tumors of the nodular or superficial type, curettage with electrodesiccation is the most common mode of treatment. Cryosurgery is also a useful method for treating superficial basal cell carcinoma.

For larger tumors, conventional surgical excision or Mohs micrographic surgery is recommended. The margins for surgical excision should range from 2 to 4 mm for nodular basal cell carcinoma. However, for ill-defined lesions, lesions of the sclerosing or infiltrating type, or areas where a 2- to 4-mm surgical margin would not be cosmetically acceptable, it is recommended that Mohs surgery be performed. Mohs surgery has been shown to achieve success rates close to 99% for basal cell carcinoma, and should be the first-choice therapy for recurrent lesions (Table 5-3). Also, it is advocated that Mohs surgery be used for removing lesions located in regions with higher chances for recurrence, such as the nose, ear, and periorbital regions.

REFERENCES AND RECOMMENDED READING

Recently published papers of particular interest have been highlighted as:
• Of interest
•• Of outstanding interest

1. Balin AK, Lin AN, Pratt L: Actinic keratoses. *J Cutan Aging Cosmetic Dermatol* 1988, 1:77–86.

2. Kwa RE, Campana K, Moy RL: Biology of cutaneous squamous cell carcinoma. *J Am Acad Dermatol* 1992, 26:1–26.

3.• Callen JP: Possible precursors to epidermal malignancies. In *Cancer of the Skin.* Edited by Friedman RJ, Rigel DS, Kopf AW, Harris MN, Baker D. Philadelphia: WB Saunders; 1991:27–34.

4. Dodson JM, DeSpain J, Hewitt JE, Clark DP: Malignant potential of actinic keratoses and the controversy over treatment. *Arch Dermatol* 1991, 127:1029–1031.

5. Mostow EN, Johnson TM: Malignant transformation from actinic keratoses to squamous cell carcinomas. *Arch Dermatol* 1992, 128:560–561.

6.•• Beacham BE: Common skin tumors in the elderly. *Am Fam Physician* 1992, 46:163–168.

7.•• Cohen PR: Bowen's disease: squamous cell carcinoma in situ. *Am Fam Physician* 1991, 44:1325–1329.

8.• Chute CG, Chuang T-Y, Bergstralh EJ, Su WD: The subsequent risk of internal cancer with Bowen's disease. *JAMA* 1991, 266:816–819.

9.•• Johnson TM, Rowe DE, Nelson BR, Swanson NA: Squamous cell carcinoma of the skin (excluding lip and oral mucosa). *J Am Acad Dermatol* 1992, 26:467–484.

10. Edwards MJ, Hirsch RM, Broadwater JR, Netscher DT, Ames FC: Squamous cell carcinoma arising in previously burned or irradiated skin. *Arch Surg* 1989, 124:115–117.

11. Smoller J, Smoller BR: Skin malignancies in the elderly. Diagnosable, treatable, and potentially curable. *J Gerontol Nurs* 1992, 18:19–24.

12. Moller R, Reymann F, Hou-Jensen K: Metastases in dermatological patients with squamous cell carcinoma. *Arch Dermatol* 1979, 115:703–705.

13. Moy RL, Zitelli JA: Mohs micrographic surgery for treatment of skin cancer in the elderly. *Ger Med Today* 1989, 8:98–107.

14.•• Preston DS, Stern RS: Nonmelanoma cancers of the skin. *N Engl J Med,I>* 1992, 327:1649–1662.

15. Lang PG, Maize JC: Basal cell carcinoma. In *Cancer of the Skin*. Edited by Friedman RJ, Riegel DS, Kopf AW, Harris MN, Baker D. Philadelphia: WB Saunders; 1991:35–73.

16. Goldberg LH, Rubin HA: Management of basal cell carcinoma. *Postgrad Med* 1989, 85:57–63.

17. Roenigk RK, Ratz JL, Bailin PL, Wheeland RG: Trends in the presentation of basal cell carcinoma. *J Dermatol Surg Oncol* 1986, 12:860–865.

18.•• Rowe DE, Carroll RJ, Day CL: Prognostic factors for local recurrence, metastasis and survival rates in squamous cell carcinoma of the skin, ear and lip. *J Am Acad Dermatol* 1992, 26:976–990.

19.• Rowe DE, Carroll RJ, Day CL: Long-term recurrence rates in previously untreated (primary) basal cell carcinoma: implications for patient follow-up. *J Dermatol Surg Oncol* 1990, 15:315–328.

Benign and Malignant Pigmented Lesions

6

Arthur J. Sober
Raymond L. Barnhill

> ### *Key Points*
>
> • The incidence rate of cutaneous melanoma is increasing dramatically.
>
> • Early diagnosis usually results in cure of the patient.
>
> • Routine physical examination should include inspection of the skin, especially of the torso in men and the back and lower legs in women.
>
> • Individuals at increased risk of developing melanoma are those with large numbers of nevi, clinical atypical moles, a personal or family history of melanoma, skin that tans poorly, and freckles.
>
> • Most melanomas can be detected using the *ABCDE* rule: *A*ssymetry, *B*order irregularity, *C*olor variation, *D*iameter >6mm, and *E*nlargement.

Cutaneous melanoma is the most common cause of death from diseases developing initially in the skin [1•]. Because the frequency of cutaneous melanoma is increasing among white populations, it is imperative that the general physician be able to examine the skin in a discerning manner. The primary goal is to distinguish suspicious pigmented lesions from the myriad of other pigmented lesions on the skin.

Although a high proportion of melanomas are thought to be related to excessive sun exposure during childhood and adolescence, approximately 10% of cutaneous melanomas seem to have a genetic basis. Cutaneous melanomas that appear to follow a dominant inheritance pattern have been recognized for many years, and a linkage to chromosome 9 has recently been proposed.

NATURAL HISTORY

There are four distinct types of cutaneous melanoma which differ in clinical appearance, histologic appearance, and biologic behavior (Figs. 6-1 through 6-4). Three of these tend to exhibit horizontal growth in the superficial skin for extended periods of time (radial growth phase), during which surgical removal is usually curative. These types are the superficial spreading, lentigo maligna, and acral lentiginous melanoma [2] (Table 6-1).

These have relatively prolonged periods of evolution, during which they are either entirely intraepidermal or micro-invasive into the dermis with a negligible capacity for metastasis. Approximately 1 to 30 years may elapse before deeper invasion occurs with the attendant increased risk for metastasis via the lymphatics or the blood stream [2]. The fourth type, nodular melanoma, has no apparent radial growth phase and tends to rapidly invade the dermis from onset (Fig. 6-4; Table 6-1). Nodular melanoma appears to have capacity to metastasize from early in its development.

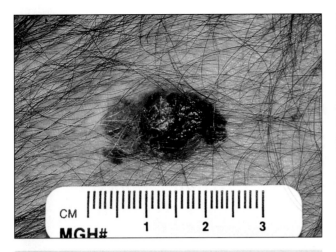

FIGURE 6-1 Superficial spreading melanoma is characterized by irregular borders and variation in color (blue color on left side).

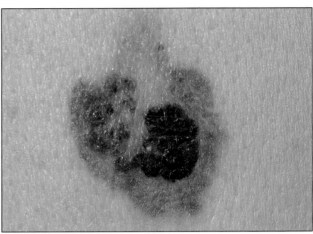

FIGURE 6-2 Superficial spreading melanoma shows irregular borders, variation in pigment pattern, and partial regression (whitish areas at 12 o'clock position).

The proportion of melanomas that arise *de novo* in apparently normal skin has been estimated to be anywhere from 30% to 70%. Conversely, the number of melanomas arising in pre-existing nevi also has been estimated to vary from 30% to 70%. Most authors believe that between 30% and 40% of melanomas arise in pre-existing nevi and the rest *de novo*.

Cutaneous melanoma spreads in three ways: within the adjacent skin, via the lymphatics to regional nodes, and via the blood stream to many visceral organs. In general, nodal presentation with metastatic disease occurs earlier than visceral presentation. The internal organs most frequently involved with metastatic disease are liver, lung, bone, and brain. Long disease-free intervals are not unusual with cutaneous melanoma so that 5 years disease-free survival does not necessarily represent cure. Thirteen percent of recurrences occur between 5 and 10 years and occasional

recurrences occur thereafter, especially with thinner tumors. Approximately 6% of patients with cutaneous melanoma will develop a second primary tumor during their lifetime. This figure is considerably higher in patients with familial melanoma, 30% of whom may develop a second primary tumor.

DIAGNOSIS

Clinical suspicion of cutaneous melanoma may be enhanced by applying the pneumonic *ABCDE: A*, asymmetry which refers to the lack of mirror image symmetry when the two halves of the lesion are compared; *B*, border irregularity; *C*, color variation; *D*, diameter >6 mm; and *E*, enlargement [3•]. Although certain melanomas may lack one or more of these features, or uncommonly all, their presence, especially in combination, should raise suspicion

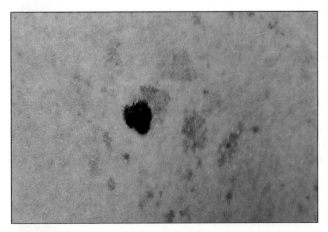

FIGURE 6-3 Early melanoma arising in markedly sun-damaged skin shows raised, dark-brown plaque with irregular border arising adjacent to a flat brown lesion.

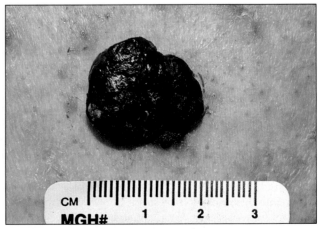

FIGURE 6-4 Nodular melanoma seen here is a brown-black nodule with no flat surrounding pigmentation.

TABLE 6-1 CLINICAL FEATURES OF MALIGNANT MELANOMA

Type	Site	Average age at diagnosis, y	Duration of known existence, y	Color
Lentigo maligna melanoma	Sun-exposed surfaces, particularly malar region of cheek and temple	70	5–20* or longer	In flat portions, shades of brown and tan predominant, but whitish gray occasionally present; in nodules, shades of reddish brown, bluish gray, bluish black
Superficial spreading melanoma	Any site (more common on upper back in men and on lower leg in women)	40–50	1–7	Shades of brown mixed with bluish red (violaceous), bluish black, reddish brown, and often whitish pink, and the border of lesion is at least in part visibly and/or palpably elevated
Nodular melanoma	Any site	40–50	Months to less than 5	Reddish blue (purple) or bluish black; either uniform in color or mixed with brown or black
Acral lentiginous melanoma	Palm, sole, nail bed, mucous membrane	60	1–10	In flat portions, dark brown predominantly; in raised lesions (plaques) brown-black or blue-black predominantly

*For much of this time (the precursor stage) active growth is confined to the epidermis.
Adapted from Sober and Koh [2]; with permission.

for melanoma [4]. Benign pigmented lesions may at times have one or more of these features, but by becoming aware of the clinical characteristics of the common benign pigmented lesions, most can be distinguished (Figs. 6-5 through 6-12 and Table 6-2). Those features most frequently present in early melanoma are increase in size and change in color. Increase in height correlates with deeper penetration within the skin and is a sign of more advanced disease, as are bleeding, pain, and ulceration. Itching in a pigmented lesion may raise suspicions because this symptom is present in approximately one quarter of patients with early melanomas.

Not everyone is at equal risk for developing melanoma. Those at greatest risk tan poorly, burn easily, freckle, have blonde or red hair, and blue or gray eyes, and have increased numbers of nevi [5,6]. Also at risk are those with a prior cutaneous melanoma, a positive family history of melanoma, and those who are immunosuppressed. Individuals who have had severe sunburns in childhood and adolescence also appear to have increased risk for development of melanoma later in life. Table 6-3 lists the factors associated with increased risk for development of melanoma. Increased regular surveillance would be appropriate for individuals with an elevated risk.

The best time to diagnose cutaneous melanoma is during the general physical examination. A complete skin examination of the patient should be performed in a room with bright lighting. A 5 to 10 power hand lens is also helpful in appreciating the differences noted in Figures 6-1 through 6-3 and Tables 6-1 and 6-2. Patients with a suspicious lesion should be considered for biopsy to establish the diagnosis [7], referred to a dermatologist for an additional opinion, or if suspicion is low-grade, given a follow-up appointment for reevaluation.

FIGURE 6-5 Solar lentigo (lentigines) results from chronic solar exposure. The face and back of the hands are the most common sites. Pigmentation is reticulate when magnified.

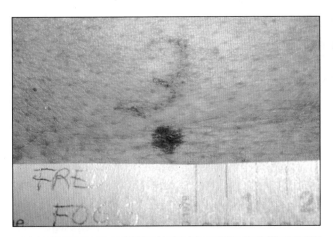

FIGURE 6-6 Lentigo is a flat (macular), sharply bordered medium- to dark-brown lesion that can vary in size from 2 mm to greater than 1 cm.

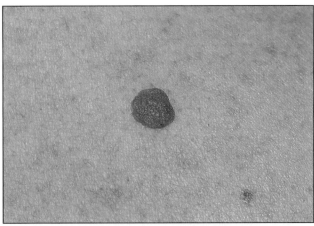

FIGURE 6-7 Dermal nevus is a flesh-colored papule or nodule usually with regular borders.

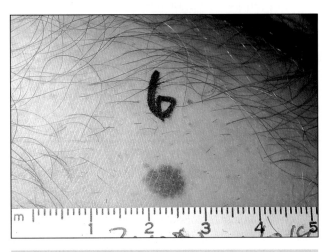

FIGURE 6-8 Compound nevus can be papillomatous or dome-shaped with smooth, well-demarcated borders. Colors may vary from light to very dark brown to flesh colored.

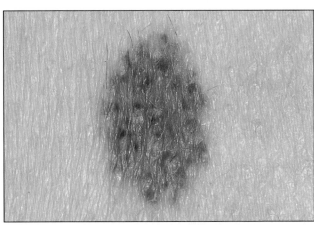

FIGURE 6-9 Congenital, melanocytic nevi are compound nevi present from birth. The size may range from less than 1 cm to greater than 144 in². Many will also have prominent dark hairs emerging from the nevus.

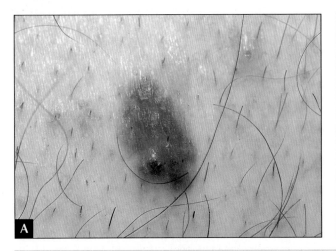

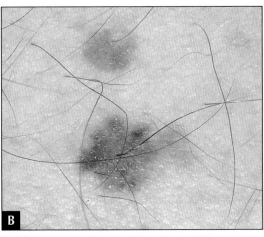

FIGURE 6-10 A, B, Dysplastic nevi, in contrast to benign acquired nevi, show more variable mixtures of tan, brown, and red or pink coloration, have irregular and sometimes hazy borders, are often 6 mm or larger, and may be present in great numbers.

Assessment

The most important evaluation in establishing the diagnosis of cutaneous melanoma is a biopsy of the lesion itself. Numerous studies have shown that a punch or incisional biopsy does not adversely affect outcome [7]. Total excisional biopsy with narrow margins is the procedure of choice, however, and can usually be performed under local anesthesia on an outpatient basis. This procedure provides the pathologist with the entire specimen for both diagnostic and prognostic purposes.

The prognosis of the patient with localized disease is directly related to the primary tumor thickness measured in millimeters from the granular cell layer of the epidermis to the deepest tumor cell. A second prognostic system depends on determining the anatomic level within the skin of the primary tumor, using Clark's levels of invasion: level I, intraepidermal (in situ); level II, into papillary dermis; level III, filling papillary dermis; level IV, into reticular dermis; and level V, into subcutaneous fat. Survival based

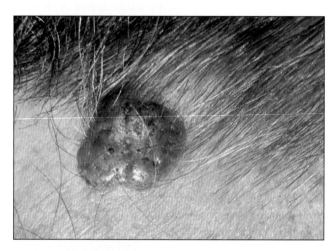

FIGURE 6-11 Seborrheic keratosis is a very common benign lesion which typically appears as a waxy "stuck-on" plaque. When highly pigmented or inflamed, differentiation from melanoma may be difficult. These lesions are typically multiple.

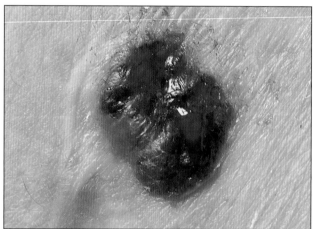

FIGURE 6-12 Pigmented basal cell carcinomas may appear as nodules such as this one or as barely raised plaques. In contrast to melanoma, which occurs more in fair-complexioned individuals with blue or gray eyes and lighter-colored hair, the pigmented basal cell carcinoma typically occurs in dark-complexioned individuals with dark brown or black hair and brown eyes.

TABLE 6-2 PIGMENTED LESIONS TO BE DISTINGUISHED FROM MELANOMA

Hemangioma

Reddish-brown or purple nodule. May blanch with compression (glass microscope slide), indicating its vascular nature

Subungual hematoma

Traumatic bleeding below the nail typically has maroon discoloration. A curved clear area is seen as the nail grows out

Tattoo

May be of medical origin (blue or green dots in a geometric pattern) or traumatic (pigmentation is irregularly dispersed and may appear black)

Blue nevus

Blue-gray, well-demarcated, stable 2–3 mm to 1 cm lesion. Occurs most often on hands, feet, and buttocks. The pigment is brown melanin, which appears blue because of the location in the mid-dermis

Pigmented dermatofibroma

Usually not pigmented, this firm, button-like fibrous response to injury may occasionally present with increased pigmentation. Dermatofibromas will ``dimple'' downward with lateral compression

TABLE 6-3 FACTORS THAT INCREASE RISK OF MELANOMA DEVELOPMENT

Greatly increase

Large numbers of nevi (>50 nevi ≥ 2 mm)
Clinically atypical moles in individuals with 2 family members with melanoma
Persistently changing pigmented lesion

Moderately increase

History of prior melanoma
Family history of melanoma
Clinically atypical nevi, nonfamilial melanoma
Light-complexioned whites versus blacks, Asians, or dark-complexioned whites

Modestly increase

Easily sunburned, poor at tanning
Freckles
Transplant suppression

on Clark's level is also shown in Table 6-4. Favorable prognostic factors are as follows:

Female sex
Patient age under 50 years
Clinically localized disease
Primary tumor located on arms and legs (other than hands and feet)
Thin primary tumor ≤ 0.75 mm)
Clark level II

Factors considered to be unfavorable are as follows:
Male sex
Patient age over 50 years
Evidence of metastases
Primary tumor located on head and neck, torso, or hands and feet
Thick primary tumor (> 1.70 mm)
Clark level IV or V
Ulcerated primary tumor
High mitotic rate of primary tumor
Presence of microscopic satellites

A variety of multifactorial models exist to further refine prediction of outcome, but these are beyond the scope of this chapter [8].

In the absence of positive signs or symptoms, patients with localized disease do not warrant extensive "high-tech" diagnostic investigations. A baseline chest radiograph is sufficient for individuals with low-risk disease, and for those at higher risk for recurrent disease, annual chest radiographs are recommended.

TREATMENT

Table 6-5 summarizes the treatment for primary melanoma [9•,10•]. In some centers, patients with localized disease who have primary tumors thicker than 1.50 mm undergo elective lymph nodal dissection if a single defined drainage pathway can be determined. The value of elective nodal dissection versus close observation followed by delayed dissection if nodes become clinically palpable is currently undergoing investigation by randomized clinical trial [11].

At present, there are no adjuvant therapies of proven value to lower risk of recurrence in patients with high-risk disease. Many agents are currently under investigation, including α-interferon, various tumor vaccines, and various types of monoclonal antibody therapy [12••].

The treatment for isolated metastatic disease is surgical excision, if possible. Some patients, especially those with lymph nodal and soft tissue disease, may have long disease-free intervals following surgery [13]. Such patients should be staged carefully before surgical treatment. Patients in whom metastatic disease cannot be surgically eliminated are candidates for palliative forms of therapy. At the present time, there is no highly successful form of chemotherapy or radiation therapy for metastatic cutaneous melanoma. Current treatment protocols usually involve multiple drugs, and referral to a medical oncologist is appropriate. Radiation therapy is palliative for metastasis to brain or bone.

ROLE OF THE GENERALIST

Most melanomas are detected either by the patient, patient's family members, or the family physician. As cutaneous melanoma can occur in relatively young individuals (mean age of melanoma is between 40 and 50 years), the early detection and subsequent cure of the patient translates into a gain of many years of productive life. In addition to early diagnosis, the generalist has an important role to play in primary and secondary prevention.

TABLE 6-4 FIVE-YEAR SURVIVAL RATES FOR LOCALIZED MELANOMA	
Thickness, *mm*	**5-Year Survival, %**
< 0.76	96
0.76–1.49	87
1.50–2.49	75
2.50–3.99	66
≥ 4.00	47
Clark level	
II (Into papillary dermis)	95
III (Filling papillary dermis)	82
IV (Into reticular dermis)	71
V (Into subcutaneous fat)	49

TABLE 6-5 SURGICAL GUIDELINES FOR PRIMARY TUMOR MANAGEMENT IN PATIENTS WITH LOCALIZED MELANOMA*		
Tumor thickness, *mm*	**Excision margin, *cm***	**Closure**
< 1.0	1.0	Primary
1.0–4.0	2.0	Primary
> 4.0	3.0†	Primary, flap, or graft

*These guidelines are arbitrary. They should be modified for individual patients, depending on overall assessment of prognosis. †Margins < 3 cm may be necessary to achieve primary closure.

PATIENT EDUCATION

Because there is no highly effective therapy for advanced melanoma, the cornerstone of decreasing melanoma mortality is based on a combination of early diagnosis and primary prevention. Primary prevention currently focuses on reducing the overall exposure of the population, especially those at increased risk, to sunlight from as early in life as possible. The three ways in which this is best done are avoidance of the most intense rays of the midday sun (10 a.m. to 2 p.m. eastern standard time or 11 a.m. to 3 p.m. daylight savings time), use of clothing cover-up such as a t-shirt with sleeves and a hat with a broad brim, and use of sunblocks with a high sun protection factor. Current recommendations suggest the use of a broad spectrum blocker so that both UVA (long wave) and UVB (sunburn) are reduced.

Identification of patients at increased risk is important so that they can be enrolled in a regular follow-up program and can be educated in self-examination. The American Cancer Society and the Skin Cancer Foundation have both published aids for patient education in learning self-examination. Every 6 to 8 weeks is a reasonable frequency for patients to check their own skin. The *ABCDE* warning signs should be part of the patient's health knowledge base. In addition, first-degree relatives of patients with melanoma or with clinically atypical moles should undergo skin examination (*see* Table 6-2 for features of clinically atypical moles).

REFERENCES AND RECOMMENDED READING

Recently published papers of particular interest have been highlighted as:
• Of interest
•• Of outstanding interest

1.• Koh HK: Cutaneous melanoma. *N Engl J Med* 1991, 325:171–182.

2. Sober AJ, Koh HK: Melanoma and other pigmented skin lesions. In *Harrison's Principles of Internal Medicine*, Edited by Isselbacher KJ, *et al.* New York: McGraw-Hill: 1994:1867–1871.

3.• Friedman RJ, Rigel DS, Kopf AW, *et al.*: *Cancer of the Skin.* Philadelphia: WB Saunders; 1991.

4. Sober AJ, Fitzpatrick TB, Mihm MC Jr, *et al.*: Early recognition of cutaneous melanoma. *JAMA* 1979, 242:2795–2799.

5. Rhodes AR, Weinstock MA, Fitzpatrick TB, *et al.*: Risk factors for cutaneous melanoma. *JAMA* 1987, 258:3146–3154.

6. MacKie RM, Aitchison TC, Freudenberger T: A personal risk factor chart for cutaneous melanoma. *Lancet* 1989, ii:487–490.

7. Lederman JS, Sober AJ: Does biopsy type influence survival in clinical stage I cutaneous melanoma? *J Am Acad Dermatol* 1985, 13:983–987.

8. Clark WH Jr, Elder DE, Guerry D IV, *et al.*: Model predicting survival in stage I melanoma based on tumor progression. *J Natl Cancer Inst* 1989, 81:1893–1904.

9.• Veronesi U, Cascinelli N: Narrow excision (1 cm-margin): a safe procedure for thin cutaneous melanoma. *Arch Surg* 1991, 126:438–441.

10.• Ho VC, Sober AJ: Therapy for cutaneous melanoma: an update. *J Am Acad Dermatol* 1990, 22:159–176.

11. Veronesi U, Adamus J, Bandiera DC, *et al.*: Delayed regional lymph node dissection in stage I melanoma of the skin of the lower extremities. *Cancer* 1982, 49:2420–2430.

12.•• Balch CM, Houghton AN, Milton GW, *et al.*: *Cutaneous Melanoma*, edn 2. Philadelphia: JB Lippincott; 1992.

13. Markowitz JS, Cosimi LA, Carey RW, *et al.*: Prognosis after initial recurrence of cutaneous melanoma. *Arch Surg* 1991, 126:703–708.

SELECT BIBLIOGRAPHY

Kelly JW, Rivers JK, MacLennan R, *et al.*: Sunlight: a major factor associated with development of melanocytic nevi in Australian school children. *J Am Acad Dermatol* 1994, 30:40–48.

Newton JA, Bataille V, Griffiths K, *et al.*: How common is the atypical mole syndrome phenotype in apparently sporadic melanoma? *J Am Acad Dermatol* 1993, 29:989–996.

Common Cutaneous Tumors 7

Tissa R. Hata
Kenneth A. Arndt

Key Points

- Common tumors of the skin are often difficult to recognize as "common," unless one can make an accurate diagnosis.
- Treatment hinges on the pathology and natural history of the lesion.
- Seborrheic keratosis is the most common benign tumor in adulthood.
- Dermatofibromas are characterized by the "dimple" sign.
- Sebaceous hyperplasia is often mistaken for basal cell carcinoma.
- Fibrous papules of the nose and angiofibromas seen in tuberous sclerosis are similar both clinically and histologically.
- Painful tumors are characterized by the acronym "*LEND AN EGG.*"

SEBORRHEIC KERATOSES

Seborrheic keratoses are benign lesions that are sometimes referred to as barnacles because of their "stuck on" appearance on the surface of the skin (Figs. 7-1 through 7-3). They are the most common benign tumor encountered in the older patient, and their number increases with age. Their onset is usually in patients aged in their late twenties to early thirties. These tumors are less common in native Americans and blacks.

Seborrheic keratoses may have several different appearances. Most typically they are raised brown waxy or greasy plaques with a verrucous surface, often containing small white inclusions which correspond to horn cysts seen on histopathologic examination. The second type is somewhat more difficult to recognize, and may be confused with lentigo maligna. These slightly raised waxy brown plaques often demonstrate variation in color, consisting of shades of brown or black. Even for dermatologists, this type of seborrheic keratosis is difficult to assess and may require biopsy for definitive diagnosis. Irritated seborrheic keratoses have a surrounding area of erythema, and may be associated with lesional swelling, bleeding, and oozing. Multiple seborrheic keratoses occurring in an eruptive manner may be a sign of internal malignancy, known as the sign of Leser-Trélat. The most common malignancy alleged to be associated with this is adenocarcinoma of the gastrointestinal tract [1].

Microscopically, these lesions display hyperkeratosis, acanthosis, and papillomatosis. Interspersed are multiple horn cysts or pseudo–horn cysts that show sudden and complete keratinization with only a very thin granular layer.

Seborrheic keratoses have a benign clinical course, but often the patient complains either of their unsightly appearance or of irritation of the lesion. Treatment by cryosurgery with liquid nitrogen is often sufficient to remove these lesions, but caution should be taken to ensure that the lesion is truly a seborrheic keratosis and not a lentigo maligna or melanoma. If the clinician is unsure of the

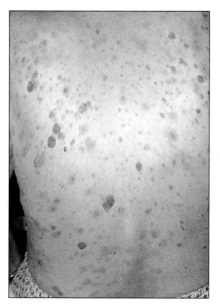

FIGURE 7-1 Seborrheic keratoses widely distributed on the trunk.

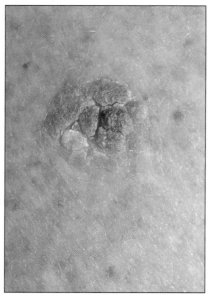

FIGURE 7-2 Seborrheic keratosis showing verrucous changes.

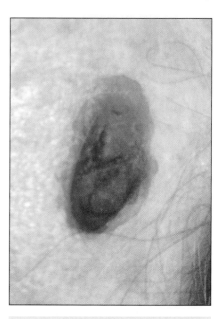

FIGURE 7-3 Seborrheic keratosis showing pigmentary variation.

diagnosis, treatment with gentle curettage and a hemostatic agent (Monsel's solution or aluminum chloride solution) applied to the base will provide a histologic specimen and effectively remove the keratosis. Surgical excision is strongly discouraged.

DERMATOSIS PAPULOSA NIGRA

Dermatosis papulosa nigra, which most often occurs on the faces of Hispanics and blacks, consists of 1- to 5-mm, stuck on–appearing, brown-black papules (Fig. 7-4). Histologically, these lesions are seborrheic keratoses, but they often have a different clinical presentation. The most typical areas of predilection are the malar regions and the forehead. They are of no medical consequence, but often the patient wishes to have them removed for cosmetic reasons.

Treatment is often limited to gentle curettage alone; electrodesiccation or freezing with a cotton-tipped swab is also effective but increases the risk of pigmentary sequelae. Vigorous treatment with liquid nitrogen or electrosurgery may cause postinflammatory hypopigmentation or hyperpigmentation of dark-skinned individuals, and should be avoided.

ACROCHORDONS

Acrochordons are soft, pedunculated, skin-colored polypoid papules, ranging from 1 to 5 mm in diameter, that are most commonly found on the neck, axillae, groin, and trunk (Fig. 7-5), although they can appear almost anywhere. They have a benign course, and removal is usually requested because of irritation in and around the lesion or for cosmesis.

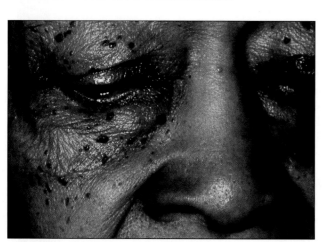

FIGURE 7-4 Dermatosis papulosa nigra.

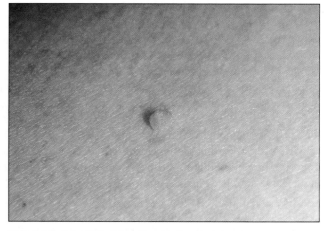

FIGURE 7-5 Skin tags.

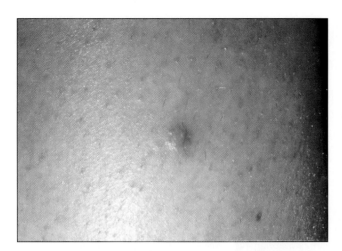

FIGURE 7-6 Dermatofibroma.

Histologically, these lesions have a connective tissue stalk composed of loose collagen fibers with numerous dilated capillaries, with overlying papillomatosis, hyperkeratosis, and acanthosis in the epidermis.

Treatment consists of removal with Gradle scissors, cryosurgery with liquid nitrogen, or gentle electrodesiccation. Most patients are able to tolerate these procedures without anesthesia. However, for large acrochordons, the use of local anesthesia is usually necessary.

DERMATOFIBROMAS

Dermatofibromas are usually pea-sized nodules that often occur on the lower legs or forearms and are associated with overlying hyperpigmentation (Fig. 7-6). These lesions are usually fixed within the skin but move freely over underlying tissues. They may be depressed or slightly elevated. A characteristic clinical sign is the "dimple" sign: on pinching, the dermatofibroma characteristically dimples into the skin. These lesions are very common. They may be noticed by the patient after minor trauma or an insect bite, but the relation of these incidents to the induction of lesions is unclear. Dermato fibromas are quite rare in children, and usually occur in adults. The etiology of these lesions is unknown.

Histologically, the dermatofibroma consists of spindle cells or histiocytes in association with collagen that is irregularly arranged in a storiform pattern. The overlying epidermis often shows elongation of the rete in a "dirty fingers" pattern. The best treatment for the dermatofibroma is usually none at all; the clinician should simply reassure the patient that these lesions are benign. However, for cosmetic reasons, surgical excision, tangential excision (shaving the lesion flat but leaving the base), or cryosurgery with liquid nitrogen can be performed.

Any dermatofibroma that is rapidly growing should be excised completely to rule out other causes, particularly dermatofibrosarcoma protuberans, which is a malignant soft tissue sarcoma. Primary excision of these tumors is usually inadequate, with a 40% recurrence rate with less than 1-cm margins [2], and excision by Mohs surgery is the treatment of choice [3].

SEBACEOUS HYPERPLASIA

Lesions of sebaceous hyperplasia often occur on the face as umbilicated or lobular yellow to orange-yellow papules of 2 to 5 mm in diameter (Fig. 7-7). They are often thought to be basal cell carcinomas because of their shared characteristics of translucency, telangiectasia, and central indentation. Sebaceous hyperplasia papules are most frequently located on the temples, cheeks, and forehead. They are usually first noted in patients who are aged over 40 years. Histologically, these lesions are composed of an enlarged sebaceous gland that consists of numerous lobules surrounding a centrally located wide sebaceous duct.

Sebaceous hyperplasia lesions do not require treatment unless the patient requests it for cosmetic purposes. They can be treated successfully with gentle electrodesiccation or electrofulguration if there is no doubt of the diagnosis. Alternative methods include the application of acids, cryosurgery, and carbon dioxide laser ablation. If there is any doubt, tangential excision or gentle curettage will also remove the lesion and provide a histologic specimen for examination.

HYPERTROPHIC SCARS AND KELOIDS

The hypertrophic scar is defined as a fibrous, thickened, firm reddish-brown plaque (Figs. 7-8 through 7-10) not overgrowing the boundaries of an original injury and often demonstrating partial resolution over 1 or several years. The keloid is an exuberant version of the hypertrophic scar that spreads well beyond the limits of the original scar and

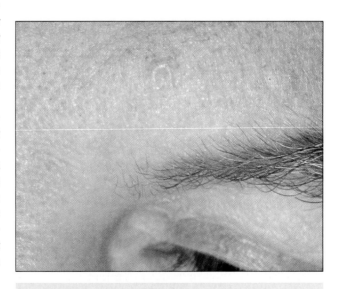

FIGURE 7-7 Sebaceous adenoma.

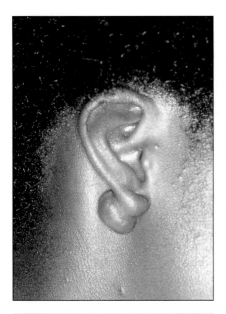

FIGURE 7-8 Ear keloid.

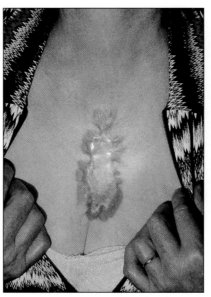

FIGURE 7-9 Presternal keloid.

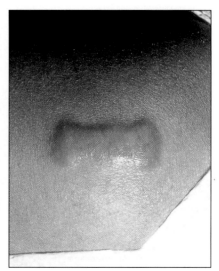

FIGURE 7-10 Hypertrophic scar. Note that the lesion does not extend out of the area of previous trauma.

shows no improvement with time. Keloids more often are accompanied by symptoms of itching or pain. Common sites for keloids are the sternal region, the neck and shoulders, the deltoid area, and the earlobes; a less common site is the trunk.

Histologically, the keloid or hypertrophic scar is composed of thick, highly compacted, hyalinized bands of collagen in a whirled or nodular pattern.

Effective treatment of keloids is quite difficult. The most effective therapy is prevention! First-line treatment is usually injection with an intralesional steroid such as triamcinalone acetonide, 10 to 40 mg/ml every 4 to 6 weeks, on one or several occasions, which flattens and softens the keloids. Other various treatment approaches are listed in Table 7-1.

TABLE 7-1 TREATMENT OF KELOIDS

Intralesional steroids
Cryosurgery with liquid nitrogen alone or in combination with intralesional steroids*[†]
Pressure dressings[†]
Silicone gel dressings[‡]
Excision and injection of intralesional steroids[†]
Excision and radiotherapy[§]
Ultrasound[†]
Laser surgery[¶]
Adhesive zinc tapes[†]
Topical retinoic acids[**]
Intralesional injection of interferon γ [††]

Data from *Ceilley and Babin [4]; [†]Datubo-Brown [5•]; [‡]Hirshowitz *et al.* [6]; [§]Darzi *et al.* [7•]; [¶]Sherman and Rosenfeld [8]; [**]Haas and Arndt [9]; [††]Granstein *et al.* [10•].

CHONDRODERMATITIS NODULARIS HELICIS

Chondrodermatitis lesions are typically small, very tender red nodules commonly occurring on the outer helix of the ear in older men (Fig. 7-11). They may be single or multiple, are typically 2 to 6 mm in diameter, and often present as erythematous red nodules firmly attached to the underlying cartilage. The surface may be covered with an adherent crust that on removal reveals a central ulceration.

The etiology is unclear; however, pressure or chronic trauma, particularly over skin altered by actinic exposure, is believed to be important in their evolution. Histologically, the epidermis of these lesions shows an ulcer filled with necrotic dermal debris and covered with a crust. The dermis in the center of the lesion shows degenerated collagen

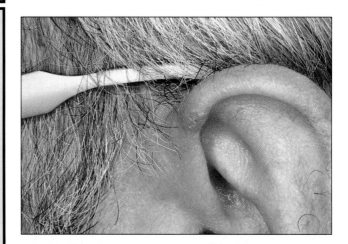

FIGURE 7-11 Chondrodermatitis nodularis helicis.

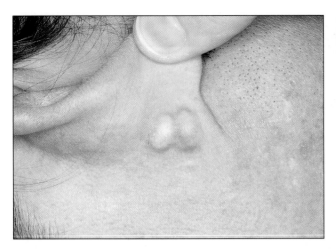

FIGURE 7-12 Epidermal inclusion cyst.

TABLE 7-2 TYPES OF CYSTS	
Epidermoid	Branchial cleft cyst
Eruptive vellus hair cyst	Thyroglossal duct cyst
Dermoid cyst	Thymic cyst
Trichilemmal cyst	Cutaneous ciliated cyst
Steatocystoma	Digital mucous cyst
Median raphe cyst	Omphalomesenteric duct
Bronchogenic cyst	cyst

Data from Golitz and Poomeechaiwong [14].

surrounded by granulation tissue. The perichondrium is often thickened, and focal degeneration of the cartilage itself may occur.

Treatment options include injection of intralesional corticosteroids [11•], excision along with the underlying cartilage [11•], electrodesiccation and curettage [12], and carbon dioxide laser surgery [13].

EPIDERMAL INCLUSION CYSTS

Epidermal inclusion cysts are lesions that are typically 0.5 to 2 cm in size and are most commonly seen on the face, neck, and trunk (Fig. 7-12). These lesions are freely movable over underlying structures, but they are often connected to the overlying skin by a central punctum. The content of the cyst is usually a pasty, cheesy material that is formed of macerated keratin and cheesy, fatty material.

There are many different types of cysts (Table 7-2), but the ones most commonly confused with epidermal inclusion cysts are trichilemmal cysts, or pilar cysts (Table 7-3). It may be impossible to differentiate clinically between the appearance of epidermal inclusion cysts and that of trichilemmal cysts, however, clinical differentiation is often not important because the treatment regimens are identical.

Treatment of inflamed cysts is by intralesional injection of corticosteroids. Once the inflammation has subsided, the lesions can be excised. Drainage of a cyst may provide relief or cure; however, because the wall of the cyst remains, the lesion may recur.

LIPOMAS

Lipomas are soft subcutaneous nodules approximately 1 to 2 cm in diameter that commonly occur on the posterior trunk, abdomen, forearm, buttocks, and thighs. They usually arise as solitary lesions but may also be multiple. Frequently, lipomas are first noted between the fourth and fifth decades of life and are most common in women. The skin overlying these benign tumors is freely movable, and no textural or pigmentary changes are evident. Lipomas are usually asymptomatic, as opposed to a painful variant, the angiolipoma (Table 7-4). Painful tumors of the skin can be characterized using the acronym *LEND AN EGG* (Table 7-5).

Several syndromes are associated with multiple lipomas occurring in adult life. Madelung's disease refers to the occurrence of multiple large, painless, coalescent lipomas around the neck, shoulders, and upper arms, most commonly occurring in older men [16]. Dercum's disease, or adiposis dolorosa, occurs primarily in obese menopausal women and presents as symmetric, tender, circumscribed fatty deposits that are often associated with weakness and psychiatric disturbances [17].

Lipomas may be left untreated unless they are cosmetically bothersome or painful. The most effective treatment

TABLE 7-3 EPIDERMAL INCLUSION CYSTS VERSUS TRICHILEMMAL CYSTS		
	Inclusion cyst	**Trichilemmal cyst**
Clinical appearance	Identical	Identical
Location	Face, scalp, neck, trunk	90% on scalp
Histopathology	Cystic structure with wall of true epidermis containing a granular layer, filled with horny material arranged in laminated layers	Cystic structure derived from the middle portion of the hair follicle, with a wall of epidermis without a granular layer or visible intercellular bridging. Palisade arrangement of cells peripherally
Inheritance	Unknown	May be autosomal dominant

TABLE 7-4 LIPOMAS VERSUS ANGIOLIPOMAS		
	Lipomas	**Angiolipomas**
Symptoms	Asymptomatic	Painful
Groups affected	Frequently first noted between the 4th and 5th decades; most common in women	Typically arise in young adults
Histologic findings	Surrounded by a connective tissue capsule; contains normal fat cells similar to those found in the subcutaneous tissue	Similar to those for lipoma, except for an increase in vascular tissue often containing fibrin within the capillaries
Appearance	Identical	Identical

TABLE 7-5 PAINFUL TUMORS	
Leiomyoma	Angiolipoma
Eccrine spiradenoma	Neurilemmoma
Neuroma	Endometrioma
Dermatofibroma	Glomus tumor
	Granular cell tumor

Data from **Naversen** *et al.* [15•].

growths are of little but cosmetic consequence. However, they may be mistaken for dermal nevi or basal cell carcinoma. Table 7-6 compares fibrous papules with the angiofibromas of tuberous sclerosis.

No treatment is necessary for the isolated fibrous papule of the nose. However, if excision is indicated, tangential excision is usually the treatment of choice. It will remove the lesion with good results and will also provide tissue for histologic examination. Laser surgery with the carbon dioxide or argon laser has been shown as effective in treating angiofibromas of tuberous sclerosis.

for lipomas is excision, although liposuction has also been reported to be effective [18].

FIBROUS PAPULES OF THE NOSE

The fibrous papule is a dome-shaped, often singly occurring skin-colored papule, 1 to 3 mm in diameter, that is most often located on the nose. Lesions can also occur on the forehead, cheeks, chin, and neck. These benign

MILIA

Milia are firm white papules 1 to 2 mm in diameter that often give the appearance of containing a grain of sand or a pearl immediately beneath the epidermis (Fig. 7-13). These lesions can occur either spontaneously, secondary to an associated disease state (*eg*, bullous pemphigoid, dystrophic epidermolysis bullosa, or porphyria cutanea tarda), or after trauma.

TABLE 7-6 FIBROUS PAPULES VERSUS ANGIOFIBROMAS		
	Fibrous papule	**Angiofibroma**
Age group affected	Middle aged adults	Children
Inheritance	Acquired	Autosomal dominant
Clinical appearance	Usually singly occurring; most often located on the nose, but may also occur on the forehead, cheeks, chin, and neck	Multiple; often occur on the nasolabial folds, cheeks, and chin; associated cutaneous findings include periungual fibromas, shagreen patch, and ash leaf macules*
Histologic findings	Papular lesions with a localized area of fibrosis and vascular proliferation in the upper portion of the dermis	*Same as* fibrous papule
Internal associations	None	Mental retardation, seizures, retinal phakomas, renal angiomyolipomas, cardiac rhabdomyomas
Treatment of fibrous papule or angiofibroma	Tangential excision, argon or CO_2 laser	*Same as* fibrous papule

Data from Fitzpatrick *et al.* [19].

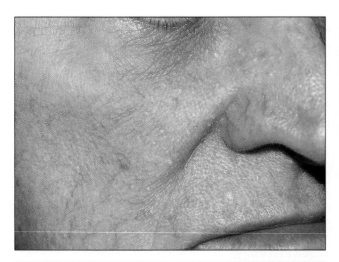

FIGURE 7-13 Milia.

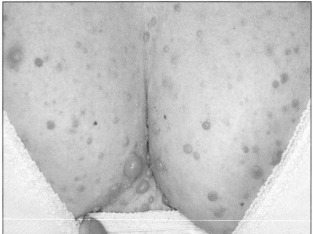

FIGURE 7-14 Neurofibroma.

Histologically, they represent miniature epidermal inclusion cysts and are derived from the lowest portion of the infundibulum of vellus hairs. Treatment is by incision with a no. 11 blade scalpel and expression of the cyst contents.

NEUROFIBROMAS

Neurofibromas may appear as soft, skin-colored pedunculated or sessile polyps (Fig. 7-14). They are often confused with acrochordons or as skin-colored lesions mistaken for nevi. Frequently, these tumors exhibit "buttonholing," which occurs when the soft tumor is invaginated into the skin by pressure with a finger. They can be solitary or multiple, and if they are multiple, the syndrome of neurofibromatosis must be considered.

Neurofibromas are benign nerve sheath tumors composed of thin wavy collagen fibers in association with spindle cells with slightly wavy nuclei and slender elongated cytoplasmic processes that extend in various directions. These lesions are usually well circumscribed but not encapsulated. Treatment is by either tangential excision or surgical excision. Superficial ablation procedures, such as defocused carbon dioxide laser surgery, may also be useful for flattening lesions.

SYRINGOMAS

Syringomas are multiple skin-colored to yellow papules usually occurring on the lower eyelids and cheeks (Fig. 7-15), although they may occur in any location. Their typical diameter is 2 to 3 mm, and they usually occur in women in the second or third decade of life. One association of syringomas has been made in patients with Down's syndrome: there is a 39% occurrence rate in these patients [20].

Histologically, these lesions represent adenomas of the intraepidermal eccrine ducts. They are embedded in a fibrous stroma and consist of small ducts whose walls are lined by two rows of epithelial cells. The ducts often possess small, comma-like tails, which give them the characteristic tadpole appearance. Treatment is usually by gentle electrolysis, laser ablation, or cautious cryotherapy.

CHERRY ANGIOMAS

Cherry angiomas are one of the most common benign skin tumors. Their onset is in early adult life, and they increase in number with age. Lesions can occur anywhere, but the trunk is the most common site (Fig. 7-16). They most often appear as nonblanching, bright red, smooth dome-shaped lesions one to several millimeters in diameter.

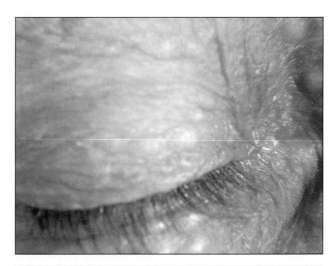

FIGURE 7-15 Periorbital syringoma.

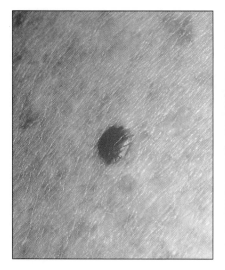

FIGURE 7-16 Cherry hemangioma.

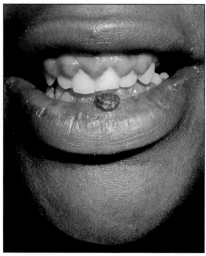

FIGURE 7-17 Pyogenic granuloma.

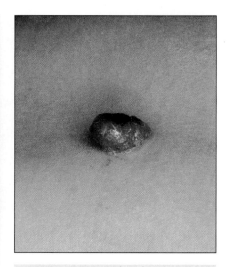

FIGURE 7-18 Pyogenic granuloma of pregnancy.

Histologically, they are composed of numerous moderately dilated capillaries lined by flattened endothelial cells. The epidermis is thinned and often surrounds most of the angioma in a collarette.

These lesions respond well to electrosurgery or laser surgery [21].

PYOGENIC GRANULOMAS

Pyogenic granulomas are small, solitary erythematous growths, either sessile or pedunculated, that are most commonly seen on an exposed surface such as the hands, forearms, face, or mouth (Figs. 7-17 and 7-18). Typically, these lesions begin as small erythematous papules that rapidly enlarge and become pedunculated. They are quite common in children, although all age groups are affected. There is often a history of trauma to the area preceding the appearance of the pyogenic granuloma. This lesion tends to be friable and bleeds easily, and it commonly recurs after treatment.

Histologically, pyogenic granulomas are composed of circumscribed lesions covered by a flattened epidermis that forms an epidermal collarette around the lesions, in association with a lobular capillary proliferation and an edematous stroma.

Treatment is usually most effective if the lesion is first curetted, and the base is then destroyed by electrofulguration. Laser ablation and excision also are effective.

WHEN TO REFER

Although each case is individually different, there are certain rules which one can apply to decide if referral is appropriate. In general, pigmented lesions should be referred unless one is 100% sure of the diagnosis. Differentiation from melanoma is difficult even for the best of dermatologists. If the lesion is behaving in an atypical manner, for example by continuing to enlarge, becoming multiple, bleeding, or becoming painful, this is a signal to refer. Also, referral is appropriate if the lesion is not responding to conventional treatment.

REFERENCES AND RECOMMENDED READING

Recently published papers of particular interest have been highlighted as:

• Of interest

•• Of outstanding interest

1. Sperry K, Wall J: Adenocarcinoma of the stomach with eruptive seborrheic keratosis: the sign of Leser-Trélat. *Cancer* 1980, 45:2434–2437.

2. Roses DF, Valensi Q, LaTrenta G, *et al.*: Surgical treatment of dermatofibrosarcoma protuberans. *Surg Gynecol Obstet* 1986, 162:449–452.

3. Robinson JK: Dermatofibrosarcoma protuberans resected by Mohs surgery. *J Am Acad Dermatol* 1985, 12:1093–1098.

4. Ceilley RI, Babin RWQ: The combined use of cryosurgery and intralesional injections of suspensions of fluorinated adrenocorticosteroids for reducing keloids and hypertrophic scars. *J Dermatol Surg Oncol* 1979, 5:54–56.

5.• Datubo-Brown DD: Keloids: a review of the literature. *Br J Plast Surg* 1990, 43:70–77.

6. Hirshowitz B, Ullmann Y, Har-Shai Y, *et al.*: Silicone occlusive sheeting (SOS) in the management of hypertrophic and keloid scarring, including the possible mode of action of silicone, by static electricity. *Eur J Plast Surg* 1993, 16:5–9.

7.• Darzi MA, Chowdri NA, Kaul SK, *et al.*: Evaluation of various methods of treating keloids and hypertrophic scars: a 10-year follow-up study. *Br J Plast Surg* 1992, 45:374–379.

8. Sherman R, Rosenfeld H: Experience with the Nd:YAG laser in the treatment of keloid scars. *Ann Plast Surg* 1988, 21:231–235.

9. Haas AA, Arndt KA: Selected therapeutic applications of topical tretinoin. *J Am Acad Dermatol* 1986, 15:870–877.

10.• Granstein RD, Rook A, Flotte TJ, *et al.*: A controlled trial of intralesional recombinant interferon-gamma in the treatment of keloidal scarring. *Arch Dermatol* 1990, 126:1295–1302.

11.• Coldiron BM: The surgical management of chondrodermatitis nodularis chronica helicis. *J Dermatol Surg Oncol* 1991, 17:902–904.

12. Kromann N, Hoyer H, Reymann F: Chondrodermatitis nodularis chronica helicis treated with curettage and electrocauterization. *Acta Derm Venereol (Stockh)* 1983, 63:85–87.

13. Taylor MB: Chondrodermatitis nodularis chronica helicis: successful treatment with the carbon dioxide laser. *J Dermatol Surg Oncol* 1991, 17:862–864.

14. Golitz L, Poomeechaiwong S: Cysts. In *Pathology of the Skin.* Edited by Farmer ER, Hood AF. Norwalk: Appleton & Lange; 1990:513–529.

15.• Naversen DN, Trask DM, Watson FH, *et al.*: Painful tumors of the skin: "LEND AN EGG." *J Am Acad Dermatol* 1993, 28:298–300.

16. Ruzicko T, Vieluf D, Landthaler M, *et al.*: Benign symmetric lipomatosis Launois-Bensaude. *J Am Acad Dermatol* 1987, 17:663–674.

17. Palmer ED: Dercum's disease: adiposis dolorosa. *Am Fam Physician* 1981, 24:155–157.

18. Coleman WP: Noncosmetic applications of liposuction. *J Dermatol Surg Oncol* 1988, 14:1085–1090.

19. Fitzpatrick TB, Szabo G, Hori Y, *et al.*: White leaf-shaped macules. *Arch Dermatol* 1968, 98:1–6.

20. Carter DM, Jegasothy BV: Alopecia areata and Down's syndrome. *Arch Dermatol* 1976, 112:1397–1399.

21. Arndt KA: Argon laser therapy of small vascular lesions. *Arch Dermatol* 1982, 118:220–224.

Psoriasis

Karen Simpson
Nicholas J. Lowe

> ### *Key Points*
> - Increased epidermal proliferation, aberrant keratinocyte differentiation, and inflammatory abnormalities characterize psoriasis.
> - Clinical diagnosis can be made by careful examination of skin lesions in most patients. Skin biopsies are occasionally needed.
> - Management should commence with topical therapy and patient education for those patients with localized disease. More severely affected patients should be referred to a dermatologist.
> - Psoriasis is a chronic relapsing disease, and treatment toxicity should always be considered and monitored.

Psoriasis is a chronic skin disease usually characterized by discrete erythematous papules and plaques covered by a silvery white scale. Some patients develop sterile pustules, while others develop total body or erythrodermic psoriasis. Patients with psoriasis are concerned with cosmetic disfigurement and the resultant social isolation that the disease may cause. Associated itching and pain resulting from fissuring of the lesions may also be present.

Approximately 2% of the US population is affected. Psoriasis is an inherited disorder, and current investigations are attempting to localize the gene responsible for the disease. The onset is frequently in early adult life, but the disease may be seen first in childhood or old age. When psoriasis occurs earlier in life, there is often an associated family history of psoriasis. In contrast, psoriasis that appears for the first time later in life (*eg*, in the fifth decade) often lacks a family history [1]. Arthritis is seen in approximately 10% of patients with psoriasis, and it may occasionally occur before skin manifestations.

The primary physician should be able to treat mild and localized psoriasis. An understanding of the pathophysiology of the disease, and knowledge of the different treatment modalities available will facilitate collaboration with a dermatologist for those patients with moderate and severe psoriasis.

DIAGNOSIS

There are several forms of psoriasis: plaque, guttate, erythrodermic, and pustular. In addition, distinct manifestations of psoriasis may depend on body location (*eg*, the scalp, nails, palms, or soles).

Plaque Psoriasis

The most classic form is plaque psoriasis. Clinically, patients with plaque psoriasis present with well-marginated, erythematous, elevated papules that coalesce into plaques. If it has not previously been treated by the patient, thick, silvery scaling will be seen (Fig. 8-1). The differential diagnosis of plaque psoriasis includes

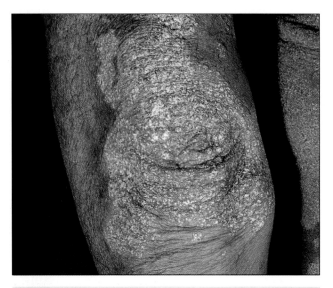

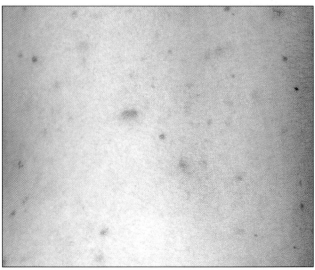

FIGURE 8-1 Plaque psoriasis.

FIGURE 8-2 Guttate psoriasis.

nummular eczema and cutaneous T-cell lymphoma (Table 8-1). Removal of this scale reveals punctate bleeding points known as Auspitz's sign. Mucous membranes are rarely involved.·

Histologically, the epidermis is thickened, and immature nucleated cells are seen in the horny layer. An accompanying dilation of the subepidermal blood vessels and infiltration with mononuclear cells accounts for erythema. Neutrophils are often seen within the stratum corneum, forming characteristic micropustules.

Guttate Psoriasis

Another clinical type is guttate psoriasis (Fig. 8-2), which presents with small, discrete, erythematous papular lesions that may appear suddenly after an upper respiratory tract infection. This form is often associated with *Streptococcus pyogenes* infection, but it is not serotype specific [2]. The differential diagnosis of guttate psoriasis includes pityriasis rosea, parapsoriasis guttata, and secondary syphilis. Table 8-2 lists some distinguishing characteristics.

Erythrodermic Psoriasis

An exfoliative or erythrodermic form of psoriasis shows generalized erythema without any characteristic lesions

(Fig. 8-3). This form must be differentiated from Sézary syndrome and pityriasis rubra pilaris (Table 8-3).

Pustular Psoriasis

An uncommon but serious variation is generalized pustular psoriasis (Fig. 8-4), which is often accompanied by systemic symptoms. The patient has sudden onset of fever and arthralgias, followed by the eruption of 2- to 3-mm sterile pustules on erythematous skin. The original pustules may resolve in a few days; however, the patient continues to experience new waves of fever followed by the formation of new pustules. Patients with this type of psoriasis usually require hospitalization and intensive treatment. At times, generalized pustular psoriasis is life threatening.

Localized pustular psoriasis of the palms and soles (Fig. 8-5) may also be seen without characteristic lesions of psoriasis elsewhere.

Scalp Psoriasis

Scalp psoriasis may accompany any form of psoriasis, or it may be the only visible sign of psoriasis. It may at times be difficult to distinguish from seborrheic dermatitis. Some distinguishing features of these conditions appear in Table 8-4.

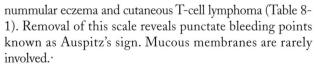

	TABLE 8-1 DIFFERENTIAL DIAGNOSIS OF PLAQUE PSORIASIS		
	Plaque psoriasis	**Nummular eczema**	**Cutaneous T-cell lymphoma**
Lesion	Sharply marginated erythematous plaques; silvery scale	Erythematous, vesicular; scale present often	May be identical to plaque psoriasis; varying thickness; little or no scale
Location	Symmetric	May be asymmetric	Asymmetric
Diagnosis	Skin biopsy	Skin biopsy	Skin biopsy
Pruritus	Usually not pruritic	Yes	Yes

TABLE 8-2 DIFFERENTIAL DIAGNOSIS OF GUTTATE PSORIASIS

	Guttate psoriasis	Pityriasis rosea	Parapsoriasis guttata	Secondary syphilis
Lesion	Fine maculopapules; silvery scale	Small, thin oval plaques; fine scale at periphery of plaque	Fine maculopapules; silvery scale	Papules or small plaques; usually fine but may be marked
Location	Entire body	Trunk in "Christmas tree" pattern; initial single plaque (herald patch)	Mainly on trunk	Trunk, palms, soles, mouth
Pruritus	Yes	Usually mild	Uncommon	Usually none
Course	Abrupt onset; occasional spontaneous recovery in 6 wk	Spontaneous resolution, generally in 6–8 wk; may be longer	Chronic	Resolves with therapy
Diagnosis	Skin biopsy	Skin biopsy	Skin biopsy	Serologic tests for syphilis, skin biopsy

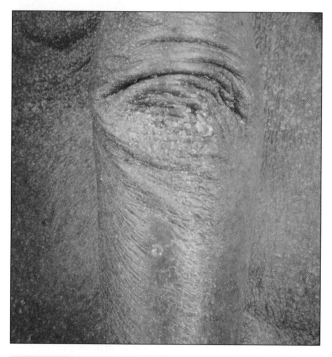

FIGURE 8-3 Erythrodermic psoriasis.

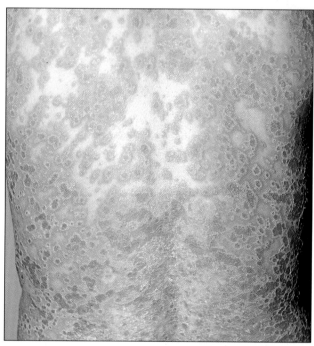

FIGURE 8-4 Generalized pustular psoriasis.

TABLE 8-3 DIFFERENTIAL DIAGNOSIS OF ERYTHRODERMIC PSORIASIS

	Erythrodermic psoriasis	Pityriasis rubra pilaris	Sézary syndrome
Lesion	Whole body erythema and scaling	Discrete papules; areas of generalized erythema; islands of normal skin; perifollicular lesions	Same as erythematous psoriasis
Location	Whole body	Whole body; thick, smooth yellow palms and soles	Whole body
Pruritus	Severe	Severe	Extreme
Diagnosis	Skin biopsy	Skin biopsy	Minimum 5% Sézary cells (abnormal lymphocytes)

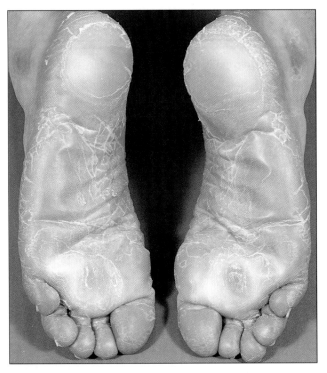

FIGURE 8-5 Pustular psoriasis of the soles.

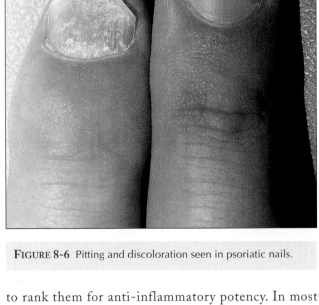

FIGURE 8-6 Pitting and discoloration seen in psoriatic nails.

Nails often show punctate pitting and a characteristic discoloration of the nail surface that resembles an oil spot (Fig. 8-6). Subungual collections of keratotic material are also common and can be confused with tinea unguium. Fungal infections can be distinguished clinically by their usual lack of nail pitting. A scraping of the keratotic material placed in 10% potassium hydroxide may reveal fungal hyphae.

TOPICAL THERAPY

Topical Steroids

Topical corticosteroids are widely used, especially for ambulatory patients, because they are relatively easy to apply. The ability of topical steroids to produce vasoconstriction, with resultant pallor of the skin, has been used

to rank them for anti-inflammatory potency. In most patients with psoriasis, the more potent steroids are usually required to produce a good response. Topical steroids are sometimes effective in clearing psoriasis and may be used in certain situations (*eg,* for exposed and unsightly areas of psoriasis and flexural psoriasis); however, caution is needed in their use. Table 8-5 lists some commonly used steroid preparations.

With the exception of the face, skin fold areas, and genitals, treatment begins with a superpotent corticosteroid preparation (group 1), followed by the use of a less potent preparation to maintain the improvement achieved. Some of the superpotent steroids may not be used for longer than 2 weeks or at dosages of greater than 50 g/wk.

Fluorinated steroids should be avoided on the face, genitals, and skin fold areas because they are more likely

	Scalp psoriasis	Seborrheic dermatitis
Lesion	Discrete patches; may be raised	Diffuse with fine scale; erythematous areas not raised
Location	Scalp; rarely on face; common on elbows, knees, and extremities	Scalp; common on face, chest, and upper back; rarely on elbows, knees, and extremities
Course	Waxing and waning; increased severity with stress; may respond to sunlight; winter flare-up common	Same

TABLE 8-4 DIFFERENTIAL DIAGNOSIS OF SCALP PSORIASIS

to cause skin atrophy. Group 6 steroids can be used on a short-term basis in these areas (no longer than 2 or 3 weeks). Group 7 steroids may be used for extended periods on the face and skin fold areas with little risk of atrophy. Most patients prefer creams; however, ointments are used when there is thick psoriatic scale. Solutions are used for scalp lesions. An example of patient instructions for the use of topical steroids is given in Table 8-6.

Maintenance therapy with pulse "weekend" steroids has proven to be clinically beneficial and well tolerated [3•]. Once plaques are clear or nearly clear, relapse rates may be kept to a minimum with the use of three consecutive applications 12 hours apart, once a week.

Side effects

Side effects seen with potent topical steroids include skin atrophy, rebound worsening of psoriasis after discontinuation

---

TABLE 8-5 POTENCY RANKING OF SOME COMMONLY USED BRAND-NAME CORTICOSTEROIDS*

Group 1

Ultravate cream 0.05% (*a*: Westwood-Squibb; Buffalo, NY)

Ultravate ointment 0.05% (*a*: Westwood-Squibb)

Temovate cream 0.05% (*b*: Glaxo Dermatology; Research Triangle Park, NC)

Temovate ointment 0.05% (*b*: Glaxo Dermatology)

Diprolene cream 0.05% (*c*: Schering-Plough; Kenilworth, NJ)

Diprolene ointment 0.05% (*c*: Schering-Plough)

Psorcon ointment 0.05% (*d*: Dermik Laboratories; Blue Bell, PA)

Group 2

Cyclocort ointment 0.1% (*e*: Lederle; Wayne, NJ)

Diprolene AF cream 0.05% (*c*: Schering-Plough)

Diprosone ointment 0.05% (*f*: Schering-Plough)

Elocon ointment 0.1% (*g*: Schering-Plough)

Florone ointment 0.05% (*h*: Dermik)

Halog cream 0.1% (*i*: Westwood-Squibb)

Lidex cream 0.05% (*j*: Syntex; Palo Alto, CA)

Lidex gel 0.05% (*j*: Syntex)

Lidex ointment 0.05% (*j*: Syntex)

Maxiflor ointment 0.05% (*h*: Herbert Laboratories; Irvine, CA)

Topicort cream 0.25% (*k*: Hoechst-Roussel; Sommerville, NJ)

Topicort gel 0.05% (*k*: Hoechst-Roussel)

Topicort ointment 0.25% (*k*: Hoechst-Roussel)

Group 3

Aristocort A ointment 0.1% (*l*: Fujisawa Pharmaceutical; Deerfield, IL)

Cyclocort cream 0.1% (*e*: Lederle)

Cyclocort lotion 0.1% (*e*: Lederle)

Diprosone cream 0.05% (*f*: Schering-Plough)

Florone cream 0.05% (*h*: Dermik)

Lidex E cream 0.05% (*j*: Syntex)

Halog ointment 0.1% (*i*: Westwood-Squibb)

Maxifor cream 0.05% (*h*: Herbert Laboratories)

Valisone ointment 0.1% (*m*: Cheesebrough Ponds; Research Triangle Park, NC)

Group 4

Cordran ointment 0.05% (*n*: Schering-Plough)

Elocon cream 0.1% (*g*: Schering-Plough)

Kenalog cream 0.1% (*l*: Westwood-Squibb)

Synalar ointment 0.025% (*o*: Syntex)

Westcort ointment 0.2% (*p*: Westwood-Squibb)

Group 5

Cordran cream 0.05% (*n*: Oclaussen Pharmaceutical; San Rafael, CA)

Diprosone lotion 0.05% (*f*: Schering-Plough)

Kenalog lotion 0.1% (*l*: Westwood-Squibb)

Locoid cream 0.1% (*q*: Ferndale; Ferndale, MI)

Synalar cream .025% (*m*: Syntex)

Valisone cream 0.1% (*n*: Ferndale)

Westcort cream 0.2% (*p*: Westwood-Squibb)

Group 6

Alcovate cream 0.05% (*r*: Glaxo Dermatology)

Alcovate ointment 0.05% (*r*: Glaxo Dermatology)

Aristocort cream 0.1% (*l*: Fujisawa)

Desowen cream 0.05% (*s*: Owen/Galderma; Fort Worth, TX)

Synalar solution 0.01% (*o*: Syntex)

Synalar cream 0.01% (*o*: Syntex)

Tridesilon cream 0.05% (*s*: Miles Pharmaceutical; Elkhart, IN)

Valisone lotion 0.05% (*m*: Ferndale)

Group 7

Topicals with hydrocortisone, dexamethasone, flumethalone, prednisolone, and methylprednisolone

*Group 1 is the superpotent category; potency descends with each group, to group 7, which is least potent (2 and 3, potent steroids; 4 and 5, midstrength steroids; 6 and 7, mild steroids). There is no significant difference between agents in groups 2 through 7; the compounds simply are arranged alphabetically. However, within group 1, Temovate cream or ointment is more potent than Diprolene cream or ointment and Psorcon ointment.

a—halobetasol; b—clobetasol propionate; c—betamethasone dipropionate (optimized vehicle); d—diflorasone diacetate (optimized vehicle); e—amcinonide; f—betamethasone dipropionate; g—mometasone furoate; h—diflorasone diacetate; i—halcinonide; j—fluocinonide; k—desoximetasone; l— triamcinolone acetonide; m—betamethasone valerate; n— flurandrenolide; o—fluocinolone acetonide; p—hydrocortisone valerate; q—hydrocortisone butyrate; r— alclometasone dipropionate; s—desonide.

These are often very effective preparations, but they have to be used with care

Apply only small amounts twice daily to psoriatic skin, unless advised otherwise by your physician; rub them well into your psoriasis

Unless specified by your doctor, do not continue treatment after the psoriasis has cleared; this can lead to skin thinning

Do not apply any steroid to the face or skin folds unless you are specifically advised to do so by your physician

If any new skin irritation, skin bruising, ulcers, or skin infections occur, stop using the corticosteroid until you have checked with your physician

of steroid use, a tendency to convert "stable" psoriasis to "unstable" (erythrodermic or pustular) types, significant skin absorption, systemic steroid effects in patients with extensive psoriasis, and the possibility of rosacea-like syndrome after long-term use of potent steroids on the face.

After an initially good response, steroid resistance often occurs. The clinician should discontinue the steroid temporarily and switch to a different topical agent, such as anthralin or calcipotriene, if there are no contraindications. If a different topical agent is not effective or is contraindicated, the clinician should refer the patient to a dermatologist.

Sunlight

Many patients with milder psoriasis experience an improvement in their psoriasis with exposure to sunlight; however, they must take care not to get sunburned because this may cause a Koebner reaction with worsening of their psoriasis in the sunburned areas.

Coal Tar Preparations

Goeckerman described the combination of ultraviolet (UV) light and coal tar in 1925 [4]. Numerous modifications of this treatment have been proposed. Crude coal tar application may be no more effective than petrolatum when combined with aggressive erythemogenic UVB (290 to 320 nm) therapy for psoriasis. However, suberythemogenic UVB plus 1% crude coal tar or a coal tar extract in oil has proved to be more effective than suberythemogenic UVB plus petrolatum [5•]. Thus, coal tars themselves are probably therapeutic and enhance the effect of suberythemogenic UVB.

Although tar used alone has some beneficial effect in treating psoriasis, it is generally used as adjunctive therapy. Some commercial purified tar preparations available for body and scalp psoriasis are:

Aquatar gel (Herbert Laboratories; Irvine, CA)
Baker's P & S Plus gel (Baker Cummins; Miami, FL)

Estar tar gel (ICN Pharmaceuticals; Costa Mesa, CA)
Fototar tar cream (Westwood-Squibb; Buffalo, NY)
Psorigel (Owen/Galderma; Fort Worth, TX)
T-Derm tar oil (Neutrogena; Los Angeles, CA)
T-Derm tar and salicylic acid scalp lotion (Neutrogena)

Liquor carbonis detergens is available as an alternative to crude coal tar, usually in 5% to 20% concentrations in cream, ointment, or oil. Balnetar and Doak oil are available as additives for bathwater. One possible treatment for localized psoriasis is a combination of tar and topical steroids. The patient may apply a purified tar at night and allow it to dry for a minimum of 10 to 15 minutes before going to bed. This will minimize staining. Once or twice during the day, a steroid cream or ointment is then applied to the localized lesions.

Folliculitis is a possible side effect of the use of tar products. If folliculitis occurs, a less occlusive base or a lower concentration of crude coal tar can be used. The purified tar preparations listed in Table 8-7, provided with instructions for patients' use, present less risk of folliculitis.

Anthralin

Anthralin is trihydroxyanthracene, an aromatic compound with three benzene rings that has been used topically for psoriasis since the 19th century. It is available commercially in creams and ointments. The use of 0.1% anthralin for at least 8 hours daily improves psoriasis. The relapse rate is increased by the addition of topical corticosteroids to the regimen. Interestingly, the application of much higher concentrations (1% and above) of anthralin, which are washed off after 10 to 60 minutes, improves psoriasis and makes outpatient psoriasis treatment with anthralin practical. This is known as as short-contact anthralin therapy.

TABLE 8-7 INSTRUCTIONS FOR PATIENTS USING COAL TAR PRODUCTS FOR PSORIASIS

Many of these products can be messy and stain your clothing and furnishings

Apply small amounts and rub them well into the skin; use old or stained garments as clothing after applying the coal tars

Many purified tar gels, lotions, creams, and oils will cease staining your clothes after they have been on the skin for several minutes

Avoid any sun exposure of coal tar–treated skin unless advised by your physician; your physician may advise sun or ultraviolet treatments after you apply the coal tar, but these have to be done with your physician's advice to avoid skin burning

If skin infections, infections around hairs, increased redness of the skin, or stinging or smarting of the skin occurs, stop using the coal tar until you have checked with your physician

The patient gradually increases the time the anthralin is left on the skin, as long as no irritation occurred with the previous contact time. The patient starts using anthralin for 10 minutes and reaches a maximum contact time of 60 minutes. Caution is needed to avoid skin irritation. Anthralin may also stain adjacent skin reddish-brown, and clothing may be stained purple.

Anthralin is often very effective, but patients resent the staining of skin and clothing. Careful instruction and good physician–patient rapport are helpful when anthralin is prescribed (Table 8-8). Anthralin is best used by physicians familiar with its use.

Vitamin D Analogues

Calcipotriol (1,24-dihydroxyvitamin D_3), which will be known as calcipotriene in the United States, is a promising new topical treatment that has been recently approved by the Food and Drug Administration. Several studies with calcipotriol ointment have shown approximately 70% improvement after a 3-month course of therapy [6–8]. It is used extensively in several countries, including Denmark, New Zealand, the United Kingdom, and Canada.

Calcipotriol ointment has been shown to be significantly superior to betamethasone valerate and anthralin in recent clinical trials [9•]. Long-term use is not likely to cause skin atrophy.

This agent may cause skin irritation when applied to the face and skin fold areas, so these areas must be avoided. Patients should apply it sparingly to psoriatic lesions while avoiding surrounding normal skin. Side effects include local perilesional skin erythema and irritation, as well as facial dermatitis in approximately 5% of patients, even when the agent is not applied to the face [8]. This may have been caused by accidental transference of the drug from the hands to the face.

Scalp Treatment

Scalp psoriasis is often frustrating to treat, both from the clinician's and the patient's points of view. Different regimens may be used according to the severity of the psoriasis, and whether the hair is color treated, blond, or gray.

Mild, diffuse scalp psoriasis

Mild, diffuse scalp psoriasis may be easily confused with seborrheic dermatitis, especially if no other signs of psoriasis are present. Mild scalp psoriasis often responds well to regular shampooing with tar or salicylic acid preparations, which may be alternated with an antifungal shampoo if needed (ketoconazole). The use of tar must be avoided with color-treated, blond, or gray hair because it will cause discoloration of the hair. At night, phenol and saline solutions, for example, P & S liquid (Baker-Cummins) or Keralyt gel (Westwood-Squibb) or a steroid in an oil base such as Dermasmoothe (Hill Dermaceuticals, Orlando, FL), applied to the scalp, will help loosen scale. This effect is intensified with occlusion (eg, wearing a shower cap to bed). Application of midpotency steroid lotions or sprays during the day can be useful [10]. A high-powered shower nozzle may also be helpful in removing some of the scale when patients shampoo their hair.

Ketoconazole theoretically acts by depleting the surface yeast contaminants, which are thought to activate the complement cascade in psoriatic skin, leading to leukocyte chemotaxis [11].

Localized plaque scalp psoriasis

Local application of tar, anthralin, or salicylic acid compounds is often useful. Again, tar should not be used with light-colored hair or color-treated hair. Anthralin can also cause discoloration in these cases, although red hair tends to tolerate the anthralin without much discoloration.

TABLE 8-8 SOME AVAILABLE ANTHRALIN PREPARATIONS WITH USUAL CONCENTRATIONS

Form of preparation	Product	Concentrations, %
Paste	Formulated by pharmacist in Lassar's paste (best used under dermatologist's supervision)	0.1–5.0
Ointment	Anthra-Derm*; (Dermik Laboratories, Blue Bell, PA)	0.1, 0.25, 0.5, 1.0
Cream	Drithocream*†; (Dermik Laboratories)	0.1, 0.25, 0.5
	Drithocream*†; (Dermik Laboratories)	0.1, 0.25, 0.5, 1.0
	Drithoscalp; (Dermik Laboratories)	0.5
	Anthranol†; (Stiefel Laboratories, Coral Gables, FL)	0.1, 0.2, 0.4
	Psoradrate†; (Eaton, UK)	0.1, 0.2
Stick	Anthra-Derm†; (Brocades, UK)	0.5, 1.0
Future options: Solutions, Gels, Tapes, Possibility of effective anthralin analogues		

*Available in the United States and Canada; †available in the United Kingdom.

Ultrapotent corticosteroid lotions or aerosols may be used during the day. Occasional use of intralesional steroids may be useful; however, several precautions should be followed. Injections should not be given more frequently than every 4 to 6 weeks because skin atrophy, folliculitis, and systemic effects from the corticosteroid can result with repetitive use. At each treatment session, no more than 2 mL of triamcinolone at a concentration of 3 to 5 mg/mL should be used. Treatment regimens for mild psoriasis may be followed in between injections [10•].

Extensive, severe scalp psoriasis

Treatment of extensive, severe scalp psoriasis can be a particularly arduous task and often requires day care or hospitalization under a dermatologist's supervision. The first step should be a home treatment regimen. A tar or salicylic acid gel or lotion, or a combination may be applied by the patient at night.

Examples of available preparations are provided below:

•*Steroid preparations*
Aristocort lotion (Fujisawa Pharmaceutical; Deerfield, IL)
Cordran lotion (Oclaussen Pharmaceutical; San Rafael, CA)
Cyclocort lotion (Lederle; Wagner, NJ)
Dermasmoothe lotion (Hill Dermaceuticals)
Diprolene lotion (Schering-Plough, Kenilworth, NJ)
Diprosone lotion (Schering-Plough)
Diprolene gel aerosol (Schering-Plough)
Lidex gel (Syntex; Palo Alto, CA)
Temovate lotion (Glaxo Dermatology; Research Triangle Park, NC)
Valisone lotion (Cheeseborough Ponds; Research Triangle Park, NC)
•*Purified tar preparations*
Bakers P & S Plus gel (Baker-Cummins)
Estar tar gel (ICN Pharmaceuticals)
Fototar tar cream (Westwood-Squibb)
Psorigel (Owen/Galderma)
T-Derm tar and salicylic acid scalp lotion (Neutrogena)
•*Salicylic acid preparations*
Keralyt gel (Westwood-Squibb)
•*Other*
P & S liquid (Baker Cummins)

These formulations should be rubbed well into the scalp and then covered with a plastic or a paper shower cap. In the morning, the patient should wet the scalp and rub in a shampoo containing tar, salicylic acid, or ketoconazole, wrapping the scalp in a damp warm towel afterward. The towel should be left on for 15 to 30 minutes. The patient should shower off this initial shampoo and continue shampooing until the cream or gel preparations have been removed. The scalp may then be treated with a single application of a high-potency corticosteroid lotion such as Temovate lotion (Glaxo Dermatology), Lidex solution (Syntex), or Diprolene lotion (Schering-Plough) [10•].

If response to this therapy is slow, referral to a dermatologist is indicated. Short-contact anthralin may be added to the regimen for home treatment. If this fails, day care or hospital scalp treatment may be needed. For truly incapacitating scalp psoriasis that does not respond to topical treatment regimens, systemic treatment may be indicated. This should be done under a dermatologist's supervision.

SYSTEMIC TREATMENT

Systemic treatment is indicated only for severe or incapacitating psoriasis. This includes generalized pustular psoriasis, exfoliative psoriasis, severe psoriatic arthropathy, and extensive psoriasis (> 20% body surface area). Systemic treatments include psoralen photochemotherapy and the administration of methotrexate, retinoids, cyclosporine, or systemic corticosteroids. These systemic treatments are best used by dermatologists familiar with their effects.

PREVENTION

Although nothing can be done to decrease the chance of getting psoriasis, several things can be done to decrease the chance of exacerbating the disease. Stress (physical and emotional) in the patient's life should be minimized. Although this may be easier said than done, psychological support from the treating physician, the psychiatrist or psychologist, and support groups are important measures [12•]. Cautious sun exposure and careful topical therapy can prevent relapse in many patients for prolonged periods. An excellent resource for patients with psoriasis is the National Psoriasis Foundation, which provides information on the latest treatment modalities and educational materials (PO Box 9009, Portland, Oregon 97207).

REFERENCES AND RECOMMENDED READING

Recently published papers of particular interest have been highlighted as:
• Of interest
•• Of outstanding interest

1. Schmitt-Egenolf M, Boehncke W-H, Christophers E, *et al.*: Type I and type II psoriasis show a similar usage of T-cell receptor variable regions. *J Invest Dermatol* 1991, 97:1053–1056.

2. Funk J, Langeland T, Schrumpf E, *et al.*: Psoriasis induced by interferon alpha. *Br J Dermatol* 1991, 125:463–465.

3.• Katz H, Prawer S, Medansky R, *et al.*: Intermittent corticosteroid maintenance treatment of psoriasis: a double-blind multicenter trial of augmented betamethasone diproprionate ointment in a pulse dose treatment regimen. *Dermatologica* 1991, 183:269–274.

4. Goeckerman WH: The treatment of psoriasis. *Northwest Med* 1925, 24:2–9.

5.• Lowe N: Tars, keratolytics, and emollients. In *Practical Psoriasis Treatment*, edn 2. Edited by Lowe N. St. Louis: Mosby; 1993:45–57.

6. Kato T, Rokugo M, Terui T, *et al.*: Successful treatment of psoriasis with topical application of active vitamin D$_3$ analogue, 1,24-dihydroxycholecalciferol. *Br J Dermatol* 1986, 115:431–433. 1993:45–57.

7. Kragballe K: Treatment of psoriasis by the topical application of the novel cholecalciferol analogue calcipotriol. *Arch Dermatol* 1989, 125:1647–1652.

8. Morimoto S, Yoshikawa K, Kozuka T, *et al.*: An open study of vitamin D$_3$ treatment in psoriasis vulgaris. *Br J Dermatol* 1986, 115:421–429.

9.• Murdoch D, Clissold S: Calcipotriol: a review of its pharmacological properties and therapeutic use in psoriasis vulgaris. *Drugs* 1992, 43:415–429.

10.• Lowe N: Therapy of scalp psoriasis. In *Practical Psoriasis Treatment*, edn 2. Edited by Lowe N. St. Louis: Mosby; 1993: 207–217.

11. Rosenberg E, Belew P: Role of microbial factors in psoriasis. In *Proceedings: The Third International Symposium.* Edited by Katz SI. New York: Grune & Stratton; 1982:343–344.

12. •Koo J: Emotional and psychological aspects of psoriasis. In *Practical Psoriasis Treatment*, edn 2. Edited by Lowe N. St. Louis: Mosby; 1993:23–31.

SELECT BIBLIOGRAPHY

Baker H: Psoriasis. In *Textbook of Dermatology*, edn 4. Edited by Rook A, Wilkinson DS, Ebling FJG, *et al.* Oxford: Blackwell Scientific Publications; 1986:1469–1532.

Christopher E, Krueger GS: Psoriasis. In *Dermatology in General Medicine*, edn 3. Edited by Fitzpatrick TB, Eisen AZ, Wolff K, *et al.* New York: McGraw-Hill; 1987:461–491.

Lowe NJ, ed.: *Practical Psoriasis Therapy*, edn 2. St. Louis: Mosby; 1993.

Morison WL: Management of psoriasis vulgaris. In *Phototherapy and Photochemotherapy of Skin Disease*, edn 2. Edited by Morison WL. New York: Raven Press; 1991:53–93.

Roenigk HH, Maibach HI, eds: *Psoriasis*, edn 2. New York: Marcel Dekker; 1991.

The Eczemas 9

Terrence Hopkins
Richard A.F. Clark

Key Points

- Eczema is dermal inflammation. It is associated with epidermal edema that can sometimes appear as vesiculation.

- Acute, subacute, and chronic eczema do not refer to chronicity but rather to clinical and histologic manifestations of eczema.

- The eczemas are categorized by clinical appearance or location, etiologic cause, or associated conditions.

- Although management varies according to the type of eczema, certain basic principles apply, such as the need for topical steroids in acute eczema or hydration, moisturizers, and nonsteroidal topical medication in subacute and chronic eczema.

The terms *dermatosis*, *dermatitis*, and *eczema* are often loosely applied to inflammatory skin disorders; therefore, they should be clearly defined to limit confusion and enable classification of the eczemas. The term *dermatosis* refers to the entire spectrum of skin disorders, varying from inflammatory to neoplastic. Dermatitis relates to all inflammatory disorders of the skin, such as sunburn, contact dermatitis, and psoriasis. Finally, *eczema*, or *eczematous dermatitis* embraces only those dermatitis conditions that are associated with intraepidermal edema (spongiosis), which is often manifested clinically as vesiculation.

Eczema is defined by its clinical and histologic characteristics; however, the clinical manifestations of eczema can vary during the disease evolution. Often, the clinical characteristics of eczema are subdivided into three stages: acute, subacute, and chronic (Figs. 9-1 through 9-4). These stages frequently overlap within a given patient; nevertheless, general topical therapy can be tailored to the most prominent stage of eczema present (Fig. 9-1).

Six general histopathologic findings often occur in eczematous dermatitis: in the epidermis, spongiosis (intraepidermal edema), acanthosis (thickening of the epidermis), and parakeratosis (retention of nuclei within the cells of the stratum corneum); in the dermis, blood vessel dilatation, infiltration of lymphocytes and monocytes, and edema. The exact histopathologic pattern depends on the stage of clinical evolution.

A particular type of eczema can be classified by etiology, clinical pattern, or associated phenomena that distinguish it from the group.

CONTACT DERMATITIS

Contact reactions can be separated into three major categories: allergic contact dermatitis, irritant contact dermatitis, and contact urticaria. Each category is defined by its time of onset, specific immunologic mechanism or mechanisms, and inciting agents (Table 9-1).

ATOPIC DERMATITIS

Atopic dermatitis is a chronic relapsing, pruritic dermatitis that usually occurs in individuals with a personal or family history of atopy (food allergy or allergic asthma, rhinitis, or conjunctivitis). The onset is usually in childhood, but the disease may persist in adults. In older patients in whom a diagnosis of atopic dermatitis is being entertained for the first time, a childhood history should be ascertained [4•]. If the patient does not have a childhood history of this condition, he or she may have another eczema or an eczematous reaction to a medication or an underlying malignancy.

Much evidence suggests that IgE-mediated immediate and late-phase reactions play a role in the development of atopic dermatitis. In addition, recent evidence has suggested that an immunologic dysregulation may cause overactivation of a variant delayed-type hypersensitivity reaction distinct from classic delayed-type hypersensitivity. House dust mite antigen, molds, pollens, animal dander, and other proteinaceous aeroallergens, as well as certain foods, may precipitate flares of eczema in these patients [5]. Important questions include those about the home environment, including the presence of pets, and those about disease variation with the season or with travel.

The distribution of eczema varies with age, but a characteristic distribution is usually seen by the age of 3 or 4 years (Fig. 9-5). Atopic dermatitis is usually associated with other manifestations of atopy and can be complicated by cutaneous infection as well as a variety of other problems (Table 9-2). Herpes simplex infection may begin as a cold sore and then become generalized and complicated by ocular involvement. Therefore, when pustules form on these patients, both a Gram stain and Tzanck preparation should be performed. In adult patients who give a history of no previous atopy, an itemization of medications and exposures and a thorough

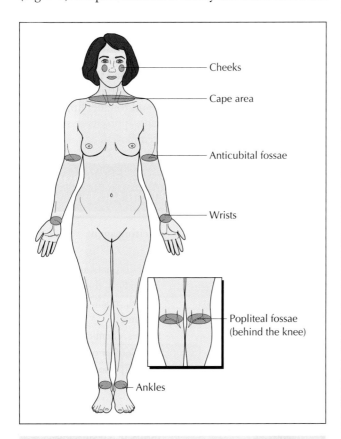

FIGURE 9-5 Characteristic distribution of eczema in older children and adults with atopic dermatitis.

TABLE 9-2 ATOPIC DERMATITIS

Variants
Infants
   Involves the face, scalp, extensor surfaces
Older children
   Tends to localize to flexural areas, especially antecubital and popliteal fossae
Adults
   Usually involves the flexural areas, but may be localized to the hands and feet only
Erythroderma (any age)
   Generalized flare
Neurodermatitis or prurigo nodularis (older children and adults)
   Excoriations or excoriated nodules on the extremities

Potential allergens
Dust mite antigen, animal dander, cockroach, molds
Pollens
Foods (especially in children younger than 5 y)

Associated conditions
Atopic diathesis (*ie*, allergic asthma, rhinitis, or dermatitis): familial inheritance
Xerosis, ichthyosis vulgaris, keratosis pilaris
Eye findings
   Periorbital dermatitis, allergic or vernal conjunctivitis
   Posterior cataracts, keratoconus, glaucoma
Postinflammatory hypo- or hyperpigmentation
White dermatographism

Complications
Cutaneous infections
   Viral: herpes simplex, vaccinia, molluscum contagiosum, papillomavirus infection
   Bacterial: *Staphylococcus aureus* infection
   Fungal: dermatophyte infection
Exoliferative erythroderma
Growth retardation and weight loss
Mental and emotional dysfunction

Laboratory findings
Blood eosinophilia
Increased serum IgE level
Positive reaction to immediate hypersensitivity testing

physical examination, including lymph node palpation and an abdominal examination, are appropriate.

IgE levels are not diagnostic but may help guide the diagnosis. Prick skin testing and patch testing may be indicated in patients with recalcitrant disease. The treatment is outlined in Figure 9-1; however, the use of systemic steroids should be avoided. Some success has been seen with psoralen-UVA photochemotherapy and immunomodulatory agents.

HAND AND FOOT DERMATITIS

Table 9-3 categorizes hand and foot eczema. Irritant hand and foot dermatitis usually appears on the palms and soles, respectively (Fig. 9-6), and often occurs in adults with a history of atopic dermatitis. Allergic contact dermatitis usually appears on the dorsal surfaces of the hands and feet (Fig. 9-6). Allergic contact dermatitis, however, can be superimposed on irritant contact dermatitis [6,7•]. Patch testing can be useful for documenting allergic contact. Nummular eczema appears as coin-shaped lesions in a mirror image distribution over the trunk and extremities, including the hands and feet, in middle-aged adults. There is no known pathogenesis. Asteatotic eczema is a form of eczema that is derived from dry skin and often has the appearance of "cracked porcelain" (eczema craquelé). Usually seen in elderly patients during the winter, it most commonly affects the hands, feet, and lower extremities. Stress can be associated with the development or the recurrence of hand and foot eczema, especially pompholyx, in which patients develop deep-seated vesicles bilaterally and symmetrically over the sides of the fingers, over the thenar and hypothenar eminences, or along the sides of the feet.

When confronted with a patient who has hand and foot eczema, the physician should ask about wet work (eg, cleaning, bartending, cooking, and nursing) and exposure to potential contact allergens [6,7•]. Bacterial infections are a common complication of hand dermatitis and should be excluded when vesiculopustular formation is present.

Dermatophyte infection should be considered when vesiculation occurs on the feet. Psoriasis can masquerade as recalcitrant hand and foot dermatitis associated with sterile pustules.

The treatment of hand dermatitis follows the outline in Figure 9-1. In addition, the patient should avoid wet work or any inciting chemical or chemicals. For difficult cases, tar soaks, followed by the application of a layer of diiodohydroxyquinone cream and a potent topical steroid ointment, can be tried. This treatment is aided by occlusion with

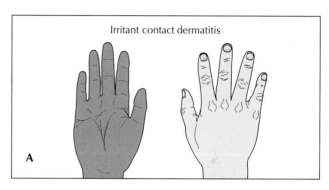

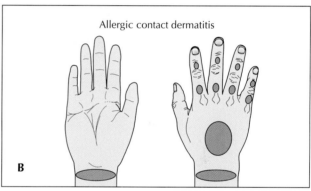

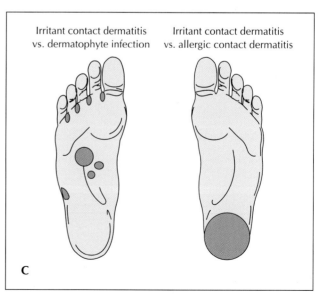

FIGURE 9-6 The location of eczema on the hands and feet may help distinguish irritant contact dermatitis from allergic contact dermatitis or dermatophyte infection.

Endogenous factors	**Exogenous factors**
Nummular eczema	Irritant contact
Xerosis (dry skin)	Soaps, detergents
Atopic dermatitis	Chemicals (especially solvents)
	Cold air
	Friction
	Allergic contact
	Chemicals
	Foods
	Plants
	Metals

TABLE 9-3 HAND AND FOOT ECZEMA

cotton or vinyl gloves for several hours or overnight. Oral antibiotics are used for bacterial superinfection.

SEBORRHEIC DERMATITIS

Seborrheic dermatitis is a common waxy, scaling, superficial eczematous dermatitis showing a predilection for areas of increased sebaceous gland activity (ie, seborrheic areas) (Fig. 9-7 and Table 9-4). Seborrheic dermatitis affects approximately 3% of the general population. In AIDS or AIDS-related complex, the incidence of seborrheic dermatitis ranges from 20% to 80%. It is more common in men than in women and appears to be associated with an oily complexion (ie, the seborrheic diathesis). Seborrheic dermatitis was historically found in two major age groups: infants in the first 3 months of life and persons 40 to 70 years of age. However, in patients with AIDS, severe seborrheic dermatitis can be seen at any age.

Pityrosporum ovale, a saprophyte found in the seborrheic areas of normal adults, may be an important inciting factor. It grows exuberantly on patients with AIDS [8]. The disease also has a predilection for patients with neurologic disorders, such as mental retardation, parkinsonism, cerebrovascular trauma, facial nerve palsy, syringomyelia, and quadriplegia; patients with alcoholism; patients with endocrinologic disease; and patients receiving neuroleptic drugs. Treatment of seborrheic dermatitis is outlined in Table 9-5.

NEURODERMATITIS

Neurodermatitis is characterized by skin changes that occur because of itching, scratching, and rubbing. It is associated with many conditions that predispose the patient to a habitual itch-scratch cycle, including insect bites, drug reactions, atopic dermatitis, contact dermatitis, photodermatitis, other chronic eczematous conditions, lichen planus, cutaneous T-cell lymphoma, other malignancies, AIDS, metabolic causes of pruritus, and stress or psychiatric disorders. Patients with this condition classically have pruritus out of proportion to the appearance of the lesion.

Clinically, neurodermatitis is characterized by excoriations, erythematous excoriated papules, plaques with increased skin markings (lichenification), or fibrous nodules. In addition, changes in pigmentation may be present. It is more commonly observed in middle-aged women than in men. The acute form is commonly associated with insect bites. The subacute form often presents as widespread excoriations (Fig. 9-8). The chronic forms, well

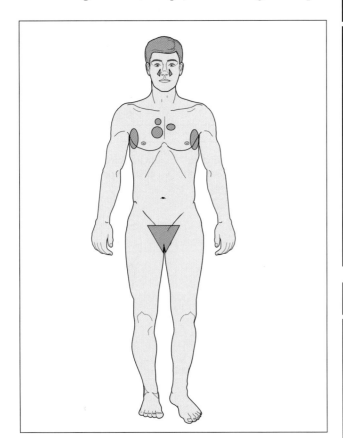

FIGURE 9-7 Seborrheic dermatitis has a predilection for the seborrheic areas of the body.

TABLE 9-4 CLINICAL VARIANTS OF SEBORRHEIC DERMATITIS

Scalp	Forehead, cheeks, chin: diffuse or plaques
Pityriasis sicca: dandruff without inflammation	
Inflammatory: often extends beyond the hairline onto the postauricular area	**Otitis externa**
	Flexural
Facial	Axillary
Eyebrows	Inframammary
Marginal blepharitis	Umbilical
Conjunctivitis	Intergluteal
Nasolabial fold	Groin
Beard area: often follicular	**Generalized**
	Erythroderma

TABLE 9-5 TREATMENT OF SEBORRHEIC DERMATITIS

Scalp

Antidandruff shampoo (tar, selenium sulfide, zinc pyrithione, salicylic acid)

Glucocorticoid lotion

Glaborous skin

Topical steroids (1%–2% hydrocortisone) twice daily

Topical ketoconazole cream (2%) twice daily

Tar preparations (LCD 5% or 10% in Aquaphor [Biersdorf, Norwalk, CT]) at bed time

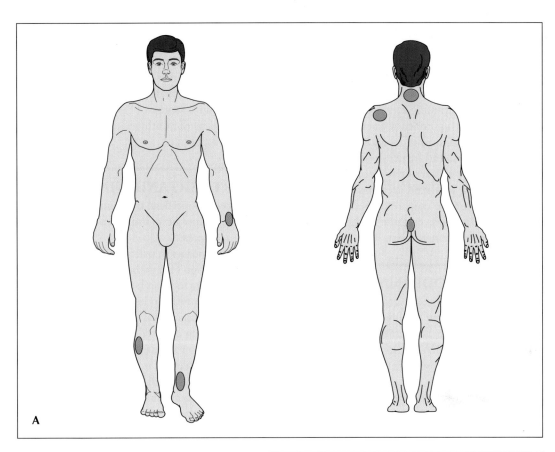

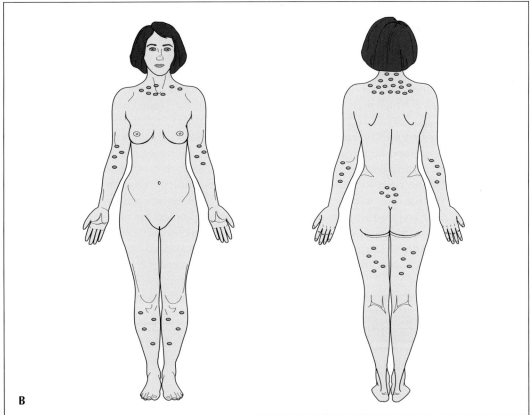

FIGURE 9-8 Neurodermatitis has characteristic locations when it presents as chronic eczema (*panel A*; lichen simplex chronicus) or subacute eczema (*panel B*; neurotic excoriations).

known as lichen simplex chronicus and prurigo nodularis, present as localized plaques or nodules (Fig. 9-8). If no etiology is obvious, a thorough history taking and physical examination for underlying illness are indicated [9].

The treatment of this condition is based initially on preventing patients from continuing to rub or scratch. This outcome can be achieved in a number of ways, among them cutting the patient's nails; administering antipruritics (topical and systemic) or topical and intralesional glucocorticoids; using tar products or barrier systems such as an occlusive dressing over a localized area; and having the patient undergo a psychiatric consultation. Alternative modalities have been tried; however, these methods are best handled by an experienced dermatologist.

ERYTHRODERMA

The terms *erythroderma* and *exfoliative dermatitis* are commonly used synonymously in the literature. Both terms imply the widespread dilation of cutaneous blood vessels associated with inflammation. When increased epidermal cell proliferation causes marked scaling, *exfoliative dermatitis* is the preferred term.

Clinically, patients have generalized erythema with or without scaling. Involvement of the hair and nails may result in alopecia and nail dystrophy. The condition may be acute or chronic. An underlying malignancy should be sought in chronic forms [10].

In adults, preexisting skin disease, (*eg*, psoriasis, atopic dermatosis, stasis dermatitis, contact dermatitis, and seborrheic dermatitis), drug allergy, and underlying malignancy (internal malignancy, leukemia, lymphoma, and cutaneous T-cell lymphoma) can lead to erythroderma. Therefore, close examination of the skin, as well as lymph node palpation and abdominal examination, is important. In a variable but substantial number of patients described, no cause was found [10]. Except when secondary to atopic dermatitis, seborrheic dermatitis, or ichthyosiform erythroderma, erythroderma will usually occur in individuals over 40 years old. Men appear to be affected about twice as often as women.

Metabolic complications of erythroderma are shown in Table 9-6. In acute erythroderma, patients usually need to be followed up closely and are usually hospitalized. These patients can become hypothermic very easily, as manifested

TABLE 9-6 METABOLIC COMPLICATIONS OF ERYTHRODERMA	
Skin dysfunction	Complication
Loss of permeability barrier	Xerosis, water loss, dehydration
Marked scaling	Protein loss, hypoalbuminemia
Increased vasopermeability	Edema
Marked vasodilation	Chills, hypothermia, high-output cardiac failure

by chills. A high-output cardiac failure state may occur. Thus, fluid and electrolyte levels should be monitored closely. Associated liver function abnormalities may indicate underlying drug hypersensitivity or internal malignancy.

The treatment is described in Figure 9-1. Underlying disease should be sought [11•], and any suspected medications should be discontinued. A dermatologic consultation is strongly suggested.

INTERTRIGO AND DIAPER DERMATITIS

Intertrigo is a superficial traumatic dermatitis that occurs in skin folds. Diaper dermatitis is an irritant contact secondary to urine and feces.

Intertrigo occurs in patients of all ages. Most adults who acquire intertrigo tend to be obese, diabetic, or both. Intertrigo also occurs more in hot and humid environments.

Clinically, intertrigo begins as well-marginated, diffuse erythema confined to areas within skin folds. When the rubbing between apposed skin surfaces continues, maceration and frank erosions compound the dermatitis. If the area is left untreated, it will become superinfected with bacteria or yeast. Candida superinfected intertrigo usually involves the inframammary area, the genitocrural area, or the scrotum and can extend to the buttock in the patient receiving long-term broad-spectrum antibiotics. Often, patients become sensitized to topical agents being used to treat the intertrigo.

Diaper dermatitis affects convex surfaces in closest contact with the wet diaper. Inadequate cleansing, frequent loose stools, high environmental temperature, and occlusive rubber or plastic pants are frequent contributing factors. With the use of disposable diapers, diaper dermatitis has markedly decreased in the United States [12]. Infants, however, still develop candida infection and nonspecific intertrigo.

The differential diagnosis of inguinal eruptions is vast (Table 9-7). However, the clinician should concentrate on the most common possibilities. Treatment is tailored to the underlying etiology. Concerted efforts should be made to preserve good hygiene and encourage weight loss. To reduce maceration, powders free of cornstarch can be used. Antibacterial and antifungal creams may also be helpful. A low-potency topical steroid cream may be used along with appropriate antimicrobial therapy until the acute inflammation has resolved. Gentian violet may be effective in patients with mixed superinfections in whom conventional therapy fails.

STASIS DERMATITIS

Stasis dermatitis is eczema secondary to venous hypertension of the lower extremity. This condition has a predilection for middle-aged to elderly women with venous incompetence or an inadequate calf pump. It is also seen in patients who have had deep venous thromboses.

The exact mechanism for the development of eczematous skin changes in patients with venous hypertension remains obscure; however, trauma, rubbing, scratching, and topical steroid use can perpetuate and exacerbate the condition.

Clinically, the dermatitis can begin rapidly or insidiously. A rapid onset of stasis dermatitis is usually associated with deep venous thrombosis. The lower leg becomes erythematous, warm, and eczematous. This process can progress proximally from the ankle. The skin can be seen in any of the classically described stages of eczema. Frequent flares of acute dermatitis are often precipitated by the application of topical medications and moisturizers. Recurrent inflammation in the dermis and subcutaneous tissue results in repeated erythrocyte extravasation, with hemosiderin deposition in the dermis and sclerosis of the subcutaneous tissue. Together, these changes give the skin a woody appearance called *liposclerosis* [13••]. As liposclerosis becomes established, edema no longer accumulates around the ankle and lower leg but rather proximal to the sclerosis. The skin of the lower leg is prone to ulceration; however, not all ulcerations are secondary to venous incompetence. Diagnosis and treatment of the ulcers are geared toward the potential etiology. However, basic principles of wound care must be kept in mind. The general treatment of stasis dermatitis consists of leg elevation, the use of support stockings, the administration of diuretics as necessary, the use of end-diastolic pneumatic compression boots, the administration of low- or intermediate-potency corticosteroids in a petrolatum base, the application of petrolatum after a bath or shower, and the use of systemic antibiotics for cellulitis.

TABLE 9-7 DIFFERENTIAL DIAGNOSIS OF INTERTRIGO IN ADULTS

Fungal
Candida (especially in obesity and diabetes)
Dermatophyte
Deep fungal (blastomycosis, actinomycosis, trichomycosis)

Bacterial
Staphylococcal or streptococcal (toxic shock syndrome)
Pseudomonas aeruginosa
Corynebacterium minutissimum (erythrasma)

Venereal diseases
Lymphogranuloma venereum
Granuloma inguinale

Skin diseases
Psoriasis or impetigo herpetiformis
Contact dermatitis
Acrodermatitis enteropathica
Migratory epidermal necrolysis (glucagonoma)
Short bowel syndrome
Darier's disease
Pemphigus foliaceus, subcorneal pustular dermatosis
Benign familial pemphigus (Hailey-Hailey disease)
Pemphigus vegetans

REFERENCES AND RECOMMENDED READING

Recently published papers of particular interest have been highlighted as:
• Of interest
•• Of outstanding interest

1.• Grevelink S, Dedee FM, Olsen EA: Effectiveness of various barrier preparations in preventing and/or ameliorating experimentally produced toxicodendron dermatitis. *J Am Acad Dermatol* 1992, 27:182–188.

2.• Hogan D, Dannaker C, Maibach H: The prognosis of contact dermatitis. *J Am Acad Dermatol* 1990, 23:300–307.

3.• Hamann C: Natural rubber latex protein sensitivity in review. *Am J Contact Dermatitis* 1993, 4:4–21.

4.• Larsen FS: Atopic dermatitis: a genetic-epidemiologic study in a population-based twin sample. *J Am Acad Dermatol* 1993, 28:719–723.

5. Adinoff AD, Tellez P, Clark RAF: Atopic dermatitis and aeroallergen contact sensitivity. *J Allergy Clin Immunol* 1988, 81:736–742.

6. Epstein E: Dermatitis: practical management and current concepts. *J Am Acad Dermatol* 1984, 10:395–424.

7.• Wall L, Gebauer KA: Occupational skin disease in Australia. *Contact Dermatitis* 1991, 24:101–109.

8. Wikler JR, Nieboer C, Willemze R: Quantitative skin cultures of pityrosporum yeasts in patients seropositive for the human immunodeficiency virus with and without seborrheic dermatitis. *J Am Acad Dermatol* 1992, 27:37–39.

9. Kantor GR, Lookingbill DP: Generalized pruritus and systemic disease. *J Am Acad Dermatol* 1983, 9:375–382.

10. Thestrup-Pederson K, Halkier-Sorenson L, Sogaard H, Zachariae H: The Red Man syndrome. *J Am Acad Dermatol* 1988, 18:1307–1312.

11.• Bakels V, van Oostveen J, Gordijn R, *et al.*: Diagnostic value of T-cell receptor beta gene rearrangement analysis on peripheral blood lymphocytes of patients with erythroderma. *J Invest Dermatol* 1991, 97:782–786.

12. Seymour JL, Keswick BH, Hanifin JM, *et al.*: Clinical effects of diaper types on the skin of normal infants and infants with atopic dermatitis. *J Am Acad Dermatol* 1987, 17:988–997.

13•• Phillips TJ, Dover JS: Leg ulcers. *J Am Acad Dermatol* 1991, 24:965–987.

SELECT BIBLIOGRAPHY

Cooper KD: Atopic dermatitis: recent trends in pathogenesis and therapy. *J Invest Dermatol* 1994, 102:128–137.

Hopkins T, Clark RAF: The other eczemas. In *Dermatology*, edn 3. Edited by Moschella SL, Hurley HJ. Philadelphia: WB Saunders; 1992: 465–504.

Katsambas A, Antonion CH, Frangouli E, *et al.*: A double-blind trial of treatment of seborrheic dermatitis with 2% ketoconazole cream with 1% hydrocortisone cream. *Br J Dermatol* 1989, 121(3):353–357.

Kay J, Gawkrodger DJ, Mortimer MJ, Jaron AG: The prevalence of childhood atopic eczema in a general population. *J Am Acad Dermatol* 1994, 30:35–39.

Acne Vulgaris and Related Diseases 10

Guy F. Webster

Key Points

- Acne is a two-stage disease, with comedonal and inflammatory stages.
- Cleanliness, dirt, and diet have no role in acne pathogenesis or management.
- Comedonal and papular inflammatory acne may be treated topically.
- Isotretinoin should be reserved for therapy-resistant, disfiguring (usually nodular) acne.
- Long-term oral antibiotic therapy is safe and effective for most inflammatory acne patients.

ACNE VULGARIS

Acne vulgaris is an extraordinarily common disease, with nearly every individual affected at some time in their life. The process is centered around the pilosebaceous units of the face, upper back, and chest and is a true multifactorial condition (Table 10-1). The primary lesion is termed a *comedo* and results from the impaction and distention of the follicle with improperly desquamated follicular epithelium. Instead of being shed as small particles, the epithelium produces large sheets, not unlike scales, which are shed into the follicle and result in an impaction. Another factor in the development of acne is the onset of sebum secretion that follows the puberal surge of androgen levels, which not only further distends the follicle but also provides nutrition for *Propionibacterium acnes*, an anaerobic diphtheroid that lives within the follicle. Although of very little infectious potential, *P. acnes* is very inflammatory and in certain individuals provokes a vigorous inflammatory and immune response. The patients with the most severe acne may reasonably be said to be hypersensitive to *P. acnes* in a classical immunologic sense (Fig. 10-1) [1,2•,3•].

Some patients are predisposed to severe acne because of an underlying hormonal abnormality (Fig. 10-2). It was once thought incorrectly that everyone with severe acne was hyperandrogenic: this is clearly not true, and in fact hyperandrogenism is common only in a small subset of patients with acne, namely adult women with therapeutically resistant acne.

Treatment

Acne vulgaris is a very treatable disease. Using currently available drugs and techniques, the patient whose disease cannot be well controlled is rare.

Because of the many misconceptions about acne, no discussion of its treatment would be complete without a section on patient instructions (Table 10-2). Whatever treatment is chosen, there are several instructions that generally apply. Above all, patients should be instructed not to pop their pimples. Manipulation of acne lesions can force inflammatory comedonal contents into the tissue and prolong inflammation, producing a scar where none would have formed. A second very important issue is that acne is not caused by dirt or bad hygiene.

TABLE 10-1 ETIOLOGIC FACTORS IN ACNE

Major
Comedo formation
Sebum secretion-*Propionibacterium acnes* populations
Hypersensitivity to *P. acnes*

Minor
Hyperandrogenism

Excessive or vigorous face washing can have the same effect as squeezing pimples and generally results in more severe skin disease.

The role of cosmetics in causing acne is a matter of some debate. In the past it was certain that many cosmetics, especially oily ones, could cause comedones to form. In recent years acnegenic components have been eliminated from most cosmetics, and makeup can be judiciously applied. Finally, diet has no known influence on the acne process.

Comedonal Acne

The comedo is the primary acne lesion [1,3•]. It may be present as a visible blackhead or whitehead, or exist as a microcomedo at the center of an inflammatory lesion. Reduction in follicular plugging is a major goal of acne therapy and a key to long-lasting remission. In the past,

agents that induced desquamation (peeling agents) were used to accomplish this goal. For the past decade or so most dermatologists have favored using topical vitamin A (tretinoin), usually in a cream form. The medication is very safe and does not produce detectable changes in circulating vitamin A levels. The single adverse effect that may be expected is mild irritation of the skin to which it is applied. The skin will be somewhat reddish and perhaps have the appearance of being windburned, and patients often complain of an associated dryness. When this occurs, topical moisturizing lotions may be applied. These lotions should be noncomedogenic (*ie*, not induce acne).

Inflammatory Acne

Most patients have a significant number of inflammatory papules in addition to comedones. Although topical tretinoin will eventually reduce the number of inflammatory lesions, this does not happen quickly. Patients with inflammatory acne should receive either topical or systemic antibiotic treatment. The more mild and superficial the inflammatory lesion, the more suitable the patient is for topical therapy (Table 10-3). Benzoyl peroxide in 2.5% to 10% concentrations is of great value; however, a percentage of the population is severely irritated by this medication. Combination products of benzoyl peroxide and erythromycin seem to be better tolerated and quite effective. Other topical products include clindamycin phosphate and erythromycin preparations. Although lotions and gels

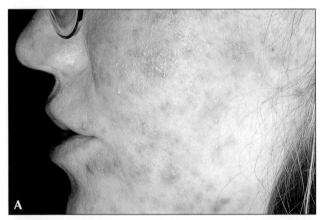

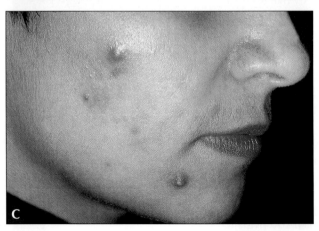

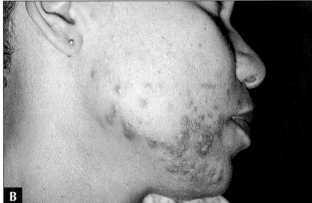

FIGURE 10-1 **A**, Severe papulopustular acne in a young woman. A few closed comedones are present. Scaling resulted from overvigorous washing. **B**, Papulonodular acne. Note the severe hyperpigmentation that may result in dark-skinned patients. **C**, Patients may have very few lesions and still be badly disfigured.

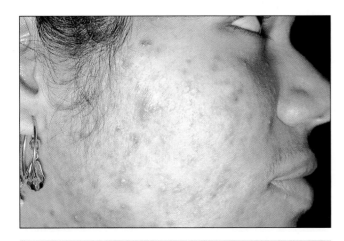

Figure 10-2 Papulopustular acne in a woman with polycystic ovaries. Note facial hirsuitism.

TABLE 10-2 PATIENT INSTRUCTIONS

Clean *gently* (dirt has no role in the acne process)
No popping, picking, or emptying of lesions
Diet has no role in acne
Minimize but do not eliminate cosmetics

are available, I generally prefer topical antibiotics in aqueous or alcoholic solutions.

Systemic treatment for acne should be considered when a large body-surface area is involved (for example, the face and the back or when acne in any area is more severe than superficial papules or pustules). Patients may be treated safely and successfully for many years using typical oral regimens. Systemic antibiotics appear to work through two mechanisms: suppression of *P. acnes* populations, and direct inhibition of components of the inflammatory response (Table 10-4). The tetracyclines and erythromycin are most commonly used and are generally well tolerated. Typical dosages are found in Table 10-5. Penicillins and cephalosporins are of little benefit in treating acne. In general, erythromycin and tetracycline are adequate for mild-to-moderate acne, but more severe disease requires doxycycline or minocycline for improvement. Although many doctors recommend minocycline for the most severe forms of acne, I find doxycycline to be as effective and significantly less expensive. The incidence of photosensitivity while taking the drug is a consideration with the use of doxycycline. For this reason, patients should be counseled to avoid sun exposure and to use sunscreens liberally.

Application of topical tretinoin is a useful adjunct to oral antibiotic therapy. Its use should be considered in most patients with acne who are taking systemic or topical antibiotics.

Patients whose disease is predominantly composed of deep nodules that result in scars or patients who have significant acne that is refractory to oral antibiotic therapy should be considered for isotretinoin treatment. Isotretinoin (13-*cis*-retinoic acid) is a metabolite of vitamin A that has profound effects on the skin. In the majority of patients isotretinoin will produce a permanent cure of their acne after a 6-month treatment period. This cure is accomplished through a suppression of sebum secretion, a change in the formation of comedones by the follicular epithelium, and a modulation of the follicular inflammatory response. Isotretinoin is an extraordinarily important and useful drug that has greatly changed the course of severe acne. At this time there is little reason for a patient to be significantly disfigured because of acne.

Unfortunately, the great benefits of isotretinoin are balanced by a significant side-effect profile. The side effects of all oral retinoids are identical to the effects of chronic

TABLE 10-3 TOPICAL ACNE THERAPY

Benzoyl peroxide—cream, 2.5% to 10.0% one to two times daily
Erythromycin or clindamycin, 2% solution one to two times daily
Benzoyl peroxide–erythromycin gel (Benzamycin; Dermik, Collegeville, PA) one to two times daily
Retin-A (Ortho, Raritan, NJ), 0.025% to 0.1% gel or cream one to two times daily

TABLE 10-4 ANTI-INFLAMMATORY ACTIVITY OF ANTIBIOTICS IN ACNE

Decreased *Propionibacterium acnes* stimulus
Decreased *P. acnes* chemotactic factor production
Inhibition of neutrophil motility
Inhibition of chronic acne inflammation

TABLE 10-5 ORAL ANTIBIOTICS IN ACNE

Commonly used treatments
Tetracycline (250 to 500 mg bid to qid)
Erythromycin (250 mg bid to qid)
Doxycycline (50 to 100 mg qd to bid)
Minocycline (50 to 100 mg qd to bid)

Occasionally used treatments
Trimethoprim-sulfamethoxazole (single or double strength qd to bid)
Ciprofloxacin (500 mg bid or tid)

bid—Twice a day; qd—every day; qid—four times a day; tid—three times a day.

vitamin A intoxication. Dryness of the skin and mucous membranes is expected, with the lips, nasal mucosa, and conjunctiva most severely affected. Some patients note a thinning of scalp hair, which tends to be reversible. Few patients complain of muscle and joint pain, and a syndrome of diffuse idiopathic skeletal hyperostosis has been reported in a few patients on long-term retinoid treatment. This latter condition is usually asymptomatic. Decreased night vision is rarely noticed, but can be measured in a significant number of patients. An elevation in triglyceride levels is seen in about one third of patients, and increases of two to three times normal levels are not rare. These elevations usually resolve with modification in diet or dosage, and on the whole seem to be well tolerated. In very rare instances an elevation in liver transaminases has been noted, as has the release of creatinine kinase from skeletal muscle, a process which may be exercise-related.

The most serious concern regarding oral retinoid treatment is the potential for birth defects [4,5]. Women of childbearing age must take extreme care to avoid conception while taking the drug, because the birth of a normal child is extremely unlikely. There is no adverse effect on subsequent pregnancies. The manufacturer of Accutane (Roche, Nutley, NJ) has gone to great lengths to see that proper counseling is given before the treatment is instituted in women. It is recommended that these guidelines be scrupulously followed. Isotretinoin has no adverse effects on male fertility.

Typical isotretinoin dosages are between 0.5 and 1.0 mg/kg/d. Lower dosages may have some benefit, but are associated with an increased frequency of relapse following discontinuation of treatment. Lower dosages do produce fewer side effects, but also necessitate a longer period of treatment than 5 or 6 months.

Other treatments for acne are occasionally used. Some women have significant elevations of circulating androgens that worsen their acne. Normalization of androgen levels, using low-progestin oral contraceptives or low daily dosages of oral corticosteroids, may aid the control of acne. Likewise, spironolactone is occasionally used because of its ability to block the binding of testosterone to sebaceous gland receptors. Neither of these maneuvers is usually enough to completely control severe acne alone or in combination with oral antibiotics. Oral corticosteroids in anti-inflammatory dosages (*eg*, 30 or 40 mg/d) are sometimes used for severe exacerbations of inflammatory acne: situations where this is appropriate are very rare.

ROSACEA

Rosacea is a chronic skin problem that is usually limited to the central portions of the face. It occurs most commonly in fair-skinned adults, often those who have had significant acne as children. Severity is very variable, with manifestations that range from red cheeks and telangiectasia to crops of pustules and inflammatory nodules (Fig. 10-3). Follicular

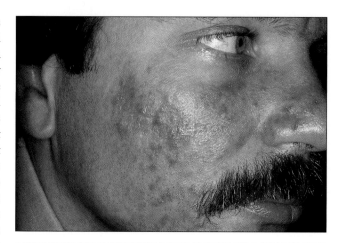

FIGURE 10-3 Papular rosacea.

impaction (comedones) are not a part of rosacea. Left untreated, the most severe cases may trigger a sebaceous hyperplasia, particularly on the nose, a reaction which is termed *rhinophyma* (Fig. 10-4).

It is sometimes difficult to distinguish rosacea from the malar eruption of lupus erythematosus (LE). No single criterion is suitably sensitive or specific. Both diseases occur in similar age groups, and both may have prominent telangiectasia. If papules or pustules are present, the diagnosis is usually rosacea. Small, white, atrophic scars favor LE. Erythema that waxes and wanes over several hours is more likely to be seen in rosacea. A confluent induration favors LE. To complicate matters, some LE patients may also develop rosacea. Evaluation by a dermatologist is often required.

The cause of rosacea is not known. It is certain that individuals with abnormal vascular reactivity on their cheeks, that is, people who flush and blush readily, tend to get rosacea. Compounds that promote facial redness, such as alcohol and spicy food, can exacerbate the rosacea process. There is also clearly a role for the follicular bacterium *P. acnes* in the pustular and nodular forms of the disease. It has long been suspected that the *Demodex* mite that is a normal inhabitant of the sebaceous glands has some role in rosacea. Although that is a widely held belief, supporting evidence is scanty, and treatment with antiparasitic drugs is of no proven benefit.

Many patients with rosacea also have evidence of chronic blepharitis, dry eyes, or recurrent styes. This is certainly part of the rosacea process and may be seen in up to 50% of patients. Treatment of the rosacea with systemic medication usually produces a great improvement in symptoms.

Rosacea is treated by two general approaches. Low-potency corticosteroids may be used alone or in combination with 3% precipitated sulfur. This treatment seems to work best in patients whose rosacea is predominantly vascular. A major problem with topical corticosteroid therapy for rosacea is the tendency of facial skin to accommo-

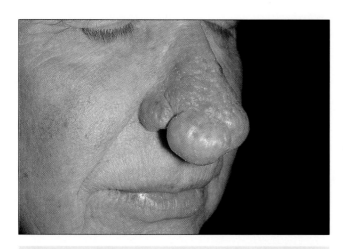

FIGURE 10-4 Rhinophyma, a sebaceous hyperplasia triggered by the rosacea process.

date to the corticosteroid, requiring an increase in drug potency for the same clinical effect. This phenomenon has a great potential to lead to the use of inappropriately strong steroids on the face, which invariably results in a worsening of the rosacea and a severe, potentially permanent, facial atrophy. Topical antibiotics are of some use in treating rosacea and are very safe, but in the hands of most dermatologists are not completely effective in more than moderately severe disease.

Systemic therapy for rosacea is often the most satisfactory, especially in disease with a significant papulopustular component. Tetracyclines are generally superior to erythromycin, although both are effective. I prefer to use doxycycline, 100 mg, one to three times daily, in most situations. Patients who report significant conjunctival symptoms often benefit greatly from systemic treatment.

REFERENCES AND RECOMMENDED READING

Recently published papers of particular interest have been highlighted as:
- Of interest
- • Of outstanding interest

1. Kligman AM: An overview of acne. *J Invest Dermatol* 1974, 62:268–287.

2.• Webster GF: Inflammatory acne. *Int J Dermatol* 1990, 29:313–317.

3.• Pochi PE, and Members of Consensus Panel: Report of the consensus conference on acne classification. *J Am Acad Dermatol* 1991, 24:1–6.

4. Rothman KF, Pochi PE: Use of oral and topical agents for acne in pregnancy. *J Am Acad Dermatol* 1988, 19:431–442.

5. Dai WS, Hsu M-A, Itri LM: Safety of pregnancy after discontinuation of isotretinoin. *Arch Dermatol* 1989, 125:362–365.

Pruritus 11

Seth G. Kates
Jeffrey D. Bernhard

Key Points

- Pruritus, which is the most common dermatologic complaint, has an extensive differential diagnosis.

- Pruritus can be present with diagnostic or nondiagnostic skin eruptions, or without skin eruptions.

- A positive diagnosis is frequently based on careful patient history, physical examination, and, if necessary, laboratory evaluation.

- Primary dermatologic conditions associated with pruritus include inflammatory conditions, infestations or infections, and neoplastic conditions.

- Systemic disorders associated with pruritus include drug reactions, hepatobiliary, endocrinolgic, and hematologic disorders.

- Management of pruritus is best achieved by alleviating the underlying cause, but if this is not possible, many other treatments are available.

Pruritus, or itching, is defined as the sensation that provokes the urge to scratch. It is the most common dermatologic symptom. Itching can be described as deep or superficial, can provoke a desire to rub or scratch the skin, and can be associated with specific eruptions, nonspecific rashes (*eg*, excoriations), or no eruption whatsoever. It can arise from a primary dermatologic etiology; a complication of pharmacologic therapy; an underlying psychogenic pathology; or a systemic cause, including infection, metabolic disorders, malignancy, hematologic disease, and senescence. Pruritus is a symptom of underlying systemic disease in an estimated 10% to 50% of patients [1]. When a patient complains of pruritus, there is a rational way to assemble the myriad of etiologies into finite groups, to evaluate the patient in a cost-effective and thoughtful manner, and to then correct the underlying cause or treat the pruritus [2••].

The history and physical examination are crucial in the evaluation of a patient with pruritus. The history must include duration, quality (*eg*, burning, tingling, crawling), intensity (*eg*, nocturnal wakening), location, aggravating factors (*eg*, after exposure to water, while at work, in the sun), time of day, careful drug history, and general review of symptoms. A primary eruption, if present, can frequently be diagnostic to the trained eye. A secondary eruption consisting of excoriations, changes caused by rubbing, or cutaneous infection can indicate an obscured primary eruption or an underlying systemic etiology [3] (Fig. 11-1).

PRURITUS WITH CUTANEOUS ERUPTION

Pruritus is a very common feature of dermatologic conditions; therefore, the differential diagnosis of itching with a rash is complex (Table 11-1). It becomes easier if the quality of the cutaneous eruption can be characterized and if the

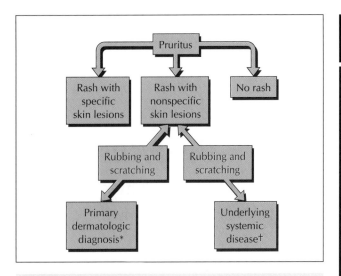

FIGURE 11-1 Clinical algorithm for evaluation of pruritus. *See Table 11-2; †see Table 11-3. (For a more extensive algorithm, see Champion [3].)

TABLE 11-1 MOST COMMON PRIMARY SKIN ERUPTIONS THAT ITCH

Inflammatory conditions	Infestations or infections
Atopic eczema	Scabies
Contact allergic and irritant dermatitis	Pediculosis
	Arthropod bites
Urticaria	Parasitic infestations
Dermatitis herpetiformis	Varicella
Bullous pemphigoid	Cutaneous fungal infections
Lichen planus	Impetigo
Photosensitivity reactions	**Neoplastic**
Psoriasis	Mycosis fungoides
Drug hypersensitivity reactions	Urticaria pigmentosa (mastocytosis)

Adapted from Bernhard [1]; with permission.

distribution can be appreciated. An urticarial eruption, if transient, can signify urticaria from many causes or, if the lesions are of a longer duration, can signify an urticarial vasculitis or an early form of bullous pemphigoid. Vesicular, bullous, or pustular lesions can be diagnostic of different conditions. The presence of excoriations in a flexural pattern in a patient with a history of seasonal allergies or asthma (although not primary lesions) strongly suggests the diagnosis of atopic eczema (Fig. 11-2). Multiple excoriations and erythematous papules on the lower extremities or arms in a patient with a pet at home, even during the winter, frequently result from flea bites, although patients generally protest the diagnosis (Fig. 11-3).

Drugs can cause either a primary cutaneous eruption or itching without any other cutaneous effects. The pruritus from drugs can be localized, as in a fixed drug eruption, or diffuse. The itching can result from hypersensi-

tivity to the drug itself or from complications from medications such as estrogen-induced cholestasis. Table 11-2 is a partial list of common medications that can cause pruritus, although any drug can cause pruritus through idiosyncratic mechanisms, no matter how long the drug has been used.

PRURITUS WITHOUT RASH

Pruritus secondary to underlying systemic pathology is frequently generalized, although some conditions are associated with a localized presentation. Table 11-3 provides a partial list of systemic disorders associated with pruritus.

Diabetes Mellitus

Diabetes mellitus was once thought to be a cause of diffuse pruritus, but more recently it has been recognized as a

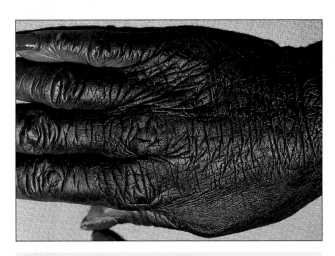

FIGURE 11-2 Lichenification of the skin resulting from chronic scratching in a patient with atopic dermatitis.

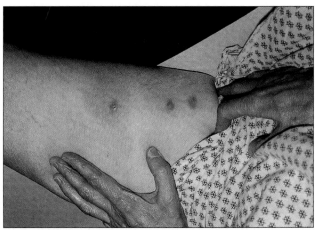

FIGURE 11-3 Typical "breakfast, lunch, dinner" configuration of insect bites.

TABLE 11-2 DRUGS ASSOCIATED WITH PRURITUS

Opiates and opiate derivatives
Phenothiazines
Tolbutamide
Erythromycin estolate
Anabolic steroids
Estrogens
Progestins
Testosterone
Aspirin
Quinidine
Vitamin B complex
Psoralens with ultraviolet A radiation
Antimalarials

Adapted from Bernhard [4•]; with permission.

TABLE 11-3 SYSTEMIC DISORDERS ASSOCIATED WITH PRURITUS

Hepatobiliary disorders
Primary biliary cirrhosis
Biliary obstruction
Cholestasis during pregnancy

Endocrine disorders
Hyperthyroidism
Hypothyroidism
Diabetes mellitus
Carcinoid syndrome
Adrenal insufficiency

Hematologic disorders
Polycythemia vera
Iron deficiency
Paraproteinemia
Waldenström's macroglobulinemia

Renal disorders
Chronic renal failure
Chronic hemodialysis

Malignant disorders
Lymphoma
Leukemia

Visceral carcinoma
Central nervous system tumors
Mycosis fungoides
Multiple myeloma

Parasitic infestations
Hookworm
Onchocerciasis
Ascariasis
Trichinosis

Infections
HIV*
Hepatitis B virus

Psychogenic states
Psychogenic pruritus
Delusions of parasitosis
Neurotic excoriations

Senescense

Aquagenic pruritus

Data from Shapiro and coworkers [5], and Liautaud and coworkers [6].
Adapted from Bernhard [4•]; with permission.

frequent cause of localized pruritus, especially of the anogenital area [7]. Diffuse pruritus in diabetes is usually associated with chronic renal failure.

Chronic Renal Failure and Chronic Hemodialysis

Pruritus is usually a late finding in patients with renal failure and rarely heralds its onset. It is frequently most marked in patients during or immediately after dialysis and can affect up to 75% of patients [8]. Pruritus can be both generalized and persistent, as well as localized and intermittent. The precise molecule or molecules responsible for itching in chronic renal failure are not known. Pruritus is not a feature of acute renal failure. Other factors in chronic renal failure that may contribute to pruritis include secondary hyperparathyroidism [9], xerosis, and hypermagnesemia [10] (Fig. 11-4).

Cholestasis

Pruritus is a hallmark of obstructive liver disease. The pathophysiology of the itching is unclear, and although elevated bile salts have been implicated, doubt that bile salts are responsible is increasing [11]. Itching is unusual in infective hepatitis or hemolytic anemias, although it is common in drug-induced cholestasis. It is commonly the presenting complaint in primary biliary cirrhosis [12].

Polycythemia Vera and Aquagenic Pruritus

Case series have disclosed greater than 50% incidence of pruritus in patients with polycythemia vera [13,14]. It typically occurs after bathing, and is frequently described as severe and prickling, lasting for 15 to 60 minutes. The skin examination is normal, and the history and quality of the pruritus is very similar to those of aquagenic pruritus. Aquagenic pruritus of the elderly most commonly occurs in women and is described as a prickling pruritus lasting approximately 15 minutes after bathing. Xerosis is some-

times present. No underlying systemic abnormality exists. Because water-induced pruritus can precede the onset of polycythemia vera by several years, long-term follow-up is suggested [15]. The pruritus of polycythemia vera frequently improves with treatment.

Malignancies

Patients with Hodgkin's disease can have associated pruritus as the presenting complaint. Frequently, the pruritis can have bizarre patterns that are localized or diffuse and occasionally migratory. Severe pruritus may portend a poor prognosis [16]. Pruritus can also be severe in cutaneous T-cell lymphoma, in which it is frequently associated with a rash. Itching occurs in internal occult malignancies, especially multiple myeloma, adenocarcinoma, and squamous cell carcinoma. However, the actual incidence is probably rare.

Senescence

Pruritus in the elderly is extremely common and increases in incidence with age. Although it is important to rule out an underlying systemic etiology, a large number of patients are left with advancing age as the only etiology. Xerotic or winter itch, or dry skin with fine cracking, is common in the elderly.

TABLE 11-4 LABORATORY EVALUATION OF A PRURITIC PATIENT*
Routine screening tests
Complete blood count with differential
Liver function
Thyroid function panel
Renal panel and urine
Blood glucose
Chest radiograph
Other tests, as indicated by above, or by history and physical examination
Stool for occult blood
Stool for ova and parasites
Papanicalaou smear
Serum protein electrophoresis
Erythrocyte sedimentation rate
Serum iron and ferritin
Blind skin biopsy with or without immunoflorescence
Additional radiologic or serologic investigations
*As indicated by history and physical examination. *Adapted from* Bernhard [1]; with permission.

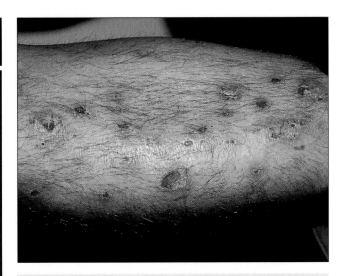

FIGURE 11-4 Excoriations in a patient with chronic renal failure on dialysis.

Age-related degenerative changes in cutaneous nerve endings may cause "phantom" pruritus in elderly patients in whom no other explanation exists for itching [17].

EVALUATION

The evaluation of a patient presenting with pruritus should proceed in a logical manner. The history, review of systems, and physical examination should provide a differential diagnosis. An initial laboratory evaluation should include a complete blood count with differential, liver function tests with a chemistry battery, thyroid function studies, and a chest radiograph (Table 11-4). Further studies can be performed but should be tailored to the patient's history. Performing a very large panel of laboratory studies with a small pretest index of suspicion is generally not helpful and can be misleading. Therefore, if the test results are negative initially, the patient can be treated symptomatically and re-evaluated at regular intervals (Table 11-4). If a primary cutaneous eruption is present, a dermatology consultation is indicated. Beware of allowing patients to fall out of contact when they are sent for evaluation because the collaborative efforts of the dermatologist and primary care physician may be required to make a diagnosis over time.

TREATMENT

Ideally, the best way to treat pruritus is to identify the underlying etiology and to correct it. Commonly, no underlying etiology is found during the initial evaluation, and treatment must be instituted for symptomatic relief [18].

Emollients are the easiest, least expensive, and most reliably successful treatments. They can be curative in patients with xerosis, atopic dermatitis, aquagenic pruritus of the elderly, and many other disorders. They can be compounded with 0.25% menthol, 0.125% phenol, or both, which may increase their efficacy. Cool soaks or a cool shower before bed can also be very effective.

Low-potency topical corticosteroids can be used, although their use should be restricted over the long term, especially when there is no definite diagnosis. Similarly, high-potency corticosteroids should be avoided unless a clear inflammatory condition is being treated. Systemic corticosteroids have no role in the treatment of pruritus of undetermined origin.

Aside from their soporific effect, H_1-blocking antihistamines are not particularly effective unless a histamine disorder, such as urticaria, is present. Again, caution should be used in the dispensing of these agents if the etiology of the pruritus is unclear. Drugs that work both peripherally and centrally, although more effective, can be very sedating. The newer nonsedating agents are not usually effective for the treatment of generalized pruritus, which is to be expected. H_2-blockers alone or in combination with H_1-blockers add little, if at all, to the treatment of pruritus.

Cholestyramine, activated charcoal, psoralens plus ultraviolet A or ultraviolet B light, and aspirin can be effective in the treatment of specific types of pruritus. It is important to remember that, in all cases of pruritus in which a cause has not been identified or in cases in which an etiology has been determined but appropriate treatment has failed, periodic re-evaluation is required.

References and Recommended Reading

Recently published papers of particular interest have been highlighted as:

• Of interest

•• Of outstanding interest

1. Bernhard JD: Itching as a manifestation of noncutaneous disease. *Hosp Pract* 1987, 22:81–95.

2.•• Bernhard JD: *Mechanism and Management of Pruritus*. New York: McGraw Hill; 1994.

3. Champion RH: Generalized pruritus. *Br Med J* 1984, 289:751–753.

4.• Bernhard JD: Pruritus: Pathophysiology and clinical aspects. In *Dermatology*, edn 4. Edited by Moschella SL, Hurley HJ. Philadelphia: WB Saunders; 1992:2042–2047.

5. Shapiro RS, Samorodin C, Hood AF: Pruritus as a presenting sign of acquired immunodeficiency syndrome. *J Am Acad Dermatol* 1987, 16:1115–1117.

6. Liautaud B, Pape JW, DeHovitz JA, *et al.*: Pruritic skin lesions. A common initial presentation of acquired immunodeficiency syndrome. *Arch Dermatol* 1989, 125:629–632.

7. Neilly JB, Martin A, Simpson N, MacCuish AC: Pruritus in diabetes mellitus: investigation of prevalence and correlation with diabetes control. *Diabetes Care* 1986, 9:273.

8. Gilchrest BA, Stern R, Steinman TI, *et al.*: Clinical features of pruritus among patients undergoing maintenance hemodialysis. *Arch Dermatol* 1982, 118:154–156.

9. Massry SG, Popovtzer MM, Coburn JW, *et al.*: Intractable pruritus as a manifestation of secondary hyperparathyroidism in uremia. Disappearance of itching after subtotal parathyroidectomy. *N Engl J Med* 1968, 279:697–700.

10. Graf J, Kovarik J, Stumjmvoll HK, *et al.*: Disappearance of uremic pruritus after lowering dialysate magnesium concentration. *Br Med J* 1979, ii:1478–1479.

11. Jones EA, Bergasa NV: Hypothesis. The pruritus of cholestasis: From bile acids to opiate agonists. *Hepatology* 1990, 11:884–887.

12. Ghent CN, Carruthers SG: Treatment of pruritus in primary biliary cirrhosis with rifampin. Results of a double-blind, crossover, randomized trial. *Gastroenterology* 1988, 94:488–493.

13. Berlin NI: Diagnosis and classification of the polycythemias. *Semin Hematol* 1975, 12:339–351.

14. Fjellner B, Hagermark O: Pruritus in polycythemia vera: Treatment with aspirin and possibility of platelet involvement. *Acta Derm Venereol (Stockh)* 1979, 59:505–512.

15. Kligman AM, Greaves MW, Steinman H: Water-induced itching without cutaneous signs. Aquagenic pruritus. *Arch Dermatol* 1986, 122:183–186.

16. Feiner AS, Mahmood J, Wanner SF: Prognostic importance of pruritus in Hodgkin's disease. *JAMA* 1978, 240:2738–2740.

17. Bernhard JD: Phantom itch, pseudophantom itch, and senile pruritus. *Int J Dermatol* 1992:856–857.

18. Bernhard JD: Pruritus: advances in treatment. *Adv Dermatol* 1991, 6:57–71.

Leg Ulcers 12

Jeffrey B. Pardes
Vincent Falanga

Key Points

- Venous ulcers occur frequently in areas affected by lipodermatosclerosis, which is manifest in its acute phase by redness, scaling, induration, and intense pain on the medial aspect of the leg.

- Biopsies of the edge of venous ulcers heal to the original margin.

- The androgenic steroid stanozolol is an effective treatment for acute lipodermatosclerosis and for ulcers caused by cryofibrinogenemia.

- Compressive bandages should not be used without first ensuring that there is adequate arterial flow in the lower extremities.

- Patients with cholesterol embolization generally have palpable pulses in the lower extremities.

- Topical agents should be avoided in patients with venous disease because of their frequent potential for sensitization.

- Although bacterial organisms are cultured from chronic ulcers regularly, systemic antibiotics should only be prescribed if cellulitis is present.

- Occlusive dressings help leg ulcers by decreasing pain, stimulating granulation tissue, and causing painless débridement.

Ulceration of the lower extremity is an increasingly common clinical problem as our population ages, and it is responsible for significant morbidity. Noninflammatory vascular disease is responsible for the vast majority of leg ulcers, with venous disease accounting for nearly 75% of cases [1]. Arterial and neuropathic disease are responsible for most other cases of leg ulcers. Table 12-1 lists many causes of leg ulcers that should be considered in a differential diagnosis.

DIAGNOSIS

Because most leg ulcers are the result of structural abnormalities in large vessels, knowledge of the vascular system is important. Physicians should look for the presence of venous, arterial, or neuropathic disease in any patient who presents with a leg ulcer. A comprehensive evaluation is required. In a given patient, ulcers may be caused by a combination of factors. The gross appearance of the lower extremities should be noted: leg deformities or scars may provide clues about past pathologic processes or surgical intervention that may have led to structural damage in the vascular or nervous system, thereby contributing to ulcer development. Typical venous, arterial, or neuropathic ulcers are often easy to diagnose. Table 12-2 illustrates features of the history and physical examination that help distinguish between the three most common causes of leg ulcers. It should be noted that the presence, quality, or intensity of pain within an ulcer is not sufficiently specific for a diagnosis,

TABLE 12-1 CLASSIFICATION OF LEG ULCERS

Vascular (noninflammatory)
Venous disease
Arterial disease
  Atherosclerosis
  Buerger's disease
Cholesterol emboli
Antiphospholipid antibody syndrome
Hemoglobinopathies

Vascular (inflammatory)
Vasculitis
  Chronic hypersensitivity angiitis
  Polyarteritis nodosa
  Necrobiosis lipoidica diabeticorum
  Wegener's granulomatosis
  Connective tissue disease
    Systemic lupus erythematosus
    Rheumatoid arthritis
    Scleroderma
Cryofibrinogenemia, cryoglobulinemia

Neuropathic
Diabetes mellitus
Hansen's disease
Syringomyelia

Neoplastic
Squamous cell carcinoma
Basal cell carcinoma
Cutaneous lymphoma
Kaposi's sarcoma
Metastases

Infectious
Bacterial
Mycotic
Mycobacterial
Syphilitic gumma

Physical
Factitial
Postirradiation

Pyoderma gangrenosum

although arterial ulcers are generally more painful than venous ulcers, and neuropathic ulcers are often painless.

COMMON CAUSES OF LEG ULCERS

Venous Ulcers

Venous disease and ulceration are more frequent in older women than in men, even when the greater longevity of women is taken into account [1]. A characteristic finding in patients with venous disease is the presence of dermatitis in the affected extremity (Fig. 12-1). In addition to the typical clinical features of venous disease, which include hyperpigmentation surrounding the ulcer (Table 12-2; Figs. 12-2 and 12-3), the physician often obtains a history of intense pain, redness, and scaling preceding the development of the ulcer. These clinical features suggest the diagnosis of lipodermatosclerosis. The acute phase of lipodermatosclerosis does not occur in every patient who develops a venous ulcer, and is often misdiagnosed as morphea or a cellulitis unresponsive to antibiotic treatment [2••]. Chronic lipodermatosclerosis often results in depression and induration on the medial aspect of the leg (Fig. 12-4). It may cause the lower leg to assume a shape similar to an inverted bottle. A palpa-

TABLE 12-2 DISTINGUISHING FEATURES OF SELECTED LEG ULCERS

Feature	Venous	Arterial	Neuropathic
History	Previous deep venous thrombosis or vein stripping	Risk of atherosclerosis	Diabetes or neurologic disease
Symptoms	Dull leg pain, heaviness, relief with leg elevation	Claudication; pain with leg elevation	None or paresthesias
Ulcer location	Medial and lateral malleoli	Toes or areas of pressure	Malleolar or plantar surfaces
Ulcer appearance	Shallow, irregular exudative	Deep, regular, dry, necrotic, exposed tendons	Deep, often surrounded by callus
Associated findings	Edema, venous dermatitis (scaling, redness, hyperpigmentation), venous dilatation, lipodermatosclerosis	Xerosis, fissures, alopecia, dependent rubor, decreased pulses	Evidence of deformity, muscle atrophy, sensory deficit

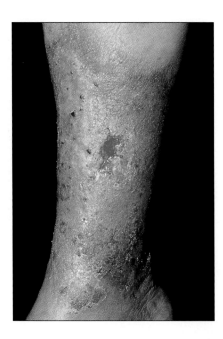

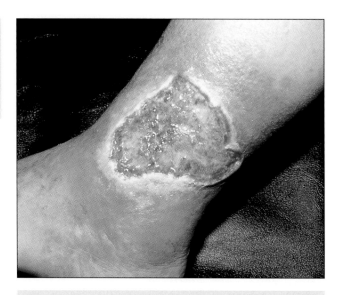

FIGURE 12-1 Marked pruritus in the setting of venous dermatitis led to ulcer development.

FIGURE 12-2 Venous ulcer with surrounding dermatitis.

ble abrupt transition is detectable between the indurated and the normal skin, reminiscent of a cliff drop. We stress clinical recognition of lipodermatosclerosis because biopsy incisions in the indurated skin may not heal and may become venous ulcers. However, if a biopsy does become necessary, direct immunofluorescence studies of the ulcer's edge will show the presence of pericapillary fibrin [1]. Interestingly, after biopsy specimens are obtained from the edge of venous ulcers, remaining tissue heals up to the original margin [3].

Arterial Ulcers

Patients with known risk factors for atherosclerosis and the cutaneous findings displayed in Table 12-2 often have arterial ulcers (Fig. 12-5). With advanced arterial disease, elevation of the leg for less than 1 minute leads to limb pallor; return of the elevated leg to a dependent position results in diffuse erythema. It is important to realize that palpable distal pulses do not absolutely exclude the presence of arterial disease. Doppler ultrasonography is a quick, effective method of measuring systolic blood pressure in the leg and of excluding arterial insufficiency. The ratio of the ankle systolic blood pressure to the brachial systolic blood pressure (ankle–brachial index) is a widely used parameter [4]. The presence of an index greater than 0.8 is a reliable indicator that significant arterial disease is not present in a given patient. Figure 12-6 demonstrates the method of

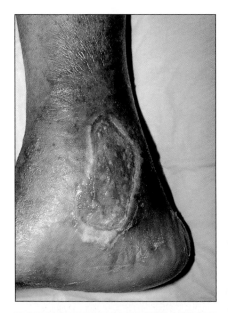

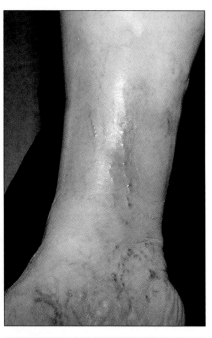

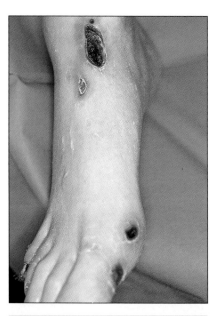

FIGURE 12-3 Venous ulcer overlying the medial malleolus. Ulcers in this location are difficult to heal.

FIGURE 12-4 Lipodermatosclerosis.

FIGURE 12-5 Arterial ulcers covered by necrotic eschar. Notice the presence of alopecia.

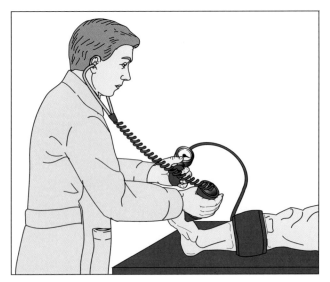

FIGURE 12-6 Method of obtaining ankle systolic blood pressure.

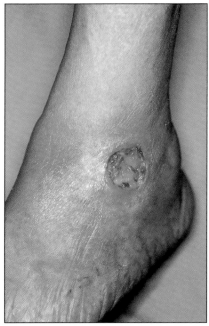

obtaining the ankle systolic blood pressure. Patients with suspected arterial disease should be evaluated further for corrective vascular surgery. Up to 20% of patients have combined venous and arterial disease (Fig. 12-7).

Neuropathic Ulcers

Patients with neuropathies (*eg*, from diabetes mellitus) often have considerable leg deformity. This deformity is the result of constant trauma from loss of or alteration in sensory function and failure to maintain normal neurologic impulses to the musculature of the lower extremity [5]. The development of new pressure points unaccustomed to pressure can lead to the findings shown in Table 12-2. Ulcers developing as a result of pressure are often surrounded by a callus and are typically larger than suggested by the overlying skin defect: subcutaneous tissue may be necrotic with little clinical evidence. In patients with diabetes, vascular deficits may combine with the neuropathy to produce complex ulcers (Figs. 12-8 and 12-9).

LESS COMMON CAUSES OF LEG ULCERS

Patients often present with ulcers whose appearance and location are atypical for vascular and neuropathic etiologies, leading to consideration of less common causes of ulceration. Table 12-3 suggests a diagnostic framework in which to view leg ulcers that are not caused by large arterial disease, venous insufficiency, or neuropathy.

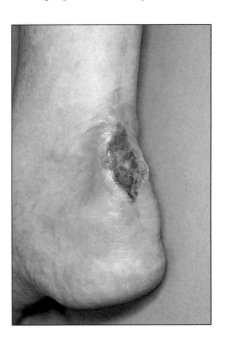

FIGURE 12-8 Neuropathic ulcer overlying the Achilles tendon region after previous surgery in that location.

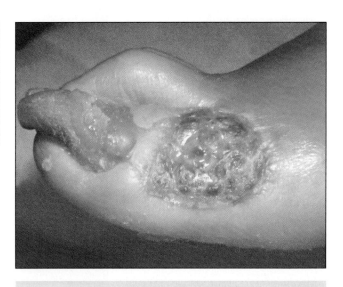

FIGURE 12-9 Distal ulcer in a patient with diabetes and severe arterial disease.

TABLE 12-3 DIFFERENTIAL FEATURES OF SELECTED CAUSES OF LEG ULCERS

Finding	Cryoproteins	Cholesterol emboli	Antiphospholipid antibody syndrome	Vasculitis	Pyoderma gangrenosum
Pulses	+	+	+	+	+
Purpura	+	+	+	+	-
Livedo reticularis	+	+	+	+	-
Punched-out ulcer	-	-	-	-	-
Eschar over ulcer	+	+	+	+	+
Undermined edges	-	-	-	-	+
Violaceous edges	+	-	-	-	+
Cribriform healing	-	-	-	-	+
Raynaud's phenomenon	+	-	+/-	+/-	-
Intractable pain	+	-	+	-	-
Associated diseases	Carcinoma, infections, connective tissue disease, embolic processes	Atherosclerosis	Systemic lupus erythematosus and other connective tissue diseases, recurrent abortions	Connective tissue disease, neoplasia	Inflammatory bowel disease, rheumatoid arthritis, IgA gammopathy

+—common; -—uncommon; +/-—sometimes.

Physicians should look for several cutaneous symptoms that may provide clues to the etiology of the ulceration. Purpura, which represents extravasation of blood into the skin, suggests the possibility of inflammatory vascular disease (ie, vasculitis). Livedo reticularis, a fixed reddish-blue mottling of the skin in a netlike pattern, is often prominent on the lower extremities. Livedo reticularis is commonly seen in association with underlying vascular occlusion, connective tissue disease, or vasculitis. The following sections discuss selected causes of leg ulcers that are less common, but often prove to be diagnostic dilemmas for the physician.

Cryoproteinemia

Cryofibrinogenemia may occur either as a primary disease or in association with underlying connective tissue disease, neoplasm, acute infection, or thromboembolic disorders [6,7]. Characteristically, ulcers caused by cryofibrinogenemia are exquisitely painful. During our examination of patients with this condition, we have repeatedly observed that they constantly rub the surrounding skin in an effort to get pain relief. The skin surrounding the ulcers is often a violaceous color and may show purpura and livedo reticularis (Figs. 12-10 and 12-11). Histologically, intravascular fibrin thrombi are typically seen in the dermis. The use of

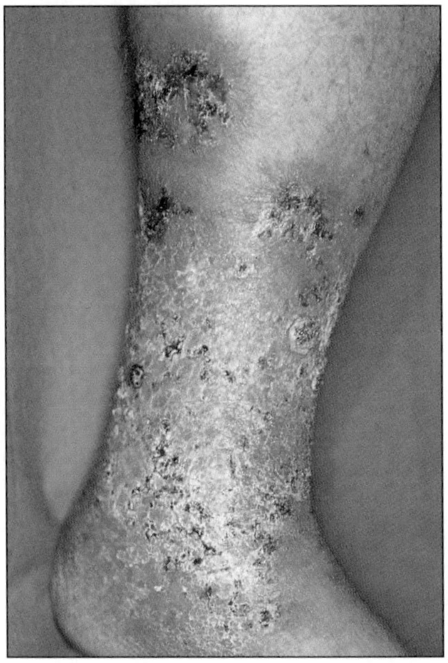

FIGURE 12-10 Multiple, crusted necrotic ulcers with surrounding erythema in a patient with cryofibrinogenemia.

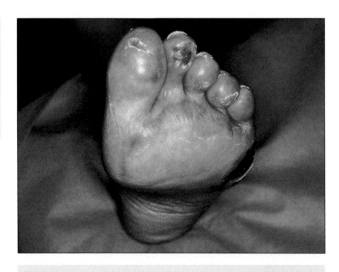

FIGURE 12-11 Distal purpura and necrotic toe ulcers in a patient with cryofibrinogenemia secondary to lymphoblastic leukemia.

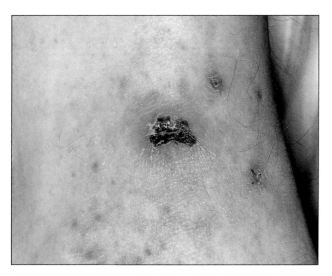

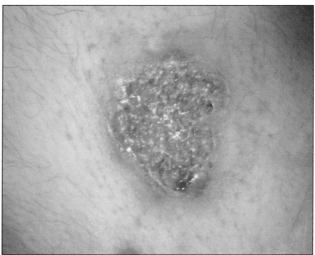

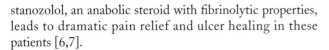

FIGURE 12-12 Necrotic ulcer and purpura secondary to cholesterol emboli.

FIGURE 12-13 Pyoderma gangrenosum. Note the violaceous borders and evidence of cribriform healing.

stanozolol, an anabolic steroid with fibrinolytic properties, leads to dramatic pain relief and ulcer healing in these patients [6,7].

Cholesterol Emboli

Ulcers due to cholesterol emboli typically occur when atheromatous material is dislodged from the abdominal aorta. Cholesterol embolization often occurs after anticoagulant therapy, vascular surgery, or arteriography. Patients may be quite ill, with nonspecific findings including fever, central nervous system changes, sudden arterial hypertension, and myalgia [8]. Leg ulcers due to cholesterol emboli may be associated with extensive livedo reticularis, purpura, and characteristic purple toes (Fig. 12-12). Cholesterol clefts within arterioles are the expected histopathologic finding, but serial subsectioning of biopsy material may be necessary for detection. Interestingly, despite extensive atherosclerotic disease, distal pulses are readily palpable in patients with cholesterol emboli.

Antiphospholipid Antibody Syndrome

Patients with antiphospholipid antibody syndrome develop vascular thromboses, recurrent fetal loss, and thrombocytopenia. The syndrome is not restricted to patients with systemic lupus erythematosus. Positive or reactive testing for Venereal Disease Research Laboratory (test), anticardiolipin antibody, and lupus anticoagulant help confirm the diagnosis of this syndrome [9]. Leg ulcers, livedo reticularis, and purpura are not uncommon in these patients.

Pyoderma Gangrenosum

Rapidly enlarging ulcers with violaceous, undermined edges and cribriform healing (ie, with sievelike perforations of the re-epithelializing wound bed) are typical of pyoderma gangrenosum (Figs. 12-13 and 12-14). Many patients develop ulcers at sites of trauma (pathergy), and lesions often begin as pustules. Although often idiopathic, pyoderma gangrenosum may be associated with ulcerative colitis, rheumatoid arthritis, IgA gammopathies, and multiple myeloma [10]. Mycotic and atypical mycobacterial infection must be excluded. Histology does not aid the diagnosis.

Factitial Ulcers

Manipulation of the skin by the patient can result in the development of leg ulcers that are often atypical in appearance. Such ulcers have odd geometric or linear shapes (Fig. 12-15).

Necrobiosis Lipoidica Diabeticorum

Necrobiosis lipoidica diabeticorum refers to characteristic circumscribed, atrophic, yellow-brown patches that rarely

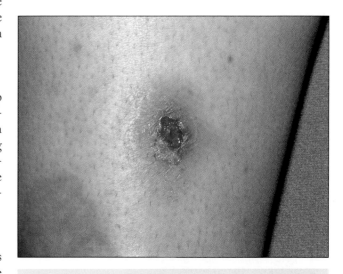

FIGURE 12-14 Healing pyoderma gangrenosum in a patient with Behçet's syndrome. Previously healed hypopigmented plaque is also present.

ulcerate (Fig. 12-16). Patients with necrobiosis lipoidica diabeticorum either have diabetes, will develop diabetes, or have a strong family history of diabetes.

Neoplasia

A chronic ulcer that is refractory to treatment may be caused by a cutaneous neoplasm. The most common neoplasms arising from a venous ulcer are basal cell carcinoma and rarely, squamous cell carcinoma [11]. The physician should be particularly suspicious of ulcers with exuberant granulation tissue, which is a presentation common in basal cell carcinoma.

TREATMENT

Certain fundamental principles are followed in the treatment of any leg ulcer. Correction of or improvement in underlying illnesses that impair wound healing should be undertaken. Common systemic diseases in which this approach is feasible are diabetes mellitus, anemia, nutritional deficiency, systemic hypertension, and congestive heart failure. Systemic agents that may impair wound healing include corticosteroids and other immunosuppressive drugs, nonsteroidal anti-inflammatory medications, and antineoplastic drugs. Topical agents, including antiseptics and various home remedies (*eg*, soap), may have a deleterious effect on wound healing. The damage caused by antiseptics is often overlooked [3,12].

Chronic wounds often become infected and have copious malodorous drainage. Although bacterial organisms are cultured from chronic ulcers regularly, we do not prescribe antibiotics unless signs of cellulitis are present. Topical antibiotics have little effect in patients with venous ulcers

who also have a high frequency of allergic contact dermatitis. Moreover, the use of topical antibiotics leads to the development of resistant organisms [3].

The goals of ulcer treatment include cleansing of the wound bed, stimulation of granulation tissue formation, and re-epithelialization.

Cleansing

Irrigation of ulcers with normal saline or water, followed by gentle patting, is recommended. The use of antiseptic solutions (*eg*, hydrogen peroxide or povidone-iodine) is not recommended because of their toxicity to the cells within the wound bed. Hydrogen peroxide is also quite ineffective in the presence of serum.

Granulation Tissue Formation
Occlusive dressings

Occlusive dressings include hydrocolloids, hydrogels, and films. Occlusive dressings promote painless débridement and granular tissue formation, and they also reduce pain associated with the ulcer [3]. They should not be used in the presence of cellulitis, but any fear of causing infection with the use of these agents is unwarranted. Patients must be warned that within a few days of the application of an occlusive dressing, a foul-smelling and considerable exudate may occur. This is not a sign of infection and is expected, particularly with hydrocolloid dressings, which melt into the wound and form a brown or green exudate (Fig. 12-17). Occlusive dressings should be removed and changed only when they start to peel away from the wound, a process that may take days to occur. With the continued use of these dressings, the initial, exudative phase of occlusive therapy is generally followed by

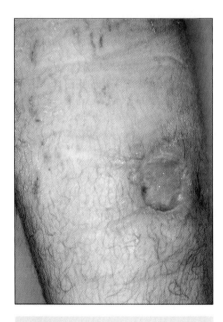

FIGURE 12-15 Factitial ulcer. Proximal, crusted linear excoriations were produced with a stick in an attempt to manipulate the ulcer that was under an Unna boot.

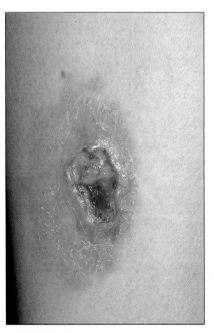

FIGURE 12-16 Necrobiosis lipoidica diabeticorum with ulceration.

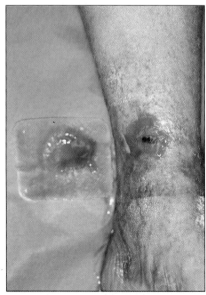

FIGURE 12-17 Removal of a hydrocolloid dressing demonstrates the expected brown exudate several days after dressing application.

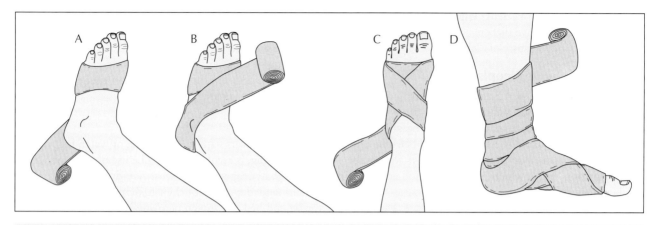

FIGURE 12-18 Unna boot application.

less exudate production. Hasty removal of an occlusive dressing may disrupt fragile, nascent epithelium.

Vitamin A derivatives

Vitamin A or retinoic acid is particularly useful in immunosuppressed patients with ulcers. In this setting, ulcers typically have poor granulation tissue. The once-daily application of retinoic acid lotion to the wound bed often promotes good granulation tissue. The skin surrounding the ulcer should be protected from the irritant action of retinoic acid with petrolatum. If irritation does develop, alternate-day therapy may be better tolerated.

SPECIFIC TREATMENTS

Venous Ulcers

The main goal of therapy is improved venous return and treatment of edema. Specifically, bed rest and leg elevation are recommended, but this may be not practical advice for all patients. Compressive occlusive therapy with an Unna boot or tight, self-adherent bandages is highly efficacious in controlling edema and promoting ulcer healing [12]. Compressive bandages, such as the Unna boot, should be changed weekly. Figure 12-18 demonstrates the method of Unna boot application. It is important to exclude arterial disease before compression therapy is used.

Arterial Ulcers

Referral to a physician skilled in determining the feasibility of vascular reconstruction is recommended for patients with arterial ulcers. If patients are not eligible for bypass procedures, conservative management includes cessation of smoking, weight loss, reduction of systemic blood pressure, and treatment of hyperlipidemia.

Neuropathic Ulcers

Diseases underlying the neuropathy that causes these ulcers should be treated. Patients should examine or should have a

trained person examine their legs and feet periodically to prevent the development of new ulcers. Educating the patient about the avoidance of external pressure on the ulcer is essential to ulcer healing. Often, neuropathic ulcers contain deep necrotic tissue, akin to the configuration of an iceberg under the surface of a body of water. Thus, deep débridement and a high index of suspicion for osteomyelitis are often necessary [5,13]. Treatment with pressure-relief hydrocolloid dressings has proved to be useful.

Therapies for Less Common Leg Ulcers

Treatments useful for selected rarer causes of leg ulcers are found in Table 12-4.

TABLE 12-4 UNCOMMON CAUSES OF LEG ULCERS AND SPECIFIC RECOMMENDED THERAPIES	
Disease process causing ulcer	**Treatment**
Cholesterol embolization	No effective treatment
Antiphospholipid antibody syndrome*	Intralesional or systemic corticosteroids
Pyoderma gangrenosum*	Corticosteroids (intralesional or systemic [orally or intravenous pulse])
	Sulfones, clofazimine, cyclosporine
Cryofibrinogenemia*	Stanozolol
	Directed at underlying disease
Vasculitis associated	Steroids
Neoplasia	Excision and referral
Infection	Microbial chemotherapy
Factitial*	Physical occlusion with bandages (Unna boot)

*In the absence of arterial insufficiency, compression therapy may be helpful. The concomitant presence of venous disease should be treated with compression.

Systemic Agents

Stanozolol is an anabolic steroid that has shown promise in the treatment of patients with ulcers caused by cryofibrinogenemia [7]. Similarly, patients with acute lipodermatosclerosis often respond dramatically to stanozolol (at a dosage of 2 to 4 mg twice a day). This agent should not be used in patients with arterial hypertension, congestive heart failure, renal failure, prostatic hypertrophy or cancer, lipid disorders, and liver function test abnormalities.

Ulcers That Fail to Heal

On occasion, despite proper treatment and the development of good granulation tissue, ulcers do not re-epithelialize. Split-thickness skin grafting (eg, with pinch grafts or keratome sheets) can be used in refractory cases as a rapid method of wound closure (Fig. 12-19). When an ulcer does not heal, the diagnosis must be reconsidered. The possibility that the ulcer has a factitial or neoplastic component should be considered. Inquiry about the use of topical or systemic agents that can adversely affect wound healing is very important in such cases. Hospitalization may be necessary to gain control over topical treatment.

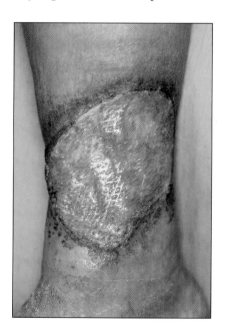

FIGURE 12-19
Split-thickness skin graft applied to a venous ulcer.

REFERENCES AND RECOMMENDED READING

Recently published papers of particular interest have been highlighted as:
- Of interest
- • Of outstanding interest

1. Katz MH, Falanga V, Eaglstein WH: Leg ulcers: a wound-healing model. In *Recent Advances in Dermatology*. Edited by Champion RH, Pye RJ. Edinburgh: Churchill Livingstone; 1992: 199–218.

2.•• Kirsner RS, Pardes JB, Eaglstein WH, Falanga V: The clinical spectrum of lipodermatosclerosis. *J Am Acad Dermatol* 1993, 28:623–627.

3. Falanga V, Eaglstein WH: A therapeutic approach to venous ulcers. *J Am Acad Dermatol* 1986, 14:777–784.

4. Yao ST, Hobbs JT, Irvine WT: Ankle systolic pressure measurements in arterial disease affecting the lower extremities. *Br J Surg* 1969, 56:676–679.

5. Boulton AJM: The diabetic foot. *Med Clin North Am* 1988, 72:1513–1530.

6. Falanga V, Kirsner RS, Eaglstein WH, *et al*.: Stanozolol in treatment of leg ulcers due to cryofibrinogenemia. *Lancet* 1991, 338:347–348.

7. Kirsner RS, Eaglstein WH, Katz MH, *et al*.: Stanozolol causes rapid pain relief and healing of ulcers caused by cryofibrinogenemia. *J Am Acad Dermatol* 1993, 28:71–75.

8. Falanga V, Fine MJ, Kapoor WN: The cutaneous manifestations of cholesterol crystal embolization. *Arch Dermatol* 1986, 122:1194–1198.

9. Stephens CJM: The antiphospholipid syndrome: clinical correlations, cutaneous features, mechanisms of thrombosis and treatment of patients with the lupus anticoagulant and anticardiolipin antibodies. *Br J Dermatol* 1991, 125:199–206.

10. Matis WL, Ellis CN, Griffiths CEM, Lazarus GS: Treatment of pyoderma gangrenosum with cyclosporine. *Arch Dermatol* 1992, 128:1060–1064.

11. Harris B, Eaglstein WH, Falanga V: Basal cell carcinoma arising in venous ulcers and mimicking granulation tissue. *J Dermatol Surg Oncol* 1993, 19:150–152.

12. Mayberry JC, Moneta GL, Taylor LM, Porter JM: Fifteen-year results of ambulatory compression therapy for chronic venous ulcers. *Surgery* 1991, 109:575–581.

13. LoGerfo FW, Coffman JD: Current concepts: vascular and microvascular disease of the foot in diabetes. *N Engl J Med* 1984, 311:1615–1619.

SELECT BIBLIOGRAPHY

Cheatle TR, Sarin S, Coleridge Smith PD, Scurr JH: The pathogenesis of skin damage in venous disease: a review. *Eur J Vasc Surg* 1991, 5:115–123.

Falanga V: Occlusive wound dressings: why, when, which? *Arch Dermatol* 1988, 124:872–877.

Falanga V, Moosa HH, Nemeth AJ, *et al*.: Dermal pericapillary fibrin in venous disease and venous ulceration. *Arch Dermatol* 1987, 123:620–623.

Phillips TJ, Dover JS: Leg ulcers. *J Am Acad Dermatol* 1991, 25:965–987.

Photosensitivity 13

Yardy Tse
Henry W. Lim

Key Points
- Evaluation of photosensitive patients should include history, physical examination, and photobiologic studies.
- Polymorphous light eruption is the most common idiopathic photodermatosis.
- Solar urticaria is characterized by development of urticaria after exposure to sunlight.
- Photoallergy and phototoxicity require the concomitant presence of photosensitizers and radiation.
- Chronic actinic dermatitis consists of a spectrum of chronic photosensitivity disorders, known previously under other terminologies.

Solar radiation can be classified according to wavelength (Table 13-1). Ultraviolet (UV)C is absorbed in the atmosphere and does not reach the surface of the earth. Common side effects of sun exposure, ranging from sunburn to skin cancers, are the result of acute and chronic exposure to UVB (Fig. 13-1). UVA may potentiate the photocarcinogenic effect of UVB and is responsible for the development of most types of photoallergy and phototoxicity. UV light may also induce the development of idiopathic dermatoses (*eg*, polymorphous light eruption [PMLE], solar urticaria, and chronic actinic dermatitis [CAD]), and exacerbate other disorders, such as lupus erythematosus, pellagra, pemphigus, and Hartnup disease (for porphyrias, *see* Werth and McKinley Grant, Cutaneous Manifestations of Endocrine and Metabolic Disorders).

APPROACH TO THE PATIENT WITH PHOTOSENSITIVITY

A detailed history must be obtained when evaluating patients with photosensitivity. Particular attention should be paid to 1) age at onset of the eruption; 2) length of exposure, and whether reaction is immediate or delayed (Table 13-2); 3) persistence of reactions (recurrent or chronic); 4) seasonal variation; and 5) the effect of window glass (which blocks out most UVB). Questioning with regard to exposure to photosensitizers, either systemic or topical (the latter including sunscreens, cosmetics, plants or occupational agents), is essential. Current systemic medication, as well as medication to which the patient was exposed at the time of the initial episode of photosensitivity, should be reviewed. A history of exposure to oral contraceptives or ingestion of ethanol is important in patients who may have porphyria. Of particular interest in the review of systems is multiple organ involvement in connective tissue disease (*ie*, arthralgia, oral ulcers, hair loss, and neurologic symptoms associated with the hepatic porphyrias).

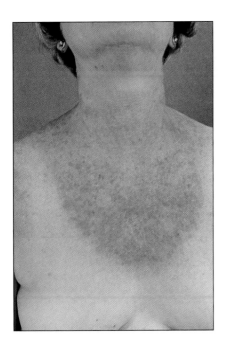

Figure 13-6
Phototoxicity presenting as erythema on the upper chest, with sharp cutoff at areas covered by clothing.

Persistent light reactivity usually begins as a photocontact dermatitis, but patients remain exquisitely sensitive to sunlight for many years. Photopatch tests in these patients are usually positive, although negative results have been observed. In contrast to photoallergy to topical agents, photo testing reveals lowered MEDs to UVB, UVA, or visible light. A skin biopsy specimen of persistent light reactivity demonstrates a spongiotic dermatitis with a lymphohistiocytic infiltrate.

Patients with photosensitive eczema present with an eczematous eruption, lowered MED to UVB, and negative photopatch tests. Histopathologic findings are similar to those seen with persistent light reactivity.

Like patients with persistent light reactivity, patients with actinic reticuloid also have lowered MEDs to UVB, UVA, or visible light. Photopatch tests may be either positive or negative. Diagnosis of actinic reticuloid is confirmed by histologic evidence of atypical mononuclear cells in the epidermis and dermis, changes which are indistinguishable from those seen in cutaneous T-cell lymphoma.

The pathophysiology of CAD is only partially understood [13,14]. It has been postulated that the carrier protein which binds the photoallergen is altered by UV radiation, resulting in the formation of a neoantigen (an altered carrier protein) which initiates a delayed hypersensitivity response. Sensitivity to contact allergens such as *Compositae oleoresins*, fragrances and lichens, an impaired ability to repair tissue damage induced by oxygen-free radicals, and possible persistence of photoallergens in the skin, have all been postulated to play a role in the pathogenesis of CAD.

Management of patients with CAD consists of restriction of UV light exposure, with the use of broad-spectrum sunscreens and topical corticosteroids for symptomatic relief. If these are ineffective, PUVA, hydroxychloroquine, azathioprine, or cyclosporin A are efficacious in some patients [15–17].

PHOTOAGGRAVATED DERMATOSES

Photoaggravated dermatoses are a group of heterogeneous diseases which share the common feature of being induced or exacerbated by exposure to sunlight. Photoaggravation occurs in only a minority of affected patients; for the most part, the action spectra have not been clearly defined. Selected examples of these dermatoses are described below.

Lupus Erythematosus

Photosensitivity is one of the 11 major criteria in the diagnosis of systemic lupus erythematosus (SLE). One third to one half of all patients with SLE are photosensitive. New cutaneous lesions with the morphologic, histologic, and immunofluorescence characteristics of LE may develop after exposure to solar or artificial UV light. The action spectrum for induction of cutaneous lesions in LE includes both UVA and UVB wavelengths [18•].

The pathogenic role of UV radiation is uncertain, but evidence exists to suggest that it can act as a stimulus to immune complex formation. UV light has been shown to increase the immunogenicity of DNA, induce expression of nuclear and cytoplasmic antigens on keratinocyte cell membranes, induce expression and release of proinflammatory factors from keratinocytes, and enhance the activity of a clastogenic factor found in lymphocytes of LE patients [19–22].

TABLE 13-7 SPECTRUM OF CHRONIC ACTINIC DERMATITIS			
Clinical entity	**MED**	**Photopatch test**	**Histology**
Persistent light reactivity	↓ UVB, UVA, visible	+	Spongiotic dermatitis, lymphohistiocytic infiltrate
Photosensitive eczema	↓ UVB	−	Spongiotic dermatitis, lymphohistiocytic infiltrate
Actinic reticuloid	↓ UVB, UVA, visible	±	Atypical mononuclear cells in dermis and epidermis

+—positive; - —negative; ↓—decreased; ±—positive in some patients. MED—minimal erythema dose; UV—ultraviolet.

TABLE 13-8 PHOTOAGGRAVATED DERMATOSES

Acne vulgaris	Herpes simplex
Atopic dermatitis	Lupus erythematosus
Bloom's syndrome	Pellagra
Darier's disease	Pemphigus foliaceus
Disseminated superficial actinic porokeratosis	Pemphigus erythematosus
Benign familial pemphigus (Hailey-Hailey disease)	Transient acantholytic dermatosis
	Hartnup disease

Pellagra

Pellagra results from a deficiency of niacin or its precursor, the essential amino acid tryptophan. It is characterized by the triad of dermatitis (erythema, desquamation, hyperpigmentation), gastroenteritis, and encephalopathy. Prominent skin changes are precipitated by sun exposure, with a tendency to appear in the spring and summer and to improve in the winter.

Niacin, in the form of nicotinamide, is necessary for the synthesis of nicotinamide adenine dinucleotide (NAD) and NAD phosphate. A deficiency of niacin causes decreased availability of these cofactors, which appear to be essential for oxidation and reduction reactions to repair epidermal damage after UV exposure.

Hartnup Disease

Hartnup disease, inherited as an autosomally recessive trait, is a disorder of tryptophan absorption from the gastrointestinal tract and renal tubule. Clinically, it is characterized by pellagralike photosensitivity dermatitis, cerebellar ataxia, and mental retardation. The pellagralike dermatitis appears to be the result of a defect in niacin production due to the decreased tryptophan absorption.

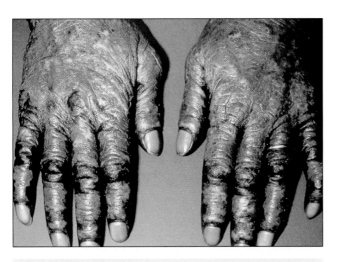

FIGURE 13-7 Lichenification and excoriation on the dorsum of the hands of a patient with chronic actinic dermatitis.

Pemphigus Foliaceus and Pemphigus Erythematosus

Pemphigus foliaceus and erythematosus are chronic, autoimmune, blistering dermatoses characterized by deposition of intercellar IgG throughout the epidermis. Sun exposure has been shown to induce cutaneous lesions [23].

REFERENCES AND RECOMMENDED READING

Recently published papers of particular interest have been highlighted as:
- Of interest
- • Of outstanding interest

1. Parrish JA, Levine MJ, Morison WL, et al.: Comparison of PUVA and beta-carotene in the treatment of polymorphous light eruption. Br J Dermatol 1979, 100:187–191.

2. Hölzle E, Plewig G, von Kries R, Lehmann P: Polymorphous light eruption. J Invest Dermatol 1987, 88:32s–38s.

3.• Hönigsmann H: Polymorphous light eruption. In Clinical Photomedicine. Edited by Lim HW, Soter NA. New York: Marcel Dekker; 1993:167–180.

4. Molin L, Volden G: Treatment of polymorphous light eruption with PUVA and prednisolone. Photodermatol 1987, 4:107–108.

5. Murphy GM, Logan RA, Lorell CR et al.: Prophylactic PUVA and UVB therapy in polymorphic light eruption—a controlled trial. Br J Dermatol 1987, 116:531—538.

6. Leenutaphong V, Hölzle E, Plewig G: Pathogenesis and classification of solar urticaria: a new concept. J Am Acad Dermatol 1989, 21:237–240.

7. Neittaanmaki H, Jaaskelainen T, Harvima RJ, Fraki JE: Solar urticaria: demonstration of histamine release and effective treatment with doxepin. Photodermatol 1989, 6:52–55.

8. Kobza Black A: Oral beta-carotene therapy in actinic reticuloid and solar urticaria. Failure to demonstrate a photoprotective effect against long-wave UV and visible radiation. Br J Dermatol 1973, 88:157–166.

9. Addo HA, Sharma SC: UVB phototherapy and photochemotherapy (PUVA) in the treatment of polymorphic light eruption and solar urticaria. Br J Dermatol 1987, 116:539–547.

10.• DeLeo VA: Photoallergy. In Clinical Photomedicine. Edited by Lim HW, Soter NA. New York: Marcel Dekker, 1993:227–239.

11. Gange RW, Lim HW: Photobiology and pathophysiology of cutaneous responses to electromagnetic radiation. In Pathophysiology and Dermatologic Diseases, edn 2. Edited by Soter NA, Baden HP. New York: McGraw Hill, 1990:395–423.

12.• Lim HW, Morison W, Kamide R, et al.: Chronic actinic dermatitis: an analysis of 51 patients evaluated in the United States and Japan. Arch Dermatol 1994, 130:1284–1289.

13. Norris PG, Hawk JLM: Chronic actinic dermatitis: a unifying concept. Arch Dermatol 1990, 126:376–378.

14. Addo HA, Sharma SC, Ferguson J, et al.: A study of compositae plant extract reactions in photosensitivity dermatitis. Photodermatol 1985, 2:68–79.

15. Yokel B, Morison WL: PUVA therapy of chronic photosensitive eczema. Arch Dermatol 1990, 126:1283–1285.

16. Haynes HA, Bernhard JD, Gange RW: Actinic reticuloid: response to combination treatment with azathioprine, hydroxychloroquine, and prednisone. J Am Acad Dermatol 1984, 10:947–952.

17. Norris PG, Camp RDR, Hawk JLM: Actinic reticuloid: response to cyclosporine. *J Am Acad Dermatol* 1989, 21:301–309.

18.• Lehmann P, Hölze E, Kind P, *et al.*: Experimental reproduction of skin lesions in lupus erythematosus by UVA and UVB radiation. *J Am Acad Dermatol* 1990, 22:181–187.

19. Lee LA, Norris DA: Mechanisms of cutaneous tissue damage in lupus erythematosus. *Immunol Series* 1989, 46:359–386.

20. Furukawa F, Kashihara-Sawami M, Lyons MB, Norris DA: Binding of antibodies to the extractable nuclear antigens SS-A/Ro and SS-B/La is induced on the surface of human keratinocytes by ultraviolet light (UVL): implications for the pathogenesis of photosensitive cutaneous lupus. *J Invest Dermatol* 1990, 94:77–85.

21. Golan TD, Elkon KB, Gharavi AE, Krueger JG: Enhanced membrane binding of autoantibodies to cultured keratinocytes of systemic lupus erythematosus patients after ultraviolet B/ultraviolet A irradiation. *J Clin Invest* 1992, 90:1067–1076.

22. Steinberg AD, Gourley MF, Klinman DM, et al.: NIH conference. Systemic lupus erythematosus. *Ann Intern Med* 1991, 115:548–559.

23. Deschamps P, Pedailles S, Michel M, Leroy D: Photoinduction of lesions in a patient with pemphigus erythematosus. *Photodermatol* 1984, 1:38–41.

24. Hawk JLM, Norris PG: Abnormal responses to ultraviolet radiation: idiopathic. In *Dermatology in General Medicine*, edn 4. Edited by Fitzpatrick TB, Eisen AZ, Wolff K, *et al.* New York: McGraw Hill; 1993:1661—1677.

Collagen-Vascular Diseases 14
Jeffrey P. Callen

Key Points

- Cutaneous disease is a common feature of lupus erythematosus, dermatomyositis, and sclerodermoid syndromes.
- The skin changes can be the initial feature of these disorders and the most prominent feature.
- Recognition of subsets of cutaneous lupus erythematosus can aid in the prognostic prediction.
- Dermatomyositis, while predominantly a disease of the skin and muscle, can be associated with multisystem changes.
- Appropriate testing to evaluate for malignancy should occur in the patient with dermatomyositis.
- Any treatment of these disorders should be tailored to the specific findings in each disorder.

The term *collagen-vascular diseases* is widely used to encompass systemic disorders with prominent musculoskeletal abnormalities. These disorders have been linked to immunologic aberrations. There is frequent cutaneous involvement, and in fact, many of the diseases were described and named based on the dermatologic findings. In this chapter, we discuss the three more common types of these disorders in which skin disease is an important feature: lupus erythematosus, dermatomyositis, and sclerodermoid syndromes.

LUPUS ERYTHEMATOSUS

Lupus erythematosus is a multisystem disorder that spans from a relatively benign, self-limited cutaneous eruption to a severe, often fatal, systemic disease. The American College of Rheumatology has developed a set of criteria to be used for the classification of systemic lupus erythematosus (SLE) (Table 14-1) [1]. When a patient meets four or more of the criteria either concurrently or serially during any period of observation, the patient is classified as having SLE.

In the 1940s and 1950s, dermatologists first recognized that most of their patients with chronic, scarring, discoid lupus erythematosus (DLE) lesions had few, if any, systemic findings, whereas those with photosensitivity, malar erythema, or both frequently had systemic disease. They also recognized a middle group in whom the skin lesions were more transient, resolved without scarring, and in whom there was frequent, non–life-threatening systemic disease. The classification of cutaneous subsets was stressed by Gilliam and Sontheimer [2], who proposed that patients be classified into two groups by the type of skin disease present: those that are histopathologically lupus erythematosus specific or those that are not histopathologically specific (Table 14–2).

TABLE 14-1 CRITERIA FOR THE DIAGNOSIS OF SYSTEMIC LUPUS ERYTHEMATOSUS*

Malar rash

Discoid lupus erythematosus lesions

Photosensitivity, by history or observation

Oral ulcers, usually painless, observed by physician

Nonerosive arthritis involving two or more joints

Serositis and pleuritis or pericarditis

Renal disorder: proteinuria (> 500 mg/d) or cellular casts

Central nervous system disorder: seizures or psychosis (absence of known cause)

Hematologic disorder: hemolytic anemia, leukopenia (< 4000/mm^3) or thrombocytopenia (< 10,000/mm^3)

Immunologic disorder: positive lupus erythematosus preparation, abnormal titer of antinative DNA and anti-Sm, false-positive result on VDRL test

Antinuclear antibody

*If four or more criteria are present serially or simultaneously during any observation, the patient is said to have systemic lupus erythematosus.

VDRL—Venereal Disease Research Laboratory.

From Tan and coworkers [1]; with permission.

TABLE 14-2 A CLASSIFICATION OF MUCOCUTANEOUS LESIONS IN LUPUS ERYTHEMATOSUS

LE-specific histopathology

Chronic cutaneous LE

  Discoid LE (widespread vs localized)

  Hypertrophic or verrucous LE

  Palmar or plantar LE

  Oral discoid LE

  LE panniculitis

SCLE

  Polymorphous light eruption-like lesions

  Annular lesions

    Oriental SCLE (annular erythema of primary Sjögren's syndrome)

  Papulosquamous lesions (photosensitive psoriasis?)

  Neonatal LE

  C2-deficient LE-like syndrome

  Drug-induced SCLE

Acute cutaneous LE

  Malar erythema

  Photosensitivity dermatitis

  Generalized erythema

LE-nonspecific histopathology

Vasculopathy

  Urticaria

  Vasculitis

  Livedo reticularis or leg ulcerations

Mucosal lesions

Nonscarring alopecia

Bullous LE or epidermolysis bullosa acquisita

Associated mucocutaneous problems

  Mucinous infiltrations

  Porphyrias

  Lichen planus

  Psoriasis

  Sjögren's syndrome

  Squamous cell carcinomas

LE—lupus erythematosus; SCLE—subacute cutaneous LE.

Chronic cutaneous lupus erythematosus can be manifested in several clinical variations. The commonest subset is that with DLE lesions [3]. These patients may be classified as having localized DLE, when lesions are only on the head and neck, or widespread DLE, when lesions are on other body surfaces as well as on the head and neck. Other, less common forms of chronic cutaneous lupus erythematosus include hypertrophic or verrucous (wartlike) lesions, lesions on the palms or soles, oral discoid lupus erythematosus, and lupus panniculitis (lupus profundus).

The discoid lupus erythematosus lesion is characterized by erythema; telangiectasia; adherent scale, varying from fine to thick; follicular plugging; dyspigmentation; and atrophy and scarring (Fig. 14-1). The lesions are usually sharply demarcated and can be round, thus giving rise to the term *discoid* (or disklike). The presence of scarring or atrophy is the characteristic that separates these lesions from those of subacute cutaneous lupus erythematosus (SCLE). The differential diagnosis most often includes papulosquamous diseases, such as psoriasis, lichen planus, secondary syphilis, superficial fungal infection, polymorphous light eruption, and sarcoidosis. Histopathologic examination is usually very helpful in confirming a diagnosis, and only rarely is immunofluorescence microscopy necessary.

Hypertrophic or verrucous DLE is a unique subset in which an unusual lesion occurs [4]. The thick, adherent scale is replaced by massive hyperkeratosis, and the lesions look like warts or squamous cell carcinomas (Fig. 14-2). These lesions usually occur in the setting of other, more typical DLE lesions. These patients tend to have

chronic disease, to have few systemic symptoms or laboratory findings, and to be extremely difficult to treat with conventional therapy.

The DLE-SLE subset defines a small group of patients (approximately 5% to 10%) who by the nature of their selection have systemic disease in association with scarring cutaneous disease. Patients who progress from pure cutaneous disease into this group are characterized by widespread DLE, the presence of clinically appreciable periungual telangiectasias, persistent elevated sedimentation rates, leukopenia, and positive antinuclear antibody (ANA). These patients with DLE-SLE rarely have renal disease,

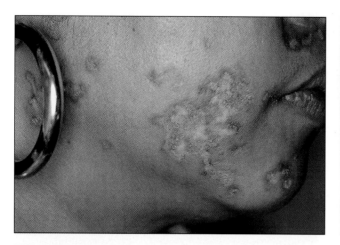

FIGURE 14-1 Discoid lupus erythematosus. This young black woman demonstrates multiple features of discoid lupus erythematosus, including follicular plugging, scarring, atrophy, and dyspigmentation.

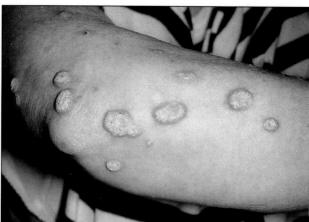

FIGURE 14-2 Hypertrophic (verrucous) lupus erythematosus. These wart-like lesions were present in a patient with typical discoid lupus erythematosus elsewhere. They simulate warts, keratoacanthoma, or squamous cell carcinoma.

and even when they do, it is most often transient and mild. DLE-SLE is a distinct lupus erythematosus subset because of its relatively benign, albeit chronic, course.

Subacute cutaneous lupus erythematosus is a skin lesion that has all the features of DLE without the scarring or atrophy [5•]. Patients whose major cutaneous manifestation is SCLE lesions have been classified as having a subset called SCLE. However, a patient in the SCLE subset can also have scarring lesions of DLE or can have lesions generally associated with SLE, such as a malar rash or vasculitic lesions. Many of the SCLE patients (approximately 50%) fulfill four or more of the American College of Rheumatology criteria for SLE; thus, some authorities have not recognized these patients as forming a distinct subset.

Subacute cutaneous lupus erythematosus skin lesions are of at least two types: annular or papulosquamous. Annular

SCLE lesions are characterized by erythematous rings with central clearing (Fig. 14-3). Often a slight scale is present. Lesions of annular SCLE must be differentiated from other figurate erythemas. Papulosquamous SCLE lesions are characterized by plaques and papules with scale (Figs. 14-4 and 14-5). The differential diagnosis of papulosquamous SCLE lesions includes psoriasis and lichen planus. In both annular and papulosquamous SCLE, the lesions often begin as erythematous papules or plaques in a photosensitive distribution (Fig. 14-6). SCLE may be associated with Sjögren's syndrome, idiopathic thrombocytopenic purpura, cutaneous vasculitis, or deficiency of the second component of complement (C2d). SCLE has also been reported to be induced by hydrochlorothiazide.

Malar erythema is the classic butterfly rash from which the name *lupus erythematosus* (wolflike redness) was coined

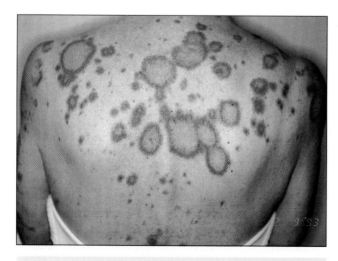

FIGURE 14-3 This erythematosus, annular lesion lacks scarring or atrophy yet represents a histologically specific pattern of lupus erythematosus.

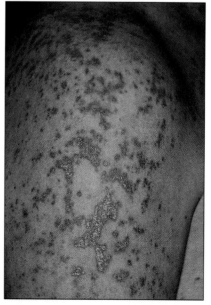

FIGURE 14-4 Subacute cutaneous lupus erythematosus, papulosquamous variant. This patient developed an exquisitely photosensitive eruption with minimal sun exposure.

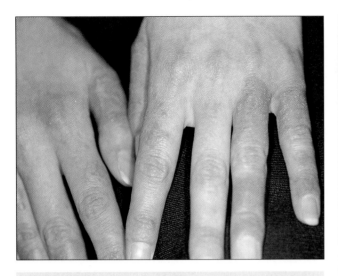

FIGURE 14-5 Lichen planus–like lesions of subacute cutaneous lupus erythematosus.

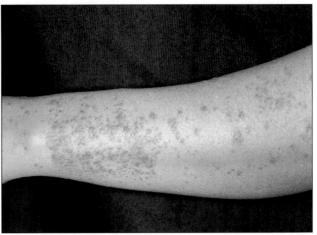

FIGURE 14-6 Erythematous papular lesion of polymorphous light eruption representing a clinical picture similar to that seen in subacute cutaneous lupus erythematosus.

(Fig. 14-7). The rash is induced by sun exposure, usually by ultraviolet B light ranging from 290 to 320 nm. Patients with an active malar butterfly rash usually have active systemic disease, but no specific organ system is involved.

Livedo reticularis, pyoderma gangrenosum–like leg ulcerations, or both may occur in patients with antiphospholipid antibodies (anticardiolipin and lupus anticoagulant) [6•]. Many such patients have lupus erythematosus, but some have primary antiphospholipid antibody syndrome. These patients have arterial occlusions, which can result in transient ischemic attacks, cerebrovascular accidents, and recurrent fetal loss; venous occlusion, which can result in thrombophlebitis, renal or hepatic vein occlusion, or pulmonary embolism; thrombocytopenia; and cardiac valvular vegetations and dysfunction.

Laboratory Abnormalities in Patients With Cutaneous Lupus Erythematosus

The ANA is a system that represents many antibodies to multiple substrates [7••]. The frequency of a positive ANA correlates with the substrate used. The reported pattern of the ANA may also correlate with specific antibodies; however, except when interpreted by experts, the ANA pattern is not highly specific. Table 14-3 represents the frequency of these antibodies in the subsets discussed. Antinative (double-stranded) DNA correlates with active SLE and, in particular, active renal disease. Anti-Ro (SS-A) was initially described in patients with ANA-negative lupus erythematosus and Sjögren's syndrome. However, it is also present in mothers who have babies with neonatal lupus erythmatosus, individuals with cutaneous vasculitis associated with SCLE, those with C_2 deficient lupus erythematosus syndromes, and patients with hydrochlorothiazide-induced SCLE. Therapy should not be based solely on these laboratory abnormalities.

Cutaneous immunofluorescence was applied as a diagnostic and prognostic tool that led to a better understanding of lupus erythematosus. Lesional immunofluorescence may be helpful when the clinical and histopathologic diagnosis is in question. However, one must realize that normal facial skin can demonstrate 10% to 20% false-positive reactions [8•]. The use of noninvolved, "nonexposed" skin in the lupus band test is believed to correlate with active renal disease. Refined antibody testing has reduced the need for immunofluorescence testing.

Therapy for Cutaneous Lupus Erythematosus

Before therapy is begun, the clinician must evaluate the patient thoroughly to determine the extent of disease and to be able to reassure the patient of the benign nature of the process. Table 14-4 lists the testing that should be ordered, and Table 14-5 the therapeutic options available.

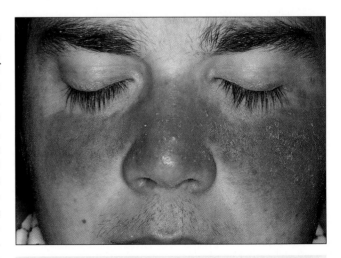

FIGURE 14-7 Systemic lupus erythematosus. This young man has a very typical butterfly eruption of systemic lupus erythematosus.

Test	DLE	HLE	DLE/SLE	SCLE	NLE	ACLE
ANA	5–10	5	75	50–75	60–90	95
Anti-ssDNA	35	25	75	20–50	?	90
Anti-nDNA	< 5	< 5	10	10	10–50	70
Anti-RNP (U_1RNP)	< 5	25	?	10	?	40
Anti-Sm	< 5	5	5	10	?	25
Anti-Ro (SS-A)	5	5–10	5	40–95	90	30
Anti-La (SS-B)	5	5	5	15	15–20	10

*All numbers given are percentages.

ACLE—acute cutaneous lupus erythematosus; ANA—antinuclear antibody; DLE—discoid lupus erythematosus; HLE—hypertrophic lupus erythematosus; nDNA—native DNA; NLE—neonatal lupus erythematosus; RNP—ribonucleoprotein; SCLE—subacute cutaneous lupus erythematosus; SLE—systemic lupus erythematosus; ssDNA—single-stranded DNA.

Photosensitivity is a major factor in all types of cutaneous lupus erythematosus. Almost all SCLE patients are photosensitive, and approximately 60% to 75% of SLE patients demonstrate photosensitivity. This reaction is induced by ultraviolet B light, but in some individuals, ultraviolet A light (320 to 360 nm) can be involved as well [9••]. Therefore, one of the most important therapeutic manipulations is the use of sunscreens and sun avoidance. Sunscreens with a sun protective factor of at least 15 are to be used every day. Topical corticosteroids should be prescribed in conjunction with other agents. The specific agent used is chosen based on the clinical lesion and area of the body affected. The prescribing physician must remember that these agents can produce atrophy, which is also a sign of the disease. Lesions that do not respond to topical agents can be injected intralesionally with a corticosteroid, such as triamcinolone acetonide (3 to 4 mg/mL).

Antimalarial agents form a mainstay of systemic therapy of cutaneous lupus erythematosus. The mechanism of action of these agents is unknown, but it may relate to photoprotection, immunomodulation, or both. The agents available include hydroxychloroquine hydrochloride and

TABLE 14-4 EVALUATION OF THE PATIENT WITH CUTANEOUS LUPUS ERYTHEMATOSUS

Standard testing

Careful history and physical examination

Skin biopsy for routine histology

Complete blood count with differential and platelet count

Serum multiphasic analysis

Antinuclear antibody

Serological tests

Antinative DNA

Anti-RNP (U_1RNP)

Anti-Ro (SS-A)

Erythrocyte sedimentation rate

Urinalysis

Total hemolytic complement (if abnormal, C3, C2, C4 levels)

Creatinine clearance

Optional tests

Serum protein electrophoresis

Circulating immune complexes

Immunofluorescence skin biopsy

Antiphospholipid antibodies

RNP—ribonucleoprotein.

TABLE 14-5 THERAPEUTIC AGENTS USED TO TREAT CUTANEOUS LUPUS ERYTHEMATOSUS

Standard therapy

Sunscreens

Topical corticosteroids

Intralesional corticosteroids (avoid atrophy)

Antimalarials

    Hydroxychloroquine: potential ocular toxicity

    Chloroquine: potential ocular toxicity

Alternatives

Dapsone (best for bullous lupus erythematosus, vasculitis)

Auranofin (oral gold)

Accutane (13-*cis*-retinoic acid)

Clofazimine

Low-dose cytotoxic agents, *eg*, azathioprine or methotrexate

Systemic corticosteroids (poorly effective for chronic lesions)

Interferon (recombinant interferon α)

chloroquine phosphate. Chloroquine and hydroxychloroquine may be associated with retinopathy. Hydroxychloroquine is given orally in a dosage of 200 to 400 mg/d.

DERMATOMYOSITIS

Dermatomyositis is a condition that combines an inflammatory myopathy with a characteristic cutaneous disease. This disorder is related to polymyositis, which has similar features to the muscle disease caused by dermatomyositis but lacks the characteristic cutaneous findings. These disorders are of unknown etiology, but immune-mediated muscle damage is believed to be an important pathogenetic mechanism. Dermatomyositis appears to be characterized by an increased frequency of internal malignancy, whereas the association with malignancy in patients with polymyositis is less well resolved. Both dermatomyositis and polymyositis may occur in children, and both disorders are associated with morbidity and occasional mortality; therefore, a prompt and aggressive approach to therapy is indicated.

Bohan and Peter [10] suggested the use of five criteria to define the entities of polymyositis and dermatomyositis and also suggested a classification system. The criteria include:

Proximal symmetric muscle weakness that progresses over a period of weeks to months
Elevated serum levels of muscle-derived enzymes
Abnormal electromyographic results
Abnormal muscle biopsy results
The presence of cutaneous disease compatible with dermatomyositis

The following system of classification has been useful in differentiating groups of patients:

Dermatomyositis
Polymyositis
Myositis with malignancy
Childhood myositis
Overlap syndromes with other collagen vascular disease and myositis
Inclusion body myositis
Dermatomyositis-sine-myositis (amyopathic dermatomyositis)

Clinical Manifestations

The characteristic and possibly pathognomonic cutaneous features of dermatomyositis are the heliotrope rash and Gottron's papules. Several other cutaneous features that occur in patients who have dermatomyositis are characteristic of the disease despite not being pathognomonic and include malar erythema, poikiloderma in a photosensitive distribution, violaceous erythema on the extensor surfaces, and periungual and cuticular changes.

The heliotrope rash consists of a dark lilac discoloration or a violaceous to dusky erythematous rash with or without edema in a symmetric distribution involving periorbital skin

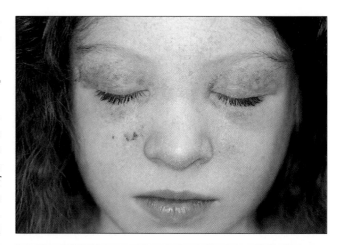

FIGURE 14-8 Dermatomyositis. This young girl developed inflammatory myopathy in conjunction with a very typical heliotrope eruption around the eyelids and typical lesions elsewhere on her body.

(Fig. 14–8). Gottron's papules are found over bony prominences, particularly over the metacarpal-phalangeal joints, the proximal interphalangeal joints, or the distal interphalangeal joints (Fig. 14–9). They may also be found over bony prominences, such as the elbows, knees, and feet. Nail fold changes consist of periungual telangiectasias and a characteristic cuticular change with hypertrophy of the cuticle and small, hemorrhagic infarcts within this hypertrophic area (Fig. 14–10). Poikiloderma can occur within Gottron's papules or on exposed skin, such as the extensor surfaces of the arm or "V" of the neck (Fig. 14–11).

Dermatomyositis-sine-myositis is diagnosed when typical cutaneous disease is present without clinical weakness and with normal serum muscle enzyme levels. A small subset of patients never develop myositis, despite having prominent cutaneous changes [11•]. A larger group exists in whom the myositis resolves with therapy,

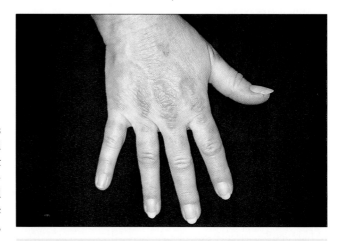

FIGURE 14-9 Gottron's papules. Typical erythematous to violaceous lesions over the bony prominences on the extensor surfaces of the hands.

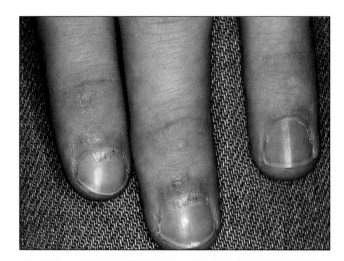

FIGURE 14-10 Cuticular hypertrophy, splinter hemorrhages, and periungual telangiectasias are present in this patient with dermatomyositis.

and the skin disease becomes the most important feature of the disease.

Clinical and laboratory abnormalities suggestive of muscle disease are characteristic features of dermatomyositis and polymyositis. Even in patients who initially have only skin disease, myositis often eventually follows. The myopathy affects mainly proximal muscle groups of the shoulder and pelvic girdle muscles, and the disease is usually symmetric. Initial complaints include weakness, fatigue, an inability to climb stairs, an inability to raise the arms for actions like hair grooming or shaving, an inability to rise from a squatting or sitting position, or a combination of these features. The progression of disease is variable but usually occurs over a period of weeks to months. An inability to swallow and symptoms of aspiration may reflect the involvement of striated muscle of the pharynx or upper esophagus. Dysphagia often signifies a rapidly

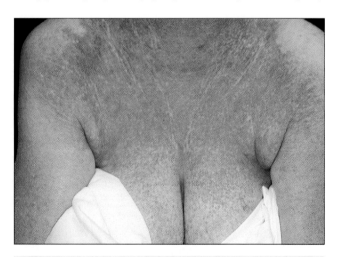

FIGURE 14-11 Poikilodermatous eruption in the photosensitive distribution is present in this woman with dermatomyositis.

progressive course and may be associated with a poor prognosis.

The laboratory abnormalities are enzyme elevations, disturbances of electrical action, histopathologic changes, or all of these. Muscle enzyme levels are frequently elevated in patients with inflammatory myopathy. The enzymes that are commonly elevated are creatine kinase, aldolase, lactic dehydrogenase, and serum transaminases. Creatine kinase determination seems to be the most practical and available test for measuring activity of muscle disease. Occasionally, patients may have normal muscle enzyme levels, and in these individuals, the measurement of creatine excretion in the urine may be reflective of active muscle disease.

Electromyography characteristically shows sharp or positive waves, insertional irritability, fibrillation, and short polyphasic motor units. Innervation remains intact; thus, neuropathic changes do not occur. Muscle biopsy specimens show typical features, including II fiber atrophy, necrosis, regeneration, centralization of the nuclei, and a lymphocytic infiltrate in a perifascicular or perivascular region. Other assessments that may be used are various imaging techniques, in particular, magnetic resonance imaging. In children, levels of von Willebrand factor VIII–related antigen or neopterin may predict a more severe dermatomyositis variant with vasculopathy. However, the use of these tests, particularly the von Willebrand factor VIII–related antigens, adds little to the information obtained with enzyme testing and clinical examination [12•].

Dermatomyositis and polymyositis are multisystem disorders, as is reflected by the high frequency of other clinical features in patients with these diseases. Arthralgias and arthritis may be present in up to 25% of patients with inflammatory myopathy. Esophageal disease, as manifested by dysphagia, is estimated to be present in 15% to 50% of patients with inflammatory myopathy. The dysphagia can be of two types: proximal dysphagia or distal dysphagia. Pulmonary disease occurs in dermatomyositis, and polymyositis, in approximately 15% to 30% of patients. Cardiac disease may also occur in patients with polymyositis, as manifested by myocarditis or pericarditis. Calcinosis of the skin or muscle is unusual in adults but may occur in up to 40% of children with dermatomyositis.

Myositis and Malignancy

The issue of the relationship of dermatomyositis and polymyositis to malignancy remains controversial. The frequency of malignancy in dermatomyositis has varied from 6% to 60% in various studies. This variation is probably related to differing methodology. In 1992, Siguregeirsson and coworkers [13••], in a well-controlled study, clearly documented the increased frequency of malignancy in patients with dermatomyositis over that in the general population. Although polymyositis patients had a slight increase in cancer frequency, it was not highly significant and could be explained by the more aggressive cancer search in these patients. Malignancies may occur before the onset of myositis, concurrently with myositis, or after the onset of dermatomyositis. In addition, the myositis may follow the course of the malignancy (a paraneoplastic course) or its own course independent of the treatment of the malignancy. Siguregeirsson and coworkers also suggested that ovarian cancer might be overrepresented in their group. Other investigators have also reported this finding [14•]. Studies demonstrating benefits of cancer surgery on myositis as well as those showing no relationship of the myositis and malignancy have been reported.

Evaluation

The diagnosis of myositis is one of exclusion (Table 14-6). A complete history should be taken, with particular attention to drugs or toxins that may be involved [15•]. It should include a history of previous malignancies, previous travel, changes in diet, and any symptoms of associated phenomena, such as dysphagia, dyspnea, or arthritis. A thorough review of systems is necessary, which will aid in the evaluation of patients with dermatomyositis for malignancies.

Course and Therapy

Several general measures are helpful in treating patients with dermatomyositis and polymyositis. Bed rest is often valuable in the individual with progressive weakness; however, this measure must be combined with a range-of-motion exercise program to prevent contractures. Nutrition is important because of a negative nitrogen balance that exists in inflammatory myopathy. This feature of treatment is particularly important in children. Patients who have evidence of dysphagia should have the head of their bed elevated and should avoid eating meals before retiring.

The mainstay of therapy for dermatomyositis is the use of systemic corticosteroids. Traditionally, prednisone is given in a dosage of 0.5 to 1 mg/kg/d as the initial therapy [16•]. Approximately 25% to 30% of patients with dermatomyositis or polymyositis do not respond to systemic corticosteroids or develop significant steroid-related side effects. In these patients, immunosuppressive agents (methotrexate, azathioprine, cyclophosphamide, chlorambucil, or cyclosporine) may be an effective means of inducing or maintaining a remission [17•]. The most recent therapeutic maneuver for immunosuppressive-resistant dermatomyositis is the use of intravenous immunoglobulin. Dalakas and coworkers [18••] demonstrated that the myopathy as well as the cutaneous disease improved with this therapy.

Therapy for cutaneous disease in patients with dermatomyositis is often difficult because even though the myositis may respond to treatment with corticosteroids, immunosuppressives, or both, the cutaneous lesions often persist. Although cutaneous disease may be of minor importance in patients with serious fulminant myositis, in many patients cutaneous disease becomes an important aspect of their disorder. Most patients with cutaneous lesions are photosensitive [19]; thus, as in patients with lupus erythematosus, the daily use of a sunscreen with a sun protective factor of at least

15 is recommended. Some may require a broader-spectrum sunscreen. Hydroxychloroquine in dosages of 200 to 400 mg/d is effective in approximately 80% of patients treated as a means of partially controlling their cutaneous disease and allowing a decrease in the corticosteroid dosage [20]. In some patients, the use of low-dose methotrexate has been effective.

TABLE 14-6 EVALUATION OF THE PATIENT WITH MYOSITIS

Careful history

Previous malignancy

Associated symptoms

History of toxins, infections, travel, drug intake, bovine collagen implants, or breast augmentation surgery

Complete physical examination

Dermatologic evaluation

Pelvic and breast examinations in women

Rectal examination in men

Evaluation of muscle disease

Creatine kinase or phosphokinase, aldolase, urinary creatine EMG (if results of laboratory tests are normal)

Muscle biopsy (if EMG and laboratory results are abnormal)

MRI/MRS

Skin disease evaluation

Biopsy

Routine laboratory studies

Complete blood count, serum multiphasic analysis, urinalysis

Chest radiograph

Thyroid function

Stool hematest

Electrocardiogram

Papanicolaou smear, mammography in women

Pulmonary function tests

Esophageal studies

Manometry

Cineradiography

Optional

Holter monitor

Echocardiogram

Autoantibody studies, *eg,* Jo-1, PM, Ku, Mi-2

Viral serologies

Further testing

Based on abnormalities discovered in above tests

EMG—electromyography. MRI—magnetic resonance imaging; MRS—magnetic resonance spectroscopy.

The prognosis of dermatomyositis and polymyositis varies greatly, depending on the series of patients studied. Factors that affect the prognosis include the patient's age, the type and severity of myositis, the presence of dysphagia, the presence of an associated malignancy, duration of disease prior to treatment, and the response to corticosteroid therapy. The fact that therapy alters prognosis seems to be well established by retrospective reports on the benefits of corticosteroids and immunosuppressives.

SCLERODERMA

Scleroderma is a term used to describe a specific clinical disease spectrum represented by cutaneous involvement, multisystem involvement, or both. In addition, several disorders are associated with sclerodermoid changes (Table 14-7). Scleroderma is a disorder of unknown cause and pathogenesis that can be subdivided into two major categories: localized scleroderma and systemic sclerosis.

Localized Scleroderma

Localized scleroderma refers to primary involvement of the skin, with minimal if any systemic features. Only rarely have patients with localized scleroderma developed systemic sclerosis or SLE. Three major types of localized scleroderma exist: morphea, generalized morphea, and linear scleroderma. Morphea is manifested by indurated dermal or subcutaneous plaques (Fig. 14-12). The disease is commonest in young women. Morphea sometimes overlaps or coexists with another cutaneous condition known as *lichen sclerosus et atrophicus*. In contrast, a small number of patients develop numerous and larger lesions, which coalesce (Fig. 14-13). These individuals are said to have *generalized morphea*. Patients with morphea usually have a benign course, characterized by softening of their lesions with time.

TABLE 14-7 SCLERODERMA AND SCLERODERMOID CONDITIONS

Localized scleroderma

Morphea (dermal, subcutaneous and pransclerotic variants)
Linear scleroderma
Generalized morphea

Systemic sclerosis (scleroderma)

Limited (acrosclerosis, CREST variant)
Diffuse
Overlap with another collagen vascular disease (lupus erythematosus or dermatomyositis)
Mixed connective tissue disease

Idiopathic syndromes possibly related to scleroderma

Eosinophilic fasciitis
Eosinophilia myalgia syndrome

Mucinoses

Scleredema
Scleromyxedema (lichen myxedematosus or papular mucinosis)

Chemical or drug-induced sclerosis

Polyvinylchloride
Silicone (breast implants, injectable) or collagen injections
Bleomycin
Spanish rapeseed oil

Metabolic

Porphyria cutanea tarda
Carcinoid syndrome

Immunologic

Chronic graft-vs-host disease

Vibratory injury

CREST—calcinosis, Raynaud's phenomenon, esophageal dysmotility, sclerodactyly, and telangiectasia.

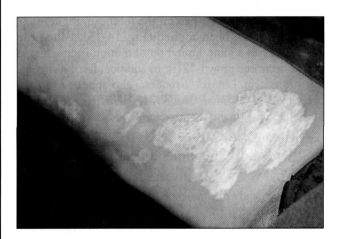

FIGURE 14-12 Morphea. Note discrete sclerotic plaques.

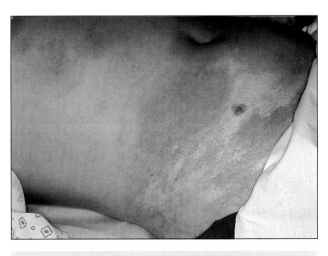

FIGURE 14-13 Generalized morphea. Note coalescent plaques of induration on the trunk.

A syndrome characterized by eosinophilia, myalgia, cutaneous sclerosis, neuropathy, and pulmonary dysfunction developed in patients taking contaminated L-tryptophan. Some of the features closely mimic eosinophilic fasciitis, but the patients often fail to respond to therapy and may have progressive debilitation, or death may even occur [24•].

Mixed Connective Tissue Disease

Mixed connective tissue disease is an overlap syndrome that is frequently characterized by cutaneous sclerosis with features of another collagen-vascular disease, such as lupus erythematosus or inflammatory myopathy. Patients with this disease commonly possess high levels of anti–U_1 ribonucleoprotein antibodies. Despite this antibody marker, follow-up of the patient presumed to have mixed connective tissue disease usually allows classification within one of the more traditional categories.

REFERENCES AND RECOMMENDED READING

Recently published papers of particular interest have been highlighted as:
• Of interest
•• Of outstanding interest

1. Tan EM, Cohen AS, Fries JF, et al.: The 1982 revised criteria for the classification of systemic lupus erythematosus. *Arthritis Rheum* 1982, 25:1271–1277.

2. Gilliam JN, Sontheimer RD: Distinctive cutaneous subsets in the spectrum of lupus erythematosus. *J Am Acad Dermatol* 1981, 4:471–475.

3. Callen JP: Chronic cutaneous LE. *Arch Dermatol* 1982, 118:412–416.

4. Spann CR, Callen JP, Klein JB, et al.: Clinical, serologic and immunogenetic studies in patients with chronic cutaneous (discoid) lupus erythematosus who have verrucous and/or hypertrophic skin lesions. *J Rheumatol* 1988, 15:256–261.

5.• David-Bajar KM: Subacute cutaneous lupus erythematosus. *J Invest Dermatol* 1993, 100:2S–8S.

6.• Petri M: Antiphospholipid antibodies: lupus anticoagulant and anticardiolipin antibody. *Curr Probl Dermatol* 1992, 4:171–201.

7.•• Sontheimer RD, McCauliffe DP, Zappi E, et al.: Antinuclear antibodies: clinical correlations and biologic significance. *Adv Dermatol* 1991, 7:3–53.

8.• Fabré VC, Lear S, Reichlin M, et al.: Twenty percent of biopsy specimens from sun-exposed skin of normal young adults demonstrate positive immunofluorescence. *Arch Dermatol* 1991, 127:1006–1011.

9.•• Lehmann P, Hölzle E, Kind P, et al.: Experimental reproduction of skin lesions in lupus erythematosus by UVA and UVB radiation. *J Am Acad Dermatol* 1990, 22:181–187.

10. Bohan A, Peter JB: Polymyositis and dermatomyositis. *N Engl J Med* 1975, 292:344–347.

11.• Stonecipher MR, Jorizzo JL, White WL, et al.: Cutaneous changes of dermatomyositis in patients with normal muscle enzymes: dermatomyositis sine myositis? *J Am Acad Dermatol* 1993, 28:951–956.

12.• Guzmán J, Petty RE, Malleson PN: Monitoring disease activity in juvenile dermatomyositis: the role of von Willebrand factor and muscle enzymes. *J Rheumatol* 1994, 21:739–743.

13.•• Siguregeirsson B, Lindelöf B, Edhag O, et al.: Risk of cancer in patients with dermatomyositis or polymyositis. *N Engl J Med* 1992, 326:363–367.

14.• Cherin P, Piette JC, Herson S, et al.: Dermatomyositis and ovarian cancer: a report of 7 cases and literature review. *J Rheumatol* 1993, 20:1897–1899.

15.• Cukier J, Beauchamp RA, Spindler JS, et al.: Association between bovine collagen implants and a dermatomyositis or polymyositis-like syndrome. *Ann Intern Med* 1993, 118:920–928.

16.• Fafalak RG, Peterson MGE, Kagen LJ: Strength in polymyositis and dermatomyositis: best outcome in patients treated early. *J Rheumatol* 1994, 21:643–648.

17.• Sinoway P, Callen JP: Chlorambucil: an effective corticosteroid sparing agent for patents with recalcitrant dermatomyositis. *Arthritis Rheum* 1993, 36:319–324.

18.•• Dalakas MC, Illa I, Dambrosia JM, et al.: A controlled trial of high-dose intravenous immune globulin infusions as a treatment for dermatomyositis. *N Engl J Med* 1993, 329:1993–2000.

19. Callen JP: Photodermatitis in a 6-year-old child. *Arthritis Rheum* 1993, 36:1483–1485.

20. Woo TY, Callen JP, Voorhees JV, et al.: Cutaneous lesions of dermatomyositis are improved by hydroxychloroquine. *J Am Acad Dermatol* 1984, 10:592–600.

21.• Uziel Y, Krafchik BR, Siverman ED, et al.: Localized scleroderma in childhood: a report of 30 cases. *Sem Arthr Rheum* 1994, 23:328–340.

22. Steen VD, Ziegler GL, Rodnan GP, et al.: Clinical and laboratory associations of anticentromere antibody in patients with progressive systemic sclerosis. *Arthritis Rheum* 1984, 27:125–131.

23. Siebold JR, Furst DE, Clements PJ: Why everything (or nothing) seems to work in the treatment of scleroderma. *J Rheumatol* 1992, 19:673–676.

24.• Swygert LA, Back EE, Auerbach SE, et al.: Eosinophilia-myalgia syndrome: mortality data from the US national surveillance system. *J Rheumatol* 1993, 20:1711–1717.

SELECT BIBLIOGRAPHY

Bohan A, Peter JB, Bowman RL, et al.: A computer-assisted analysis of 153 patients with polymyositis and dermatomyositis. *Medicine* 1977, 56:255–286.

Callen JP: Lupus erythematosus. In *Clinical Dermatology*, rev 19. Edited by Demis DJ. Philadelphia: JB Lippincott; 1992: 5–1,1–28.

Callen JP, Tuffanelli DL, Provost TT: Collagen-vascular disease: an update. *J Am Acad Dermatol* 1993, 28:477–484.

Campbell PM, Leroy EC: Raynaud phenomenon. *Semin Arthritis Rheum* 1986, 16:92–103.

Falanga V: Localized scleroderma. *Med Clin North Am* 1989, 73:1143–1156.

Lee LA, David KM: Cutaneous lupus erythematosus. *Curr Probl Dermatol* 1989, 1:161–200.

Targoff IN: Dermatomyositis and polymyositis. *Curr Probl Dermatol* 1991, 3:131–180.

Urticaria and Other Reactive Dermatoses

Carol L. Kulp-Shorten

15

Key Points

- Urticaria, erythema multiforme, and erythema nodosum represent hypersensitivity phenomena.
- Laboratory testing should be directed by pertinent history and physical examination findings.
- With all hypersensitivity states, the ideal treatment is identification and elimination of the antigenic stimulus.
- An etiology cannot be determined in more that 75% of cases of chronic urticaria (urticaria greater than 6 weeks' duration).
- Herpes simplex virus infections are responsible for the majority of erythema multiforme cases in the United States.
- Oral contraceptives are a leading cause of erythema nodosum.

URTICARIA

General Considerations

Urticaria and angioedema are transient reactive erythemas to substances systemically distributed. Raised evanescent erythematous wheals secondary to superficial dermal edema are known as urticaria (Fig. 15-1), whereas angioedema develops when the deep dermal, subcutaneous, or submucosal layers are involved (Fig. 15-2). Individual lesions arise suddenly, rarely persist for longer than 12 to 24 hours, and are intensely pruritic.

Urticarial reactions are common: they are experienced by 20% to 25% of the population at least once during a lifetime [1]. Patients may experience urticaria alone (40%), angioedema alone (10%), or combined urticaria and angioedema (50%) [2••]. The final endpoint in the pathogenesis of urticaria centers on the local increased permeability of capillaries and postcapillary venules secondary to mediators such as histamine, kinins, prostaglandins, complement, and leukotrienes. Extravasation of protein-rich fluid produces the characteristic wheals.

Classification

There are many ways to classify urticaria. One schema involves the duration of an attack. Acute urticaria is often IgE mediated, evolves over days to weeks, and then completely resolves. Episodes persisting longer than 6 weeks are termed chronic urticaria. Approximately 50% of patients with urticaria alone will be free of lesions within 1 year, whereas 20% have involvement for more than 20 years. Of patients who have both urticaria and angioedema, 75% continue to have episodes for more than 5 years and 20% continue to have them for more than 20 years [3••].

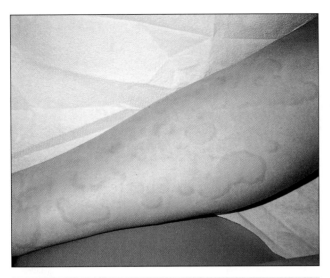

FIGURE 15-1 Erythematous wheals typical of urticaria.

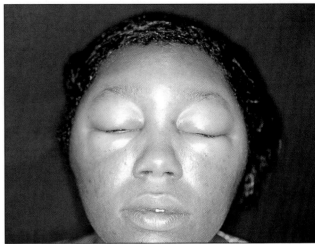

FIGURE 15-2 Periorbital angioedema with deep dermal and subcutaneous edema.

Urticaria can also be classified with respect to etiology, that is, as immunologic, nonimmunologic, or idiopathic urticaria (Table 15-1). IgE-dependent (type I hypersensitivity) mechanisms are often involved in urticarial reactions

---

TABLE 15-1 CLASSIFICATION OF URTICARIA

Immunologic

IgE dependent (type I hypersensitivity)
    Specific antigen sensitivities
    Physical urticarias
Complement mediated (type III hypersensitivity)
    Hereditary angioedema
    Acquired C1 esterase inhibitor deficiency (lymphomas, myelomas, systemic lupus erythematosus)
    Serum sickness
    Urticarial vasculitis

Nonimmunologic

Direct mast cell degranulators
    Opiates
    Polymyxin
    Tubocurarine
    Radiocontrast dye
Indirect mast cell degranulators via arachidonic acid pathway alteration
    Aspirin
    Nonsteroidal anti-inflammatory drugs
    Tartrazine (yellow food dye)
    Benzoate (food preservative)

Idiopathic

ie, etiology cannot be determined

---

to food, drugs, therapeutic agents, infections, inhalants, and venoms. IgE is also believed to play a role in many of the physical urticarias (Table 15-2). Deficiency of the inhibitor of the activated first component of the complement system (C1 esterase inhibitor) may be hereditary (autosomal dominant) or may be acquired with systemic disease. Direct degranulators cause the release of histamine from mast cells, whereas indirect degranulators exert their effects via alteration of arachidonic acid metabolism. Unfortunately, an etiology cannot be determined in more than 75% of cases of chronic urticaria, so the designation *idiopathic* is used [4•].

Diagnosis and Evaluation

Urticaria and angioedema are usually easily diagnosed. As mentioned previously, however, the etiology of chronic urticaria often remains obscure. Patients with acute urticaria often do not present for evaluation because the cause is readily apparent. The physician is often faced with the frustration of evaluating the patient with chronic urticaria. A detailed history will establish a pattern of occurrence, relationship to physical agents, medication usage, and concomitant infection or underlying disease. Physical examination may reveal the characteristic small wheals (1 to 2 mm) with large erythematous flares of cholinergic urticaria. These lesions usually develop with exercise. Simple provocative tests can be performed in patients suspected of having a physical urticaria [5] (Table 15-2 and Fig. 15-3). A recent report by Barlow and coworkers [6••] documents a high incidence (71%) of physical urticarias in patients with urticaria. One hundred and thirty-five chronic urticaria patients were specifically tested for immediate dermatographism, delayed-pressure urticaria and, when indicated by the history, for cholinergic and/or cold urticaria. Fifty patients (37%) had delayed-pressure urticaria, 30 (22%) had immediate dermatographism, 15

TABLE 15-2 PROVOCATIVE TESTING OF
PHYSICAL URTICARIAS

Urticaria	Diagnostic test
Dermatographism	Stroke skin with firm pressure
Pressure	Apply a 15-lb weight for 20 min, with inspection at 4–8 h
Solar	Perform phototesting with ultraviolet light and fluorescent light
Familial cold	Expose to cold air for 20–30 min (ice-cube test results are negative)
Acquired cold	Place a plastic-wrapped ice cube on the skin for 5 min
Cholinergic	Exercise; mecholyl skin test
Aquagenic	Apply 35°C water compress on the upper body skin for 30 min
Vibratory	Apply vortex vibration to forearm for 5 min

(11%) had cholinergic urticaria, and 3 (2%) had cold urticaria. Lin and Schwartz [7•] also report three patients seropositive for HIV antibody with cold urticaria. These patients had no AIDS-defining illness and two of them were taking zidovudine at the time of onset of urticaria.

Skin biopsy is not helpful unless urticarial vasculitis is suspected (ie, if wheals last longer than 24 hours or resolve with purpura or hyperpigmentation). Laboratory testing should be directed by the history and physical examination findings, but most patients with chronic urticaria probably warrant a basic evaluation with a complete blood count and differential, measurement of the erythrocyte sedimentation rate, and urinalysis.

Treatment

The ideal treatment for urticaria is identification and elimination of its cause. However, because the etiology is often obscure, symptomatic treatment is usually necessary. Antihistamines are considered the mainstay of therapy. Although the classic (H_1) antihistamines are effective, their use is limited by central nervous system effects such as sedation, anticholinergic effects such as dry mouth, and inconvenient dosing. Most of these agents must be used every 4 to 6 hours. Representative H_1 antagonists include chlorpheniramine maleate (Chlor-Trimeton; Schering Plough, Liberty Corner, NJ), diphenhydramine hydrochloride (Benadryl; Parke Davis, Morris Plains, NJ), cyproheptadine hydrochloride (Periactin; Merck & Co., West Point, PA), hydroxyzine hydrochloride (Atarax; Roerig, New York, NY), and clemastine fumarate (Tavist; Sandoz, East Hanover, NJ). Cyproheptadine hydrochloride is said to be the drug of choice for acquired cold urticaria [5].

New second-generation H_1 antihistamines have recently been developed. These agents have the advantage of low affinity for brain H_1 receptors, producing less sedation and no potentiation of alcohol or benzodiazepines. Dosing schedules are also convenient, ie, daily to twice daily. Terfenadine (Seldane; Merrell Dow, Kansas City, MO), astemizole (Hismanal; Janssen, Titusville, NJ), and loratadine (Claritin; Schering, Kenilworth, NJ) are available in the United States, whereas cetirizine (Reactin; Pfizer, New York, NY) awaits Food and Drug Administration approval. Clinical efficacy studies have established the superiority of these agents to placebo and their comparability to the traditional H_1 antagonists [8,9•]. The safety profile for these agents is good, although astemizole and terfenadine may interact with ketoconazole, itraconazole, or erythromycin to produce cardiac side effects. These agents should also be avoided in patients with underlying hepatic dysfunction [8].

Histamine$_2$ antihistamines, such as cimetidine hydrochloride (Tagamet; SmithKline Beecham, Deerfield, IL) and ranitidine hydrochloride (Zantac; Glaxo, Research Triangle Park, NC), may also be beneficial in the treatment of urticaria when they are combined with an H_1 blocker. The tricyclic antidepressant doxepin hydrochloride (Sinequan; Roerig, New York, NY) has activity against both histamine receptors and may be initiated in doses of 10 to 25 mg twice daily. In general, systemic corticosteroids have no place in the regular therapy for chronic urticaria because of their unacceptable risk-to-benefit ratio. Finally, avoidance of aspirin, nonsteroidal anti-inflammatory drugs, narcotics, and benzoates may help control urticaria in some patients.

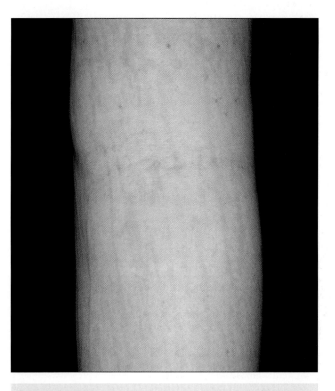

FIGURE 15-3 Dermatographism can be demonstrated by stroking the skin with firm pressure.

Erythema Multiforme

General Considerations

Erythema multiforme (EM) is a reactive hypersensitivity erythema that targets mucosal as well as cutaneous surfaces. The mucocutaneous syndrome can be broadly subdivided into EM minor and EM major (Stevens-Johnson syndrome). This discussion focuses on EM minor (80% of all EM cases); for Stevens-Johnson syndrome, *see* Liang-Federman and Kerdel, Life-Threatening Dermatoses.

Erythema multiforme is a benign, self-limited, and frequently recurrent host immune response to an antigenic stimulus. This hypersensitivity reaction develops 7 to 14 days after initial exposure and is probably both humoral and cell mediated [10,11]. Young adults are the primary target, although 20% of cases develop in children and teenagers [11].

Etiology

The possible etiologic agents of EM are innumerable, but they can be grouped into the categories of infections, medications, collagen vascular disease, and neoplasms. Table 15-3 lists the most common etiologic agents in each of these categories. In the United States, herpes simplex virus (HSV) infection (Fig. 15-4) and medications are the

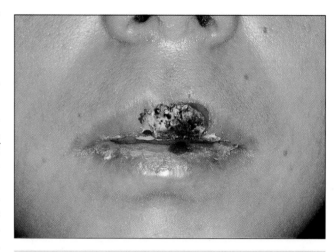

FIGURE 15-4 Herpes labialis of the upper lip with erythema multiforme erosions of the lower lip.

most common causes, with HSV infection probably responsible for more than 50% of all EM cases [10]. Use of the polymerase chain reaction technique has shown HSV to also be an overwhelming etiologic agent of childhood EM [12•].

Clinical Presentation

Erythema multiforme begins as an acral eruption characterized initially by fixed erythematous macules that may progress to papules and urticarial plaques, 1 to 2 cm in diameter (Figs. 15-5 and 15-6). The characteristic lesion with targetlike appearance (central blister and purpura or necrosis) is not always seen. The palms and soles are commonly involved (Fig. 15-7), and lesions often progress to involve the trunk over a 1-week period (Fig. 15-8). Resolution then proceeds over a 1- to 2-week period, with postinflammatory hyperpigmentation but no scarring typical. This eruption may be completely asymptomatic or

TABLE 15-3 SOME ETIOLOGIC AGENTS ASSOCIATED WITH ERYTHEMA MULTIFORME

Infections

Herpes simplex
Mycoplasma pneumoniae infection
Mononucleosis
Yersinia infections
Tuberculosis
Deep fungal infections (*eg*, histoplasmosis and coccidioidomycosis)

Medications

Penicillins
Sulfonamides
Phenytoin
Barbiturates

Neoplasms*

Lymphoproliferative disorders
Solid tumors
Dysproteinemias

Connective tissue disease*

Systemic lupus erythematosus
Rheumatoid arthritis

*These associations are rare.

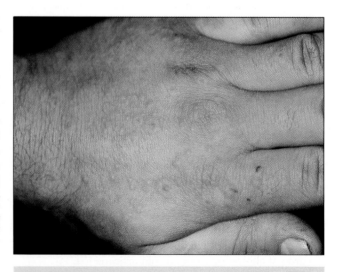

FIGURE 15-5 Urticarial papules and targetlike lesions on the dorsum of the hand, in a patient with erythema multiforme.

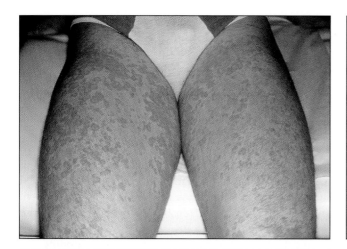

FIGURE 15-6 Urticarial papules and plaques on the thighs of a patient with erythema multiforme.

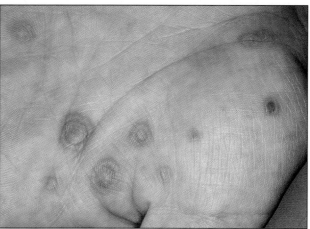

FIGURE 15-7 Classic target-like palmar lesions in a patient with erythema multiforme minor.

associated with itching and burning, and it has a tendency to develop in areas of trauma or ultraviolet exposure (isomorphic phenomenon) [11,13]. Mucosal involvement occurs in 20% to 45% of EM minor cases and is usually mild, with erosions of the oral mucosa as a common feature (Fig. 15-9) [11]. Constitutional symptoms are usually absent, and hospitalization is usually avoidable.

Evaluation

Evaluation of the EM patient centers on identification of the etiologic agent, which is often possible with a thorough history and physical examination, including a medication history and review of symptoms for infectious processes. No specific laboratory abnormality is present with EM minor, although an elevated erythrocyte sedimentation rate, mild leukocytosis, or both may be encountered. Laboratory testing is not always necessary if the etiologic agent is apparent from the history and physical examination findings. The choice of laboratory tests should be directed by

these findings. Table 15-4 provides a partial list of suggested tests. Skin biopsy often reveals the characteristic hydropic degeneration of basal keratinocytes with mixed dermal infiltrate [10,11] but is not helpful in pinpointing the etiology.

Treatment

Treatment of EM minor centers on the removal or treatment of the etiologic agent, or both, and on symptomatic care. Antihistamines, oatmeal baths, and emollients with menthol may help symptoms of itching. Topical corticosteroids may also help symptoms but have little other benefit [14]. Oral lesions may be treated with a 1:1 mixture of diphenhydramine elixir and attapulgite

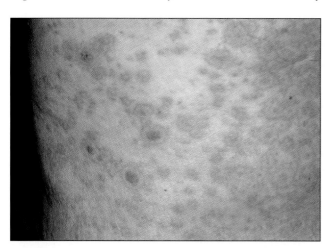

FIGURE 15-8 Trunk involvement in a patient with erythema multiforme.

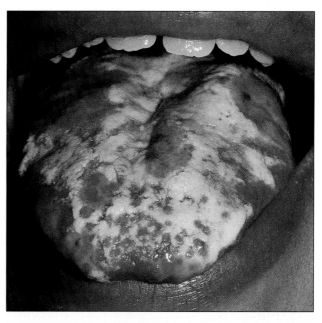

FIGURE 15-9 Oral mucosal erosions in a patient with erythema multiforme minor.

Table 15-4 Laboratory evaluation in erythema multiforme

Complete blood count with differential
Liver function tests
Urinalysis
Erythrocyte sedimentation rate
Anti-streptolysin O titer
Chest roentgenography
Viral cultures or titers
Cold agglutinins

(Kaopectate; Upjohn, Kalamazoo, MI). The use of systemic corticosteroids, although common, is controversial. If the EM is HSV associated, the patient should be counseled about the risk of recurrent EM with future episodes of HSV infection. Sunscreens and sun avoidance should be recommended in herpes labialis-associated EM. Oral acyclovir (Zovirax; Burroughs Wellcome, Research Triangle Park, NC), given episodically for infrequent recurrences of HSV infection (200 mg five times a day for 5 days) or as a long-term suppressive regimen for frequent recurrences (400 mg twice daily), may prevent EM if the HSV episode can be aborted. Even without treatment, EM minor is benign and self-limited within 2 to 6 weeks.

Erythema Nodosum

General Considerations

Erythema nodosum (EN) is a reactive hypersensitivity process in which the target of the inflammatory reaction is the subcutaneous fat (panniculitis). EN is the most common cause of inflammatory nodules on the lower extremities [15].

As with other reactive erythemas, EN develops as the host mounts an immune response to an antigenic stimulus. Both humoral and cell-mediated immune mechanisms probably play a role in the pathogenesis of EN. Circulating immune complexes (type III hypersensitivity) are postulated to participate in this process because patients often present with a serum sickness-like syndrome [16].

Etiology

Multiple agents may play an antigenic role in the development of EN. Table 15-5 summarizes the most common etiologic associations. Infections, sarcoidosis, medications, and pregnancy head the list in the United States today. In the 1950s, tuberculosis was the primary infectious trigger for EN, but infection with group A β-hemolytic streptococci is most common today. Yersinia infections remain an important etiologic agent in Europe [15]. Of the medications listed, oral contraceptives are the leading trigger, and often the physician neglects to obtain a history of their use in the female patient presenting with EN. Finally, with respect to inflammatory bowel disease, the patient with ulcerative colitis is much more likely to develop EN than the patient with Crohn's disease.

Clinical Presentation

The typical patient with EN is usually a woman who presents with the sudden development of multiple tender, red, warm nodules (1 to 5 cm in diameter) on the pretibial surfaces (Fig. 15-10). These nodules are not suppurative and do not ulcerate. After a 3- to 6-week course, the nodules eventuate into a bruise without scar formation. Atypical presentations include subcutaneous nodules on the trunk, arms, calves, or face. Patients may present with a serum sickness–like syndrome with associated findings of fever, chills, malaise, leukocytosis, and arthropathy.

Evaluation

As with any disease process, evaluation of the EN patient begins with a thorough history and physical examination to pinpoint a possible etiologic factor. A thorough medication history, including information on the use of oral contraceptives, must be obtained, and women need to be questioned about the possibility of pregnancy. A biopsy is not always necessary with the classic presentation, but if a biopsy is performed, an adequate specimen that includes subcutaneous fat is paramount. Usually this requires an incisional wedge biopsy. Histopathologic changes include septal inflammation of the subcutaneous

Table 15-5 Etiologic agents of erythema nodosum

Infections
Group A β-hemolytic streptococcus infections
Chlamydial infections
Deep fungal infections
Tuberculosis
Yersinia infections
Medications
Oral contraceptives
Sulfonamides
Bromides
Systemic conditions
Sarcoidosis
Inflammatory bowel disease
Behçet's syndrome
Lymphoreticular malignancy
Reiter's disease
Pregnancy

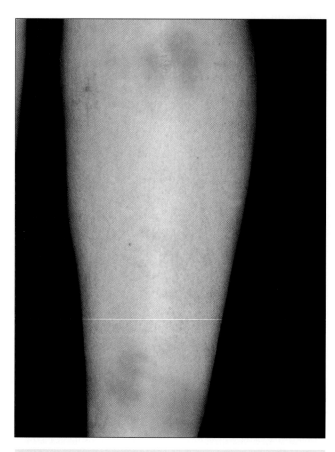

FIGURE 15-10 Tender subcutaneous inflammatory nodules of the pretibium that are typical of erythema nodosum.

tissue with possible granuloma formation. Vasculitis and fat necrosis are not seen [16]. The selection of laboratory tests should be directed by the history and physical examination findings. Table 15-6 provides a partial listing of suggested tests.

Treatment

Treatment of EN centers on the removal or treatment of the etiologic agent, or both. Supportive therapy includes bed rest, the use of an elastic support bandage, leg eleva-

TABLE 15-6 LABORATORY EVALUATION IN ERYTHEMA NODOSUM

Chest roentgenography
Urinalysis
Throat culture
Complete blood count with differential
Erythrocyte sedimentation rate
Anti-streptolysin O titer or anti-DNAase titer
Pregnancy test
Plus/minus intradermal tests for tuberculosis, histoplasmosis, or coccidioidomycosis

tion, and the use of nonsteroidal anti-inflammatory agents. Many clinicians favor the use of aspirin (650 mg three times a day) or indomethacin (50 mg two to three times a day). The use of potassium iodide (300 mg three times a day) or supersaturated potassium iodide (0.3 mL three times a day) is often beneficial [17], as may be colchicine (0.6 mg twice a day). Patients should be warned of possible gastrointestinal side effects with all of these agents. Finally, some physicians advocate a 2-week systemic corticosteroid taper. In patients given systemic corticosteroids, the physician needs to exclude underlying fungal or mycobacterial disease before administration of these agents is started.

ACKNOWLEDGMENTS

I thank Dr. Jeffrey P. Callen for supplying the clinical photographs for this manuscript and also for his editorial suggestions. I also thank Ms. Sandy Lingle for her secretarial assistance.

REFERENCES AND RECOMMENDED READING

Recently published papers of particular interest have been highlighted as:
• Of interest
•• Of outstanding interest

1. Jorizzo JL: Urticaria. In *Dermatological Signs of Internal Disease.* Edited by Callen JP and Jorizzo JL. Philadelphia: WB Saunders; 1988:59–69.

2.•• Soter NA: Urticaria: current therapy. *J Allergy Clin Immunol* 1990, 86:1009–1014.

3.•• Kulp-Shorten CL, Callen JP: Urticaria and angioedema. In *Conn's Current Therapy.* Edited by Rakel RE. Philadelphia: WB Saunders; 1993:827–828.

4.• Sibbald RG, Cheema AS, Lozinski A, *et al.*: Chronic urticaria: evaluation of the role of physical, immunologic, and other contributory factors. *Int J Dermatol* 1991, 30:381–386.

5. Casale TB, Sampson HA, Hanifin J, *et al.*: Guide to physical urticarias. *J Allergy Clin Immunol* 1988, 82:758–763.

6.•• Barlow RJ, Warburton F, Watson K, *et al.*: Diagnosis and incidence of delayed pressure urticaria in patients with chronic urticaria. *J Am Acad Dermatol* 1993, 29:954–958.

7.• Lin RY, Schwartz RA: Cold urticaria and HIV infection. *Br J Dermatol* 1993, 129:465–467.

8. Monroe EW: Chronic urticaria: Review of nonsedating H$_1$ antihistamines in treatment. *J Am Acad Dermatol* 1988, 19:842–849.

9.• Sharpe GR, Shuster S: The effect of cetirizine on symptoms and wealing in dermographic urticaria. *Br J Dermatol* 1993, 129:580–583.

10. Huff JC: Erythema multiforme. *Dermatol Clin* 1985, 3:141–152.

11. Ledesma GN, McCormack PC: Erythema multiforme. *Clin Dermatol* 1986, 4:70–80.

12.• Weston WL, Brice SL, Jester JD, *et al.*:Herpes simplex virus in childhood erythema multiforme. *Pediatrics* 1992, 89:32–34.

13. Fitzpatrick JE, Thompson PB, Aeling JL, *et al.*: Photosensitive recurrent erythema multiforme. *J Am Acad Dermatol* 1983, 9:419–423.

14. Tonnesen MG: Erythema multiforme. In *Conn's Current Therapy*. Edited by Rakel RE. Philadelphia: WB Saunders; 1993:812–814.

15. White JW: Erythema nodosum. *Dermatol Clin* 1985, 3:119–127.

16. Jorizzo JL: Erythema nodosum. In *Dermatological Signs of Internal Disease*. Edited by Callen JP, Jorizzo JL. Philadelphia: WB Saunders; 1988:76–79.

17. Horio T, Danno K, Okamoto H, *et al.*: Potassium iodide in erythema nodosum and other erythematous dermatoses. *J Am Acad Dermatol* 1983, 9:77–81.

SELECT BIBLIOGRAPHY

Champion RH: Urticaria: then and now. *Br J Dermatol* 1988, 119:427–436.

Chan H-L, Stern RS, Arndt KA, *et al.*: The incidence of erythema multiforme, Stevens-Johnson syndrome, and toxic epidermal necrolysis. *Arch Dermatol* 1990, 126:43–47.

Kalivas J, Breneman D, Tharp M, *et al.*: Urticaria: clinical efficacy of cetirizine in comparison with hydroxyzine and placebo. *J Allergy Clin Immunol* 1990, 86:1014–1018.

Monroe EW: The role of antihistamines in the treatment of chronic urticaria. *J Allergy Clin Immunol* 1990, 86:662–665.

Simons FER: Recent advances in H1-receptor antagonist treatment. *J Allergy Clin Immunol* 1990, 86:995–999.

Small Vessel Vasculitis and Neutrophilic Dermatoses

16

Jamie A. Alpert
Joseph L. Jorizzo

Key Points

- Necrotizing venulitis is characterized by palpable purpura clinically and by leukocytoclastic vasculitis pathologically.

- Patients evaluation can involve histopathologic confirmation of the diagnosis, determination of the extent of disease, and attempting to uncover and underlying etiology.

- Sweet's syndrome is characterized by inflammatory cutaneous plaques with a neutrophilic vascular reaction pathologically.

- Behçet's disease is characterized by oral aphthae and various combinations of genital aphthae, synovitis, cutaneous pustular vasculitis, and meningoencephalitis.

- Pyoderma gangrenosum belongs in this category of disease because the histopathologic findings in early lesions (controversial) may represent a neutrophilic vascular reaction.

NECROTIZING VENULITIS

Clinical Features

The hallmark of necrotizing venulitis is the palpable purpuric papule. However, there is a spectrum of clinical presentation [1]. Lesions begin as erythematous macules and progress to palpable purpura. They usually occur in crops on dependent sites (Fig. 16-1). The papules are usually less than 1 cm in diameter, and they often become confluent to form plaques, which may ulcerate. They are often asymptomatic but may be pruritic or painful. Frequently, patients have associated serum sickness–like symptoms, such as arthralgias, arthritis, myalgias, and fever.

Patients may have internal involvement, presumably resulting from circulating immune complex–mediated vessel damage [2]. Systemic involvement may include involvement of the renal glomeruli, resulting in proteinuria or hematuria; involvement of the neurologic system with focal, diffuse, central, or peripheral neurologic impairment: synovial involvement with polyarthritis; involvement of the gastrointestinal tract with associated abdominal pain or gastrointestinal bleeding; and involvement of the cardiovascular system or the respiratory tract with pericarditis or pleuritis [2,3••]. An algorithm for patient evaluation is shown in Figure 16-2.

Histopathology

Leukocytoclastic vasculitis is a disease that affects postcapillary venules in the dermis. Its histopathologic features include 1) endothelial swelling, 2) invasion of neutrophils into blood vessels, 3) leukocytoclasia, 4) extravasation of erythrocytes, and 5) fibrinoid necrosis of blood vessel walls [4]. Positive direct immunofluores-

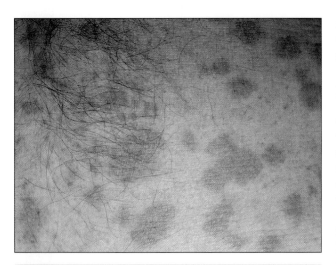

FIGURE 16-1 Necrotizing venulitis. Note the typical palpable purpura.

relapsing [7]. There have been reports of death associated with diffuse or proliferative glomerulonephritis, as well as from pulmonary, neurologic, and gastrointestinal bleeding [2]. The course of the underlying disease may also affect prognosis (*eg*, collagen vascular disease).

No treatment of necrotizing vasculitis has ever been subjected to the scrutiny of a double-blind, prospective trial. The course can be variable, further complicating the assessment of therapies. In patients in whom there is a recognized cause, removal of that cause can eradicate the disease (*eg*, drug-induced, or herpes simplex virus infection).

Systemic corticosteroids are used if there is systemic involvement or severe progressive cutaneous ulcerating lesions. Prednisone (1 mg/kg/d) given as a single morning dose is the most commonly enforced regimen. Split dosing increases the effectiveness, but it also increases the side effects. Every-other-day dosing is suboptimal for treating immune complex–mediated disease.

Corticosteroids should be tapered slowly because rebound may occur if tapering is done too quickly. Pulse therapy (1 g/d) of methylprednisolone sodium succinate (Solu-Medrol; Upjohn, Kalamazoo, MI) over 3 to 5 days has been reported to be beneficial, and this treatment can be used in life-threatening cases [2]. It is necessary to monitor for cardiac arrhythmias and sudden electrolyte

cence has been identified for IgG, IgM, IgA, C3, C4, C1q, and fibrin. However, results are inconsistent and are usually positive only in early lesions [5,6].

Prognosis and Therapy

The prognosis depends on the presence and severity of internal involvement. The course may be acute, chronic, or

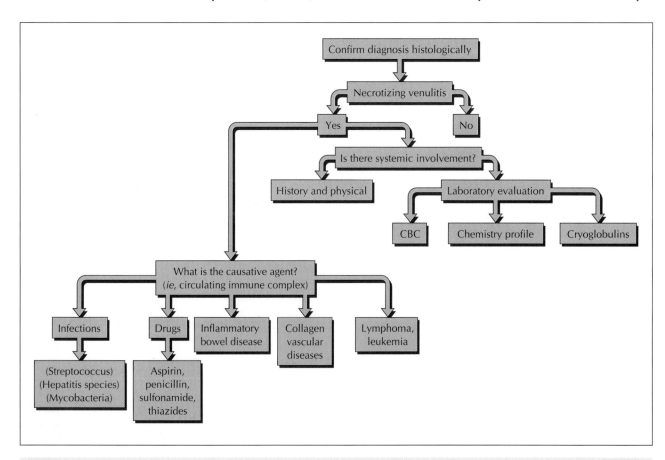

FIGURE 16-2 Patient evaluation procedure for necrotizing vasculitis. CBC—complete blood count.

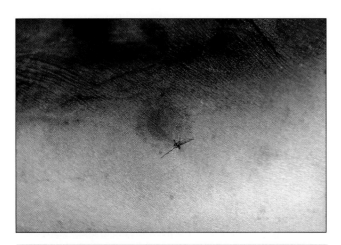

FIGURE 16-3 Sweet's syndrome: an erythematous plaque on a patient who has no underlying disease after an extensive work-up.

shifts if pulse therapy is used [2]. Cyclophosphamide and azathioprine, which have been successfully used in large vessel vasculitis, are usually not necessary for small vessel necrotizing vasculitis [2]. Low-dose weekly methotrexate may have a role in treating this disease.

Patients with cutaneous lesions only may not require therapy. Antihistamines have been used but are not helpful in our opinion [2]. Oral colchicine has been reported to be effective in doses of 0.6 mg orally two or three times daily [2]. Nonsteroidal anti-inflammatory drugs may be beneficial in treating serum sickness–like symptoms, but they do little for the cutaneous lesions. Oral dapsone therapy may also be helpful [2].

SWEET'S SYNDROME

Clinical Features

Sweet's syndrome is characterized by recurrent episodes of inflammatory cutaneous plaques, fevers, arthralgias, and neutrophilia and by histologic evidence of neutrophilic dermal inflammation occurring in the absence of infection. Cutaneous findings include erythematous, well-marginated inflammatory plaques varying from 1 to 3 cm in diameter (Fig. 16-3). Usually no epidermal change is seen; however, some vesicle or pustule formation can occur, as can postinflammatory desquamation. Occasionally, there is associated epidermal necrosis. Lesions can occur anywhere on the body but are usually limited to the trunk, face, and upper extremities. Usually, lesions occur in crops over a 1- to 2-month period. Signs and symptoms associated with this syndrome include fever, myalgia, arthralgia, headache, dyspepsia, and conjunctivitis. Mucosal involvement is unusual. Systemic involvement often lags behind the cutaneous eruption by 7 to 10 days.

Sweet's syndrome is often associated with other systemic diseases, such as acute myelogenous leukemia, ulcerative

colitis, or even leukemia and lymphoma. There are no specific laboratory abnormalities, but there is often neutrophilia, an increased white blood cell count (> 20,000 cells/mL), and an elevated erythrocyte sedimentation rate (50 to 100 mm/h).

Histopathology

The characteristic histopathologic findings in specimens from patients with Sweet's syndrome are a dense, diffuse neutrophilic infiltrate with leukocytoclasia; dermal edema; and endothelial swelling. However, no fibrinoid necrosis is seen. There have been reports of involvement of the panniculus, but this is unusual [7,8].

Patient Evaluation

It is important to distinguish Sweet's syndrome from diseases such as erythema multiforme, erythema annulare centrifugum, erythema elevatum diutinum, granuloma facile, erythema nodosum, bromoderma, and pustular vasculitis associated with Behçet's disease. Infection should be excluded clinically and histologically. In addition, associated diseases (*eg*, leukemia and other myeloproliferative disorders, malignancy, ulcerative colitis, Sjögren syndrome, rheumatoid arthritis, and systemic lupus erythematosus) should be excluded.

Prognosis and Therapy

The lesions of Sweet's syndrome normally remit spontaneously in several weeks to months. Usually 50% of patients have at least one recurrence [6]. The most effective treatment is the use of systemic corticosteroids, but these agents are often not required. No prospective, double-blind assessment of this or any other treatment has been performed. The usual doses required range from 30 to 80 mg of prednisone per day, which is then tapered over several weeks [9••,10]. Other therapies have been tried, including indomethacin, potassium iodide, colchicine, dapsone, and oral isotretinoin. The effect of these drugs on neutrophil migration may at least partially explain their benefit [8,11].

PUSTULAR VASCULITIS: BEHÇET'S DISEASE

Behçet's disease is a multisystem disease named after and first described by a Turkish dermatologist. It is characterized by oral aphthae and two of the following systemic or mucocutaneous findings: 1) genital aphthae, 2) synovitis, 3) posterior uveitis, 4) cutaneous pustular vasculitis, and 5) meningoencephalitis. It is important to exclude inflammatory bowel disease and other autoimmune disease [12,13]. There are no pathognomonic laboratory tests; the diagnosis is made on clinical criteria only [13]. Behçet's disease is common in the Middle East and Japan and rare in the United States and Northern Europe. The disease usually affects young adults and rarely children [13].

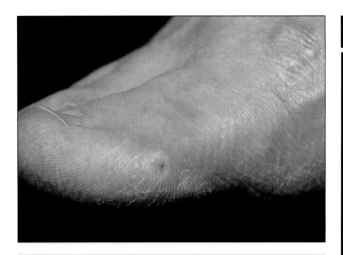

FIGURE 16-4 Behçet's disease: pustular vasculitis. An indistinguishable lesion can be seen in bowel bypass syndrome.

Clinical Features

Behçet's disease has an extremely variable course. Morbidity depends on the development of ocular manifestations. Death is rare and usually occurs from neurologic or large vessel vascular disease. The cutaneous findings are varied. However, only pustular vasculitis and erythema nodosum–like nodules should be accepted as diagnostic criteria (Fig. 16-4). Follicular-based or acneiform lesions should not be included [13].

Behçet's disease has a number of ocular manifestations [13]. However, posterior uveitis is the principal ophthalmic cause of major morbidity. The posterior uveitis represents a retinal vasculitis that may result in blindness [6]. The associated arthritis is asymmetric, nonerosive, and oligoarthritic [13,14]. Meningoencephalitis is the principal neurologic manifestation [13]. There are a multitude of diffuse, focal, central, and peripheral neurologic associations [2]. Neurologic involvement usually occurs later in the disease process. Vascular involvement includes aneurysm, arterial occlusion, venous occlusion, and varices and can be fatal [15]. The vascular lesions are not always vasculitis and do not always respond to medical therapy.

Histopathology

Biopsy specimens from aphthae or from pustular vasculitis lesions show fully developed leukocytoclastic vasculitis or a neutrophilic vascular reaction.

Patient Evaluation

It is important to remember that 20% of the normal population has oral aphthae [16]. Clinical criteria for Behçet's disease must be met, and inflammatory bowel disease must be excluded. It is essential to exclude herpes virus infection by culture, histologic examination, or polymerase chain reaction from mucocutaneous lesions in patients suspected of having Behçet's disease. Periodic ophthalmologic exami-

TABLE 16-1 TREATMENT OF BEHÇET'S DISEASE
Mucosal lesions only
Topical corticosteroids
Intralesional corticosteroids
Viscous lidocaine
Mucocutaneous disease or more severe mucosal disease
Oral colchicine, 0.6 mg orally, two to three times daily. (monitor for neutropenia)
Oral dapsone
Oral thalidomide
Oral corticosteroids (limited because of long-term side effects)
Possible low-dose weekly methotrexate
Mucocutaneous disease and ocular or neurologic symptoms
Oral corticosteroids
Immunosuppressive therapy
Azathioprine
Methotrexate
Cyclosporine

nation is also required. Rheumatologic and neurologic consultations are often appropriate as well.

Prognosis and Therapy

The clinical course is variable. The mucocutaneous and arthritic manifestations usually precede any neurologic manifestations [2]. There is chronic morbidity due to mucosal ulcerations and joint aches, but the mortality rate is low in patients without ophthalmic or neurologic involvement [13]. Death is usually due to central nervous system complications, vascular disease, or less frequently, bowel perforation or cardiopulmonary disease [17].

Palliative therapies are delineated in Table 16-1 [18,19,20•].

PYODERMA GANGRENOSUM

Clinical Features

Pyoderma gangrenosum is a cutaneous ulcerative disease of unknown etiology. The lesions start as tender papules or pustules and evolve into ulcers with raised, characteristic, undermined borders with a dusty purple hue (Fig. 16-5 and 16-6). There is destruction of the skin down to subcutaneous fat, with associated granulation tissue and necrotic purulent material at the base of the ulcer. One lesion or many lesions may be present. The lesions demonstrate pathergy and may expand in an explosive fashion if the

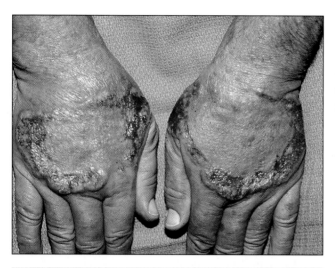

FIGURE 16-5 Bullous pyoderma gangrenosum: atypical lesions are common in patients with myleodysplastic syndrome.

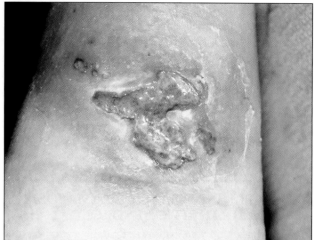

FIGURE 16-6 Pyoderma gangrenosum: typical clinical presentation.

borders are traumatized by débridement or by mechanical manipulation [5]. Pyoderma gangrenosum is a diagnosis of exclusion [21] (Table 16-2).

Histopathology

The classic histopathologic findings in specimens from pyoderma gangrenosum lesions are controversial. Findings are usually nonspecific, with specimens showing chronic inflammatory changes. The debate focuses on whether early lesions show a neutrophilic infiltrate or primarily a lymphocytic infiltrate [22]. The degree of vessel involvement may range from none to endothelial swelling to fibrinoid necrosis. The histopathologic findings obviously depend on the stage of the ulcer. Findings from early lesions of pyoderma gangrenosum resemble those from lesions of pustular vasculitis associated with Behçet's disease and show a neutrophilic vascular reaction [6].

Bullous pyoderma gangrenosum and Sweet's variant associated with myeloproliferative disease show predominantly a neutrophilic inflammatory infiltrate. More fully developed lesions show extensive tissue necrosis with surrounding mild inflammatory cell infiltrate with associated foreign body giant cells [22,23].

Patient Evaluation

It is essential to exclude other dermatoses, as outlined in the clinical section. This may be accomplished with a deep incisional biopsy specimen with routine histology, with special stains for mycobacteria, bacteria, and fungi, and with a second biopsy specimen for culture of these organisms. It is important to evaluate the patient for the following underlying conditions: ulcerative colitis, regional enteritis, hepatitis (chronic persistent or chronic active), paraproteinemia, myeloproliferative disease, and rheumatoid and seronegative arthritis [23,24].

Prognosis and Therapy

The most important aspect of treatment and prognosis is to identify the disease process correctly. The spread of the disease may be rapid, with significant local tissue destruction. Local care may consist of preventing bacterial overgrowth and gentle débridement. Aggressive déebridement will lead to extension and flaring of existing ulcers (*ie*, pathergy). Intralesional corticosteroids have been used for mild localized disease. However, debate surrounds the effectiveness of this approach [25]. Systemic corticosteroids are the treatment of choice for most patients. Initially, very aggressive

TABLE 16-2 ETIOLOGIES OF ULCERS THAT CAN RESEMBLE PYODERMA GANGRENOSUM
Infections
Bacterial
Fungal
Mycobacterial
Rheumatologic disease
Systemic lupus erythematosus
Rheumatoid vasculitis
Behçet's disease
Wegener's granulomatosis
Factitial ulceration
Bromoderma or iododerma
Malignant neoplasm
Squamous cell carcinoma

therapy with 1 mg/kg/d is usually necessary. If there is continued expansion of lesions, a doubling of the dosage may be necessary. Pulse corticosteroids (1 g/d) are effective but require close monitoring [22]. Maintenance therapy is often required. Rebound may occur if corticosteroids are tapered too quickly. Dapsone and sulfapyridine have also been used, in dosages of 100 to 300 mg/d and 3 g/d, respectively, for maintenance therapy [25]. Azathioprine, cyclophosphamide, clofazimine, and antibiotics such as rifampin and minocycline have also had some beneficial effect.

BOWEL-ASSOCIATED DERMATOSIS-ARTHRITIS SYNDROME

Bowel bypass syndrome consists of cutaneous lesions that are pustular vasculitis associated with signs and symptoms similar to those of serum sickness. This syndrome has also been reported in people who have not had bypass surgery, such as those with inflammatory bowel disease or a blind loop due to another surgical procedure [2].

Clinical Features

The lesions associated with bowel bypass syndrome begin as small macules; they then evolve into papules and blossom into pustules on purpuric bases. They can range in size from 0.5 to 1.5 cm. Usually, they are located on the upper body, not the legs. Pathergy may be important in clinical distribution. Each cycle of lesions lasts for more than 2 weeks, and often recovery occurs over a 1- to 7-month period [26]. The lesions may be associated with fevers, myalgias, flulike syndromes, or gastrointestinal upset. Patients may have arthralgias and a nonerosive polyarthritis.

Histopathology

The histopathologic changes seen in specimens from the early lesions of pustular vasculitis associated with bowel-associated dermatosis-arthritis syndrome have been described as identical to the vessel changes associated with Behçet's disease and as similar to those seen in Sweet's syndrome [26,27].

Patient Evaluation

Patients with pustular vasculitis lesions with histologically confirmed neutrophilic vascular reactions must be distinguished from those with Behçet's disease, disseminated gonococcemia, or meningococcemia [2].

A complete history taking and physical examination are essential. It is important to exclude blind loops of bowel and inflammatory bowel disease with appropriate radiologic assessments, endoscopic evaluation; or both. If bowel disease has been excluded, Behçet's disease must also be eliminated.

Prognosis and Therapy

The bowel bypass syndrome usually resolves with correction of bowel anatomy. If the underlying condition is inflammatory bowel disease, progress depends on the prog-

nosis of the underlying bowel disease. Therapy has included the use of multiple antibiotics, such as tetracycline, metronidazole, and erythromycin [26]. Systemic corticosteroids have been used in patients with refractory conditioning and thalidomide has been useful [18].

REFERENCES AND RECOMMENDED READING

Recently published papers of particular interest have been highlighted as:
• Of interest
•• Of outstanding interest

1. Sams WM Jr, Thorne EG, Small P, *et al.*: Leukocytoclastic vasculitis. *Arch Dermatol* 1976, 112:219–226.

2. Jorizzo JL, Solomon AR, Zanolli MD: Neutrophilic vascular reaction. *J Am Acad Dermatol* 1988, 19:983–1005.

3.•• Jorizzo JL: Classification of vasculitis. *J Invest Dermatol* 1993, 100:106F–100F.

4. Winklemann RK, Ditto WB: Cutaneous and visceral syndromes of necrotizing or "allergic" angiitis: A study of 38 cases. *Medicine* 1964, 43:59–89.

5. Schroeter AL, Copeman PWM, Jordon RE, *et al.*: Immunofluorescence of cutaneous vasculitis associated with systemic disease. *Arch Dermatol* 1971, 104:254–259.

6. Dambuyant C, Thivolet J: Antigenic similarities within circulating immune complexes in patients suffering from cutaneous vasculitis. *Dermatologica* 1981, 162:429–437.

7. Ekenstam EA, Callen JP: Cutaneous leukocytoclastic vasculitis: clinical and laboratory features of 82 patients seen in private practice. *Arch Dermatol* 1984, 120:484–489.

8. Su WPD, Liu HNH: Diagnostic criteria for Sweet's syndrome. *Cutis* 1987, 37:167–174.

9.•• Vondendriesch P: Sweets syndrome acute neutrophilic dermatosis. *J Am Acad Dermatol* 1994, 31:535–560.

10. Storer JS, Nesbitt LT, Galen WK, DeLeo VA: Sweet's syndrome. *Int J Dermatol* 1983, 22:8–12.

11. Hoffman GS: Treatment of Sweet's syndrome (acute febrile neutrophilic dermatosis) with indomethacin. *J Rheumatol* 1977, 4:201–206.

12. Jorizzo JL, Hudson RD, Schmalstieg FC: Bowel associated syndrome, immune regulation, circulating immune complexes, neutrophil migration and colchicine therapy. *J Am Acad Dermatol* 1984, 10:205–214.

13. Jorizzo JL, Rogers RS: Behçet's disease: an update based on the International Conference held in Rochester, Minnesota. *J Am Acad Dermatol* 1989, 23:738–741.

14. Yurkakul S, Yuzici H, Tuzan Y, *et al.*: The arthritis of Behçet's disease: a prospective study. *Ann Rheum Dis* 1983, 42:1505–1515.

15. Shimizu T, Ehrlich GE, Goro I, *et al.*: Behçet's disease. *Semin Arthritis Rheum* 1979, 8:223–260.

16. Rogers RS III: Recurrent aphthous ulcers: clinical characteristics and evidence for immunopathogenesis. *J Invest Dermatol* 1977, 69:499–509.

17. Schreiner DT, Jorizzo JL: Behçet's disease and complex aphthosis. *Dermatol Clin* 1987, 4:769–778.

18. Jorizzo JL, Schmalstieg FS, Solomon AR: Thalidomide effects in Behçet's syndrome and pustular vasculitis. *Arch Intern Med* 1986, 146:878–881.

19. Nassenblatt RB, Palestine AG, Chan CC, *et al.*: Effectiveness of cyclosporin therapy for Behçet's disease. *Arthritis Rheum* 1985, 28:671–679.

20•. Jorizzo JL: Behçet's disease: and update based on international conference, Paris. *J Eur Acad Dermatol Veneral* 1994, 3:215–223.

21. Spiers EM, Hendricks SL, Jorizzo JL, Solomon AR: Sporotrichosis masquerading as pyoderma gangrenosum. *Arch Dermatol* 1986, 122:691–694.

22. Su WP, Schroeter AL, Perry HO, Powell FC: Histopathologic and immunopathologic study of pyoderma gangrenosum. *J Cutan Pathol* 1986, 13:323–330.

23. Stathel GM, Abbott LG, McGuiness AE: Pyoderma gangrenosum in association with regional enteritis. *Arch Dermatol* 1987, 95:375–380.

24. Green LK, Herbert AA, Jorizzo JL, Solomon AR: Pyoderma gangrenosum and chronic persistent hepatitis. *J Am Acad Dermatol* 1985, 13:892–897.

25. Johnson RB, Lazarus GS: Pulse Therapy: Therapeutic efficacy in treatment of pyoderma gangrenosum. *Arch Dermatol* 1982, 118:76–84.

26. Ely PH: The bowel bypass syndrome: A response to bacterial peptidoglycans. *J Am Acad Dermatol* 1980, 2:473–487.

27. Jorizzo JL, Schmalstieg FC, Dinehart SM, *et al.*: Bowel associated dermatosis-arthritis syndrome: Immune complex-mediated vessel damage and increased neutrophil migration. *Arch Intern Med* 1984, 144:738–740.

Drug Eruptions 17

Paul I. Oh
Neil H. Shear

Key Points

- Rashes are a common adverse effect of drug therapy.
- Clinical features of the rash may suggest a drug reaction.
- Drugs are not the only cause of such rashes, and a stepwise clinical approach is needed.
- The propensity to develop severe reactions may be based on genetic differences in drug metabolism.

It is well known that drugs are a common cause of skin rashes. In the Boston Collaborative Drug Surveillance Program [1], the frequency of cutaneous adverse reactions varied from 0% to 5.1%, depending on the drug in question. In clinical practice the situation is somewhat more enigmatic as patients present with a rash, and one or more drugs are considered in the differential etiology. The clinician therefore requires a systematic approach to the following aspects of the problem: 1) rashes in general, 2) adverse drug reactions, 3) determination of causation, and 4) current and future management of the patient. An overview of types of drug eruptions is given in Figure 17-1.

TYPES OF DRUG ERUPTIONS

Exanthematous Eruptions

Exanthematous eruptions are the most common rashes seen by physicians and are known by the synonyms *morbilliform*, scarlatiniform and toxic erythema [2••,3–5]. The term maculopapular is used widely, but should be discouraged because of a lack of specificity. Any drug may cause these reactions. Repeated administration of the same drug in the future will most likely cause a similar syndrome, rather than a more accelerated or severe reaction. The major differential diagnosis for these rashes, particularly in children, are viral exanthems. Exanthematous eruptions start as erythematous macules and papules on the trunk, become confluent, and later spread symmetrically to the face and limbs.

Simple eruptions (Fig. 17-2) usually occur within 1 week of beginning therapy, especially if the patient has been previously sensitized, and resolve within 7 to 14 days. A common scenario is the occurrence of a generalized rash in almost all patients with infectious mononucleosis who are treated with ampicillin. A similar reaction occurs in approximately 50% of HIV-infected patients who are exposed to aromatic amines such as sulfonamide antibiotics [6•]. Many other antibiotics, with or without concurrent viral infections, have been associated with simple rashes.

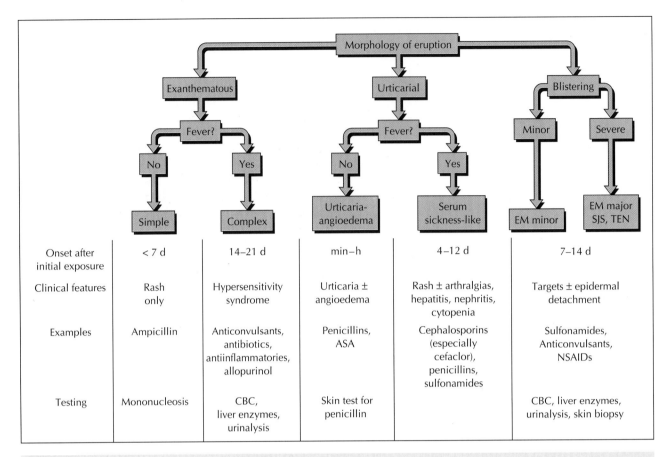

Onset after initial exposure	< 7 d	14–21 d	min–h	4–12 d	7–14 d
Clinical features	Rash only	Hypersensitivity syndrome	Urticaria ± angioedema	Rash ± arthralgias, hepatitis, nephritis, cytopenia	Targets ± epidermal detachment
Examples	Ampicillin	Anticonvulsants, antibiotics, antiinflammatories, allopurinol	Penicillins, ASA	Cephalosporins (especially cefaclor), penicillins, sulfonamides	Sulfonamides, Anticonvulsants, NSAIDs
Testing	Mononucleosis	CBC, liver enzymes, urinalysis	Skin test for penicillin		CBC, liver enzymes, urinalysis, skin biopsy

FIGURE 17-1 Algorithm to aid the clinical diagnosis of drug rashes. ASA—acetylsalicylic acid; CBC—complete blood count; EM—erythema multiforme; NSAIDs—nonsteroidal anti-inflammatory drugs; SJS—Stevens-Johnson syndrome; TEN—toxic epidermal necrolysis.

Complex rashes (Fig. 17-3) occur as a part of a *hypersensitivity syndrome* that is characterized by delayed onset of an exanthema (with or without pruritus) in association with fever, lymphadenopathy, and possibly hepatitis, nephritis, thyroiditis, and hematologic abnormalities [7]. The frequencies of these other findings is shown in Table 17-1. The syndrome usually begins with fever at 2 to 3 weeks from initial drug exposure, but an onset as long as 3 months into therapy has been reported. The major groups of drugs associated with hypersensitivity syndromes are the anticonvulsants (phenytoin, carbamazepine, and phenobarbital), antibiotics (sulfonamides), anti-inflammatories (gold and nonsteroidal anti-inflammatory drugs [NSAIDs] such as piroxicam), and allopurinol. There may be cross reactivity among different medications, and patients should therefore be advised about potentially hazardous drugs for the future. For example, in the case of anticonvulsants, 80% of patients who have had a hypersensitivity response to any one of phenytoin, phenobarbital, or carbamazepine will react to the other two in a similar way if exposed. The preferred choice for future treatment would then be an agent such as valproic acid. The propensity to develop a reaction is inherited. Genetic differences in drug-metabolizing enzymes result in insufficient clearance of toxic intermediates. Direct relatives of a patient who has had

a hypersensitivity reaction may have a dramatically increased risk of having a similar response when compared with the general population. Thus, counseling of family members is a crucial part of the assessment.

Urticarial Eruptions

Urticarial rashes are characterized by pruritic red wheals of varying sizes that can occur with any medication. When deep dermal and subcutaneous tissues are also swollen, the

TABLE 17-1 MANIFESTATIONS OF ANTICONVULSANT HYPERSENSITIVITY SYNDROME

Symptom	Incidence, %
Fever	100
Skin rash	87
Hepatitis	51
Eosinophilia	30
Nephritis	11
Pneumonitis	9
Atypical lymphocytosis	6

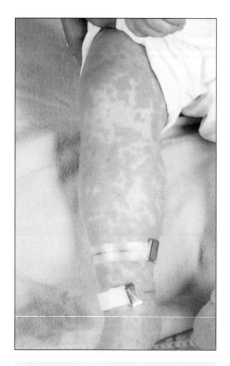

FIGURE 17-2 Exanthematous eruption caused by amoxicillin. There were no systemic symptoms, and no evidence of Epstein–Barr virus infection.

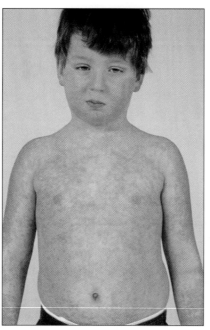

FIGURE 17-3 Generalized erythematous eruption associated with fever, lymphadenopathy, and nephritis. Hypersensitivity syndrome to phenobarbital was confirmed by *in vitro* testing.

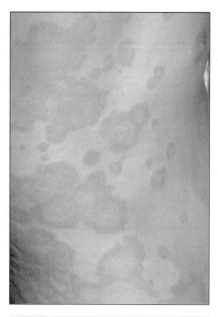

FIGURE 17-4 Itchy, red raised plaques that last for less than 24 hours are characteristic of urticaria. The annular morphology is commonly seen and often misdiagnosed as erythema multiforme. This reaction was caused by cloxacillin and confirmed by skin testing to penicillin.

reaction is known as angioedema. Angioedema may involve mucous membranes and be part of an anaphylactic reaction. There are several mechanisms for urticarial eruptions that are distinguished by their time course and accompanying features [2••,3–5].

Immunoglobulin E-dependent *urticaria* occurs within minutes to hours of drug exposure and is typified by immediate reactions to penicillins or acetylsalicylic acid (ASA) (Fig. 17-4). Combinations of the drug or metabolite with IgE bound to the surfaces of cutaneous mast cells lead to activation, degranulation, and release of vasoactive mediators such as histamine, leukotrienes, and prostaglandins. The resulting vasodilatation and increased vascular permeability lead to hive formation. *Angioedema* may occur in the absence of urticaria, but the two are often seen together in drug reactions. Idiopathic chronic recurrent urticaria can be confused with drug reactions unless the timing of reactions (*eg* occurrence of hives independent of drug exposure) is examined carefully. True urticaria usually resolves within 24 hours.

Immune complex disease, such as serum sickness reactions, are characterized by urticarial rashes, palpable purpura, or ulcerations, in association with fever, arthralgias, and possibly a combination of hepatitis, nephritis, hematologic or neurologic abnormalities that occur 4 to 12 days after exposure. Penicillins, cephalosporins, sulfonamides, animal-derived sera such as antivenom and antilymphocyte globulins, and streptokinase are common causative agents. Circulating immune complexes that

subsequently cause complement activation are thought to be one of the major pathogenic factors in these reactions. Circulating immune complexes have not been demonstrated in all the associated drugs (*eg*, antibiotics). The term *serum sickness–like reaction* (Fig. 17-5) has therefore been

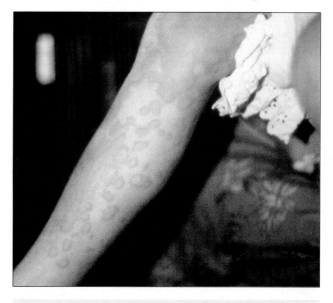

FIGURE 17-5 Annular urticarial plaques that last for more than 24 hours and are associated with fever and arthralgias are characteristic of serum sickness–like reactions. This patient had received cefaclor therapy for pharyngitis.

Classification	EM minor	EM major	SJS	TEN
Epidermal detachment, *% of body surface area*	<10	<10	<10	>30
Typical targets	Yes	No	No	No
Atypical targets	Raised	Flat	Flat	Flat
Macules	No	No	Yes	Yes
Mucous membrane involvement	No	Yes	Yes	Yes
Severity	+	++	+++	++++
Likelihood of drug etiology	+	++	+++	++++

EM—erythema multiforme; SJS—Stevens-Johnson syndrome; TEN—toxic epidermal necrolysis; +—low; ++++—high.

used in reference to these drug reactions. These reactions are associated with urticarial plaques, arthralgia, and fever. Nephritis is rare. Patients usually improve with supportive care in 5 to 7 days. Cefaclor is a common cause.

Urticarial reactions may also result from nonimmunologic activation of inflammatory mediators. Drugs such as ASA, NSAIDs, radiographic dyes, and opiates may directly cause release of histamine from mast cells independent of IgE, or activate complement and arachidonic acid pathways.

There are few laboratory tests that are helpful in the diagnosis of drug-induced urticaria or angioedema. Radioallergosorbent testing (RAST), if available, may help define the IgE-dependence of the reaction. At present, skin testing is of value for investigating suspected immediate hypersensitivity reactions to penicillins, but for other drugs no well-verified tests are available.

Blistering Eruptions

Eruptions associated with blisters or bullae encompass a spectrum from erythema multiforme (EM) to more serious reactions such as Stevens-Johnson syndrome (SJS) and toxic

epidermal necrolysis (TEN). These reactions can all be caused by drugs, but whereas TEN is almost always related to a drug exposure, EM and SJS have also been associated with infectious diseases such as *Mycoplasma pneumoniae* and herpes simplex. A recent international consensus conference [8•] proposed a standardized classification system for these eruptions, based on the presence or absence of target lesions and percentage of epidermal detachment as shown in Table 17-2. Classification may be further aided by the use of a photographic atlas illustrating the various types of lesions.

Bullous EM is characterized by both typical targets (red or bluish lesions with a regular round shape, well-defined border, and at least three different concentric zones, usually occurring on the limbs; Fig. 17-6) and atypical targets (round edematous, palpable lesions with only two zones and a poorly defined border; Fig. 17-7). Sulfonamide-induced EM is the best characterized of the drug eruptions in this category (Fig. 17-8). The reaction to this drug occurs 7 to 14 days after initiation of therapy and may be associated with fever or other constitutional symptoms. Other drugs that have been associated with EM include penicillins, phenytoin, carbamazepine, phenobarbital, rifampin, thiazides, and NSAIDs such as phenylbutazone. The same drugs may cause the more severe SJS, in which hemorrhagic bullae, erosions, and crusts appear in the mouth, on the lips and other mucous membranes, and where more prominent systemic features such as myalgias and arthralgias occur. A very severe disease course is associated with ocular involvement and possibly respiratory and renal pathology. Complete blood counts, liver enzymes, chest x-ray, and urinalysis should be performed to evaluate internal organ involvement. A skin biopsy may also be of value. Treatment is supportive, and the use of corticosteroids is still controversial.

Toxic epidermal necrolysis or Lyell's syndrome is the most serious cutaneous drug reaction (Fig. 17-9). The onset is generally acute and, in adults, drugs such as sulfonamides, barbiturates, NSAIDs (phenylbutazone, piroxicam), allopurinol, carbamazepine, and phenytoin are the most frequent cause of the reaction. It is important to emphasize that the scalded skin syndrome that occurs in children secondary to group 2 staphylococcal infections is a

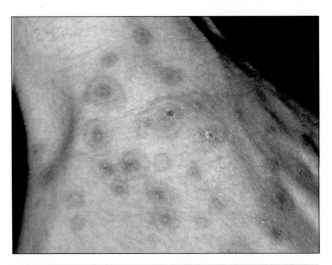

FIGURE 17-6 Typical target lesions with three concentric rings. This patient had a preceding mycoplasma infection.

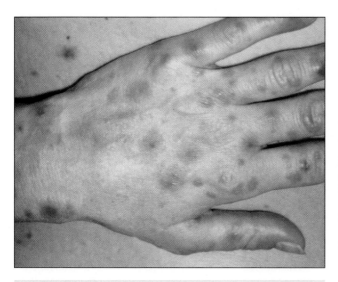

FIGURE 17-7 Inflammatory papules and blisters with surrounding erythema are characteristic of atypical targets. These lesions are usually found in severe blistering reactions to drugs, including erythema multiforme, Stevens-Johnson syndrome, and toxic epidermal necrolysis.

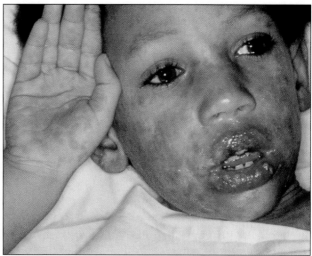

FIGURE 17-8 Mucosal erosions and atypical targets characteristic of a bullous drug eruption. The minor amount of blistering on the skin suggests a diagnosis of erythema multiforme rather than Stevens-Johnson syndrome. The diagnosis of drug reaction was not confirmed for this patient, and the differential diagnosis included both a sulfonamide reaction and post-mycoplasma erythema multiforme.

distinct entity and is not drug metabolizing. The clinical features, pathology, etiology, and prognosis are quite different. True TEN does occur in children as a potentially lethal drug-induced disease. The typical course consists of generalized tender erythema of the skin followed by extensive epidermal necrosis and sloughing of any area of skin or mucous membranes. This widespread denudation leads to a marked loss of fluids and electrolytes and also predisposes to pneumonia and septicemia. Mortality as high as 30% has been reported as a result of these complications. Investigations should include assessment for internal organ involvement (liver, kidney, or hematologic) as in hypersensitivity syndromes, and skin biopsies may be helpful. Treatment should take place in a specialized burn unit and be mainly supportive, but if the patient survives the acute phase of the illness the prognosis is generally favorable, with complete regeneration of the epidermal surfaces within a few weeks.

Photosensitivity

Photosensitive eruptions are produced by an interaction with the drug or its metabolite, and light energy. The drug itself may have been administered topically or orally, and the rash usually appears in sun-exposed areas such as the face, neck, arms, back of hands, and anterior thighs. Three major mechanisms can be considered in the pathogenesis of these reactions (Fig. 17-10) [2••,3–5], and the most common drugs are listed in Table 17-3.

Phototoxic reactions are the most frequent of the photosensitivity responses (Fig. 17-11). Reactions are not immunologic, and may occur on first exposure to the drug if an adequate dose of both drug and light are present. These reactions resemble sunburns and are caused by a lowered sun-sensitivity threshold. Ultraviolet light activates the drug

and the energy that is subsequently emitted damages adjacent tissue. The most commonly implicated medications include chlorpromazine, tetracyclines, psoralens, NSAIDs such as piroxicam and benoxaprofen, sulfonamides, and amiodarone. Appropriate sun protection such as clothing, hats, and use of sunscreens may be preventative.

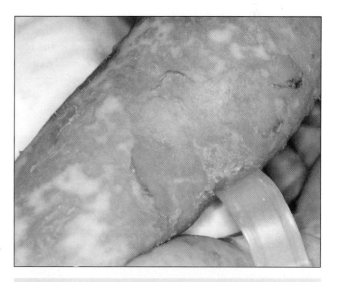

FIGURE 17-9 Painful erythema, blistering, and sloughing skin are caused by toxic epidermal necrolysis. This patient reacted to phenobarbital given for febrile seizures. The skin disease was associated with neutropenia, fever, lymphadenopathy, and pulmonary infiltrates. Supportive treatment was provided in a burn unit. The patient survived, but developed extensive postinflammatory hyperpigmentation.

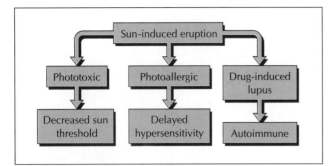

FIGURE 17-10 Algorithm of photosensitive eruptions.

TABLE 17-3 DRUGS CAUSING PHOTOSENSITIVITY

Drug	Incidence	Main reaction
Amiodarone	High	Phototoxic
Chlorpromazine	Medium	Photoallergic
Nalidixic acid	High	Phototoxic
NSAIDs (eg, ketoprofen, naproxen, piroxicam, tiaprofenic acid)	Low	Phototoxic
Protriptyline	High	Phototoxic
Psoralens	High	Phototoxic
Sulfonamides (both antibiotics and sulfonylureas)	Low	Photoallergic
Tetracyclines		
Doxycycline	Medium	Phototoxic
Tetracycline	Low	Phototoxic
Thiazide diuretics	Medium	Photoallergic

NSAIDs—nonsteroidal anti-inflammatory drugs.

Photoallergic eruptions are delayed hypersensitivity responses similar to contact dermatitis, and therefore occur only after initial sensitization. Light acts on the drug or drug metabolite to form a hapten that binds with a tissue antigen. Upon repeat light exposure, a cellular reaction with lymphocytic infiltration results that manifests with a variety of possible morphologies ranging from lichenoid papules to eczema. Hydrochlorothiazide, NSAIDs, and sulfonamides are the drugs most frequently involved.

Drug-induced lupus erythematosus is occasionally seen during treatment with hydralazine, procainamide, isoniazid, alphamethyldopa, and β-blockers such as acebutolol. Patients may develop facial rashes, as seen in systemic lupus erythematosus, but other organ involvement such as nephritis is less common. There may be a genetic predisposition to this condition, as is the case with the slow-acetylator phenotype and isoniazid.

Fixed-Drug Eruptions

Fixed-drug eruptions consist of a solitary or a few sharply demarcated erythematous lesions, usually involving the face or genitalia (Fig. 17-12). As the name would imply, drugs are the only known etiologic agent, but the pathogenesis remains unknown. They recur in the same location with repeat drug exposures and are associated with burning or

pruritus. Once the acute inflammation resolves over 2 to 3 weeks, there is often residual local hyperpigmentation. Pathology of the lesion may be reported as showing features of erythema multiforme, but the two conditions should not be confused. Many drugs have been implicated but the most frequently reported ones are listed in Table 17-4 [2••,3–5].

Contact Dermatitis

For certain drug preparations, topical application leads to local sensitization [2••,3–5]. Upon repeat exposure, redness, pruritus, and a papular eruption, followed by edema and vesiculation, may develop as a result of lymphocytic infiltration. Systemic exposure in the future might lead to flare-ups at the sites of previous reactivity, but more generalized eruptions might also be induced. In sensitized persons, the reaction usually becomes evident 6 to 48 hours after contact.

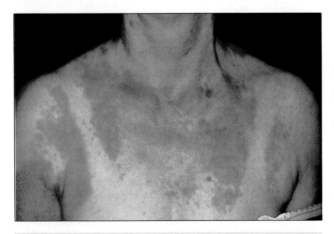

FIGURE 17-11 Erythema and scaling in sun-exposed areas. The patient was taking chlorpromazine.

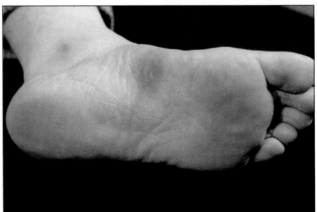

FIGURE 17-12 Well-demarcated red oval of fixed drug eruption, caused by phenolphthalein.

TABLE 17-4 DRUGS CAUSING FIXED DRUG ERUPTIONS	
Antibiotics	Benzodiazepines
Sulfonamides	Chloral hydrate
Tetracyclines	
Penicillins	**NSAIDs and analgesics**
Erythromycin	Acetylsalicylic acid
Nystatin	Phenylbutazone
Metronidazole	Ibuprofen
	Acetominophen
Sedatives and hypnotics	
Barbiturates	**Phenolphthalein**
Opiates	

NSAIDs—nonsteroidal anti-inflammatory drugs.

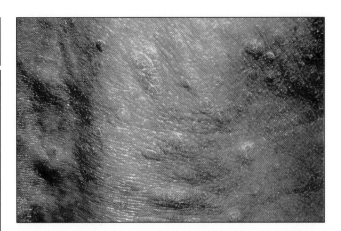

FIGURE 17-13 Purple-red plaques with striated surface show pathologic features of lichen planus-like drug eruption. Drug-induced etiology can be inferred from the pathological features. The patient was receiving intramuscular gold therapy for rheumatoid arthritis.

The most commonly implicated drugs for contact dermatitis include topically applied local anesthetics, antihistamines, antibiotics (*eg*, penicillin, sulfonamides, and neomycin), and corticosteroids. Sometimes the reaction is induced by other components of the cream or lotion rather than the drug itself. The differential diagnosis includes primary irritant contact dermatitis that is nonimmunologic and other forms of dermatitis (*eg*, nummular).

The causal agent of contact dermatitis can often be identified through a careful history, but skin testing may be of benefit when there is uncertainty. In patch testing, components of the topical agent including the drug itself, preservatives such as paraben esters, fragrances, and any other excipients are each applied separately to a small area of skin and left in place for 48 hours. Development of a typical lesion of contact dermatitis is considered positive and confirms the diagnosis [9].

Other Eruptions

Lichenoid cutaneous reactions (Fig. 17-13) that are identical to lichen planus have been reported in association with gold, antimalarials, β-blockers, and captopril. The mechanism by which these agents produce this reaction is unknown.

Erythema nodosum is a panniculitis that is characterized by tender subcutaneous erythematous nodules, usually located over the anterior portion of the lower extremities. It has occasionally been associated with medications such as oral contraceptives, sulfonamides, salicylates, bromides, iodides, and gold, but is most commonly related to infections such as streptococcus, fungi, and tuberculosis, or to chronic granulomatous diseases such as sarcoidosis. The pathogenesis is unknown.

Vasculitis may be confined to the skin or be part of a more generalized multiorgan process such as polyarteritis nodosa. Cutaneous necrotizing vasculitis presents with

palpable purpuric lesions, usually over the lower extremities. Although it is believed that immune mechanisms such as immune complex formation are involved in drug-induced vasculitis, the exact pathogenesis is unknown. The following drugs have been associated with vasculitic reactions: sulfonamides, NSAIDs such as phenylbutazone and indomethacin, propylthiouracil, and phenytoin. In addition, almost all antibiotics have been linked to a case of vasculitis.

Drug-induced bullous pemphigoid and pemphigus are occasionally seen, and are similar in appearance to the idiopathic conditions. Bullous pemphigoid has been reported with a number of drugs, many of which have in common the presence of a sulfur group (*eg*, frusemide, penicillamine, and sulfasalazine). Pemphigus has been seen with medications containing a thiol group in the molecule in over 80% of cases (*eg*, penicillamine, captopril, and gold sodium thiomalate), as well as with antibiotics such as penicillin and cephalosporins.

APPROACH AND MANAGEMENT

The approach to diagnosing drug eruptions is the same as that used for adverse drug reactions in general (Table 17-5) [10•]. Drug reactions occur in complicated clinical scenarios that often entail exposures to multiple agents, but a systematic, stepwise approach that examines each component of the reaction in turn can lead the clinician to the correct diagnosis. Accurate recognition of the rash may require the aid of a dermatologist and possibly a skin biopsy. References such as *A Guide to Drug Eruptions* [2••] provide a quick cross-index between rashes and particular medications as well as a listing of relevant literature. Figure 17-3 illustrates a simple algorithm to follow in order to differentiate among the various types of eruptions, which highlights distinguishing clinical features and key investigations.

TABLE 17-5 STEPS IN THE APPROACH TO A SUSPECTED ADVERSE DRUG REACTION

- Clinical diagnosis of the adverse event (a dermatology consult is often helpful)
- Analysis of drug exposure (timing, consideration of multiple drugs, patient factors, underlying or coexisting diseases)
- Differential diagnosis of skin rash
- Literature search (a clinical pharmacist can be of great help)
- Confirmation (*in vivo* or *in vitro* testing or challenge, where possible)
- Advice to patient (which drug, likelihood of reaction, future risks, safe medications for future use, possible genetic predisposition)
- Reporting to state or federal regulators and drug manufacturer of severe or unusual reactions

Treatment of drug eruptions may simply involve stopping and avoiding the offending agent. Symptomatic care could include topical corticosteroids and oral antihistamines for pruritus. In some of the more severe hypersensitivity reactions, such as SJS, TEN, or vasculitis, systemic corticosteroids or other immunosuppressive therapy might be indicated. It might also be helpful to determine serum concentrations of a drug to confirm exposure and possibly establish a dose–response relationship. Most other testing is either experimental, not readily available, or of limited utility. There are decision aids in the form of questionnaires or computerized spreadsheets with databases to work through the problems of adverse reactions [11•], but these are also not generally available. Physicians should follow a thoughtful, comprehensive, clinical approach to the diagnosis and management of adverse cutaneous drug reactions.

REFERENCES AND RECOMMENDED READING

Recently published papers of particular interest have been highlighted as:
- Of interest
- •• Of outstanding interest

1. Bigby M, Jick S, Jick H, *et al.*: Drug-induced cutaneous reactions. A report from the Boston Collaborative Drug Surveillance Program on 15 438 consecutive inpatients, 1975 to 1982. *JAMA* 1986, 256:3358–3363.

2.•• Bruinsma W: *A Guide to Drug Eruptions*, edn 5. Oosthuizen: The File of Medicines; 1990.

3. Wintroub BU, Stern R: Cutaneous drug reactions: pathogenesis and clinical classification. *J Am Acad Dermatol* 1985, 13:167–179.

4. Kaplan AP: Drug-induced skin disease. *J Allergy Clin Immunol* 1984, 74:573–579.

5. Breathnach SM, Hintner H: *Adverse drug reactions and the skin.* Oxford: Blackwell Scientific Publications; 1992.

6.• Coopman SA, Johnson RA, Platt R, Stern RS: Cutaneous disease and drug reactions in HIV infection. *N Engl J Med* 1993, 328:1670–1674.

7. Shear NH, Spielberg SP: Anticonvulsant hypersensitivity syndrome. *J Clin Invest* 1988, 89:1826–1832.

8.• Bastuji-Garin S, Rzany B, Stern RS, *et al.*: Clinical classification of cases of toxic epidermal necrolysis, Stevens-Johnson syndrome, and erythema multiforme. *Arch Dermatol* 1993, 129:92–96.

9. Bruynzeel DP, van Ketel WG: Patch testing in drug eruptions. *Seminar Dermatol* 1989, 8:196–203.

10.• Shear NH: Diagnosing cutaneous adverse reactions to drugs. *Arch Dermatol* 1990, 126:94–97.

11.• Naranjo CA, Shear NH, Lanctot KL: Advances in the diagnosis of adverse drug reactions. *J Clin Pharmacol* 1992, 32:897–904.

SELECT BIBLIOGRAPHY

Breathnach SM, Hintner H: Adverse drug reactions and the skin. Oxford: Blackwell Scientific Publications; 1992.

Prussick R, Knowles S, Shear NH: Cutaneous drug reactions. *Current Prob Dermatol* 1994, 6:81-124.

Life-Threatening Dermatoses 18
Grace S. Liang-Federman
Francisco A. Kerdel

Key Points
- Dermatologic disorders with manifestations that usually remain confined to the skin may on rare occasions become so widespread that they result in systemic complications.
- Conditions such as psoriasis, pemphigus, and erythematous drug reactions must be managed aggressively to limit morbidity and reduce associated mortality.
- Systemic diseases such as streptococcal or staphylococcal infections, rickettsial and meningococcal infections, and coagulopathies leading to purpura fulminans can first be recognized by changes in the skin.
- Rapid intervention with systemic therapies must be combined with treatment of the skin to reverse systemic disease processes.

The skin is an ideal organ for the direct examination and rapid availability of tissue samples, allowing us easy access to diagnostic clues for various disorders. Although true dermatologic emergencies are fortunately rare, when they do arise, prompt recognition and immediate intervention can be life saving. The life-threatening dermatoses can be divided into two categories: disorders that are primary skin conditions with potential systemic complications, and systemic disorders that have prominent manifestations in the skin. Immunocompromised patients represent a subset of patients who are susceptible to a host of other unusual skin conditions, especially those that are infectious (Table 18-1). In these patients the clinical presentation can be greatly modified by unpredictable inflammatory responses, making skin findings atypical or nonspecific.

PRIMARY SKIN DISORDERS WITH POTENTIAL SYSTEMIC COMPLICATIONS

Toxic Epidermal Necrolysis

Toxic epidermal necrolysis (TEN), or acute disseminated epidermal necrosis, is a fulminant desquamating process that begins as a generalized morbilliform or confluent erythema and rapidly progresses to extensive bullae formation with exfoliation (Fig. 18-1). The skin lesions are typically painful, and mucosal involvement can be extensive. Loss of nails is not uncommon, but the scalp is usually spared. Patients are often febrile, and the acute phase may be associated with multiple complications, including fluid and electrolyte imbalances, and sepsis. These latter complications result in a mortality rate of 25% to 70%.

The majority of TEN cases have been associated with the intake of various drugs; antibiotics, antiseizure medications, nonsteroidal antiinflammatory drugs, and allopurinol are commonly implicated. Skin lesions appear between 2 to 21 days after the ingestion of a given agent and become generalized within 24 to 48

TABLE 18-1 CHARACTERISTICS OF LIFE-THREATENING DERMATOSES IN IMMUNOCOMPROMISED PATIENTS
Ecthyma gangrenosum
Disseminated candidiasis
Varicella-zoster virus infections
Disseminated herpes simplex virus infections
"Deep fungal" infections
Cryptococcus, histoplasmosis, *Aspergillus*, *Rhizopus*, mucormycosis, protothecosis, *Coccidioides*, *Paracoccidioides*, *Blastomyces*
Tuberculosis and atypical mycobacterial infections
Nocardia and Actinomyces infections
Kaposi's sarcoma
Bacillary angiomatosis

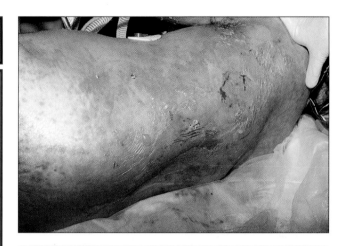

FIGURE 18-1 Toxic epidermal necrolysis: widespread areas of desquamation on the back with erythema.

hours. Laboratory tests may yield findings such as prerenal azotemia, elevated liver enzyme levels, disseminated intravascular coagulation, and, rarely, pancreatitis. Neutropenia, lymphopenia, anemia, and thrombocytopenia portend a poor prognosis. Histopathologic analyses of skin biopsy specimens show full-thickness epidermal necrosis with a minimal-to-absent dermal mononuclear cell infiltrate.

The management of TEN should ideally be undertaken in a burn unit or intensive care setting where fluid and electrolyte levels can be closely monitored, and careful attention can be paid to nutritional support. Ophthalmologic consultation is essential to prevent long-term sequelae, including xerophthalmia, visual impairment, and even blindness from conjunctival, corneal, and lacrimal duct damage. Skin care should be aimed at rapid healing and prevention of infection. Areas not affected should be handled carefully to minimize progression. Some authors advocate stripping the necrotic epidermis and placing xenografts, homografts, or skin substitutes while the patient is receiving general anesthesia. Silver nitrate irrigation, 0.5%, or frequent dressing changes may be as effective. Corticosteroids should not be administered because they may increase the frequency of medical complications, mask signs of impending sepsis, and impair wound healing. Likewise, prophylactic antibiotic use is not recommended, although careful monitoring for secondary skin infection and vigorous pulmonary toilet are essential. *Staphylococcus aureus* is a common skin pathogen found early in the course of the disease whereas *Pseudomonas aeruginosa* infection may develop at later stages. The role of other treatment modalities such as plasmapheresis, cyclophosphamide therapy, and hyperbaric oxygen application have yet to be defined [1••,2].

Erythema Multiforme Major

Erythema multiforme (EM) is considered by some authors to be related to TEN in that the entities may represent ends of a spectrum of hypersensitivity disorders [3]. EM minor accounts for 80% of EM cases and is characterized by

targetlike plaques with dusky centers and "multiform" urticarial, annular, solid, and bullous plaques often involving the palms, soles, and distal extremities. EM minor is commonly associated with an antecedent history of herpes simplex virus infection. In EM major or Stevens-Johnson syndrome, which constitutes the other 20% of EM cases, skin involvement is extensive and is associated with involvement of at least two mucosal surfaces as well as prominent systemic symptoms (Fig. 18-2). Most cases are sporadic, lasting 3 to 6 weeks, but recurrent cases have been reported. EM major is commonly associated with drugs or infection with *Mycoplasma pneumoniae*, and less often with herpes simplex virus infection. The treatment of EM major depends on the severity of disease and on the underlying condition. If involvement is extensive, TEN-like management may be required [4••].

Staphylococcal Scalded Skin Syndrome

Toxic epidermal necrolysis must be distinguished from another disease characterized by extensive sloughing of the

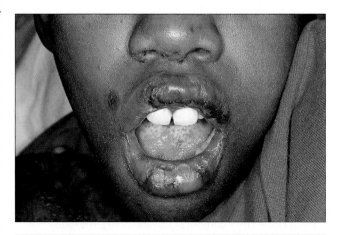

FIGURE 18-2 Erythema multiforme major (Stevens-Johnson syndrome) with severe involvement of the oral mucosa.

TABLE 18-2 CONDITIONS ASSOCIATED WITH EXFOLIATIVE ERYTHRODERMA

Condition	Diagnostic clues
Psoriasis	Family history, skin biopsy
Dermatitis: atopic, contact, seborrheic	Eosinophilia, increased IgE
Drug induced	History
Cutaneous T-cell lymphoma (mycosis fungoides)	Skin biopsy: atypical lymphocytes
Lymphoma, leukemia	Skin or lymph node biopsy, CBC, chest radiograph
Pityriasis rubra pilaris	Clinical presentation, skin biopsy
Underlying malignancy	Radiographic studies, tissue biopsy
Icthyosis	Family history, skin biopsy

CBC—complete blood count.

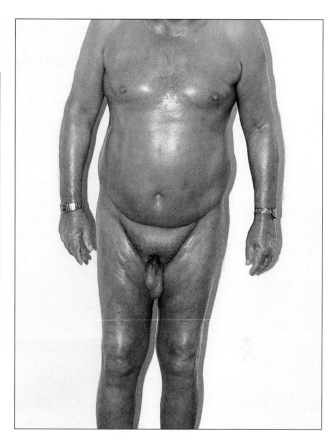

FIGURE 18-3 Diffuse erythroderma secondary to psoriasis.

skin, staphylococcal scalded skin syndrome (SSSS) [5•]. Most patients with SSSS are children under 5 years of age; in this setting the condition runs a benign course. However, when SSSS occurs in adults, especially those with impaired renal function, the condition has a worse prognosis. Patients present with a faint, scarlatiniform erythema and superficial desquamation, often with periorificial and flexural accentuation. Mucous membrane involvement is not prominent, but an occult focus of staphylococcal infection may be present in the nose, conjunctiva, or umbilicus.

Staphylococcal scalded skin syndrome is the result of an exfoliating toxin produced by *S. aureus* phage II; therefore, the skin lesions of SSSS are usually sterile. Frozen-section examinations of the blister roof or skin biopsy specimens can be used to distinguish SSSS from the more serious TEN. In SSSS, the split occurs subcorneally within the stratum granulosum, whereas a subepidermal split is seen in TEN. Cytodiagnosis (Tzanck smear) can also be helpful. In SSSS there are broad epithelial cells with small nuclei, whereas in TEN there are cuboidal cells with large nuclei and inflammatory cells. A prompt diagnosis allows rapid treatment of the staphylococcal focus with antibiotics to reduce the amount of toxin present. Careful attention to skin hygiene and abundant application of emollients are also indicated.

Exfoliative Erythrodermas

Exfoliative erythroderma is a generalized erythematous scaling eruption that may be secondary to a variety of conditions (Table 18-2). Despite attempts to determine the cause of the erythroderma, approximately 40% of cases remain of idiopathic origin. Patients may have associated peripheral edema, alopecia, nail dystrophy, lymphadenopathy, hepatosplenomegaly, and impaired temperature regulation.

A diagnostic evaluation should include multiple skin biopsies, with particular attention paid to the possibility of cutaneous T-cell lymphoma. In these cases, examinations for malignant cells in the circulation (Sézary cells) and for lymph node or systemic involvement are essential. Patients with psoriasis (Figs. 18-3 and 18-4) may have family histo-

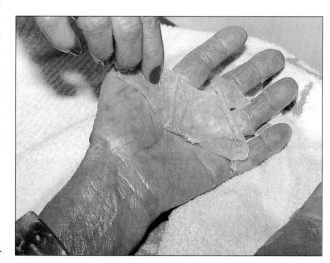

FIGURE 18-4 Desquamation of a thick keratoderma of the palm in a patient with psoriasis.

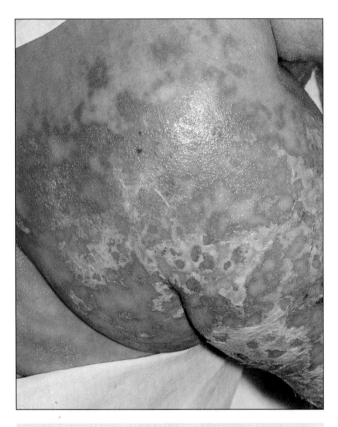

FIGURE 18-5 Generalized pustular psoriasis (Von Zumbusch type): "lakes of pus" with moist red plaques on the shoulder and back.

ries of psoriasis or classic nail changes. Patients with atopic dermatitis may have severe pruritus and lichenification, peripheral eosinophilia, and elevated serum IgE levels. The erythroderma of pityriasis rubra pilaris usually has a distinct salmon-pink hue with islands of spared skin and a yellowish keratoderma of the palms and soles. Histories of drug or contact allergy should be sought.

Patients with erythroderma should be treated according to the underlying process. In cases with no discernible cause, conservative measures are recommended, including whirlpool baths, emollient application, mid-potency topical steroid administration, and occlusive dressings [6•].

Pustular Psoriasis

Patients with the Von Zumbusch type of pustular psoriasis present with fulminant widespread erythema, with crops of sterile subcorneal pustules that coalesce into "lakes of pus" (Fig. 18-5). The oral mucosa and tongue may be involved, and the patient is usually febrile. The condition may be associated with hypocalcemia, hypoalbuminemia, and leukocytosis. Fluid and protein loss, cardiac failure, and sepsis are not unusual complications [7•]. A similar generalized form of pustular psoriasis can occur during pregnancy (impetigo herpetiformis), typically appearing before the sixth month of pregnancy and often recurring in subsequent pregnancies.

Treatment begins with hospitalization and conservative measures such as bedrest and sedation, topical emollient application, and maintenance of fluid and electrolyte balance. Provocative agents such as lithium, β-blockers, antimalarials, and salicylates should be discontinued. The discontinuation of systemic corticosteroid therapy or discontinuation of the widespread use of potent topical steroids under occlusion have precipitated generalized pustular psoriasis; therefore, their use in patients with psoriasis should be avoided. Phototherapy, the topical application of coal tar, and anthralin use are relatively contraindicated, and PUVA (psoralens and ultraviolet A light therapy) should be used only with extreme caution. Systemic agents such as methotrexate, etretinate, dapsone, hydroxyurea, and cyclosporin-A should be given according to the severity of the disease. In the case of impetigo herpetiformis, systemic steroid administration and general supportive measures are recommended. (*See* Simpson and Lowe, Psoriasis.)

Pemphigus and Pemphigoid

Severe cases of pemphigus vulgaris (and less often, bullous pemphigoid) can lead to extensive cutaneous denudation. Before corticosteroids were available for treatment use, the disease carried a mortality rate in excess of 50%. Paraneoplastic pemphigus is a recently described entity associated with antibodies against desmoplakin-I [8]. This disease is associated most often with reticuloendothelial malignancies and has a particularly poor prognosis.

SYSTEMIC DISORDERS WITH PROMINENT CUTANEOUS MANIFESTATIONS

Toxic Shock and Associated Syndromes

Toxic Shock Syndrome (TSS) has an incidence rate of 3 to 14 per 100,000 women of menstrual age and a mortality rate of 2%. It is most often seen in association with menstruation, and 98% of affected women have reported having used tampons at the onset of the disease. The incidence of this disease appears to be decreasing with the discontinued use of some super-absorbency tampons. Postoperative wound infections, superficial skin infections, and postpartum complications are less common predisposing causes of TSS [9,10].

Clinical features of TSS include fever (>40°C), hypotension, and a diffuse nontender erythroderma that appears within the first 24 hours and leads to a generalized desquamation after 7 to 10 days, most prominently on the hands and feet. Mucosal involvement may manifest as a strawberry tongue or as conjunctival, oropharyngeal, or vaginal hyperemia. The patient can have a sore throat, myalgias, gastrointestinal symptoms, and renal failure, and central nervous system changes such as headaches, dizziness, confusion, and agitation.

TSS is thought to be caused by exotoxins (*eg*, TSST-1) produced by a phage group I strain of *Staphylococcus aureus*. Blood cultures, however, are only rarely positive for staphylococcal organisms, and there may not be actual infection but only colonization of the responsible strain as a part of the patient's local flora. Failure to eradicate the organisms or lack of development of antibodies against the endotoxin may cause recurrences of TSS at rates of as high as 30%.

Prompt recognition and early intervention are essential. Tampon removal, drainage of pus, and debridement or irrigation of wounds serve to reduce bacterial load. Aggressive fluid replacement, and if necessary, the administration of systemic adrenergic agents, should be undertaken to maintain adequate blood pressure. The use of antistaphylococcal antibiotics is recommended to eliminate the focus of staphylococcal organisms, but these agents do not actually alter the immediate course of TSS. The antibiotics of choice are penicillinase-resistant penicillins (oxacillin or nafcillin), or first-generation cephalosporins, vancomycin, or clindamycin in penicillin-allergic patients.

Staphylococcal-induced TSS must be differentiated from streptococcal toxic shock–like syndrome (TSLS), or "toxic strep syndrome," which is caused by pyrogenic exotoxins (M types 1 and 3) produced by group A *Streptococcus*. TSLS is a fulminant disease that can be seen in association with cellulitis or other soft-tissue infections. Clinical features include fever, hypotension, mental status changes, toxin-induced renal impairment (distinct from poststreptococcal glomerulonephritis), and a variety of cutaneous changes such as swelling, erythema, bullae, scarletiniform rash, and desquamation. Unlike in TSS, blood cultures are often positive for streptococcal organisms [11•,12].

The recommended treatment for TSLS is similar to that for TSS. Fluid and electrolyte support, surgical debridement, and antibiotic therapy (high-dose penicillin or clindamycin) must be initiated promptly.

Kawasaki Syndrome

Kawasaki syndrome or mucocutaneous lymph node syndrome is an idiopathic, acute disease resembling toxic shock syndrome [13,14•,15]. It primarily affects children and adolescents, with 95% of patients being less than 5 years of age. Clinical criteria for diagnosis include fever lasting 5 or more days; bilateral conjunctivitis; oropharyngeal mucous membrane inflammation manifested by diffuse erythema, fissured lips, or strawberry tongue; edema and erythema of distal extremities with periungual desquamation; a diffuse erythematous rash that may be scarlatiniform, morbilliform, or macular; and cervical lymphadenopathy measuring greater than 1.5 cm (Table 18-3). Early histopathologic changes show vasculitis involving arterioles, venules, and capillaries.

Although the initial febrile course is self-limited, approximately 1.5% of patients die of late cardiac complications, especially coronary artery aneurysm and myocardial infarction. Treatment to prevent coronary artery

TABLE 18-3 CLINICAL CRITERIA FOR THE DIAGNOSIS OF KAWASAKI SYNDROME
Fever lasting ≥5 d
Bilateral conjunctivitis
Oropharyngeal mucous membrane inflammation
Distal extremity edema, erythema, desquamation
Diffuse erythematous rash
Cervical lymphadenopathy >1.5 cm

lesions and to reduce systemic inflammation entails giving aspirin (100 mg/kg/d for 14 days, then 3–5 mg/kg/d) with intravenous gammaglobulin in a single infusion of 2 g/kg over 10 hours [16].

Purpura Fulminans

Disseminated intravascular coagulation (DIC) can result in the sudden onset of extensive petechiae, purpura, hemorrhagic bullae, and severe skin necrosis due to generalized cutaneous thromboses (Fig. 18-6). Patients have various signs of hemolysis, bleeding, and thromboembolism. Most cases of purpura fulminans are fatal within 2 to 3 days of onset and can be seen in association with severe infections (especially gram-negative septicemia, streptococcal and staphylococcal sepsis, and acute varicella infections), obstetric complications, malignancies, trauma, snake bites, and giant hemangiomas (Kasabach-Merritt syndrome). Patients with congenital or acquired protein C and protein S deficiencies may be particularly predisposed to developing purpura fulminans.

Characteristic laboratory findings show consumption of platelets and clotting factors with decreased fibrinogen and increased fibrin degradation products. Skin biopsy specimens show intravascular thrombi, hemorrhage, and necrosis.

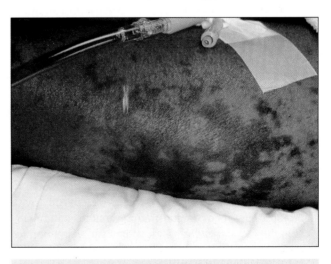

FIGURE 18-6 Purpura fulminans in a patient with acute meningococcemia: large areas of purpura and petechiae on the lateral trunk. (*Courtesy of* A. Blauvelt, MD).

The first objective of therapy is to treat the underlying condition and transfuse with blood, platelets, and fresh frozen plasma as indicated. Extensive cutaneous necrosis can be treated with skin debridement and grafting. Debate over the role of heparin and other agents such as aspirin, dipyridamole, and ε-aminocaproic acid in controlling consumption coagulopathy is still controversial [17••].

Meningococcemia

Septicemia and meningitis from *Neisseria meningitidis* (especially types A, B, and C) carry an overall mortality rate of 10% to 50%. Severe meningococcal infection is most common in children, but epidemics can occur in adults living in close contact—such as in military barracks. Cutaneous eruptions may be the first clue to early diagnosis, although in about 25% of cases there will be no skin findings. Early skin lesions are morbilliform, urticarial, or discrete macules and papules. Characteristic petechiae and purpura appear later and are caused by organisms within capillary walls and by DIC. Late purpuric lesions are the result of immune complex–mediated vasculitis. Nodules, bullae, ulcers, and even full-blown purpura fulminans may develop.

The diagnosis is confirmed by the detection of *N. meningitidis* organisms in blood cultures or cerebrospinal fluid. Treatment should begin promptly with the intravenous administration of high-dose benzyl penicillin, chloramphenicol, or ceftriaxone. Exposed persons in close contact with the patient should be given prophylactic treatment with rifampin [18,19].

Rocky Mountain Spotted Fever

The recognition of the most severe rickettsial infection, Rocky Mountain spotted fever (RMSF), is imperative because untreated cases carry a reported mortality rate of up to 80%. The disease is caused by *Rickettsia rickettsii* and is transmitted by the wood tick, *Dermacentor andersoni*, in the western United States, and mainly by *D. variabilis* in the eastern United States [20•].

Approximately 3 to 12 days after a tick bite, patients have the sudden onset of fevers, chills, malaise, headache, myalgias, and arthralgias. Two to six days later a maculopapular eruption characteristically appears on the wrists, ankles, and forearms, spreads to the palms and soles, and then extends centrally to the trunk and face. The rash soon becomes petechial and more confluent. Large ecchymoses and acral gangrene are not unusual. Patients appear severely ill and can have myocarditis, hepatitis, renal failure, and neurologic changes. The diagnosis can be established with skin biopsy specimens demonstrating vasculitis and organisms in the vascular endothelium when using immunofluorescent staining. Serologic studies are valuable in confirming the diagnosis of RMSF, but results do not become reliably positive for 6 to 10 days after the onset of clinical symptoms. Tetracycline, doxycycline, and chloramphenicol are effective when administered early. The use of sulfon-

TABLE 18-4 OTHER SYSTEMIC DISEASES WITH PROMINENT CUTANEOUS MANIFESTATIONS
Angioedema (hereditary and allergic)
Systemic lupus erythematosus or neonatal lupus
Dermatomyositis
Relapsing polychondritis
Vasculitis
Behçet's disease
Cholesterol emboli
Systemic mastocytosis
Histiocytosis X
Graft-versus-host disease

amides is contraindicated because they may actually enhance rickettsial infection. Other life-threatening disorders that have prominent manifestations in the skin are listed in Table 18-4.

CONCLUSION

Life-threatening skin conditions can have multiple morphologic patterns, and the differential diagnosis is often extensive. Establishing a diagnosis may be difficult, but it is important for the clinician to be familiar with these entities because the skin may offer the first clues to recognition of a severe systemic illness. Important information can be rapidly obtained through the performance of skin biopsies and other tests such as Tzanck smears and tissue cultures. Prompt intervention with systemic therapy and local skin care is imperative in such cases.

REFERENCES AND RECOMMENDED READING

Recently published papers of particular interest have been highlighted as:
• Of interest
•• Of outstanding interest

1.•• Roujeau JC, Chosidon O, Saiag P, Guillaume JC: Toxic epidermal necrolysis (Lyell syndrome). *J Am Acad Dermatol* 1990, 23:1039–1058.

2. Avakian R, Flowers FP, Araujo OE, Ramos-Caro FA: Toxic epidermal necrolysis: a review. *J Am Acad Dermatol* 1991, 25:69–79.

3. Bastuji-Garin S, Rzany B, Stern RS, *et al.*: Clinical classification of cases of toxic epidermal necrolysis, Stevens-Johnson syndrome, and erythema multiforme. *Arch Dermatol* 1993, 129:92–96.

4.•• Brice SL, Huff JC, Weston WL: Erythema multiforme. In *Current Problems in Dermatology*, edn 2. Edited by Weston WL. Chicago: Year Book; 1990:5–25.

5.• Resnick SD: Staphylococcal toxin-mediated syndromes in childhood. *Semin Dermatol* 1992, 11:11–18.

6.• Wilson DC, Jester JD, King LE: Erythroderma and exfoliative dermatitis. *Clin Dermatol* 1993, 11:67–72.

7.• Zelickson BD, Muller SA: Generalized pustular psoriasis: a review of 63 cases. *Arch Dermatol* 1991, 127:1339–1345.

8. Anhalt GJ, Kim SC, Stanley JR, *et al.*: Paraneoplastic pemphigus: an autoimmune mucocutaneous disease associated with neoplasia. *N Engl J Med* 1990, 323:1729–1735.

9. Reingold AL, Hargrett NT, Dan BB, *et al.*: Nonmenstrual toxic shock syndrome: a review of 130 cases. *Ann Intern Med* 1982, 96:871–874.

10. Reingold AL: Toxic shock syndrome: an update. *Am J Obstet Gynecol* 1991, 165:1236–1239.

11.• The Working Group on Severe Streptococcal Infections: Defining the group A streptococcal toxic shock syndrome. *JAMA* 1993, 269:390–391.

12. Wood TF, Potter MA, Jonasson O: Streptococcal toxic shock-like syndrome: the importance of surgical intervention. *Ann Surg* 1993, 217:109–114.

13. Gersony WM: Diagnosis and management of Kawasaki disease. *JAMA* 1991, 265:2699–2703.

14.• Wortmann DW: Kawasaki syndrome. *Semin Dermatol* 1992, 11:37–47.

15. Leung DYM, Meissner HC, Fulton DR, *et al.*: Toxic shock syndrome toxin-secreting *Staphylococcus aureus* in Kawasaki syndrome. *Lancet* 1993, 342:1385–1388.

16. Newburger JW, Takahashi M, Beiser AS, *et al.*: A single intravenous infusion of gamma globulin as compared with four infusions in the treatment of acute Kawasaki syndrome. *N Engl J Med* 1991, 324:1633–1639.

17.•• Francis RB. Acquired purpura fulminans. *Semin Thromb Hemostasis* 1990, 16:310–325.

18. Wong VK, Hitchcock W, Mason WH: Meningococcal infections in children: a review of 100 cases. *Pediatr Infect Dis J* 1989, 8:224–1227.

19. Klein NJ, Heyderman RS, Levin M: Management of meningococcal infections. *Br J Hosp Med* 1993, 50:42–49.

20.• Weber DJ, Walker DH: Rocky Mountain spotted fever. *Infect Dis Clin North Am* 1991, 5:19–35.

SELECT BIBLIOGRAPHY

Frieden IJ, Resnick SD: Childhood exanthems, old and new. *Pediatr Clin North Am* 1991, 38:859–887.

Kerdel FA: Life-threatening dermatoses. In *The Dermatological Signs of Internal Disease*, edn 2. Edited by Callen JP, Jorizzo J, Greer KE, *et al.* Philadelphia: WB Saunders; In press.

Krusinski PA, Flowers FP, eds: *Life Threatening Dermatoses*. Chicago: Year Book; 1987.

Levine N: Management of life-threatening dermatoses. *Emerg Med Clin North Am* 1985, 3:747–763.

Phillips TJ, Dover JS: Recent advances in dermatology. *N Engl J Med* 1992, 326:167–178.

Cutaneous Manifestations of Internal Malignancy

19

Philip R. Cohen

> **Key Points**
> - Cutaneous metastases are directly related to the tumor.
> - Genodermatoses with malignant potential are a clinical feature of a cancer-associated inherited disorder.
> - Cutaneous paraneoplastic syndromes are indirectly secondary to the neoplasm.
> - Mucocutaneous reactions to antineoplastic agents are caused by treatment of the malignancy.
> - Appropriate evaluation and treatment of an individual should be undertaken when a mucosal or skin lesion that may be a dermatologic manifestation of an internal malignancy is discovered.

Lesions of the skin and mucosa may be manifestations of internal malignancy. Systemic neoplasms may initially present with cutaneous metastases; alternatively, metastatic tumor involvement of the skin may reflect progressive or recurrent cancer. There are several inherited dermatoses in which patients may subsequently develop disease-related neoplasms. The mucocutaneous manifestations of these conditions may suggest or establish the diagnosis of a genodermatosis with malignant potential. There are also several dermatologic conditions that may precede, occur concurrently with, or follow the discovery of an associated internal malignancy. The identification of a cutaneous paraneoplastic syndrome should prompt an appropriate investigation for an asymptomatic neoplasm in a previously cancer-free individual, or a diligent search for a progressing or a recurring malignancy in an oncology patient. Once the diagnosis of an internal malignancy has been established, patients are often treated with systemic chemotherapeutic drugs. Therefore, adverse mucocutaneous reactions to antineoplastic agents may occur in these individuals. This chapter provides a brief overview of cutaneous manifestations of internal malignancy: cutaneous metastases, genodermatoses with malignant potential, cutaneous paraneoplastic syndromes, and mucocutaneous reactions to antineoplastic agents.

CUTANEOUS METASTASES

Cutaneous metastases may be the initial manifestation of an undiagnosed malignancy in a previously cancer-free individual or the cutaneous stigmata of tumor progression or recurrence in an oncology patient [1••]. However, a recently published retrospective study noted cutaneous involvement of internal malignancy at the time of presentation in merely 1.3% of 7316 patients; in fact, skin involvement was the first sign of cancer in only 59 patients (0.8%) [2•].

Solid Tumors

The malignancies that occur most frequently in the general population account for the cancers that most commonly metastasize to the skin. These include pulmonary and colon carcinoma, melanoma, and tumors of the oral cavity, kidney, and stomach in men. In women, carcinomas of the breast, colon, lung, and ovary, followed by melanoma, are the malignancies that most often have skin metastases [1••].

The morphology, pattern, and distribution of these lesions can be variable. The clinical presentation can range from bound-down, indurated sclerodermoid skin changes (Fig. 19-1) to dermal papules or subcutaneous nodules (with or without ulceration) (Fig. 19-2) or to inflammatory patches or plaques of erythema (Fig. 19-3). Carcinoma metastatic to the skin often presents with skin lesions that overlie the site of the underlying neoplasm. The scalp and the umbilical region (Sister Joseph's nodule) are two of the more frequent sites of distant metastases. Less commonly, metastatic carcinoma may occur in a subungual location and mimic an acute paronychia [3] or may present in a dermatomal distribution and mimic a varicella-zoster virus infection [4]. When the possibility of a cutaneous metastasis is suspected, a biopsy of the lesion for microscopic evaluation should be considered in order to confirm the diagnosis.

Patients with solid tumors, as well as leukemias, lymphomas, and sarcomas, may present with or develop skin lesions. This particularly affects patients with Stewart-Treves syndrome, which is characterized by lymphangiosarcomas that appear in the lymphedematous upper extremity of patients approximately 10 years after they have been treated for breast cancer by means of radical mastectomy with or without local radiotherapy.

Leukemia Cutis

Leukemia cutis is characterized by the infiltration of leukemic cells into the skin; the lesions may also be referred to as either chloromas (because the presence of granulocyte myeloperoxidase may result in a green appearance of the gross specimen) or granulocytic sarcomas (when the cutaneous leukemic infiltrate is composed of immature cells of the granulocytic series) (Fig. 19-4) [5]. Although leukemia cutis may present as gingival hypertrophy in acute monocytic leukemia and acute myelomonocytic leukemia, or as erythroderma or bullous lesions in chronic lymphocytic leukemia, it most commonly appears as papules and nodules. The onset of leukemia cutis is generally a poor prognostic sign: 37 of 42 patients in one series died within 1 year after their leukemic infiltrates had been detected.

Lymphoma Cutis

Lymphoma cutis may be either cutaneous T-cell lymphoma (mycosis fungoides), Hodgkin's lymphoma, or non-Hodgkin's (cutaneous B-cell) lymphoma. **Cutaneous T-cell lymphoma** typically presents as either erythematous

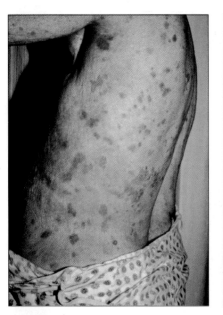

FIGURE 19-1 Carcinoma en cuirasse is characterized by the erythematous area of confluent induration secondary to neoplasm on the left flank; red tumor nodules and plaques of metastatic breast carcinoma are also present. (*From* Cohen [1••]; with permission.)

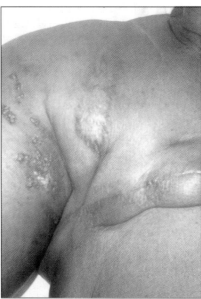

FIGURE 19-2 Papules in the mastectomy scar and ipsilateral edematous arm of a woman with recurrent breast carcinoma. (*From* Cohen [1••]; with permission.)

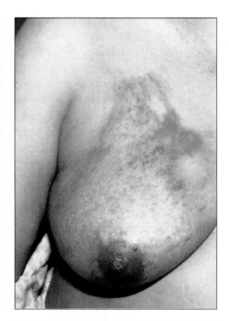

FIGURE 19-3 Carcinoma erysipelatoides is a morphologic pattern of metastatic carcinoma (often involving the lymph vessels) that appears as sharply demarcated areas of erythema that mimic an erysipelas infection. (*From* Cohen [1••]; with permission.)

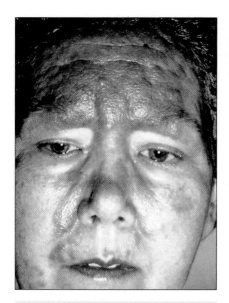

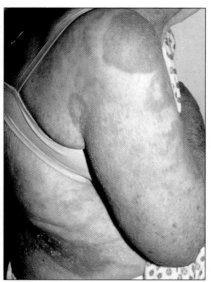

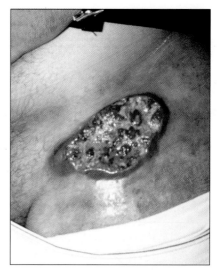

FIGURE 19-4 Leukemia cutis on the face of a 52-year-old white woman with chronic myelomonocytic leukemia that presented as extensive asymptomatic blue-gray to purple infiltrated plaques. (*From* Cohen and coworkers [5]; with permission.)

FIGURE 19-5 Cutaneous T-cell lymphoma appearing as erythematous patches and plaques, which have been present for several years, on the right shoulder, arm, and back of an elderly white woman. (*From* Cohen [1••]; with permission.)

FIGURE 19-6 A large ulcer with a granulation tissue–like base and advancing, indurated borders and surrounding erythema on the left inguinal area that demonstrated recurrent Hodgkin's disease on microscopic evaluation of a lesional biopsy. (*From* Cohen [1••]; with permission.)

patches (Fig. 19-5), lichenoid plaques, or tumor nodules; Sézary syndrome refers to cutaneous T-cell lymphoma with pruritus, exfoliative erythroderma, and abnormal mononuclear cells (mycosis cells or Sézary cells) circulating in the blood. Depending on the extent of disease, patients with cutaneous T-cell lymphoma often receive, either sequentially or concurrently, several of the available treatment modalities: conventional or electron-beam radiotherapy, extracorporeal or routine photochemotherapy, interferon alpha, retinoids (oral isotretinoin or etretinate), and systemic or topical chemotherapy [1••].

Cutaneous involvement of **Hodgkin's disease** is uncommon. The skin lesions usually appear as papules or nodules; dermal infiltration, erythroderma, plaques, tumors, and ulcers are other clinical morphologies (Fig. 19-6). Although the specific skin lesions often respond to systemic chemotherapy, local radiotherapy, or both, the prognosis for the patient is generally poor because cutaneous Hodgkin's disease usually reflects hematogenous dissemination in patients with advanced disease [1••].

Non-Hodgkin's lymphomas of the skin are also uncommon and can either present with the skin as the primary site of involvement (often in patients with an early clinical stage of lymphoma, and therefore, a prolonged disease-free survival) or develop in the skin as a secondary site of dissemination (in patients with advanced clinical stages of disease associated with a poor prognosis). Cutaneous lesions of non-Hodgkin's lymphoma typically appear as a solitary nodule or a few nonulcerating tumors on the head and neck. When the disease is limited to the skin, local treatment (excision or

radiotherapy) may be curative; if the lymphoma is extracutaneous, systemic polychemotherapy (with or without adjuvant local treatment) is necessary [1••].

GENODERMATOSES WITH MALIGNANT POTENTIAL

Inherited disorders with dermatologic manifestations are referred to as genodermatoses [6••]. Some genodermatoses are associated with the potential for subsequent development of a disease-related malignancy (Table 19-1) [6••,7•,8,9]. The individual genodermatoses with malignant potential may be inherited in an autosomal dominant, an autosomal recessive, or an X-linked pattern. The detection of disease-associated cutaneous features should enable the physician to suspect the systemic condition. Once the diagnosis of a genodermatosis with malignant potential has been confirmed, the patient should be appropriately screened and periodically followed up for disease-associated neoplasms. In addition, the members of the patient's family should be evaluated for the genodermatosis. Both the patient and the patient's family should receive genetic counseling, as well. The cutaneous features of some of the autosomal dominant genodermatoses with malignant potential are briefly summarized in the following section.

Nevoid Basal Cell Carcinoma Syndrome

Cutaneous findings that may be present in patients with nevoid basal cell carcinoma syndrome are basal cell carci-

TABLE 19-1 GENODERMATOSES WITH MALIGNANT POTENTIAL

Genodermatosis	Inheritance	Predominant malignancies
Ataxia telangiectasia	AR	Lymphoma, leukemia
Bloom's syndrome	AR	Leukemia
Bruton's sex-linked agammaglobulinemia	XL	Leukemia, lymphoma
Chédiak-Higashi syndrome	AR	Lymphoma
Cowden's syndrome (multiple hamartoma syndrome)	AD	Breast carcinoma, thyroid carcinoma
Dyskeratosis congenita	XL	Squamous cell carcinoma of the skin, mucosa, and esophagus; pancreatic carcinoma; Hodgkin's lymphoma; leukemia
Fanconi's anemia	AR	Leukemia
Gardner's syndrome	AD	Colon adenocarcinoma
Hemochromatosis	AR	Hepatocellular carcinoma
Howel-Evans syndrome (tylosis)	AD	Esophageal carcinoma
Muir-Torre syndrome	AD	Colorectal carcinoma, genitourinary carcinoma
Multiple endocrine neoplasias IIB or III (multiple mucosal neuroma syndrome)	AD	Medullary carcinoma of thyroid, pheochromocytoma
Neurofibromatosis 1 (von Recklinghausen's disease)	AD	Neurofibrosarcomas, brain tumors, neuroblastomas, pheochromocytoma, medullary thyroid carcinoma, melanoma, Wilms' tumor, rhabdomyosarcoma, leukemia
Nevoid basal cell carcinoma syndrome (Gorlin's syndrome)	AD	Basal cell carcinomas, medulloblastoma, fibrosarcoma of the jaw
Peutz-Jeghers syndrome	AD	Reproductive organ neoplasms, colon adenocarcinoma
Porphyria cutanea tarda	AD	Hepatocellular carcinoma
Tuberous sclerosis (Bourneville's disease)	AD	Cardiac rhabdomyoma, astrocytoma, glioblastoma
von Hippel-Lindau	AD	Cerebellar and spinal hemangioblastomas, pheochromocytoma, hypernephroma
Werner's syndrome (adult progeria)	AR	Sarcomas, meningiomas
Wiskott-Aldrich syndrome	XL	Leukemia, lymphoma

AD—autosomal dominant; AR—autosomal recessive; XL—X-linked. *From* Cohen [6••]; with permission.

nomas, café au lait macules, dermal calcinosis, epithelial cysts, fibromas, lipomas, milia, and palmoplantar pits (Fig. 19-7). The basal cell carcinomas often mimic the appearance of benign nevi and continue to develop throughout the patient's life. In addition to calcification of the falx cerebri and odontogenic keratocysts of the jaw, several skeletal anomalies (most commonly involving the ribs and vertebrae) are also present in these patients (Fig. 19-8) [6••].

Gardner's Syndrome

The presence of colonic polyposis in individuals with multiple epidermoid cysts, desmoid tumors, fibromas, or osteomas characterizes Gardner's syndrome (Fig. 19-9). Dental anomalies, ocular pigmentation of the fundi, and polyps of the small intestine and stomach are additional features of this syndrome. Because malignant transformation of the colonic polyps occurs in all patients with Gardner's syndrome, prophylactic colectomy is recommended [6••].

Howel-Evans Syndrome

Howel-Evans syndrome is the association of hereditary palmar and plantar hyperkeratosis (tylosis) with the development of esophageal carcinoma. Since the original description of this syndrome in 1958, only a small number of additional families with this condition have been reported. Nonfamilial, acquired keratosis of the palms and soles, however, has been observed in several individuals with an associated bronchial, esophageal, or pulmonary malignancy [6••].

Muir-Torre Syndrome

The association of sebaceous tumors (adenomas, epitheliomas, and carcinomas) and an internal malignancy (most commonly colorectal carcinomas proximal to the splenic flexure and genitourinary neoplasms) is defined as the Muir-Torre syndrome (Fig. 19-10) [7•,10]. Because these sebaceous lesions are rare, the detection of even one Muir-Torre syndrome–associated cutaneous tumor warrants an

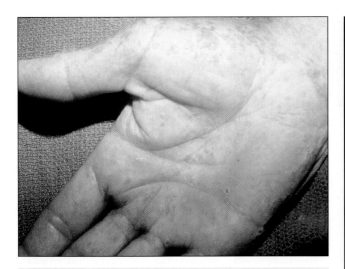

FIGURE 19-7 Pits in the palm of a patient with nevoid basal cell carcinoma syndrome. (*From* Cohen [6••]; with permission.)

initial evaluation and periodic assessment for malignancy in that individual [8]. Keratoacanthoma is another skin lesion that has been observed in at least 20% of patients with this syndrome.

Neurofibromatosis Type 1

The gene responsible for neurofibromatosis type 1 (*NF1*) has recently been mapped to band 11.2 of the long arm of chromosome 17. The phenotypic expression of this disease is variable; some individuals with NF1 are severely affected, whereas others have minimal skin or systemic stigmata. Café au lait macules (Fig. 19-11*A*), axillary or inguinal "frecking" (referred to as Crowe's sign) (Fig. 19-11*B*, and neurofibromas (Fig. 19-11*C*) are cutaneous manifestations of neurofibromatosis type 1 [9]. Other diagnostic criteria for neurofibromatosis type 1 are disease-specific osseous lesions, optic

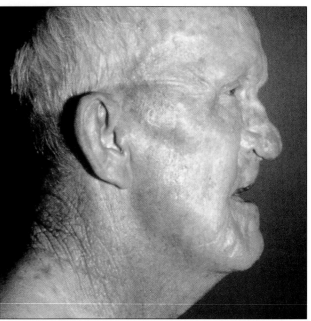

FIGURE 19-8 Frontal bossing, hypertelorism, and prognathism are nevoid basal cell carcinoma syndrome–associated skeletal anomalies that can be observed on the lateral view of this patient; multiple prior surgical sites from which basal cell carcinoma was removed are also demonstrated. (*From* Cohen [6••]; with permission.)

gliomas, pigmented hamartomas of the iris (Lisch nodules), and a first-degree relative with the condition [6••].

Peutz-Jeghers Syndrome

Macular hyperpigmentation and polyposis of the gastrointestinal tract (stomach, small intestine, colon, and rectum) defines Peutz-Jeghers syndrome. The pigmented macules either are present at birth or appear in childhood. They may

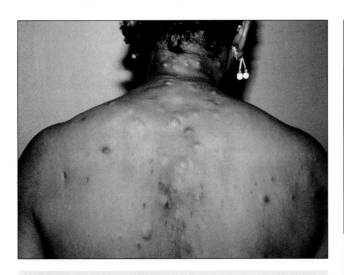

FIGURE 19-9 Multiple epidermoid cysts on the back of a black woman with Gardner's syndrome. (*From* Cohen [6••]; with permission.)

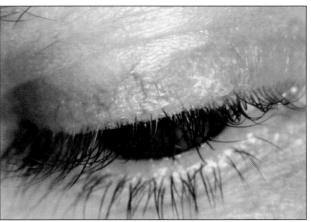

FIGURE 19-10 A diagnosis of the Muir-Torre syndrome was made when a sebaceous carcinoma (the hyperkeratotic nodule on the medial upper eyelid) was discovered in a young man who had previously been successfully treated for Hodgkin's lymphoma. (*From* Cohen [10]; with permission.)

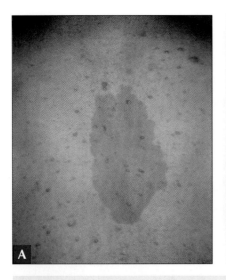 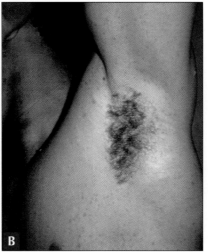 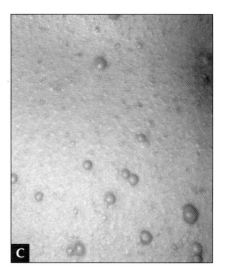

FIGURE 19-11 Café au lait macules (*panel A*), Crowe's sign (freckling in the axilla) *panel B*) and neurofibromas (*panel C*) are cutaneous features of neurofibromatosis type 1. (*From* Cohen [6••]; with permission.)

be located on the acral skin, buccal mucosa, face, gums, hard palate, and lips; they are most frequently periorificial. Whereas the facial lesions may fade as the patient becomes older, the mucosal pigmentations persist [6••].

CUTANEOUS PARANEOPLASTIC SYNDROMES

Cutaneous paraneoplastic syndromes are a group of dermatoses that appear either before, concurrent with, or after an associated malignancy [11••]; the syndromes, their clinical characteristics, and their associated malignancies are summarized in Table 19-2 (Figs. 19-12 through 19-17) [11••,12,13•,14,15,16•,17,18•,19•]. In addition, some of these dermatoses may be observed in cancer-free individuals, either in association with a systemic disease or as an isolated dermatologic condition.

Criteria for Defining Cutaneous Paraneoplastic Syndromes

The criteria for establishing a causal relationship between a dermatosis and a malignant internal disease were initially proposed by Curth in 1976 [11••]. They included:

- The two conditions begin simultaneously (*ie*, dermatomyositis)
- The two conditions follow a parallel course (*eg*, malignant acanthosis nigricans)
- In certain syndromes, neither the course nor the onset of one of the two conditions is dependent on the course or onset of the other condition because the two conditions are part of a genetic syndrome (*eg*, Gardner's syndrome)
- A specific tumor (*ie*, adenocarcinoma in malignant acanthosis nigricans) occurs in connection with a specific dermatosis
- The dermatosis is usually not common (*ie*, erythema gyratum repens)

- The associated tumor is found in a high percentage of cases of the dermatosis

The criteria for defining a cutaneous paraneoplastic syndrome have been modified since Curth's original description. For example, the last three criteria are not essential for a mucocutaneous condition to be a paraneoplastic syndrome [11••]. In addition, the third criterion (genetic syndromes that may be associated with an internal malignancy) is more appropriately classified as "genodermatoses with malignant potential" [6••].

Evaluation for Associated Malignancy

Although a cutaneous paraneoplastic syndrome may initially appear in an individual with an established diagnosis of cancer (and thereby may be the heralding sign of recurrent neoplastic disease), it often precedes or coincides with the clinical detection of the related neoplasm. Therefore, once the diagnosis of a potential cutaneous paraneoplastic syndrome is confirmed, an appropriate systemic evaluation for an underlying neoplasm should be considered in a cancer-free individual and a search for possible recurrent or metastatic disease should be performed in a patient with a known history of malignancy. The initial work-up should include a detailed medical history, a complete physical examination, and routine screening laboratory tests. Subsequent studies should then be directed by the abnormalities discovered during the patient's preliminary evaluation, with an emphasis placed on detecting malignancies that are especially prevalent in association with that individual's specific cutaneous paraneoplastic syndrome [11••].

Etiology

The etiology of many of these dermatoses remains undetermined. However, recent studies have suggested that the cutaneous paraneoplastic syndromes are likely to be caused

Cutaneous paraneoplastic syndrome	Clinical characteristics	Site or type of associated malignancies
Acanthosis nigricians (see Fig. 19-12)	Flexural (axillae and posterior neck) verrucous, velvety-textured, hyperpigmented epidermal hyperplasia	Intraabdominal (stomach)
Acquired ichthyosis	Diffuse rhomboid scales with free edges	Hodgkin's lymphoma
Amyloidosis	Purpura; macroglossia, tongue papules, or both; periocular purpura, waxy papules, or both	Myeloma, Hodgkin's lymphoma, kidney
Bazex's syndrome (acrokeratosis paraneoplastica)	Erythematous, scaling papulosquamous lesions on the fingers, toes, ears, and nose; nail dystrophy; palmoplantar keratoderma	Squamous cell carcinomas of the upper aerorespiratory tract or a neoplasm with cervical lymph node metastases in white men older than 40 y
Bowen's disease	Erythematous plaque on a photodistributed or non–sun-exposed site	Controversial (age-associated neoplasms)
Bullous pemphigoid	Erythematous-based, subepidermal tense bullae on flexor thighs and forearms	Controversial (lung, larynx, breast, gallbladder, kidney, bladder, ovary, uterus, rectum, prostate, cervix, thyroid, stomach)
Dermatitis herpetiformis	Pruritic papulovesicles on the elbows and knees, upper back, and buttocks	Lymphoma (gastrointestinal and nongastrointestinal), lung, small intestine, bladder
Dermatomyositis	Periocular heliotrope rash, Gottron's papules, periungual telangiectasias, poikiloderma	Age-associated neoplasms
Epidermolysis bullosa acquisita	Adult-onset, subepidermal blisters at trauma sites	Controversial (myeloma, lung, lymphoma, chronic lymphocytic leukemia)
Erythema annulare centrifugum	Expanding, annular erythema with a raised edge, peripheral scale, and central clearing	Lung, lymphoma (Hodgkin's and non-Hodgkin's), histiocytosis, prostate
Erythema gyratum repens	Advancing erythematous rings with "wood grain" or striped appearance	Lung, esophagus, uterus, cervix, breast, stomach
Erythroderma and exfoliative dermatitis	Generalized erythema with or without scaling	Lymphoma (cutaneous T-cell and Hodgkin's), chronic lymphocytic leukemia, acute and chronic myelogenous leukemia, uterus, lung, stomach, prostate, thyroid, liver, larynx
Erythromelalgia [12,13•]	Severe burning pain, erythema, and warmth of the distal extremities relieved by cold exposure, elevation of the extremity, or both	Polycythemia vera, essential thrombocythemia, agnogenic myeloid metaplasia, chronic myelogenous leukemia
Extramammary Paget's disease (see Fig. 19-13)	Erythematous, exudative plaque located on the vulva, perianal area, penis, scrotum, or groin	Cutaneous adnexal carcinoma; internal malignancies: breast, uterus, rectum, bladder, vagina, or prostate
Florid cutaneous papillomatosis	Verrucous papillomas on the trunk and the extremities	Intraabdominal (stomach, bladder, bile ducts, ovary, uterus)
Glucagonoma syndrome	Necrolytic migratory erythematous patch, glossitis, angular stomatitis	α-Cell pancreatic carcinoma (glucagonoma)
Hypertrichosis lanuginosa acquisita	Generalized pale, fine-textured hair growth	Lung, colorectal, breast, uterus, bladder, lymphoma
Hypertrophic pulmonary osteoarthropathy [14] (see Fig. 19-14)	Clubbing of fingers and toes with tender swelling of the distal arms, legs, and adjacent joints	Lung, mediastinal tumors, sarcomas
Multicentric reticulohistiocytosis	Papules, nodules, and rapidly progressive, debilitating polyarthritis	Breast, lymphoma, cervix, stomach, ovary, colon, lung, pleura, acute myelogenous leukemia

Paraneoplastic pemphigus	Polymorphous pruritic papules and blisters; cutaneous and painful mucosal erosions	Lymphoma, chronic lymphocytic leukemia, sarcoma, lung, thymoma
Pemphigus vulgaris	Intraepidermal bullae of the skin, oral blisters and erosions	Lymphoreticular (Kaposi's sarcoma), thymus, breast, skin
Pityriasis rotunda	Noninflammatory, geometrically perfect circular patches of scales	Liver
Porphyria cutanea tarda	Early: photodistributed subepidermal vesicles, skin fragility, facial hypertrichosis, and hyperpigmentation	Controversial (liver)
	Late: scarring, milia, sclerodermoid changes, calcinosis cutis, alopecia	
Pruritus (*see* Fig. 19-15)	Excoriations, prurigo nodularis, lichen simplex chronicus	Lymphoma (Hodgkin's and cutaneous T-cell), polycythemia vera
Pyoderma gangrenosum (*see* Fig. 19-16)	Papulopustule that develops into a nodule that ulcerates with an irregular, violaceous, undermined border	Hematologic malignancies
Sign of Leser-Trélat	Seborrheic keratoses (may be pruritic)	Stomach, lymphoma, breast, lung
Sweet's syndrome (acute febrile neutrophilic dermatosis) [15,16•]	Tender, erythematous pseudovesicular plaques on the arms, head, and neck	Acute myelogenous leukemia
Tripe palms [17,18•,20] (*see* Fig. 19-17)	Thickened, velvet- or moss-textured, honeycombed or cobbled palms with pronounced dermatoglyphics	Lung, stomach
Trousseau's syndrome	Thrombophlebitis (often superficial and migratory)	Pancreas, lung, stomach
Vasculitis [19•]	Palpable, nonblanchable purpura; erythematous nodules	Leukemia (hairy cell and myelogenous), myeloma, lymphoma, myelodysplastic syndrome

From Cohen [11••]; with permission.

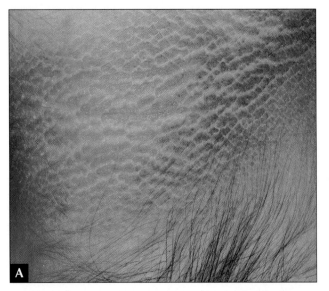
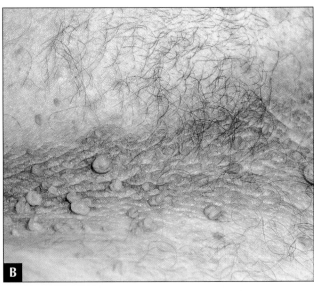

FIGURE 19-12 Malignancy-associated acanthosis nigricans commonly appears as hyperpigmented, velvet-textured hyperplasia of the epidermis in the flexural areas, such as the axilla (*panel A*), and the posterior neck (*panel B*), of patients with intraabdominal neoplasms. (*Panel A courtesy of* D. Hazelrigg, Evansville, IN; *Panel B courtesy of* K. Greer, Charlottesville, VA.)

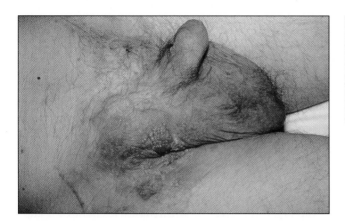

FIGURE 19-13 Extramammary Paget's disease, a cutaneous adenocarcinoma that appears as a pruritic, erythematous, dermatitis-like plaque, is often associated with an underlying adnexal carcinoma or an underlying internal malignancy, frequently of the digestive system (when perianal in location) or the genitourinary organs (when at a penile, scrotal, or groin location). (*From* Cohen [11••]; with permission.)

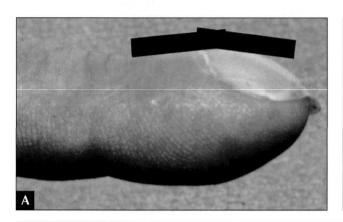

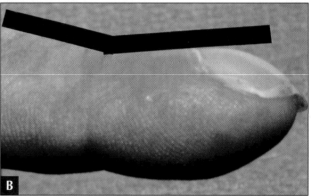

FIGURE 19-14 Clinical indicators of clubbing are Lovibond's profile sign (*panel A*) and Curth's modified profile sign (*panel B*). Clubbing is present when the angle between the curved nail plate and the proximal nail fold (which is normally less than or equal to 160°) exceeds 180° (*panel A*) or the angle between the middle and the terminal phalanx at the interphalangeal joint (which is normally about 180°) is reduced to less than 160° (*panel B*). (*From* Cohen [11••]; with permission.)

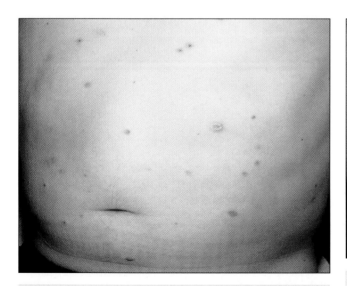

FIGURE 19-15 Although paraneoplastic pruritus (which may appear as excoriated papules and prurigo nodules) has most frequently been associated with Hodgkin's disease, it is also a common symptom in patients who have either cutaneous T-cell lymphoma or polycythema vera. (*From* Cohen [11••]; with permission.)

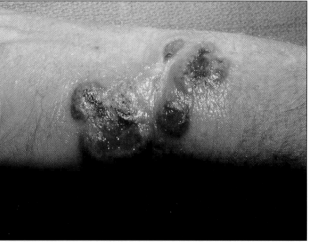

FIGURE 19-16 Hematologic malignancies, and rarely solid tumors, may be associated with "atypical" or "bullous" pyoderma gangrenosum, which often begins as a painful erythematous papule or pustule and subsequently develops into a bullous nodule that frequently breaks down and forms an ulcer with violaceous, irregular, undermined borders and a boggy, necrotic base. (*From* Cohen [11••]; with permission.)

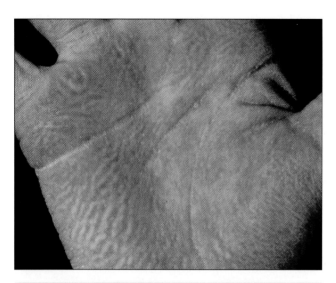

FIGURE 19-17 Pulmonary and gastric carcinomas are the most common neoplasms in patients with malignancy-associated tripe palms, which can appear as thickening of the palms with moss-like, velvet-textured exaggeration of the palmar dermato-glyphics. (*From* Cohen and coworkers [20]; with permission.)

directly by a cytokine secreted by the tumor; alternatively, the tumor may participate indirectly by inducing accessory cells to secrete the causative factor. The investigation of patients with these malignancy-associated dermatoses may provide additional insight not only into the biologic behavior of their underlying neoplasms but also into the pathogenesis of these conditions when they occur in a paraneoplastic setting or as an idiopathic disorder [11••].

MUCOCUTANEOUS REACTIONS TO ANTINEOPLASTIC AGENTS

Mucocutaneous reactions may be observed in patients receiving cancer chemotherapy (Tables 19-3 and 19-4) [21••,22,23]. Some of these reactions are primarily associated with a specific malignancy or the administration of a specific agent. Most of these reactions, however, are related neither to a specific neoplasm nor to a particular medication. The severity of these reactions can range from an incidental asymptomatic clinical observation to a life-threatening or drug-limiting toxicity. Certain reactions are dose dependent (either single or cumulative dose), whereas others represent hypersensitivity reactions that are not influenced by the quantity administered. Some of these reactions can be adequately managed symptomatically and will resolve after chemotherapy has been completed; alternatively, other reactions require either reduction of the dose of the chemotherapeutic agent or discontinuation of the drug.

Alopecia

One of the most frequently observed cutaneous reactions to the use of chemotherapeutic agents is alopecia (Fig. 19-18).

Because the antineoplastic drugs affect actively proliferating hair follicles, an anagen effluvium occurs; the hair loss is dose dependent and reversible once the chemotherapy has been discontinued. The most common site of involvement is the scalp; the chemotherapy-induced alopecia is often only partial because 10% to 15% of the hairs on the scalp are not in the proliferating (anagen) stage at any specific time. With long-term therapy, patients may also experience loss of axillary, facial, and pubic hair [21••,22].

Stomatitis

Stomatitis or mucositis is also a common adverse mucocutaneous side effect of antineoplastic therapy. Symptoms can range from mild to dose limiting (Fig. 19-19) [22]. The rapid replication rate of the mucosal epithelium of the conjunctiva, gastrointestinal tract, oral cavity, perianal region, urethra, and vagina makes these tissues extremely susceptible to the direct cytotoxic effect, the immunosuppressive (infectious) effects, and the myelosuppressive (bleeding) effects of the chemotherapeutic drugs. Symptoms (burning and reddening) often begin shortly after administration of the agent, and erosions or ulcerations appear within 1 to 5 days. Within 2 weeks after stopping the drug, healing has usually occurred. Supportive treatment is the mainstay of therapy. Often, symptomatic relief can be provided by "swishing and swallowing" 5 to 15 mL of the following solution (Powell's mouthwash) three to four times daily: tetracycline (7500 mg), hydrocortisone powder (1500 mg), nystatin oral suspension (100,000 U/mL x 180 mL), and diphenhydramine cough syrup with minimal alcohol (to a total volume of 3750 mL or 1 gal) [21••].

TABLE 19-3 MUCOCUTANEOUS REACTIONS TO CANCER CHEMOTHERAPY
Common
Alopecia
Stomatitis
Less common
Acral erythema
Extravasation injuries
Hyperpigmentation (*see* Table 19-4)
Inflammation of actinic keratoses
Radiation interactions
Rare
Hypersensitivity reactions
Neutrophilic eccrine hidradenitis
Reactive erythemas
Vasculitis
From Cohen [21••]; with permission.

Pattern of hyperpigmentation	Associated chemotherapeutic agent
Generalized (nonspecific)	
Mucous membranes	Busulfan, doxorubicin
Nails	Bleomycin, cyclophosphamide, daunorubicin, doxorubicin, fluorouracil
Skin	Bleomycin, busulfan, carmustine (topical), cyclophosphamide, daunorubicin, doxorubicin, fluorouracil, hydroxyurea, mechlorethamine (topical), methotrexate, mithramycin, mitomycin, thiotepa
Teeth	Cyclophosphamide
Specific	
Flag sign of chemotherapy (hair)	Methotrexate
Flagellate hyperpigmentation (see Fig. 19-21)	Bleomycin
Serpentine supravenous hyperpigmentation	Fluorouracil, fotemustine

From Cohen [21••]; with permission.

Less Common Reactions to Chemotherapy

Less common reactions to chemotherapeutics are listed in Table 19-3 [21••,22,23]. Chemotherapy-induced acral erythema (also referred to as hand-foot syndrome or palmar-plantar erythrodysesthesia) is most frequently associated with the administration of either cytarabine, doxorubicin, or fluorouracil. It presents as painful macular reddening primarily involving the palms and soles and may progress to blister formation before superficial desquamation and reepithelialization of the involved skin (Fig. 19-20) [23]. Extravasation injuries, which may be caused by several of the antineoplastic drugs, can range in severity from phlebitis to chemical cellulitis with or without tissue necrosis. Generalized and specific patterns of mucocutaneous hyperpigmentation secondary to chemotherapeutic agents are summarized in Table 19-4 and illustrated in Figure 19-21 [21••,22]. Inflammation of previously asymptomatic actinic keratoses may follow the systemic administration of several different chemotherapeutic drugs (Fig. 19-22); this reaction neither requires discontinuation of the agent nor contraindicates future use of the medication. Photosensitivity, radiation enhancement (drugs act synergistically with radiation), radiation recall (inflammatory response in tissues previously irradiated), and reactivation of ultraviolet light–induced erythema (in patients who have received either intramuscular, intravenous, or oral methotrexate) are four types of interactions that have been observed between chemotherapeutic agents and either ionizing or ultraviolet radiation [21••,22].

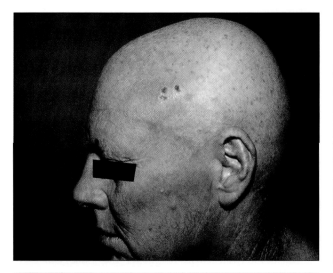

FIGURE 19-18 Alopecia of the scalp following treatment with systemic chemotherapy; cutaneous lesions of a concurrent disseminated varicella-zoster virus infection appear as erythematous-based crusted erosions. (*From* Cohen [21••]; with permission.)

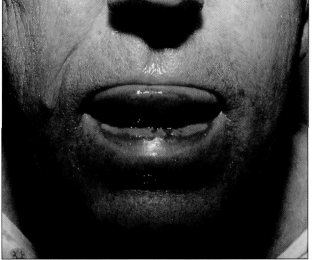

FIGURE 19-19 The mucosal erosions of the tongue and lower lip are secondary to treatment of this man's metastatic colon carcinoma with fluorouracil. (*From* Cohen [21••]; with permission.)

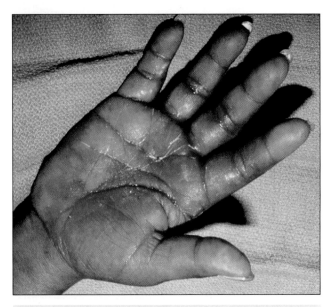

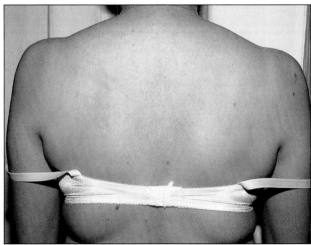

FIGURE 19-21 The "flagellate" (whip-like), linear, hyperpigmented streaks (which are most prominent in this patient over the scapulae and the posterior shoulders) that appeared after treatment with systemic bleomycin are a specific pattern of chemotherapy-induced hyperpigmentation. (*From* Cohen [21 • •]; with permission.)

FIGURE 19-20 Chemotherapy-induced acral erythema lesions characterized by tender, red palms and fingers with superficial desquamation. (*From* Cohen [23]; with permission.)

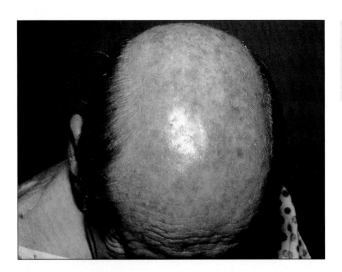

FIGURE 19-22 Multiple actinic keratoses on the scalp of a man with metastatic colon carcinoma that became inflamed 1 week after systemic chemotherapy with continuous-infusion fluorouracil and daily interferon alpha was started. (*From* Cohen [21 • •]; with permission.)

REFERENCES AND RECOMMENDED READING

Recently published papers of particular interest have been highlighted as:

• Of interest

•• Of outstanding interest

1.•• Cohen PR: Cutaneous metastases. *Am Fam Physician*, in press.

2.• Lookingbill DP, Spangler N, Sexton FM: Skin involvement as the presenting sign of internal carcinoma: a retrospective study of 7316 cancer patients. *J Am Acad Dermatol* 1990, 22:19–26.

3. Cohen PR, Buzdar AU: Metastatic breast carcinoma mimicking an acute paronychia of the great toe: case report and review of subungual metastases. *Am J Clin Oncol (CCT)* 1993, 16:86–91.

4. Manteaux A, Cohen PR, Rapini RP: Zosteriform and epidermotropic metastasis: report of two cases. *J Dermatol Surg Oncol* 1992, 18:97–100.

5. Cohen PR, Rapini RP, Beran M: Infiltrated blue-gray plaques in a patient with leukemia: Chloroma (granulocytic sarcoma) [off-center fold]. *Arch Dermatol* 1987, 123:251–254.

6.•• Cohen PR: Genodermatoses with malignant potential. *Am Fam Physician* 1992, 46:1479–1486.

7.• Cohen PR, Kohn SR, Kurzrock R: The association of sebaceous gland tumors and internal malignancy: the Muir-Torre syndrome. *Am J Med* 1991, 90:606–613.

8. Cohen PR: Sebaceous carcinoma of the ocular adnexa and the Muir-Torre syndrome [letter]. *J Am Acad Dermatol* 1992, 27:279–280.

9. Cohen PR: Neurofibromatosis type 1. *N Engl J Med* 1993, 329:1549.

10. Cohen PR: Muir-Torre syndrome in patients with hematologic malignancies. *Am J Hematol* 1992, 40:64–65.

11.•• Cohen PR: Cutaneous paraneoplastic syndromes. *Am Fam Physician* 1994, 50:1273–1282.

12. Kurzrock R, Cohen PR: Erythromelalgia: review of clinical characteristics and pathophysiology. *Am J Med* 1991, 91:416–422.

13.• Kurzrock R, Cohen PR: Paraneoplastic erythromelalgia. *Clin Dermatol* 1993, 11:73–82.

14. Cohen PR: Hypertrophic pulmonary osteoarthropathy and tripe palms in a man with squamous cell carcinoma of the larynx and lung: report of a case and review of cutaneous paraneoplastic syndromes associated with laryngeal and lung malignancies. *Am J Clin Oncol (CCT)* 1993, 16:268–276.

15. Cohen PR, Talpaz M, Kurzrock R: Malignancy-associated Sweet's syndrome: review of the world literature. *J Clin Oncol* 1988, 6:1887–1897.

16.• Cohen PR, Kurzrock R: Sweet's syndrome and cancer. *Clin Dermatol* 1993, 11:149–157.

17. Cohen PR, Kurzrock R: Malignancy-associated tripe palms. *J Am Acad Dermatol* 1992, 27:271–272.

18.• Cohen PR, Grossman ME, Silvers DN, Kurzrock R: Tripe palms and cancer. *Clin Dermatol* 1993, 11:165–173.

19.• Kurzrock R, Cohen PR: Vasculitis and cancer. *Clin Dermatol* 1993, 11:175–187.

20. Cohen PR, Grossman ME, Almeida L, Kurzrock R: Triple palms and malignancy. *J Clin Oncol* 1989, 7:669–678.

21.•• Cohen PR: Cancer chemotherapy-associated mucocutaneous reactions. In *Medical Oncology: A Comprehensive Board Review. University of Texas MD Anderson Cancer Center.* Edited by Pazdur R. Huntington, NY; PRR 1993; 491–500.

22. Kerker BJ, Hood AF: Chemotherapy-induced cutaneous reactions. *Semin Dermatol* 1989, 8:173–181.

23. Cohen PR: Acral erythema: a clinical review. *Cutis* 1993, 51:175–179.

Select Bibliography

Callen JP: Skin signs of internal malignancy. *Australas J Dermatol* 1987, 28:106–114.

Cohen PR, Kurzrock R, eds: Cutaneous paraneoplastic syndromes. *Clin Dermatol*, 1993, 11:1–187.

Cohen PR, Kurzrock R: Genodermatoses with malignant potential. *Dermatol Clin* 1995, 13:1–230.

Hood AF: Cutaneous side effects of cancer chemotherapy. *Med Clin North Am* 1986, 70:187–209.

Poole S, Fenske NA: Cutaneous markers of internal malignancy: I. Malignant involvement of the skin and the genodermatoses. *J Am Acad Dermatol* 1993, 28:1–13.

Poole S, Fenske NA: Cutaneous markers of internal malignancy: II. paraneoplastic dermatoses and environmental carcinogens. *J Am Acad Dermatol* 1993, 28:147–164.

Worret W-IF: Skin signs and internal malignancies. *Int J Dermatol* 1993, 32:1–5.

Immunobullous Diseases 20

Grant J. Anhalt

Key Points

- Autoantibody-mediated skin diseases are infrequent but have significant morbidity and mortality.
- Diagnoses are established by histologic examination of lesions and immuno-fluorescent examination of perilesional skin and serum.
- The most common disease is bullous pemphigoid, manifest by pruritic skin blisters in the elderly.
- The most serious disorder is pemphigus vulgaris, manifest by painful erosions of the mouth and skin.
- Oral corticosteroids, immunosuppressive agents, and select other drugs are used to control these diseases.

Although immunobullous diseases are not common, they are the cause of significant morbidity and mortality, hence their importance in a specialty that predominantly deals with less serious disorders. Additionally, study of the autoantibodies that cause these diseases has provided critical reagents for identifying important cell adhesion molecules [1••]. This chapter concentrates on practical points for recognition and diagnoses of immunobullous disorders. Prompt identification is important because in these disorders early therapeutic intervention can greatly reduce morbidity. The disorders covered are presented in approximate order of their prevalence and not in terms of their traditional immunopathologic categories.

BULLOUS PEMPHIGOID

Clinical Presentation

By far the most common bullous disease and the one most likely to be seen in a general medical practice is bullous pemphigoid (BP) [2], although its precise incidence or prevalence is not known. BP is primarily a disease of the elderly, with the vast majority of patients over 60 years of age at the time of eruption. With the aging of the general population in this country, the incidence seems to be increasing. It occurs very rarely in children or young adults.

The cutaneous eruption can have a prolonged prodrome manifested by very pruritic urticarial patches and plaques, or the condition may erupt rather abruptly with pruritus and blisters (Figs. 20-1 through 20-3). The blistering eruption primarily affects the trunk and flexures of the extremities. Unlike other

false-negative result, as the immunoreactants will only be weakly detected. Biopsy specimens immersed in formalin cannot be used for detection of immunoreactants. The immunofluorescent transport media is a stable solution of ammonium sulfate. Once the specimens are immersed in the transport media they are stable for weeks and can be mailed or transported to a laboratory without concern for stability. This transport media is inexpensive to prepare and should be available without cost from any laboratory that performs the test. Because the detection of autoantibodies in the serum can be negative in almost 50% of cases, this test is not critical for the diagnosis; demonstration of tissue-bound antibodies alone is often sufficient.

Therapy

Fortunately, BP is usually relatively easy to manage; anticipated morbidity is low, and mortality is rare. The disease is very responsive to oral corticosterioids (Table 20-1). The physician can anticipate that approximately one half of patients will experience a remission, and one half will require chronic therapy.

Despite this fact, a minority of patients with BP will have disease activity that will require prohibitively large doses of corticosteroids, and a second steroid-sparing agent is indicated [5]. The most effective drug in this scenario is azathioprine, 1 to 3 mg/kg/d. It has a high rate of success, does not produce significant neutropenia, and is generally well tolerated. Use of azathioprine carries with it a small increase in incidence of lymphoreticular malignancies, but in an elderly patient the risk for this event would often be expected to peak beyond the expected life span of the patient. Some patients are intolerant of azathioprine because of nausea or hepatotoxic reactions, and alternative drugs must be considered. These drugs include, in decreasing order of efficacy, cyclophosphamide, methotrexate, cyclosporine, dapsone, and gold therapy. Cyclophosphamide is effective, but the risk of neutropenia or hemorrhagic cystitis in the elderly is very high. Cyclosporine is extremely expensive and difficult to monitor in most cases. The response to methotrexate, dapsone, and gold therapy is unpredictable.

Rarer Variants of Pemphigoid

Herpes gestationis or gestational pemphigoid

Pruritic skin eruptions in the second or third trimester of pregnancy are relatively common, and most are caused by unknown factors (*eg*, pruritic urticarial papules and plaques of pregnancy). Rarely, a blistering eruption that is immunopathologically identical to BP can occur, and this eruption is called *herpes gestationis*. The disease resolves after delivery, often will flare with the return of menses or in the immediate postpartum period, and can be reproduced by challenge with oral estrogen. The incidence of disease is estimated at one in every 50,000 births, so a physician would not expect to see many cases.

Cicatricial Pemphigoid

Cicatricial pemphigoid is a serious disease of the elderly with peak incidence occurring in the sixth or seventh decade. Unlike BP, in which skin is involved and mucosal lesions are absent, cicatricial pemphigoid has scarring blisters that predominantly affect mucous membranes, and skin lesions are rare. Mucosal blisters and erosions are immunopathologically similar to BP [6•], but recurrent scarring may lead to profound morbidity or mortality. If lesions are found only on the gingiva or buccal mucosa, no serious morbidity will ensue. However, involvement of other structures can be disastrous. Specifically, if not aggressively treated, scarring of the conjunctiva leads to blindness, esophageal scarring leads to stenosis and asphyxiation from food, and laryngeal stenosis can also lead to asphyxiation. The physician must be alert to patients with chronic oral ulcerations or erosions or chronic conjunctival inflammation. Diagnosis is established by histologic and direct immunofluorescence (IF) examination of affected mucosa or conjunctiva. Lesions restricted to the oral cavity are treated with topical steroids, intralesional triamcinolone injections, or oral dapsone with variable response. If the eyes, esophagus, or larynx is involved, aggressive treatment with cyclophosphamide or prednisone for a period of 18 to 24 months will induce a remission in the majority of cases [7]. Early diagnosis is critical to a good prognosis.

PEMPHIGUS VULGARIS

Clinical Presentation

Pemphigus vulgaris (PV) is less common than BP but is a serious form of bullous disease. It is most common in middle-aged patients, but young adults and the elderly are also affected. The disease has a specific immunogenetic basis. The genes that encode this susceptibility appear to be overrepresented in the Jewish population, especially those of Eastern European origin. The incidence is highest in this population, although every race and ethnic group is affected

TABLE 20-1 DRUG REGIMEN FOR TREATMENT OF BULLOUS PEMPHIGOID
• Initial dosage of 0.5–0.75 mg/kg/d prednisone
• After a few weeks, slow taper of oral steroids, switch to alternate-day regimen
• Over 3–6 mo, dosage may be reduced by increments every 2–3 wk
• Drug may be discontinued after this time
• In case of recurrence Severe: low-dose prednisone, 5–10 mg every other day Mild: combination of potent topical steroid (fluocinonide 0.5% cream, three times daily) or intralesional injections with triamcinolone suspension (10 mg/cc) for limited areas

to some extent. PV usually presents with slowly progressive ulcerations of the oropharynx that often are misdiagnosed for weeks or months. Later, fragile cutaneous blisters and erosions occur on the head and neck, then spread acrally (Fig. 20-8). Without intervention, progressive skin loss and poor oral intake because of pain cause progressive debilitation, sepsis, and death. Prior to the introduction of oral corticosteroids, the mortality of this disease was 50% at 2 years and 100% at 5 years. The presence of persistent cutaneous and oral erosions should be a clinical red flag that prompts consideration of a serious immunobullous disease such as PV.

Diagnostic Techniques

The following is known about the pathophysiology of the disease, and this knowledge forms the basis for diagnostic maneuvers: 1) PV is an autoimmune disease caused by IgG autoantibodies against a cell-adhesion molecule of squamous epithelium (skin and mucosa); 2) binding of the antibody to the cell surface causes cell–cell detachment, resulting in an intraepidermal blister; and 3) there is a good correlation between levels of circulating autoantibodies and disease activity. Therefore, the diagnosis is established by fulfilling the following criteria: 1) clinically, there are erosions or blisters on both skin and mucous membranes; 2) histologically, there is an intraepidermal blister caused by epithelial

cells detaching from each other (Fig. 20-9); 3) direct IF shows IgG bound to the cell surface of affected oral epithelium or skin (Fig. 20-10); and 4) circulating antibodies that bind to the cell surface of squamous epithelium on frozen sections of skin or esophagus are detectable. Unlike BP, circulating antibodies are always

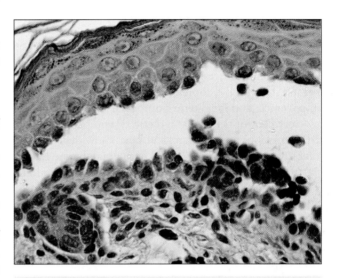

FIGURE 20-9 Histologic examination of the edge of a blister in pemphigus vulgaris shows a blister that forms just above the lower-most cells of the epidermis. Pemphigus, therefore, is a disorder in which the blister is intraepidermal. Note the epidermal cells have detached and rounded up and are floating free in the blister cavity. This loss of cell-cell detachment (acantholysis) is characteristic of all forms of pemphigus.

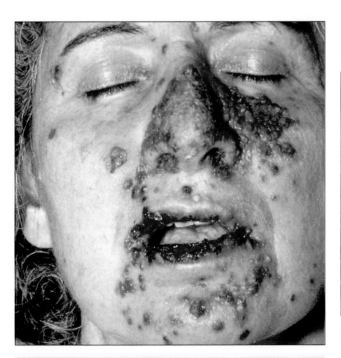

FIGURE 20-8 A typical presentation for pemphigus vulgaris. Note the mucosal lesions on the tongue and the lips. After these intraoral lesions have been present for a period of weeks or months, blisters and erosions start to appear on the central part of the face and then spread acrally. The combination of cutaneous and oral blistering must alert the clinician to the possibility of a serious immunobullous disease, such as pemphigus vulgaris.

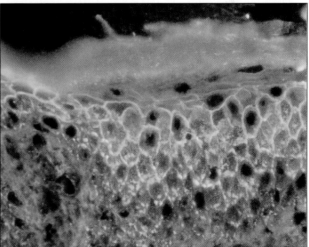

FIGURE 20-10 Direct immunofluorescence from perilesional skin in pemphigus vulgaris shows immunoglobulin G and complement components bound to the surface of the epithelial cells. Binding of the antibody to the cell surface adhesion molecules that are the target antigens in this disease cause the cell–cell detachment seen in the previous figure. It is easy to note the difference between the intraepidermal blistering disorders (pemphigus) and the subepidermal blistering disorders (pemphigoid) on the basis of these two criteria.

detectable. Given the fact that the disease is potentially life-threatening, circulating autoantibodies must be demonstrated to fulfill the diagnostic criteria. Again, these criteria can be fulfilled by performing a biopsy on the edge of a blister for histology, and on adjacent perilesional skin for direct IF, and by obtaining a serum tube for indirect IF.

Therapy

Therapy must be directed at reducing autoantibody synthesis because as long as significant amounts of antiepithelial antibodies are present the disease will persist. Unlike BP, topical treatments are of secondary importance, and long-term improvement will only occur by treatment of the hematopoietic system. Again, unlike BP, remissions are very rare, and most individuals require therapy for life (Table 20-2). Approximately one half of patients will respond well to oral corticosteroids alone. Maintenance therapy with low-dose, alternate-day corticosteroids is required in all patients [8]. Patients that have resistant disease or are intolerant of corticosteroids should receive a second steroid-sparing agent. In decreasing order of efficacy these agents are cyclophosphamide [9•], azathioprine, chlorambucil, methotrexate, and gold. Management of difficult cases of PV is best handled by physicians with experience in its treatment.

Rarer Variants of Pemphigus
Pemphigus foliaceus and paraneoplastic pemphigus

Pemphigus foliaceus (PF) is a superficial form of pemphigus that is differentiated by two major criteria: 1) clinically, lesions are superficial and mucous membranes are never affected; and 2) histologically, cell-cell detachment occurs only in the most superficial layer of the epidermis. Otherwise, direct and indirect IF features of PV and PF are virtually identical.

In contrast to PV, PF has far less morbidity and only very rare mortality, so therapy is generally less problematic. It is important to note that certain drugs have been shown to induce PF and, less commonly, PV. Implicated drugs include D-penicillamine, gold sodium thiomalate, and angiotensin-converting enzyme inhibitors such as captopril and enalapril.

Paraneoplastic pemphigus

Paraneoplastic pemphigus is a recently described bullous disease associated with specific neoplasms [10]. These neoplasms include non-Hodgkin's lymphomas, chronic lymphocytic leukemia, thymomas, Castleman tumors, and Waldenström's macroglobulinemia. The presence of persistent mucosal erosions and a polymorphous skin eruption in patients with these neoplasms should prompt referral for evaluation of this syndrome. Treatment is difficult and when the syndrome is associated with malignant neoplasms, the mortality rate is approximately 90%.

DERMATITIS HERPETIFORMIS

Clinical Presentation, Diagnosis, and Therapy

Dermatitis herpetiformis is a rare IgA-mediated skin disease. It presents with intense pruritic papules and

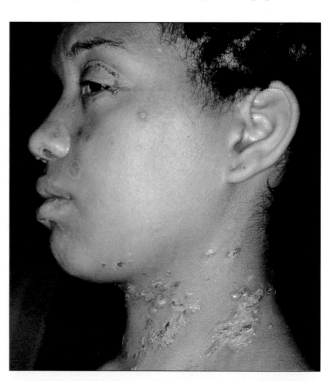

FIGURE 20-11 This young woman presented with a high fever, cerebritis, and blistering erosions of mucous membranes and flexural areas of the skin. She was subsequently found to have subepidermal blisters with dense IgG and complement components in the epidermis. This case was of epidermolysis bullosa acquisita that presented in a patient with bullous systemic lupus erythematosus. This presentation is typical for the inflammatory variety of epidermolysis bullosa acquisita seen in the context of acute lupus erythematosus. Once again, the combination of both mucosal and cutaneous blistering is a critical clinical feature of an evolving serious immunobullous disease.

TABLE 20-2 TREATMENT OF PEMPHIGUS VULGARIS IN VARYING CASES
50% Of patients diagnosed respond well to oral corticosteroids alone (prednisone, 1 mg/kg/d) tapered slowly over 6–9 mo
All patient responders require maintenance therapy with low-dose, alternate-day corticosteroids
Patients with resistant disease or intolerance to corticosteroids should receive a second steroid-sparing agent (*ie*, cyclophosphamide, azathioprine, chlorambucil, methotrexate, or gold)

vesicles distributed symmetrically over the shoulders, extensor elbows, and knees and on the scalp and sacrum. Peak incidence is in young adults; it is associated with a specific immunogenetic inheritance and asymptomatic gluten-sensitive enteropathy [11]. The disease affects white people and is extraordinarily rare in black people. The burning pruritus is typically disproportionate to the severity or extent of the skin lesions. Diagnosis is based on histologic evidence of coalescent subepidermal vesicles filled with neutrophils and granular IgA deposition in the upper dermis of perilesional skin. Circulating antibodies are not detectable. A dramatic elimination of pruritus within 24 to 48 hours of treatment with oral dapsone is an accepted clinical diagnostic sign. However, individuals who are glucose-6-phosphate-dehydrogenase-(G6PD)–sensitive cannot receive dapsone or massive hemolysis could ensue. Complete elimination of gluten from the diet for a period of months to years will reduce or eliminate maintenance requirements for dapsone, but complete avoidance of gluten is very difficult in North American diets.

VERY RARE BULLOUS DISEASES

Epidermolysis Bullosa Acquisita

This disease is an autoimmune disease that may mimic BP. Inflammatory blisters on mucous membranes and skin or trauma-induced blisters on the extremities are typical for this condition. IgG and complement components are present along the basement-membrane zone, but the target antigen is type VII collagen, and the subepidermal blister is actually located in the uppermost zone of the dermis [12]. Similar autoantibodies to type VII collagen and inflammatory blistering are seen in bullous systemic lupus erythematosus (Fig. 20-11).

Linear IgA Dermatitis

Linear IgA dermatitis, previously referred to as chronic *bullous disease of childhood*, presents as pruritic blisters on the trunk and extremities. It can occur in infants, young children, and adults. Subepidermal blisters are seen, and linear IgA is deposited along the basement membrane in contrast to the granular IgA deposition of dermatis herpetiformis.

REFERENCES AND RECOMMENDED READING

Recently published papers of particular interest have been highlighted as:

• Of interest

•• Of outstanding interest

1.•• Stanley JR: Cell adhesion molecules as targets of autoantibodies in pemphigus and pemphigoid, bullous diseases due to defective epidermal cell adhesion. *Adv Immunol* 1993, 53:291–325.

2. Anhalt GJ, Morrison L: Pemphigoid: bullous, gestational and cicatricial. In *Bullous Diseases.* Edited by Provost TT, Weston WL. St. Louis: Mosby-Year Book; 1992:63–112.

3. Lui Z, Diaz DA, Troy JL, *et al.*: A passive transfer model of the organ-specific autoimmune disease, bullous pemphigoid, using antibodies generated against the hemidesmosomal antigen BP180. *J Clin Invest* 1993, 92:2480–2488.

4. Fine JD, Briggaman RA, Gammon WR: Laboratory approach to the evaluation of vesiculbullous disorders. In *Topics in Clinical Dermatology: Bullous Diseases.* Edited by Fine JD. New York: Igaku-Shoin; 1993:3–22.

5. McDonald CJ: Cytotoxic agents for use in dermatology. *J Am Acad Dermatol* 1985, 12:753–775.

6.• Chan LS, Yancey KB, Hammerberg C, *et al.*: Immune mediated subepidermal blistering diseases of mucous membranes. *Arch Dermatol* 1993, 129:448–455.

7. Jabs DA, Anhalt GJ: Cicatricial pemphigoid. In *Current Therapy in Dermatology*, edn 2. Edited by Farmer ER, Provost TT. Philadelphia: BC Decker; 1988:56–57.

8. Morrison L, Anhalt GJ: Pemphigus. In *Current Therapy in Allergy and Immunology.* Edited by Liechtenstein L, Fauci A. Philadelphia: BC Decker; 1988:186–189.

9.• Pandya AG, Sontheimer RD: Treatment of pemphigus vulgaris with pulse intravenous cyclophosphamide. *Arch Dermatol* 1992, 128:1626–1630.

10. Anhalt GJ, Kim SC, Stanley JR, *et al.*: Paraneoplastic pemphigus: an autoimmune mucocutaneous disease associated with neoplasia. *New Engl J Med* 1990, 323:1729–1735.

11. McCord M, Hall III RP: IgA mediated autoimmune blistering diseases. In *Topics in Clinical Dermatology: Bullous Diseases.* Edited by Fine JD. New York: Igaku-Shoin; 1993:97–120.

12. Gammon WR, Fine JD, Briggaman RA: Autoimmunity to type VII collagen: features and role in basement membrane injury. In *Topics in Clinical Dermatology: Bullous Diseases.* Edited by Fine JD. New York: Igaku-Shoin; 1993:75–98.

Cutaneous Manifestations of Endocrine and Metabolic Disorders 21

Victoria P. Werth
Lynn McKinley-Grant

Key Points

- There are many inflammatory and infectious skin dermatoses associated with diabetes mellitus. Prevention, evaluation, and treatment of infected leg and foot ulcers are particularly important concerns.
- The presence of xanthomas indicates the need for evaluation of serum cholesterol and triglyceride levels.
- Hyperandrogenemia, as manifest by hirsutism, acne, and androgenetic alopecia, can indicate either ovarian or adrenal pathology, and may warrant screening tests for elevated hormone levels.
- Porphyria cutanea tarda has recently been found to be associated with hepatitis C infection in some individuals, and can be aggravated by alcohol use and various medications.
- Other metabolic diseases affecting the skin include amyloidosis, hemochromatosis, cutis calcinosis, and acrodermatitis enteropathica.

ENDOCRINE DISORDERS

Diabetes Mellitus Disorders

Many inflammatory and infectious skin dermatoses are seen in patients with diabetes mellitus (Table 21-1). None are pathognomonic of diabetes, as is the case with granuloma annulare, but their occurrence should lead the clinician to consider whether diabetes is present (Fig. 21-1). In addition, the vascular changes seen in diabetics result in secondary cutaneous changes.

Inflammatory dermatoses

Necrobiosis lipoidica diabeticorum occurs in three in every 1000 diabetics, but only two thirds of those affected will eventually have diabetes. Clinically, erythematous to yellowish papules and plaques, atrophic in the center, occur most often on the legs (Fig. 21-2). About one third of these lesions ulcerate. Treatment includes topical and intralesional corticosteroid therapy, but care must be taken because the lesions are atrophic and tend to ulcerate.

Diabetic dermopathy is manifest by multiple, discrete, brown, slightly atrophic macules on the anterior lower legs. The origin of this condition is unknown, but it is seen in about 50% of patients with diabetes. No known therapy exists for this disorder. The bullous eruption of diabetes (bullous diabeticorum) is represented by the spontaneous formation of painless, tense blisters on the feet, lower legs, and occasionally, arms and hands, in patients with long-standing diabetes. The lesions heal in 2 to 5 weeks without scarring and can recur over a period of several years. The diagnosis can be made only after traumatic and chemical causes are excluded, cultures are sterile, and both uropor-

severe atherosclerosis is present, revascularization may be necessary to heal an ulcer.

Evaluation of infected leg and foot ulcers

Purulent discharge or the presence of two or more of the signs and symptoms of inflammation (induration, redness, warmth, and tenderness) usually suggests infection. Cultures should be obtained from most soft tissue infections to select the appropriate specific antibiotic treatment. Swabs of purulent discharge are unreliable because anaerobes are inhibited by cotton swab and because the culture does not distinguish between pathogens and colonization [3]. Possible methods of specimen collection for quantitative assessment of bacteria in the wound include curettage specimen, biopsy, or needle aspiration. The curettage specimen is obtained after the surface of an open wound is cleaned with saline-soaked gauze, betadine, or alcohol. A sterile dermal curette or scalpel blade is used to scrape tissue from the base and edges of the ulcer [4••].

Organisms causing ulcers

Ulcers are commonly colonized by *Staphylococcus aureus*. Aerobic gram-negative bacilli are commonly isolated, including *Proteus, Escherichia coli, Klebsiella-Enterobacter* species, and *Pseudomonas*. Obligate anaerobes may also be important pathogens in these infections.

Treatment of infected leg and foot ulcers

Treatment of mild infections should include oral dicloxacillin, erythromycin, cephalexin, or clindamycin for 1 to 2 weeks. If gram-negative bacilli are involved, trimethoprim-sulfamethoxazole, amoxicillin-clavulanate, or ciprofloxacin should be administered. If the infection has a foul odor or the gram-stained smear shows several types of organisms, obligate anaerobes may be present. In these cases, clindamycin alone or metronidazole and an anti-staphylococcal drug should be given [4••]. If the infection does not respond in 2 to 3 days, parenteral treatment should be given and the wound cultures used to determine therapy. Local care of ulcers should include elevation of the feet; local débridement of any eschar; soaks with saline; application of antimicrobial ointments, such as polysporin or bacitracin; and a nonadherent dressing. Once the infection is cleared, a whole range of new wound-care dressings is available to expedite healing. It is important to avoid desiccation of the wound, often caused by using wet-to-dry dressings.

Xanthomas and Dysproteinemias

Xanthomas can occur with or without elevated blood lipids. When a hyperlipidemia is present, the type of hyperlipidemia can be predicted from the type of xanthoma present (tuberous, tendon, eruptive, or planar; Table 21-2) [5]. Secondary causes of the hyperlipidemia must be sought. Xanthelasmas, and xanthomas associated with various

TABLE 21-2 CLINICAL DISORDERS IN WHICH XANTHOMAS OCCUR	
Xanthoma	**Clinical disorders**
Tuberous	Types II and III hyperlipoproteinemia
Tendon	Types IIa, IIb, and III hyperlipoproteinemia
	Obstructive liver disease
	Hypothyroidism
	Diabetes mellitus
	Cerebrotendinous xanthomatosis
Eruptive	Types I, IV, and V hyperlipoproteinemia
	Diabetes mellitus
	Pancreatitis
	Hypothyroidism
	Nephrotic syndrome
	Medications: isotretinoin, estrogen, glucocorticoids
Xanthoma striatum palmare	Type III, IV hyperlipoproteinemia
	Biliary cirrhosis
	Diabetes mellitus

dysproteinemias, inflammatory skin disorders, and lipid storage disease can occur in the setting of normal blood lipid levels [6].

Tuberous xanthomas appear as yellow-to-red grouped papules and nodules, often located on elbows, extensor forearms, knuckles, palms, knees, heels, and buttocks. This condition is particularly associated with increased serum cholesterol levels but can be seen with increased very-low-density lipoprotein (triglyceride-rich) and intermediate-density lipoprotein levels.

Tendinous xanthomas are deep, firm, variably sized nodules with normal overlying skin that are present in tendons, ligaments, and fascia. They occur in the Achilles tendons and extensor tendons of the knees, elbows, and dorsa of the hands, and can be painful. The differential diagnosis includes rheumatoid nodules and gouty tophi. These xanthomas are seen with hypercholesterolemia.

Eruptive xanthomas are 1- to 4-mm erythematous papules usually found on the buttocks and extensor thighs, knees, and arms (Fig. 21-8). They may be pruritic and often occur in response to trauma. This form of xanthoma occurs with hypertriglyceridemia.

Planar xanthomas include several discrete entities. Xanthelasmas are yellow infiltrative macules and papules found on the eyelids. These are associated with increased serum cholesterol in 50% of people, and those under 40 to 50 years of age are particularly at risk. Xanthoma striatum palmare occurs as yellow, soft, often linear patches in the creases of the palms and fingers. This condition is associ-

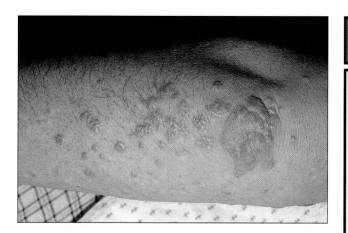

FIGURE 21-8 Eruptive xanthomas in a diabetic patient whose blood glucose level is poorly controlled. Note yellow papules and plaques on the extensor surface of the elbow and arm. (*Courtesy of* B. Witmer.)

TABLE 21-4 DERMATOLOGIC DISEASES ASSOCIATED WITH THYROID DISEASE
Dermatitis herpetiformis
Alopecia areata
Pemphigus foliaceus and vulgaris
Bullous pemphigoid
Herpes gestationis
Dermatomyositis
Lupus erythematosus, chronic cutaneous and systemic
Scleroderma
Vitiligo
Pustulosis palmoplantaris
Sweet's syndrome
Urticaria
Cowden's disease

ated with increased triglyceride or intermediate-density lipoprotein levels. Extensive, yellow-orange infiltrative plaques on the face, neck, upper trunk, and arms are seen in association with several dysproteinemias, including myeloma, lymphomas, chronic leukemias, cryoglobulinemias, Waldenström's macroglobulinemia, and benign monoclonal gammopathy.

Evaluation and treatment of xanthomas

A skin biopsy helps confirm the diagnosis of xanthoma if the diagnosis is uncertain. The clinical appearance of xanthelasma is usually distinctive enough to render a biopsy unnecessary. Any patient with xanthomas deserves serum cholesterol and serum fasting triglyceride level testing to screen for hyperlipidemia. Any abnormalities need further evaluation as to the type of hyperlipidemia, any possible secondary causes, and then treatment of the secondary cause or the primary disorder.

Control of the hyperlipidemia leads to rapid resolution of eruptive xanthomas and slower regression of tuberous xanthomas. Tendinous xanthomas and xanthelasmas seldom resolve with treatment.

Thyroid Disorders

Many nonspecific findings occur in the skin, hair, and nails in hyperthyroidism and hypothyroidism (Table 21-3) [7]. Other findings are more specific, as discussed later. In addition, many dermatologic diseases, such as vitiligo, are associated with thyroid disease (Table 21-4, Fig. 21-9).

Pretibial myxedema is seen in 0.5% to 4% of patients with Graves' disease, and rarely, in patients with Hashimoto's thyroiditis. Bilateral, asymmetric, pink to purple-brown firm plaques and nodules occur most frequently on the lower legs (Fig. 21-10*A*). The lesions may exhibit hypertrichosis or become verrucous (Fig. 21-10*B*). Pretibial myxedema is often associated with exophthalmos

TABLE 21-3 NONSPECIFIC GENERAL DERMATOLOGIC FINDINGS IN HYPERTHYROIDISM AND HYPOTHYROIDISM		
	Manifestations	
Affected area	**Hyperthyroidism**	**Hypothyroidism**
Skin	Warm, moist, smooth	Cold, pale, decreased sweating
Hair	Facial, palmar erythema	Xerosis, ichthyosis, keratoderma
Nail	Generalized hyperhidrosis	Carotenemia (yellow palms, soles, nasolabial folds)
	Increased pigmentation (palms, soles, oral mucosa)	Poor wound healing
	Pruritus	Dry, course, brittle
	Fine, soft	Diffuse thinning
	Diffuse, nonscarring alopecia	Loss of lateral third of eyebrows
	Plummer's nails (concave contour with distal onycholysis)	Thick, brittle
		Longitudinal striations
		Slow growth

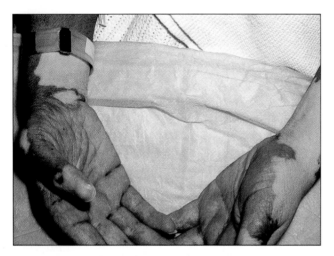

FIGURE 21-9 Vitiligo in a patient with hypothyroidism. Note hypopigmented patches on the wrists and hands.

(Fig. 21-11), and results from the accumulation of hyaluronic acid in the dermis and sometimes the subcutaneous tissue. The diagnosis is confirmed with a skin biopsy. If the patient is not known to have thyroid disease, thyroid function tests should be obtained. This process is most often found in euthyroid patients whose hyperthyroidism has been treated with surgery or radioactive iodine. Treatment with topical or intralesional corticosteroids is sometimes effective.

Thyroid acropachy is seen in 0.1% to 1% of patients with Graves' disease and rarely in those with Hashimoto's thyroiditis. It consists of digital clubbing, soft-tissue swelling of the hands and feet, and periosteal proliferation of the shafts of the fingers, toes, and other distal long bones (Fig. 21-12). It is often associated with exophthalmos or pretibial myxedema and most often occurs after treatment

of the thyroid disease. No treatment is necessary, and the findings may slowly resolve.

Generalized myxedema occurs in patients with hypothyroidism and is manifest as diffusely edematous, waxy, and firm skin. Patients often have a puffy appearance, with thickening of the lips, a broad nose, and macroglossia. These changes result from dermal deposition of acid mucopolysaccharides in the skin. Thyroid hormone replacement generally leads to resolution of the cutaneous changes.

Adrenal Cortex Disorders

Skin disorders are associated with several hypersecretion syndromes of the adrenal, including those in which increased cortisol (Cushing's syndrome), androgens (virilization), and estrogens (feminization) occur. In addition, adrenocortical failure results in skin changes.

Cushing's syndrome results from an increase in endogenous cortisol production from an adrenal tumor or from exogenous glucocorticoids. The associated cutaneous findings include increased fat deposition in the supraclavicular fossae, upper back, and abdomen. The face is round and puffy, and the skin is thinned, leading to easy bruising and delayed wound healing (Fig. 21-13). Other changes include acne, facial erythema, lanugo hair, and hair loss [8].

Hyperandrogenemia can lead to hirsutism, acne, and androgenetic alopecia (Figs. 21-14 and 21-15). Other cutaneous signs include loss of breast tissue and clitoral enlargement. The sources of elevated androgens include the adrenal and ovary glands [9]. Ovarian causes of increased androgens include polycystic ovarian syndrome, insulin resistance, and ovarian tumors. Adrenal causes include Cushing's disease, androgen-producing tumors, and congenital adrenal hyperplasia. Some drugs can cause hirsutism by a mechanism unrelated to androgens. These

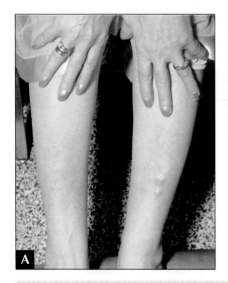
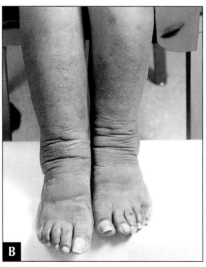
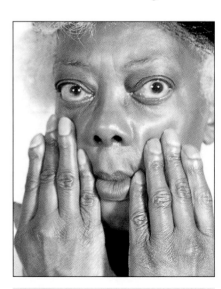

FIGURE 21-10 **A**, Pretibial myxedema. Note pink nodules on legs with diffuse, nonpitting edema. **B**, Nonpitting edema with prominent hair follicles and "cobblestone" pattern to lesions on legs. (*Courtesy of* F. Sterling; Philadelphia, PA.)

FIGURE 21-11 Graves' ophthalmopathy. Prominent proptosis of the eyes is seen. (*Courtesy of* F. Sterling.)

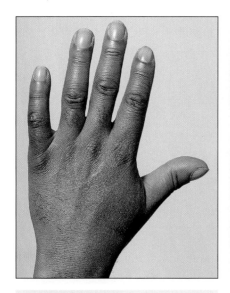

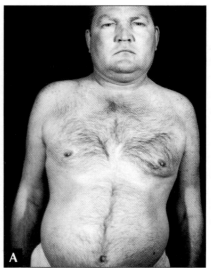

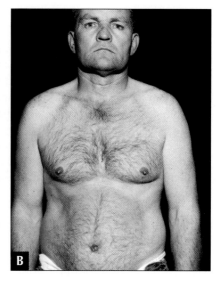

FIGURE 21-12 Thyroid acropachy with clubbing of the digits. (*Courtesy of* F. Sterling.)

FIGURE 21-13 Cushing's disease, before (*panel A*) and after (*panel B*) bilateral adrenalectomy. There is truncal obesity and cushingoid facies before surgery. (*Courtesy of* F. Sterling.)

drugs include minoxidil, diazoxide, phenytoin, glucocorticoids, and cyclosporine.

In evaluating patients for hyperandrogenemia, it is important to obtain a history, including the age and rapidity of onset, other symptoms of virilism, other symptoms of Cushing's disease, drug history, and menstrual history. The physical examination should evaluate the amount and distribution of hair, clitoral enlargement, presence of acne refractory to treatment, pelvic and abdominal exam, skin qualities, and muscle strength. Screening tests should include a total and free serum testosterone and dehydroepiandrosterone sulfate (DHEAS) level. If the total testosterone level is greater than 200 ng/dL or the DHEAS level is over 700 μg/dL, then evaluation should include pelvic ultrasound, and computed tomography or magnetic resonance imaging of the adrenals, in search of tumors. Free testosterone level is a more sensitive indicator of hyperandrogenism than total testosterone level. Intermediate elevations of DHEAS level suggest an adrenal etiology of hyperandrogenemia and can be evaluated with an corticotropin stimulation test to detect mild, late-onset congenital adrenal hyperplasia [10••]. Intermediate elevations of testosterone can be seen with hyperandrogenemia of adrenal or ovarian cause. If menstrual dysfunction exists with other signs of hyperandrogenism,

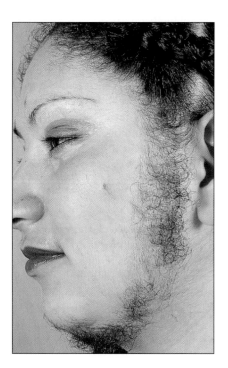

FIGURE 21-14 Hirsutism in a patient with ovarian thecoma. There is prominent facial hair, especially in the beard and mustache areas.

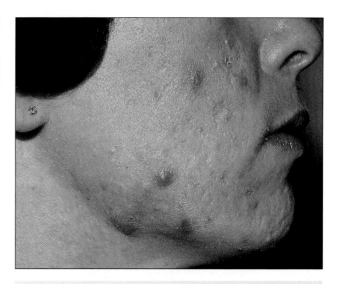

FIGURE 21-15 Acne in a patient with hyperandrogenemia. There are active erythematous cysts, as well as many areas with pitted scarring owing to previous acne lesions. (*Courtesy of* B. Witmer.)

then a serum prolactin level and luteinizing hormone–follicle-stimulating hormone ratio should be checked. If the serum prolactin level is greater than 20 ng/dL, then a prolactinoma should be excluded with magnetic resonance imaging or computed tomography. Mild prolactin elevations have been reported in up to 30% of women with polycystic ovary disease. If the luteinizing hormone–follicle-stimulating hormone ratio is greater than three, polycystic disease should be suspected, and a gynecologic consult and ultrasound of the ovaries should be obtained. If symptoms of Cushing's syndrome exist, a dexamethasone suppression test should be performed: 1 mg of dexamethasone given at midnight and the morning serum cortisol level measured. If the cortisol level is greater than 0.5 μg/dL, then Cushing's syndrome must be ruled out.

Treatment of hyperandrogenemia

First, any medications that may be contributing to the condition must be stopped. Polycystic ovary disease can be treated with low-dose oral contraceptives. Insulin resistance has been treated with oral contraceptives or a long-acting luteinizing hormone-releasing hormone analogue. Ovarian tumors are treated with surgery, and Cushing's disease is treated with pituitary surgery. Androgen-producing tumors are treated with surgery. Congenital adrenal hyperplasia is treated with small evening doses of prednisone (2.5 to 5.0 mg) for 1 year. During treatment, the serum testosterone or DHEAS level should be obtained every 3 months to assess the effectiveness of therapy. After treatment ends, glucocorticoids should be restarted after serum androgen levels increase or if the patient becomes symptomatic. Idiopathic hirsutism is usually ovarian in etiology and can be treated with oral contraceptives. Other therapy includes antiandrogens that work mainly at the end-organ tissue level, and these can be used alone or with other therapies. These agents include spironolactone, 50 to 200 mg/d, and flutamide, neither of which is approved for use in hyperandrogenemia. Mild symptoms of hyperandrogenemia can be treated directly with such treatments as bleaching, depilation, epilation, and electrolysis to treat increased facial hair.

Adrenocortical failure

Adrenocortical failure can result from autoimmunity, chronic infections, bilateral tumors, or vasculitis. Secondary failure can result from hypopituitarism. The findings include hyperpigmentation of the skin, especially involving the oral mucosa and palmer creases (Fig. 21-16). Nevi darken and flat pigmented macules called lentigos can develop. Body hair can decrease. Fifteen percent of patients, usually those with autoimmune disease, develop vitiligo.

Multiple endocrine neoplasia

The multiple endocrine neoplasia type 3 syndrome includes mucosal neuromas, bumpy lips, pheochromocytoma, and medullary thyroid carcinoma. The mucosal neuromas involve the tongue, lips, buccal mucosa, and other sites. The

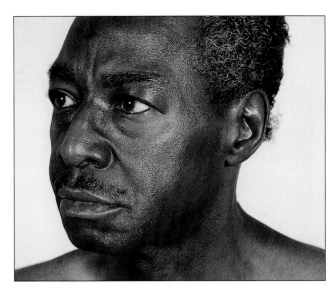

FIGURE 21-16 Addison's disease. There is marked hyperpigmentation of the face. (*Courtesy of* B. Witmer.)

neuromas begin in the first decade of life, and the syndrome is inherited in an autosomal dominant fashion [11]. Pituitary gland disorders, such as acromegaly, Cushing's disease, and panhypopituitarism each have associated skin findings (Table 21-5).

METABOLIC DISORDERS

Porphyrias

The porphyrias are a group of defects in heme synthesis that affect the skin, the nervous system, and the gastrointestinal system. Only two porphyrias do not have photodermatoses: acute intermittent porphyria and aminolevulinic acid dehydrase deficiency. The diagnostic test for porphyria depends on the type of porphyria present.

Porphyria cutanea tarda, the most common porphyria, involves decreased production of the enzyme uroporphyrinogen decarboxylase. Variegate porphyria, which results from a defect in protoporphyrin oxydase, presents with the same skin lesions as porphyria cutanea tarda but also causes gastrointestinal and neurological symptoms. Clinically, these patients present with bullae, erosions, scarring, hyperpigmentation and hypopigmentation, and sclerodermoid changes of sun-exposed areas of the hands, face, and legs (Fig. 21-17). Hypertrichosis of the face is common (Fig. 21-18). Porphyria cutanea tarda is associated most frequently with excessive alcohol intake. In addition, several drugs may exacerbate the disease (*eg*, estrogens). Hemochromatosis, carcinomas, lymphomas, and chronic renal failure may also be associated with porphyria cutanea tarda [12]. Recently, multiple reports of porphyria cutanea tarda, HIV infection [13•] and hepatitis C antibodies [14] have been published. HIV, hepatitis antigen and anti-hepatitis C virus should be checked as part of a routine evaluation.

TABLE 21-5 PITUITARY GLAND DISORDERS

Affected area	Manifestations
Acromegaly	
Skin	Enlarged hands, feet
	Thickened eyelids
	Cutis verticis gyrata
	Hypertrichosis
	Hyperhidrosis
	Skin tags
	Acanthosis nigricans
	Abscesses: axillae, buttocks
	Hyperpigmentation
Mouth	Macroglossia
Nail	Thick, hard
Hair	Loss of body hair
	Scalp hair fine, silky
Cushing's disease	
Skin	Hyperpigmentation
	Changes of hypercorticism (Cushing's syndrome)
Panhypopituitarism	
Skin	Dry, smooth, soft, pale
	Fine wrinkles
Hair	Hair loss: axillae, pubic, beard
	Scalp hair: fine, dry, thin

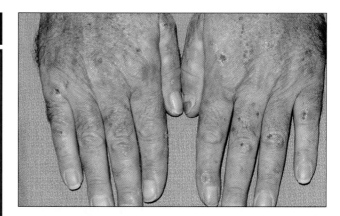

FIGURE 21-17 Bullae and erosion on the dorsal surface of the hands resulting from porphyria cutanea tarda.

The diagnosis of porphyria cutanea tarda can be suggested by demonstration of pink coral fluorescence of the urine with a Wood's lamp; however, a 24-hour urine specimen is required to measure uroporphyrins and coproporphyrins. The treatment is to remove any drugs, which exacerbate the disease. Iron stores are removed by repeated phlebotomy [15].

Erythropoietic porphyria is a rare porphyrin disorder that presents in childhood with severe photosensitivity, even through window-glass, resulting initially in erythematous urticarial plaques. Chronic erythropoietic porphyria leads to scarring, very thick skin over the finger joints, severe photodamage, and atrophy of the rim of the ears. Patients can also develop liver involvement, and rarely even fatal cirrhosis. The diagnosis is made through measurement of erythrocyte protoporphyrin and fecal protoporphyrin levels. The urine does not fluoresce. Treatment includes administration of oral β-carotene, antimalarials, antihistamines, and cholestyramine. To prevent photosensitivity in all porphyrias, physical sunscreens, protective clothing, and sun avoidance are advised [16].

Amyloidosis

Amyloidosis is a group of disorders in which amyloid is deposited in tissue. The classification of amyloidosis is as follows: primary localized cutaneous amyloidosis (which includes papular or lichen amyloidosis, macular amyloidosis, and nodular amyloidosis), secondary localized cutaneous amyloidosis, systemic immunoglobulin-related amyloidosis, and familial amyloidosis [12]. All types of amyloid have the same biochemical configuration and appear as an amorphous eosinophilic material on routine pathologic staining. When tissue is stained with Congo red, a green birefringent appears under a polarizing microscope.

Primary systemic amyloidosis can present with skin findings early in the disease. Spontaneous purpuric lesions develop in areas of trauma, body folds, eyelids, sides of the nose, neck, axilla, umbilicus, and the anogenital region. The hemorrhage results from amyloid infiltration in blood vessel walls. Macroglossia, mucosal lesions, waxy translucent papules, sclerodermoid plaques, alopecia, and bullous lesions may occur [17]. Patients with these findings should have serum and urine immunoelectrophoresis, and an evaluation for end-organ involvement.

The cutaneous types of amyloidosis do not need a systemic evaluation. Lichen or papular amyloid consists of

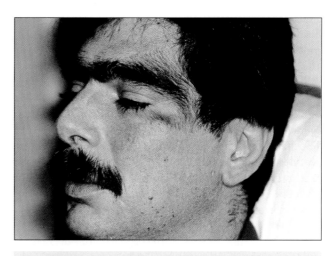

FIGURE 21-18 Hypertrichosis of the lateral forehead resulting from porphyria cutanea tarda.

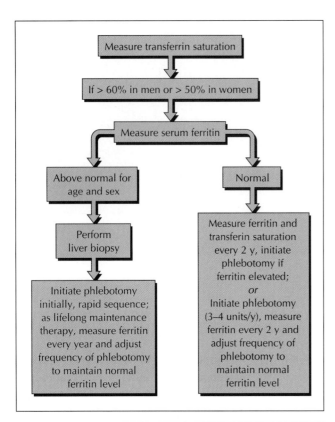

FIGURE 21-19 Protocol for hemochromatosis screening and treatment. (*From* Edwards and Kushner [19]; with permission.)

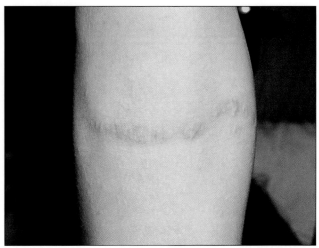

FIGURE 21-20 Cutis calcinosis due to renal failure and secondary hyperparathyroidism. Note yellow-white, firm papules in a linear distribution on the arm.

very pruritic papules and plaques on the shins of adults and can be treated with topical steroids. Macular amyloid presents with reticulated hyperpigmentation on the trunk and extremities [18]. Nodular amyloid is rare, with waxy brown yellow nodules occurring anywhere. Secondary localized cutaneous amyloidosis can occur in previous areas of inflammation, such as near basal cell carcinomas.

Hemochromatosis

Hemochromatosis is an inborn error of intestinal iron absorption. The dermatologic manifestations are a distinct gray-to-brown coloration of the face, extensor surfaces of the forearms, dorsum of the hand, and genital areas. Mucosal hyperpigmentation is also seen. It occurs mostly in men and is rarely seen in homozygous persons under the age of 20 years. Xerosis, diabetes, endocrine failure, heart failure, and arthropathy are also seen. Recently, a screening test that detects hemochromatosis before symptoms appear was described (Fig. 21-19) [19]. This test would measure transferrin saturation and serum ferritin levels. Therapy with phlebotomy can remove iron and lead to an improvement in liver function.

Cutis Calcinosis

There are three main types of calcium deposits in the skin: metastatic calcinosis (hypercalcemia or hyperphosphatasemia), dystrophic cutis calcinosis (no metabolic disorder), and idiopathic calcinosis (no metabolic disorder) [20]. There are two causes of metastatic calcinosis: hypercalcemia or hyperphosphatasemia, or deficient end-organ response to parathyroid hormone. Clinically, these conditions occur in normal skin as subcutaneous nodules or plaques around the joints. Linear cutaneous nodules and plaques can also be present. The differential diagnosis for metastatic calcinosis includes secondary hyperparathyroidism, uremia, vitamin D toxicity, milk alkali syndrome, and sarcoidosis (Fig. 21-20). Dystrophic cutis calcinosis occurs in areas of previous trauma or inflammation. This condition occurs in two types: localized and generalized. The localized type occurs in areas of trauma and old inflammation, such as acne cysts and calcium infusion [21]. A generalized type of dystrophic calcinosis is found in hereditary disorders, such as pseudoxanthoma elasticum, Ehlers-Danlos syndrome, or Werner's syndrome. Calcinosis is also seen in dermatomyositis and

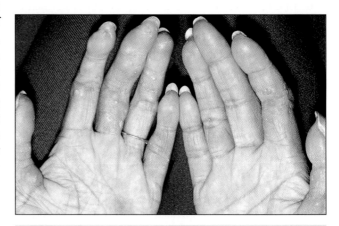

FIGURE 21-21 Cutis calcinosis in a patient with scleroderma. Note firm, whitish papules on the fingers.

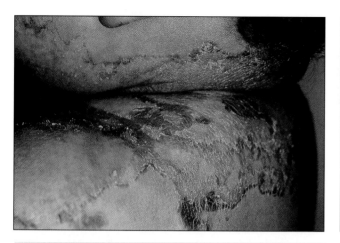

FIGURE 21-22 Acrodermatitis enteropathica in a child. Note desquamating, eczematous eruption on the neck and upper back.

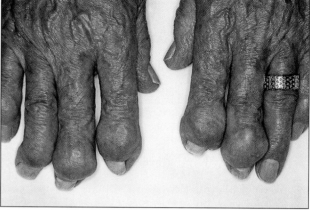

FIGURE 21-23 Gouty tophi of hands. Note white to skin-colored firm papules on distal interphalangeal joints of hands.

scleroderma, but only rarely in lupus erythematosus (Fig. 21-21). Idiopathic cutis calcinosis occurs most commonly in the scrotum and is asymptomatic. Treatment of calcinosis cutis is generally directed toward the underlying metabolic disorder, or the lesion is excised.

Acrodermatitis Enteropathica

Two types of acrodermatitis enteropathica exist: an autosomal recessive disorder and an acquired zinc deficiency. The clinical findings are similar in adults and children, and present with early acral and periorificial erythema and scale with serpiginous borders, alopecia, gastrointestinal symptoms, anorexia, immune dysfunction, growth retardation, and central nervous system symptoms (Fig. 21-22).

Borderline zinc deficiency can occur in patients with any malabsorption disorder, liver disease, chronic alcohol abuse, those on total parenteral nutrition, and those with other nutritional deficiencies. Recently, cases of acrodermatitis enteropathica have been described in anorexia nervosa [22•] and immunodeficiency syndrome [23•]. Response to treatment is very rapid, with lesions clearing in approximately 10 days with oral zinc sulfate, 250 mg, administered once or twice a day. The diagnosis of zinc deficiency is most accurately made by obtaining a serum concentration of zinc. Before the level is drawn, consultation should be made with the laboratory that will interpret the results. Urine and hair concentrations of zinc are not reliable methods of measuring zinc levels.

Gout

Gout is a disorder of uric acid, where there is either a defect in absorption and production, or a defect in excretion of the acid. It results in a group of diseases that are caused by the deposit of monosodium urate monohydrate crystals in the tissues around the joints of the extremities, the ears, and the kidney.

A positive family history is present in some patients with gout. Gout is commoner in men and in patients taking thiazide diuretics. Acute gouty arthritis commonly involves the first metatarsal of the foot. Patients can develop tophaceous gout, in which deposits in the subcutaneous tissues of the skin, gouty nephropathy, and urolithiasis occur (Figs. 21-23 and 21-24). Therapy for acute gouty arthritis is discussed in the rheumatology section, but nonsteroidal anti-inflammatory agents and antiurate agents are used as preventive therapy. Allopurinol is probably the best inhibitor of the enzyme xanthine oxidase, and thus inhibits uric acid production and prevents tophaceous gout. Many patients develop an allergy to allopurinol. Patients with maculopapular eruptions and not life-threatening dermatoses can be desensitized to allopurinol by use of an oral desensitization method, but this method should be used with extreme caution [24•].

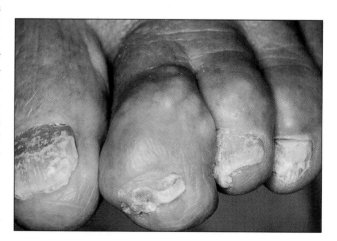

FIGURE 21-24 Gouty tophi of feet. Note yellow- to skin-colored firm papules on distal joints of feet. Nail changes are typical of onychomycosis.

References and Recommended Reading

Recently published papers of particular interest have been highlighted as:

• Of interest

•• Of outstanding interest

1. Oursler JR, Goldblum OR: Blistering eruption in a diabetic. *Arch Dermatol* 1991, 127:247–252.

2. Johnson MP, Ramphal R: Malignant external otitis. *Rev Infect Dis* 1990, 12:173–180.

3. Wheat LJ, Allen SD, Henry M, *et al.*: Diabetic foot infections. Bacteriologic analysis. *Arch Intern Med* 1986, 146:1935–1940.

4.•• Lipsky BA, Pecoraro RE, Wheat LJ: The diabetic foot: soft tissue and bone infection. *Infect Dis Clin North Am* 1990, 4:409–432.

5. Parker F: Xanthomas and hyperlipidemias. *J Am Acad Dermatol* 1985, 13:1–30.

6. Feingold KR, Castro GR, Ishikawa V, *et al.*: Cutaneous xanthoma in association with paraproteinemia in the absence of hyperlipidemia. *J Clin Invest* 1989, 83:796–802.

7. Heymann WR: Cutaneous manifestations of thyroid disease. *J Am Acad Dermatol* 1992, 26:885–902.

8. Werth VP: Management and treatment with systemic glucocorticoids. *Adv Dermatol* 1993, 8:81–103.

9. Sperling SC, Heimer WL: Androgen biology as a basis for the diagnosis and treatment of androgenic disorders in women. *J Am Acad Dermatol* 1993, 26:669–683.

10.•• Sperling SC, Heimer WL: Androgen biology as a basis for the diagnosis and treatment of androgenic disorders in women: II. *J Am Acad Dermatol* 1993, 26:901–916.

11. Khairi MRA, Dexter RN, Burzynski NJ, Johnston CC: Mucosal neuroma, pheochromocytoma and medullary thyroid carcinoma: multiple endocrine neoplasia, type 3. *Medicine* 1965, 54:89–112.

12. Finkel LJ: Cutaneous mucinoses and amyloidosis. In *J Dermatology*, edn 3. Edited by Moschella S, Hurley HJ. Philadelphia: WB Saunders; 1992:1597–1604.

13.• Blauvelt A, Harris H, Hogan D, *et al.*: Porphyria cutanea tarda and human immunodeficiency virus. *Int J Dermatol* 1992, 31:474–479.

14. LaCour J, Bodokh I, Castanet J, *et al.*: Porphyria cutanea tarda and antibodies to hepatitis C virus. *Br J Dermatol* 1993, 128:121–123.

15. Paslin D: The porphyrias. *Int J Dermatol* 1992, 31:517–539.

16. Parker F: Disorders of metabolism. In *Dermatology*, edn 3. Edited by Moschella S, Hurley HJ. Philadelphia: WB Saunders; 1992:1667–1678.

17. Robert C, Aractin G, Prost S, Verola C: Bullous amyloidosis: report of three cases and review of the literature. *Medicine* 1993, 72:38–44.

18. Bourke JF, Berth-Jones J, Burns DA: Diffuse primary cutaneous amyloidosis. *Br J Dermatol* 127:641–644.

19. Edwards C, Kushner J: Screening for hemochromatosis. *N Engl J Med* 1993, 328:1616–1620.

20. Orlow S, Watsky K, Bolognia J: Skin and bones II. *J Am Acad Dermatol* 1991, 25:447–462.

21. Werth S, Latour D, Wilson D: Yellow plaques and ulcerations in a cardiac transplant patient. *Arch Dermatol* 1992, 128:547–552.

22.• Voorhees A, Riba M: Acquired zinc deficiency in association with anorexia nervosa. *Pediatr Dermatol* 1992, 9:268–271.

23.• Reichel M, Mauro T, Ziboh V, *et al.*: Acrodermatitis enteropathica in a patient with the acquired immunodeficiency syndrome. *Arch Dermatol* 1992, 128:415–416.

24.• Fam AG, Lewtaf J, Stein J, Patton TW: Desensitization allopurinol in patients with gout and cutaneous reactions. *Am J Med* 1992, 93:299–302.

Select Bibliography

Decastro M, Sanchez J, Herrera JF, *et al.*: Hepatitis C virus antibodies and liver disease in patients with porphyria cutanea tarda. *Hepatology* 1993, 17:551–557.

Fatourechi V, Pajouhi M, Fransway AF: Dermopathy of Graves' disease (pretibial myxedema)—review of 150 cases. *Medicine* 1994, 73:1–7.

Meola T, Lim HW: The porphyrias. *Dermatol Clin* 1993, 11:583–596.

Reiber GE, Pecoraro RE, Koepsell TD: Risk factors for amputation in patients with diabetes mellitus: a case control study. *Ann Intern Med* 1992, 117:97–105.

Rosenfield RL, Lucky AW. Acne, hirsutism, and alopecia in adolescent girls. Clinical expressions of androgen excess. *Endocrinol Metab Clin North Am* 1993, 22:507–532.

Stevens B, Fleischer A, Piering F, Crosby D: Porphyria cutanea tarda in the setting of renal failure. *Arch Dermatol* 1993, 129:337–339.

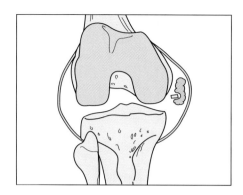

RHEUMATOLOGY

VI

In the Rheumatology section of *Current Practice of Medicine*, we have emphasized common conditions encountered by primary care physicians, but also have included the latest contributions of laboratory medicine. Chapters discussing back and neck pain, regional pain syndromes, fibromyalgia, osteoarthritis, and metabolic bone diseases provide current knowledge and references pertaining to these subjects. A chapter on sports medicine, co-authored by the team physician of the Sacramento Kings and a primary care physician, was included because of the growing importance of this field.

Chapters on the use of diagnostic tests in rheumatic disease and their application to diagnosis and differential diagnosis integrate new knowledge of antiphospholipid antibodies. These tests have added an entirely new dimension to our understanding of systemic lupus erythematosus. The remarkable specificity of cANA antibody for Wegener's granulomatosis and microscopic polyarteritis is discussed in a chapter on vasculitis. The expanding spectrum of infectious organisms capable of triggering a "reactive" arthritis now includes type A *Streptococcus* and *Giardia* species. The efficacy of combinations of remittive agents in the treatment of rheumatoid arthritis is covered, as is the importance of specific crystal identification in the diagnosis and differential diagnosis of monarthritis syndromes.

Throughout the text, we have attempted to emphasize the practical without eliminating scientific principles where these apply. We look forward to feedback from our readers.

Section Editor
Daniel J. McCarty

Diagnostic Tests in Rheumatic Disease

W. Watson Buchanan

1

Key Points

- Diagnosis of the 100 or more forms of arthritis and allied conditions essentially is based on pattern recognition.
- Synovianalysis is important in confirming the diagnosis of crystal-induced arthritis and excluding joint infection. It is a technique that family practitioners should be able to perform.
- Synovial biopsy can be performed by needle but is best performed by arthroscopy or arthrotomy, which permits direct visualization and a more generous tissue size.
- Muscle biopsy, electromyography, and serum muscle enzyme tests all have limitations in evaluating disease of skeletal muscle. Tests for rheumatoid and antinuclear factors commonly are performed in investigation of arthritic and connective tissue diseases, as are other procedures, such as assays or serum complement components, lupus anticoagulant, cryoglobulins, and acute phase reactants.
- Not only must the family doctor be aware of what information can be obtained by routine black and white radiographs, but also the many new musculoskeletal imaging methods: nuclear medicine, ultrasonography, computed tomography, and magnetic resonance.

"The diagnosis of disease is often easy; often difficult; and often impossible" [1].

Although diagnosis is the cornerstone of medical science, its precise definition and ascertainment are less clear. Many strategies have been employed to arrive at a diagnosis. Defining probabilities, although of interest to biostatisticians, is probably rare in the clinical situation. Similarly, algorithmic approaches, although frequently used in teaching and as therapeutic guidelines, have not proven popular with clinicians. Diagnosis of rheumatic disease is based on a gestalt method of pattern recognition [2].

ARTHROCENTESIS

Arthrocentesis has been aptly described as liquid biopsy of the joint. With the exception of the hip and sacroiliac joints, which require fluoroscopic guidance for aspiration, most peripheral joints can be aspirated easily. The site of injection for each joint was well described by Doherty and coworkers [3••], and the technique was described by Gatter and Schumacher [4••].

Technique

It is convenient to mark the site of injection using a ball-point pen with the point withdrawn. Drapes are unnecessary, as are masks and gowns. Rubber gloves, which need not be sterile, are mandatory to protect the physician. The skin should be cleaned with a detergent, such as povidone-iodine (Betadine, Purdue Frederick Co., Norwalk, CT). The area of skin to be punctured and the subcutaneous tissues should then be anesthetized with 1% or 2% lidocaine hydrochloride (Xylocaine,

RHEUMATOID FACTOR TESTS

Rheumatoid factors are autoantibodies to antigenic determinants of the Fc portion of IgG molecules. The most commonly used tests for IgM rheumatoid factors are the bentonite and latex agglutination tests and the Waaler-Rose, or sheep cell, agglutination test (Fig. 3).

Rheumatoid factor test results are positive in many chronic inflammatory and infectious diseases (Table 2), but high titers are found particularly in rheumatoid arthritis. Persistently high titers in this disease usually auger a poor prognosis and are frequently associated with vascular and granulomatous complications. Rheumatoid factors transfused into healthy persons, however, are without ill effect.

Test findings for rheumatoid factor may remain negative during the first year of rheumatoid arthritis, and indeed a proportion of patients remain seronegative for the whole course of their illness. These seronegative patients tend to have milder disease and rarely develop systemic complications. Patients who are seronegative for rheumatoid factor by classic tests may, however, be shown to have IgG and IgM antiglobulins.

ANTINUCLEAR AND ANTICYTOPLASMIC ANTIBODIES

The most practical and convenient method of screening for antinuclear antibodies is the indirect immunofluorescence technique, in which suspected serum is incubated with cryostat sections of rodent liver or kidney or with proliferating cells in tissue culture that have larger nuclei. The antibodies are detected by applying standardized fluorescent conjugates of antihuman \gamma globulin. The giant mitochondria of the parasite *Crithidia luciliae* contain pure circular native DNA and thus serve as a convenient substrate in tests for anti-DNA antibodies.

The different patterns of staining that have been identified in different disease states are summarized in Table 3. The presence of antibodies to native or double-stranded DNA is specific for systemic lupus erythematosus (SLE) and is the most powerful criterion for diagnosis [7••]. Occasionally, anti-DNA antibodies are found in patients with rheumatoid arthritis, but these patients, although manifesting systemic features, such as pleurisy, do not develop the serious complications of SLE, and their clinical course is similar to that of rheumatoid arthritis. Antibodies to single-stranded DNA are found in many diseases and are thus of no practical value. Anti-DNA antibody–DNA complexes play a role in the development of lupus glomerulonephritis. When these complexes are being laid down in the kidney, low serum levels of total complement and complement components C3 and C4 can be expected. Anti-DNA antibodies cross-react with cardiolipin, which accounts for the false-positive Venereal Disease Research Laboratory Test reactions.

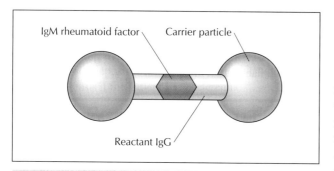

FIGURE 3 Principle of rheumatoid factor tests. The reactant IgG may be either of human origin, as in the latex or bentonite fixation tests, or of rabbit origin, as in the sheep cell agglutination test. The carrier particles are latex or bentonite or sheep cells. These agglutination tests identify only IgM rheumatoid factor.

TABLE 2 DISEASES ASSOCIATED WITH POSITIVE TEST FINDINGS FOR IgM RHEUMATOID FACTOR AND CONNECTIVE TISSUE DISEASES	
Arthritis	**Viral diseases**
Rheumatoid arthritis*	Infectious mononucleosis
Juvenile rheumatoid arthritis†	Rubella
Systemic lupus erythematosus	Cytomegalovirus infection
Progressive systemic sclerosis	Influenza
Dermatomyositis and polymyositis	
Sjögren's syndrome*	**Chronic inflammatory diseases of unknown etiology**
Seronegative spondyloarthropathies‡	Sarcoidosis
Gout, especially tophaceous	Chronic liver disease
	Chronic interstitial pulmonary fibrosis
Chronic bacterial infections	
Subacute bacterial endocarditis	**Other conditions**
Syphilis	Waldenström's macroglobulinemia
Tuberculosis	Polyclonal cryoglobulinemia
Leprosy	**Parasitic infections**

*Often in very high titers.
†Rheumatoid factor test results are negative in patients with disease onset of < 5 y, are 5%–10% positive in patients with disease onset of 5–10 y, and gradually reach adult levels in those developing disease between 10 and 15 y previously.
‡Despite a seronegative designation, 10%–15% of patients have positive test results but in low titer.

TABLE 3 ANTINUCLEAR ANTIBODY IMMUNOFLUORESCENT PATTERNS, ANTIGENIC DETERMINANTS, AND DISEASE ASSOCIATIONS

Pattern	Antigen	Disease
Homogeneous	DNA histone	SLE, rheumatoid arthritis, drug-induced SLE, CAH
Peripheral (rim, ring, shaggy)	Native DNA	SLE
Speckled	Soluble nonhistone nuclear proteins	PSS, Sjögren's syndrome, SLE, liver disease, tuberculosis
Nucleolar	Small nucleolar-weight nuclear RNA	Sjögren's syndrome, PSS
Centromeric	Histone-like proteins of kinetochore	PSS (especially CREST)

CAH—chronic active hepatitis; CREST—calcinosis, Raynaud's phenomenon, esophageal dysmotility, sclerodactyly, and telangiectasia (a variant of progressive systemic sclerosis); PSS—progressive systemic sclerosis; SLE—systemic lupus erythematosus.

The lupus anticoagulant is an antibody to phospholipid and is associated with thrombotic episodes that occur in SLE (Table 4) [8••].

Antibodies to nonhistone nuclear proteins and RNA-protein complexes occur in many connective tissue diseases (Table 5) [9]. Patients exposed to certain drugs (Table 6) may develop a lupus-like syndrome. In this syndrome, antibodies to histone are present, but neurologic and renal complications do not occur. The syndrome disappears when the medication is discontinued.

Cryoglobulins may be found in SLE and other connective tissue diseases, causing vasculitis and glomerulonephritis. Monoclonal cryoglobulins in multiple myeloma and Waldenström's macroglobulinemia often cause hyperviscosity syndrome.

ERYTHROCYTE SEDIMENTATION RATE

The erythrocyte sedimentation rate (ESR), which is measured by the Westergren, the Wintrobe, or the zeta method, is a marker of tissue inflammation. As such, it has a high sensitivity but low specificity. Changes in serial readings are of limited value in rheumatoid arthritis but are more useful in polymyalgia rheumatica and temporal arteritis. Decreased values are found in hyperviscosity syndromes and in sickle cell anemia. The latter is particularly important because an ESR of 20 mm or more in the first hour should alert the physician to possible infection. Iron-deficiency anemia also results in a decreased ESR because the hypochronic microcytic erythrocytes do not sink as fast as normal erythrocytes. The ESR is frequently increased, up to 40 mm in the first hour, in osteoarthritis. Plasma viscosity correlates well with the ESR, and now that the plasma viscosity procedure can be automated, it may well supersede the time-honored ESR screening test. The C-reactive protein value is especially useful in monitoring infection, especially in SLE and other connective tissue diseases, which normally have relatively low values [9]. The C-reactive protein value correlates well with disease activity in rheumatoid arthritis

TABLE 4 CLINICAL CONSEQUENCES OF ANTIPHOSPHOLIPID ANTIBODIES*

Thrombosis in both veins and arteries
Bleeding (less common)
Thrombocytopenia
Fetal loss

*Antiphospholipid syndrome can occur in systemic lupus erythematosus or other connective tissue diseases or it may occur in the absence of any autoimmune disease. Both lupus anticoagulant and anticardiolipin antibodies are antiphospholipid antibodies.

TABLE 5 ANTIBODIES TO NONHISTONE NUCLEAR PROTEINS, RNA-PROTEIN COMPLEXES, AND CYTOPLASMIC ANTIGENS

Antigen	Disease
Ro (SS-A)	Sjögren's syndrome, SLE
La (SS-B)	Sjögren's syndrome, SLE
Sm	SLE
Rana	Rheumatoid arthritis
Scl-70	PSS
Jo-1	Polymyositis
nRNP	MCTD; also SLE, PSS, DLE
Mitochondria	SLE, PBC

DLE—discoid lupus erythematosus; MCTD—mixed connective tissue disease; PBC—primary biliary cirrhosis; PSS—progressive systemic sclerosis; SLE—systemic lupus erythematosus.

TABLE 6 DRUG-INDUCED LUPUS

Implicated drugs	Possible causes
Hydralazine	Anticonvulsants
Procainamide	Antibiotics
Chlorpromazine	Antithyroidal agents
Isoniazid	Oral contraceptives
Penicillamine	

and as a result has become popular in monitoring treatment of the disease [10••]. Haptoglobin, transferrin, and ceruloplasmin have all been used as outcome measures to assess drug efficacy in clinical therapeutic trials [11].

RADIOLOGY

Despite recent advances in imaging technology, much can still be learned from black and white plain radiographs. It is useful to have a routine for examining black and white films, as shown in Table 7. Looser's zones may be apparent in patients with osteomalacia (Fig. 4).

New musculoskeletal imaging methods include nuclear medicine, ultrasonography, computed tomography, and MR imaging. In these cost-conscious times, the relative costs of these procedures are worth keeping in mind. Tomography is no more expensive than is plain radiography, but isotope bone scanning and computed tomography are six times as expensive, and MR imaging costs 12 times as much. The clinical usefulness of these various modalities is summarized in Table 8.

TABLE 7 ROUTINE FOR EXAMINING BLACK AND WHITE FILMS*
1. Check the black and white film for film density; the fingers, when placed behind the black part of the film, should not be visible
2. Examine the soft tissues for swellings, calcification, tophi, and foreign bodies; it may be possible to diagnose joint effusions and inflamed bursae (*eg*, Achilles bursitis); thickening of tendons may be seen in conditions such as xanthomatosis, and synovial hypertrophy may be evident as a bulge at the margin of a joint, such as the anterior aspect of the ankle
3. Assess joint space narrowing, which is indicative of cartilage loss; calcification, such as that in chondrocalcinosis, may be evident; it should be noted that cartilage loss may occur with a relatively normal joint space
4. Consider bone density next; juxtaarticular osteoporosis is normal; interpretation in inflammatory joint disease of juxtaarticular osteoporosis is subject to high interobserver error; generalized osteoporosis is more readily appreciated but merely indicates loss of bone substance and can be caused by severe conditions (*eg*, hyperparathyroidism and osteomalacia); pseudofractures

*The radiologic features of the common diseases affecting peripheral joints are covered elsewhere.

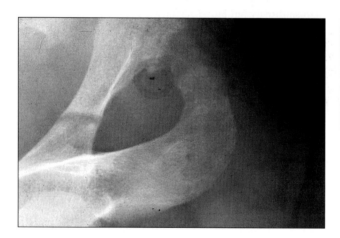

FIGURE 4 Typical pseudofracture or Looser's zone (also known as Milkman's fracture) in osteomalacia. Note how the lucent area is orientated at right angles to the cortex. Pseudofractures tend to occur in characteristic sites of increased stress (*eg*, inner margins of the proximal femora) and are typically bilateral and symmetric. They may precede other radiologic changes of osteomalacia, and true fractures may occur through them.

TABLE 8 CLINICAL USEFULNESS OF VARIOUS IMAGING MODALITIES

Radionuclide bone scanning

General

Can scan the whole body with technetium phosphonate

Gallium- and indium-labeled leukocytes are particularly useful in identifying infection

Infection

Useful for early detection, especially in children

Can identify difficult problems (*eg*, epiphyseal osteomyelitis)

Can differentiate septic arthritis from osteomyelitis

Bone disease

Useful in the early detection of avascular necrosis of bone and in Legg-Calvé-Perthes disease in children

Subtle stress fractures can be identified (*eg*, of the pars interarticularis), as can conditions such as shin splints; ideal for scanning for metastases in bone (will determine whether solitary or multiple)

Useful also in primary tumors of bone, especially asteroid osteoma, which may be small (typical "hot" center, with a halo of low uptake or "ring" sign)

Benign tumors on the whole are "cold" and malignant tumors are "hot" on bone scans; the exception is multiple myeloma, which is "cold"

Metabolic bone disease and Paget's disease

Demonstrates generalized uptake in bone in these conditions

Ultrasonography

Soft tissue swellings

Can identify soft tissue swellings (*eg*, Baker's cysts) and differentiate them from popliteal aneurysms

Shoulder joint disease

Can identify tendon tears and ruptures and inflamed bursae

Joint aspiration

Can identify synovial effusions and aid in their aspiration (*eg*, hip joint aspiration)

Computed tomography

Bone pathology

Ideal for identifying changes in bone

Facilitates evaluation of subtle fractures (*eg*, in the pelvis) and identifies fragments within joints

Joint disease

Useful in assessing changes in the cervical spine in rheumatoid arthritis, the sacroiliac joints in the seronegative spondyloarthropathies, septic arthritis affecting deep articulations (*eg*, the hip joint) and mediastinal involvement in sternoclavicular hyperostosis

Low back pain

Provides cross-sectional display of vertebral bodies, intervertebral disks, bony canal, thecal sacs and segmental nerves, and dural and epidural spaces

Particularly useful in the diagnosis of spinal stenosis

Can identify apophyseal joint disease

Combined with myelography, can visualize the subarachnoid space and its contents

Bone tumors

Extremely useful in assessing both benign and malignant tumors of bone, especially in the assessment of bone changes

Magnetic resonance imaging

General

Noninvasive

No radiation exposure

No side effects

Spinal disease

Fast overtaking computed tomography and myelography in the assessment of spinal disk disease; enhancement with gadolinium provides improved soft tissue images

Proving to be extremely useful in the assessment of changes in the cervical spine in rheumatoid arthritis and in infections of the spine

Peripheral joints

Has proven to be superior to arthrography and ultrasonography in the assessment of soft tissues in the shoulder and knee joints

Bone disease

The most sensitive imaging modality in the diagnosis of early avascular necrosis

Also useful in the diagnosis of infiltrative bone marrow diseases (*eg*, multiple myeloma and Gaucher's disease) and in the diagnosis of osteomyelitis

References and Recommended Reading

Recently published papers of particular interest have been highlighted as:
• Of interest
•• Of outstanding interest

1. Latham PM: *The Collected Works (1789–1879)*. London: The Sydenham Society; 1876–1878.

2. Balint GP, Buchanan WW, Harden RM, *et al.*: Punched-card aid in rheumatological diagnosis. *Br J Rheumatol* 1987, 26:46–50.

3.•• Doherty M, Hazelman BL, Hutton CW, *et al.*: *Rheumatology Examination and Injection Techniques*. London: WB Saunders; 1992.

4.•• Gatter RA, Schumacher HR: *A Practical Handbook of Joint Fluid Analysis*, edn 2. Philadelphia: Lea & Febiger; 1991.

5.•• Dalakas MC: Polymyositis, dermatomyositis, and inclusion body myositis. *N Engl J Med* 1991, 325:1487–1498.

6. Fraser DD, Frank JA, Dalakas M, *et al.*: Magnetic resonance imaging in the idiopathic inflammatory myopathies. *J Rheumatol* 1991, 18:1693–1700.

7. Wallace DJ, Hahn BH, eds.: *Dubois' Lupus Erythematosus*, edn 4. Philadelphia: Lea & Febiger; 1993.

8. Asherson RA, Cervera R: The antiphospholipid syndrome: a syndrome in evolution. *Ann Rheum Dis* 1992, 51:147–150.

9. Pepys MB, Lanham JG, de Beer FC: C-reactive protein in SLE. *Clin Rheum Dis* 1982, 8:91–103.

10.•• Bellamy N, Buchanan WW: Clinical evaluation in rheumatic diseases. In *Arthritis and Allied Conditions*, edn 12. Edited by McCarty DJ, Koopman WJ. Philadelphia: Lea & Febiger; 1993:15–178.

11.•• Crues JV III, ed.: *MRI of the Musculoskeletal System*. New York: Raven Press; 1991.

12.•• Markisz JA, ed.: Musculoskeletal Imaging: MRI, CT, nuclear medicine, and ultrasound. In *Clinical Practice*. Boston: Little, Brown and Company; 1991.

Select Bibliography

Bellamy N: *Colour Atlas of Clinical Rheumatology*. Lancaster, England: Kluwer Academic Publishers Group; 1985.

Berquist TH, ed.: *MRI of the Musculoskeletal System*. New York: Raven Press; 1990.

Brostoff J, Scadding GK, Male D, Roitt IM: *Clinical Immunology*. London: Gower Medical Publishing; 1991.

Brower AC: *Arthritis in Black and White*. Philadelphia: WB Saunders; 1988.

Churg A, Churg J: *Systemic Vasculitides*. New York: Igaku-Shoin Medical Publishers; 1991.

Dieppe PA, Bacon PA, Bamji AN, Watt I: *Atlas of Clinical Rheumatology*. Oxford: Oxford University Press; 1986.

Docherty P, Mitchell MJ, MacMillan L, *et al.*: Magnetic resonance imaging in the detection of sacroiliitis. *J Rheumatol* 1992, 19:393–401.

Gardner DL: *Pathological Basis of the Connective Tissue Disorders*. Philadelphia: Lea & Febiger; 1992.

Greenspan A: *Orthopedic Radiology: A Practical Approach*, edn 2. New York: Raven Press; 1992.

Manaster PJ: *Skeletal Radiology Handbooks in Radiology Series*. Chicago: Mosby Yearbook; 1989.

Milgram JW: *Radiologic and Histologic Pathology of Nontumorous Diseases of Bones and Joints*, vols 1 and 2. Northbrook, IL: Northbrook Publishing Company; 1990.

Quencer RM, ed.: *MRI of the Spine*. New York: Raven Press; 1991.

Resnick D, Niwayama G, eds.: *Diagnosis of Bone and Joint Disorders*, vols 1–6, edn 2. Philadelphia: WB Saunders; 1988.

Roitt I, Brostoff J, Male D: *Immunology*. London: Gower Medical Publishing; 1985.

Stoller DW: *Magnetic Resonance Imaging in Orthopaedics and Sports Medicine*. Philadelphia: JB Lippincott; 1993.

Tedorescu M, Froelich C, eds.: *Advanced Immunoassays in Rheumatology*. Boca Raton: CRC Press; 1994.

Weston WJ, Palmer DG: *Soft Tissues of the Extremities: A Radiologic Study of Rheumatic Disease*. New York: Springer-Verlag; 1978.

Rheumatoid Arthritis 2

Daniel J. McCarty

Key Points

- Accurate diagnosis of inflammatory polyarthritis is important for prognosis.
- Radiographic bony erosion, articular capsular distention, and ligamentous laxity or rupture in early disease are signs of a poor prognosis.
- Articular damage (ashes) and inflammation (fire) both limit function; most damage in rheumatoid arthritis is irreversible and occurs disporportionately in the early years of the disease.
- Early treatment is most successful in restoring normal joint function as inflammatory changes are reversible.
- Drug combinations guided by serial evaluation often are needed for disease control.
- The generalist's role is to make an early *referral*, to *reinforce* the treatment program prescribed by the rheumatologist, and to *review* the results periodically.

The treatment of rheumatoid arthritis, found in approximately 0.3% of the United States population, occupies approximately half the time of practicing rheumatologists. The clinical syndrome denoted by the term rheumatoid arthritis has grown progressively more restricted because other conditions that superficially resemble it have been recognized as distinctive [1•].

Twin studies provided the first proof of the heritability of rheumatoid arthritis. Subsequent studies have shown not only a hereditary predisposition for seropositive rheumatoid arthritis but also genetic determinants for both the severity and the pattern of disease (*eg*, nodules, sicca syndrome). Current notions about etiology envision an infectious agent or agents triggering a harmful immunologic reaction in a genetically primed host [2•]. This putative agent has thus far eluded detection. Problems in treating rheumatoid arthritis are listed in Table 1 (*see* Treatment).

DIAGNOSIS

The revised American College of Rheumatology diagnostic criteria for rheumatoid arthritis provide for classification of patients under clinical investigation. They are not meant to define the disease in patients seen in everyday practice. A tentative classification of chronic polyarthritis is shown in Figure 1 [3•].

Rheumatoid factor positivity (RF+) is nearly always associated with bony erosions, and these two features are the hallmarks of rheumatoid arthritis. Vasculitis, nodules, sicca features, and Felty syndrome (splenomegaly with neutropenia) are found in subsets of seropositive rheumatoid arthritis patients. Patients consistently negative for rheumatoid factor (RF-) are diagnosed as having seronegative polyarthritis. This group includes patients with a potpourri of different syndromes, including adult juvenile rheumatoid arthritis and remitting seronegative synovitis with pitting edema (RS_3PE).

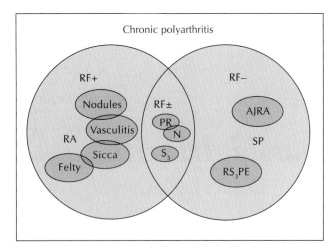

FIGURE 1 A working classification of chronic polyarthritis. It is important to classify each patient because of differences in prognosis between the various syndromes. *RF+*, *RF–*, and *RF±* refer to results of tests for IgM rheumatoid factor. Adult juvenile rheumatoid arthritis (AJRA) and remitting seronegative symmetrical synovitis with pitting edema (RS₃PE) are examples of subsets of seronegative polyarthritis (SP). Nodules, vasculitis, sicca syndrome, and Felty syndrome may develop in subsets of patients with rheumatoid arthritis (RA). Palindromic rheumatism (PR), nodulosis (N), and seronegative symmetric synovitis of the wrists (S₃) are recognizable syndromes included in the ambiguous category of RF±.

A few patients with seropositive rheumatoid arthritis occasionally test negative for rheumatoid factor. In other patients, rheumatoid factor test results change from positive to negative, either spontaneously or while the patient is receiving remission-inducing agents. These patients are shown as *RF±* in Figure 1.

Rheumatoid Nodulosis

Patients with this uncommon variant of rheumatoid nodulosis are usually seropositive. Radiologists often incorrectly diagnose gout because of the presence of punched-out bony lesions and soft tissue nodules. Twenty-two of the 28 reported cases have been men [3•]. All patients have had acute intermittent attacks of palindromic rheumatism.

Palindromic Rheumatism

Palindromic rheumatism is much more common than is rheumatoid nodulosis. Acute gout-like attacks develop quickly near one joint. Pain and disability last from 1 day to 1 week, at which time all symptoms disappear and the patient is perfectly well. Sometimes attacks stop altogether, but often they eventually fail to resolve completely, and a fixed symmetric (rheumatoid) arthritis supervenes. At this point the palindromic attacks usually stop, but they can coexist with fixed rheumatoid arthritis. Attacks are usually periarticular, and few joint fluids or synovial membranes have been examined. Approximately 20% of rheumatoid arthritis cases have a palindromic onset. Tests for rheumatoid factor are usually negative in palindromic rheumatism but become positive as the syndrome converts to rheumatoid arthritis.

Seronegative Polyarthritis

A few patients with seronegative polyarthritis develop positive tests for rheumatoid factor over time. Some seronegative adult patients show the clinical features of juvenile rheumatoid arthritis, including rash and fever, and the characteristic involvement of larger joints, such as the wrist, shoulder, and knee, with lesser involvement of the small hand joints and the forefoot. Involvement is often more asymmetric than that found in adult seropositive disease.

Remitting Seronegative Symmetric Synovitis with Pitting Edema

The syndrome of RS₃PE occurs predominantly in white men (with a male-to-female ratio of 4:1) [3•]. The onset is usually acute, with symmetric swelling and pain of the wrists, carpal joints, flexor tendon sheaths, and small hand joints, accompanied by pitting edema of the dorsum of the hand (boxing-glove hand). The elbows, shoulders, hips, knees, and ankles also may be involved, as may the joints in the feet.

Pitting edema over the feet or pretibial area may or may not be present. In most patients, the inflammation fails to respond to nonsteroidal antiinflammatory drugs (NSAIDs). Bony erosions do not occur. Persistent RF–, mild anemia, elevated erythrocyte sedimentation rate (ESR), and decreased serum albumin levels are the rule. The edema is exquisitely sensitive to small daily doses of prednisone (*eg*, 10 mg). Hydroxychloroquine (200 to 400 mg daily) and salicylate, given in doses sufficient to produce therapeutic blood levels, are predictably effective and are the treatment of choice. Remission is invariably maintained even after all drugs have been stopped, unlike in rheumatoid arthritis, where disease recrudescence almost invariably occurs when remittive agents are withdrawn. Certain features of RS₃PE resemble those of polymyalgia rheumatica, but severe flexor tenosynovitis and pitting edema do not occur in patients with polymyalgia rheumatica.

Symmetric Synovitis of Wrists and Carpal Joints

Another distinctive group of elderly patients with rheumatoid arthritis–like illness also has been identified. Symmetric synovitis of the wrists and carpal joints is the main clinical feature, but the severity of synovitis is much milder than that in RS₃PE [3•]. The onset of joint involvement is often gradual, and there is no pitting edema. Again, men predominate, but approximately half of these patients are RF+. The response to hydroxychloroquine and aspirin is uniformly excellent, but unlike the symptoms of RS₃PE, some evidence of low-grade inflammation often persists. Most patients who are initially RF+ become permanently RF– while receiving these drugs. More than half of these patients type as HLA-B8DR3, the classic autoimmune haplotype. This syndrome, *S₃* in Figure 1, also appears to be distinct from seropositive rheumatoid arthritis.

Rheumatoid Arthritis

Approximately 80% of adult patients with chronic polyarthritis treated at referral center clinics are consistently RF+. Most develop radiographic evidence of bony erosions within the first 2 years of disease (Fig. 2). Subsets of this group develop extraarticular features as well, such as nodules (Fig. 3), vasculitis, sicca features, and Felty syndrome.

NATURAL HISTORY

All reported series of patients with rheumatoid arthritis treated at referral centers show a gloomy outcome with respect to function (morbidity) and mortality. Patients die 5 to 10 years earlier than their normal life expectancy. They die of heart disease, cancer, and infection, as does the general population [3•]. The radiographic rate of joint destruction is disproportionately greater in the first 2 years of the disease [4], possibly because muscular weakness and deformity have not yet combined to produce enforced rest (Fig. 4). Rheumatoid nodulosis, which is rare, is not associated with increased mortality and causes relatively little morbidity. Palindromic rheumatism that does not progress to rheumatoid arthritis may continue indefinitely or may remit.

Most cases of seronegative polyarthritis are relatively easy to treat, but a minority do not respond to any drug. Morbidity in seronegative polyarthritis is much less than that in rheumatoid arthritis, and patients with seronegative polyarthritis do not have a decreased life expectancy.

CLINIMETRICS

It is vitally important to record meaningful data on the degree of synovitis at every visit of a patient with rheumatoid arthritis or seronegative polyarthritis [5•]. Duration (in hours) of stiffness on arising, proximal interphalangeal joint circumference (in millimeters), grip strength (in millimeters of mercury), ESR, and C-reactive protein level are easily obtained and recorded. With successful treatment, each of these values should move toward normal. Standardized questionnaires, such as the Health Assessment Questionnaire (HAQ) or the Arthritis Impact Measurement Scale (AIMS), have become popular because they provide serial

outcome measurements. A modified HAQ (MHAQ), developed at Vanderbilt University, is shown in Figure 5.

TREATMENT

As indicated in Table 1, treatment of rheumatoid arthritis and seronegative polyarthritis is entirely empirical. The classic approach used a pyramid (Fig. 6) [6]. Ostensibly safer drugs and simpler measures were given to all patients initially. Drugs of increasingly greater risk were reserved for patients who did not respond, but it is now clear that a disproportionate amount of irreversible damage occurs in the first few years of disease as the clinician and the patient climb the pyramid one unsuccessful step at a time. It is equally clear that drugs deemed effective in short-term controlled therapeutic trials

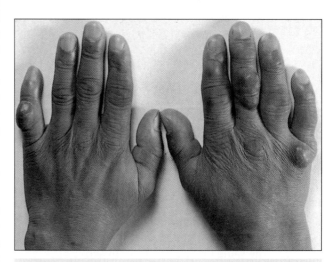

FIGURE 3 Synovial soft tissue swelling is seen at the ulnar styloid of the left hand. There is more diffuse swelling of the radiocarpal joint on the right. Firm rheumatoid nodules are adjacent to and overlying some proximal interphalangeal and metacarpophalangeal joints of both hands. (*From* Schumacher and Gall [18]; with permission.)

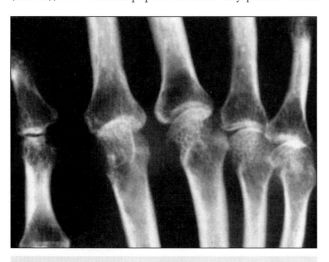

FIGURE 2 Erosions typical of rheumatoid arthritis, at the radial sides of the metacarpals at the metacarpophalangeal joints. (*From* Schumacher and Gall [18]; with permission.)

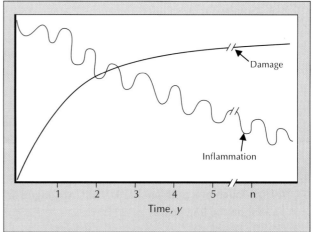

FIGURE 4 Joint damage is both irreversible and cumulative. Although inflammation often gradually subsides over time it does not go away completely. (*From* McCarty [1•]; with permission.)

(up to 1 year) have been woefully inadequate in controlling the ravages of rheumatoid arthritis over long periods [7]. All long-term observational studies show this outcome [8•].

This manifest failure has led some rheumatologists to invert the pyramid, using potent agents early in the course of the disease, often in combination, to suppress synovitis [9].

Activities and Lifestyle Index

The questions below concern your daily activities. Please try to answer each question, even if you do not think it is related to you or any condition you may have. There are no right or wrong answers. Please answer exactly as you think or feel.

Please check (✔) the **ONE** best answer for your abilities:

1. **AT THIS MOMENT,** are you able to:

	Without **ANY** Difficulty	With **SOME** Difficulty	With **MUCH** Difficulty	**UNABLE** To Do
a. Dress yourself, including tying shoelaces and doing buttons?	1	2	3	4
b. Get in and out of bed?	1	2	3	4
c. Lift a full cup or glass to your mouth?	1	2	3	4
d. Walk outdoors on flat ground?	1	2	3	4
e. Wash and dry your entire body?	1	2	3	4
f. Bend down to pick up clothing from the floor?	1	2	3	4
g. Turn regular faucets on and off?	1	2	3	4
h. Get in and out of a car?	1	2	3	4

2. **How do you feel TODAY compared to ONE MONTH AGO?** *Please check (✔) only one.*
___Much better today than one month ago
___Better today than one month ago
___The same today as one month ago
___Worse today than one month ago
___Much worse today than one month ago

3. **Which of the following best describes you TODAY?**
Please check (✔) only one.
___I can do everything I want to do.
___I can do most of the things I want to do, but have some limitations.
___I can do some, but not all, of the things I want to do, and I have many limitations.
___I can hardly do any of the things I want to do.

4. **How SATISFIED are you with your ability to do your usual activities?**
Please check (✔) only one.
___Very Satisfied
___Somewhat Satisfied
___Somewhat Dissatisfied
___Very Dissatisfied.

5. **When you get up in the morning, do you feel stiff?**
_____ Yes _____ No

6. **If you answer "Yes," how long is it until you are as limber as you will be for that day?**

_____ minutes or _____ hours

7. **How much pain have you had because of your condition IN THE PAST WEEK? Place a mark on the line below to indicate how severe your pain has been:**

NO PAIN |——————————————————| PAIN AS BAD AS IT COULD BE

8. **How much trouble have you had with your stomach or gastrointestinal (GI) tract (including nausea, heartburn, bloating, pain, etc.) IN THE PAST WEEK? Place a mark on the line below:**

NO GI TROUBLE |——————————————————| A LOT OF GI TROUBLE

9. **How much of a problem has UNUSUAL fatigue or tiredness been for you OVER THE PAST WEEK? Place a mark on the line below:**

FATIGUE IS NO PROBLEM |——————————————————| FATIGUE IS A MAJOR PROBLEM

FIGURE 5 Modified Health Assessment Questionnaire (MHAQ) developed at Vanderbilt University by Pincus and Callahan.

TABLE 1 PROBLEMS IN TREATING RHEUMATOID ARTHRITIS
Disease definition: Nonspecific criteria
Etiology: Unknown
Pathogenesis: Only partially defined
Prognosis: Requires skill and experience in early disease
Course: Synovitis fluctuates but is lifelong
Evaluation: Often confounded by comorbidities, including psychologic factors
Therapy: Empirical

Success at this point reverses the disability completely. My own results using this approach in 90 patients with seropositive rheumatoid arthritis followed for at least 1 year are shown in Figure 7.

Role of the Generalist

A detailed physical, radiologic, and laboratory assessment of each patient should be performed by a rheumatologist. This initial assessment is important to provide the best estimate of prognosis. Erosive disease evident within a few months of disease onset, distended joint capsules, and ruptured ligaments are all clues to aggressive disease. The first duty of the generalist is appropriate referral of the patient while the disease effects are still reversible (Table 2). It is important that the same rheumatologist see the patient periodically in follow-up to assess progress and to suggest appropriate changes in therapy. The consultant cannot, however, provide the primary physician with a stereotypic protocol that, if followed, will guarantee success.

The generalist should understand the deranged physiology and the goals of therapy so that he or she can reinforce the need for compliance with the program. The last responsibility of the generalist is to monitor the results of therapy in the patient at regular intervals (no less than annually). Is the rheumatologist getting adequate results? Serial use of the MHAQ and of radiographs of small flat parts that are usually involved, such as the hands and forefeet, will suffice. The problems of confounding illnesses [10] and psychologic factors [11] on overall function are often missed by the consultant.

Patient Education

Most patients have only a vague notion of the nature of rheumatoid arthritis and how it differs from other forms of arthritis. Many believe they are destined to become crippled. They are often unaware that the intensity of their symptoms may fluctuate spontaneously. Anxiety and depression may result from fear and ignorance of what the future may hold and the inability to judge from day to day whether the disease is improving or worsening. Patients with rheumatoid arthritis often become discouraged if the initial steps taken by the physician are not immediately successful. The patient is often unaware of the role he or she must play in following the prescribed program.

The patient should be told that rheumatoid arthritis is a chronic, lifelong disease for which no cure exists but that various measures, in the aggregate, can nearly always lead to satisfactory control. Relief of symptoms, preservation of joint function, and a reasonable lifestyle are three realistic goals for all patients. With early combination drug therapy, remission [12] is achieved (Table 3) in many patients, but lifelong therapy is still needed. Patients must understand that treatment with disease-suppressive agents generally does not provide overnight relief of symptoms. Initial disappointment with therapy may lead the patient to seek a cure through quackery.

Rest

Inflamed articular tissues are often ischemic, and this abnormality is intensified by exercise [13,14]. The potent antiinflammatory effect of rest splints on wrist synovitis in rheumatoid arthritis was shown many years ago [15]. Splints increase the sensation of stiffness, which should be explained to the patient. The antiinflammatory effect of a stroke is another example of the relationship between motion and synovitis. "Burned-out" rheumatoid arthritis does not occur. The combination of deformed unstable joints and weakened muscles produces enforced rest with a corresponding decrement in joint inflammation. The patient's physical activity should not be increased in tandem with decreasing synovial inflammation. Irreversible loss of function due to structural damage to cartilage, bone, tendon, and capsule is cumulative (damage = inflammation $\times$ intensity $\times$ time). Irreversible damage can occur relatively rapidly (in several months).

Exercise

A balance is needed between adequate rest and sufficient movement to maintain range of motion [16•]. All joints should

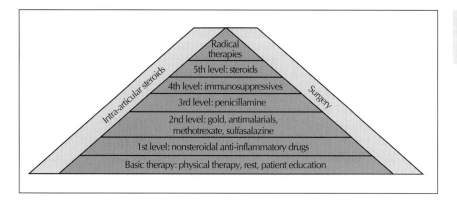

FIGURE 6 The therapeutic pyramid for rheumatoid arthritis (*From* McCarty [1•]; with permission.)

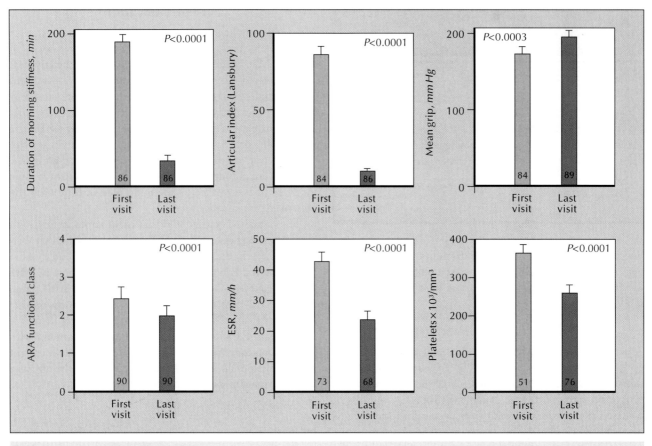

FIGURE 7 Results of therapy in 90 patients with seropositive rheumatoid arthritis (women-to-men ratio = 3:1). The data available at the first and last visit are shown for each variable. Disease duration at first visit was 8.6±0.9 (SEM) years, and the duration of treatment was 7±0.5 (SEM) years. All patients were taking a nonsteroidal drug at the time of the first visit, and 38% were taking prednisone. At the time of last visit, 79% were taking a nonsteroidal drug, and 19% were taking prednisone; 82% were taking antimalarials, 71%, methotrexate, and 60%, azathioprine; 48 patients were receiving all three drugs in combination. ARA—American Rheumatism Association; ESR—erythrocyte sedimentation rate.

be moved through a full range of active motion once daily. Sleep should be in a position as near to anatomic as possible. A consultation with a physical therapist is invaluable early in the course of rheumatoid arthritis or seronegative polyarthritis to train the patient in optimum technique for range-of-motion exercises. Do not worry about muscular strength. The muscles moving inflamed joints become weak rapidly but will return to normal, albeit slowly, when the inflammation subsides. Aerobic conditioning using an exercise bicycle is of great value once synovitis in knees and hindfoot has been controlled.

Modalities

Hot or cold application may relieve pain or muscle spasm, but modalities in general are at best worthless and at worst harm-

---

TABLE 2 THE "4 R's": ROLE OF THE GENERALIST IN TREATMENT OF RHEUMATOID ARTHRITIS AND SERONEGATIVE POLYARTHRITIS

Refer patient to rheumatologist early before irreversible damage has occurred

Reinforce the basic program of rest and exercise and monitor the patient's drug program

Return the patient periodically to the rheumatologist for reassessment of prognosis and treatment program

Review the goals of the therapeutic program with the patient annually; if goals are not being met consider obtaining a second opinion

---

TABLE 3 REMISSION OF RHEUMATOID ARTHRITIS*

1. Duration of morning stiffness <15 min
2. No fatigue
3. No joint pain
4. No joint tenderness or pain on motion
5. No swelling in joints or tendon sheaths
6. ESR <30 mm/h for women, <20 mm/h for men

*American College of Rheumatology definition. Five of six criteria must exist for at least 2 months.
ESR—erythrocyte sedimentation rate.
(From Pinals and coworkers [12]; with permission.)

ful if the demand for blood by the inflamed tissue is increased out of proportion to any increase in local flow. Cold applications are preferred for intense inflammation because local hyperemia is already maximal.

Shoes and Orthotics

Because rheumatoid arthritis affects the small joints of the hands and feet predominantly, the metatarsophalangeal (MTP) joints are usually involved. The transverse arch collapses, and weight is borne by MTP joints 2, 3, and 4 instead of 1 and 5 as in a healthy forefoot. An orthopedic shoe with a 1/8 medial wedge to correct ankle eversion, if present, and with a metatarsal bar to shift weight bearing behind the inflamed MTP joints is often needed. Molded inserts may be useful, and a double toe box may be needed for a patient with dorsal subluxation of the proximal phalange ("cocked-up") toe deformity.

The cervical spine is often involved in rheumatoid arthritis. A soft collar with velcro straps to hold the neck in mid-anatomic position is often helpful symptomatically. This collar acts as a splint for the inflamed cervical facet joints.

Crutches and canes are often useful, although they often cause a flare in the upper extremity joints. Platform crutches of the Canadian type shift the weight to the forearm and are very useful. Axillary crutches should be avoided. Patients must be carefully taught how to use crutches. Their chief use in my practice is to obtain rest after joint injection with triamcinolone hexacetonide.

A crippled patient may need many specialized appliances, from raised toilet seats to hand rails in the home, lift chairs, motorized wheel chairs, and bathtub bars. Consultation with an occupational therapist or, in the most severe cases, with a physiatrist is often helpful.

Drug Therapy

Successful suppression of rheumatoid joint inflammation is almost routine with rational use of available agents. Aspirin or other NSAIDs and microcrystalline corticosteroid esters injected intrasynovially are useful initially because their action is immediate. I routinely use enteric-coated aspirin in doses individually tailored to produce serum salicylate levels of 20 to 30 mg/dL. Local intrasynovial injections of microcrystalline triamcinolone hexacetonide are used to correct flexion deformities and to debulk the total body inflammatory load. This compound is the drug of choice for intrasynovial use because it is the most sparingly soluble of this class of drugs. I routinely splint upper extremity joints for 3 weeks after injection, with removal of the splint for one full range of motion daily, and instruct patients to avoid weight bearing for 6 to 8 weeks in lower extremity joints by using crutches. In a controlled study [17], fully 88% of upper extremity synovial structures were still in complete remission nearly 2 years after injection. I believe that the results of injection of lower extremity joints are even better, but no controlled data are available.

There is no point in waiting to assess the effectiveness of an NSAID in treating severe inflammation of multiple joints in rheumatoid arthritis. Used alone, it will be inadequate. A remission-inducing agent prescribed early in the course of

treatment can always be stopped in the unlikely event of satisfactory control by aspirin or another NSAID. Use of various remittive agents alone or in combination constitutes the art of rheumatology.

The serial use of sensitive parameters reflecting rheumatic inflammatory activity, joint and overall function, and radiographic assessment (Fig. 8) is essential to manage rheumatoid arthritis. A progressive decline in the number of inflamed joints and in the intensity of inflammation in each affected joint should be expected. Patients in prolonged remission need to see a rheumatologist only every 2 or 3 years.

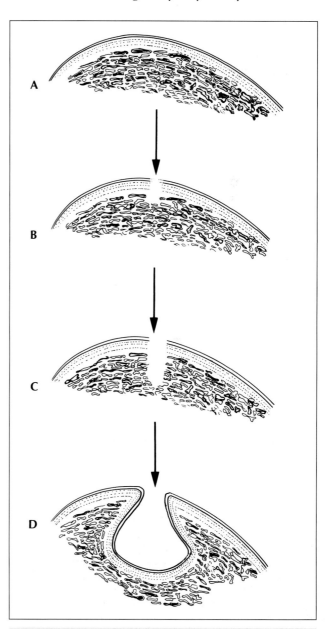

FIGURE 8 The natural radiographic history of a pocket erosion with successful suppression of inflammation. **A**, A normal cortical and trabacular bone. **B**, The earliest detectable lesion is a break in the bony cortex followed by **C**, loss of spongy bone to produce a pocket erosion. Rarely, these pockets are filled in with new bone and disappear. **D**, Most often, they become recorticated with the reformed cortical bone outlining the erosive pocket. (*From* McCarty [1 •]; with permission.)

Fully 60% of the 90 patients with rheumatoid arthritis whose treatment results are shown in Figure 7 have remained in complete and sustained remission (Table 3). Most did not progressively lose function because of rheumatoid arthritis. Many had concomitant comorbidities, such as fibromyalgia, osteoarthritis, coronary artery disease, and emotional depression, that often confounded functional evaluation. Results were best if the patient was treated early in the disease before much irreversible change had occurred. Approximately half of the patients (48 of 90) were treated with a combination of low-dose methotrexate (approximately 7.5 mg/wk), azathioprine (50 to 100 mg/d), and hydroxychloroquine (200 to 400 mg/d) after debulking of the disease in large joints with triamcinolone hexacetonide plus rest. Most were also taking salicylate to produce a therapeutic level of 20 to 30 mg/dL in the serum.

The rationale of combination drug therapy is analogous to that of tuberculosis or cancer therapy. If a single agent is used to treat rheumatoid arthritis, the response is usually incomplete and is lost after approximately 2 years of treatment in most cases. I hypothesize that the loss of response is due to clonal expansion of resistant cells. The use of multiple agents simultaneously appears to slow or prevent this phenomenon. Whether this is the mechanism or not, the use of drug combinations empirically produces excellent suppression of synovitis.

Adverse effects of combination therapy have been surprisingly few. Herpes zoster has been noted frequently (18 of 90 cases). Bacterial infections were not a problem. Nausea, vomiting, or a flu-like reaction often resulted in azathioprine withdrawal. "Methotrexate lung" occurred in three elderly women. Reversible mild bone marrow suppression occurred in three patients. There were no fatalities. No ocular toxicity due to hydroxychloroquine was found even after decades of daily use. Apparently the risk of retinal toxicity with daily doses of 6.5 mg/kg body weight or less is zero. Some ophthalmologists no longer recommend periodic eye examinations if the patient is taking the drug in these doses.

The long-term use of prednisone, even in low daily doses (5 to 10 mg), is not advisable. Bone loss in postmenopausal women is significant. More ominous is accelerated atherogenesis, which occurs in patients of either gender taking prednisone for many years. The only virtues of prednisone are its low cost and its rapidity of action. It is almost never needed in patients receiving combination remittive drug therapy. The six steps necessary for successful therapy for seropositive rheumatoid arthritis are summarized in Table 4.

REFERENCES AND RECOMMENDED READING

Recently published papers of particular interest have been highlighted as:
• Of interest

1. • McCarty DJ: The treatment of rheumatoid arthritis. In *Arthritis and Allied Conditions: A Textbook of Rheumatology*, edn 12. Edited by McCarty DJ, Koopman WJ. Malvern, PA: Lea & Febiger; 1993:877–886.

TABLE 4 SIX STEPS TO SUCCESSFUL THERAPY FOR SEROPOSITIVE RHEUMATOID ARTHRITIS
1. Accurate diagnosis and prognosis
2. Precise assessment, initial and serial, using clinical, radiographic, and laboratory variables
3. Explain pathophysiology and basic program to patient
4. Use whatever drugs it takes to control synovitis
5. Monitor serially for drug effectiveness and for side effects with gradual dose reduction after sustained remission
6. Never completely withdraw therapy from a patient in remission

2. • Salmon M: The immunogenetic component of susceptibility to rheumatoid arthritis. *Curr Opin Rheumatol* 1992, 4:342–347.

3. • McCarty DJ: The clinical picture of rheumatoid arthritis. In *Arthritis and Allied Conditions: A Textbook of Rheumatology*, edn 12. Edited by McCarty DJ, Koopman WJ. Malvern, PA: Lea & Febiger; 1993:781–809.

4. Buckland-Wright JC, Clarke GS, Walker SR: Erosion number and area progression in the wrists and hands of rheumatoid patients: a quantitative microfocal radiographic study. *Ann Rheum Dis* 1986, 48:25–29.

5. • Bellamy N, Buchanan WW: Clinical evaluation in the rheumatic diseases. In *Arthritis and Allied Conditions: A Textbook of Rheumatology*, edn 12. Edited by McCarty DJ, Koopman WJ. Malvern, PA: Lea & Febiger; 1993:151–180.

6. Smythe CJ: Therapy of rheumatoid arthritis: a pyramidal plan. *Postgrad Med* 1972, 51:31–93.

7. Pincus T: Rheumatoid arthritis: disappointing long term outcomes despite successful short term clinical trials. *J Clin Epidemiol* 1988, 41:1037–1041.

8. • Harris ED Jr.: Rheumatoid arthritis: pathophysiology and implications for therapy. *N Engl J Med* 1990, 322:1272–1289.

9. Wilske KR, Healey LA: Remodeling the pyramid: a concept whose time has come. *J Rheumatol* 1989, 16:565–567.

10. Berkanovic E, Hurwicz ML: Rheumatoid arthritis and comorbidity. *J Rheumatol* 1990, 17:888–892.

11. Hagglund KJ, Haley WE, Reveille JD, *et al.*: Predicting individual differences in pain and functional impairment among patients with rheumatoid arthritis. *Arthritis Rheum* 1989, 31:851–858.

12. Pinals RS, Baum J, Bland J, *et al.*: Preliminary criteria for clinical remission in rheumatoid arthritis. *Bull Rheum Dis* 1982, 32:7–10.

13. Simkin PA: Synovial physiology. In *Arthritis and Allied Conditions: A Textbook of Rheumatology*, edn 11. Edited by McCarty DJ. Philadelphia: Lea & Febiger; 1989:207–221.

14. Blake DR, Unsworth J, Ourthwaite JM: Hypoxic-reperfusion injury in the inflamed human joint. *Lancet* 1989, i:289–293.

15. Gault SJ, Spyker JM: Beneficial effect of immobilization of joints in rheumatoid and related arthritides: a splint study using sequential analysis. *Arthritis Rheum* 1969, 12:34–44.

16. • Gerber LH: Exercise and arthritis. *Bull Rheum Dis* 1990, 39:1–9.

17. McCarty DJ: Treatment of rheumatoid joint inflammation with triamcinolone hexacetonide. *Arthritis Rheum* 1972, 15:157–173.

18. Schumacher HR, Gall EP: *Rheumatoid Arthritis*. Philadelphia: JB Lippincott; 1988.

Differential Diagnosis of Systemic Collagen Vascular Diseases: Nosology and Overlap Syndromes

Robert W. Lightfoot, Jr.

> ### Key Points
> - The history and physical examination are more valuable than laboratory tests in differentiating the connective tissue diseases.
> - For diagnosing an illness, the rheumatoid factor and antinuclear antibody tests should be ordered simultaneously.
> - The combination of history, physical examination, and laboratory tests may permit reasonable assessment for prognosis and management even if they do not provide a specific diagnosis.
> - When the serologic tests do not suggest any connective tissue disease but the history and physical examination do, suspect a vasculitis syndrome.
> - In atypical vasculitis syndromes, mimickers such as cholesterol emboli or atrial myxomas must be considered.

The systemic collagen vascular diseases include an array of syndromes with shared manifestations, many of which are listed in Table 1. Frequently, these manifestations present in unique clusters that permit the diagnosis of a specific disease entity, such as systemic lupus erythematosus (SLE), scleroderma, or dermatomyositis. At other times, patients present with permutations of these manifestations that do not allow for delineation of a single diagnostic entity, leading to the diagnosis of an overlap syndrome. In perhaps no other specialty are clinical stigmata as crucial to the categorization of disease as in this subset of rheumatic diseases. Therefore, the first step in their diagnosis is a well-taken history, including a review of systems, and a well-performed physical examination. Diagnostic criteria for several of these diseases, developed by the American College of Rheumatology, rely predominantly on clinical manifestations. Although occasionally serologic tests provide a specific diagnosis, serologic testing should be done in most patients only after the presence or absence of these clinical features has been established.

PATHOPHYSIOLOGY

No single mechanism explains the pathophysiology of these diseases. The two features most often shared by these illnesses are autoimmune phenomena and vasculitis. The best-understood collagen vascular disease is SLE, in which autoantibodies, especially those to DNA, combine with their antigens in the plasma or in tissue to cause immune complex vasculitis and glomerulitis. A similar vasculitis seems to involve muscles in childhood dermatomyositis but is not apparent in the adult form of the disease. In some instances, autoantibodies cause disease by binding to their antigens. One example is the thromboembolic diathesis seen in the antiphospholipid syndrome, which can accompany any of these diseases and is most notably seen in SLE. Another is congenital heart block in children born of mothers with circulating anti–SS-A (anti-Ro), which can occur in any of these diseases.

TABLE 1 CLINICAL MANIFESTATIONS OF COLLAGEN VASCULAR DISEASES					
Manifestation	Systemic lupus erythematous	Systemic sclerosis	Polymyositis/ dermatomyositis	Rheumatoid arthritis	Sjögren's syndrome
Arthritis	3+	1–2+	0–1+	4+	1–2+
Pleurisy	3+	0	0	1+	0
Raynaud's phenomenon	2+	3–4+	1+	1+	0
Central nervous system involvement	3+	0	0	0	2+
Neuropathy	1+	0	0	1+	2+
Sicca symptoms	1–2+	1+	0–1+	2+	3+
Myositis	2+	2+	4+	1+	2–3+
Glomerulitis	4+	0	0	0	1+
Renovascular disease	0	2–3+	0	0	0
Pulmonary infiltrates	1+	2–3+	2+	2+	1–2+
Esophageal dysmotility	1+	4+	2+	0	1+
Skin Sclerodactyly	1+	4+	2+	0	0
Rash	3+	0	2–3+	0	0

Although autoantibodies often are found in polymyositis/ dermatomyositis (PM/DM), there is little understanding of their role in the immunopathology of these diseases. This immunologic heterogeneity prevents a simple immunoserologic approach to distinguishing these diseases from one another and underscores the need for the careful clinical assessment mentioned in the previous paragraphs.

CLINICAL FEATURES

Spectrum of Organ System Involvement

Table 1 lists the relative involvement of various organ systems in the major collagen vascular diseases. The systemic vasculitides are not shown because their symptoms tend to be much less specific than those of the five conditions listed. Combinations of the clinical features shown in Table 1 have higher positive predictive values in diagnosing these syndromes than does any combination of laboratory tests. Thus, renal disease is rare in PM/DM but is seen in 50% of patients with SLE and in 20% of those with systemic sclerosis (SSc). In SLE, the nephritis is an immune complex glomerulitis and is closely associated with the presence of hypocomplementemia, circulating fragments of activated complement components, and antibodies to native DNA (nDNA). In SSc, the nephritis results from noninflammatory narrowing of renal arteries and arterioles, with resulting renal ischemia, renin release, and activation of the angiotensin system. In both diseases, renal failure and hypertension can result.

Arthritis can occur in SLE, rheumatoid arthritis (RA), Sjögren's syndrome, SSc, and PM/DM. However, it is seldom an outstanding feature except in RA and SLE. In the former, it can be both deforming and erosive with time, whereas in SLE, it is rarely erosive or deforming. In acute SSc, fibrinous tendon friction rubs can often be heard or felt in the vicinity of an involved wrist or foot. Although the joint fluid in RA often contains many thousands of neutrophilic leukocytes, in SLE

and other collagen vascular diseases, the fluid contains fewer leukocytes and a lower percentage of neutrophils.

Raynaud's phenomenon can occur in any condition that narrows distal arteries, including embolic conditions (atrial myxomas, cholesterol emboli), necrotizing vasculitides (SLE, RA, cryoglobulinemia), vascular trauma (occupational use of vibrating instruments), and the noninflammatory intimal proliferation of SSc. It is an extremely common early manifestation of the latter condition, occurring in more than 90% of cases. It occurs in 50% of SLE patients but is much less common in those with RA, PM/DM, and Sjögren's syndrome.

Dryness of the mouth or eyes (sicca syndrome or Sjögren's syndrome) can occur in any of the collagen vascular diseases and may be associated with the presence of anti–SS-A (anti-Ro) antibodies, anti–SS-B (anti-La) antibodies, or both.

Mild fibrosis of the lower lung fields can occur in occasional patients with RA, SLE, Sjögren's syndrome, or PM/DM, but more extensive and progressive fibrosis is common in SSc. Lung involvement in RA and SLE also can include acute or chronic pleural inflammation, whereas this finding is very rare in SSc. Pulmonary rheumatoid nodules occur in a few RA patients who have rheumatoid factors, but they are not seen in those with the other collagen vascular diseases.

Cutaneous involvement in these diseases can include the classic rashes of discoid and subacute cutaneous lupus; the infarcted lesions of cutaneous vasculitis in RA, SLE, and Sjögren's syndrome; and the progressive contractural cutaneous fibrosis of SSc.

Weight of Clinical Feature in Diagnostic Criteria Sets

It is thus important that the qualitative features of the organ system involvement listed in Table 1 be discerned as well as the degree of involvement. Having ascertained the extent and type of system involvement by the history taking, physical examination, and initial routine testing of blood and urine, the clinician can make a priori diagnostic estimations of the likelihood of one of these diseases. Thus, a patient with acute pleurisy, moderately inflamed joints, and a sun-sensitive malar rash can be suspected of having SLE with a considerable degree of certainty. On the other hand, a patient with severe Raynaud's phenomenon and generalized puffiness and tenderness of the hands and wrists is more likely to have SSc. In many patients the overlap of the manifestations in Table 1 will be sufficient to muddle the diagnosis. At this point the serologic tests may offer powerful diagnostic and prognostic information.

Although it is ideal to make an unequivocal diagnosis, rheumatologists frequently are faced with establishing a prognosis on the basis of clinical findings and the results of routine laboratory and serologic tests in patients in whom the precise diagnosis may remain unclear for several years. The following questions should be asked: 1) What is the likely natural history of the process present? 2) Is there a therapy that can alter this course? 3) Given the risks of the course, are the risks of leaving the condition untreated greater than the risks of the therapy proposed? A useful exercise is to ask whether additional tests are likely or unlikely to yield more diagnostic information and whether this information will change the therapy already planned.

Let us see how these characteristics affect the use of the two most important laboratory tests in rheumatology, the history taking and the physical examination. Imagine that a patient has severe Raynaud's phenomenon, dysphagia, and mild arthralgias but lacks all of the remaining features in Table 1. The weights of the three findings are examined across the rows in Table 1. The values in each row are ordinal rather than quantitative. Raynaud's phenomenon is slightly suggestive of SLE, less so of RA and PM/DM, and strongly suggestive of SSc. The same is true for the dysphagia resulting from esophageal dysmotility. Arthralgias, reflecting possible underlying arthritis, are more common in RA and SLE, less

so in SSc and Sjögren's syndrome, and even less so in PM/DM. If the weight in each of the three rows (arthritis, Raynaud's phenomenon, and esophageal symptoms) is considered, SSc is the most likely diagnosis.

When the above process suggests that two diagnoses are equally likely, only the natural evolution of the disease may reveal the true diagnosis; however, substantial diagnostic and prognostic information may be gained from the rational use of serologic tests.

DIAGNOSTIC LABORATORY FEATURES

The autoantibody tests used frequently in the diagnosis of the collagen vascular diseases are shown in Table 2 [1••]. When a collagen vascular disease is suspected, the two serologic tests initially ordered are those for rheumatoid factor (RF) and antinuclear antibody (ANA). In the discussion that follows, it should be evident that both of these tests should always be ordered in the initial work-up of a patient because the information derived from either test alone is extremely nonspecific.

Rheumatoid Factor

Rheumatoid factor findings are positive in 80% of patients with RA. RF is also found in many diseases in which chronic immunostimulation occurs, such as chronic sarcoidosis, chronic fungal or parasitic infections, lymphomas, and chronic liver and lung inflammation, and in a small percentage of patients intentionally hyperimmunized for public health reasons. RF is seen in 70% of patients with subacute bacterial endocarditis and disappears with cure of the infection. RF in low titer is also found in 10% to 15% of those older than 70 years of age. As is evident in Table 2, RF also occurs in 15% to 70% of patients with nonrheumatoid collagen vascular diseases. It is relatively sensitive for RA but extremely nonspecific when used alone in the differential diagnosis.

	Sensitivity, %				
Serologic test	Systemic lupus erythematosus	Systemic sclerosis	Polymyositis/dermatomyositis	Rheumatoid arthritis	Sjögren's syndrome
Antinuclear antibody	95	70	30	15–20	70
Rheumatoid factor	30	30	15	80	70
Antiribonucleoprotein	35	?	?	0	0
Antihistone	70	0	0	0	0
Anti-nDNA	50	0	0	0	0
Anti-Sm	40	0	0	0	0
Anti–SS-A (anti-Ro)	35	0	0	0	65
Anti–SS-B (anti-La)	15	0	0	0	55
Anti-Jo-1	0	0	30 (polymyositis)	0	0
Anti-PM-1	0	±0	50	0	0
Anticentromere	0	17	0	0	0
Anti–Scl-70	0	30	0	0	0
Antinuclear	0	1	1	0	10

nDNA—native DNA.

TABLE 2 SEROLOGIC MANIFESTATIONS OF COLLAGEN VASCULAR DISEASES

Antinuclear Antibody

Antinuclear antibody is found in 95% or more of patients with SLE and is thus very sensitive in detecting this condition. However, it is also found in 1% of normal blood donors; 17% of patients hospitalized for conditions other than SLE; 80% or more of patients who have received for more than 5 months drugs such as procainamide, isoniazid, phenothiazines, phenytoin, and other agents known to induce ANA; and 33% of

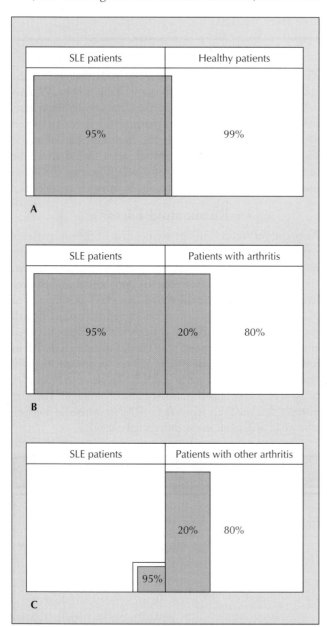

FIGURE 1 The sensitivity, specificity, and predictive value of a laboratory test. In each panel, the left hand box represents the disease being sought (in this case systemic lupus erythematosus [SLE]); the right-hand box, the comparison population; and the crosshatched area, patients testing positive. **A**, Antinuclear antibody (ANA) findings in SLE patients and in healthy people. **B**, ANA findings in SLE and rheumatoid arthritis (RA) populations. **C**, ANA findings in SLE and RA, with adjustments for the actual prevalence of the two diseases in the population. When the low prevalence of SLE and the relatively high prevalence of RA are accounted for, it is seen that most positive ANA findings in these two tested populations occur in RA patients.

normal relatives of SLE patients. It, too, is seen in 10% to 15% of people older than 70 years of age. The significance of these incidences is depicted in Figure 1.

Use of Rheumatoid Factor and Antinuclear Antibody in Clinical Practice

The relative sensitivities and specificities of ANA and RF for the collagen vascular diseases are expressed in Table 2. In Figure 2, Venn diagrams depict the relationships of these two tests in RA and SLE. If a patient presents with a persistent, predominantly symmetric large and small joint polyarthritis of the upper and lower extremities, row one in Table 1 suggests SLE and RA as the most likely diagnoses. If both the ANA and the RF findings are positive, either disease may be present, as indicated in Figure 2. Virtually all of the RA patients with a positive ANA result are among the 80% who have RF as well. In patients with classic appearing RA who have ANA but lack RF, SLE should be highly suspected. The disease in such patients may behave like RA for many years, but complications such as thrombocytopenia, central nervous system disease, and glomerulitis often supervene, suggesting that the illness was SLE all along. In a population of 100,000 people, 2000 (2%) should have RA. Of these 2000, 1600 (80%) have RF, among whom 320 (20%) also should have ANA. In the same population, 50 (0.05%) have SLE, of whom 48 (95%) have ANA, among whom 14 (30%) also should have RF. There should be 23 such doubly seropositive patients with RA in a physician's practice for every one with SLE (320 to 14). Clearly, a finding classic for SLE, such as a nasal septal perforation, mucosal ulcers, or a classic butterfly rash, can be a much more powerful diagnostic test than either of these standard serologic tests.

Because each of these serologic tests provides relatively nonspecific information when done alone, it can be argued persuasively that these tests should always be performed together in attempting a differential diagnosis in such patients. The possible results of this approach can be seen in Figure 3.

What, then, is learned from performing these two tests? The most powerful diagnostic information derives when the ANA finding is negative, which suggests very strongly that

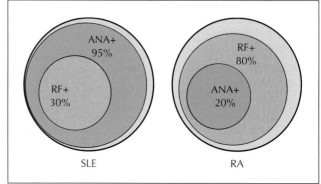

FIGURE 2 Venn diagrams showing the relationships of rheumatoid factor positivity (RF+) and antinuclear antibody positivity (ANA+) in systemic lupus erythematosus (SLE) and rheumatoid arthritis (RA).

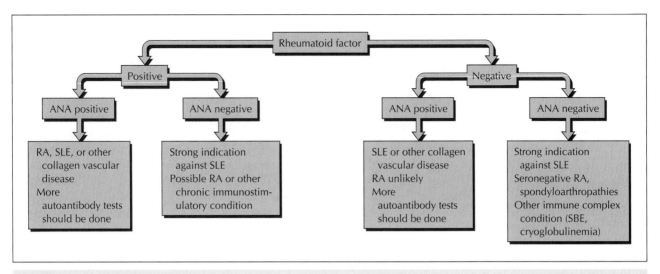

FIGURE 3 Information derived from initial serologic testing. ANA—antinuclear antibody; RA—rheumatoid arthritis; SBE—subacute bacterial endocarditis; SLE—systemic lupus erythematosus.

SLE is not present. A positive ANA finding is nonspecific in the absence of compelling clinical information suggesting SLE. It simply suggests that if clinically indicated, additional, more specific tests for antibodies to nuclear antigens should be performed.

Role of Other Autoantibody Tests in Differential Diagnosis and Prognosis

Since the development of the ANA test in the 1950s, various nuclear and cytoplasmic antigens have been discovered; testing for antibodies to them may permit additional differentiation of the collagen vascular diseases. As indicated in the previous paragraphs, the presence of a positive ANA finding primarily indicates to the clinician that additional tests for autoantibodies may be needed. The most relevant of these tests appear in Table 2.

Anti-native DNA antibodies

Antibodies to nDNA (anti-nDNA) occur in 50% of SLE patients, predominantly in those who are at risk for serious organ system involvement, especially immune complex glomerulitis. Moreover, anti-nDNA is quite specific for SLE (Table 2). This test would be a logical follow-up for the arthritis patient described earlier if the ANA finding were positive. An unequivocally positive anti-nDNA result is virtually diagnostic of SLE. Incidentally, antibodies to single-stranded DNA are of little diagnostic value. They are nonspecific, occurring in many inflammatory states. Although testing for these antibodies has been recommended by some investigators to monitor the disease activity in SLE, these tests have never been proven to be superior to the sedimentation rate, clinical parameters, or more conventional features of disease activity in following SLE.

Anti-Smith antibodies

Antibodies to the Sm antigen, a protein antigen within the nucleus, are also highly specific for SLE, although they are found in only approximately 40% of patients with this condi-

tion. A patient with an unexplained illness who has either anti-nDNA or anti-Sm antibodies should be considered to have SLE until proven otherwise. Pragmatically, the clinician ordering the test should never abbreviate the term for this antibody as "anti-Sm" because this designation is often mistaken for "anti-SM" and the test performed is for anti–smooth muscle antibodies.

Antibodies to ribonucleoprotein

Antibodies to ribonucleoprotein are also common in the collagen vascular diseases. In the 1960s, a subset of patients was described in whom antiribonucleoprotein was the dominant autoantibody. These patients tended to lack immune complex nephritis and often had features of Raynaud's phenomenon, early edematous scleroderma of the fingers, and elements of myositis. This overlap syndrome was called mixed connective tissue disease. Some investigators now question whether the distinction of this complex as a separate nosologic entity is of practical value because many of these patients' conditions appear to differentiate ultimately into SSc. At the same time that mixed connective tissue disease was described, a group of SLE patients was identified who also had antiribonucleoprotein antibody and a much lower incidence of immune complex nephritis, proteinuria, or end-stage renal disease. Whatever name is given to this poorly differentiated overlap syndrome early, the presence of antiribonucleoprotein antibody identifies a group of patients at low risk for developing lupus nephritis but at significant risk for ultimately developing classic SSc. Anti-Sm and antiribonucleoprotein are grouped by many diagnostic laboratories under the term *anti-ENA* (extractable nuclear antigens) and titered simultaneously.

Anti–SS-A and anti–SS-B antibodies

Anti–SS-A and anti–SS-B are antibodies that were initially reported to occur predominantly in patients with Sjögren's syndrome, whether the condition was primary or in association with another collagen vascular disease, such as RA or SLE. Lupus patients with anti–SS-B antibody are less likely to develop immune complex nephritis. Women with anti–SS-A antibody, whatever their primary diagnosis, are predisposed to deliver infants with congenital heart block. There is debate over whether SS-A and SS-B are nuclear or cytoplasmic antigens, probably because their location varies in different cell lines. Many cell substrates used in ANA testing give cytoplasmic staining with sera containing anti–SS-A. This staining is often read as "spindle" or "smooth muscle type" by technicians. The practitioner should be aware that such an interpretation is often a clue to the presence of anti–SS-A. Most of the 5% of SLE patients who are ANA negative have anti–SS-A antibody. This antibody is strongly associated with a unique form of cutaneous lupus known as subacute cutaneous lupus.

Other antinuclear antibodies

Anti–PM-1 is associated with PM/DM with the sensitivity and specificity shown in Table 2, and anti–Jo-1 is seen especially in PM patients with a propensity to pulmonary fibrosis.

Scleroderma-related antibodies

A unique subset of ANAs is seen in variants of SSc. As detailed elsewhere in this text, SSc may be broadly subdivided into two forms. In the limited form, which is more subtle and chronic in nature, skin changes are largely confined to the face and distal extremities, telangiectasias become prominent with time, serious renal or cardiac involvement is rare, and isolated pulmonary hypertension may occur late. In its full form, this syndrome is called CREST (calcinosis of the skin, Raynaud's phenomenon, esophageal dysmotility, sclerodactyly, and telangiectasia). The more diffuse form of SSc is generally more rapidly progressive, and serious renal and cardiac involvement and extensive cutaneous involvement may occur very early. The subsets of ANAs seen in SSc include anticentromere and antinucleolar antibodies, as well as antibodies to the topoisomerase Scl-70 nuclear antigen (anti–Scl-70) [2]. The relationships of these antibody subsets to the clinical forms of SSc are shown in Figure 4.

Clinical utility of autoantibody subjects

Knowing the associations described previously and depicted in Table 2, the clinician may not actually need to establish a precise diagnosis. An ANA-positive patient who has arthralgias but lacks anti-DNA, anti-Sm, and the autoantibodies of SSc may or may not have SLE. This patient is unlikely,

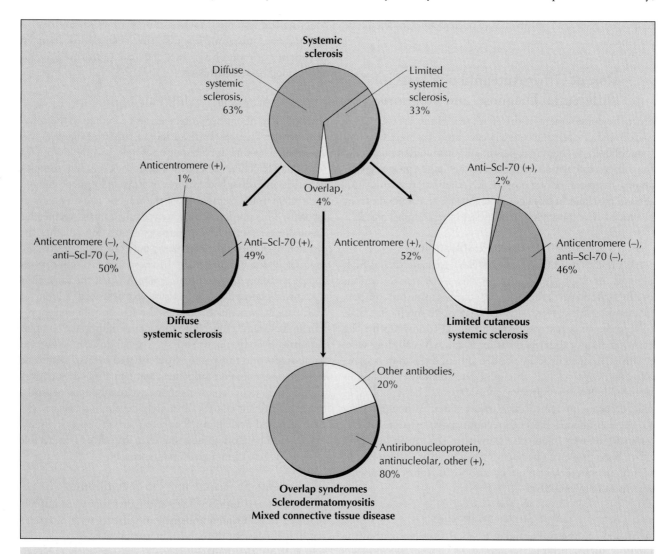

FIGURE 4 Relationships of autoantibody subsets to the different forms of scleroderma (*Adapted from* Smiley [2]; with permission).

however, to develop immune complex nephritis, such as that which occurs in SLE. If anti–SS-B is present, nephritis is even less likely. Similarly, the absence of anti–Scl-70 in the same patient makes progressive scleroderma unlikely. Antiribonucleoprotein in such a patient suggests that 1) some form of collagen vascular disease is present, 2) immune complex nephritis is somewhat unlikely, and 3) the disease may differentiate into SSc ultimately. Thus, with the use of the data in Table 2, either a diagnosis or a considerable assessment of prognosis should be possible in most patients with collagen vascular diseases.

The most cost-effective approach to ordering the previously described tests is to use the clinical features listed in Table 1 to determine the most likely diseases and then to order the appropriate subset of autoantibody tests. These steps can be expressed algorithmically, as shown in Figure 5. If arthralgia and pleurisy dominate, the SLE part of the algorithm should be used first. If Raynaud's phenomenon, dysphagia, and skin changes dominate, the SSc part of the algorithm is preferable. If the clinical features are indeterminate, the indeterminate part of the algorithm shown for PM/DM should be pursued. If the first series of tests does not successfully aid in the diagnosis, the clinician should order the additional tests shown in the algorithm.

APPROACH TO DIAGNOSIS

As stated earlier, despite their many dissimilarities, the collagen vascular diseases have in common the occurrence of vasculitis. They share this characteristic with many other syndromes in which inflammation of the vessels is the dominant feature. These diseases are collectively called the vasculitis syndromes. The most common classic vasculitis syndromes are listed in Figure 6 in order of the diameter of the typical vessel involved. These syndromes should be suspected whenever evidence of unexplained organ ischemia is present, when unexplained systemic symptoms of inflammation (*eg*, fever,

sweats, weight loss) are present, and when one of the conventional collagen vascular diseases discussed earlier is suspected. An algorithm for assisting in the diagnosis is shown in Figure 7. This algorithm serves to determine if features of one of the conventional collagen diseases are present and if clinical criteria set for one of the classic vasculitic syndromes is present (these criteria have recently been published by the American College of Rheumatology [3,4••]) and assist in determining the involvement of different organ systems, such as the skin, the central and peripheral nervous systems, the lungs, the sinuses, and the upper airways. As is the case for the other collagen vascular diseases, a thorough history taking and physical examination are important.

The next diagnostic step is to use conventional laboratory studies to determine which organs are involved. At the same time, serologic tests should be performed to look for the collagen vascular diseases already mentioned.

If neither typical autoantibodies for the collagen vascular diseases, the other serologic features mentioned in the preceding paragraph, nor the clinical criteria for one of the classic vasculitic syndromes are present, diseases that mimic vasculitis must be ruled out. These diseases are listed in Table 3 along with the tests that aid in their detection.

By the end of the algorithm shown in Figure 7, the clinician has one of the following: a diagnosis of one of the specific collagen vascular diseases shown in Table 1, a diagnosis of one of the other vasculitis syndromes (Fig. 6), a diagnosis of one of the mimickers of the previously mentioned diseases (Table 3), or an estimation of the extent of organ system involvement and sufficient serologic data to assess the prognosis for various system involvements.

WHEN TO REFER

If the preceding approaches have not yielded a diagnosis, the clinician must aggressively seek evidence of vasculitis by performing either angiographic or biopsy studies. Biopsy spec-

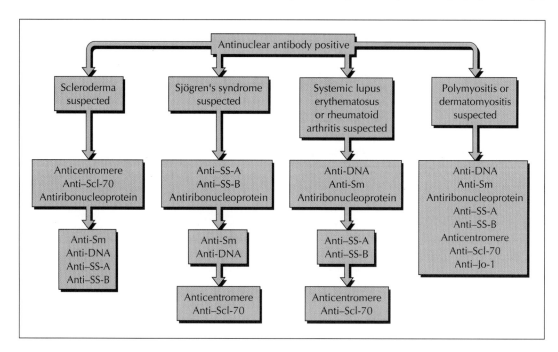

FIGURE 5 Algorithm depicting the most efficient stepwise approach to requesting tests for autoantibodies when collagen vascular diseases are suspected. When the diagnosis is less clear or when systemic symptoms are severe, ordering all tests at once is preferable, as in suspected polymyositis or dermatomyositis.

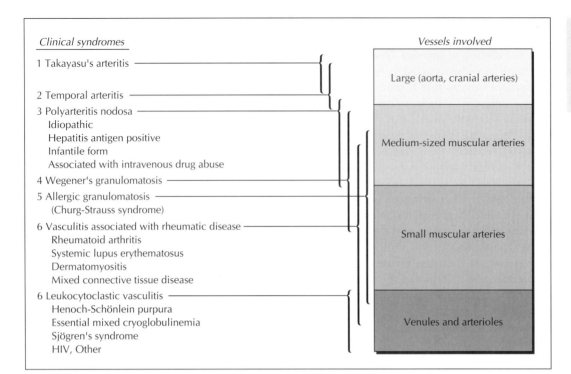

FIGURE 6
Classification
of vasculitis
syndromes and
spectrum of the
vessels involved.

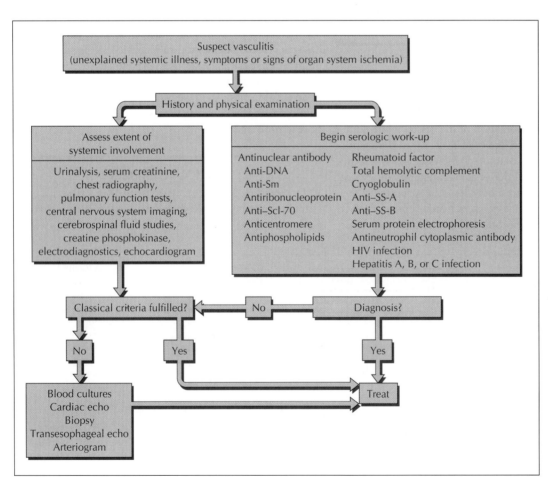

FIGURE 7 Algorithm for differentially diagnosing suspected vasculitis syndromes.

TABLE 3 DETECTING MIMICKERS OF VASCULITIS

Condition	Diagnostic test
Atrial myxoma	Lesion biopsy, transesophageal echocardiography
Cholesterol embolism	Lesion biopsy, transesophageal aortography
Ergot poisoning	History
Phenylpropanolamine toxicity	History, drug screen
Hypertensive arteritis	History, blood pressure evaluation
Subacute bacterial endocarditis	Blood cultures, transesophageal echocardiography

imens of skin lesions suspected on clinical grounds to be vasculitic often do show nonspecific vasculitis. However, in the cholesterol emboli syndrome and in atrial myxomatous embolization, such a biopsy specimen may show cholesterol clefts characteristic of the former or myxoid emboli suggestive of the latter. It is generally fruitless to perform blind biopsies of various organs. A directed biopsy is much more likely to yield diagnostic information. Thus, if there is pulmonary involvement and other causes cannot be identified, lung biopsy may be necessary. Usually, transbronchial or transthoracic needle biopsy does not produce adequate tissue in these diseases, and open lung biopsy is often the best procedure. If the creatine phosphokinase level is elevated, unilateral electromyography is indicated, which should include the proximal extremity and the paraspinal muscles. The most electrically abnormal group identifies the site from which the biopsy specimen should be taken on the side opposite the one on which electromyography was performed, avoiding the artifact caused by electromyography needles. Obviously, if urinalysis results are consistent with renal involvement, needle biopsy of the kidney is in order.

If central nervous system, cardiac, or gastrointestinal involvement is suggested by the signs and symptoms, angiography of the clinically involved organ systems is indicated because biopsy of these organs is usually neither sensitive nor feasible.

Most vasculitis is probably limited to the skin, often results from the use of a medication, is seen by primary care physicians, never gets into series published from academic institutions, does not threaten to cause serious visceral involvement, and requires minimal systemic therapy. At the opposite end of the spectrum is SLE or polyarteritis nodosa, which can cause significant damage to multiple organ systems, is often fatal if left untreated, and generally necessitates aggressive multidrug immunosuppressive therapy, which is best directed by a consultant rheumatologist. Specific aspects of such therapy can be found in the respective chapter in this text dealing with those syndromes.

REFERENCES AND RECOMMENDED READING

Recently published papers of particular interest have been highlighted as:

• Of interest

•• Of outstanding interest

1.•• Tan EM: Auto-antibodies in systemic lupus erythematosus. In *Arthritis and Allied Conditions*, edn 12. Edited by McCarty DJ, Koopman WJ. Malvern, PA: Lea & Febiger; 1993:1179–1184.

2. Smiley JD: The many faces of scleroderma. *Am J Med Sci* 1992, 304:319–333.

3. Hunder GG, Arend WP, Bloch DA, *et al.*: The American College of Rheumatology 1990 criteria for the classification of vasculitis: introduction. *Arthritis Rheum* 1990, 33:1065–1067.

4.•• Churg A, Churg C, eds.: *Systemic Vasculitides*. New York: Igaku-Shoin; 1991.

SELECT BIBLIOGRAPHY

Elstein AS, Shulman LS, Sprafka SA: *Medical Problem Solving: An Analysis of Clinical Reasoning*. Cambridge, MA: Harvard University Press; 1978.

Ingelfinger JA, Mosteller F, Thibodeau LA, Ware JH: *Biostatistics in Clinical Medicine*. New York: Macmillan; 1983.

McCarty DJ, Koopman WJ, eds.: *Arthritis and Allied Conditions*, edn 12. Malvern, PA: Lea & Febiger; 1993.

Sox HC, Blatt MA, Higgins MC, Marton KI: *Medical Decision Making*. Stoneham, MA: Butterworths; 1988.

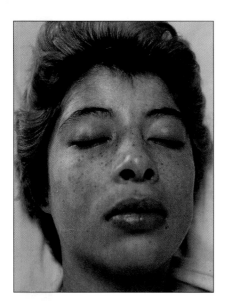

consider an initial consultation with a rheumatologist, who may aid in determining the treatment plan, providing prognostic information, and gaining epidemiologic information, which may further our knowledge of the incidence, prevalence, and pathophysiology of the disease.

Systemic lupus erythematosus is a disease of exacerbations and remissions. Some patients may have completely symptom-free intervals; however, almost all patients will experience constitutional symptoms and arthralgias or arthritis during the course of their illness. Patients therefore should be counseled regarding the proper balance of rest and exercise, whereas those with deformities may require active consultation from physiatrists, with specific programs of occupational and physical therapy. Splinting of affected joints (Fig. 2) may be required for protection at rest or during certain activities. A well balanced diet is important for all individuals with chronic disease. In SLE, diet may need modification relative to disease activity (*eg*, a low-salt diet in patients with nephritis or myocarditis) or to complications of therapy, such as corticosteroids (*eg*, a diabetic diet for a patient with hyperglycemia). Although not all lupus patients exhibit photosensitivity, it is best to caution against direct sun exposure in general and to insist on the use of sun screens to avoid sun-provoked disease flares.

are included. Using these criteria, early diagnosis may be facilitated and should lead to the search for early organ involvement, such as renal disease, prior to the development of organ dysfunction. Patients with mild disease may be readily treated by a primary care physician; nevertheless, it is appropriate to

---

TABLE 1 CRITERIA FOR THE CLASSIFICATION OF SYSTEMIC LUPUS ERYTHEMATOSUS (SLE)*	
Criterion	**Definition**
Malar rash	Fixed erythema, flat or raised, over the malar eminences, tending to spare the nasolabial folds
Discoid rash	Erythematous, raised patches with adherent keratotic scaling and follicular plugging; atrophic scarring may occur in older lesions
Photosensitivity	Skin rash as a result of unusual reaction to sunlight, by patient history or physician observation
Oral ulcers	Oral or nasopharyngeal ulceration, usually painless, observed by a physician
Arthritis	Nonerosive arthritis involving two or more peripheral joints, characterized by tenderness, swelling, or effusion
Serositis	Pleuritis—convincing history of pleuritic pain or rub heard by a physician or evidence of pleural effusion; or pericarditis—documented by electrocardiography or rub or evidence of pericardial effusion
Renal disorder	Persistent proteinuria greater than 0.5 g/d or greater than 3 g/d if quantitation not performed; or cellular casts—may be erythrocyte, hemoglobin, granular, tubular, or mixed
Neurologic disorder	Seizures—in the absence of offending drugs or known metabolic derangements, *eg*, uremia, ketoacidosis, or electrolyte imbalance; or psychosis—in the absence of offending drugs or known metabolic derangements, *eg*, uremia, ketoacidosis, or electrolyte imbalance
Hematologic disorder	Hemolytic anemia—with reticulocytosis; or leukopenia—less than 4000/mm^3 on two or more occasions; or lymphopenia—less than 1500/mm^3 on two or more occasions; or thrombocytopenia—less than 100,000/mm^3 in the absence of offending drugs
Immunologic disorder	Positive lupus erythematosus cell preparation; or anti-DNA—antibody to native DNA in abnormal titer; or anti-Sm—presence of antibody to Sm nuclear antigen; or false-positive serologic test for syphilis known to be positive for at least 6 mo and confirmed by Treponema pallidum immobilization or fluorescent treponemal antibody absorption test
Antinuclear antibody	An abnormal titer of antinuclear antibody by immunofluorescence or an equivalent assay at any point in time and in the absence of drugs known to be associated with drug-induced lupus syndrome

*For the purpose of identifying patients in clinical studies, a person shall be said to have SLE if any four or more of the 11 criteria are present, serially or simultaneously, during any interval of observation.
From Tan and coworkers [23]; with permission.

Musculoskeletal Features

Musculoskeletal involvement in SLE is characteristically nonerosive and nondeforming. Therapy is aimed at symptomatic relief. Aspirin in antiinflammatory doses or nonsteroidal antiinflammatory drugs are appropriate as initial therapy. A 1- to 2-week trial of a medication is sufficient to determine therapeutic efficacy; if no benefit is noted, another agent, generally from a different chemical class, should be substituted. The potential complications, including epigastric discomfort or frank gastrointestinal bleeding and renal insufficiency, should be monitored.

A patient may have musculoskeletal disease that closely resembles rheumatoid arthritis, including chronic synovitis and even bony erosions. Low doses of corticosteroids may be necessary to achieve initial remission. Such patients also may be candidates for treatment with a disease-modifying antirheumatic drug (Table 2). Although the primary care physician should monitor chronic therapy with these agents, the initial decision regarding the particular regimen and regular reassessments of efficacy and toxicity should be made by a rheumatologist.

Constitutional Symptoms, Rash, and Serositis

In addition to their value in the management of chronic lupus arthritis, antimalarials are particularly effective as steroid-spar-

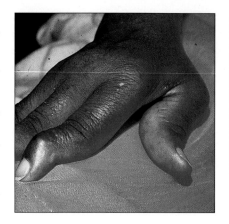

FIGURE 2 The "lupus hand," with reducible swan neck deformity and ulnar deviation resulting from chronic inflammation of tendons and periarticular tissues.

ing agents in the treatment of chronic constitutional symptoms, such as fever; severe malaise; skin manifestations, including alopecia (Fig. 3), discoid lupus rash (Fig. 4), subacute cutaneous lupus, and cutaneous vasculitis (Fig. 5); and recurrent pleuritis or pericarditis. In a Canadian study of patients whose disease was in remission, continued hydroxychloroquine therapy was associated with 2.5 times fewer exacerbations of SLE than were observed among patients in whom the drug was discontinued [1•]. No difference in steroid dose was observed in the two groups; however, all patients began the study with their disease in remission. An

TABLE 2 DISEASE-MODIFYING ANTIRHEUMATIC DRUGS USED IN THE TREATMENT OF CHRONIC ARTHRITIS IN SYSTEMIC LUPUS ERYTHEMATOSUS		
Agent	**Dosage**	**Comments**
Antimalarials		
Hydroxychloroquine	Started at 200 mg twice daily and reduced to once daily if an initial beneficial result is obtained	Ophthalmologic examinations at regular intervals to detect retinal toxicity are essential
Immunosuppressives		
Methotrexate	Generally started at 7.5 mg/wk, with incremental increases by 2.5 mg/wk (up to 15–20 mg/wk), to achieve a beneficial response or if flare occurs after an initial good response; orally once per week to control chronic synovitis	Elevated hepatic transaminases frequently result, but actual histologic damage is uncommon
Azathioprine	2–2.5 mg/kg/d (usually 100–150 mg/d) as a single daily dosage	Leukopenia is the most common side effect that may necessitate a reduction in dose; chronic therapy may result in a macrocytic anemia usually responsive to folic acid, and elevated hepatic transaminases and alkaline phosphatase may also occur
Injectable gold		
Aurothiomalate	Weekly to induce remission of chronic synovitis, then reduced to monthly	May result in proteinuria or occasionally microscopic hematuria; systemic lupus erythematosus versus drug-induced leukopenia may be difficult to differentiate
Aurothioglucose	Begin with a test dose of 10–25 mg, then continue with 50 mg/wk; as response is achieved (usually after 500–1000 mg), increase interval between doses to 2–4 wk	None
Oral gold		
Auranofin	Begin with 3 mg twice daily, increase to three times daily if complete response is not achieved after 1–2 mo	Mild diarrhea is a common side effect; monitoring for proteinuria, leukopenia, thrombocytopenia, and hepatic dysfunction is necessary

Australian study of SLE patients beginning hydroxychloroquine therapy found that the probability of discontinuing this agent by 12 or 24 months was 8% or 24%, respectively. Treatment was generally terminated for lack of efficacy, with no ocular toxicity noted [2].

Renal Disease

Despite advances in diagnosis and treatment, nephritis remains the most frequent manifestation resulting in both mortality and morbidity among patients with SLE. The clinical course of lupus nephritis has been well characterized. Progression from mild or mesangial (class II) involvement to focal proliferative (class III) and diffuse proliferative (class IV) nephritis has been well documented. The clinical severity of this disease generally parallels the severity of histologic disease; deterioration in renal function or significant increases in proteinuria may signal such histologic progression, with its accompanying poor prognosis. Renal function may deteriorate progressively in the absence of serologic evidence of disease activity, probably as a result of prior flares of nephritis, whereas glomerular sclerosis, interstitial fibrosis, and tubular atrophy ensue.

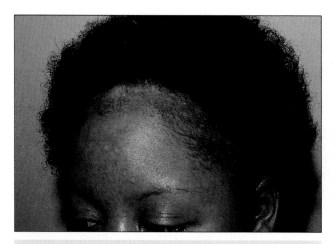

FIGURE 3 Frontal and temporal alopecia in a patient with active lupus. With remission, hair growth returns.

The overall goals of management are to preserve renal function and minimize the complications of proteinuria, including hypoalbuminemia with edema, hyperlipidemia, and hypertension. Despite the absence of controlled studies documenting their efficacy, corticosteroids are accepted therapy for active disease. Treatment includes prednisone in moderate (30–60 mg/d) to high (> 60 mg/d) oral dosages or pulse intravenous methylprednisolone (1000 mg/d for 3 d); these corticosteroids are used especially to reverse progressive azotemia. Controversies regarding management remain, however.

Serologic abnormalities

Should serologic abnormalities, such as hypocomplementemia and the presence of antibodies to double-stranded DNA, be treated in the absence of concomitant clinical manifestations, such as proteinuria, active urinary sediment, or azotemia?

Several studies have shown that the duration of remission is longer and the severity of renal flares milder among subsets of SLE patients in whom decreased complement levels were normalized and anti–double-stranded DNA antibody titers reduced. Nevertheless, many cases have been reported in which abnormal serologies reversed spontaneously without treatment. In 39 SLE patients followed for nearly 10 years, maintenance of normal total hemolytic complement (CH50) was associated with significantly better renal function and patient survival [3]. Two caveats exist, however, in that normal CH50 was maintained in only 17 patients throughout the study, and a significant survival difference was not observed until after 5 years of follow-up.

Practically, in the individual patient, treatment strategy should take into account the mimetic nature of SLE. To try to minimize steroid dosage and its associated complications, it may be appropriate during an initial episode of serologic abnormalities to serially measure them without changing therapy. If repeated abnormal valves occur, especially if clinical nephritis ensues, it would be prudent to institute therapy.

Indications for renal biopsy

Generally, the class of histologic renal lesion in subsets of SLE patients may be predicted based upon the severity of

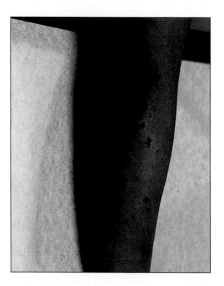

FIGURE 4 Discrete and confluent discoid lupus lesions in a characteristic location over the elbow in a patient with systemic lupus erythematosus.

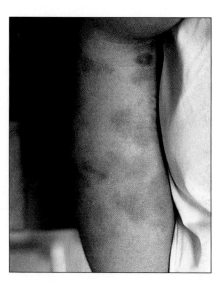

FIGURE 5 Erythematous tender nodules of the skin and subcutaneous tissue. Biopsy of the lesions showed characteristic lymphocytic infiltration of the dermis and perivascular inflammation.

renal manifestations, especially those related to the degree of hematuria, cylindruria, proteinuria, including the nephrotic syndrome, and azotemia. In an individual patient, however, class IV nephritis may be accompanied only by hypocomplementemia and mild proteinuria, whereas patients with class III disease have been reported with nephrotic range proteinuria and azotemia. This finding has led some investigators to suggest that renal biopsy does not provide added benefit to clinical variables in predicting outcome or response to therapy. Distinguishing diffuse proliferative from membranous nephropathy in a patient with nephrotic syndrome and inconclusive features suggesting inflammatory activity (eg, mild serologic abnormalities or mildly active urinary sediment) may be an indication for biopsy; more aggressive immunosuppressive treatment may be planned for patients with class IV disease, whereas conservative measures such as sodium restriction and antihypertensive therapy may be stressed for patients with class V disease because it is less likely to progress to renal failure.

The concept of identifying histologic features of activity versus chronicity provides a possible basis for determining therapy [4]. Renal biopsy may be of practical use, therefore, in disclosing irreversible damage such as sclerotic glomeruli and tubular atrophy, especially in the patient with significant azotemia yet minimal features of disease activity (Fig. 6). Protracted aggressive immunosuppressive therapy may be avoided in such patients by placing emphasis on controlling blood pressure to prolong renal function [5•]. Recent studies have addressed the issue of specific histologic features associated with poor outcome. Some have found that a high chronicity index is associated with decreased survival [6], whereas others have failed to find such an association [7,8].

Maintenance therapy

Is prolonged maintenance therapy with intravenous cyclophosphamide indicated in patients with diffuse proliferative nephritis or will short courses (eg, monthly for six doses) provide a

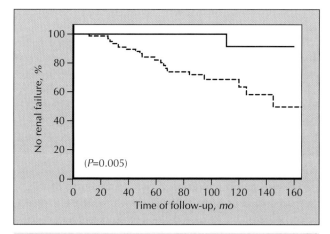

FIGURE 6 Probability of maintaining life-supporting renal function in patients with active lupus nephritis identified as being at high risk (*broken line*) or low risk (*solid line*), according to the presence of chronic histologic changes. (*From* Austin and coworkers [4]; with permission.)

therapeutic benefit while sparing toxicity, especially the long-term risk of malignancy?

A prospective study of the efficacy of steroids and immunosuppressive agents, including azathioprine and both oral and intravenous cyclophosphamide in nephritis, has now been extended to approximately 10 years, although many of the patients discontinued taking their medications after 4 to 7 years. Regimens containing cyclophosphamide resulted in a significantly reduced probability of progression to renal failure. Again, the major differences among the treatment groups were apparent only after 5 to 6 years [9]. Initial recommendations for the intravenous cyclophosphamide regimen, designed to minimize bladder and bone marrow toxicity, were three monthly infusions of cyclophosphamide escalating in dose from 0.5 to 0.75 to 1 g/m^2, followed by a maintenance dose every 3 months for an indefinite period. Patients with a resolution of initial serum creatinine elevations within 48 weeks had a low risk for renal failure, suggesting that short-term treatment may be sufficient for some patients [10•].

Plasmapheresis, which is still experimental, has been used as an adjunct to pharmacologic therapy for lupus patients with refractory nephritis. No positive effect of plasmapheresis on serum creatinine or other features of disease exacerbation were noted in 86 patients [11]. Clearly, this expensive, invasive modality should be reserved for highly controlled conditions under the direction of a rheumatologist or nephrologist.

Despite careful follow-up and aggressive therapy, some patients with lupus nephritis progress to end-stage renal disease, either as a direct consequence of an episode of active nephritis or because of the slow progression of glomerular sclerosis, interstitial fibrosis, and tubular atrophy. When renal failure occurs in this setting, chronic maintenance hemodialysis or peritoneal dialysis should be instituted. Renal transplantation in carefully selected patients, especially those who are seronegative with respect to antinuclear and anti-DNA antibodies, has been shown in one study to be highly successful, with recurrent nephritis developing in only one allograft [12••].

Neuropsychiatric Disease

Neuropsychiatric abnormalities have been described in 10% to 20% of series of SLE patients. The features are highly variable, with the most common being seizures and organic brain syndrome (Table 3). Differential diagnosis may be difficult, often necessitating a distinction between SLE activity and functional psychiatric disorders, metabolic disturbances, central nervous system infection, or side effects of steroid therapy. No diagnostic gold standard exists; however, the presence of disease activity in other systems and titers of antilymphocyte antibodies or antiribosomal P antibodies may be helpful. Both anatomic and functional studies have been proposed as methods for identifying neuropsychiatric SLE (Table 4); however, most of these studies tend to confirm focal clinical neurologic abnormalities already apparent on physical examination.

High-dose oral or intravenous corticosteroid therapy is the accepted standard for severe neuropsychiatric features such as obtundation or coma, transverse myelitis, and focal neurologic

TABLE 3 NEUROPSYCHIATRIC MANIFESTATIONS OF SYSTEMIC LUPUS ERYTHEMATOSUS
Neurologic manifestations
Seizures
Obtundation, coma
"Lupus" headache
Cerebral or retinal vasculitis
Stroke
Transverse myelitis
Ascending polyneuropathy
Mononeuritis multiplex
Peripheral neuropathy
Psychiatric manifestations
Organic brain syndrome
Affective disorders, emotional lability
Diminished concentration, memory impairment
Progressive dementia
Hallucinations, delirium

TABLE 4 DIAGNOSTIC MEASURES IN NEUROPSYCHIATRIC SYSTEMIC LUPUS ERYTHEMATOSUS
Immunologic measures
Serum lymphocytotoxic antibodies
Antiribosomal P protein antibodies
Antineuronal antibodies
Specialized testing measures
Computed tomography of brain, spinal cord
Single photon emission computed tomography
Positron-emission tomography
Magnetic resonance imaging
Phosphorus-31 nuclear magnetic resonance spectroscopy
Central nervous system angiography

abnormalities in a specific cerebrovascular distribution. Cyclophosphamide may be added. Manifestations of organic brain syndrome may respond to corticosteroids; however, psychotropic agents may be equally efficacious. Similarly, seizures may be controlled with anticonvulsant therapy, thereby avoiding the chronic side effects of steroids.

A feature of the central nervous system that has received considerable attention recently is chronic progressive dementia, which may result from the antiphospholipid antibody syndrome with its predisposition to thrombosis. Recurrent cerebrovascular accidents also have been attributed to antiphospholipid antibodies, both as a consequence of in situ thrombosis and as embolic phenomena from mitral and aortic valve vegetations [13••]. Such features must be distinguished from active neuropsychiatric disease, and long-term anticoagulant therapy should be instituted. Similarly, SLE patients with thrombosis anywhere in the body should be investigated for the presence of circulating lupus anticoagulant or anticardiolipin antibodies; if these features are found, long-term treatment with anticoagulants is in order. Some of these patients have little or no clinical evidence of classic systemic lupus.

New Therapies

Several drugs have been introduced for specific manifestations of SLE, especially when these features prove refractory to conventional therapy, such as steroids and standard immunosuppressive drugs. Anecdotal reports of the benefit of intravenous immunoglobulins for severe lupus nephritis have appeared in recent years [14]. Similarly, intravenous immunoglobulin therapy was reported to be successful in treating persistent thrombocytopenia in five of seven SLE patients [15]. Although immediate results may be positive, repeated episodes of thrombocytopenia are also common.

Danazol, a low-potency androgenic steroid, has been effective in some patients as maintenance therapy for thrombocytopenia, and it has been used in patients with chronic autoimmune hemolytic anemia in SLE [16].

Several drugs appear to be useful in controlling persistent cutaneous manifestations of SLE, such as subacute cutaneous lupus, bullous lupus, and cutaneous vasculitis. Among these agents are dapsone [17], isotretinoin [18], and interferon-α-2a [19]. The immunosuppressive agent azathioprine, used for many years as a steroid-sparing and remission-maintaining agent for the systemic features of SLE, also is useful in controlling recalcitrant cutaneous manifestations [20]. The aforementioned successes are all case reports; controlled studies are needed. Use of these agents for SLE manifestations is best directed by a dermatologist or rheumatologist.

Immunotherapy tailored to the abnormalities associated with specific features of SLE is a hope of the future. Improvement after the administration of monoclonal anti-CD4 to an SLE patient with unresponsive nephritis [21] suggests the need for controlled clinical trials of such agents and reinforces the need for such patients to be referred to centers performing clinical and epidemiologic research on SLE.

Dietary manipulation may provide the most cost-effective and least toxic therapy for patients with SLE. As survival in this disease improves and late morbidity and mortality from cardiovascular complications predominate, preventive measures become increasingly important. Lipid abnormalities should be treated initially with an appropriate diet; if this approach fails, lipid-lowering agents should be instituted. Similarly, elevated blood pressure should be rigidly controlled with diet or antihypertensive agents.

Dietary supplementation with large amounts of fish oil (eicosapentaenoic acid) has been shown to have a beneficial effect on both lipid levels and blood pressure and may decrease the risk of coronary artery disease. Fish oil has also been shown to have an anti-inflammatory effect by replacing arachidonic acid in the formation of inflammatory mediators. It has been postulated that dietary supplementation with fish oil may prevent the tissue damage resulting from immune

TABLE 5 CLINICAL FEATURES OF SJÖGREN'S SYNDROME
Sicca syndrome: keratoconjunctivitis sicca, dry mouth
Parotid gland enlargement
Associated rheumatic disease: rheumatoid arthritis, systemic lupus erythematosus
Lymphocytic interstitial pneumonitis
Interstitial nephritis, renal tubular acidosis
Primary biliary cirrhosis
Chronic atrophic gastritis
Sensory neuropathy
Lymphoma, pseudolymphoma
Severe shortness of breath and chronic cough

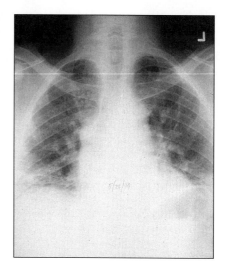

FIGURE 7 Chest roentgenography showing bilateral infiltrates in a patient with Sjögren's syndrome.

complex deposition and the ensuing inflammation in a lupus flare. Walton and coworkers [22•] found a significant benefit of a fish oil regimen when compared with placebo, with no toxicity noted. Others have not observed a benefit, but most have studied few patients for a short time. A large, controlled study of longer duration is necessary to clarify the potential of fish oil in the management of SLE.

SJÖGREN'S SYNDROME

Sjögren's syndrome may exist as a manifestation of SLE and other rheumatic disorders or as a disease of its own. Classically, individuals with primary Sjögren's syndrome and, to a lesser extent, those with SLE plus Sjögren's syndrome produce autoantibodies to Ro(SS-A) and La(SS-B) antigens. The pathologic features of lymphocyte and plasma cell infiltration of salivary and lacrimal glands, as well as other exocrine glands and systemic organs such as the lungs and kidneys, lead to most of the clinical features (Table 5).

Symptoms of the sicca syndrome are treated with conservative measures, including artificial methylcellulose tears, frequent oral fluids, and occasionally artificial saliva preparations. Frequent dental care, with attention to periodontal disease, is essential.

Pulmonary symptoms are a result of dryness of the tracheobronchial tree, with secondary infection developing. Lymphocytic interstitial pneumonitis (LIP) is characterized by cough, dyspnea, hypoxia, and infiltrates on chest radiography (Fig. 7). Bronchoscopy with bronchoalveolar lavage or even open lung biopsy may be necessary to rule out opportunistic infection. LIP is generally a steroid-sensitive lesion; treatment should begin with a prednisone dosage of at least 1 mg/kg/d, followed by slow tapering as symptoms and radiologic evidence of infiltrates are monitored.

The pathologic abnormality of Sjögren's syndrome may progress to pseudolymphoma or even true malignant lymphoma. The former may respond to corticosteroids and cyclophosphamide, whereas the latter should be treated with a regimen determined via oncologic consultation, taking into consideration the organs involved and the extent of disease.

REFERENCES AND RECOMMENDED READING

Recently published papers of particular interest have been highlighted as:
• Of interest
•• Of outstanding interest

1• The Canadian Hydroxychloroquine Study Group: A randomized study of the effect of withdrawing hydroxychloroquine sulfate in systemic lupus erythematosus. *N Engl J Med* 1991, 324:150–154.

2. Morand EF, McCloud PI, Littlejohn GO: Continuation of long term treatment with hydroxychloroquine in systemic lupus erythematosus and rheumatoid arthritis. *Ann Rheum Dis* 1992, 51:1318–1321.

3. Latman PS, Glicklich D, Sablay LB, *et al.*: Effect of long-term normalization of serum complement levels on the course of lupus nephritis. *Am J Med* 1989, 87:132–138.

4. Austin HA III, Klippel JH, Balow JE, *et al.*: Therapy of lupus nephritis: controlled trial of prednisone and cytotoxic drugs. *N Engl J Med* 1986, 314:614–619.

5.• Ginzler EM, Felson DT, Anthony JM, Anderson JJ: Hypertension increases the risk of renal deterioration in systemic lupus erythematosus. *J Rheumatol* 1993, 20:1694–1700.

6. Nossent HC, Henzen-Logmans SC, Vroom TM, *et al.*: Contribution of renal biopsy data in predicting outcome in lupus nephritis: analysis of 116 patients. *Arthritis Rheum* 1990, 33:970–977.

7. Edworthy SM, Bloch DA, McShane DJ, *et al.*: A "state model" of renal function in systemic lupus erythematosus: its value in the prediction of outcome in 292 patients. *J Rheumatol* 1989, 16:29–35.

8. Schwartz MM, Bernstein J, Hill GS, *et al.*: Predictive value of renal pathology in diffuse proliferative lupus glomerulonephritis: Lupus Collaborative Study Group. *Kidney Int* 1989, 36:891–896.

9. Steinberg AD, Steinberg SC: Long-term preservation of renal function in patients with lupus nephritis receiving treatment that includes cyclophosphamide versus those treated with prednisone only. *Arthritis Rheum* 1991, 34:945–949.

10.• Levey AS, Lan S-P, Corwin HL, *et al.*: Progression and remission of renal disease in the Lupus Nephritis Collaborative Study. *Ann Intern Med* 1992, 116:114–123.

11. Lewis EJ, Hunsicker LG, Lan S-P, *et al.*: A controlled trial of plasmapheresis therapy in severe lupus nephritis. *N Engl J Med* 1992, 326:1373–1379.

12.•• Goss GA, Cole BR, Jendrisak MD, *et al.*: Renal transplantation for systemic lupus erythematosus and recurrent lupus nephritis: a single-center experience and a review of the literature. *Transplantation* 1991, 52:805–810.

13.•• Stephens CJM: The antiphospholipid syndrome: clinical correlations, cutaneous features, mechanism of thrombosis, and treatment of patients with the lupus anticoagulant and anticardiolipin antibodies. *Br J Dermatol* 1991, 125:199–210.

14. Akashi K, Nagasawa K, Mayumi T, *et al.*: Successful treatment of refractory systemic lupus erythematosus with intravenous immunoglobulins. *J Rheumatol* 1990, 17:375–379.

15. Maier WP, Gordon DS, Howard RF, *et al.*: Intravenous immunoglobulin therapy in systemic lupus erythematosus-associated thrombocytopenia. *Arthritis Rheum* 1990, 33:1233–1239.

16. Chan AC, Sack K: Danazol therapy in autoimmune hemolytic anemia associated with systemic lupus erythematosus. *J Rheumatol* 1991, 18:280–282.

17. Holtman JH, Neustadt DH, Klein J, Callen JP: Dapsone is an effective therapy for the lesions of subacute cutaneous lupus erythematosus and urticarial vasculitis in a patient with C2 deficiency. *J Rheumatol* 1990, 17:1222–1225.

18. Shornick JK, Formica N, Parke AL: Isotretinoin for refractory lupus erythematosus. *J Am Acad Dermatol* 1991, 24:49–52.

19. Nicolas J-F, Thivolet J, Kanitakis J, Lyonnet S: Response of discoid and subacute cutaneous lupus erythematosus to recombinant interferon α 2A. *J Invest Dermatol* 1990, 95:142S–145S.

20. Callen JP, Spencer LV, Burress JB, Holtman J: Azathioprine: an effective, corticosteroid-sparing therapy for patients with recalcitrant cutaneous lupus erythematosus or with recalcitrant cutaneous leukocytoclastic vasculitis. *Arch Dermatol* 1991, 127:515–522.

21. Hiepe F, Volk H-D, Apostoloff E, *et al.*: Treatment of severe systemic lupus erythematosus with anti-CD4 monoclonal antibody. *Lancet* 1991, 338:1529–1530.

22.• Walton AJE, Snaith ML, Locniskar M, *et al.*: Dietary fish oil and the severity of symptoms in patients with systemic lupus erythematosus. *Ann Rheum Dis* 1991, 50:463–466.

23. Tan EM, Cohen AS, Fries JF, *et al.*: The 1982 revised criteria for the classification of systemic lupus erythematosus (SLE). *Arthritis Rheum* 1982, 25:1271–1277.

SELECT BIBLIOGRAPHY

Older SA, Boumpas DT, Austin HA III: Management of lupus nephritis: I. Pathogenesis; clinical, histologic evaluation. *J Musculoskel Med* 1991, 8:35–48.

Older SA, Boumpas DT, Austin HA III: Management of lupus nephritis: II. Emerging utility of cytotoxic therapy. *J Musculoskel Med* 1991, 8:74–84.

Talal N, Moutsopoulos HM, Kassan SS, eds.: *Sjögren's Syndrome: Clinical and Immunological Aspects.* New York: Springer-Verlag; 1987.

Sclerosing Syndromes

Bashar Kahaleh

Key Points

- Primary and secondary Raynaud's can be easily identified by careful history, physical examination, and selected serologic tests.
- Undifferentiated connective tissue syndrome, rather than mixed connective disease, is a preferable term for describing the early overlap syndrome.
- Cutaneous fibrosis, digital infarcts, and lung fibrosis imply the diagnosis of scleroderma.
- The term *limited scleroderma* replaced the term CREST, and diffuse scleroderma is associated with poor prognosis.
- More promising therapy for scleroderma is becoming available, yet attention to individual organ involvement is the best approach to therapy.

Human sclerosing syndromes are defined histopathologically by increased connective tissue matrix accumulation in association with a low-grade inflammatory process. Vascular involvement with symptoms and signs of vascular injury is generally present. Sclerosis leads to dysfunction of the involved organ, manifested clinically by chronic, progressive organ insufficiency. Examples of human sclerosing syndromes include pulmonary interstitial fibrosis, cirrhosis, retroperitoneal and mediastinal fibrosis, Peyronie's disease, palmar or plantar fasciitis, and Dupuytren's contracture. Scleroderma (systemic sclerosis) and the overlap syndromes represent the most explicit examples of diffuse multisystem sclerosing syndromes of unknown etiology. The clinical expression of the disease begins with symptoms of vascular instability (Raynaud's phenomenon), a transition stage (undifferentiated or mixed connective tissue disease [MCTD]), and a later stage of widespread tissue fibrosis (scleroderma).

Treatment

No single therapeutic intervention has been proven to erase human tissue fibrosis; approaches directed at both the pathophysiologic and clinical expression of the disease are recommended. Early clinical detection and therapeutic intervention in the presclerotic stages is the most promising approach to these devastating disorders.

RAYNAUD'S PHENOMENON

The classic triphasic color changes of pallor, cyanosis, and rubor are rarely seen sequentially in the same patient: current definitions do not require all three colors for diagnosis [1•]. Biphasic color change of pallor and cyanosis is commonly noted.

Primary Raynaud's phenomenon or Raynaud's disease is a benign condition with negligible consequences and reflects most cases. An association with fibromyalgia, prolapsed mitral valve, migraine headache, irritable bowel syndrome, and heightened anxiety has been reported. Secondary Raynaud's phenomenon or Raynaud's

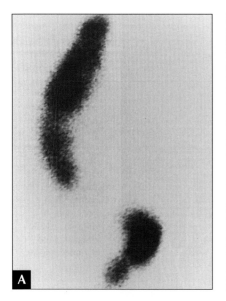

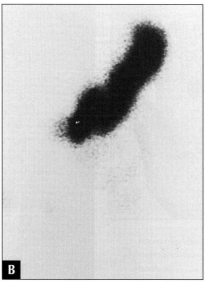

FIGURE 5 Gastric emptying scans of a 47-year-old patient with a 3-year history of diffused scleroderma. **A,** The view at 60 minutes shows that 98% of the activity is in the esophagus, which is compatible with a marked delay in esophageal transit time. Note dilatation of the esophagus. **B,** The view at 120 minutes shows that most of the administered activity is still in the stomach, with minimal activity noted in the C loop of the duodenum and upper jejunum. The findings are consistent with a severe delay in gastric emptying.

ventilatory defect with impairment in gas exchange is very common. An isolated reduction in diffusion capacity may indicate the presence of pulmonary hypertension. High-resolution computed tomographic scans (HRCT) (Fig. 7) are much more sensitive than is routine chest radiography (Fig. 8) for the evaluation of interstitial pulmonary fibrosis. Up to 75% of patients with normal chest radiographs have an abnormal HRCT scan. Gallium lung scanning (Fig. 9) and bronchoalveolar lavage are promising tools for detecting alveolitis.

Pulmonary artery spasm is seen early, but diffuse, fixed, intimal proliferation in the pulmonary arterioles is found in established disease. The 2-year cumulative survival rate is only 40% in patients with pulmonary hypertension compared with 88% in patients without hypertension.

Renal hypertensive crisis was once the leading cause of mortality in scleroderma. A 92% mortality rate was reduced to 44% after the introduction of angiotensin-converting enzyme (ACE) inhibitors [8•]. At risk are older men with congestive heart failure and patients with rapidly progressive diffuse disease of less than 3 years' duration. The onset of renal crisis is abrupt, with the occurrence of headache, blurred vision, hypertension with retinopathy and papilledema, and oliguria and sudden death.

Course

The course of scleroderma is extremely variable; early detection of organ involvement and thoughtful therapeutic intervention are essential for patient survival. Variables that predict poor survival include older age, reduced renal function, anemia, reduced pulmonary diffusing capacity, and reduced total serum protein level. These parameters may be useful in identifying patients at risk for shortened survival [9•]. Scleroderma remains a lethal rheumatic disorder. The cumulative survival rates are 80% at 2 years, 50% at 8 years, and 30% at 12 years after disease onset.

Differential Diagnosis

Many conditions may mimic scleroderma skin disease (Table 7) but are distinguished by the lack of the classic scleroderma visceral involvement, the absence of Raynaud's

TABLE 6 INVESTIGATIONS OF SCLERODERMA SYSTEMIC INVOLVEMENT
Heart
Resting and exercise electrocardiogram
24-Hour Holter monitor
Echocardiogram and Doppler studies
Thallium perfusion scan
Lung
Chest radiogram
High-resolution computed tomography scan
Gallium lung scan
Pulmonary functions with diffusion studies
Bronchoalveolar lavage
Technetium aspiration scan

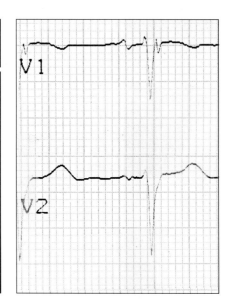

FIGURE 6 Electrocardiogram of a 39-year-old patient with a 2-year history of diffuse scleroderma. Note the poor anterior R wave progression and the ventricular conduction delay. This pattern is common in scleroderma heart disease without large coronary vessel disease.

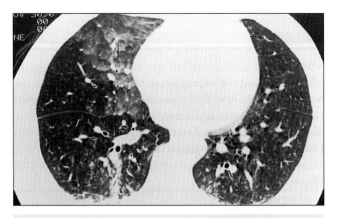

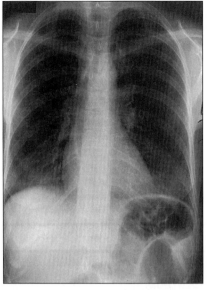

FIGURE 8 A chest radiogram of a 45-year-old patient with a 3-year history of diffused scleroderma. Note the basilar interstitial changes consistent with pulmonary fibrosis.

FIGURE 7 Parenchymal lung disease as detected by a high-resolution computed tomography scan of a 34-year-old patient with a 6-month history of diffused scleroderma. Alveolitis is suggested by the thickened septal lines and the ground glass appearance of the interstitium.

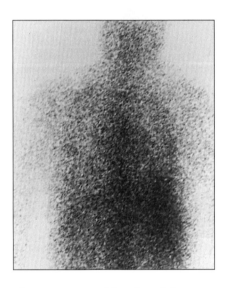

FIGURE 9 Gallium scan of a 68-year-old patient with a 1-year history of diffused scleroderma. Note the slight increase in activity over the entire lung field, particularly in the right lung. This finding is compatible with inflammatory lung disease.

TABLE 7 DIFFERENTIAL DIAGNOSIS OF SCLERODERMA
Eosinophilic fasciitis
Eosinophilia myalgia syndrome
Scleredema
Scleromyxedema
Progeria
Porphyria cutanea tarda
Reflux dystrophy
Bleomycin and other drug-induced fibrosis
Carcinoid syndrome
Amyloidosis
Phenylketonuria

phenomenon and hand and feet cutaneous involvement, frequent neuropathy and myalgia, and characteristic clinical features of their own. An increased incidence of scleroderma in patients with chronic graft-versus-host disease and gold, coal, and silica miners and in patients exposed to organic solvent is reported.

The possibility that silicone breast implants may predispose to the development of scleroderma has been raised by anecdotal case reports. There is still insufficient information to indicate that implants are a cause of systemic sclerosis or other rheumatic diseases and that removal of implants alter the course of existing disease or prevent the occurrence of new disease.

Treatment

Consultation with a rheumatologist experienced in caring for scleroderma is helpful in assessing prognosis and formulating a treatment plan. Supportive measures consist of patient and family counseling and avoidance of exposure to cold and trauma. Physical therapy is an important adjunct in management and should include active and passive range-of-motion exercises and heat to improve circulatory flow and impede

contractions caused by fibrotic skin and joints. Penile implants are helpful in impotence.

No drug or combination of drugs (Table 8) is of proven value in adequately controlled prospective trials [10•]. Use of antiinflammatory agents and corticosteroids has been disappointing. Because of potent side effects, corticosteroid use should be restricted to patients with myositis. Long-term steroid therapy has no place in the treatment of scleroderma.

Musculoskeletal

Prompt improvement in the clinical and biochemical parameters of inflammatory myositis is achieved with the use of 1 mg/kg/d of prednisone in divided dosages. Steroid-resistant cases may respond to azathioprine (2.5 mg/kg/d) or methotrexate (25 mg weekly). Arthralgia, arthritis, and tenosynovitis respond adequately to nonsteroidal antiinflammatory agents.

Gastrointestinal tract

Symptomatic esophageal reflux is best managed by avoiding recumbent position after meals, elevation of the head of the bed, and the regular use of antacids. Other agents used to treat

Polymyositis and Dermatomyositis

Robert L. Wortmann

6

> ### Key Points
> - Polymyositis and dermatomyositis are two diseases that can be classified as idiopathic inflammatory myopathies.
> - Patients with any idiopathic inflammatory myopathy have weak proximal muscles, elevated serum creatine kinase levels, eletromyographic changes of myopathy, and inflammatory changes in skeletal muscle.
> - The differential diagnosis of proximal muscle weakness is extensive.
> - The test used to diagnose these diseases (muscle enzymes, electromyography, and muscle histology) are by themselves nonspecific; diagnoses are made, in part, by excluding other recognized causes of muscle weakness.
> - Treatment is largely empiric and begins with glucocorticoids. Modalities other than medications also are important in treatment.

It is appropriate to use the term *idiopathic inflammatory myopathy* to represent the entire group of conditions (Table 1) [1] that satisfy specific criteria (Table 2) [2] and to reserve the terms *polymyositis* and *dermatomyositis* for more specific condition subsets [2,4•].

CLINICAL FEATURES

Clinical features of the idiopathic inflammatory myopathies include those listed in Table 2 [2]. Symmetric proximal muscle weakness predominates. Although strength may be normal at the time of presentation, virtually all patients develop significant weakness during the course of their illness. Myalgias and muscle tenderness may be present, and atrophy and fibrosis may develop. Weakness is associated with elevated levels of serum creatine kinase and other enzymes of skeletal muscle origin (aldolase, aspartate aminotransferase, alanine aminotransferase, lactate dehydrogenase), electromyographic changes consistent with an inflammatory myopathy, and skeletal muscle histology characteristic of an inflammatory process. These manifestations can occur in various combinations or patterns, and no single feature is diagnostic or specific. Consequently, the diagnosis of an idiopathic inflammatory myopathy is made when these features are recognized in combination and other causes for them can be excluded.

Polymyositis in Adults

The clinical characteristics of polymyositis in the adult are representative of the fundamental features of all idiopathic inflammatory myopathies. Typically, the onset is insidious, occurring over 3 to 6 months, and no precipitating event can be identified. Weakness initially involves the muscles of the shoulder and pelvic girdles, with weakness of the latter slightly more common. Distal weakness is uncommon initially and only develops in severe cases. Weakness of neck flexor muscles occurs in approximately half of the patients. Ocular muscles are virtually never involved, and bulbar muscle weakness is rare. Dysphagia may develop secondary to esophageal dysfunction or cricopharyngeal obstruction. Pharyngeal muscle weakness may cause dysphonia and difficulty in swallowing.

Patients may experience morning stiffness, fatigue, anorexia, weight loss, and fever. Arthralgias are not uncommon, but frank synovitis is rare. Raynaud's phenomenon may occur, and periorbital edema may be observed. The findings in the neurologic portion of the physical examination are normal, except for motor function results. Interstitial pneumonitis may cause dyspnea, a nonproductive cough, and hypoxemia. Additional pulmonary manifestations also may include interstitial fibrosis, with dry rales or crackles heard on chest auscultation, and fibrotic changes on chest radiograph. Aspiration pneumonia may complicate the disease course in patients with esophageal dysmotility, swallowing difficulties, or dysphonia. Cardiac involvement is unusual, although heart block, supraventricular arrhythmia, or cardiomyopathy may develop, causing syncope, palpitations, or congestive heart failure.

The creatine kinase level is elevated in almost every patient with polymyositis at some time during the course of the illness. Normal creatine kinase levels may be found very early in the disease course, at times during active disease when circulating inhibitors of creatine phosphokinase activity may be present, or in advanced cases when significant muscle atrophy has occurred [5]. In most patients, the creatine kinase level is an indicator of disease severity. Levels of other muscle enzymes (aldolase, aspartate aminotransferase, alanine aminotransferase, lactate dehydrogenase) are found to be elevated in most cases. The erythrocyte sedimentation rate is normal in half of the patients with polymyositis and is higher than 50 mm/h (Westergren's method) in only 20% of patients.

The triad of classic electromyographic changes in idiopathic inflammatory myopathies includes 1) increased insertional activity, fibrillations, and sharp positive waves, 2) spontaneous, bizarre high-frequency discharges, and 3) polyphasic motor unit potential of low amplitude and short duration. These changes are not specific and only help to confirm the diagnosis. In larger series, the complete triad is found in approximately 40% of patients [4•]. In contrast, 10% of patients may have completely normal study findings. Electromyographic abnormalities may have a variable distribution and may be present only in the paraspinal muscles in a few patients.

Although the histopathology of polymyositis is well described, no specific change is pathognomonic. In the typical case, muscle fibers are found in different stages of necrosis and regeneration. The inflammatory cell infiltrate is predominantly focal and endomysial, although perivascular accumulations also may be seen. However, wide variations in histology can be observed within the tissue of an individual patient as well as among patients. In some cases, lymphocytes accompanied by fewer macrophages are found surrounding and invading nonnecrotic fibers. In others, degeneration is seen in the absence of inflammatory cells in the immediate area, or the only recognized change is type 2 fiber atrophy. Over time, destroyed fibers are replaced by fibrous connective tissue and fat.

Dermatomyositis in Adults

The clinical features of dermatomyositis include all of those described for polymyositis plus cutaneous manifestations [6].

TABLE 1 CLASSIFICATION OF IDIOPATHIC INFLAMMATORY MYOPATHIES
Polymyositis
Dermatomyositis
Myopathy with myositis-specific autoantibody
Inclusion body myositis
Polymyositis or dermatomyositis of childhood
Myositis with malignancy
Myositis with associated collagen vascular disease

TABLE 2 CRITERIA FOR THE DIAGNOSIS OF IDIOPATHIC INFLAMMATORY MYOPATHY
Symmetric weakness of the limb-girdle muscles and anterior neck flexors, progressing over weeks to months, with or without dysphagia or respiratory muscle involvement
Skeletal muscle histology showing evidence of necrosis of type 1 and 2 muscle fibers, phagocytosis, regeneration with basophilia, large sarcolemmal nuclei and prominent nucleoli, atrophy in a perifascicular distribution, variation in fiber size, and an inflammatory exudate
Elevation in serum levels of skeletal muscle enzymes (creatine kinase, aldolase, aspartate aminotransferase, alanine aminotransferase, and lactate dehydrogenase)
Electromyographic triad of short, small, polyphasic motor units; fibrillations, positive waves, and insertional irritability; and bizarre high-frequency discharges
Dermatologic features, including a lilac (heliotrope) discoloration of the eyelids with periorbital edema; a scaly, erythematous dermatitis over the dorsa of the hands, especially over the metacarpophalangeal and proximal interphalangeal joints (Gottron's sign); and involvement of the knees, elbows, medial malleoli, face, neck, and upper torso
(*From* Bohan and Peter [1]; with permission.)

These cutaneous manifestations comprise periungual erythema; erythematous lesions around the nail beds that scale, become hyperpigmented, or become depigmented; "machinist's hands" (indicated by a darkened, "dirty" appearance and horizontal lines across the lateral and palmar aspects of the fingers); nailfold capillary changes; digital infarcts; palpable, white-centered petechiae; livedo reticularis; and Raynaud's phenomenon. They may vary and may antedate the onset of weakness by more than 1 year. The severity of the rash and muscle weakness do not always coincide. More characteristic skin changes include heliotrope (lilac) discoloration of the eyelids (Fig. 1); an erythematous rash over the face, neck, and upper torso (Fig. 2); and Gottron's sign, which is pink to violaceous scaling typically found over the knuckles, elbows, and knees (Fig. 3). The rash may change from one type to another during the course of the disease.

The muscle histopathology of adult dermatomyositis may be identical to that of polymyositis. However, fiber invasion is rare, and a perivascular distribution of inflammatory cells is the rule. Perifascicular atrophy may also be observed.

Myopathy with Myositis-Specific Autoantibodies

A group of circulating autoantibodies has been described exclusively in patients with inflammatory myopathies, and these autoantibodies have been termed *myositis-specific autoantibodies*. These autoantibodies are directed at cytoplasmic antigens involved in protein synthesis, are present in genetically restricted groups of patients, and may indicate a clinical subset of patients with specific patterns of disease [7,8•].

The most common myositis-specific antibody, anti–Jo-1, is directed at histidyl–transfer RNA synthetase. Patients with anti–Jo-1, as well as those with antibodies directed at other transfer RNA synthetases (anti–PL-7, anti–PL-12, anti-OJ, anti-EJ), tend to be younger adults with polymyositis and a high prevalence of interstitial lung disease, arthritis, and fever. In contrast, patients with antibodies directed against signal recognition particles (a ribonucleoprotein complex that mediates the translocation of nascent polypeptides across the endoplasmic reticulum) have a very acute onset of severe myositis with distal muscle involvement and cardiac abnormalities. Neither group generally responds well to therapy. Other myositis-specific antibodies are anti-KJ, anti-Fer, anti-Mas, and anti–Mi-2.

Inclusion Body Myositis

The actual incidence of inclusion body myositis is unknown, but this recently described condition probably accounts for 15% to 28% of all inflammatory myopathies [3]. It generally affects elderly persons, and its symptoms may be identical to those of polymyositis. Myalgia and muscle tenderness are usual. As the muscle weakness becomes severe, atrophy develops and deep tendon reflexes diminish. In some patients, disease progression is slow and steady. In others, it seems to plateau, leaving the patient with fixed weakness. Current therapies appear to have limited or no effect in most patients with this problem [9,10•].

Inclusion body myositis may differ from classic polymyositis in several ways. These differences have allowed diagnostic

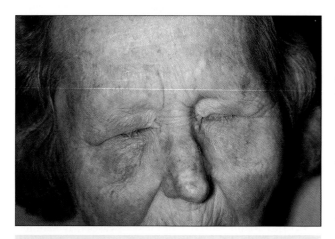

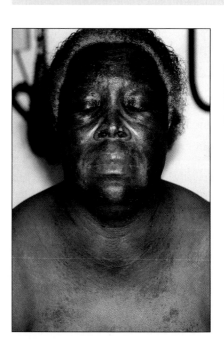

FIGURE 1 Heliotrope rash over eyelids and cheeks of patient with dermatomyositis.

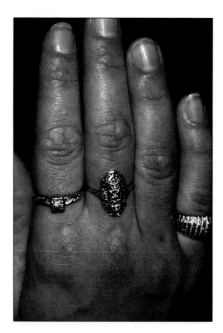

FIGURE 2 Rash on face, neck, and upper chest of patient with dermatomyositis.

FIGURE 3 Gottron's sign. Note the pink patches over knuckles in this patient with dermatomyositis.

criteria to be proposed (Table 3). Although the weakness may be proximal and symmetric in distribution, it may also be focal, distal, or asymmetric. Creatine kinase levels are often minimally elevated, and they may be normal. Electromyographic changes are myopathic, but features consistent with neurogenic or mixed neurogenic and myopathic changes are found in half of patients. Finally, the diagnosis is defined primarily by pathology, with characteristic changes seen with light and especially electron microscopy.

Juvenile (Childhood) Dermatomyositis

Although a disease similar to adult polymyositis occasionally is encountered in children, dermatomyositis is more common in this age group. Juvenile dermatomyositis differs from the adult form because of the coexistence of vasculitis, ectopic calcification, and lipodystrophy [11]. Classically, the child develops cutaneous manifestations followed by muscle weakness. Involved muscles are tender and swollen to palpation. The rash is typically erythematous and occurs on the malar region and the extensor surfaces of the elbows, knuckles, and knees. These lesions are often scaling, and they may become pigmented or depigmented. Complete remission can occur in some children with little or no therapy. In severe cases, especially if vasculitis is present, the disease course may be devastating despite therapy.

Myositis and Malignancy

The association of myositis and malignancy has long been recognized, but questions still remain about the frequency of the association and whether the risk is higher for patients with dermatomyositis. It is clear that the types of malignancy and the organs involved in patients with myositis are those expected for the age and gender of the patient [12]. The relationship between the malignancy and myositis can vary widely. The malignancy can develop before, at the same time as, or after the myositis. Occasionally, malignancy and myositis seem to follow a parallel course, but more commonly the two appear to have only a temporal relationship, with one developing within 1 year of the other. Treatment of the neoplastic process has no predictable effect on the muscle disease.

Myositis with Other Collagen Vascular Diseases

Muscle weakness is often a manifestation of collagen vascular disease. Some examples of collagen vascular diseases that may be associated with myopathy include allergic granulomatosis, giant cell arteritis, polyarteritis nodosa, polymyalgia rheumatica, and Wegener's granulomatosis. The myopathy may dominate the clinical picture of some patients with systemic lupus erythematosus, mixed connective tissue disease, scleroderma, and Sjögren's syndrome. In some patients, the weakness may be accompanied by enzyme, electromyographic, and histologic changes identical to those in polymyositis. In others, enzyme levels and electromyographic findings may be entirely normal. Weakness also may be a significant feature in rheumatoid arthritis and vasculitic syndromes (hypersensitivity and leukocytoclastic vasculitis).

DIFFERENTIAL DIAGNOSIS

Although the idiopathic inflammatory myopathies are relatively rare diseases, many diseases can cause muscle weakness [13•,14]. Patients with one of many diseases may manifest some, if not all, of the criteria for the diagnosis of polymyositis (see Table 2). Consequently, these conditions must be excluded before the diagnosis of an inflammatory myopathy can be made. The diseases and conditions that can be confused with an idiopathic inflammatory myopathy can be divided into categories, as shown in Table 4.

DIAGNOSTIC TESTING

Physical Examination

Abnormalities found in patients with inflammatory muscle disease are typical of those noted in patients with most other myopathies and are generally limited to the motor component of the examination, with weakness found to be distributed symmetrically in proximal muscles. Objective measurement of strength is very useful in assessing disease severity and must be done to establish a baseline for monitoring the effect of therapy. The most commonly used muscle strength grading system is shown in Table 5.

The timed-stands test is helpful in following disease progression and in fine tuning therapy [15]. This test has been standardized for men and women of various ages and has been

---

TABLE 3 DIAGNOSTIC CRITERIA PROPOSED FOR INCLUSION BODY MYOSITIS*

Pathologic criteria

Electron microscopy
  Microtubular filaments in the inclusions
Light microscopy
  Lined vacuoles
  Intranuclear inclusions, intracytoplasmic inclusions, or both

Clinical criteria

Proximal muscle weakness (insidious onset)
Distal muscle weakness
Electromyographic evidence of a generalized myopathy (inflammatory myopathy)
Elevation in muscle enzyme levels (creatine phosphokinase, aldolase, or both)
Failure of muscle strength to improve with a high-dose corticosteroid regimen (at least 40–60 mg/d for 3–4 mo)

From Calabrese *et al.* [2]; with permission.
*Definite inclusion body myositis is the pathologic electron microscopy criterion and the first clinical criterion plus one other clinical criterion. Probable inclusion body myositis is the first pathologic light microscopy criterion and the first clinical criterion plus three other clinical criteria. Possible inclusion body myositis is the second pathologic light microscopy criterion plus any three clinical criteria.

Toxic or drug-related myopathies

Causes: alcohol, D,L-carnitine, chloroquine, cimetidine, clofibrate, cocaine, colchicine, danazol, gemfibrozil, glucocorticoids, heroin, hydralazine, ipecac, levodopa, lovastatin, D-penicillamine, phenytoin, procainamide, rifampin, sulfonamides, valproic acid, vincristine, zidovudine

Infections

Viral causes: adenovirus, coxsackievirus, cytomegalovirus, echovirus A9, Epstein-Barr virus, hepatitis B virus, HIV, influenza A and B viruses, mumps virus, rubella virus, varicella-zoster virus

Bacterial causes: *Borrelia burgdorferi* (Lyme spirochete), *Clostridium welchii*, *Mycobacterium* species, including the causative agents of leprosy and tuberculosis, *Mycoplasma pneumoniae*, *Rickettsia* species, *Staphylococcus* species, and *Streptococcus* species

Fungal causes: *Cryptococcus* species

Parasitic causes: *Schistosoma* species, *Toxoplasma* species, and *Trichinella* species

Cancer-related myopathies

Cachexia

Polymyositis

Dermatomyositis

Disseminated carcinomatosis

Paraneoplastic syndrome

Eaton-Lambert syndrome

Myasthenia gravis

Carcinoid syndrome

Metabolic myopathies

Primary disorders of metabolism

Disordered glycogen metabolism, including myophosphorylase deficiency (McArdle's disease), phosphofructokinase deficiency, and acid maltase deficiency

Disordered lipid metabolism, including carnitine deficiency (inherited and acquired) and fatty acid acyl coenzyme A dehydrogenase deficiency

Myoadenylate deaminase deficiency

Mitochondrial myopathies

Endocrine disorders	Metabolic-nutritional disorders	Electrolyte disorders
Acromegaly	Uremia	Hypernatremia
Hypothyroidism	Hepatic failure	Hyponatremia
Hyperthyroidism	Malabsorption	Hyperkalemia
Hyperparathyroidism	Periodic paralysis	Hypokalemia
Cushing's disease	Vitamin D deficiency	Hypercalcemia
Addison's disease	Vitamin E deficiency	Hypocalcemia
Hyperaldosteronism		Hypophosphatemia
Carcinoid syndrome		Hypomagnesemia

Neurologic diseases

Muscular dystrophies	Denervating conditions	Proximal neuropathies
Duchenne's muscular dystrophy	Spinal muscular atrophies	Diabetic amyotrophy
Becker's muscular dystrophy	Amyotrophic lateral sclerosis	Guillain-Barré syndrome
Facioscapulohumeral muscular dystrophy	Neuromuscular junction disorders	Acute intermittent porphyria
Limb-girdle muscular dystrophy	Myasthenia gravis	
	Eaton-Lambert syndrome	

Other conditions

Sarcoidosis

Fibromyalgia

TABLE 5 OBJECTIVE SCHEME FOR GRADING MUSCLE STRENGTH	
Grade	**Description**
5	Normal power resistance
4	Power is decreased, but muscle contraction is possible against resistance
3	Muscle contraction against gravity only
2	Muscle contraction is possible only when gravity is eliminated
1	Contraction without motion
0	No contraction

validated using Cybex dynamometric muscle testing. It uses a stopwatch to measure the time required for the patient to stand up 10 times from a chair.

Laboratory Testing

Serum enzymes

Damage or injury to skeletal muscle may cause increased serum levels of creatine kinase, aldolase, aspartate aminotransferase, alanine aminotransferase, and lactate dehydrogenase. High levels of these enzymes are found in the inflammatory myopathies but are not specific for these diseases. In fact, elevated levels of serum creatine kinase may not be the result of a disease at all. They may be caused by the following:

Racial differences: The normal values for black men are higher than those for other populations and may be above the value listed as the upper limit of normal for some laboratories.

Trauma: Sharp trauma occurs with intramuscular injection, electromyographic needle evaluation, or muscle biopsy. Blunt trauma occurs with heavy body contact or bruising injuries.

Exercise: Higher levels may be caused aerobic exercise, including long distance running and aerobic dancing, especially in physically untrained individuals, and isometric exercise or weight lifting.

Physiologic factors: Fever and seizures may be responsible.

Medications: Narcotics and barbiturates may spuriously raise levels by retarding the elimination of creatine phosphokinase from the blood.

TABLE 6 CREATINE PHOSPHOKINASE ISOENZYMES REVEAL THE TISSUE OF ORIGIN OF ENZYME IN SERUM	
Isoenzyme	**Source**
MM	Skeletal muscle
MB	Cardiac muscle
	Embryonal muscle
	Regenerating muscle
BB	Smooth muscle
	Brain and spinal cord

Not all creatine kinase in the blood is derived from skeletal muscle. Diseases of or damage to cardiac muscle, smooth muscle, or brain also can elevate serum levels. The tissue origin of creatine phosphokinase can be established by determining its isoenzymes (Table 6). In cases of inflammatory myopathy, the creatine kinase level is generally the most sensitive indicator of disease activity and is most useful to follow during the course of the illness.

Autoantibodies

Circulatory autoantibodies can be detected in many patients with inflammatory muscle disease. Patients with myositis associated with another collagen vascular disease have autoantibodies specific for the associated condition (Table 7). Specific myositis-associated autoantibodies are present in some patients, as discussed previously [7,8•].

Electromyography

Electromyography is a valuable technique that can be used to determine the classification, distribution, and severity of conditions affecting skeletal muscles. The triad of characteristic changes observed in patients with inflammatory muscle disease are not specific, can occur with other myopathic processes, and may vary greatly from muscle to muscle, from patient to patient, and with disease severity and duration. Electromyographic studies are perhaps most useful in differentiating between myopathic and neuropathic conditions and in identifying the area of abnormality most suitable for muscle biopsy.

Muscle biopsy

If muscle biopsy is used appropriately, information obtained from it may prove invaluable in establishing the diagnosis.

TABLE 7 AUTOANTIBODIES IN COLLAGEN VASCULAR DISEASES	
Disease	**Autoantibody**
Systemic lupus erythematosus	Anti–double-stranded DNA
	Anti-Sm
	Anti-ENA
	Anti–SS-A (Ro)
	Anti–SS-B (La)
	Antihistone
Sjögren's syndrome	Anti–SS-A (Ro)
	Anti–SS-B (La)
Mixed connective tissue disease	Anti-RNP
Scleroderma	Anti-Scl-70
	Anti-PM-Scl
	Anti-Ku
CREST	Anticentromere
Wegener's granulomatosis	Anti-neutrophil cytoplasmic antibodies
Polyarteritis nodosa	Anti-neutrophil cytoplasmic antibodies

CREST—calcinosis cutis, Raynaud's phenomenon, esophageal dysfunction, sclerodactyly, and telangiectasia; ENA—extractable nuclear antigen.

Four types of evaluation can be performed on muscle tissue: histologic testing, histochemistry, electron microscopic evaluation, and assays of enzyme activities or other chemicals. These techniques should be used with specific questions in mind rather than employed routinely.

Either percutaneous needle biopsy or an open surgical technique can be used. The method selected varies somewhat with the analyses desired and should be agreed on prospectively by the physician ordering the test, the individual who will perform the biopsy, and the pathologist. Careful definition of the biopsy site helps to ensure optimal results. Ideally, the area selected is not too severely involved. The most involved areas may be too necrotic or scarred to give meaningful information. Electromyography may be helpful in selecting the site. However, electromyographic needles can traumatize tissue. Because most myopathies have a symmetric distribution, electromyography can be performed on one side of the body, and the biopsy specimen can be taken from the comparable abnormal area on the other side.

Forearm ischemia exercise testing

Forearm ischemia exercise testing is useful in screening patients for glycogen storage diseases and myoadenylate deaminase deficiency [16]. These conditions are primary metabolic myopathies that may mimic polymyositis [13•]. The protocol for the test is illustrated in Figure 4. A normal response to ischemic exercises is at least a threefold rise over baseline levels for venous lactate and ammonia. In individuals with a glycogen storage disease (except acid maltase deficiency), ammonia levels increase normally, but lactate levels remain at baseline. In contrast, lactate levels increase, but ammonia levels do not change in individuals with myoadenylate deaminase deficiency.

TREATMENT

Although the term idiopathic inflammatory myopathy encompasses various conditions, the initial therapeutic approach applied to each diagnostic category is generally the same. The treatment of the inflammatory myopathies remains empiric [3,4•,17••]. Before drug treatment is initiated, the diagnosis must be accurate, and the patient's clinical status needs to be objectively evaluated. Pretreatment testing of the strength of individual muscle groups and timed-stands testing provide valuable information for assessing the results of treatment [15]. A physical therapist is invaluable for performing muscle group strength testing and instructing the patient in an exercise program. Exercise programs that take into account the amount of inflammatory activity are important for good outcome [18]. Bed rest is important, and active range of motion is to be avoided during intervals of severe inflammation. Passive motion is encouraged during these intervals in an effort to maintain range of motion and prevent contractures. With patient improvement, the program moves to active-assisted exercise and then to active exercises.

Glucocorticoids remain the standard first-line drugs for patients with an idiopathic inflammatory myopathy. Initially, prednisone is given in a single dosage of 1 to 2 mg/kg/d (with

a usual arbitrary maximum of 100 mg). In severe cases, the daily dose is divided or intravenous methylprednisolone is substituted. Once instituted, daily high-dose prednisone is continued until strength improves. Clinical improvement may be noted in the first weeks or gradually over 3 to 6 months. This variability relates, at least in part, to the timing of the treatment. The sooner after disease onset prednisone is given, the faster and more effectively it may work [19••]. Serial evaluations of muscle strength should be performed, and creatine phosphokinase levels should be measured during treatment. Ideally, the initial steroid dosage is maintained until strength and creatine phosphokinase values have normalized for 4 to 8 weeks. Although creatine phosphokinase levels are a useful monitor, muscle strength is much more important. Once remission is apparent, the prednisone dosage can be tapered gradually by reducing the daily dosage by approximately 10 mg/mo. As the taper continues, therapy may be changed to an alternate-day schedule.

If a patient fails to respond to glucocorticoid therapy after 6 weeks or has had some improvement but the level of strength has reached a plateau, azathioprine or methotrexate should be added. The usual dose of azathioprine is 2 to 3 mg/kg (with the usual maximum of 150 mg/d in a single oral dosage). Azathioprine is the only drug to have been tested in a blinded, controlled trial. The combination of azathioprine and prednisone was shown to be superior to prednisone alone in patients whose disease had plateaued while they were taking prednisone alone [20]. Methotrexate is usually given on a weekly schedule at doses ranging between 5 and 15 mg orally

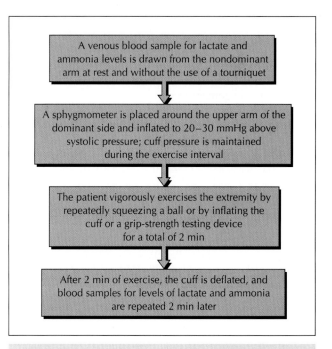

FIGURE 4 Protocol for forearm ischemic exercise testing. Normal results are a threefold or greater increase from baseline in ammonia and lactate levels. False-positive results can occur because of a submaximal exercise effort due to poor compliance, pain, weakness, or malignancies. Therefore, any abnormal result must be confirmed with the appropriate enzyme analysis in muscle tissue.

or 15 and 50 mg intravenously. Measurements of serum aspartate aminotransferase and alanine aminotransferase levels should be performed before methotrexate therapy is initiated to minimize confusion due to potential hepatic toxic effects of the medication. Pulmonary function tests should be performed in those with evidence of interstitial pulmonary fibrosis for similar reasons.

Other immunosuppressive agents and treatment modalities have been used in steroid-resistant disease [21,22•,23]. Hydroxychloroquine can be used to treat the cutaneous lesions of dermatomyositis, but it has no recognized effect on the myositis. Cyclophosphamide, chlorambucil, and cyclosporine have been used. Additional treatments that have been used include plasmapheresis, lymphopheresis, total body or total lymph node radiation, and the administration of intravenous gamma globulin. Controlled trials involving more patients are definitely needed to prove benefit for any of these measures.

ROLE OF GENERALIST

Early recognition of the syndromes described in this chapter, especially those with an insidious onset, is important to make a firm diagnosis and begin appropriate therapy. Consultation with a rheumatologist is often useful if an idiopathic inflammatory myopathy is suspected. The consultant should coordinate the work-up and initial evaluation, perform serial clinical evaluations, and suggest the appropriate drug program. Experience is helpful in this regard. The consultant also should be expected to provide a reasonable prognosis.

REFERENCES AND RECOMMENDED READING

Recently published papers of particular interest have been highlighted as:
• Of interest
•• Of outstanding interest

1. Bohan A, Peter JB: Polymyositis and dermatomyositis. Part I. *New Engl J Med* 1975, 292:344–347.

2. Calabrese LH, Mitsumoto H, Chou SM: Inclusion body myositis presenting as treatment-resistant polymyositis. *Arthritis Rheum* 1987, 30:397–403.

3. Plotz PH, Rider LG, Targoff IN: Myositis: immunologic contribution to understanding cause, pathogenesis, and therapy. *Ann Intern Med* 1995, 122: 715–724.

4.• Wortmann RL: Inflammatory diseases of muscle. In *Textbook of Rheumatology*. Edited by Kelly WN, Harris E, Ruddy S, *et al.* Philadelphia: WB Saunders; 1993:1159–1182.

5. Kagen LJ, Aram S: Creatinine kinase activity inhibitor in sera from patients with muscle disease. *Arthritis Rheum* 1981, 30:213–217.

6. Euwer RL, Sontheimer RD: Dermatologic aspects of myositis. *Curr Opin Rheumatol* 1994, 6:583–589.

7. Targoff IN: Immune manifestations of inflammatory muscle disease. *Rheum Dis Clin North Am* 1994, 20: 857–880.

8.   Love LA, Leff RL, Fraser DD, *et al.*: A new approach to the classification of idiopathic inflammatory myopathy: myositis-specific autoantibodies define useful homogeneous patient groups. *Medicine* 1991, 70:360–374.

9. Leff RL, Miller FW, Hicks J, *et al*: The treatment of inclusion body myositis: a retrospective review and a randomized, prospective trial of immunosuppressive therapy. *Medicine* 1993, 72:225–235.

10.• Sayers ME, Chou SM, Calabrese LH: Inclusion body myositis: analysis of 32 cases. *J Rheumatol* 1992, 19:1385–1389.

11. Rider LG, Miller FW: New perspectives on the idiopathic inflammatory myopathies of childhood. *Curr Opin Rheumatol* 1994, 6:575–582.

12. Sigargeirsson B, Lindeloff B, Edhog O, *et al.*: Risk of cancer in patients with dermatomyositis or polymyositis: a population based study. *N Engl J Med* 1992, 326:363–367.

13.• Wortmann RL: Metabolic diseases of muscle. In *Arthritis and Allied Conditions*, edn 12. Edited by McCarty DJ, Koopman WJ. Malvern, PA: Lea & Febiger; 1993:1895–1912.

14. Wortmann RL: Proximal muscle weakness of unknown etiology. In *Rheumatology*, edn 1. Edited by Klippel JH, Dieppe P. London: Gower Medical Publishing; 1993:6:15.1–15.3.

15. Csuka ME, McCarty D: A rapid method for measurement of lower extremity muscle strength. *Am J Med* 1985, 78:77–81.

16. Valen PA, Nakayama DA, Veum J, *et al.*: Myoadenylate deaminase deficiency and forearm ischemic exercise testing. *Arthritis Rheum* 1987, 30:661–668.

17.•• Dalakas MC: Polymyositis, dermatomyositis and inclusion body myositis. *N Engl J Med* 1991, 325:1487–1498.

18. Hicks JE: Comprehensive rehabilitative management of patients with polymyositis and dermatomyositis. In *Polymyositis and Dermatomyositis*. Edited by Dalakas MC. Boston: Butterworths; 1988:293–317.

19.•• Joffee MM, Love LA, Leff RL, *et al.*: Drug therapy of idiopathic inflammatory myopathies: predictors of response to prednisone, azathioprine, and methotrexate and a comparison of their efficacy. *Am J Med* 1993, 94:379–387.

20. Bunch TW: Prednisone and azathioprine for polymyositis: long-term follow-up. *Arthritis Rheum* 1981, 24:45–48.

21. Wortmann RL: Idiopathic inflammatory diseases of muscles. In *Treatment of the Rheumatic Diseases: Companion to the textbook of Rheumatology*. Edited by Weisman MA, Weinblatt MC. Philadelphia: WB Saunders, 1995: 201–216.

22.• Oddis CV: Therapy of inflammatory myopathy. *Rheum Dis Clin North Am* 1994, 20:899–918.

23. Dulakas MC: Current treatment of the inflammatory myopathies. *Curr Opin Rheumatol* 1994, 6:595–601.

SELECT BIBLIOGRAPHY

Fafalak RG, Peterson MGE, Kagen LJ: Strength in polymyositis and dermatomyositis: best outcome in patients treated early. *J Rheumatol* 1994, 21:643–648.

Koh ET, Seow A, Ong B, *et al.*: Adult onset polymyositis/dermatomyositis: clinical and laboratory features and treatment response in 75 patients. *Ann Rheum Dis* 1993, 52:857–861.

Sayers ME, Chou SM, Calabrese LH: Inclusion body myositis: analysis of 32 cases. *J Rheumatol* 1992, 19:1385–1389.

Targoff IN: Autoantibodies associated with polymyositis and dermatomyositis. *Clin Aspects of Autoimmunity* 1993, 5:5–18.

Vasculitis 7

David W. Puett
John S. Sergent

Key Points
- Vasculitis refers to blood vessel injury resulting from inflammation.
- Vasculitis affects blood vessels of all sizes and can occur in any vascularized tissue.
- Vasculitis is classified into types based on clinical and histologic differences.
- The different vasculitis types vary widely in their prognosis and therapeutic requirements.

CLASSIFICATION

Vasculitis refers to an inflammatory disruption of blood vessels. It occurs in vessels of all sizes and is thus responsible for a wide spectrum of disease states. Characteristics used to distinguish different vasculitis types are listed in Table 1, and Table 2 provides a widely accepted classification scheme for the primary vasculitis syndromes. Information from patient history, examination, and laboratory and imaging studies is necessary to categorize a suspected vasculitis and rule out a pseudovasculitis syndrome (Table 3).

EVALUATION AND DIAGNOSIS

Clinical Evaluation

Vasculitis should be suspected in any patient who presents with an unexplained systemic illness or signs and symptoms of organ ischemia. The coincident involvement of several organs, the presence of mononeuritis multiplex, or palpable purpura strongly suggests vasculitis. Constitutional symptoms, such as fever, fatigue, and weight loss, as well as muscle and joint aches, are present in most patients, although frank joint inflammation is unusual unless the vasculitis accompanies a systemic rheumatic disease. The primary vasculitis syndromes differ in their tendency to affect people of a particular sex, age, and ethnic background. Although much overlap exists, such demographic clues can be helpful (Table 4).

Laboratory Studies

Patients with vasculitis typically manifest nonspecific laboratory features of chronic inflammation, including an elevated erythrocyte sedimentation rate (ESR), anemia of chronic disease, and leukocytosis. In addition, specific serologic tests often can help establish the diagnosis. Antinuclear antibodies, rheumatoid factors, complement levels, and cryoglobulins are indicative of autoimmune activity and should be checked in most patients with suspected vasculitis.

The recent discovery of antineutrophil cytoplasmic antibodies (ANCA) has provided a valuable serologic marker [1]. A diffuse cytoplasmic pattern (C-ANCA)

sion from aortic coarctation or renal artery stenosis, and chest pain from cardiac ischemia or aortic aneurysm dissection. The diagnosis is usually established by aortic angiography (Fig. 2).

The inflammatory phase of the illness may respond to corticosteroids and typically resolves within several years. However, slowly progressive vessel stenosis is not unusual and may require late surgical revascularization.

Medium vessel necrotizing vasculitis

Polyarteritis nodosa can affect any organ but commonly produces mononeuritis multiplex (80%), renal disease (75%), and skin lesions (50%) [5]. Diagnosis is confirmed by biopsy or arteriography (Fig. 3).

This disease carries a poor prognosis, with most untreated patients dying in less than 1 year, primarily from renal disease. Corticosteroids have improved the 5-year survival rate from 10% to approximately 50%, and alkylating agents such as daily oral cyclophosphamide provide additional benefit.

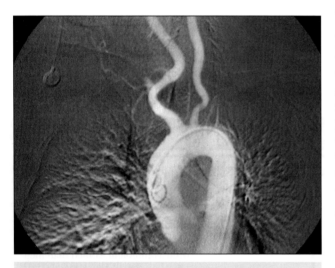

FIGURE 2 Digital subtraction angiography of the aortic arch from a patient with Takayasu's arteritis. Note occlusion of the subclavian arteries.

Small vessel granulomatous vasculitis

Wegener's granulomatosis classically involves the respiratory tract (100%) and kidney (85%) in young adults [6••]. Fever, fatigue, and weight loss are common, but patients usually seek medical attention for respiratory tract symptoms, which may include sinusitis, shortness of breath, hemoptysis, and chest pain. Patients often experience musculoskeletal pains (70%), ocular disease (50%), skin lesions (30%), and peripheral neuropathy (15%).

Laboratory studies show the nonspecific findings of chronic inflammation. Ninety percent of patients have renal disease, manifested by an abnormal urinary sediment and a moderate azotemia that may progress rapidly. Imaging studies can show severe pansinusitis, often with bony destruction, and changing pulmonary infiltrates that may cavitate (Fig. 4).

In more than 90% of patients, C-ANCA is present at the time of diagnosis. Granulomatous inflammation will be found on biopsy of involved lesions in the respiratory tract in 90% of patients. Although vasculitis occasionally can be seen in the kidney (< 10%), most renal biopsy specimens (80%) show a segmental necrotizing glomerulonephritis without vasculitis.

Untreated Wegener's granulomatosis has a poor prognosis. Patients typically die within several months after diagnosis, usually of renal failure or pulmonary hemorrhage. Treatment with corticosteroids and cyclophosphamide has markedly improved survival. Prednisone (1 mg/kg/d in a divided dosage for several weeks during the initiation of daily oral cyclophosphamide) results in improvement in up to 90% of patients and disease remission in as many as 75%. The cyclophosphamide dose is adjusted to keep the leukocyte count at greater than 3000 and is typically continued for 1 to 2 years after disease remission. However, recurrence occurs in approximately 50% of patients, and mortality remains in the 10% to 25% range. The relationship between the C-ANCA titer and disease activity is unpredictable, and clinical findings are much more important for monitoring patients than are changes in the C-ANCA titer.

Churg-Strauss vasculitis (allergic granulomatosis and angiitis) is a systemic necrotizing vasculitis occurring in middle-aged adults with a pre-existing history of allergic rhinitis,

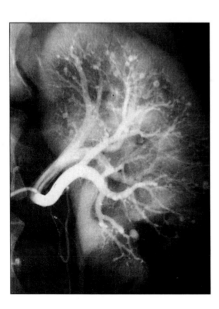

FIGURE 3 Angiogram of the renal circulation from a patient with polyarteritis nodosa. Note the multiple aneurysms.

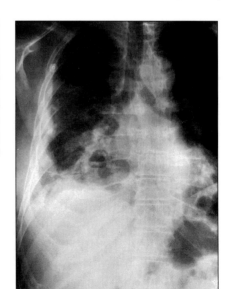

FIGURE 4 Chest radiograph from a patient with Wegener's granulomatosis. Note the multiple lung nodules, many with cavitation.

sinusitis, asthma, or other chronic lung disease [7]. Its onset is usually heralded by several months of progressive worsening of respiratory tract symptoms, followed by an abrupt appearance of renal disease, mononeuritis multiplex, skin lesions, and abdominal pain.

Marked eosinophilia (5000–20,000 cells/μL) is present in most untreated patients, and the diagnosis is established by lung biopsy. The disease responds to high-dose corticosteroids in most cases, although relapses often occur months to years later.

Small vessel leukocytoclastic vasculitis

Leukocytoclastic vasculitis is a histopathologic description of inflammation involving arterioles and postcapillary venules. It most commonly reflects a hypersensitivity response following exposure to a triggering antigen, usually a drug but occasionally an infection [8]. Leukocytoclastic vasculitis is also the pathologic process in the syndromes recognized as Schönlein-Henoch purpura [9] and essential cryoglobulinemia (Table 5), and it can occur in association with systemic inflammatory diseases and rarely some malignancies (Table 6).

Physical examination usually reveals a palpable purpura (Fig. 5), and patients frequently complain of joint pains, although frank arthritis is unusual. A stocking and glove sensory neuropathy may be seen. In severe cases, visceral disease is present, usually affecting the kidney or gut. These visceral injuries are more common in Schönlein-Henoch purpura and cryoglobulinemia than in hypersensitivity angiitis due to drugs.

Evaluation should include a skin biopsy to confirm the diagnosis and history, physical examination, and laboratory studies to attempt to identify the offending agent or underlying disease.

Prognosis is related to severity of the illness at onset, but drug-related leukocytoclastic vasculitis is usually self-limited, lasting 4 to 6 weeks, eventually with full recovery. Therapy is best directed at treating the underlying illness or removing the offending agent (*eg*, cold avoidance in cryoglobulinemia). Supportive measures are important and may be the only treatment required, although corticosteroids or even alkylating therapy is necessary if visceral involvement is severe.

Arteritis involving multiple vessel sizes with prominent venulitis

Behçet's disease may involve vessels of all sizes, from the aorta to the postcapillary venules and large veins. The disease is diagnosed clinically by identifying the following features: recurrent stomatitis (100%), genital aphthous ulcers (75%), cutaneous vasculitis (60%), uveitis (50%), and meningoencephalitis (30%). Ischemic symptoms from large vessel involvement are seen in 10% to 30% of patients and may involve any larger artery or vein [10]. Complications from large vessel arterial involvement include aneurysm formation

TABLE 6 DISEASE ASSOCIATED WITH LEUKOCYTOCLASTIC VASCULITIS
Systemic inflammatory disease
Rheumatic disease
Rheumatoid arthritis
Systemic lupus erythematosus
Sjögren's syndrome
Gastrointestinal disease
Inflammatory bowel disease
Primary biliary cirrhosis
Malignancy
Multiple myeloma and Waldenström's macroglobulinemia
Lymphoma
Leukemia
Carcinomas

TABLE 5 DISEASES ASSOCIATED WITH CRYOGLOBULINEMIA
Malignancy
Multiple myeloma or Waldenström's macroglobulinemia (type 1)
Lymphoma or leukemia (types 2 and 3)
Systemic rheumatic diseases (type 3 > type 2)
Rheumatoid arthritis
Systemic lupus erythematosus
Sjögren's syndrome
Chronic infections (type 3 more commonly than type 2)
Bacterial
Subacute bacterial endocarditis
Abscesses
Viral
Hepatitis B and C

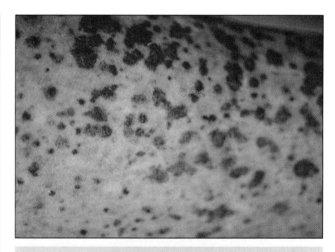

FIGURE 5 Palpable purpura on the leg from a patient with hypersensitivity vasculitis following penicillin therapy.

with possible rupture or vascular occlusion and are responsible for most deaths related to this disease. Although colchicine is effective in many patients with mucositis only, immunosuppression with corticosteroids and cytotoxic drugs is needed for vasculitis, progressive uveitis, and meningoencephalitis.

Buerger's disease is also known as thromboangiitis obliterans [11]. The clinical presentation is usually one of distal extremity ischemia (leg more common than arm) associated with marked sympathetic activity producing color changes and pain. A peripheral sensory neuropathy is common, and patients may have a history of thrombophlebitis or venous thrombosis.

The diagnosis is usually made clinically, although arteriography may show some characteristic changes, including segmental occlusions and numerous collateral vessels producing a corkscrew appearance.

Acute occlusive attacks last 1 to 4 weeks. Immunosuppressive therapy, anticoagulation, and sympathectomy have not been proven effective during the acute event or in preventing future attacks. Vasodilating agents, such as long-acting calcium channel blockers, may be beneficial, although total avoidance of tobacco products, including passive smoke inhalation, is the primary treatment. The disease course can be chronic, eventually resulting in amputation.

Limited vasculitis syndromes

In contrast to the more commonly encountered systemic involvement, isolated organ vasculitis can occur. For example, polyarteritis nodosa can be limited to the skin (cutaneous polyarteritis nodosa) and has been discovered unexpectedly in abdominal organs after surgical removal, such as vasculitic cholecystitis.

Vasculitis restricted to the central nervous system (isolated central nervous system angiitis) is also recognized [12]. Central nervous system symptoms and signs are nonspecific, and no characteristic brain computed tomography or magnetic resonance imaging findings are known. Diagnosis therefore requires a suggestive cerebral arteriogram or examination of brain tissue. Aggressive therapy using corticosteroids and cyclophosphamide is recommended, although inadequate experience is available to document the success of this approach.

Secondary Vasculitic Syndromes

Vasculitis may be secondary to systemic rheumatic diseases, infections, and malignancies (Table 7). The vasculitis syndromes associated with rheumatoid arthritis and hepatitis B are the best characterized.

Rheumatoid vasculitis occurs in 5% to 10% of patients with rheumatoid arthritis [13], and the underlying illness is almost always evident. Peripheral sensory neuropathy, necrotic skin ulcers, and nailfold and fingerpad infarcts correlate with smaller vessel involvement and may be the only findings in the milder form of rheumatoid vasculitis (Fig. 6). However, the presence of digital gangrene or mononeuritis multiplex signifies larger vessel involvement and a bad prognosis. In this group, mortality is high and is often the result of mesenteric, coronary, or cerebral vessel involvement. Renal disease is uncommon in rheumatoid vasculitis.

TABLE 7 DISEASE ASSOCIATED WITH A SECONDARY VASCULITIS

Involvement of large muscular arteries (the aorta and its branches)
Syphilis
Seronegative spondyloarthropathies

Involvement of small to medium muscular arteries
Hepatitis B and C
Systemic rheumatic diseases
   Rheumatoid arthritis
   Systemic lupus erythematosus
   Sjögren's syndrome

Involvement or arterioles and venules (leukocytoclastic vasculitis)
Drug reactions
Infections
Malignancy
Systemic inflammatory diseases

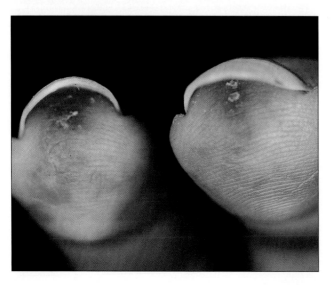

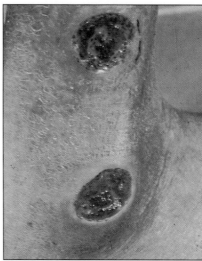

FIGURE 6 **A**, Digital infarctions and **B**, necrotic skin ulcers around the ankle of a patient with rheumatoid arthritis and small vessel vasculitis.

Therapy is tailored to the severity of presentation and includes prednisone at anti-inflammatory or immunosuppressive doses; penicillamine for mild, chronic vasculitis symptoms; and cytotoxic therapy for more aggressive disease.

Hepatitis B–associated vasculitis often presents abruptly with purpura, cyanotic or gangrenous digits, mononeuritis multiplex, or abdominal pain; it can occur at any time following exposure to the virus [14].

Hepatic enlargement and tenderness may be found, but jaundice is rare. Laboratory studies reveal an elevated ESR, a positive hepatitis B surface antigen, and elevated transaminase levels in nearly all patients. Cryoglobulins and hypocomplementemia are often seen.

Diagnosis is usually established by muscle or sural nerve biopsy. Prognosis is poor. Approximately one third of patients die from vasculitis complications, and most of the remainder are left with significant morbidity related to neurologic, renal, or liver disease.

Treatment with corticosteroids and cytotoxic agents has been disappointing, and nearly all survivors are left with a chronic active hepatitis. Attempts to clear the viral infection with antiviral agents while controlling the vasculitis by repeated plasmapheresis have been used [15]. Despite promising short-term results, the long-term success of this therapy remains unknown.

REFERENCES AND RECOMMENDED READING

Recently published papers of particular interest have been highlighted as:

• Of interest

•• Of outstanding interest

1. Kallenberg GCM, Mulder AHL, Tervaert JWC: Antineutrophil cytoplasmic antibodies: a still-growing class of autoantibodies in inflammatory disorders. *Am J Med* 1992, 93:675–682.

2.• Lie JT: Illustrated histopathologic classification criteria for selected vasculitic syndromes. *Arthritis Rheum* 1990, 33:1074–1087.

3. Huston KA, Hunder GG, Lie JT, *et al.*: Temporal arteritis: a 25-year epidemiologic, clinical, and pathologic study. *Ann Intern Med* 1978, 88:162–167.

4. Shelhamer JH, Volkman DJ, Parrillo JE, *et al.*:Takayasu's arteritis and its therapy. *Ann Intern Med* 1985, 103:125–126.

5. Travers RL, Allison DJ, Brettle RP, Hughes GRV: Polyarteritis nodosa: a clinical and angiographic analysis of 17 cases. *Semin Arthritis Rheum* 1979, 8:184–199.

6.•• Hoffman GS, Kerr GS, Leavitt RY, *et al.*: Wegener's granulomatosis: an analysis of 158 patients. *Ann Intern Med* 1992, 116:488–498.

7. Lanham JC, Elkon KB, Pusey CD, Hughes GR: Systemic vasculitis with asthma and eosinophilia: a clinical approach to the Churg-Strauss syndrome. *Medicine* 1984, 63:65–81.

8. Calabrese LH, Clough JD: Hypersensitivity and vasculitis group (HVG). *Cleve Clin Quart* 1982, 49:17–42.

9. Ilan Y, Naparstek Y: Schonlein-Henoch syndrome in adults and children. *Semin Arthritis Rheum* 1991, 21:103–109.

10. Koc Y, Gullu I, Akpek G, *et al.*:Vascular involvement in Behçet's disease. *J Rheumatol* 1992, 19:402–410.

11. Shinoya S, Ban I, Nakata Y: Diagnosis and treatment of Buerger's disease. *Surgery* 1974, 75:695–700.

12. Moore PM: Diagnosis and management of isolated angiitis of the central nervous system. *Neurology* 1989, 39:167–173.

13. Schneider HA, Yonker RA, Katz P, *et al.*: Rheumatoid vasculitis: experience with 13 patients and review of the literature. *Semin Arthritis Rheum* 1985, 14:280–286.

14. Sergent JS, Lockshin MD, Christian CL, Gocke DJ: Vasculitis with hepatitis B antigenemia: long-term observations in nine patients. *Medicine* 1976, 55:1–18.

15. Guillevin L, Lhote F, Leon A, *et al.*: Treatment of polyarteritis nodosa related to hepatitis B virus with short term steroid therapy associated with antiviral agents and plasma exchanges: a prospective trial. *J Rheumatol* 1993, 20:289–298.

SELECT BIBLIOGRAPHY

Brovet JC, Clauvel JP, Danon F, *et al.*: Biologic and clinical significance of cryoglobulins: a report of 86 cases. *Am J Med* 1974, 57:775–788.

Fan PT, Davis JA, Somer T, *et al.*:A clinical approach to systemic vasculitis. *Semin Arthritis Rheum* 1980, 9:248–304.

Jennette JC, Charles LA, Falk RJ: Antineutrophil cytoplasmic autoantibodies: disease associations, molecular biology, and pathophysiology. *Int Rev Exp Pathol* 1991, 32:193–221.

Lie JT: Vasculitis, 1815 to 1991: classification and diagnostic specificity. *J Rheumatol* 1992, 19:83–89.

Lie JT: Vasculitis simulators and vasculitis look-alikes. *Curr Opin Rheumatol* 1992, 4:47–55.

Back and Neck Pain

Muhammad A. Khan
R. Geoffrey Wilber

Key Points

- Prolonged inactivity generally worsens the pain and stiffness of the back resulting from chronic inflammation of the spine due to ankylosing spondylitis and related spondyloarthropathies.

- NSAIDs are very effective in controlling spondylitis symptoms, and daily exercises are needed to minimize deformity and preserve good posture.

- Thorough neurological examination is essential in the evaluation of patients with back or neck pain.

- Neurological loss of bowel and bladder function constitute a potential surgical emergency.

- Magnetic resonance imaging is the most sensitive test for both diagnosis and prognosis of discogenic disease, but "abnormal" results are frequently observed, even among asymptomatic patients.

- Encourage early physcial activity and minimal bed rest for patients with an episode of acute back pain.

- A supervised fitness program can help reduce pain and disability, and can improve patients' confidence and long-term compliance.

Back and neck pain, a common cause of discomfort and incapacity in the United States population [1], can result from spondylogenic causes, which can be traumatic, structural or mechanical (degenerative and discogenic), inflammatory (spondylitic), congenital, metabolic, infective, or neoplastic, or from other bone lesions; and nonspondylogenic causes, which can be neurologic, vascular, viscerogenic, or psychogenic.

By far the most common cause of back and neck pain is mechanical deterioration of the spine with age; the common term for this is *spondylosis*. This discussion is limited to the diagnosis and management of musculoskeletal pain in the back and neck arising from bones, joints, ligaments, and muscles or other soft tissue resulting from inflammation (spondylitis) or mechanical derangement (spondylosis).

SPONDYLITIS AND SPONDYLOARTHROPATHIES

Spondylitis means inflammation of the spine, and although it may result from infection, such as brucellosis, we discuss a group of diseases that are noninfectious and are associated with sacroiliitis, peripheral inflammatory arthritis, and certain extraarticular features. These disorders are referred to collectively as the *spondyloarthropathies* and include ankylosing spondylitis, Reiter's syndrome (reactive arthritis), spondyloarthritis associated with psoriasis and chronic inflammatory bowel diseases, and a form of juvenile arthritis [2–4].

The main clinical and laboratory features observed in patients with spondyloarthropathies are listed in Table 1. These diseases show a strong association with the histocompatibility antigen HLA-B27, and they seem to result from a genetically

TABLE 1 CLINICAL FEATURES OF THE SPONDYLOARTHROPATHIES

Radiographically evident sacroiliitis, with or without accompanying spondylitis

Variable inflammatory arthritis of peripheral joints

Tendency for anterior ocular inflammation (conjunctivitis and acute iritis)

Variable mucocutaneous lesions

Lack of association with rheumatoid factor or rheumatoid nodules

Increased familial incidence

Strong association with HLA-B27

determined host response to one or more environmental factors. Substantial evidence favors a direct role for HLA-B27 in enhancing genetic susceptibility [5]. Additional genetic factors that may influence disease expression or severity include putative disease susceptibility genes for psoriasis, ulcerative colitis, and Crohn's disease. Among the environmental factors suspected of triggering these diseases are infectious causes. No such trigger for ankylosing spondylitis has yet been identified; however, reactive arthritis can be triggered by enteritis resulting from certain gram-negative bacteria such as *Shigella*, *Campylobacter*, *Yersinia*, or *Salmonella*, or by genitourinary infection with *Chlamydia*. Microbial material has been found in the synovium or in the synovial fluid of some patients with reactive arthritis triggered by these bacteria, but no viable organisms have been cultured from the inflamed joints [6–9].

Ankylosing Spondylitis

Ankylosing spondylitis is a chronic systemic inflammatory disorder of undetermined etiology that primarily affects the axial skeleton; sacroiliac joint involvement is its hallmark [2,3]. The inflammation appears to originate in ligamentous and capsular sites of attachment to bones (enthesitis or enthesopathy), in articular cartilage and juxtaarticular subchondral bones and ligaments, and in the synovium of involved joints. A striking feature is a high frequency of fibrous and bony ankylosis as a consequence of the primary inflammatory process. Untreated disease gradually leads to decreased spinal mobility because of progressive ankylosis. The overall prevalence of ankylosing spondylitis is 0.2% among white populations, and it is three times less common among black populations. It is three times more common among men, and the clinical and roentgenographic features seem to evolve more slowly in women [2,3].

The disease has articular and extraarticular features (Table 2). Chronic low back pain of insidious onset is usually the first symptom, starting in late adolescence or early adulthood; onset is very uncommon in patients older than 40 years of age. The pain is dull, difficult to localize, and felt deep in the gluteal region. It may be unilateral or intermittent at first, but it generally becomes persistent and bilateral within a few months, and the lower lumbar spine area becomes stiff and painful (Fig. 1). Pain in the lumbar area may be the initial symptom. The second most common early symptom is back stiffness, which is worse in the morning and is eased by mild physical activity or a hot shower. Prolonged inactivity worsens both pain and stiffness; getting out of bed may be difficult. The pain may awaken the patient from sleep; some patients find it necessary to wake up at night to move about or exercise for a few minutes before returning to bed. Occasionally, back symptoms are absent or very mild or may consist only of back stiffness, fleeting muscle aches, or musculotendinous tender spots. The symptoms may worsen on exposure to cold or dampness, and patients with such symptoms may be misdiagnosed as having fibrositis.

Extraarticular or juxtaarticular bony tenderness may be an early feature of the disease and is due to enthesitis (inflammatory lesions of the enthesis or sites of ligamentous or tendinous attachments to bone) at costosternal junctions, spinous processes, iliac crests, ischial tuberosities, or heels. Involvement of the costovertebral and costotransverse joints and enthesitis at costosternal areas can cause chest pain that may be accentuated by coughing or sneezing, and the patient may show diminished chest expansion on full inspiration. Stiffness and pain in the cervical spine and tenderness of the spinous processes sometimes occur in the early stages of the disease but generally tend to occur much later. The reported frequency of hip joint involvement varies from 17% to 36%; it is usually bilateral, insidious in onset, and potentially more crippling than is the involvement of any other joint of the extremities. Flexion contractures of the hip are common at later stages of the disease, giving rise to a characteristic rigid gait with some flexion at the knees to maintain erect posture. Involvement of peripheral joints other than hips and shoulders is infrequent, rarely persistent or erosive, and tends to resolve without any residual joint deformity. For example, intermittent knee effusions are occasionally the first manifestation of juvenile ankylosing spondylitis. Approximately 10% of patients have temporomandibular joint pain and local tenderness. Mild constitutional symptoms, such as anorexia, malaise, and mild fever, are sometimes part of early disease and may be more common to juvenile-onset disease, especially in patients from developing countries.

Acute anterior uveitis, also called acute iritis or acute iridocyclitis (Fig. 2), occurs in 25% to 30% of patients at some time during the course of disease [2,3]. The acute inflammation is typically unilateral. Symptoms include pain, increased lacrimation, photophobia, and blurred vision; examination reveals circumcorneal congestion and increased numbers of leukocytes in the aqueous humor. Rare extraarticular complications include aortitis (leading to slowly progressive aortic valve incompetence and conduction abnormalities, sometimes requiring a pacemaker), apical pulmonary fibrosis and cavitation, amyloidosis, and IgA nephropathy [2,3,5]. The muscle wasting of some patients with advanced disease results from disuse atrophy. Neurologic involvement may be due to fracture or dislocation, atlantoaxial subluxation, or cauda equina syndrome. Because the bone is osteoporotic, fracture can follow relatively minor trauma in patients with an ankylosed spine and usually occurs in the lower cervical spine. The resultant quadriplegia is the most serious complication of ankylosing spondylitis and has a high mortality.

TABLE 2 ARTICULAR AND EXTRA-ARTICULAR MANIFESTATIONS OF ANKYLOSING SPONDYLITIS

Skeletal
  Axial arthritis
    (*eg*, sacroiliitis and spondylitis)
  Arthritis of girdle joints
    (hips and shoulders); peripheral
    joint involvement uncommon
  Others
    Enthesopathy
    Osteoporosis
    Vertebral fractures
    Spondylodiscitis
    Pseudoarthrosis

Extraskeletal
  Acute anterior uveitis
  Enteric mucosal subclinical inflammation
  Cardiovascular involvement
  Pulmonary involvement
  Cauda equina syndrome
  Amyloidosis
  Miscellaneous

Association with other diseases*
  Reactive arthritis
    (including Reiter's syndrome)
  Psoriasis
  Ulcerative colitis
  Crohn's disease
  Whipple's disease
  Other spondyloarthropathies

*Represents the secondary form of ankylosing spondylitis.
Adapted from Khan [22]; with permission.

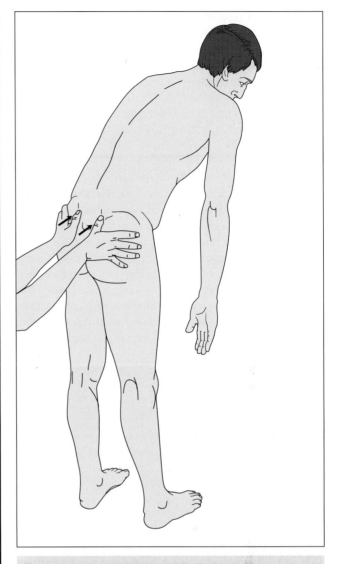

FIGURE 1 Diminished ability to fully flex the lumbar spine associated with ankylosing spondylitis; direct pressure by thumbs over sacroiliac joints elicits tenderness.

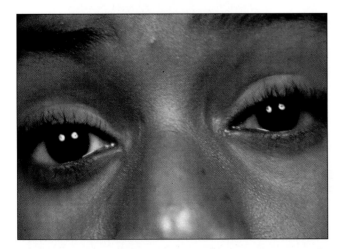

FIGURE 2 Untreated acute anterior uveitis of left eye, with circumcorneal congestion. *Adapted from* Khan [25]; with permission.

Other Spondyloarthropathies

Reiter's syndrome (reactive arthritis) is a triad of acute bacterial enteritis or nonspecific urethritis followed by acute noninfected oligoarthritis, frequently with inflammatory back pain. It occurs primarily in young men and is often associated with ocular inflammation (bilateral conjunctivitis or unilateral acute anterior uveitis) and mucocutaneous lesions [1–3]. It is self-limiting at times but can be recurrent or chronic. Genitourinary tract infection (nongonococcal urethritis) with *Chlamydia trachomatis* is the commonly recognized initiator in most patients in the United States, whereas enteric infections with *Shigella*, *Salmonella*, *Yersinia*, or *Campylobacter* are the more common triggers in patients from developing parts of the world. This syndrome can occur in an incomplete form.

Patients with Reiter's syndrome, psoriasis, ulcerative colitis, and Crohn's disease can develop ankylosing spondylitis. The reverse is also true: patients with ankylosing spondylitis more often have Crohn's disease, ulcerative disease, or psoriasis.

Ileocolonoscopic studies have disclosed bowel inflammation in many spondyloarthropathic patients without intestinal symptoms [10]. Cutaneous manifestations of psoriasis sometimes resemble those of Reiter's syndrome. Some patients with Reiter's syndrome develop psoriasis and vice versa, and some HIV-infected patients with AIDS develop severe psoriasis and even arthritis that closely resembles psoriatic arthritis and Reiter's syndrome [3].

DIAGNOSIS

The patient's history, articular and extraarticular physical findings, and roentgenographic evidence of bilateral sacroiliitis suggest a diagnosis of ankylosing spondylitis [2,3]. Various presentations, such as enthesitis and acute anterior uveitis, may antedate back pain and stiffness in some patients. Restriction of spinal mobility and decreased chest expansion support the diagnosis. The characteristic radiographic changes may evolve over many years, primarily in the axial skeleton and especially in the sacroiliac joints, but are usually present by the time the patient seeks medical attention. Radiographic evidence of sacroiliitis is required for definitive diagnosis and is the most consistent finding (Fig. 3); a simple anteroposterior roentgenogram is usually sufficient to detect it. For patients with early disease whose sacroiliac joints may be normal or show equivocal changes, quantitative bone scintigraphy may be too nonspecific to be useful. Computed tomography (CT) and magnetic resonance (MR) imaging are rarely needed. The inflammatory lesions also affect the superficial layers of the annulus fibrosus, at their attachment to the corners of the vertebral bodies, resulting in reactive bony sclerosis (seen roentgenographically as shiny corners) and subsequent bone resorption, leading to squaring of the vertebral bodies and gradual ossification of the superficial layers of the annulus fibrosus to form intervertebral bony bridging called syndesmophytes (Figs. 4 and 5). Concomitant inflammatory changes often result in ankylosis of the apophyseal joints and ossification of the spinal ligaments, ultimately resulting in complete fusion of the vertebral column (bamboo spine) (Fig. 3). Spinal osteoporosis is also frequently observed as a result of ankylosis and lack of spinal mobility.

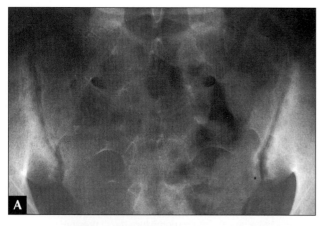
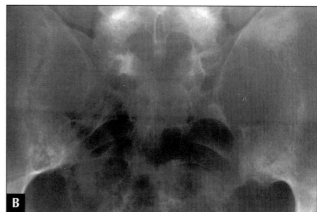
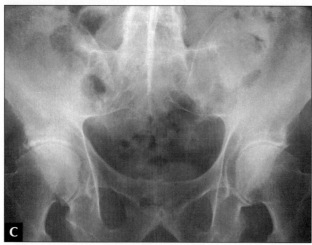
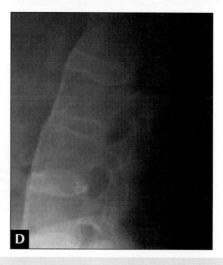

FIGURE 3 **A**, Roentgenographic changes of sacroiliitis in ankylosing spondylitis, showing early bilateral, symmetric bony erosions (postage stamp serrations) and adjacent bony sclerosis; **B**, more advanced sacroiliitis obliteration of the sacroiliac joints; **C**, complete fusion of sacroiliac joints, pubic symphysis, and the lumbar spine (bamboo spine), ossification of interspinous ligaments, and hip joint involvement; **D**, lateral view of the lumbar spine showing squaring of vertebral bodies and typical syndesmophytes.

There are no diagnostic or pathognomonic laboratory tests; most patients can be readily diagnosed by history, physical examination, and roentgenographic findings [2,3]. An elevated erythrocyte sedimentation rate (in up to 75% of patients) and a mildly to moderately elevated serum IgA concentration are common. There is no association with rheumatoid factor and antinuclear antibodies, and the synovial fluid or synovial biopsy specimens do not show distinctive features compared with other inflammatory arthropathies [2,3]. HLA-B27 typing occasionally aids diagnosis of ankylosing spondylitis or related spondyloarthropathies when used in a clinical situation in which the diagnosis is equivocal clinically and radiographically [2,3]; this is not a "screening" or "confirmatory" test for these diseases.

Differential Diagnosis

Back pain frequently results from the noninflammatory mechanical causes (Table 3), which are discussed later in this chapter; such back pain is generally aggravated by activity and relieved by rest, and chest expansion and lateral flexion of the lumbar spine are often normal. Malignancies should always be considered in the differential diagnosis of back pain, in both young and old patients. Other causes of back pain include pelvic inflammatory diseases, septic discitis, septic sacroiliitis, and Paget's disease.

Conditions that can be confused with ankylosing spondylitis include Scheuermann's disease, osteofluorosis, tuberculous spondylitis, chronic brucellosis, chondrocalci-

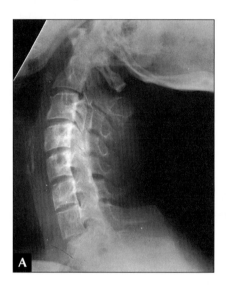 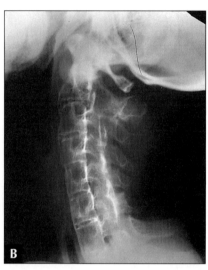

FIGURE 4 Roentgenograms of ankylosing spondylitis of the cervical spine. The lateral view shows progressive squaring and fusion of vertebral bodies anteriorly and gradual fusion of apophyseal joints posteriorly over a 12-year period. (*From* Khan [22]; with permission.)

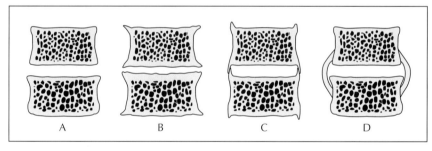

FIGURE 5 Comparison of **A**, normal vertebrae; **B**, osteophytes of spondylosis; **C**, syndesmophytes of ankylosing spondylitis; and **D**, nonmarginal syndesmophytes of psoriatic spondylitis.

| TABLE 3 DIFFERENTIAL DIAGNOSIS OF NONINFLAMMATORY BACK PAIN |||||

Degenerative	Congenital	Visceral (referred)	Neoplastic
Osteoarthritis	Dysraphic syndromes	Pancreatitis	Metastatic disease
Disk degeneration	Diastematomyelia	Pelvic disease	Primary bone tumors
or protrusion	Scoliosis	Pyelonephritis	Intradural tumors
Facet arthritis	Transitional vertebrae	Ulcer disease	Infectious
Spinal stenosis	Metabolic	Cholecystitis	Bacterial
	Osteoporosis	Aortic aneurysm	Fungal
	Hyperparathyroidism	Traumatic	Fibromyalgia
		Strain	
		Fracture	
		Spondylolisthesis or spondylolysis	

nosis, ochronosis, axial osteomalacia, and congenital kyphoscoliosis. Hyperparathyroidism can lead to irregularity of the sacroiliac joint surfaces, particularly on the iliac side, as a result of subchondral resorption and adjacent bony sclerosis; narrowing and ankylosis of the joint space do not occur, however. Sacroiliac joint changes suggesting sacroiliitis and even complete fusion of these joints are observed in some patients with long-standing paraplegia and quadriplegia. Osteitis condensans ilii, a disorder primarily of young multiparous women, is often asymptomatic, characterized by roentgenographic evidence of a triangular area of dense sclerotic bone in the iliac bones of the pelvis adjacent to the lower half of the sacroiliac joints; the joints themselves are normal. It is a self-limiting condition that shows no association with HLA-B27, and there is no evidence to indicate that it is a form of ankylosing spondylitis.

Ankylosing hyperostosis (also called Forestier's disease or diffuse idiopathic skeletal hyperostosis) is usually seen in elderly persons and is characterized by hyperostosis affecting the anterior longitudinal ligament (Fig. 6). There is no association with HLA-B27. The skeletal hyperostosis at sites of bony attachments of tendons and ligaments may be

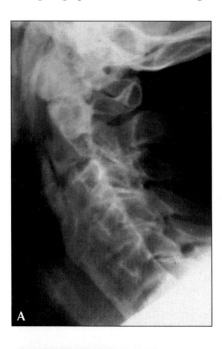 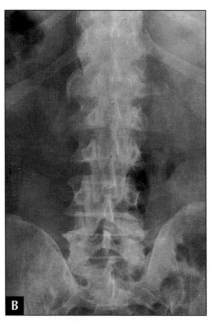

FIGURE 6 **A**, Lateral view of cervical spine showing ossification of anterior longitudinal ligament ankylosing hyperostosis (Forestier's disease). **B**, Anteroposterior view of sacroiliac joints and thoracolumbar spine, with normal sacroiliac and apophyseal joints of the lumbar spine and more prominent ossification of the longitudinal ligament in the thoracolumbar spine on the right side.

TABLE 4 DIFFERENTIATING FEATURES OF ANKYLOSING HYPEROSTOSIS (FORESTIER'S DISEASE) AND ANKYLOSING SPONDYLITIS		
Feature	**Ankylosing hyperostosis**	**Ankylosing spondylitis**
Usual age on onset, *y*	> 50	< 40
Thoracolumbar kyphosis	±	++
Limitation of spinal mobility	±	++
Pain	±	++
Limitation of chest expansion	±	++
Roentgenography		
Hyperostosis	++	+
Sacroiliac joint erosion	–	++
Sacroiliac joint (synovial) obliteration	±	++
Sacroiliac joint (ligamentous) obliteration	+	++
Apophyseal joint obliteration	–	++
Anterior longitudinal ligament ossification	++	±
Posterior longitudinal ligament ossification	+	?
Syndesmophytes	–	++
Enthesopathies (whiskerings) with erosions	–	++
Enthesopathies (whiskerings) without erosions	++	+

–, absent; ±, equivocal; +, frequently present; ++, very frequently present; ?, rarely present.
Adapted from Yagan and Khan [23]; with permission.

roentgenographically confused with ankylosing spondylitis. Table 4 lists the distinguishing features.

Radiology is generally helpful in making the differential diagnosis. For example, the degenerative changes in discovertebral junctions and apophyseal joints with adjacent osteophytes in degenerative disk disease can be well seen on roentgenography, whereas invertebral disk prolapse can be well visualized by CT, myelography, or MR imaging. The sacroiliac joints will be normal or show only some degenerative changes; the erosions and subchondral sclerosis typical of sacroiliitis will be absent. Occasionally, severe degenerative and hyperostotic changes of the sacroiliac joints, such as joint space narrowing, subchondral bone sclerosis, and capsular ossification (especially in Forestier's disease), may superficially resemble those of sacroiliitis on an anteroposterior roentgenographic view of the pelvis.

Distinguishing ankylosing spondylitis from rheumatoid arthritis is usually not difficult because involvement of the sacroiliac, apophyseal, and costovertebral joints is rare in rheumatic arthritis, whereas serologic tests for rheumatoid factor are negative and subcutaneous nodules are absent in patients with ankylosing spondylitis.

TREATMENT

Consulting a rheumatologist is helpful for determining the type of spondyloarthropathy present, assessing prognosis, and selecting optimum treatment [2,3,11–13]. There is no preventive measure or cure for ankylosing spondylitis, but most cases can be well managed according to the guidelines in Table 5 and Fig. 7. Aspirin seldom gives an adequate therapeutic response. Nonsteroidal antiinflammatory drugs (NSAIDs) should be used regularly in full therapeutic antiinflammatory doses during the active phase of the disease, and patients should be informed about this protocol because otherwise they may use the drugs occasionally and for analgesic effects only. Patients differ in response and side effects, and it is worthwhile to seek the best alternative NSAID for each. Phenylbutazone is probably the most effective NSAID for ankylosing spondylitis and offers good symptomatic relief, but because of its potentially greater risk of bone marrow toxicity, other NSAIDs are generally used, such as indomethacin, naproxen, diclofenac, or sulindac.

Sulphasalazine may be effective for treating peripheral arthritis in some ankylosing spondylitis patients whose symptoms are not adequately controlled by NSAIDs. Because of its efficacy for treating inflammatory bowel disease and psoriasis, sulphasalazine is especially useful for patients who have these associated diseases or who are intolerant to NSAIDs. Antimalarial drugs, D-penicillamine, and immunosuppressants have not been well studied as therapy for ankylosing spondylitis. Oral corticosteroids have no value for long-term management of the musculoskeletal aspects of the disease because of their serious side effects, and they do not halt disease progression. Recalcitrant enthesopathy and persistent synovitis may respond to a local corticosteroid injection.

Acute anterior uveitis can be managed with pupil dilation and use of corticosteroid eye drops. Systemic steroids or immunosuppressives may rarely be needed for patients with severe refractory uveitis. The use of total hip arthroplasty has given good results and prevents partial or total disability from severe hip disease. Vertebral wedge osteotomy may be needed to correct severe kyphosis, although it carries a relatively high risk of paraplegia. Cardiac complications may require aortic valve replacement or pacemaker implantation. Apical pulmonary fibrosis is not easy to manage; in rare cases, surgical resection is required. Radiotherapy has no role in treating patients with ankylosing spondylitis because of the high risk of leukemia and aplastic anemia. Splints, braces, and corsets are generally not helpful and are not advised. There is no special diet, and there is no evidence that specific foods initiate or exacerbate the disease.

Many patients have difficulty driving a car because of impaired neck mobility and find special wide-view mirrors very helpful. Similarly, prism glasses can improve visibility for the rare severely kyphotic patients who cannot look ahead while walking. There are many support groups for persons with ankylosing spondylitis that provide information about the disease and advice about life and health insurance, jobs, working environment, and wide-view mirrors and other useful items (Table 6).

Reactive arthritis and enteropathic arthritis vary from mild arthralgia to severely disabling conditions that render the patient bedridden for weeks [3,11]. Some patients prefer to tolerate pain and restricted movement rather than take drugs, but this attitude probably prolongs the time to full recovery.

TABLE 5 SALIENT PRINCIPLES OF MANAGING ANKYLOSING SPONDYLITIS

No cure, but most cases can be well managed; early diagnosis important

Continuity of care; recognition and early treatment of acute iritis; consultation as needed by rheumatologist, ophthalmologist, orthopedist, or other

Patient education about the disease to increase compliance

Daily exercises to preserve good posture and minimize limitation of chest expansion; appropriate sports and recreations; sleeping on firm mattress without pillows; avoidance of smoking and prevention of trauma

Supportive measures and counseling about social, sexual, and vocational aspects; patient support groups

Family counseling; family history; physical examination of relatives may disclose disease aggregation

Surgical measures; arthroplasty, correction of deformity

Adapted from Khan [24]; with permission.

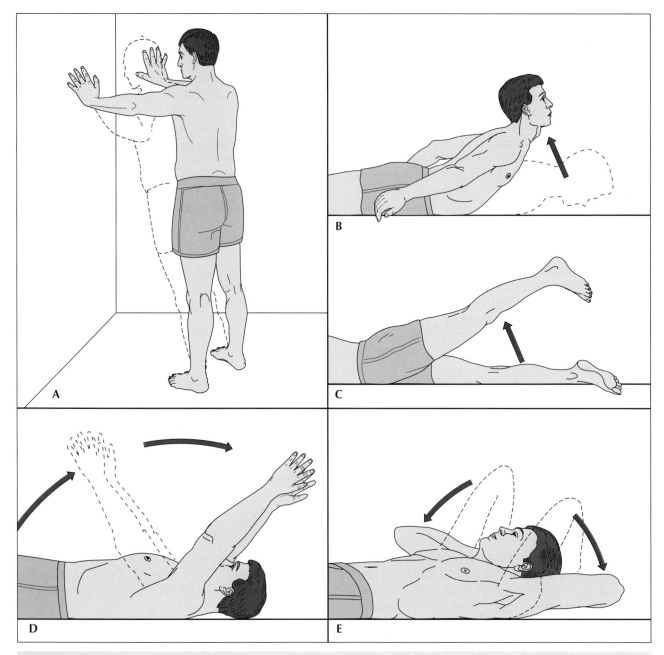

FIGURE 7 **A–E**, Regular exercises for patients with ankylosing spondylitis. To perform the corner push-up exercise (**A**) the patient stands 2 feet or more from the corner, both hands placed on the wall about 2 feet from the corner, then gently leans towards the corner keeping heels on the ground. The patient inhales and tries to straighten the spine while leaning towards the corner and exhales when coming back to the starting position. (*Adapted from* Khan [22]; with permission.)

TABLE 6 AVAILABLE SUPPORT GROUPS FOR PATIENTS WITH ANKYLOSIS SPONDYLITIS

Spondylitis Association of America
14827 Ventura Boulevard #119
Sherman Oaks, CA 91403
Phone 800-777-8189
Fax 818-981-9826
The National Ankylosing Spondylitis Society
3 Grosvenor Crescent, London SW1X 7ER, England
Phone 0171-235-9585
Fax 0171-235-5827

Response to NSAID treatment of an acute episode of arthritis varies according to severity. During recovery phase, patients should not stop treatment too rapidly. Intraarticular administration of triamcinolone hexacetamide usually gives prompt and prolonged relief from synovitis, but septic arthritis should first be excluded. Oral corticosteroids should only be used as a short course (not more than 2 or 3 months) for severe cases of reactive arthritis with many joints affected and when NSAIDs alone have not proven effective.

Physical therapy using cold pads reduces pain and edema in inflamed joints. Rest is advisable, and temporary splinting can alleviate pain at night. However, immobilization should be used carefully because muscle wasting may be a problem. During convalescence, systematic rehabilitation may be valuable.

Nonnarcotic analgesics should be used until the pain no longer inhibits full use of the muscles and joints. A comfortable pair of shoes and shoe inserts to alter weight bearing may help patients with painful feet due to inflammation of the toes or painful heels due to plantar fasciitis or calcaneal periostitis (Fig. 8).

The prognosis is usually good even in the most severe cases [2,11]. However, several follow-up studies of patients with Reiter's syndrome have demonstrated that recurrences are frequent, and a chronic form of arthritis associated with recurring tendinitis or tenosynovitis, back pains, and sacroiliitis may develop and may evolve into spondylitis. The chronic form of Reiter's syndrome causes considerable discomfort and morbidity. Rheumatologic consultation for therapeutic suggestions is useful with such patients, and they often respond well to treatment with methotrexate or azathioprine [13]. Sulphasalazine is effective for patients with enteropathic arthritis and also for those with reactive arthritis. The presence of microbial components in inflamed joints of patients with reactive arthritis raises the question of antimicrobial therapy. A 3-month course of tetracycline is associated with shorter, less severe chlamydia-induced reactive arthritis but not postenteritic reactive arthritis [6,11]. Early treatment of sexually transmitted genitourinary infections in patients with a history of reactive arthritis protects against the recurrence of arthritis [7].

Psoriatic arthropathy is first treated with an NSAID. Sulphasalazine also has been used with good results [11–13]. Treating the skin lesions with locally applied drugs is advisable; good results are achieved with psoralen-ultraviolet-light (PUVA). Often (but not always), improving the skin condition also improves the joints. Methotrexate and azathioprine are effective for treating psoriatic arthritis, especially in cases with extensive skin lesions and difficult joint disease. Cyclosporine also has been shown to be effective, although toxic. Etretinate treatment results in significant improvement but is associated with mucocutaneous side effects; it is more valuable for treating the skin lesions than the arthritis. Again, consulting a rheumatologist can be helpful [11–13].

SPONDYLOSIS

Spinal spondylosis is common, with prevalence increasing with age. When evaluating back pain, it is important to realize that there are several etiologies other than discogenic and spondylogenic that must be ruled out. Table 3 gives a differential diagnosis of noninflammatory back pain. The differential diagnosis of sciatic nerve symptoms and radiculopathy is given in Table 7. Both intraspinal and intrapelvic lesions as well as extrapelvic etiologies should be considered.

Disk Degeneration

Clinical back pain related to disk degeneration appears to increase with time [14]. Incidence of disk degeneration is 100% in autopsies of persons older than 90 years of age. Disk degeneration appears to be related to the "wear and tear" phenomenon. It is additionally accelerated by mechanical stress and idiopathic predilection. Disk degeneration occurs most markedly in the cervical disks C_5-C_6, C_4-C_5, and C_6-C_7

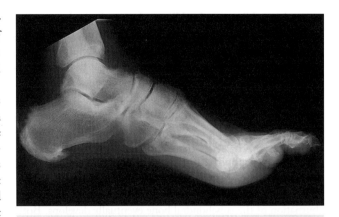

FIGURE 8 Radiographic evidence of calcaneal erosions and periostitis in a patient with chronic persistent Reiter's syndrome, with some calcium deposits in the Achilles tendon resulting from chronic inflammatory process.

[15]. In the lumbar spine, the L_4-L_5 and L_5-S_1 disks are most commonly involved [16].

Radiographic data suggest a mechanical basis for disk degeneration at these levels in both the cervical and lower lumbar spine. The primary degeneration of the disks is thought to be caused by either injury or deterioration of the disk space itself with subsequent collapse. More than 85% of the juvenile disk nucleus is water; with aging, the water content slowly but steadily decreases to approximately a 60% level in patients aged 80 years. This decrease results in diminished volume of the nucleus and narrowing of the intervertebral disk space, leading to secondary facet degeneration as well

TABLE 7 DIFFERENTIAL DIAGNOSIS OF SCIATIC NERVE SYMPTOMS AND RADICULOPATHY
Lumbosacral nerve root lesions
Disk protrusion
Spinal stenosis
Spondylolisthesis
Post laminectomy state or arachnoiditis
Spine fracture
Infection
Herpes zoster
Paget's disease
Sciatic nerve lesions
Entrapment
Trauma
Tumor
Ischemia
Lumbosacral plexus lesions
Pregnancy
Pelvic tumors
Aneurysm
Pelvic fractures
Endometriosis

Diagnostic Testing

Blood tests usually are not helpful, whereas plain radiographs often disclose signs such as disk space narrowing and osteophyte formation (*see* Fig. 9) [18,19]. Typical radiographic signs of disk abnormalities are disk space narrowing, the vacuum phenomenon within the disk spaces, end-plate sclerosis, osteophyte formation, and Schmorl's nodes. The most significant diagnostic findings in the lumbar spine for long-term prognosis of back pain are signs of Scheuermann's disease, ankylosing spondylitis, osteoporosis, bone tumors, fracture spondylolisthesis, multiple disk space narrowing, and multiple disk calcification. Of less significance are mild spondylolisthesis, kyphosis, retrolisthesis, and severe or diminished lordosis. Of no significance for prognosticating low back pain are transitional vertebrae, mildly increased lordosis, facet orientation, Schmorl's nodes, osteophytic lipping, ossicles, and single disk narrowing.

In the primary care setting the chance of significant disease requiring surgical intervention is as low as 0.2%; in most cases a 6- to 8-week trial of conservative treatment is indicated. Radiography of the spine should be ordered if the patient with back symptoms is older than 50 years or younger than 15 years; if there is history of constitutional symptoms, significant trauma, substance abuse, or malignancy; or if the pain is severe or there is neuromotor symptomatology. Radionuclide bone scan is relatively nonspecific but can be helpful when osteomyelitis, fractures or malignancy are clinically suspected and plain x-ray films are nondiagnostic.

As many as 18% of patients seen in a referral orthopedic practice have significant disease that may require surgery. Myelography is of particular benefit when looking at compressive lesions involving the nerves or spinal cord (Fig. 13). Combined with a delayed CT scan (Fig. 14), myelography can correlate compressive lesions with significant bony and soft tissue pathology with a very high degree of sensitivity. Plain CT scans often do not visualize the neuroelements and are limited to the area involved, but they are especially good for bony pathology and spinal stenosis; three-dimensional CT scans can identify extraforamenal abnormalities.

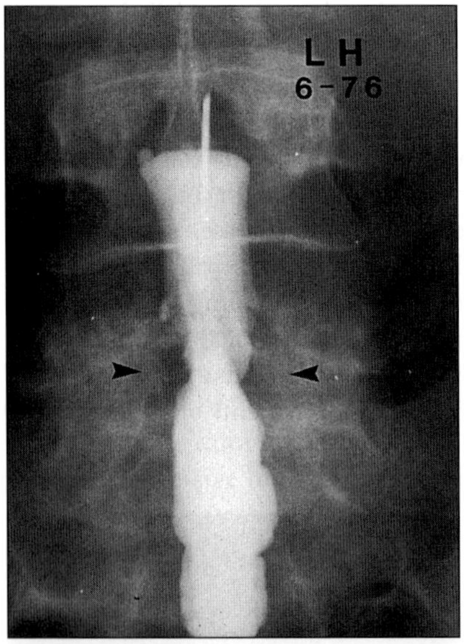

Lumbar discography remains controversial. It has a high sensitivity to interdiscal abnormalities but is relatively expensive and causes significant pain. The test is provocative for symptoms of involved levels. Potential complications include nerve injury and infection.

Magnetic resonance imaging is clearly superior for visualizing the cranial-cervical and thoracocervical junctions and for visualizing intraspinal pathology (Fig. 15). It is excellent for intradural and extradural tumors, subarachnoid cysts, arachnoids, total or partial blocks where use of dye is impaired, disk herniation, and recurrent disks, especially with gadolinium-enhanced studies, but it is only fair for bony impingement. Abnormal MR imaging scans of the spine can be observed in asymptomatic persons [20]. The sensitivity of MR imaging is equal to or greater than CT myelography for discogenic problems of the spine, and T_2-weighted images are predictors of disk degeneration and loss of water content. The cost of MR imaging is a relative

Figure 13 Water-soluble radiocontrast myelogram showing area of spinal stenosis with bilateral fourth nerve root compression (*arrows*).

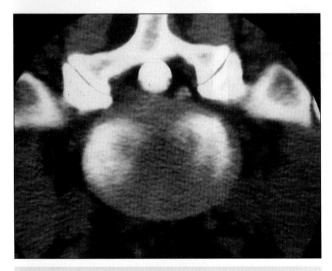

Figure 14 Area of focal spinal stenosis at the level of a unilateral side herniation of the disk between L_5-S_1 associated with deformation of the S_1 nerve root.

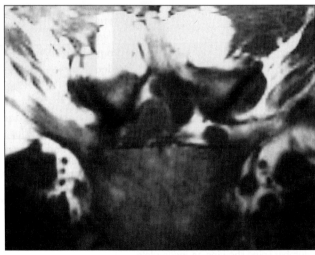

Figure 15 T_1-weighted magnetic resonance image showing large sequestered (free-fragment) disk herniation causing compression of the central dural sack.

contraindication, whereas the presence of pacemakers and ferrous implants are absolute contraindications.

Electromyography and nerve conduction studies are not indicated for simple back pain, and even when radiculopathy is present, they are not likely to add much new clinically useful information to what has been obtained by CT or MR imaging.

TREATMENT

Acute back pain is self-limited in most patients; 9 of 10 such patients will recover on their own within 6 to 8 weeks, although recurrences are common. Treatment should start with a conservative approach with nonprescription pain relievers or nonsteroidal antiinflammatory agents [Fig. 16]. Avoiding bed rest and maintaining ordinary activity as tolerated lead to the most rapid recovery [21]. Therefore, the patient should be told to stick to their regular routines as best as they can. Some clinicians use short-term treatment with antidepressants, muscle relaxants, and opioid analgesics, but these medications appear to be no more effective than nonsteroidal antiinflammatory drugs. Use of muscle relaxants should be limited for 1 to 2 weeks, and tricyclic antidepressants can be helpful in patients with chronic back pain and concommitant depression.

Exercise is helpful in patients with back pain, but controversy persists over the relative merits of bed rest versus exercise in the treatment of acute back pain. Continuing ordinary activities within the limit permitted by the pain leads to a more rapid recovery than bed rest or back mobilizing exercises; this was demonstrated in a recent controlled study [21]. Widespread use of this approach (*ie*, avoiding bed rest and maintaining ordinary activities) in managing patients with acute back pain is expected to lead to most rapid recovery and also to result in substantial monetary savings. Prolonged bed rest contributes to patient morbidity through paraspinal muscle atrophy and deconditioning. Muscle conditioning exercises, including isometric strengthening of paraspinal and abdominal muscles, are keystones to success. The low-impact exercises, such as walking, swimming, or biking, can maintain and even improve the patient's activity tolerance.

Corticosteroid and local anesthetic injections into facet joints, epidural space and trigger points remain controversial, and there is little scientific support for their long-term beneficial effect. They seem to sometimes provide short-term symptomatic relief, hopefully breaking the cycle of pain and allowing early physical therapy and other treatments to work. There is no clear scientific bases for spinal traction, acupuncture, or transcutaneous nerve stimulation for patients with back pain.

Educate the patient about proper posture, and the need to follow a regular exercise program and avoid repetitive trauma to the involved spine. This patient education can be more effectively given in group sessions based on the Swedish concept of "back schools". Some patients may need changes in their lifestyle. Wearing of abdominal lumbar support and corsets at work can cut down repetitive stress in the lumbar spine, and help avoid potential injury or re-injury in heavy manual laborers.

If the patient continues to be limited by symptoms, but shows no neurologic deficit or systemic signs, a period of 4 to 8 weeks of conservative care should be considered prior to diagnostic testing to seek the reason for the slow recovery. Spinal manipulation may help in some patients. One patient in ten may be difficult to deal with in the primary care setting and may warrant further investigation for serious disease.

Presence of neurologic deficit or systemic signs requires further workup to evaluate the degree and cause of the compressive pathology or the systemic signs, and to determine

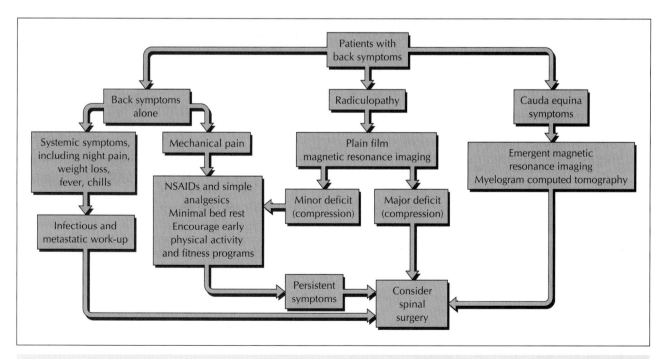

FIGURE 16 Management of patients with nonimflammatory nonsponylitic lumbar complaints. NSAIDs—nonsteroidal antiinflammatory drugs.

the prognosis. Emergency indications for surgical referral include the cauda equina syndrome with bowel and bladder dysfunction, or progressive severe motor loss of an extremity. Indications for delayed surgical intervention include persistent neuromotor deficit after 2 to 3 months of conservative management. Presence of unremitting symptoms in the absence of neurologic deficit also may be an indication for surgery if vocational and avocational activities are compromised and the patient has a favorable psychosocial profile (eg, realistic expectations and lack of depression and drug dependence).

Simple discectomy in the lumbar spine by micro or conventional techniques helps in treating radiculopathy related to disc herniation when there is no significant back pain. Fusion is indicated in patients with recurrent disc herniation or in those with severe mechanical pain at the time of their simple discectomy. Spinal stenosis is usually amenable to posterior decompression. This may be coupled with fusion as well if, at the time of the decompression, facet joints are interrupted or pars interarticularis defects are made. Other indications for fusion at the time of posterior decompression are the presence of spondylolisthesis or scoliosis. Spondylolisthesis itself is usually best treated with posterior spinal fusion, usually coupled with posterior pedicular instrumentation to improve the overall fusion rate and to maintain the spinal alignment until fusion occurs. Instrumentation of the spine can allow early postoperative mobilization of the patient with diminished pain, and may avoid the need for orthosis.

In the cervical spine, discectomy and fusion of the involved segments is preferred through an anterior approach because posterior approach carries a potentially higher risk of complications. Posterior decompressions without stabilization usually do nothing to improve neck pain, buy may have a place with isolated radiculopathy.

REFERENCES AND RECOMMENDED READING

Recently published papers of particular interest have been highlighted as:

1. Frymoyer JW, Cats-Baril WL: An overview of the incidences and costs of low back pain. *Orthop Clin North Am* 1991, 22:263–271.

2. Khan MA: Ankylosing spondylitis and related spondyloarthropathies. In *Spine: State of the Art Reviews*. Edited by Khan MA. Philadelphia: Hanley & Belfus; 1990:497–688.

3. Khan MA, ed.: Spondyloarthropathies. *Rheum Dis Clin North Am* 1992, 18:1–282.

4. Dougados M, van der Linden S, Juhlin R, *et al*.: The European Spondyloarthropathy Study Group preliminary criteria for the classification of spondyloarthropathy. *Arthritis Rheum* 1991, 34:1218–1227.

5. Feltkamp B, Khan MA, Lopez de Castro J: The pathogenic role to HLA-B27. *Immunol Today* 1996, 17:1–3..

6. Lauhio A, Lerisalo-Repo M, Lahdevirta J, *et al*.: Double-blind placebo-controlled study of three months treatment with lymecycline in reactive arthritis with special reference to Chlamydia arthritis. *Arthritis Rheum* 1991, 34:6–14.

7. Bardin T, Enel C, Cornelis F, *et al*.: Antibiotic treatment of venereal disease and Reiter's syndrome in a Greenland population. *Arthritis Rheum* 1992, 35:190–194.

8. Khan MA, Kellner H: Immunogenetics of spondyloarthropathies. *Rheum Dis Clin North Am* 1992, 18:837–864.

9. Khan MA: Pathogenesis of ankylosing spondylitis: recent advances. *J Rheumatol* 1993, 20:1273–1277.

10. Leirisalo-Repo M, Turunen U, Stenman S, *et al*.: High frequency of silent inflammatory bowel disease in spondyloarthropathy. *Arthritis Rheum* 1994, 37:23–31.

11. Toivanen A, Khan MA: Therapeutic dilemmas in ankylosing spondylitis and related spondyloarthropathies. *Rheumatol Rev* 1994, 3:21–27.

12. Amor B, Dougados M, Khan MA: Management of defractory ankylosing spondylitis and related spondyloarthropathies. *Rheum Dis Clin North Am* 1995, 21:117–128.

13. Creemers MCW, van Riel PLCM, Franssen MJAM, *et al*.: Second-line treatment in seronegative spondylarthropathies. *Semin Arthritis Rheum* 1994, 24:71–81.

14. Boden SD, Wiesel SW, Laws ER, Rothman RH: *The Aging Spine*. Philadelphia: WB Saunders, 1991.

15. Regan JJ, ed.: Cervical spine disease. In *Spine: State of Art Reviews*. Philadelphia: Hanley & Belfus; 1991.

16. Hardy RW, ed.: *Lumbar Disc Disease*, edn 2. New York: Raven Press; 1993.

17. Wilber RG, Yoo J: Diagnostic methods and therapeutic techniques. In *Painful Cervical Trauma*. Edited by Tolison CD, Satterthwaite JR. Baltimore: Williams and Wilkins; 1992.

18. Bigos S, Bowyer O, Braen G, *et al*.: Acute low back programs in adults. Agency for Health Care Policy and Research. (AHCPR) publication no. 95-0642. Clinical Practice Guideline no. 14, Public Health Servie, US DHHS, Rockville, MD, Dec. 1994.

19. Wipf JE, Deyo RA: Low back pain. *Med Clin North Am* 1995, 79: 231–246.

20. Deyo DA: Magnetic resonance imaging of the lumbar spine: terrific act or tar baby? *New Engl J Med* 1994,331:115–116.

21. Malmivaara A, Hakkinen U, Aro T, *et al*.: The treatment of acute low back pain: bed rest, excercises, or ordinary activity? *New Engl J Med* 1995, 332:351–355.

22. Khan MA: Ankylosing spondylitis. In *Spondyloarthropathies*. Edited by Calin A. Orlando: Grune and Stratton; 1984: 69–117.

23. Yagan R, Khan MA: Confusion of roentgenographic differential diagnosis between ankylosing hyperostosis (Forstier's disease) and ankylosing spondylitis. *Clin Rheumatol* 1983,2:285–292.

24. Khan MA, Skosey JL: Ankylosing spondylitis and related spondyloarthropathies. In *Immunological Diseases*, edn 4. Edited by Samter M. Boston: Little, Brown and Company; 1988:1509–1538.

25. Khan MA: Ankylosing spondylitis. In *Rheumatology*. Edited by Klippel JH, Dieppe PA. London: Mosby Year Book Europe; 1994:3.25.1–3.25.10.

SELECT BIBLIOGRAPHY

Borenstein DG, Wiesel SW, Boden SD: Low back pain: medical diagnosis and comprehensive management, edn. 2. Philadelphia: WB Saunders; 1995.

Frost H, Moffett JAK, Moser JS, Fairbank JCT: Randomised controlled trial for evaluation of fitness programme for patients with low back pain. *Br Med J* 1995, 310:151–154.

Frymoyer JW: *The Adult Spine*. New York: Raven Press, 1991.

Macnab I: Symptoms of cervical disc disorders. In *The Cervical Spine*. Cervical Spine Research Society. New York: JB Lippincott; 1989.

Von Korff M, Barlow W, Cherkin D, Deyo RA: Effects of practice style in managing back pain. *Ann Intern Med* 1994, 121:187–195.

Reiter's Syndrome and Other Forms of Reactive Arthritis

9

Peter D. Utsinger
Jennie H. Utsinger

> **Key Points**
> - Reiter's syndrome and reactive arthritis are inflammatory arthropathies primarily involving the lower extremity.
> - In Reiter's syndrome most patients are HLA-B27 positive.
> - Patient education, physical therapy, and NSAIDs are the cornerstones of treatment.

Reactive arthritis is an inflammatory rheumatic reaction to an infection remote from the joint space. The forms of reactive arthritis are listed in Table 1.

REITER'S SYNDROME

Reiter's syndrome is a seronegative (rheumatoid factor–negative) inflammatory arthritis involving primarily the ankles, knees, and feet. It is frequently asymmetric and is associated with urethritis or cervicitis, dysentery, inflammatory eye disease, and mucocutaneous diseases, including keratoderma blennorrhagica, balanitis circinata, and superficial ulcerations of the mucosa of the mouth [1]. Most patients with Reiter's syndrome have the histocompatibility antigen HLA-B27 and have had a specific gastrointestinal or genitourinary infection preceding the arthritis by 1 to 3 weeks [2,3]. Multiple gastrointestinal and genitourinary organisms have been incriminated as triggering agents. In the case of *Shigella flexneri* exposure, it has been estimated that approximately 20% of HLA-B27–positive persons will develop Reiter's syndrome compared with only 1.5% of the whole population [2].

Symptoms and Signs

Patients commonly complain of pain in their feet and heels when walking. When present, a helpful aid to diagnosis is the highly characteristic sausage appearance of the toes, known as dactylitis. This swelling extends well beyond the confines of the joint space and involves inflammation in enthesial tissue. Such swelling often is seen in the ankle. A less common characteristic is the rapid accumulation of synovial fluid; over 24 hours, a normal-appearing knee may accumulate 100 mL. A fraction of patients with Reiter's syndrome have spinal arthritis, which most commonly is isolated sacroiliitis but may progress to full-blow ankylosing spondylitis. The arthritis of Reiter's syndrome has typically been described as short lived, but many cases are remittent and intermittent or persistent. Articular destruction, however, is not common [4].

Inflammation involves both articular and extraarticular organs. The frequency of involvement of the latter is outlined in Table 2. Circinate balanitis on the glans penis or keratoderma blennorrhagica on the soles of the feet is almost always diagnostic of Reiter's syndrome.

TABLE 1 REACTIVE ARTHRITIS

Type	Characteristic
Reiter's syndrome	Asymmetric arthritis of knees, ankles, feet
Enteropathic arthritis	
Ulcerative colitis	Type 1 asymmetric arthritis of knee, ankle, hip, shoulder, wrist, elbow
Regional enteritis	Type 2 ankylosing spondylitis
Whipple's syndrome	Migratory arthritis of knees, ankles, fingers, wrists, shoulders, elbows
Bypass disease	Destructive migratory arthritis of knees, ankles, fingers
Acute rheumatic fever	Short-duration, intensely migratory, very painful arthritis beginning in the lower extremity
Poststreptococcal polyarthritis	Acute arthritis of rheumatic fever
Jaccoud's arthritis	Progressive deformity of the metacarpophalangeal joints after multiple attacks of rheumatic fever

Laboratory Studies

In the early stages of Reiter's syndrome, no specific diagnostic study is confirmatory. In most patients, the erythrocyte sedimentation rate (ESR) is elevated, and synovial fluid shows mild to moderate inflammation with no bacterial growth on routine cultures. Although 80% of Reiter's patients are HLA-B27 positive, this finding is of limited diagnostic help. Patients with persistent disease may have a hypochromic or normochromic normocytic anemia.

The radiographic characteristics of Reiter's syndrome are similar to those of ankylosing spondylitis and psoriatic arthritis. Characteristic changes include bony erosions with adjacent proliferation of bone and paravertebral ossification. Involvement of the interphalangeal joint of the great toe strongly suggests the diagnosis of Reiter's syndrome or psoriasis. Periostitis frequently is confused with osteomyelitis. Osseous proliferation of the calcaneus with a fluffy irregularity is also highly common.

Treatment

The multifactorial etiology of Reiter's syndrome has made therapeutic recommendations controversial. Because some Reiter's syndrome patients have disease triggered by *Chlamydia trachomatis* and because a chlamydial infection may be difficult to prove, an argument can be made to treat all patients with tetracycline or a tetracycline derivative. In one study, a 3-month treatment with tetracycline significantly decreased the duration of illness in reactive arthritis triggered by *C. trachomatis*.

The articular complaints of most patients are palliated by using nonsteroidal antiinflammatory drugs (NSAIDs). Many patients seem to respond best to indomethacin. Occasionally, short courses of prednisone, preferably in dosages of less than 15 mg/d, are useful. Persistent inflammation in a joint frequently responds to an injection of repository steroids. Patients with progressive joint disease recalcitrant to more conservative management or patients with systemic disease may need azathioprine or methotrexate [5]. Careful attention to physical therapy and range-of-motion exercises are important. Because there is some evidence that repeated exposure to venereal pathogens may exacerbate the disease or cause new attacks, sex education and counseling about safe sex are indicated.

TABLE 2 NONARTICULAR SYMPTOMS IN PATIENTS WITH REITER'S SYNDROME

Organ	Occurrence, %
Antecedent	
Urethritis or cervicitis	90
Diarrhea	18
Concomitant	
Eye disease	63
Back pain	72
Heel pain	56
Tendinitis	52
Balanitis	46
Stomatitis	27
Keratoderma	22
Nail lesions	6

ENTEROPATHIC ARTHRITIS

Enteropathic arthritis is associated with inflammatory bowel disease (ulcerative colitis and regional enteritis), Whipple's disease, and intestinal bypass surgery. The pathogenesis of enteropathic arthritis is unknown, but the most attractive hypothesis suggests that bacterial antigen (peptidoglycan), in association with bacterial lipopolysaccharide, accumulates in the joint, where immune mechanisms are activated. The joint does have an affinity for certain bacterial moieties, and evidence for intraarticular bacterial antigen and immune events has been documented for the enteropathic arthritides.

Inflammatory Bowel Disease

Ulcerative colitis and regional enteritis are associated with many rheumatic diseases (Table 3) [6,7]. Two arthritides are most important. Arthritis involving the appendicular skeleton is most common, usually following the onset of bowel symptoms. The activity of the arthritis often parallels that of the bowel disease. Two percent to 24% of patients with inflammatory bowel disease have such an arthritis. Inflammation usually involves only a few joints in attacks that persist from weeks to

TABLE 3 RHEUMATIC CONDITIONS REPORTED WITH INFLAMMATORY BOWEL DISEASE

Amyloidosis
Osteoarthritis
Rheumatic fever
Lumbar disk protrusion
Gout
Calcium pyrophosphate deposition disease
Psoriatic arthritis
Rheumatoid arthritis
Systemic lupus erythematosus
Discoid lupus erythematosus
Positive lupus erythematous cells
Pseudothrombophlebitis
Raynaud's phenomenon
Cryoglobulinemia
Scleroderma
Clubbing
Hypertrophic osteoarthropathy
Metabolic bone disease
Granulomatous synovitis
Granulomatous myositis
Granulomatous bone disease
Avascular necrosis of bone
Wegener's granulomatosis
Takayasu's disease
Cutaneous polyarteritis nodosa
Vasculitis myositis
Scleromalacia perforans
Common variable immunodeficiency with arthritis
Cryofibrinogenemia

From Utsinger and coworkers [16]; with permission.

months, rarely more than 5 months. The arthritis is usually asymmetrical, involving the large joints such as the knees, ankles, hips, shoulders, wrists, and elbows. Less commonly, the small joints of the hands and feet or temporomandibular joints are involved. Inflammation in the enthesial tissues of the heel, known as talalgia, is common. The arthritis tends to wax and wane, and articular damage is rare.

Laboratory findings are nonspecific and include an elevated ESR and C-reactive protein. Synovial fluid leukocyte counts, predominantly polymorphonuclear leukocytes, range from 4000 to 50,000 cells/mm^3. Radiographs show soft tissue swelling and periarticular osteoporosis; erosions are unusual [8].

The second most common arthritis associated with inflammatory bowel disease is ankylosing spondylitis. Ankylosing spondylitis complicates inflammatory bowel disease in 2% to 8% of cases. Inflammatory bowel disease patients who have the histocompatibility antigen HLA-B27 have a two hundredfold increased risk of ankylosing spondylitis but no increased risk of appendicular arthritis. Most patients with inflammatory bowel

disease have radiologic evidence of sacroiliitis without involvement of the lumbar spine. Patients with spondylitis and inflammatory bowel disease have symptoms identical to those of idiopathic ankylosing spondylitis: back pain, exacerbated by both sitting and standing, as well as pain at night. In striking contrast to peripheral arthritis, spondylitis activity is unrelated to the activity of bowel disease.

Laboratory studies are nonspecific. The ESR is normal or mildly elevated. Radiographs are indistinguishable from those of idiopathic ankylosing spondylitis and show bilateral symmetrical sacroiliac erosion, sclerosis, and spinal vertebral body erosions and syndesmophytes.

The spondylitis of inflammatory bowel disease does not respond well to any medical or surgical intervention. An important component of treatment is physical therapy emphasizing range-of-motion exercise. Patients with persistent pain may be treated with NSAIDs, of which indomethacin is often the most helpful. Some patients require corticosteroid treatment, and rarely a patient requires a single dose of radiation to palliate painful joints.

In contradistinction to axial skeletal inflammation, peripheral joint disease of inflammatory bowel disease responds well to antiinflammatory drug treatment. Recalcitrant disease may require prednisone or intraarticular injections of corticosteroids. A physical therapy program emphasizing range-of-motion and strengthening exercises is important. Surgical treatment of the underlying bowel disease promptly induces a remission, and colectomy in ulcerative colitis often results in complete remission of an associated arthritis.

Whipple's Disease

Whipple's disease is a chronic bowel disease characterized by diarrhea, weight loss, arthritis, and intestinal fat infiltration with characteristic periodic acid–Schiff (PAS) staining on histopathology [9]. Arthritis is commonly the presenting manifestation. It is frequently migratory, and in contrast to the arthritis of inflammatory bowel disease, there is no relationship to intestinal symptoms. As in inflammatory bowel disease, both sacroiliitis and ankylosing spondylitis may also be seen.

The diagnosis of Whipple's disease may be suggested by PAS-positive material in synovial fluid or in a biopsy specimen. Prolonged therapy with penicillin (500 mg four times per day), tetracycline (500 mg four times per day), or erythromycin (500 mg four times per day) frequently effects a dramatic resolution of all symptoms.

Bypass Disease

Bypass disease refers to a polysystemic illness involving primarily the joints and skin after intestinal bypass surgery (Tables 4 and 5). Arthritis usually develops within 1 year after the bypass procedure and may be either short lived or chronic; in some patients, it is lifelong [8]. It is more common in women, involves knees, ankles, fingers, wrists, shoulders, and elbows, and is nondestructive. The dermatitis consists of papulopustular eruptions strongly resembling Sweet's syndrome. Some patients have responded to short courses of tetracycline or metronidazole with decreased joint pain. NSAIDs and prednisone have also been helpful for

TABLE 4 RHEUMATIC COMPLICATIONS OF BOWEL BYPASS

Inflammatory polyarthritis	Myalgias
Tenosynovitis	Oral ulceration
Pleuritis	Superficial phlebitis
Pericarditis	Rheumatoid arthritis
Raynaud's phenomenon	Polymyositis
Paresthesias	Septic arthritis

From Clarke and coworkers [17]; with permission.

TABLE 5 CUTANEOUS MANIFESTATIONS OF BOWEL BYPASS

Macule
Pustules
Nodule
Liquefying nodule
Urticaria
Ecchymoses

From Clarke and coworkers [17]; with permission.

some patients. Reversal of the bypass procedure eliminates the arthritis and improves or eliminates the skin lesions.

ACUTE RHEUMATIC FEVER

Acute rheumatic fever is a polysystemic disease that follows an untreated or inadequately treated case of Group A, beta-hemolytic streptococcal pharyngitis [10]. The sequelae of rheumatic fever are a consequence of the immune response to the streptococcal infection [11–14]. The response occurs in approximately 3% of cases of untreated streptococcal pharyngitis. Patients who have had a prior episode of rheumatic heart disease have a 50% chance of a subsequent second episode of rheumatic fever if they do not follow a prophylactic regimen.

The arthritis of rheumatic fever is highly typical, involving several joints in rapid succession, each joint being inflamed for only a short time. Large joints are affected; usually lower extremity joints are involved before those of the upper extremity. The arthritis itself is characteristically very painful but persists for less than 7 days. On examination, the affected joints are tender, with limited motion but without striking swelling, redness, or heat. The arthritis usually remits completely after 3 weeks in an untreated patient.

Adults developing arthritis after having untreated Group A, β-hemolytic streptococcal pharyngitis rarely have extraarticular features and consequently do not fulfill Jones' criteria. They are said to have poststreptococcal polyarthritis. Jaccoud's arthritis is a rare, slowly progressive deformity of the metacarpophalangeal joints evolving after multiple severe and prolonged attacks of rheumatic fever [15]. On examination, there is ulnar deviation of the fingers and flexion of the metacarpophalangeal joints with hyperextension of the proximal phalangeal joints. There is no pain or sign of inflammation. Similar changes may involve the metatarsophalangeal and interphalangeal joints. Hand function remains excellent. Radiographs show characteristic hook-like osteophytes of the metacarpophalangeal joints.

The arthritis of acute rheumatic fever and poststreptococcal arthritis in the adult are characterized by a rapid response to aspirin (40 mg/lb/d for 2 wk, followed by 20 mg/lb/d for 4–6 wk). In patients with cardiomegaly, using aspirin may not be adequate to control symptoms or signs of congestive heart failure. These patients should be treated with corticosteroids (prednisone, 40–60 mg/d), but there is no evidence that corticosteroid treatment prevents the development of valvular heart disease. A patient with extremely severe rheumatic fever should be treated with intravenous methylprednisolone (40 mg/d). Both corticosteroids and salicylates can be tapered after 3 to 4 weeks of treatment. All patients with rheumatic fever and poststreptococcal arthritis should receive monthly injections of 1.2 MU of benzathine penicillin. Lifelong prophylaxis is indicated if they have rheumatic heart disease.

REFERENCES AND RECOMMENDED READING

Recently published papers of particular interest have been highlighted as:

• Of interest

•• Of outstanding interest

1. Paronen I: Reiter's disease: a study of 344 cases observed in Finland. *Acta Med Scand* 1948, 212(suppl):1–114.

2. Calin A, Fries JF: An "experimental" epidemic of Reiter's disease. *Ann Intern Med* 1976, 84:564–566.

3. Lerisalo M, Skyly G, Kousa M: Follow-up study on patients with Reiter's disease and reactive arthritis with special reference to HLA-B27. *Arthritis Rheum* 1985, 25:249–259.

4. Fox R, Cahn A, Gerber R: The chronicity of symptoms and disability in Reiter's syndrome: an analysis of 131 consecutive patients. *Ann Intern Med* 1979, 91:190–193.

5. Owen ET, Cohen ML: Methotrexate in Reiter's disease. *Ann Rheum Dis* 1979, 38:48–50.

6. Wright V: Seronegative polyarthritis: a unified concept. *Arthritis Rheum* 1978, 21:619–632.

7. Moll JMH: Inflammatory bowel disease. *Clin Rheum Dis* 1985, 11:87–111.

8. Utsinger PD: Systemic immune complex disease following intestinal bypass surgery: bypass disease. *J Am Acad Dermatol* 1980, 2:488–495.

9. Weiner SR, Utsinger P: Whipple's disease. *Sem Arthritis Rheum* 1986, 15:157–167.

10. Scholin J, Wesstrom G: Acute rheumatic fever in Swedish children, 1971–80. *Acta Pediatr Scand* 1985, 74:749–754.

11. Read SE, Reid SFM, Fischetti VA, *et al.*: Serial studies on the cellular immune response to streptococcal antigens in acute and convalescent rheumatic fever patients in Trinidad. *J Clin Immunol* 1986, 6:433–441.

12. Murray GC, Monteil MM, Persellin RH: A study of HLA antigens in adults with acute rheumatic fever. *Arthritis Rheum* 1978, 21:652–656.

13. Yoshinoya S, Pope RM: Detection of immune complexes in acute rheumatic fever and their relationship to HLA-B5. *J Clin Invest* 1980, 65:136–145.

14. Ayoub EM, Barrett DJ, Maclaren NK, *et al.*: Association of class II human histocompatibility leukocyte antigens with rheumatic fever. *J Clin Invest* 1986, 77:2019–2020.

15. Girgis FL, Popple AW, Bruckner FE: Jaccoud's arthropathy. *Ann Rheum Dis* 1978, 37:561–565.

16. Utsinger PD, Spalding D, Weiner SR, Clarke J: Intestinal immunology and rheumatic disease: inflammatory bowel disease and intestinal bypass arthropathy. In *Infections in the Rheumatic Disease*. Grune and Stratton; 1988: 317–343.

17. Clarke J, Weiner SR, Bassett LW, Utsinger PD: Bypass disease: clinical and experimental. *Rheumatology* 1987, 15:275–287.

SELECT BIBLIOGRAPHY

Espinozu L, Goldenberg D, Arnett A, Alaron G, eds.: *Infections in the Rheumatic Disease*, part IV. Grune and Stratton; 1988.

Espinozu L, ed.: *Rheumatic Disease Clinics of North America*. Philadelphia: WB Saunders Co.; 1991.

Wright V, Moll JMM, eds.: *Seronegative Polyarthritis*. North Molland Biomedical Press; 1976.

Arthritis Associated with Skin Disease 10

Joan M. Von Feldt
Victoria P. Werth
Monica Luchi
H. Ralph Schumacher Jr.

Key Points

- Skin lesions often can be an important clue in diagnosing an inflammatory arthritis.

- Histologic examination of skin lesions with careful attention to vessels, fascia, and deep fat is frequently necessary to help make a diagnosis of systemic disease causing inflammatory arthritis.

- The constellation of constitutional symptoms is frequently a clue to diagnosis, but there are rarely specific laboratory findings for these illnesses.

- Treatment of the skin disease frequently ameliorates the arthritis.

- Skin lesions associated with arthritis are treated with topical and systemic steroids, but occasionally immunomodulatory and cytotoxic medications are required.

Various systemic diseases often present with cutaneous lesions and arthritis. Table 1 lists some such diseases. This review focuses on a group of primary skin diseases that also may be associated with arthritis. In many instances, the skin disease is an important clue to underlying disease, such as malignancy or autoimmune disease. In many instances, the pathogenetic mechanisms of both skin and joint diseases are similar. The generalist can play a critical role in recognizing these skin-joint associations, delineating other potential systemic features, and referring refractory cases for specialty care.

PSORIASIS

Psoriasis is a common condition involving the cutaneous vasculature and the epidermis. Morphology varies, but the lesions have four prominent features: 1) they have sharply demarcated borders, 2) the surface consists of adherent silver-white scales, 3) under the scales, the skin has a glossy homogeneous erythema, and 4) the lesions exhibit the Auspitz sign; that is, when the hyperkeratotic scales are scratched from the plaque, small blood droplets appear on the erythematous surface within a few seconds. This sign is specific for plaque-type psoriasis and is absent from inverse and pustular psoriasis (Fig. 1B).

Patients with psoriasis are three times more likely to develop arthritis than are healthy persons; men and women are equally affected. The most common type of psoriasis, the patch-plaque pattern (Fig. 1), is also the most common lesion associated with psoriatic arthritis. The skin disease usually precedes the arthritis, but it follows joint involvement in as many as 20% of patients. Nail changes (Fig. 1C) have been reported to be more frequent in psoriatic patients with psoriatic arthritis. In a recent study, however, nail changes were seen in only 50% of psoriatic arthritis patients, the same as in patients with uncomplicated psoriasis [1].

TABLE 1 RHEUMATIC DISEASES WITH PROMINENT SKIN MANIFESTATIONS

Reiter's syndrome
Lyme disease
Sarcoidosis
Rheumatic fever
Rheumatoid arthritis
Systemic lupus erythematosus
Dermatomyositis
Still's disease
Antiphospholipid syndrome
Eosinophilic fasciitis
Lymphoma and leukemia
Behçet's disease
Amyloidosis
Scleroderma
Plasma cell dyscrasia with polyneuropathy, organomegaly, endocrinopathy monoclonal protein, and skin changes (POEM's syndrome)
Wegener's granulomatosis
Septic vasculitis
   Disseminated gonococcemia
   Chronic meningococcemia

Psoriatic arthritis is classified into five broad categories: oligoarthritis, symmetric polyarthritis, distal arthritis, spondyloarthropathy, and arthritis mutilans. All forms of peripheral arthritis are erosive; however, the erosions are distinct from those of rheumatoid arthritis. In psoriatic arthritis, there is frequently less osteoporosis of adjacent bone and evidence of repair at the erosion site with prominent osteophyte formation (Fig. 1D)

The most common pattern of disease is an asymmetric oligoarthritis, accounting for more than 70% of all patients with psoriatic arthritis. Periostitis may occur, and there may be diffuse sausage-like swelling of digits (dactylitis). Symmetric polyarthritis, which is clinically indistinguishable from rheumatoid arthritis, is seen in 15% of psoriatic arthritis patients. These patients lack serum rheumatoid factor or rheumatoid nodules, which are present in rheumatoid arthritis. Classic psoriatic arthritis, in which the distal interphalangeal joints are predominantly involved, accounts for fewer than 5% of psoriatic arthritis cases, although distal interphalangeal joint involvement frequently accompanies any of the other forms of psoriatic arthritis. A spondyloarthropathy resembling ankylosing spondylitis predominates in fewer than 5% of patients, although spondylitis has been reported to occur in 20% to 40% of psoriatic patients with peripheral joint involvement. Syndesmophytes in psoriatic arthritis may be nonmarginal and asymmetrical, suggesting this diagnosis. Arthritis mutilans, a severely destructive process that can cause

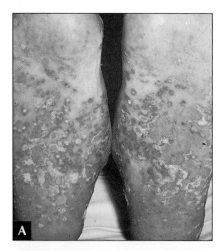

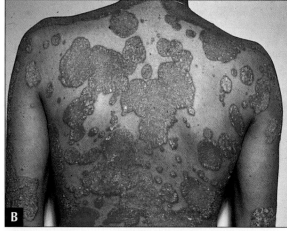

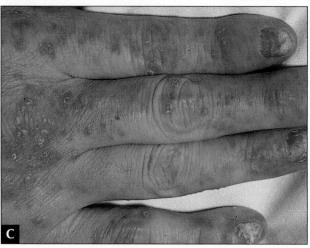

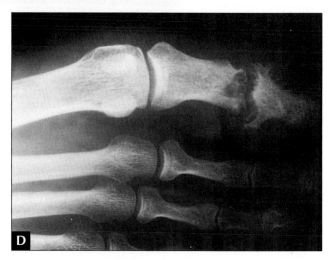

FIGURE 1 Psoriatic arthritis. **A**, Plantar pustular psoriasis. **B**, Patch-plaque pattern of psoriasis. **C**, Psoriatic lesions in a patient with distal interphalangeal arthritis and nail changes characteristic of psoriatic arthritis. **D**, Erosions of psoriatic arthritis in the interphalangeal joint of the great toe.

dissolution of phalanges, occurs in 5% of psoriatic arthritis patients. It occurs more often in patients with greater skin involvement or pustular psoriasis and in younger patients [1].

Although psoriatic arthritis is common, other arthritides can occur in psoriatic patients. Coexistence of psoriasis and seropositive rheumatoid arthritis has been documented. The frequency of psoriasis in patients with ulcerative colitis is 3.8 times greater than that in the general population; in Crohn's disease, it is 7.6 times greater [2••]. Serum uric acid is increased in one third to one half of psoriatic patients; this finding is attributed to the epidermal cell proliferation in psoriatic plaques with subsequent breakdown of nucleic acids. Gout is more common in this patient population [2••].

Treatment of psoriatic arthritis should be directed toward both skin and joint lesions. Topical treatment of the skin condition may ameliorate the peripheral arthritis. Management also includes the use of nonsteroidal antiinflammatory drugs (NSAIDs) and occupational and physical therapy [3]. Slow-acting antirheumatic drugs are usually selected for their effectiveness on both the peripheral arthritis and the psoriasis. Tables 2 and 3 highlight some of these medications and their effectiveness. Joint replacement, especially knee and hip surgery, is a useful adjunct to treat psoriatic arthritis patients. However, surgical treatment through actively diseased skin increases the risk of infection and should be avoided. Patients with uncontrolled psoriatic arthritis should be referred to a rheumatologist [3].

ACNE, HIDRADENITIS, AND RELATED SYNDROMES

Arthritis has been reported with severe acne for more than 30 years. The arthritis tends to follow the activity of the skin disease but has been reported in patients with quiescent skin lesions. Tables 4 and 5 summarize the associated findings and treatment.

The arthritis associated with acne conglobata affects large peripheral joints and is frequently episodic; many patients have associated enthesitis (inflammation of tendon insertions into bone), chest wall involvement, and sacroiliitis [4••].

Acne fulminans is a rare, acute systemic illness, presenting with highly inflammatory lesions associated with fever, weight loss, arthritis, and painful bone lesions; it is frequently seen in teen-aged boys with acne vulgaris (Fig. 2A). In a review of 41 patients, 39% had painful bone lesions, 33% had arthritis, usually of the knees, hips, or ankles, and 21% had sacroiliitis [4••,5].

Hidradenitis suppurativa is a chronic inflammatory condition of the skin and subcutaneous tissue of the axilla, groin, and perianal area. The apocrine sweat glands become occluded, with subsequent dilatation and secondary infection. The arthritis associated with hidradenitis suppurativa usually occurs in an asymmetric peripheral pattern, occasionally with axial disease (Fig. 2B).

When acne conglobata and hidradenitis suppurativa occur together along with dissecting cellulitis of the scalp, follicular occlusion triad results [5]. The arthritis accompanying this disorder is similar to that which accompanies the other skin conditions.

The acronym *SAPHO* describes the association of synovitis, acne, pustulosis, hyperostosis, and osteitis [6]. SAPHO syndrome is rarely seen in patients older than 60 years of age but occurs in children as well. The syndrome includes the sterile osteitis that is sometimes neglected in association with acne. The osteitis can be seen anywhere but most frequently involves the anterior chest wall.

TABLE 2 TREATMENT OF PSORIASIS		
Medication	**Effectiveness**	**Comments**
Topical corticosteroids	Widespread use, frequently successful	Disease can rebound after stopping medication; not recommended as isolated treatment for widespread disease
Anthralin	Benefit proven in controlled trials	Can cause straining and irritation of skin; therefore, strength and length of time of application must be individually titrated
Tar	Widespread use, frequently successful	Not useful as solitary agent; usually used with ultraviolet B light in Goeckerman regimen
Phototherapy	Widespread use, frequently successful	Ultraviolet B light therapy causes less long-term toxicity (aging of skin and risk of skin cancer) than does therapy with psoralen and ultraviolet A light
Etretinate	Benefit proven in controlled trials	Can be used with phototherapy to enhance efficacy
Methotrexate	Widespread use, frequently successful	Requires monitoring of liver function (including liver biopsy) for adverse side effects, with a frequency much greater than that in rheumatoid arthritis
Hydroxyurea	Preliminary studies report benefit in small groups of patients	Can be used with caution with underlying liver disease
Cyclosporine	Benefit proven in controlled trials	Effective treatment, but the disease recurs if medication is stopped
Topical vitamin D	Benefit proven in controlled trials	Systemic absorption limits skin area; face and intertriginous areas should be avoided.

TABLE 3 TREATMENT OF PSORIATIC ARTHRITIS

Medication	Effectiveness	Comments
Intra-articular corticosteroids	Widespread use, frequently successful	Contraindicated if psoriatic plaques overlie the joint because plaques can harbor pathogenic bacteria
Methotrexate	Widespread use, frequently successful	Most common medication to treat polyarticular disease; because of the risk of cirrhosis, requires monitoring of liver function (including liver biopsy), with a frequency much greater than that in rheumatoid arthritis
Nonsteroidal anti-inflammatory drugs	Widespread use, frequently successful	
Gold (parenteral)	Preliminary studies report benefit in small groups of patients	
Etretinate	Preliminary studies report benefit in small groups of patients	
Sulfasalazine	Benefit proven in controlled studies	Treatment of choice for inflammatory bowel disease that can accompany psoriasis
Penicillamine		
Cyclosporine	Preliminary studies report benefit in small groups of patients	Side effects preclude widespread use
Polyunsaturated ethyl ester lipids	Preliminary studies report benefit in small groups of patients	
High-dose 1,25-dihydroxyvitamin D_3	Preliminary studies report benefit in small groups of patients	
Antimalarial drugs	Avoid or use with caution	May exacerbate psoriasis
Oral corticosteroids	Avoid or use with caution	The high doses needed for arthritis can produce erythroderma and exacerbate skin condition
Azathioprine	Avoid or use with caution	Does not work well for psoriasis

Various medications that have been used to treat the acne syndromes are listed in Table 4. Retinoic acid therapies may themselves cause periostitis, especially in patients treated continuously for several years or with dosages greater than 2 mg/kg/d [4••].

PUSTULOSIS PALMARIS ET PLANTARIS

Pustulosis palmaris et plantaris is a rare chronic, relapsing pustular eruption of the palms and soles that is associated with chronic recurrent multifocal osteomyelitis and sternocosto-clavicular hyperostosis. Skin lesions are often symmetric 1- to 2-mm vesicles or pustules located on the thenar and hypothenar eminences of the hand and the instep of the foot (Fig. 3). The lesions resolve within 2 weeks. Differentiation of skin lesions from pustular psoriasis may be difficult. The sterile osteomyelitis generally begins with an insidious pain and swelling of the affected bones, most commonly at the medial ends of the clavicles and the distal metaphyses of long bones. It usually occurs in children and young adults and affects women more than men. Diagnosis is suggested by radiographs showing lytic lesions with sclerotic rims adjacent to the growth plate in the acute stage and dense sclerosis in the chronic stage. Bone scans are more sensitive than radiography in early detection. Laboratory tests show a mild leukocytosis and elevated sedimentation rate. Rare complications include premature closure of the epiphyses, bony growth abnormalities, and thoracic outlet syndrome. Recurrent exacerbations occur over months to years. Treatment with oral glucocorticoids is effective symptomatically, but relapse is common after stopping the drug [7]. Treatment attempts with antibiotics have had varied results.

PYODERMA GANGRENOSUM

Pyoderma gangrenosum is an ulcerative skin condition frequently associated with underlying systemic diseases. It is most often seen in patients with inflammatory bowel disease, many of whom have concomitant arthritis. Other associated conditions include rheumatoid arthritis, various hematologic malignancies, and monoclonal gammopathies. It has been reported in patients with systemic lupus erythematosus and Behçet's disease [8,9]. The course of the skin disease can be independent of associated bowel disease or arthritis.

Ulcers first present as painful nodules or pustules that break down to produce a painful, rapidly destructive, burrowing ulcer with surrounding erythema (Fig. 4). The lesions can be solitary or multiple and are most commonly found on the legs. Healing of the ulcers frequently results in atrophic, cribriform scars.

Many of the underlying illnesses associated with pyoderma gangrenosum can have other causes of leg ulcers, including infection, vasculitis, venous stasis, arterial insufficiency, and

TABLE 4 ACNE, HIDRADENITIS, AND RELATED SYNDROMES

Type of acne	Description	Distribution	Treatment	Associated musculoskeletal syndrome
Acne vulgaris	Inflammatory disease of pilosebaceous follicle	Face, neck, upper torso	Intralesional steroids Systemic antibiotics Benzoyl peroxide Retinoic acid Isotretinoin Débridement of lesions Topical antibiotics	— Absent
Acne conglobata	Suppurative, cystic lesions, interconnecting sinuses, scar formation	Buttocks, thighs, upper arms, face, neck, upper torso	Intralesional steroids Systemic antibiotics Benzoyl peroxide Retinoic acid Isotretinoin Débridement of lesions	Present
Acne fulminans	Inflamed, ulcerating lesions, with systemic signs of fever, weight loss	Back, chest, face	Tetracycline or erythromycin, 2 g/d Systemic corticosteroids for 5–7	Present
Hidradenitis suppurativa	Occlusion of the apocrine sweat glands with dilatation and secondary infection	Axilla, groin, perianal area	Same as for acne vulgaris plus oral antibiotics Surgical excision of apocrine glands	Present
Follicular occlusion triad	The combination of hidradenitis suppurativa, acne conglobata, and dissecting cellulitis of the scalp occur		Same as for acne conglobata and hidradenitis suppurativa	Present

TABLE 5 CLINICAL MUSCULOSKELETAL MANIFESTATIONS OF ACNE SYNDROMES

	Acne conglobata	Acne fulminans	Hidradenitis suppurativa	Isotretinoin treatment manifestations
Gender (female vs male)	1:4	1:37	1:1	1:1
Race	Black	White	Black	Any
Laboratory	Elevated ESR, elevated leukocyte count Anemia Abnormal delayed-type hypersensitivity responses	Elevated ESR, elevated leukocyte count Anemia Abnormal delayed-type hypersensitivity responses	Elevated ESR	Elevated triglyceride count
Constitutional symptoms	Absent	Present	Absent	Absent
Myositis	Absent	Present	Absent	Absent
Painful lytic bone lesions	Absent	Present	Absent	Absent
Arthralgias and myalgias	Present	Present	Present	Present
Skeletal hyperostosis	Absent	Absent	Absent	Present
Arthritis	Present	Present	Present	—

ESR—erythrocyte sedimentation rate.

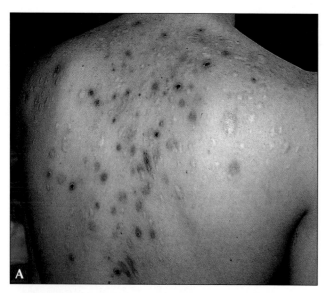

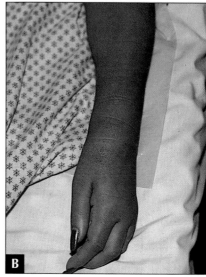

FIGURE 2
Acne-arthritis syndrome. **A**, Acne fulminans in a patient with associated arthritis. **B**, Arthritis of wrist in a patient with hidradenitis suppurativa.

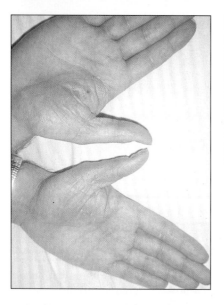

FIGURE 3
Pustulosis palmaris. Symmetric 1- to 2-mm vesicles located on the thenar and hypothenar eminences of the hand.

antiphospholipid antibody–associated thrombosis. The diagnosis is mainly one of exclusion, owing to the absence of unique features.

Treatment of pyoderma gangrenosum requires management of any underlying illness. Systemic drug therapy with corticosteroids, sulfones, and immunosuppressants, either alone or in combination, is usually required. There have been reports of successful treatment with hyperbaric oxygen therapy and cyclosporine.

PANNICULITIS

Panniculitis (Table 6) is represented by deep, nodular lesions resulting from inflammation in subcutaneous fat. The causes of panniculitis include entities that can only be differentiated by a deep biopsy of the skin, for which it is important to obtain a large amount of fat. In panniculitides with substantial fat

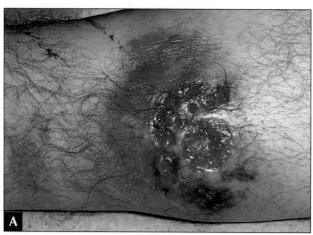

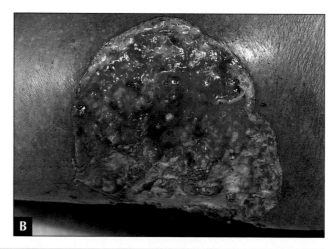

FIGURE 4 Pyoderma gangrenosum. **A**, Classic lesion in a patient with associated Crohn's disease and oligoarthritis. **B**, Lesion associated with systemic lupus erythematosus.

TABLE 6 CLASSIFICATION OF PANNICULITIS

Lobular panniculitis
Without vasculitis
  Idiopathic lobular panniculitis
    Weber-Christian panniculitis
    Rothmann-Makai panniculitis
    Histiocytic cytophagous panniculitis
  α_1-antitrypsin deficiency panniculitis
  Physical panniculitis
    Cold
    Traumatic
    Chemical
    Factitial (self-induced)
  Neonatal panniculitis
    Sclerema neonatorum
    Neonatal subcutaneous fat necrosis
  Poststeroid panniculitis
  Pancreatic panniculitis
With vasculitis
  Nodular vasculitis (erythema induratum)
  Lupus profundus
Associated with systemic disease
  Lupus erythematosus
  Sarcoidosis
  Calcifying panniculitis of renal failure (calciphylaxis)
  Lymphoma and leukemia
  Infection

Septal panniculitis
Without vasculitis
  Erythema nodosum
    Acute
    Chronic
  Scleroderma panniculitis
  Eosinophilic fasciitis
  Eosinophilia myalgia syndrome
  Necrobiosis lipoidica diabeticorum
With vasculitis
  Superficial migratory thrombophlebitis
  Polyarteritis nodosa
  Cutaneous polyarteritis nodosa

TABLE 7 CAUSES OF ERYTHEMA NODOSUM

Infections
  Streptococcus
  Yersinia
  Tuberculosis
  Coccidioidomycosis
  Histoplasmosis
  Blastomycosis
  Chlamydia
  Cytomegalovirus
  Cat scratch disease
  Neisseria gonorrhoeae
Drugs
  Sulfonamides
  Estrogen
  Oral contraceptives
Inflammatory diseases
  Inflammatory bowel disease
  Behçet's syndrome
  Sarcoidosis
Pregnancy

are ill-defined, erythematous, tender nodules on the anterior lower legs, sometimes associated with fever, malaise, and arthralgias (Fig. 5A). Nodules can be seen in other areas as well. Women are more frequently affected, and lesions gradually resolve without scarring over 3 to 6 weeks. Lofgren's syndrome is an acute presentation of sarcoidosis with fever, cough, arthralgias or arthritis, especially of the ankles, erythema nodosum, and bilateral hilar adenopathy. Similar findings may be seen with some pulmonary infections.

Helpful laboratory evaluation includes chest radiography, complete blood count, urinalysis, throat culture, antistreptolysin O titer, and intradermal skin tests for tuberculosis, coccidioidomycosis, blastomycosis, and histoplasmosis. Treatment of an underlying infection or removal of a causative medication should be the first line of therapy. Additional treatment includes rest, NSAIDs, oral potassium iodide, or systemic corticosteroids, if needed.

Weber-Christian Disease

Weber-Christian disease is a term used for idiopathic lobular panniculitis. It is seen especially in young to middle-aged women and is characterized by recurrent crops of erythematous nodules and plaques over the lower extremities but also on the arms, torso, face, breasts, and buttocks (Figs. 5B–D). The lesions regress over the course of several weeks, leaving a hyperpigmented depression. Development of skin lesions can be associated with fever, malaise, nausea, vomiting, abdominal pain, weight loss, hepatomegaly, and arthralgias. Systemic involvement of the mesentery, heart, lungs, kidneys, liver, spleen, adrenal glands, bone marrow, and central nervous system can occur. Painful osteolytic lesions have been reported. The prognosis is usually good, with gradual spontaneous reso-

necrosis, an elliptic excision is essential [10••]. The biopsy allows for classification of the condition into lobular or septal panniculitis, or both, with or without vasculitis. The diagnosis requires the expertise of a seasoned dermatopathologist because these conditions are rare. Any panniculitis other than erythema nodosum should be managed with the help of a specialist.

Erythema Nodosum

Erythema nodosum is considered a hypersensitivity reaction to one of several factors and is the most common form of panniculitis. A specific cause can be found approximately 50% of the time (Table 7). Clinically, the most common findings

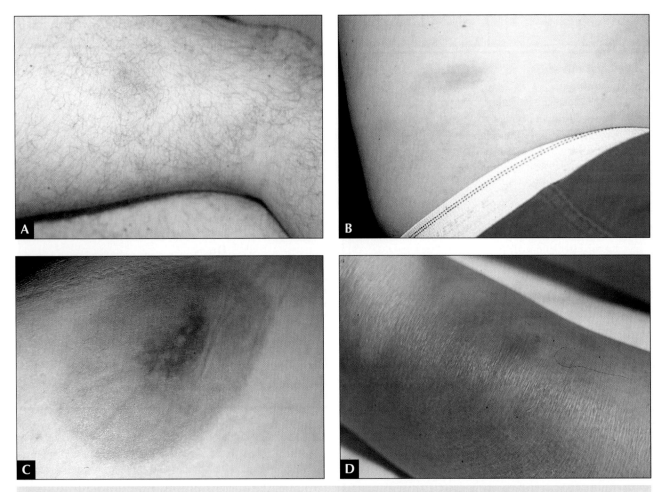

FIGURE 5 **A**, Erythema nodosum in a patient with sarcoidosis. **B** and **C**, Nodules caused by Weber-Christian panniculitis, demonstrating acute phase lesions. **D**, Area of hyperpigmentation, demonstrating the resolution phase.

lution of the attacks, but deaths have occurred because of sepsis, hepatic failure, hemorrhage, and thrombosis.

Laboratory findings are not specific and include an elevated erythrocyte sedimentation rate, leukopenia or leukocytosis, anemia, hypocomplementemia, and circulating immune complexes. Treatment options include NSAIDs, tetracycline, chloroquine, prednisone, cytotoxic agents, cyclosporine, and, for a woman without childbearing potential, thalidomide, if available.

α_1-Antitrypsin Deficiency Panniculitis

α_1-Antitrypsin deficiency panniculitis is caused by decreased levels of serine protease inhibitors and has a different clinical picture than does the panniculitis of Weber-Christian disease in that patients have multiple painful subcutaneous nodules that may ulcerate and drain. An α_1-antitrypsin level should be determined to rule out a deficiency. Relatives of affected patients should be screened. Treatment includes avoiding trauma, cigarettes, and alcohol. Dapsone, prednisone, and α_1 proteinase inhibitor have been used for therapy.

Histiocytic Cytophagic Panniculitis

Histiocytic cytophagic panniculitis is a rare variant of Weber-Christian disease characterized by multiple, recurrent, large,

tender nodules that are 2 to 10 cm in size and associated with systemic illness. The nodules can coalesce and become ecchymotic. The illness has a febrile, progressive course accompanied by hepatosplenomegaly, liver function abnormalities, and pancytopenia. Hemorrhagic death can occur secondary to hepatic failure and disseminated intravascular coagulation [11]. Splenectomy induces a short-lived remission, but recently there have been reports of success with combination chemotherapy.

Pancreatic Panniculitis

Pancreatic panniculitis is seen with several diseases of the pancreas, most often pancreatitis or carcinoma.

Of patients with carcinoma, 84% have had acinar cell carcinoma, and only 16% have had adenocarcinoma. The skin is characterized by erythematous nodules usually located on the lower legs but also seen in other areas (Fig. 6). Healing occurs with some scarring and hyperpigmentation. The skin lesions are often associated with arthralgias, especially in the ankles. Arthritis and bursitis caused by fat necrosis occur in as many as 60% of cases, and fever, osteolytic bone lesions, pleuritis, and pericarditis may occur. Fat necrosis appears to result from liberation of pancreatic enzymes and free fatty acids into the circulation and lymphatics [12]. Laboratory evaluation should include assessment of serum amylase and lipase levels because

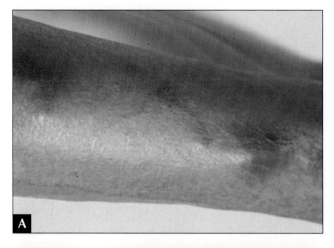

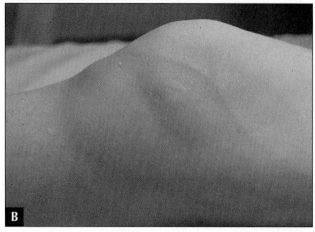

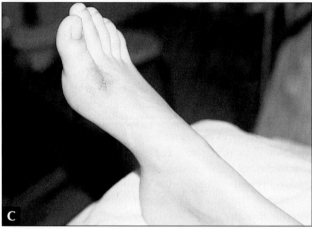

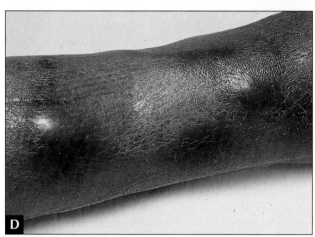

Figure 6 Pancreatic panniculitis. **A**, Skin lesions in a patient with pancreatitis. **B**, Prepatellar bursitis associated with pancreatic fat necrosis. **C**, Nodule over metatarsal phalangeal joint of great toe in pancreatitis associated with arthritis. **D**, Erythematous nodules with edema caused by pancreatic fat necrosis.

pancreatic disease is often clinically silent. Skin or synovial biopsy specimens show characteristic areas of fat necrosis. Basophilic deposits of calcium may be seen. Synovial fluid can be opalescent with lipid droplets. If the biopsy specimen is consistent with pancreatic panniculitis, computed tomography or magnetic resonance imaging of the pancreas is important. Skin and joint disease can be the first clue to pancreatic disease. Treatment of the underlying disease is the key in treating this disorder. Panniculitis also has been described in other rheumatic conditions associated with arthritis, including gout, giant cell arteritis, and familial Mediterranean fever [13].

SWEET'S SYNDROME

Sweet's syndrome, also known as acute febrile neutrophilic dermatosis, is seen most frequently in middle-aged women and is characterized by four cardinal features: fever, leukocytosis, tender red plaques, and specific histologic characteristics of a papillary dermal infiltrate of mature neutrophils and dermal edema.

The typical skin lesion is a red, sharply demarcated plaque formed by inflammatory bluish-red papules that tend to coalesce as an irregular lesion. Although solid, the lesion often has a vesicular appearance because of pronounced inflammatory

edema. There may be one lesion or many, usually asymmetrically distributed on the face, neck, and upper extremities (Fig. 7). Less commonly, lesions are found on the mucous membranes, lower extremities, or torso. The eruption tends to enlarge over several days or weeks, then resolves without scarring after weeks or months [14•]. Other common associated symptoms include myalgias, arthralgias and arthritis, iridocyclitis, and oral and genital ulcerations. Common laboratory abnormalities include an elevated sedimentation rate (> 30 mm/h), mildly elevated alkaline phosphatase levels, and transient increases in aspartate transferase and γ glutamyl transferase levels. Renal function usually remains within normal limits.

Joint symptoms range widely in severity, occurring in approximately 20% to 25% of cases and usually involving the hands, wrists, ankles, knees, and occasionally the metatarsophalangeal joints. Although the time course varies, articular changes are acute and transient, without chronicity [15].

Because of its high rate of association with coexisting conditions, Sweet's syndrome is thought to be a cutaneous marker of systemic disease [14•]. Typically, both the systemic symptoms and the skin lesions respond quickly to high doses of oral steroids. Untreated cases may remain active for months, and the skin lesions recur in approximately one third of patients.

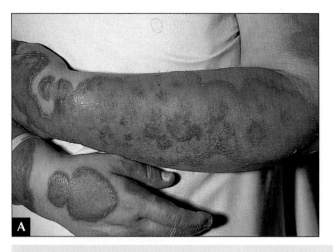

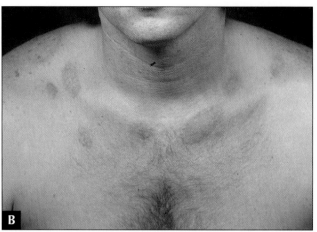

FIGURE 7 **A** and **B**, Sweet's syndrome. Typical erythematous, sharply demarcated lesions that coalesced to form large plaques in a patient with associated arthritis.

SCLEROMYXEDEMA

Scleromyxedema is a rare but distinctive cutaneous disease. Also called papular mucinosis or lichen myxedematosus, scleromyxedema is characterized by widespread waxy papular lesions and infiltrated plaques, often with induration of the skin of the hands, arms, face, torso, and legs [16,17]. This disease may be confused with scleroderma. Although skin lesions may be the sole manifestation, scleromyxedema also may be associated with various systemic features, including monoclonal gammopathy, esophageal dysmotility, Raynaud's phenomenon, telangiectasia, vascular disease, neurologic disease, decreased pulmonary diffusing capacity, and thyroid disease. These systemic findings may influence the confusion with scleroderma, but pathologic findings distinguish scleromyxedema from scleroderma.

Skin biopsy specimens show accumulation of acid mucopolysaccharides, identifiable with Alcian blue or colloidal iron stains, and large stellate or fusiform fibroblasts associated with increased and irregular bundles of collagen.

The most common musculoskeletal manifestation is a myopathy that has been reported in approximately 20 cases [17]. Most cases have the characteristic lambda-type monoclonal gammopathy. Arthritis, occasionally with erosions, carpal tunnel syndrome, and Sjögren's syndrome have been reported. There is no well-established effective therapy. Corticosteroids may be beneficial for the myopathy. Spontaneous remissions may occur. Multiple myeloma, Waldenström's disease, and lymphoma have been reported associations with cytotoxic therapy.

MULTICENTRIC RETICULOHISTIOCYTOSIS

Multicentric reticulohistiocytosis is an uncommon systemic disorder characterized by both severe mutilating polyarthritis and bead-like, copper-colored cutaneous nodules that typically begin on the hands and face. A crescent distribution around the nails is a classic virtually diagnostic presentation (Fig. 8*A*) [18]. Multicentric reticulohistiocytosis is also called lipoid dermatoarthritis, reticulohistocytosis, and normocholes-

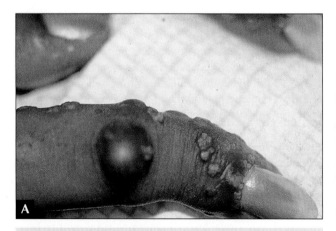

FIGURE 8 Multicentric reticulohistiocytosis. **A**, Classic crescent distribution of lesions around the nails. **B**, Arthropathy in the distal interphalangeal joints in a patient with a rapid lysis of periarticular bone, causing telescope-like shortening of the digits.

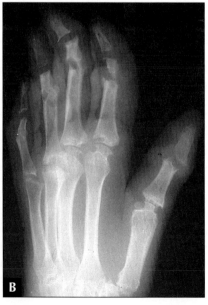

terolemic xanthomatosis. Xanthelasma are seen in approximately 30% of cases. Disease onset is usually insidious, occurring in patients aged between 11 and 71 years and most often female. Polyarthritis can occur first, and there can be systemic features, including fever and weight loss. The arthropathy most commonly involves the hands, frequently beginning in the distal interphalangeal joints with a rapid lysis of periarticular bone, causing telescope-like shortening of the digits (Fig. 8B). Any joint can be involved. Severe atlantoaxial destruction has been life-threatening.

Systemic features often complicate multicentric reticulohistiocytosis. Infiltrates can involve the larynx, lymph nodes, bone, muscle, salivary gland, and endocardium. Associated malignancies have been reported in 28% of cases. Synovial biopsy specimens and skin biopsy specimens both can show the characteristic large mononuclear or multinuclear cells, usually with homogeneous or finely granular pink cytoplasm, mixed with monocytes and lymphocytes. The exact nature of the large histiocytes has not been resolved. Cytotoxic drugs are often necessary and have been successful in some reports. NSAIDs may help joint symptoms in mild cases. Spontaneous remissions have been reported, making evaluation of anecdotal reports on therapy difficult [19].

CUTANEOUS VASCULITIS

Erythema Elevatum Diutinum

Erythema elevatum diutinum (EED) is part of the spectrum of leukocytoclastic vasculitis. The age of onset is usually between 30 and 60 years, and there is no familial history. EED occurs equally in men and women. Skin lesions include symmetric persistent brown-red to purple papules, nodules, plaques, and occasionally bullae located mainly on the extensor surfaces of the joints of the hands, elbows, and knees but also at sites of irritation, such as the palms, as well as the buttocks and shins (Fig. 9). Lesions can be pruritic or painful; cold exposure may exacerbate pain. Trauma or intradermal injection can induce lesions. Older lesions become more fibrotic and resolve with atrophy and with hypopigmentation and hyperpigmentation. There is an association of EED with hematologic malignancies, including IgA monoclonal gammopathies, IgA myeloma, polycythemia vera, hairy-cell leukemia, and mixed cryoglobulinemia. EED often occurs prior to the hematologic disorder. Other diseases associated with EED include recurrent bacterial infections (especially streptococcal), hepatitis B, HIV, rheumatic fever, prostatic carcinoma, and rheumatoid arthritis [20]. In general, the disease is chronic, and spontaneous remission is possible. Arthralgias and myalgias have been reported. Arthralgias may be persistent and severe. Ankles, knees, elbows, and shoulders are the main joints involved [21]. Early lesions show vasculitis, with mainly polymorphonuclear neutrophils in the infiltrate. Older lesions have predominantly granulation tissue and fibrosis, with occasional lipid material.

A diagnosis is made by clinical and histologic criteria. A complete blood count with differential should be performed in all patients. Routine serum protein electrophoretic pattern may not detect monoclonal gammopathies, and immunoelectrophoresis should be performed routinely in patients with EED. The treatment of choice is dapsone. Other therapies include administration of other sulfonamides, steroids (topical, intralesional, and systemic), chloroquine, and niacinamide. Phenformin is successful for treatment, but it is no longer available in the United States.

Urticarial Vasculitis

Urticarial vasculitis is thought to be a type 3 hypersensitivity reaction. It is more common in women, with a ratio of women to men of approximately 2.6:1 at a mean age of 42 years. Urticarial vasculitis is associated with collagen vascular diseases, viral infections (including hepatitis B and mononucleosis), IgA multiple myeloma, IgM gammopathy, serum sickness, drug reactions, and sun exposure. In general, the disease has a benign course. Skin lesions are urticarial, erythematous papules and plaques, sometimes mixed with palpable purpura, macular erythema, livedo reticularis,

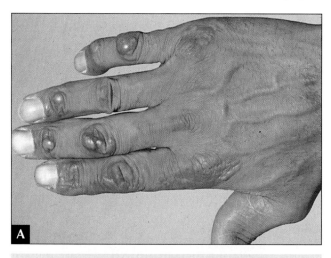

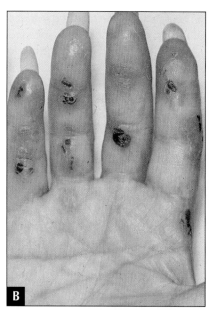

FIGURE 9 A and B, Erythema elevatum diutinum showing symmetric, persistent brown-red to purple tender papules and nodules.

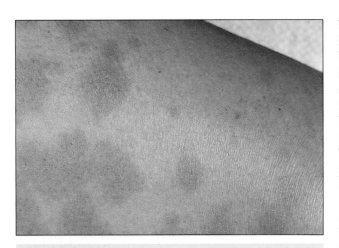

FIGURE 10 Urticarial vasculitis showing urticarial, erythematous papules and plaques, sometimes mixed with palpable purpura.

nodules, and bullae (Fig. 10). The lesions have a painful or burning quality, persist for more than 24 hours, and often resolve with purpura or hyperpigmentation. Other symptoms include fever, malaise, myalgias, hepatomegaly, splenomegaly, angioedema, arthralgias in 60% of cases, arthritis in 28% of cases, abdominal or chest pain, obstructive pulmonary disease, immune complex nephritis, episcleritis, seizures, pseudotumor cerebri, uveitis, and iridocyclitis. Joint symptoms parallel skin activity. Arthritis is usually intermittent, most commonly involving the small joints of the hands and knees, and is nondestructive.

Radiographs of the bones may show dense lesions and a positive radionucleotide scan, but no specific abnormality has been found on bone biopsy samples. The course of the disease varies, although the average duration is 3 years and depends on the associated disorders and renal involvement.

Diagnosis is made by skin biopsy showing a leukocytoclastic vasculitis in conjunction with a clinical presentation resembling urticaria. Low complement levels are found in 35% to 60% of patients. These patients are more likely to have systemic disease [22]. Circulating immune complexes are present in 15% of patients. Erythrocyte sedimentation rates are elevated in two thirds of cases. Associated rheumatic illnesses should be sought by checking antinuclear antibody titers and other serologies.

Therapy may include treatment of underlying disorders or administration of antihistamines, NSAIDs, antimalarial drugs, dapsone, colchicine, gold, oral or pulse glucocorticoids, azathioprine, and pulse cyclophosphamide.

Cutaneous Polyarteritis Nodosa

Cutaneous polyarteritis nodosa (PAN) is a cutaneous form of PAN with rare systemic features. PAN is characterized by segmental inflammation and necrosis of medium or small arteries, but cutaneous PAN involves only the small and medium arteries in the dermis and subcutaneous fat. Lesions are usually red, tender nodules varying from 5 to 20 mm, surrounded by livedo reticularis; they are most commonly found on the distal lower extremities, although the head, neck,

buttocks, and shoulders may be involved. Lesions often appear in rosette groupings, giving them a starburst appearance. Ulceration may occur secondary to vasculitis-induced ischemia, but more often lesions resolve spontaneously over several weeks, without residual scarring. A relapsing course is most common. Flares respond well to NSAIDs and steroids, but systemic therapy is not always necessary. Successful treatment with low-dose weekly methotrexate has been reported. The prognosis in most patients is good, although some patients who initially present with cutaneous PAN progress to systemic disease [23].

Both arthralgias and asymmetric polyarthritis have been described with cutaneous PAN. Arthritis is usually transient but can be associated with inflammatory effusions, although it is nonerosive and pauciarticular. It usually occurs early in the disease and most commonly involves the larger joints of the lower extremities. Symptoms usually respond to treatment of the cutaneous disease.

Henoch-Schönlein Purpura

Henoch-Schönlein purpura is seen primarily in children, but adults of any age can be affected. The classic triad of nonthrombocytopenic palpable purpura, abdominal pain, and arthritis is seen in as many as 80% of patients. Skin lesions represent leukocytoclastic venulitis and are most common over the lower extremities, occasionally accompanied by local edema (Fig. 11). The arthritis is transiently seen in the ankles and knees. Glomerulitis usually consists of microscopic hematuria without significant renal impairment; there is rare exception in some adults. Hypertension can be seen in 10% of patients. The disease is usually self-limited, with a duration of 6 to 16 weeks. Disease in adults may be more severe. Treatment usually consists of supportive, symptomatic therapy. In patients with recurrent disease, prednisone in daily doses of 1 mg/kg may be required [24].

Kawasaki's Disease

Kawasaki's disease is an acute febrile illness usually seen in young children but also in some adults. It is also known as

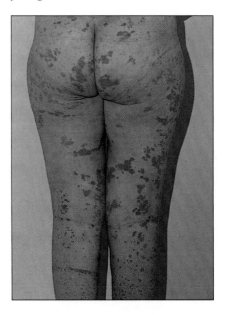

FIGURE 11 Henoch-Schönlein purpura. Palpable purpura, as seen here, is most common over the lower extremities.

mucocutaneous lymph node syndrome. The classic features are fever lasting more than 5 days, conjunctivitis, a strawberry tongue, red lips, peeling skin of the distal extremities, and lymphadenopathy (Fig. 12). Pauciarticular arthritis develops in as many as 40% of cases, most commonly involving the wrists, knees, and ankles. Occasionally, arthritis may persist beyond the convalescent phase. Although the condition is usually self-limited, 1% to 2% of patients develop clinically significant coronary aneurysms from vasculitis involvement. In addition, myocarditis and involvement of other large arteries may occur. Aspirin or other NSAIDs are helpful in the symptomatic treatment of the illness, especially if given early in the course of the disease. If coronary aneurysms are suspected, treatment with intravenous γ globulin lessens the persistence of these cardiac complications [25].

CONCLUSIONS

Although many of the conditions described in this chapter are uncommon, patients presenting with both skin and joint lesions are encountered frequently. Often, the expertise of both a consultant dermatologist and a rheumatologist is needed for differential diagnosis and appropriate therapy.

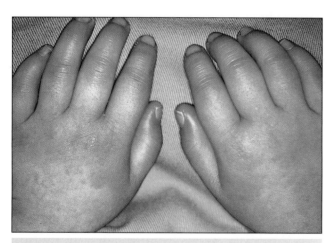

FIGURE 12 Kawasaki's disease showing diffuse swelling of the hand in a child in the acute phase.

REFERENCES AND RECOMMENDED READING

Recently published papers of particular interest have been highlighted as:
• Of interest
•• Of outstanding interest

1. Torre Alonso JC, Rodriguez Perex A, Arribas Castrillo JM, *et al.*: Psoriatic arthritis: a clinical, immunological and radiological study of 180 patients. *Br J Rheumatol* 1991, 30:245–250.
2.•• Gladman DD: Psoriatic arthritis: recent advances in pathogenesis and treatment. *Rheum Dis Clin North Am* 1992, 18:247–256.
3. Goupille P, Soutif D, Valat JP: Treatment of psoriatic arthropathy. *Semin Arthritis Rheum* 1992, 21:355–367.
4.•• Knitzer RH, White Needleman B: Musculoskeletal syndromes associated with acne. *Semin Arthritis Rheum* 1991, 20:247–255.

5. Olafsson S, Kahn MA: Musculoskeletal features of acne, hidradenitis, suppurativa, and dissecting cellulitis of the scalp. *Rheum Dis Clin North Am* 1992, 18:215–224.
6. Kahn M-F, Chamot A-M: SAPHO syndrome. *Rheum Dis Clin North Am* 1992, 18:225–246.
7. Taillandier J, Alemanni A: Coxapathie destructrice au cours de la pustulos palmo-plantaire: a propos d'un nouveau cas. *Revue du Rhumatisme* 1993, 60:257–259.
8. Ko CB, Walton S, Wyatt EH: Pyoderma gangrenosum: associations revisited. *Int J Dermatol* 1992, 31:574–577.
9. Levitt MD, Ritchie JK, Lennard-Jones JE, Phillips RK: Pyoderma gangrenosum in inflammatory bowel disease. *Br J Surg* 1991, 78:676–678.
10.•• Peters MS, Su WPD: Panniculitis. *Dermatol Clin* 1992, 10:37–57.
11. Patterson JW: Differential diagnosis of panniculitis. *Adv Dermatol* 1991, 6:309–330.
12. Smith KJ, Skelton HG, Yeager J, *et al.*: Cutaneous histopathologic, immunohistochemical, and clinical manifestations in patients with hemophagocytic syndrome: military medical consortium for applied retroviral research. *Arch Dermatol* 1992, 128:193–200.
13. Tolin BS, Esterhai JL, Allan DA, *et al.*: Pancreatic osteoarthropathy with unusually destructive sequelae. *Orthopedics* 1993, 16:473–477.
14.• Kemmett D, Hunter JAA: Sweet's syndrome: a clinicopathologic review of 29 cases. *J Am Acad Dermatol* 1990, 23:503–507.
15. Krauser RE, Schumacher HR: The arthritis of Sweet's syndrome. *Arthritis Rheum* 1975, 18:35–41.
16. Gabriel SE, Perry HO, Gleson GB: A scleroderma-like disorder with systemic manifestations. *Medicine* 1988, 67:58–65.
17. Helfrich DJ, Walker ER, Martinez AJ: Scleromyxedema myopathy: case report and review of the literature. *Arthritis Rheum* 1988, 31:1437–1441.
18. Levin RW, Schumacher HR: Multicentric reticulohistiocytosis. *Int Med Specialist* 1989, 10:148–157.
19. Rapini RP: Multicentric reticulohistiocytosis. *Clin Dermatol* 1993, 11:107–111.
20. Yiannias J, El-Azhary R, Gibson L: Erythema elevatum diutinum: a clinical and histopathologic study of 13 patients. *J Am Acad Dermatol* 1992, 26:38–44.
21. Wilkinson S, English J, Smith N, *et al.*: Erythema elevatum diutinum: a clinicopathological study. *Clin Exp Dermatol* 1992, 17:87–93.
22. Mehregan D, Hall M, Gibson L: Urticarial vasculitis: a histopathologic and clinical review of 72 cases. *J Am Acad Dermatol* 1992, 26:441–448.
23. Moreland LW, Ball GV: Cutaneous polyarteritis nodosa. *Am J Med* 1990, 88:426–430.
24. Roth DA, Wilz DR, Theil GB: Schönlein-Henoch syndrome in adults. *Q J Med* 1985, 55:145–152.
25. Burns JC, Mason WH, Giode MP, *et al.*: Clinical and epidemiologic characteristics of patients referred for evaluation of possible Kawasaki disease. *J Pediatr* 1991, 118:680–686.

SELECT BIBLIOGRAPHY

Fitzpatrick TB, Eisen AZ, Wolff K, *et al.*, eds.: *Dermatology in General Medicine*. New York: McGraw-Hill; 1993.

Klippel J, Dieppe P, eds.: *Rheumatology*. London: Mosby; 1994.

Schumacher HR Jr, ed.: *Primer on the Rheumatic Diseases*, edn 10. Atlanta: Arthritis Foundation; 1993.

Sontheimer RD, Provost T, eds.: *The Cutaneous Manifestations of Rheumatic Diseases*. Philadelphia: Lea & Febiger; 1995.

Fibromyalgia and Related Disorders 11

Don L. Goldenberg

Key Points

- Fibromyalgia is one of the most common causes of chronic generalized pain.

- The diagnosis is made in patients with chronic, diffuse pain and fatigue, and generally normal physical and laboratory examinations, with the exception of tender points at specific locations.

- Mood disturbances, more localized pain disorders (*eg*, migraine and myofascial pain), and the chronic fatigue syndrome share many clinical features and may be part of a fibromyalgia spectrum.

- Although many patients do well with education regarding their condition and simple medications to help sleep and manage pain, some patients require a more intensive multidisciplinary management program.

FIBROMYALGIA

Diagnosis

Fibromyalgia is a common cause of chronic musculoskeletal pain. It is best considered as one of several common soft tissue pain disorders, including myofascial pain syndrome, idiopathic lower back pain, muscular (tension) headaches, and chronic fatigue syndrome (CFS). These disorders primarily affect muscles and soft tissues, such as tendons and ligaments. None is associated with tissue inflammation, and the cause of the pain is not known.

Each of these conditions is controversial. Patients look well, there are no obvious findings on the physical examination, and laboratory and radiologic study findings are normal. The existence of organic illnesses has been questioned, and such disorders have often been considered to be psychogenic or psychosomatic in nature.

Rheumatologists are increasingly recognizing fibromyalgia as a discrete syndrome. Diagnostic classification criteria have been proposed, evaluated, and validated. With the use of these criteria, fibromyalgia is now the most common cause of generalized musculoskeletal pain in women between 20 and 55 years of age. Six to 10 million Americans may be affected by this syndrome [1].

Demographic and Clinical Characteristics

Fibromyalgia is 10 times more common in women. This striking gender ratio has not been explained adequately. The typical age of onset is between 30 and 50 years, and most patients are symptomatic for 5 to 10 years before the diagnosis is made. Fibromyalgia also has been reported in children and elderly patients. Approximately

50% of patients recall that symptoms began with a specific event, most often some form of physical or emotional trauma or a flu-like illness.

The cardinal manifestation of fibromyalgia is diffuse musculoskeletal pain (Table 1). Although the pain initially may be localized, often in the neck and shoulders, it eventually involves many muscle groups. Typically, patients complain of axial pain in the neck and the middle and lower back, pain in the chest wall, and pain in the arms and legs. The pain is chronic and persistent, although it usually varies in intensity. Patients often have difficulty distinguishing joint from muscle pain and may report a sensation of swelling, but the joints do not appear swollen or inflamed on objective examination.

Fatigue is present in more than 90% of patients, and in some patients it is the most distressing symptom. Patients feel very tired or even exhausted and generally do not awaken feeling refreshed. Some patients have overt insomnia; others report symptoms suggestive of pathologic sleep disturbances, such as sleep apnea or nocturnal myoclonus. However, most patients recognize only that they sleep lightly and wake up unrefreshed. In addition to complaining of generalized fatigue, patients also report muscle fatigue or weakness after modest exertion. Mood disturbances, especially depression, anxiety, and heightened somatic concern, are also common. Most patients report that the mood disturbance followed the onset of fibromyalgia. Cognitive disturbances and headaches, either of the muscular or migraine type, are also common. Patients also may have various poorly understood pain symptoms, including abdominal pain, symptoms suggestive of irritable bowel syndrome, pelvic pain, and bladder symptoms suggestive of the female urethral syndrome. True Raynaud's phenomenon has been reported in 30% to 40% of patients with fibromyalgia, a prevalence greater than that in the general population.

The only diagnostic finding on physical examination is excessive muscle tenderness, which is best determined by the palpation of predefined muscle and tendon insertions, termed *tender points* (Fig. 1). These tender points are usually bilateral and are symmetrically tender. Patients should be examined while in a sitting position, and each common tender point should be palpated with the thumb, with approximately 4 kg/cm² of pressure applied (Fig. 2). Otherwise, the musculoskeletal examination findings are unremarkable, and no evidence indicates a systemic connective tissue disease or a neurologic disease.

Diagnostic Classification Criteria

With the increased recognition of fibromyalgia as a common syndrome, investigators have proposed classification criteria for the diagnosis of fibromyalgia [2]. Studies demonstrated that fibromyalgia patients had significantly more tender points than did normal, healthy control subjects or patients with rheumatoid arthritis, osteoarthritis, or other connective tissue disorders. In 1990, the largest such diagnostic criteria study enrolled 293 fibromyalgia patients and 265 patients with

TABLE 1 CHARACTERISTICS OF PAIN IN FIBROMYALGIA
May begin in one area and then spread
Is eventually widespread
Is frequently associated with numbness, tingling, burning, and a crawling sensation
May be affected by stress, weather, exertion, and lack of sleep
Is generally chronic and not responsive to anti-inflammatory medications

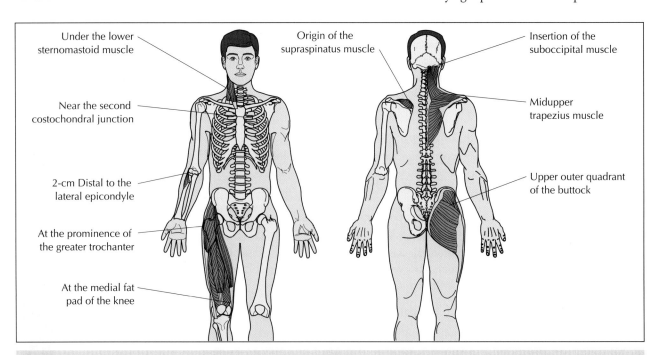

Under the lower sternomastoid muscle

Near the second costochondral junction

2-cm Distal to the lateral epicondyle

At the prominence of the greater trochanter

At the medial fat pad of the knee

Origin of the supraspinatus muscle

Insertion of the suboccipital muscle

Midupper trapezius muscle

Upper outer quadrant of the buttock

FIGURE 1 Tender points. (*Adapted from* Goldenberg [18]; with permission.)

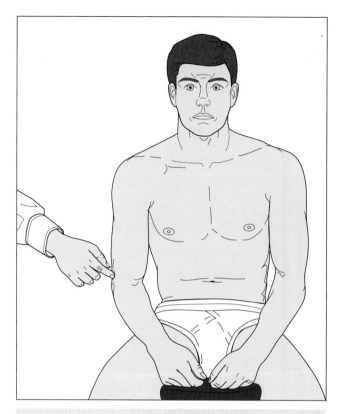

FIGURE 2 Patient being examined for a tender point.

ered subjective because they are based on patient report and there is no gold standard, such as a histologic tissue change or a laboratory measure of disease activity. Nevertheless, these criteria have been validated in broad-based population studies and are highly reliable.

Practical Guidelines for Diagnosis

The diagnosis is based largely on the patient's history, which should include details of the duration, onset, nature, and location of pain and related symptoms, such as paresthesias. Inquiry into other common features, including fatigue, sleep disturbances, headache, cognitive difficulty, and mood disturbances, is important. It is also important to spend an adequate amount of time during this initial evaluation to obtain diagnostic information and to establish a caring, empathic relationship with the patient, who may have been told by his or her rheumatologist that, "I can't find anything wrong with you" or, "It is all in your head." They may feel anger or a lack of trust because of past experience. The physician must be viewed as an ally rather than as an enemy.

The finding of multiple tender points on physical examination confirms the diagnosis (Fig. 1). The tender point examination, described in Table 2, is easy to learn and takes no more than a few minutes to perform.

A general musculoskeletal examination and a neurologic examination should be routinely performed to help exclude any obvious arthritis, connective tissue disorder, or neurologic condition (Fig. 3). Most patients have previously undergone multiple laboratory and radiologic studies, the results of which have been unrevealing. If a patient has not been previously evaluated by others or if the results of previous studies are unknown, limited laboratory testing (a complete blood count, measurement of the erythrocyte sedimentation rate and muscle enzyme levels, and assessment of thyroid function) may be warranted. However, extensive laboratory testing, often performed in chronic, poorly defined syndromes, is unnecessary and often provides confusing results. For example, the predictive value of a positive antinuclear antibody test finding in a patient without the characteristic symptoms and signs of systemic lupus erythematosus is low. Patients with fibromyalgia often are told that they may have systemic lupus erythematosus or another serious connective tissue disease based on an inappropriate interpretation of laboratory test results, especially antinuclear antibody and rheumatoid factor tests. Many patients undergo computed tomographic and

chronic rheumatic disorders, such as low back pain, neck and arm pain, osteoarthritis, and rheumatoid arthritis [2]. These control subjects were selected because they would be most difficult to distinguish from patients with fibromyalgia. More than 300 variables, including symptoms, physical findings, and laboratory and radiologic findings, were analyzed. The final recommended diagnostic criteria were simple: widespread musculoskeletal pain and excess tenderness in at least 11 of 18 predefined anatomic sites. These criteria were 80% specific and sensitive in differentiating patients with fibromyalgia from control subjects. No exclusionary criteria were proposed.

Such diagnostic criteria are especially important in clinical studies to ensure homogeneity of patients. However, in practice, it is always understood that a physician's diagnostic judgment is most important. Thus, a patient may be diagnosed with fibromyalgia without having the recommended number of tender points. Furthermore, these criteria may be consid-

---

TABLE 2 GUIDELINES FOR THE TENDER POINT EXAMINATION

Have the patient undress and sit in a comfortable position on an examination table; observe the patient during the examination.

Explain to the patient that pressure will be applied with the thumb to various areas and that if the pressure causes pain, the patient should respond verbally (Fig. 2).

Always perform a tender point examination in the same fashion, with pressure equivalent to approximately 4 kg/cm^2 applied to the muscle belly and insertion points in selected anatomic locations (the amount of pressure [force per unit area] sufficient to blanch the thumbnail is about right).

Apply the pressure gradually over a few seconds to both the right and left sides of the body.

Also examine control locations, such as over the thumbnail or the midforearm; they should not be as tender as the predefined points.

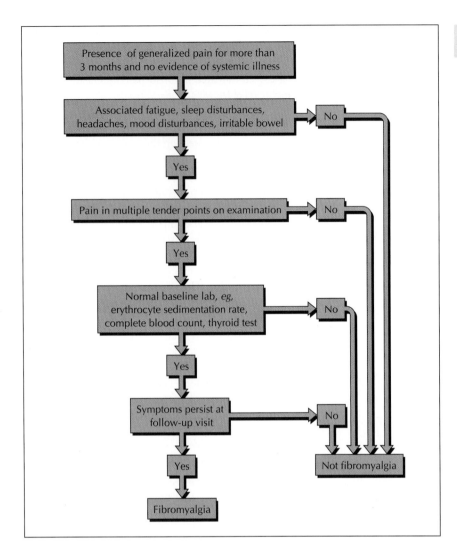

FIGURE 3 The diagnosis of fibromyalgia.

Presence of generalized pain for more than 3 months and no evidence of systemic illness

Associated fatigue, sleep disturbances, headaches, mood disturbances, irritable bowel → No

Yes

Pain in multiple tender points on examination → No

Yes

Normal baseline lab, *eg*, erythrocyte sedimentation rate, complete blood count, thyroid test → No

Yes

Symptoms persist at follow-up visit → No

Yes

Not fibromyalgia

Fibromyalgia

magnetic resonance imaging studies or electromyography and nerve conduction velocity testing, presumably in relation to the symptoms of paresthesias. Some patients have inappropriate surgery for carpal tunnel syndrome or a radiculopathy. Thus, a simple algorithm for the diagnosis of fibromyalgia is based primarily on the history and tender point examination (Fig. 3).

Differential Diagnosis

The multiple nonspecific symptoms of fibromyalgia may mimic those of many other conditions (Table 3). Probably the most common diagnostic dilemma in fibromyalgia is a psychiatric illness, particularly a somatoform or somatization disorder or major depression. Approximately 30% of fibromyalgia patients actually have major depression or anxiety disorders [3]. However, most patients do not have any current psychopathology, and they rarely meet diagnostic criteria for somatization disorders. Nevertheless, a careful psychiatric evaluation often is very useful. Any patient with obvious or suspected depression or major anxiety should undergo a structured psychiatric interview and be considered for treatment with psychotropic medications.

RELATED DISORDERS

Myofascial Pain Syndrome

Myofascial pain syndrome is closely related to fibromyalgia, and some view it as the localized form of fibromyalgia. Myofascial pain typically involves only one group of muscles, such as the left side of the neck and the left shoulder.

TABLE 3 FIBROMYALGIA MIMICS OTHER DISORDERS

Characteristic of fibromyalgia	Disorder mimicked
Chest wall pain	Cardiac disease, pulmonary disease
Abdominal pain	Gastrointestinal disease
Paresthesias	Radiculopathy, carpal tunnel syndrome
Raynaud's syndrome, arthralgias	Connective tissue disease
Weakness, myalgias	Myopathy, myositis

However, several other features distinguish it from fibromyalgia (Table 4). These characteristics of myofascial pain, such as the trigger point, have not been validated in large population-based studies [4•]. The treatment of myofascial pain has often been thought to be more curative than the treatment of fibromyalgia, primarily with the application of physical modalities, such as the use of topical injections or sprays and muscle stretching or other physical therapy. Some patients with myofascial pain have a chronic problem.

Sleep Disturbances

Most patients with fibromyalgia report sleep disturbances, and the most frequent abnormality noted on overnight polysomnography has been an early wave intrusion in the deep stages of sleep [5]. This sleep anomaly, known as α-Δ sleep, is not specific for fibromyalgia and has been demonstrated in patients with rheumatoid arthritis and other chronic pain syndromes (Fig. 4). Other sleep abnormalities, such as nocturnal myoclonus, are common in patients with either fibromyalgia or rheumatoid arthritis. Fibromyalgia, like rheumatoid arthritis, is more than a sleep abnormality. The exact relationship of any sleep disturbance to the pain and fatigue of these common disorders has yet to be determined.

Psychiatric Illness and Somatoform Disorders

Fibromyalgia cannot be viewed simply as a psychiatric disease, although mood disturbances are common and important in fibromyalgia patients [3]. Earlier descriptions of a bizarre or hysterical fibromyalgia personality led to the use of the term *psychogenic rheumatism*. However, the application of validated psychiatric criteria from the *Diagnostic & Statistical Manual of Mental Disorders*, 3rd edition to patients with fibromyalgia demonstrated that patients rarely are hysterical or meet criteria for somatization disorders. Depression and anxiety are present in 25% to 40% of patients at the time of the diagnosis of fibromyalgia. There is a greater personal and family history of depression in fibromyalgia patients than in patients with rheumatoid arthritis [6]. However, no stereotypic psychiatric or personality profile is found in patients with fibromyalgia. The frequent clustering of conditions, such as depression, migraine, irritable bowel syndrome, and CFS in patients with fibromyalgia has led to the notion that they may represent

TABLE 4 FIBROMYALGIA VERSUS MYOFASCIAL PAIN SYNDROME		
Characteristic	**Fibromyalgia**	**Myofascial pain syndrome**
Prevalence	3% to 5% of the population	Unknown
Gender	Female-to-male ratio, 10:1	Equal occurrence in men and women
Sleep disorder	Occurs in almost all patients	Often occurs
Fatigue	Occurs in almost all patients	Often occurs
Pain	Diffuse	Localized
Tenderness	Widespread	Localized
Outcome	Chronic	Self-limited (?)
Palpation	Tender point	Trigger point

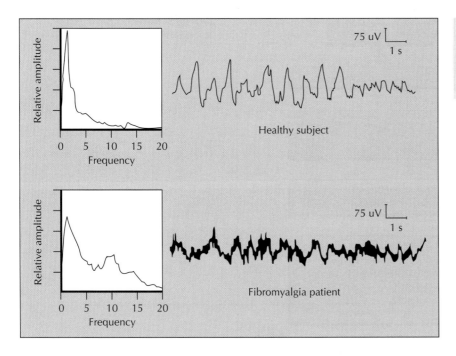

75 uV

1 s

Healthy subject

75 uV

1 s

Fibromyalgia patient

FIGURE 4 Abnormalities during restorative (nonlrapid eye movement) sleep in the fibromyalgia syndrome. (*Adapted from* Smythe and Moldofsky [19]; with permission.)

affective spectrum disorders. These common syndromes may share certain psychobiologic characteristics [6].

Chronic Fatigue Syndrome

Chronic fatigue syndrome and fibromyalgia share many demographic and clinical characteristics (Table 5). However, CFS traditionally has been believed to be caused by an infection (*eg*, a viral infection) and associated with immune dysfunction. There is no evidence that any single infectious agent is associated with CFS, despite the initial evidence indicating that Epstein-Barr virus or human herpesviruses may be causally related to CFS [7]. Probably several infectious agents may precipitate either CFS or fibromyalgia. For example, fibromyalgia has been reported to occur as a sequela of Lyme disease [8•], HIV infection, and other viral infections [9].

A striking overlap has been found in the clinical manifestations of fibromyalgia and CFS. The symptoms in these two syndromes are similar; 50% of patients with fibromyalgia reported that their illness began with a flu or viral illness [10]. Fully 75% of patients with CFS met the diagnostic criteria for fibromyalgia [11••]. Thus, these two syndromes may best be considered to be identical disorders, viewed from different perspectives, or overlapping syndromes that share psychobiologic characteristics.

TREATMENT

The treatment of fibromyalgia and related disorders should begin with education (Fig. 5). Patients and their families need to understand that these syndromes are discrete disorders, but they are not defined as true diseases leading to tissue or internal organ damage or to any cosmetic or degenerative changes. Nevertheless, patients often continue to have chronic pain and fatigue and require an altered lifestyle while they are learning to cope with their chronic symptoms. The physician must explain sensitively that this disorder is not an imagined or a psychiatric illness but that mood disturbances, such as depression and anxiety, are common and need to be treated. The intimate interaction of the mind and the body in these disorders should be discussed.

The judicious use of simple analgesics such as acetaminophen, salicylates, or nonsteroidal antiinflammatory drugs (NSAIDs) is recommended for pain as needed, but there is no evidence that therapeutic doses of NSAIDs are effective [12]. Tricyclic medications, including amitriptyline and cyclobenzaprine, have been found to be more effective than were placebo or NSAIDs in controlled trials [13,14]. These agents are generally used in very low doses (*eg*, 10–30 mg) at bedtime, and they usually decrease pain and sleep disturbances. However, only one third of patients note major clinical improvement. Thus, many patients do not continue on these medications because of side effects such as constipation or dry mouth, or the patient concludes that an initial improvement

TABLE 5 SIMILAR FEATURES OF FIBROMYALGIA AND CHRONIC FATIGUE SYNDROME

Female predominance
May be triggered by a viral-like illness or
    other stressful event
Similar symptoms
    Fatigue
    Myalgias
    Headaches
    Sleep disturbances
    Mood disturbances
Absence of laboratory abnormalities
No clear cause or pathophysiologic changes
Chronic symptoms
No highly effective medication

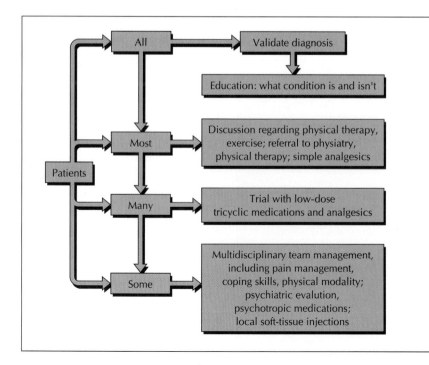

FIGURE 5 Treatment programs in fibromyalgia.

has worn off. Other central nervous system–active medications that have been used with limited success include alprazolam, carsiprodol, and other tricyclic antidepressants. No clinical trials have used therapeutic doses of these antidepressants or some of the newer antidepressants, such as fluoxetine, in the treatment of fibromyalgia or CFS. Clinical trials in CFS have included acyclovir and intravenous gamma globulin, but no major improvement was noted with these agents.

Nonmedicinal treatment found to be effective in fibromyalgia includes cardiovascular fitness training [15], electromyography biofeedback, hypnotherapy, and cognitive behavioral therapy. A multidisciplinary treatment program that uses education, physical and psychological pain management approaches, and medications is likely to be most successful in many patients. However, most patients continue to have persistent chronic pain, and the levels of pain and functional disability have been comparable to those of patients with rheumatoid arthritis [16,17]. Thus, the coping skills of each patient are important determinants of outcome and prognosis in these chronic pain syndromes.

REFERENCES AND RECOMMENDED READING

Recently published papers of particular interest have been highlighted as:
- Of interest
- • Of outstanding interest

1. Goldenberg DL: Fibromyalgia syndrome: an emerging but controversial condition. *JAMA* 1987, 257:2782–2787.
2. Wolfe F, Smythe HA, Yunus MB, *et al.*: The American College of Rheumatology 1990 Criteria for the Classification of Fibromyalgia: report of the multicenter criteria committee. *Arthritis Rheum* 1990, 33:160–172.
3. Mufson M, Regestein QR: The spectrum of fibromyalgia disorders. *Arthritis Rheum* 1993, 36:647–650.
4.• Wolfe F, Simons DG, Fricton JR, *et al.*: The fibromyalgia and myofascial pain syndromes: a preliminary study of tender points and trigger points in persons with fibromyalgia, myofascial pain syndrome, and no disease. *J Rheumatol* 1992, 19:944–951.
5. Moldofsky H: Sleep and fibrositis syndrome. *Rheum Dis Clin North Am* 1989, 15:91–103.
6. Hudson JI, Goldenberg DL, Pope HG Jr., *et al.*: Comorbidity of fibromyalgia with medical and psychiatric disorders. *Am J Med* 1992, 363–367.
7. Schluederberg A, Straus SE, Peterson P, *et al.*: Chronic fatigue syndrome research. *Ann Intern Med* 1992, 117:325–331.
8.• Dinerman H, Steere AC: Lyme disease associated with fibromyalgia. *Ann Intern Med* 1992, 117:281–285.
9. Simms RW, Zerbini CAF, Ferrante N, *et al.*: Fibromyalgia syndrome in patients infected with human immunodeficiency virus. *Am J Med* 1992, 92:368–374.
10. Buchwald D, Goldenberg DL, Sullivan JL, *et al.*: The "chronic, active Epstein-Barr virus infection" syndrome and primary fibromyalgia. *Arthritis Rheum* 1987, 30:1132–1136.
11.•• Goldenberg DL, Simms RW, Geiger A, *et al.*: High frequency of fibromyalgia in patients with chronic fatigue seen in a primary care practice. *Arthritis Rheum* 1990, 33:381–387.
12. Goldenberg DL: Treatment of fibromyalgia syndrome. *Rheum Dis Clin North Am* 1989, 15:61–71.
13. Goldenberg DL, Felson DT, Dinerman H: A randomized, controlled trial of amitriptyline and naproxen in the treatment of patients with fibromyalgia. *Arthritis Rheum* 1986, 29:1371–1377.
14. Bennett RM, Gatter RA, Campbell SM, *et al.*: A comparison of cyclobenzaprine and placebo in the management of fibrositis: a double-blind controlled study. *Arthritis Rheum* 1988, 31:1535–1542.
15. McCain GA, Bell DA, Mai FM, *et al.*: A controlled study of the effects of a supervised cardiovascular fitness training program on the manifestations of fibromyalgia. *Arthritis Rheum* 1988, 31:1135–1141.
16. Ledingham J, Doherty S, Doherty M: Primary fibromyalgia syndrome: an outcome study. *Br J Rheumatol* 1993, 32:139–142.
17. Cathey MA, Wolfe F, Kleinheksel SM, *et al.*: Functional ability and work status in patients with fibromyalgia. *Arthritis Care Res* 1988, 1:85–98.
18. Goldenberg DL: Diagnostic and therapeutic challenges of fibromyalgia. *Hosp Pract* 1989, 24:39–52.
19. Smythe HA, Moldofsky H: Contributions to understanding of the "fibrositis syndrome." *Bull Rheum Dis* 1977, 28:928–931.

SELECT BIBLIOGRAPHY

Bennett RM: Fibromyalgia and the facts. *Rheum Dis Clin North Am* 1993, 19:45–59.

Bennett RM, Goldenberg DL: The fibromyalgia syndrome. *Rheum Dis Clin North Am* 1989, 15:1–191.

Russell IJ: Musculoskeletal pain, myofascial pain syndrome, and the fibromyalgia syndrome. *J Musculoskeletal Pain* 1993, 1:1–316.

Vaeroy H, Merskey H: Progress in fibromyalgia and myofascial pain. *Pain Res Clin Management* 1993, 6:1–451.

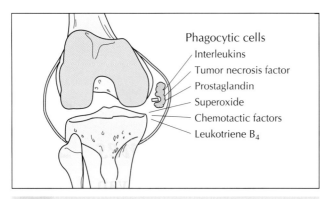

FIGURE 1 Ingestion of phlogistic crystals by phagocytic cells is followed by release of inflammatory mediators.

illness that correspond to the natural history of one of the three causes (Table 1). A history of trauma can be elicited from all patients with traumatic arthritis unless they have had impaired consciousness or mentation. However, a history of trauma may be misleading. Trauma may release crystals from articular depots into the joint space, thereby causing gout or pseudogout; blunt trauma may cause intraarticular bleeding

with microbial seeding of the joint space if the patient is bacteremic; and penetrating trauma may introduce organisms present on the skin or the penetrating object (Fig. 2). Thus, a history of trauma is necessary but never sufficient for the diagnosis of traumatic arthritis and does not obviate further evaluation. A history of fever may be elicited, but fever also occurs regularly with crystal-induced arthritis due to release of interleukins and tumor necrosis factor [2]. Antecedent medical events may be important. Both gout and pseudogout frequently occur postoperatively or after acute medical illnesses, especially cardiovascular or cerebrovascular events. Diuretics, low-dose salicylate, cyclosporine, ethambutol, pyrazinamide, cytotoxic agents, and niacin may cause hyperuricemia, which predisposes to gout. Of particular note is the frequency of gouty arthritis in transplant recipients treated with cyclosporine [3•]. Concurrent medical conditions can predispose to pseudogout or to gout (Table 2) [4•].

The historical features of chronic monarthritis also may be helpful in determining the etiology of the illness. Patients with degenerative arthritis usually describe long-standing pain and stiffness, often a distant history of trauma, and gelling phenomenon with profound stiffness lasting for several minutes after prolonged inactivity. Tuberculous arthritis often

	Cause		
Feature	**Traumatic**	**Crystal-induced**	**Septic**
Trauma	+++	+	+
Prior attacks	–	++	–
Fever (> 102°F)	–	+	++
Rigors	–	–	+
Infection elsewhere (*eg*, pneumonia, endocarditis, abscess)	–	+	++
Concurrent medical condition	–	+	+

TABLE 1 DIFFERENTIAL HISTORICAL FEATURES OF ACUTE MONARTHRITIS

-, usually absent; +, occasional; ++, frequent; +++, usual.

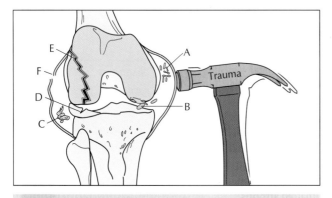

FIGURE 2 Potential consequences of joint trauma: **A**, joint hemorrhage (infection if bacteremic); **B**, release of cartilage calcium pyrophosphate crystal deposits (pseudogout); **C**, release of synovial monosodium urate crystal deposits (gout); **D**, meniscal injury; **E**, subchondral or cartilage fracture; and **F**, ligament or capsular injury.

TABLE 2 PREDISPOSING MEDICAL FACTORS TO GOUT OR PSEUDOGOUT

Gout	**Pseudogout**
Alcohol	Aging
Obesity	Hemochromatosis
Hypertension	Hyperparathyroidism
Renal failure	Hypothyroidism
Tumor (or chemotherapy)	Hypophosphatasia
Hematologic malignancy	Hypomagnesemia
Hemolysis	
Psoriasis	
Renal tubular disorders	
Acidosis	

occurs in the setting of drug or alcohol abuse, whereas fungal arthritis may be confined to certain geographic regions.

DIFFERENTIAL PHYSICAL FEATURES

Differential physical findings of acute monarthritis include characteristics of the affected joint and extraarticular features. A swollen joint with warm reddened overlying skin points toward sepsis or crystal synovitis because traumatized joints are rarely inflamed. However, inflamed joints may appear surprisingly bland. The anatomical distribution of joint involvement is important. In the nontraumatized joint, small joint distribution is typical of gout, especially if the great toe is involved (podagra). Large joint involvement is more typical of pseudogout or infection. Careful examination of other joints is important because the index joint may merely be the most prominently involved of several in a patient more appropriately classified as having polyarthritis. The sacroiliac joints deserve special attention because a pauciarticular spondyloarthritis is readily mistaken for a monarthritis. Systemic examination must include any site suggested by history as a

potential source of infection. Careful skin scrutiny is always indicated to look for tophi (Figs. 3 and 4) and characteristic skin lesions of bacterial dissemination (gonococcemia, endocarditis) (Fig. 5).

In cases of chronic monarthritis, a careful physical examination is always warranted. Palpable osteophytes, crepitance, and the absence of inflammation are characteristic of joints affected by degenerative joint disease. Joint tumors may cause nodular densities or very tense effusions, particularly in the popliteal fossa when the knee is involved. Fungal arthritis may be associated with the skin rash of erythema nodosum.

DIAGNOSTIC STUDIES

Synovial fluid analysis is the principal diagnostic study in evaluating monarthritis. However, blood studies may provide ancillary information, and radiographs may be informative. Serum uric acid determination is unreliable in the diagnosis of gout. Hyperuricemia is prevalent in patients without gout and is often absent during acute gouty attacks. Thus, hyperuricemia is neither a sensitive nor a specific indicator of gout. However,

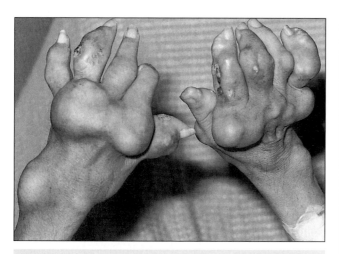

FIGURE 3 Severe tophus formation with draining tophaceous material in a patient whose gout has gone untreated for 30 years.

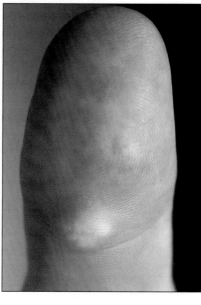

FIGURE 4 Subcutaneous tophus confirmed by aspiration and crystal identification.

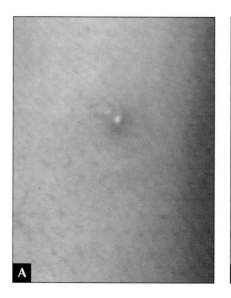

A

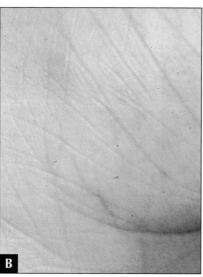

B

FIGURE 5 A, Pustular and B, macular skin lesions in a patient with gonococcal arthritis-dermatitis syndrome.

blood uric acid determination is indicated after the diagnosis is made to predict people at risk for urate nephropathy, to predict risk of recurrence, and to monitor response to hypouricemic treatment if it is indicated. In general, other blood work should be deferred until the diagnosis is established by joint fluid analysis or reserved for patients in whom no diagnosis is forthcoming after such analysis. Radiographs are important in all traumatized joints to look for evidence of fracture. Occasionally, intraarticular lipid layered over synovial fluid may be radiographically apparent. In nontraumatized joints, radiographs also may be useful. Adjacent bony lesions may suggest osteomyelitis or periarticular fractures. Gout may be suggested by soft tissue masses consistent with tophi or osseous tophi with a characteristic overhanging margin (Fig. 6). Even if classical radiographic tophi are visualized, the need for arthrocentesis remains because 5% of patients with gout also have pseudogout, and joints damaged by gout are preferential sites of seeding during bacteremia with resultant septic arthritis. Similarly, typical chondrocalcinosis strongly suggests pseudogout (Fig. 7). However, arthrocentesis must be done to evalu-

ate for coexistent gout (5% of patients with pseudogout have gout) and for joint sepsis. Lastly, monarthritis of short duration with radiographic evidence of cartilage damage and bony erosions points to septic arthritis with a pyogenic organism.

In cases of chronic arthritis, radiographs are often helpful in diagnosing degenerative joint disease. Joint tumors can be visualized directly with arthroscopy or by magnetic resonance imaging.

Synovial Fluid Analysis

Synovial fluid analysis is the keystone of differential diagnosis of acute monarthritis. It should be performed in all patients unless there is an obvious acute traumatic event with no signs of inflammation or unless the episode represents a typical recurrence in a patient for whom the diagnosis of gout or pseudogout has been established by arthrocentesis during prior attacks. In either situation, the decision not to perform arthrocentesis must be reconsidered should presumed crystal-induced disease fail to respond to treatment, and presumed traumatic arthritis must be reexamined for signs of inflammation.

Appearance

Synovial fluid analysis should include visual inspection for color, clarity, and viscosity, determination of cell counts and differential staining, microbiologic studies, and compensated polarized light microscopy for crystal identification. A bloody appearance may occur after trauma but may also be seen with pseudogout. Determination of the hematocrit of the fluid is important to distinguish gross blood from blood admixed with synovial fluid. Flecks of tophaceous material may be seen in gouty fluids. At times, joint fluids are milky with urate crystals in high concentrations (Fig. 8). After standing, a layer of fat occasionally appears at the synovial fluid surface in traumatized joints (Fig. 9). This fat may be derived from lymphatic disruption, subchondral fracture with ingress of marrow contents, or capsular injury with ingress of periarticular fat. Characteristic synovial fluid changes in monarthritis are listed in Table 3.

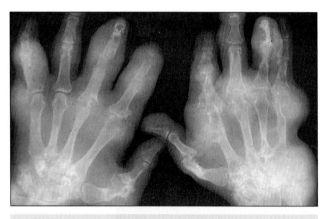

FIGURE 6 A hand radiograph of the patient in Figure 3. Note bony destructive tophi with overhanging osteophyte and soft tissue masses.

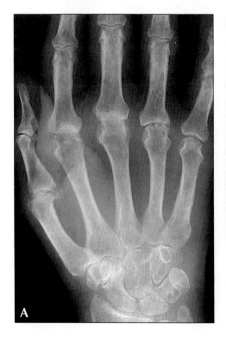

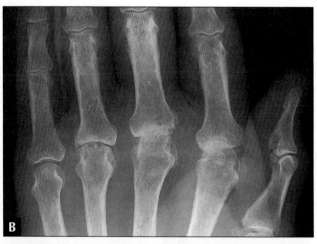

FIGURE 7 Chondrocalcinosis of the triangular fibrocartilage of the wrist. **A**, This patient also has typical secondary degenerative changes in the metacarpophalangeal joints. **B**, Note synovial calcinosis in the second metacarpophalangeal joint.

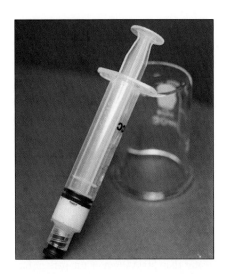

FIGURE 8 Puru-lent-appearing synovial fluid from a patient with gout. The patient was a renal transplant recipient receiving cyclosporine. The leukocyte count was 15,000 cells/cm². (*Courtesy of* Laureen Daft, BS, Medical College of Wisconsin.)

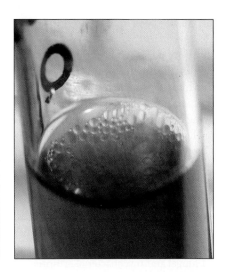

FIGURE 9 Bloody fluid from a patient with traumatic arthritis. Note the layer of fat at the fluid surface.

TABLE 3 CHARACTERISTIC SYNOVIAL FLUID CHANGES IN MONARTHRITIS						
	Appearance					
Cause	**Clear**	**Cloudy**	**Bloody**	**Opaque**	**Leukocyte count,** *cells/mm³*	**Crystals**
Traumatic	++	-	+	-	< 2000	None
Gout	-	++	-	+	> 2000	Negatively birefringent
Pseudogout	-	++	+	-	> 2000	Positively birefringent
Septic	-	+	-	++	> 50,000	None

-, almost never; +, occasional; ++, frequent.

Cell counts

Cell counts must be performed on all synovial fluids. Representative values are shown in Table 3. Leukocyte counts must be done by hand using saline diluent because the usual acetic acid diluent will cause formation of a mucin clot, cell clumping, and inaccurate results. This problem also occurs with automated cell counters, which use acetic acid as a diluent.

Crystal identification

Crystal identification requires a compensated polarized light microscope and an experienced observer. If either is unavail-able, fluid or stained slide preparations may be forwarded to a reference laboratory [5,6]. However, immediate crystal analysis is preferable [7]. Monosodium urate monohydrate crystals are typically needle-shaped and are strongly negatively birefringent. Calcium pyrophosphate dihydrate crystals are needle-shaped or parallel pipeds and are weakly positively birefringent (Fig. 10). Rarely, crystals are absent in the fluid because a sympathetic effusion in a joint or bursa adjacent to the inflammatory site was aspirated, because the attack is waning, and crystals have been cleared from the joint, or because crystals are too small to be seen by light microscopy.

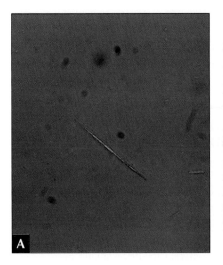

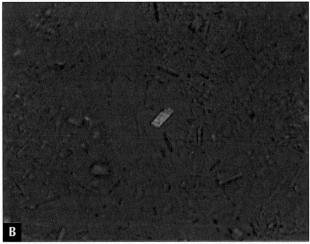

FIGURE 10 **A**, Needle-shaped urate crystals and **B**, rhomboidal calcium pyrophosphate dihydrate crystals. (*Courtesy of* Laureen Daft, BS, Medical College of Wisconsin.)

These ultramicrocrystals may be seen by electron microscopy and are less than 1 μm long [8].

Gram stain and culture are performed routinely on fluids from patients with acute monarthritis. Gram stains are less sensitive than cultures. Most septic arthritis is bacterial, and organisms are readily cultured from synovial fluid unless the patient has been receiving antibiotics. The sole exception is gonococcal arthritis, in which case synovial culture results may be negative; however, blood, urethral-cervical, rectal, or oral culture results may be positive.

In chronic infectious synovial effusions, bacterial culture results are usually negative. These fluids should be stained with KOH and cultured for fungus. An acid-fast stain and mycobacterial cultures should be performed on chronic unexplained synovial effusions. Synovial biopsies may be helpful in culture-negative cases of fungal and mycobacterial arthritis.

DIFFERENTIAL DIAGNOSIS

Referred pain, periarthritis, palindromic rheumatism, and early polyarthritis mimic monarthritis. In referred pain, active and passive joint motions are preserved, and joint effusions are absent. In periarthritis, joint swelling is absent or scant, and passive joint motion is preserved. Active motion, especially active resisted motion involving an inflamed tendon, would be painful and restricted. Palindromic rheumatism causes attacks of intense pain, swelling, and redness that typically peak in hours [9]. Inflammation is usually peri- or paraarticular. Episodes are brief (usually 2 days) and self-limited so as to mimic gout or pseudogout. Fingers and knees are the most commonly involved joints.

Uncommon crystals also may cause monarthritis. Calcium oxalate arthritis has been observed in patients on dialysis, especially if taking supplements of vitamin C, which is metabolized to oxalate (Fig. 11) [10]. These crystals are readily identified by polarized light microscopy. Microcrystalline basic calcium phosphate (hydroxyapatite and octacalcium phosphate) can produce attacks of arthritis [11], although more commonly they cause acute periarthritis or calcific tendonitis or are seen in conjunction with chronic degenerative arthritis [12]. Acute calcific periarthritis of the metatarsophalangeal

joint in premenopausal women resembles gout [13]. Liquid lipid crystals have been associated with acute attacks of monarthritis. Lastly, any polyarthritis may present as a monarthritis [14]. Long-term follow-up indicates that spondyloarthritis is the most common eventual diagnosis in cases of knee monarthritis that has evolved into systemic arthritis [15].

Treatment of acute monarthritis can begin once the diagnosis is established. Cases of traumatic arthritis should be referred to orthopedic surgeons, whereas other principle causes of acute monarthritis should be managed by primary care physicians. Because gram stains are less sensitive than cultures for bacterial arthritis, many patients with inflammatory arthritis are treated empirically with antibiotics while awaiting culture results. This is especially true if the synovial white blood count is greater than 50,000/cm or the patient has a temperature greater than 102°F. Antibiotic choice depends on identification of the site of primary infection (recalling that most joints become infected by the hematogenous route) and risk factors for gram negative infection such as intravenous drug abuse. It is important to remember that joint infections are closed space infections and adequate drainage by repeated needle aspiration or surgery is a necessary part of therapy.

Following diagnosis of the cause of monarthritis, several considerations remain. If septic arthritis is diagnosed, a careful search for a silent source of bacteremia must be made unless the septic process is a result of a penetrating injury. The search is directed by the usual anatomic distribution of pathology caused by the isolated organism. If traumatic arthritis is diagnosed, surgical considerations are important regarding repair of damaged structures, particularly menisci and ligaments. If gout is diagnosed, consideration of the correctable etiologic factors is essential. Weight reduction and limited alcohol consumption are important nonpharmacologic treatments. The clinician must be aware that pseudogout may be the presenting manifestation of several metabolic conditions that predispose to calcium pyrophosphate crystal formation. These factors are enumerated in Table 2. Some of these conditions predominantly cause crystal deposition that is clinically apparent in young persons; therefore, screening elderly patients is unnecessary (Table 4).

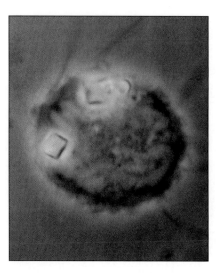

FIGURE 11
Crystals of calcium oxalate.

TREATMENT OF ACUTE AND CHRONIC MONARTHRITIS

Treatment of acute monarthritis can begin once the diagnosis is established.

TREATMENT OF CRYSTAL-ASSOCIATED ARTHRITIS

Acute gout is treated with full doses of nonsteroidal anti-inflammatory drugs (NSAIDs). Colchicine, in either oral or parenteral form, can be used as an alternative to NSAIDs but may have significant toxicity when used inappropriately. With normal kidney, liver, and bone marrow function, oral colchicine can be given at doses of 0.5 mg each hour until side effects occur or pain resolves. Oral doses should never exceed

TABLE 4 RECOMMENDED METABOLIC SCREENING IN PATIENTS WITH PSEUDOGOUT

Calcium and phosphorus
Iron and iron binding (transferrin)
Alkaline phosphatase*
Magnesium*
Thyroid-stimulating hormone

*Screen only patients younger than 55 years of age.

5 mg in 24 hours in normal individuals. Intravenous colchicine is given diluted in 20 mL of normal saline and administered slowly. Often, only a single intravenous dose is required. The total intravenous dose must not exceed 4 mg in 24 hours, and the drug should not be administered beyond 24 hours. Intravenous colchicine should be used cautiously in elderly patients. Its use is contraindicated in patients already taking oral colchicine or in those with abnormal liver, kidney, or bone marrow function. If these guidelines are not followed, severe bone marrow suppression may lead to infection and death. Patients who are unable to take NSAIDs or colchicine can be treated with intraarticular steroids. Once the acute attack has resolved, prophylactic therapy may be indicated. Uric acid–lowering agents, such as allopurinol (300 mg/d) or probenecid (1–3 g/d in divided dosages), are used most commonly. Colchicine (0.6 mg one to three times daily) may also prevent acute gouty attacks. Probenecid is not effective and should not be used in patients with renal insufficiency (creatinine, >2 mg/dL). The allopurinol dose must be reduced milligram for milligram in patients receiving azathioprine. Allopurinol or probenecid is started at least 10 days after all symptoms of the acute attack have resolved. We often continue NSAIDs or oral colchicine during hypouricemic therapy because fluxes in serum urate levels can precipitate acute gout attacks. Consultation with a rheumatologist should be obtained for gout that is refractory to the usual measures or if treatment is complicated by multiple system failures or interfering drugs.

Other types of crystal-associated arthritis are treated similarly to acute gout. NSAIDs and colchicine are most effective for acute attacks of pseudogout. Therapeutic arthrocentesis and intraarticular steroids also may be helpful. Arthritis associated with basic calcium phosphate or calcium oxalate crystals is treated with NSAIDs or intraarticular steroids. Future attacks of calcium oxalate arthritis can be diminished by decreasing ascorbate intake and increasing the efficacy of dialysis.

Treatment of chronic monarthritis also is tailored to the etiology of the illness. Degenerative joint disease is treated with analgesics, antiinflammatory drugs, and physical therapy. Fungal arthritis often responds to amphotericin B, joint drainage, and surgical debridement. Joint tumors also may require surgery. Mycobacterial joint infections usually are managed with combinations of antituberculous antibiotics.

REFERENCES AND RECOMMENDED READING

Recently published papers of particular interest have been highlighted as:
• Of interest
•• Of outstanding interest

1. Terkeltaub RA: Pathogenesis and treatment of crystal-induced inflammation. In *Arthritis and Allied Conditions*, edn 12. Edited by McCarty DJ, Koopman WJ. Philadelphia: Lea & Febiger; 1993:1819–1833.

2. Terkeltaub RA, Ginsberg MH: The inflammatory reaction to crystals. *Rheum Dis Clin North Am* 1988, 14:353–364.

3.• Burack DA, Griffith BP, Thompson ME, Kahl LE: Hyperuricemia and gout among heart transplant recipients receiving cyclosporine. *Am J Med* 1992, 92:141–146.

4.• Jones AC, Chuck AJ, Arie EA, *et al.*: Diseases associated with calcium pyrophosphate deposition disease. *Semin Arthritis Rheum* 1992, 22:188–202.

5. McGill NW, Swan A, Dieppe PA: Survival of calcium pyrophosphate crystals in stored synovial fluids. *Ann Rheum Dis* 1991, 50:939–941.

6. Lazcano O, Bilbao J, Beissner RS, *et al.*: Permanent stained preparations of synovial fluid for detection of calcium compounds using alizarin red S. *Biotech Histochem* 1992, 67:14–20.

7. Kerolus JA, Scott JT: Is it mandatory to examine synovial fluids promptly after arthrocentesis? *Arthritis Rheum* 1989, 32:271–278.

8. Bjelle A, Crocker P, Willoughby D: Ultra-microcrystals in pyrophosphate arthropathy. *Acta Med Scand* 1980, 207:89–92.

9. Guerne P-A, Weisman MH: Palindromic rheumatism: part or apart from the spectrum of rheumatoid arthritis. *Am J Med* 1992, 93:451–460.

10. Rosenthal A, Ryan LM, McCarty DJ: Arthritis associated with calcium oxalate crystals in an anephric patient treated with peritoneal dialysis. *JAMA* 1988, 260:1280–1282.

11. Schumacher HR, Smolyo AP, Tse RL, Maurer K: Arthritis associated with apatite crystals. *Ann Intern Med* 1977, 87:411–416.

12. Halverson PB, Carrera GF, McCarty DJ: Milwaukee shoulder syndrome. *Arch Intern Med* 1990, 150:677–682.

13. Fam AG, Rubenstein J: Hydroxyapatite pseudopodagra. *Arthritis Rheum* 1989, 32:741–747.

14. Gardner GC, Terkeltaub RA: Acute monarthritis associated with intracellular positively birefringent Maltese cross appearing spherules. *J Rheumatol* 1989, 16:294–296.

15. Blocka KLN, Sibley JT: Undiagnosed chronic monarthritis. *Arthritis Rheum* 1987, 30:1357–1361.

SELECT BIBLIOGRAPHY

Baker DG, Schumacher HR Jr: Acute monarthritis. *New Engl J Med* 1993, 329:1013–1020

Dieppe PA: Investigation and management of gout in the young and the elderly. *Ann Rheum Dis* 1991, 50:263–266.

Fam AG: Calcium pyrophosphate crystal deposition disease and other crystal deposition diseases. *Curr Opin Rheum* 1992, 4:574–582.

Ho G Jr: Bacterial arthritis. *Curr Opin Rheum* 1993, 5:449–453.

Scopelitis E, Martize-Osuna P: Gonococcal arthritis. *Rheum Dis Clin N Am* 1993, 19:363–377.

Endocrine and Metabolic Arthropathies 13
Alan J. Bridges

> ### Key Points
> - Endocrine and metabolic diseases are often accompanied by rheumatic symptoms and signs.
> - Diabetes mellitus is associated with limited joint mobility, neuropathy, and tendinitis.
> - Chondrocalcinosis and acute attacks of pseudogout may be seen in association with hypothyroidism, hyperparathyroidism, acromegaly, hemochromatosis, ochronosis, Wilson's disease, and dialysis-associated arthropathy.
> - Osteoporosis is associated with hyperthyroidism, hyperparathyroidism, corticosteroid excess, Wilson's disease, and dialysis-associated arthropathy.
> - Early diagnosis of the metabolic disorders is important so that therapy can be instituted prior to irreversible damage.

Some endocrine and metabolic diseases are associated with rheumatic symptoms and signs, among other clinical manifestations. For an arthropathy associated with an endocrine or metabolic disease to be diagnosed, the musculoskeletal findings must be placed in the context of other systemic and organ system abnormalities.

ENDOCRINOPATHIES

Diabetes Mellitus

Management of the common musculoskeletal manifestations associated with diabetes mellitus is listed in Table 1. Many of these disorders are associated with proliferation of fibrous tissue, which causes nerve entrapment and limited joint mobility, especially in the hands, shoulder, hip, palm, and fingers [1]. The remaining musculoskeletal manifestations of diabetes mellitus relate to long-standing small-vessel vasculopathy and diabetic neuropathy. Optimum control of the blood glucose level is important to prevent these sequelae [1]. Symptoms and disability associated with limited joint mobility should be managed with physical and occupational therapy, but the response to these treatments is often limited. Nerve entrapment, flexor tenosynovitis, and Dupuytren's contracture are managed by local corticosteroid injection or surgical decompression.

Thyroid Disease
Hypothyroidism

In primary hypothyroidism, excess mucopolypeptide tissue deposition gives rise to various musculoskeletal manifestations (Table 2). Although the relationship

TABLE 1 TREATMENT OF MUSCULOSKELETAL MANIFESTATIONS ASSOCIATED WITH DIABETES MELLITUS

Manifestation	Treatment
Diabetic syndrome of limited joint mobility (cheiroarthropathy)	Physical and occupational therapy
Diabetic stiff hand syndrome	
Adhesive capsulitis	
Neuropathic (Charcot) joints (below the knee)	Limitation of weight-bearing and pedorthic support of surrounding joint structures
Diffuse idiopathic skeletal hyperostosis	Analgesia
Carpal tunnel syndrome and other entrapment neuropathies	Local corticosteroid injection or surgical decompression
Flexor tenosynovitis	Local corticosteroid injection or surgical decompression
Dupuytren's contractures	Local corticosteroid injection or surgical decompression
Diabetic amyotrophy (acute neuropathy of a large proximal nerve)	Typically self-limiting, resolving slowly over 1–3 y

TABLE 2 MUSCULOSKELETAL MANIFESTATIONS OF HYPOTHYROIDISM

Noninflammatory myopathy
Noninflammatory synovitis
Entrapment neuropathies, including carpal tunnel syndrome
Peripheral neuropathy
Avascular necrosis
Hashimoto's thyroiditis associated with connective tissue diseases, including systemic lupus erythematosus, Sjögren's syndrome, and rheumatoid arthritis
Tenosynovitis

between this manifestation and hypothyroidism is unclear, chondrocalcinosis caused by calcium pyrophosphate dihydrate (CPPD) crystal deposition disease may be associated with hypothyroidism. Low levels of thyroid hormone may lead to myopathy or to neuropathy. Proximal muscle weakness, abnormal electromyographic and nerve conduction study results, and marked elevation of the serum creatine kinase level may be found at the time of, or may antedate, the symptoms of hypothyroidism. The arthropathy, myopathy, and neuropathy of hypothyroidism respond to treatment with thyroid hormone replacement [2]; however, subclinical pseudogout or gout may flare when thyroid replacement is begun. Nonsteroidal antiinflammatory drugs (NSAIDs) and colchicine are used to treat flares of crystalline arthropathy.

Hyperthyroidism

Thyroid acropachy is a rheumatic manifestation that occurs in 1% of patients with hyperthyroidism. Typically, patients with this disorder have been treated for hyperthyroidism by radioablation or thyroidectomy and are clinically hypothyroid or euthyroid. The clinical manifestations of thyroid acropachy include clubbing, periostitis (Fig. 1), soft tissue swelling and pain, exophthalmos, and pretibial myxedema. Long-acting thyroid stimulator is often detectable in the serum of affected patients.

Myopathy manifesting in mild to severe weakness may be found in up to 70% of patients with hyperthyroidism. Serum levels of creatine kinase are typically normal in these patients. Prolonged untreated hyperthyroidism and overtreatment with thyroid hormone replacement are associated with bone loss and subsequent osteoporosis.

Autoimmune (Hashimoto's) thyroiditis is associated with transient hyperthyroidism early in its course. During this phase, the patient often complains of diffuse stiffness and aching in the muscles and joints.

Correction of thyroid dysfunction typically is associated with improvement of the clinical manifestations of thyroid acropachy, myopathy, and diffuse myalgias and arthralgias associated with autoimmune thyroiditis [2]. NSAIDs or corticosteroids may be used to control the symptoms and inflammation associated with thyroid acropachy.

Hyperparathyroidism

Hyperparathyroidism is associated with many rheumatic manifestations, including spontaneous fractures, diffuse bone

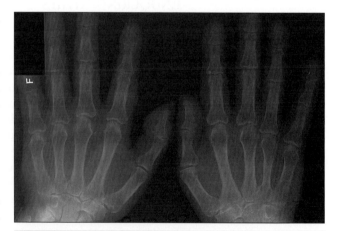

FIGURE 1 Radiograph showing the classic manifestations of thyroid acropachy: periosteal bone formation at the metacarpophalanges (left, fifth) and proximal phalanges (bilateral, second through fifth). The dense new periosteal bone is more prominent on the radial aspects of the phalanges.

and joint pain, bone cysts (brown tumor), proximal myopathy, and peripheral neuropathy. Elevated levels of parathyroid hormone accelerate bone resorption, which may lead to osteoporosis, subperiosteal bone reabsorption (Fig. 2), osteolysis (Figs. 3 and 4), bone erosions (Fig. 3), and bone cysts (Fig. 5) and if allowed to continue long enough, osteitis fibrosa cystica (Fig. 6). The bony erosions may occur in the distal interphalangeal, metacarpal, carpal, and acromioclavicular joints. Diagnosis of hyperparathyroidism is made when an elevated serum parathyroid hormone level that is disproportionate to the serum calcium level is obtained.

Crystalline arthropathy, including chondrocalcinosis, CPPD crystal disease (pseudogout) (Fig. 7), and gout are common in primary hyperparathyroidism. Secondary hyper-parathyroidism, in addition to causing the changes already discussed, may be associated with the precipitation of basic calcium phosphate crystals (apatite and related crystals) when the calcium phosphate ion product is elevated. This condition may lead to local tissue inflammation.

Resection of the hyperfunctioning parathyroid tissue is necessary in patients with hyperparathyroidism. Most of the musculoskeletal manifestations of hyperparathyroidism improve with normalization of the parathyroid hormone level. However, this effect may not be enough to reverse significant osteoporosis. Further treatment of osteoporosis may be necessary. Basic calcium crystals and CPPD crystals do not dissolve after parathyroidectomy.

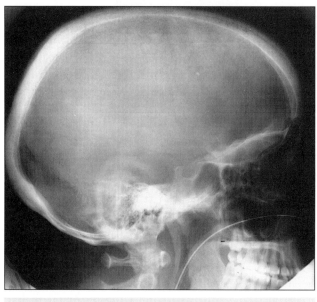

FIGURE 2 Radiograph showing subperiosteal resorption of bone, which leads to a linear lucency and focal scattered resorption of trabecular bone, giving a "salt and pepper" appearance resulting from primary hyperparathyroidism.

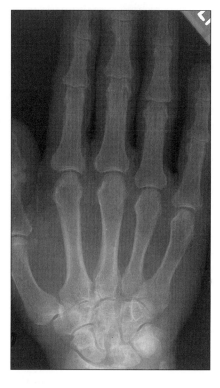

FIGURE 3 Radiograph showing subperiosteal resorption of bone in primary hyperparathyroidism, which leads to phalangeal tuft resorption (second digit), intracortical bone resorption (second through fifth proximal phalanges), and juxta-articular erosions (second and third proximal phalangeal, fifth metacarpophalangeal, and carpal bones). Multiple cysts in the carpal bones and radius suggest brown tumors.

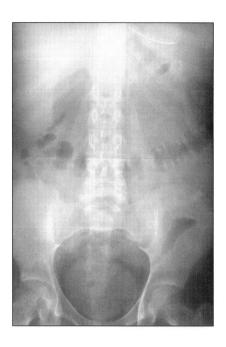

FIGURE 4 Marked subchondral bone resorption and adjacent reactive sclerosis about both sacroiliac joints are present in this patient with primary hyperparathyroidism. There is a brown tumor in the right femoral head.

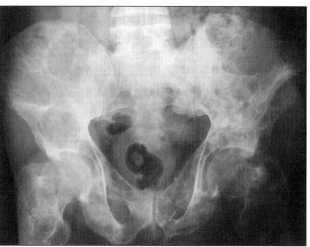

FIGURE 5 Radiograph showing widespread, well-defined bone cysts of bone tumors in a patient with primary hyperparathyroidism.

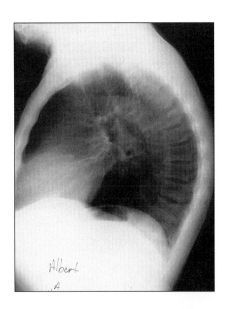

FIGURE 6
A rugger jersey
spine is evident
in this radi-
ograph of a
patient with
primary hyper-
parathyroidism.
There is marked
osteopenia of
the spine, with
band-like scle-
rosis of the
superior and
inferior margins
of the vertebral
bodies, which
suggests osteitis
fibrosa cystica.

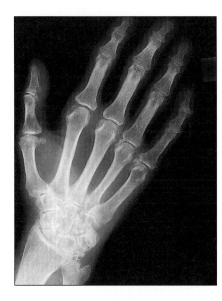

FIGURE 7
Radiograph
showing chon-
drocalcinosis of
the proximal
interphalangeal,
metacarpopha-
langeal, and
wrist joints in
a patient with
calcium
pyrophosphate
dihydrate depo-
sition disease
and primary
hyperparathy-
roidism.

Pituitary and Adrenal Gland Disorders

Acromegaly

Excess secretion of growth hormone from a pituitary adenoma leads to acromegaly, which is caused by proliferation of synovium, cartilage, bone, and other soft tissues under the influence of growth hormone and insulin-like growth factors [3]. Fifty percent to 75% of patients with acromegaly develop musculoskeletal manifestations (Table 3, Fig. 8). Carpal tunnel syndrome, usually bilateral, is a common presenting feature.

Many rheumatic manifestations of acromegaly respond to resection of the pituitary adenoma or treatment with the somatostatin analogue octreotide [3]. However, irreversible osteoarthritis typically does not respond and requires NSAIDs or surgical treatment.

Corticosteroid hormone excess or insufficiency

Hypercortisolism from Cushing's syndrome or exogenous administration of corticosteroids causes abnormalities of muscle and bone. Corticosteroid myopathy involves the proximal muscles and can mimic polymyositis. However, muscle enzyme levels are typically normal in patients with this disorder. Electromyographic study results are abnormal and are not helpful in distinguishing between polymyositis and corticosteroid myopathy. However, muscle biopsy specimens show type II fiber atrophy in patients with corticosteroid myopathy.

Osteoporosis and spontaneous fractures are a serious consequence of corticosteroid hormone excess. Avascular necrosis is more common after high-dose steroid therapy than low or moderate dose steroid therapy, but it can occur with prolonged use of more modest doses, for example, 10 to 20 mg of prednisone daily. Treatment with bolus doses of methylprednisolone (approximately 1 g) may produce a large, painful, tense knee effusion. Synovial fluid is clear and nearly acellular in these patients. Corticosteroid insufficiency from Addison's disease or prednisone withdrawal is commonly accompanied by diffuse arthralgias.

Diagnosis of Cushing's syndrome is based on the finding of elevated levels of serum and urine glucocorticoids and resistance to inhibition of adrenal cortisol secretion by dexamethasone. Treatment is directed at the cause of Cushing's syndrome and consists of resection of pituitary or nonpituitary tumor or resection of adrenal hyperplasia. Osteoporosis typically requires additional therapy to reverse the bone loss. Symptoms associated with corticosteroid insufficiency respond to replacement therapy.

TABLE 3 MUSCULOSKELETAL MANIFESTATIONS OF ACROMEGALY	
Manifestation	**Characteristics**
Arthropathy	Osteoarthritis
	Widened joint spaces
	Chondrocalcinosis
	Diffuse idiopathic skeletal hyperostosis
Soft tissue overgrowth	Ligament laxity and joint instability
	Widened intervertebral disk spaces
Noninflammatory myopathy	Muscle weakness
	Muscle pain
Neuropathy	Peripheral neuropathy
	Entrapment syndromes, *eg*, carpal tunnel syndrome

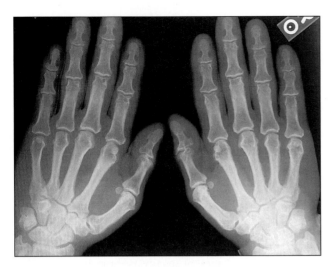

FIGURE 8 Radiograph shows findings characteristic of acromegaly: enlargement of the tuft and base of the terminal phalanges, soft tissue thickening, widening of the width of the proximal phalanges, and osteophytes of the proximal interphalangeal and metacarpophalangeal joints.

METABOLIC DISORDERS
Hemochromatosis

Idiopathic (familial) hemochromatosis is an autosomal recessive disorder characterized by excessive iron deposition in several organ systems that give rise to organ dysfunction (Table 4). It is common, occurring in 1 per 200 people; however, it is commonly undiagnosed, and many mildly affected people remain asymptomatic or minimally symptomatic [4].

Arthropathy may be the first symptom of hemochromatosis [4,5•], and the most common joint abnormality is degenerative arthritis of the knees, hips, and hands. Metacarpophalangeal and proximal and distal interphalangeal joints of the hands are characteristically involved and show bony enlargement with minimal or no soft tissue swelling. Radiographs reveal classic changes of degenerative arthritis, with nonuniform joint space narrowing, subchondral cysts and sclerosis, and osteophytosis (Fig. 9). Up to 60% of patients with hemochromatosis develop chondrocalcinosis. Presentation of chondrocalcinosis without degenerative changes or acute pseudogout is less common.

Hemochromatosis is diagnosed by measuring the serum iron level, total iron binding capacity, and serum ferritin level. The latter correlates directly with body iron stores. A serum iron level of greater than 175 µg/dL and transferrin saturation of greater than 60% suggest hemochromatosis. The diagnosis is confirmed by liver biopsy and measurement of hepatic iron content.

Preventative therapy before the onset of tissue damage and organ dysfunction is the optimal treatment. Repeated phlebotomy to remove excess iron is useful for reversing cardiomyopathy, precirrhotic liver dysfunction, and endocrinopathy, but the arthropathy of hemochromatosis does not respond to this treatment [6]. Symptomatic treatment with analgesics, NSAIDs, and physical therapy helps control pain and maintain function. Severe degenerative changes of large joints are managed by joint replacement.

Ochronosis

Ochronosis is the clinical and pathologic consequence of alkaptonuria, an autosomal recessive disorder of tyrosine metabolism with excretion of homogentisic acid in the urine. Alkaptonuria is characterized by urine that becomes black when oxidized. Tissue accumulation of homogentisic acid leads to the clinical manifestations of ochronosis (Table 5) [7]. Ochronosis develops in all persons with alkaptonuria by the age of 30 to 40 years.

Most patients with ochronosis develop spondylosis [8], and the consequent back pain and stiffness relate to degenerative disk disease and disk calcification. Degenerative disk disease can also lead to disk herniation and sciatica. In the spondylosis of ochronosis, there are few if any other manifestations of osteoarthritis of the spine.

The peripheral arthropathy of ochronosis is degenerative and involves the knees, shoulders, hips, and less commonly, the small joints [8]. Symptoms of pain and stiffness may ante-

TABLE 4 ORGAN INVOLVEMENT AND CLINICAL MANIFESTATIONS OF HEMOCHROMATOSIS	
Organ system	**Clinical manifestations**
Liver	Cirrhosis, portal hypertension, hepatoma
Pancreas	Diabetes mellitus, malabsorption
Pituitary system	Loss of libido, impotence, testicular atrophy
Skin	Hyperpigmentation, hair loss
Heart and vessels	Heart failure, dysrhythmias
Joints	Chondrocalcinosis (calcium pyrophosphate dihydrate crystal deposition disease), osteoarthritis

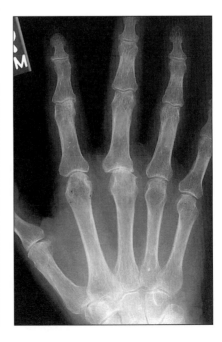

FIGURE 9 Radiograph showing degenerative changes, particularly at the second and third metacarpophalangeal joints, in a patient with hemochromatosis. Joint space narrowing, subchondral sclerosis, and cystic change are present. There is a small beak-like head at the third metacarpal head and diffuse osteopenia.

TABLE 5 MANIFESTATIONS OF OCHRONOSIS	
Organ system	**Manifestation**
Skin	Hyperpigmentation
Joints	Degenerative arthritis, chondrocalcinosis, degenerative disk disease
Kidney	Alkaptonuria, tubulointerstitial disease
Heart and vessels	Valvular disease, arteriosclerosis

date radiographic changes. Chondrocalcinosis or acute attacks of pseudogout may be seen in a few cases.

No therapy is available for the enzymatic deficiency of homogentisic acid oxidase. Diets low in phenylalanine, tyrosine, and protein may decrease urinary levels of homogentisic acid but are not effective treatments of ochronosis. Ascorbic acid administration, which decreases binding of homogentisic acid to tissue, is also ineffective. Analgesics and back braces may help control pain and improve function. Peripheral joint involvement in ochronosis is treated similarly to idiopathic osteoarthritis.

Wilson's Disease

Hepatolenticular degeneration, or Wilson's disease, is a rare autosomal recessive disorder of copper metabolism characterized by corneal pigmentation or Kayser-Fleischer rings (Table 6) [9,10].

Penicillamine is the treatment of choice for mobilizing copper from involved tissues in patients with Wilson's disease [9,10]. In dosages ranging from 1 to 4 g/d, penicillamine treatment produces symptomatic improvement over months to years. Free serum copper levels, 24-hour urine copper levels, complete blood count, and urinalysis should be monitored to assess the effectiveness of penicillamine treatment and its side effects. Free serum copper level can be expected to return to normal with successful treatment. Joint symptoms do not predictably respond to penicillamine treat-

ment and are symptomatically treated with analgesics and NSAIDs. Trientine and zinc therapy are also useful for patients with Wilson's disease.

Dialysis-Associated Arthropathy

Patients undergoing chronic dialysis for renal failure may develop disabling arthritis. Dialysis-associated arthropathy encompasses many pathologic processes that are often difficult to distinguish from one another (Table 7). Some of these processes were discussed earlier in the hyperparathyroidism section and are discussed in other chapters as well [11].

β_2-Microglobulin amyloid deposition develops in patients receiving hemodialysis or peritoneal dialysis [12,13•,14]. Symptoms typically develop after 5 years of dialysis. Radiographic features typical of spondyloarthropathy (Fig. 10) or erosive arthropathy (Fig. 11), tissue staining for amyloid by use of Congo red stain, and polarized light microscopy provide the correct diagnosis.

Aluminum toxicity from phosphate-binding antacids or dialysate fluid may cause bone pain, fracture, and myopathy [15]. In these patients, the diagnosis is based on elevated serum aluminum levels, which rise after an infusion of desferoxamine, an aluminum-binding agent.

Calcium pyrophosphate dihydrate or basic calcium phosphate crystals have been found in diseased tissues of the spine, peripheral tendons, and joints in renal failure. The clinical manifestations of such deposition appear similar to those of basic calcium phosphate or CPPD crystal deposition disease of the spine and peripheral joints.

Renal transplantation improves symptoms related to β_2-microglobulin amyloid or aluminum intoxication [16]. A change from the conventional cellulose membrane to the high-flux membrane to lower β_2-microglobulin levels may be helpful [14]. Decreasing aluminum intake and administering desferoxamine infusions are helpful treatments of aluminum intoxication and the associated musculoskeletal symptoms.

TABLE 6 MANIFESTATIONS OF WILSON'S DISEASE	
Organ system	**Manifestations**
Nervous system	Dysarthria, tremor, ataxia, psychological disturbances, headache, convulsions
Stomach and intestines	Organomegaly, abdominal pain, hepatitis, jaundice, cirrhosis, portal hypertension
Blood and blood-forming tissues	Hemolytic anemia, thrombocytopenia, leukopenia
Eyes	Kayser-Fleischer rings, cataracts, keratitis
Bone and joints	Degenerative arthritis, chondrocalcinosis, osteopenia or osteomalacia, periarticular calcifications, joint hypermobility
Kidney	Renal tubular dysfunction, renal stones
Heart and vessels	Myocarditis, myocardial fibrosis, heart failure, dysrhythmias
Endocrine system	Gynecomastia, amenorrhea, glucose intolerance, hypoparathyroidism

TABLE 7 DIALYSIS-ASSOCIATED ARTHROPATHY

β_2-Microglobulin amyloid deposition disease
    Arthropathy with large joint effusions
    Scapulohumeral periarthritis
    Spondyloarthropathy
    Entrapment neuropathy
Aluminum toxicity
Hydroxyapatite crystal deposition disease
Calcium pyrophosphate dihydrate crystal deposition disease
Secondary hyperparathyroidism
Avascular necrosis of bone
Erosive osteoarthritis

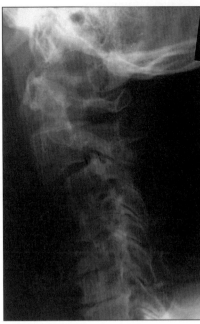

FIGURE 10
Radiograph from a patient with chronic renal failure whose condition was maintained on hemodialysis. The features are characteristic of hemodialysis spondyloarthropathy, with disk space narrowing, calcification of the disk space, erosion of the vertebral end plates at C_3-C_7, and subluxation.

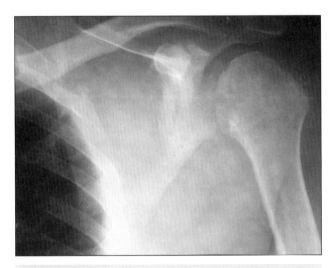

FIGURE 11 Radiograph from a patient with chronic renal failure whose condition was maintained on hemodialysis. There is marked destruction of the glenohumeral joint, with erosion, subchondral cysts, and juxta-articular calcifications.

Arthropathy of Hyperlipoproteinemia

Inherited disorders of lipid transport or lipoprotein metabolism may lead to xanthomas of soft tissues and bones and numerous musculoskeletal manifestations, including avascular necrosis of the bone [17]. Xanthomas, which may become inflamed and tender, occur along the extensor tendons, subcutaneous tissues, and periosteum in types 2, 3, and 4 hyperlipoproteinemia.

Type 2 hyperlipoproteinemia is associated with recurrent episodes of acute, migratory mono-, oligo-, or polyarthritis in 50% of patients [17]. Symmetric, inflammatory large joint involvement is typically self-limited and lasts from a few days to 2 weeks. Achilles tendinitis is common. Radiographs may be normal or may show paraarticular bone cysts that contain fat cells and fibrous tissue. A similar arthropathy may be seen in type 4 hyperlipoproteinemia and familial hypercholesterolemia [18].

The hyperlipoproteinemias are treatable by diet modification and drug therapy with lipid-lowering agents. In some cases, acute and chronic rheumatic manifestations can be abated with this treatment [17].

REFERENCES AND RECOMMENDED READING

Recently published papers of particular interest have been highlighted as:
• Of interest
•• Of outstanding interest

1. Kapoor A, Sibbitt WL Jr.: Contractures in diabetes mellitus: the syndrome of limited joint mobility. *Semin Arthritis Rheum* 1989, 18:168–180.
2. Kloppenburg M, Dijkmans BAC, Rasker JJ: Effect of therapy for thyroid dysfunction on musculoskeletal symptoms. *Clin Rheumatol* 1993, 12:341–345.
3. Lieberman SA, Bjorkengren AG, Hoffman AR: Rheumatologic and skeletal changes in acromegaly. *Endocrinol Metab Clin North Am* 1992, 21:615–631.
4. Bomford AB, Dymock IW, Hamilton EBD: Genetic haemochromatosis. *Gut* 1991, 4(suppl):S111–S115.
5.• Adams PC, Kertesz AE, Valberg LS: Clinical presentation of hemochromatosis: a changing scene. *Am J Med* 1991, 90:445–449.
6. Adams PC, Speechley M, Kertesz AE: Long-term survival analysis in hereditary hemochromatosis. *Gastroenterology* 1991, 101:368–372.
7. Gaines JJ: The pathology of alkaptonuric ochronosis. *Hum Pathol* 1989, 20:40–46.
8. O'Brien WM: Biochemical, pathologic and clinical aspects of alkaptonuria, ochronosis, and ochronotic arthropathy: review of the world literature (1584–1963). *Am J Med* 1963, 34:813–823.
9. Yarze JC, Martin P, Munoz SJ, Friedman LS: Wilson's disease: current status. *Am J Med* 1992, 92:643–654.
10. Brewer GJ, Yuzbasiyan-Gurkan V: Wilson's disease. *Medicine* 1992, 71:139–164.
11. Rubin LA, Fam AG, Rubenstein J, *et al.*: Erosive azotemic osteoarthropathy. *Arthritis Rheum* 1984, 27:1086–1094.
12. Ford PM: Arthropathies associated with renal disease including dialysis-related amyloid. *Curr Opin Rheumatol* 1992, 4:63–67.
13.• Kessler M, Netter P, Azoulay E, *et al.*: Dialysis-associated arthropathy: a multicenter survey of 171 patients receiving haemodialysis for over 10 years. *Br J Rheumatol* 1992, 31:157–162.

14. Maury CPJ: β₂-Microglobulin amyloidosis. *Rheumatol Int* 1990, 10:1–8.

15. Netter P, Kessler M, Burnel D, *et al.*:Aluminum in the joint tissues of chronic renal failure patients treated with regular hemodialysis and aluminum compounds. *J Rheumatol* 1984, 11:66–70.

16. Bardin T, LeBail-Darné JL, Zingraff J, *et al.*: Dialysis arthropathy: outcome after renal transplantation. *Am J Med* 1995, 99:245–248.

17. Careless DJ, Cohen MG: Rheumatic manifestations of hyperlipidemia and antihypelipidemia drug therapy. *Sem Arthritis Rem* 1993, 23:90–98.

18. Wysenbeek AJ, Shani E, Beigel Y: Musculoskeletal manifestations in patients with hypercholesterolemia. *J Rheumatol* 1989, 16:643–645.

SELECT BIBLIOGRAPHY

Brick JE, Brick JF, Elnicki DM: Musculoskeletal disorders: when are they caused by hormone imbalance? *Postgrad Med* 1991, 90:129–136.

Cronin ME: Rheumatic aspects of endocrinopathies. In *Arthritis and Allied Conditions: A Textbook of Rheumatology*, edn 12. Edited by McCarty DJ, Koopman WJ. Malvern, PA: Lea & Febiger; 1993:1955–1971.

Hordon LD, Wright V: Endocrine disorders. *Curr Opin Rheumatol* 1992, 4:84–89.

Infectious Arthritis 14
Frank R. Schmid

> ### *Key Points*
> - Infection of a musculoskeletal structure, although infrequent, must be considered promptly as the cause for any episode of acute inflammation of a single bone, joint, tendon, or bursa.
> - Removal and culture of infected fluid from the inflamed structure is necessary to identify the responsible bacterium.
> - Joint drainage by aspiration and lavage, or by arthroscopy or arthrectomy, is performed to reduce high intracapsular pressure and to remove phlogistic fluid.
> - A favorable outcome follows early recognition and treatment of an antibiotic-susceptible infection in a previously healthy host with an intact immune system.

Pathogens infrequently invade and cause an infectious inflammatory response of bones, joints, tendons, or bursae. When infection is due to a bacterium (Table 1), complete restoration of joint function can be expected if the problem is recognized early and treated properly. Characteristics of such an ideal bacterial infection include a previously healthy adult host with an intact immune system; involvement of a single previously normal peripheral joint, tendon, or bursa; an identifiable pathogen sensitive to a well-tolerated antibiotic; and easily accomplished needle aspiration of the infected joint. If some of these characteristics are not met, a less favorable outcome may result. Some factors in bacterial arthritis that interfere with complete recovery are:

An infant or elderly host

An immunocompromised host

Involvement of a previously damaged joint or an axial bone or joint (spine or hip)

Delayed ability or inability to identify the pathogen or detection of an antibiotic-resistant pathogen

Difficult joint drainage

Protracted inflammation despite apparently optimal therapy

Viruses, most commonly parvovirus B19, hepatitis B virus, and rubella virus and vaccine, also initiate an acute but usually self-limited polyarthritis rather than a monarthritis. Most resolve completely without treatment. Residual joint damage is rare [1••].

CLASSIC SYNDROME OF BACTERIAL ARTHRITIS

Clinical Presentation

Bacterial arthritis usually affects one or two joints. In most cases, the target joint was previously normal; occasionally, however, evidence of prior injury may be detected.

TABLE 1 FREQUENCY AND EXPECTED RESPONSE OF BACTERIAL PATHOGENS TO APPROPRIATE ANTIBIOTIC THERAPY IN UNCOMPLICATED BACTERIAL ARTHRITIS		
Bacterium	**Frequency, %**	**Response time, *wk***
Gonococci	25–50	Within 2
Staphylococci	25–50	2–6
Streptococci	10–15	2–3
Gram-negative bacilli	5–15	4–8*
Mycobacteria and fungi	2–5	Prolonged
*The host is often debilitated or immunocompromised.		

Any joint may be invaded, but the knee and the hip are attacked most frequently. In patients with a disseminated gonococcal or meningococcal infection, multiple joints are sometimes involved, often in a migratory fashion [2]. The skin over an affected joint is typically reddened and warm, and the joint is painful and distended with fluid.

Because bacteria usually enter a joint by a hematogenous route from an extraarticular site of infection, the patient may experience bacteremic symptoms of fever and chills. Bacteria lodge in the subsynovial capillary network or, less often, in paraarticular bone. From these sites, they rupture into the joint space [3,4].

Other acute arthritic disorders, such as gout, pseudogout (chondrocalcinosis), rheumatic fever, and oligoarticular syndromes associated with spondyloarthropathies, may be confused with infectious arthritis. In these conditions, however, high fever, chills, and marked leukocytosis are uncommon. Even if one of these noninfectious inflammatory syndromes exists, a superimposed infectious process should be excluded by bacterial examination and culture of synovial fluid if an infection is suspected.

Diagnostic Studies

A complete history and physical examination are essential, with a search for sites of infection elsewhere in the body from which the pathogen might have originated or to which it might have metastasized. The diagnosis can be clinched, for example, by detection of the erythema chronicum migrans of Lyme disease (a primary site of infection) or the vasculitic skin papules or microinfarcts of disseminated gonococcal disease (a metastatic site of infection) (Fig. 1), [2,5••]. In addition to examination of the skin, attention should be directed toward other possible portals of entry, such as the oropharynx, the genitourinary tract, and the gut. Culture specimens should be obtained from all obvious sites of infection, along with at least two blood specimens for cultures of aerobic and anaerobic organisms. Some microorganisms require special culture conditions. If *Neisseria gonorrhoeae* is suspected, for example, chocolate agar or a special medium and reduced oxygen incubation conditions are needed. The laboratory should be advised of the type of pathogen that is suspected clinically.

Although damage due to sepsis is not evident on early radiologic films, such films can document the extent of any prior damage and permit an estimate of the degree to which function might be restored. Other imaging techniques may be useful in special circumstances. Computed tomography is most valuable when the anatomic structures are complex or when the involved areas cannot be visualized distinctly because of adjacent or overlapping bony structures. Magnetic resonance imaging can demonstrate involvement of adjacent soft tissues. Technetium diphosphonate and gallium scintigraphy can distinguish between a soft tissue or a bony site of disease. Such scans identify which deep axial structures are involved, but they cannot indicate whether the abnormality is due to an infection.

Joint fluid examination

Examination of joint fluid is mandatory whenever infection is considered possible (Table 2). Arthrocentesis must be done at once if infection is suspected. If limited amounts of joint fluid are available, priority is given in the following order: culture, Gram's stain, and wet-mount preparation for a microscopic examination of cellular and possibly crystal contents of the fluid. These examinations can be completed with two or three drops of joint fluid [6]. Additional studies, using any remaining joint fluid, include a total leukocyte count; a differential leukocyte count; and if the patient is fasting, a synovial fluid

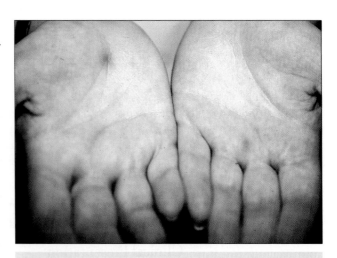

FIGURE 1 Small purpuric skin infarcts of disseminated gonococcal infection.

glucose level assessment. A decreased synovial fluid glucose value lacks specificity because low values may occur in noninfectious conditions, such as rheumatoid arthritis.

Antibiotic Treatment

Parenteral antibiotic administration should be initiated as soon as the specimens have been obtained for laboratory studies, and it should be maintained until clinical signs of active synovitis and inflammatory changes in the joint fluid revert toward normal. Infection caused by some staphylococci, particularly by Gram-negative rods, respond more slowly to antibiotic management than do infections caused by most coccal organisms (see Table 1) [7•].

Drainage

In most instances of classic peripheral joint infection, drainage is accomplished by needle aspiration of joint fluid. This procedure is performed as often as needed to reduce intracapsular pressure and remove pus. Lavage of the joint cavity with copious amounts of sterile physiologic saline or Ringer's solution facilitates more complete removal of cellular and particulate debris. Culture and leukocyte counts are needed on each specimen. Culture findings should become negative and leukocyte counts should show a serial stepwise decline if the therapy is successful. Arthroscopy allows for inspection of the articular cartilages and removal of necrotic tissue. Debris removed from the joint should be submitted for culture and histologic study. Surgical arthrotomy is withheld initially unless a deep joint,

such as the hip, in a child is involved or unless clinical or laboratory signs of inflammation have not decreased during the first week or two of antibiotic treatment [8].

Because infectious arthritis in its classic form offers a predictable response to therapy, a timetable of expected events can be constructed (Table 3). Anticipation of their occurrence aids in decision making during treatment and follow-up.

SPECIAL SITUATIONS

Lack of Identification of the Pathogen

A diagnosis of infectious arthritis is confirmed by demonstration of the etiologic agent in the synovial fluid or synovial tissue. Some microorganisms, such as spirochetes (*Borrelia* and *Treponema* species), mycobacteria, and fungi, grow slowly or require special conditions for culture. Sometimes, even common pathogens are not recovered on culture of the joint fluid, a circumstance in more than half of the cases of gonococcal arthritis. Even if an organism is not recovered from the joint, it may be cultured from the primary site of infection. Such a finding may be sufficient to initiate therapy.

Lyme disease and syphilis are examples of bacterial arthritis in which bacteria are rarely demonstrated in the patient's tissues. They share many features. Both are due to spirochetes, inoculated into the skin in Lyme disease by the bite of a species of the deer tick, *Ixodes*, and into mucous membranes in syphilis by sexual contact. After a period of days to weeks, a

TABLE 2 SYNOVIAL FLUID FINDINGS IN INFLAMMATORY ARTHRITIS

Joint fluid characteristic examined or test performed	Noninfectious finding	Infectious finding
Color	Yellow	Yellow, occasionally red or plum colored
Clarity	Turbid	Turbid, purulent
Viscosity	Reduced	Reduced
Cell count, n/mm^3	3000–50,000	10,000–> 100,000
Predominant cell type	Polymorphonuclear leukocyte	Polymorphonuclear leukocyte
Gram stain for organism	None	Positive*
Culture	Negative	Positive*

*No organism may be demonstrated in as many as 10% to 20% of cases, and negative results occur even more often in gonococcal infections.

TABLE 3 TIMETABLE FOR MONITORING THE CLASSIC SYNDROME OF BACTERIAL ARTHRITIS*

Time	Activity or outcome
0–2 h	Evaluation for possible infection
2–24 h	Initial choice of antibiotic; needle aspiration and/or lavage
24–72 h	Review of antibiotic choice; repetition of needle aspiration and lavage if needed
4–10 d	Assessment of expected decrease in joint inflammation; consideration of other antibiotic options or drainage if response is inadequate
1–4 wk	Cure of infection; outpatient planning
3 mo	Clinical and functional joint evaluation

*Major deviations from this schedule indicate unusual diagnostic problems, therapeutic problems, or both.

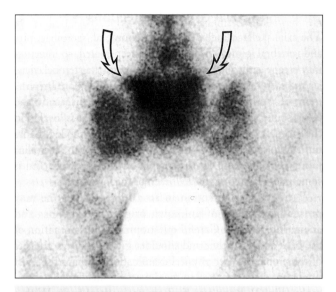

FIGURE 2 Technetium polyphosphonate scintigram showing an area of increased uptake in the vertebrae due to Staphylococcal osteomyelitis. (*From* Hendrix and Fisher [20]; with permission.)

FIGURE 3 A damaged joint resulting from synovial ischemia due to a markedly elevated intrasynovial fluid pressure, from synovial and capsular thickening, and from the erosive action of proliferative synovium.

swollen, noncompliant capsule; and by phlogistic products of the invading microorganism and the host defense system (Fig. 3). Antibiotic treatment and débridement are the logical measures to combat such tissue destruction. Because an inflammatory response may be triggered continually by antigenic fragments of the microorganism even after all viable bacteria have been eradicated by antibiotics and the bulk of the debris has been removed by drainage, nonsteroidal antiinflammatory drugs may be useful at the stage after the cause of the infection has been identified and successful treatment initiated.

WHEN TO REFER

A physician confronted with a patient in whom a diagnosis of infectious arthritis has been made or is suspected should seek the assistance of a rheumatologist (Table 5). In addition, an orthopedist or an infectious disease specialist may be needed.

TABLE 5 CONSULTANT'S ROLE IN INFECTIOUS ARTHRITIS
Rheumatologist Manager during acute episode Consultant for late complications Arthroscopy
Orthopedist Arthrotomy Joint reconstruction Arthroscopy
Infectious disease specialist Antibiotic choice Treatment of systemic infectious complications

REFERENCES AND RECOMMENDED READING

Recently published papers of particular interest have been highlighted as:
- Of interest
- •• Of outstanding interest

1.•• Smith CA: Virus-related arthritis, excluding human immunodeficiency virus. *Curr Opin Rheumatol* 1990, 2:635–641.

2. Brandt KD, Cathcart ES, Cohen AS: Gonococcal arthritis: clinical features correlated with blood, synovial fluid and genitourinary cultures. *Arthritis Rheum* 1974, 17:503–510.

3. Esterhai JL Jr., Gelb I: Adult septic arthritis. *Orthop Clin North Am* 1991, 22:503–514.

4. Nelson JD: The bacterial etiology and antibiotic management of septic arthritis in infants and children. *Pediatrics* 1972, 50:437–440.

5.•• Rahn D, Malawista S: Lyme disease: recommendations for diagnosis and treatment. *Ann Intern Med* 1991, 114:472–481.

6. Shmerling RH, Delbanco TL, Tosteson ANA, Trentham DE: Synovial fluid tests: what should be ordered? *JAMA* 1990, 264:1009–1014.

7.• Goldenberg DL: Septic Arthritis and other infections of rheumatologic significance. *Rheum Dis Clin North Am* 1991, 17:149–156.

8. Broy SB, Schmid FR: A comparison of medical drainage (needle aspiration) and surgical drainage (arthrotomy or arthroscopy) in the initial treatment of infected joints. *Clin Rheum Dis* 1986, 12:501–522.

9. Rahn DW: Lyme disease: clinical manifestations, diagnosis, and treatment. *Semin Arthritis Rheum* 1991, 20:201–218.

10.• Hughes RA, Rowe IF, Shannon D, Keats ACS: Septic bone joint and muscle lesions associated with human immunodeficiency virus infection. *Br J Rheumatol* 1992, 31:381–388.

11. Garrido G, Gomez-Reino JJ, Fernandez-Dapica P, *et al.*: A review of peripheral tuberculous arthritis. *Semin Arthritis Rheum* 1988, 18:142–148.

12. Morrissy RT: Bone and joint infection in the neonate. *Pediatr Ann* 1989, 18:33–44.

13. Yu LP, Bradley JD, Hugenberg ST, Brandt KD: Predictors of mortality in non-post-operative patients with septic arthritis. *Scand J Rheumatol* 1992, 21:142–144.

14. Petersen BH, Lee TJ, Snyderman R, Brooks GF: *Neisseria meningitidis* and *Neisseria gonorrhoeae* bacteremia associated with C6, C7 or C8 deficiency. *Ann Intern Med 1979, 90:917–920.*

15.• Gardner GC, Weisman MH: Pyarthrosis in patients with rheumatoid arthritis: a report of 13 cases and a review of the literature from the past 40 years. *Am J Med* 1990, 88:503–511.

16.•• Ruskila D, Gladman D: Musculoskeletal manifestations of infection with human immunodeficiency virus. *Rev Infect Dis* 1990, 12:223–235.

17. Ho G Jr., Mikolich DJ: Bacterial infection of the superficial subcutaneous bursae. *Clin Rheum Dis* 1986, 12:437–457.

18. Hodgson BF: Pyogenic sacroiliac joint infection. *Clin Orthop* 1989, 246:146–148.

19.• Wilson MG, Kelley K, Thornhill TS: Infection as a complication of total knee replacement arthroplasty: risk factors and treatment in sixty-seven cases. *J Bone Joint Surg [Am]* 1990, 72:878–883.

20. Hendrix RW, Fisher MR: Imaging of septic arthritis. *Clin Rheum Dis* 1986, 12:459–487.

SELECT BIBLIOGRAPHY

Espinoza L, Goldenberg D, Arnett F, Alarcon G, eds.: *Infections in the Rheumatic Diseases*. Orlando, FL: Grune & Stratton; 1988.

Osteoarthritis and Related Diseases 15

Rose S. Fife

Key Points

- Osteoarthritis is a multifactorial disease that can have different clinical patterns.
- The diagnosis of osteoarthritis usually is based on clinical and radiologic findings.
- The medical management of osteoarthritis is palliative and includes the modalities of physical and occupational therapy and mild analgesics.
- The judicious use of joint arthroplasty can be beneficial.

Osteoarthritis is the most common rheumatic disease affecting humans. It is a major cause of early retirement, and it is the second most common disease responsible for disability in the United States [1•]. Although its occurrence increases with age, osteoarthritis is not merely a normal variant of aging but a true disease process.

CLINICAL MANIFESTATIONS

Osteoarthritis is associated with loss of cartilage thickness and fibrillation of the cartilage down to bone. Several subsets of osteoarthritis have been identified (Table 1).

The large weight-bearing joints are among the most commonly involved. The knees and hips are often affected, but disease can also occur in the spine (Fig. 1).

Involvement of the proximal interphalangeal joints of the hands is referred to as Bouchard's nodes, and involvement of the distal interphalangeal joints is called Heberden's nodes (Fig. 2). Sometimes an inflammatory form of osteoarthritis occurs in the proximal and distal interphalangeal joints, producing significant pain for variable lengths of time and often resulting in significant deformities, including large Heberden's nodes. This inflammatory form of osteoarthritis of the hands tends to cluster in women in a familial distribution [2]. Ultimately, fairly good function of the involved joints is usually maintained, despite the deformities. Unlike other forms of osteoarthritis, which commonly present with symptoms in persons older than 50 years of age, this syndrome afflicts younger people, including those in the fourth decade of life.

Posttraumatic osteoarthritis is a disease subset in which a clear-cut previous injury has resulted in a lasting abnormality in a joint. This injury allows a joint, such as a knee or hip, to develop osteoarthritis at an earlier stage than it might otherwise have, and it may result in involvement of a joint that might otherwise be an uncommon site of osteoarthritis, such as the wrist, the elbow, the shoulder, or the ankle.

A relative of osteoarthritis is diffuse idiopathic skeletal hyperostosis, which is also called Forestier's disease. This condition is characterized by significant bony overgrowth of osteophytes at the edges of joints, particularly in the spine and occasionally in some appendicular joints [3]. This condition is identified radiographically

TABLE 1 CLINICAL SUBSETS OF OSTEOARTHRITIS

Involvement of large weight-bearing joints
Involvement of the hands
    Heberden's and Bouchard's nodes
    Inflammatory osteoarthritis
Posttraumatic osteoarthritis
    Injury
    Abnormal biomechanics
    Repetitive stress (*eg*, occupational)
Diffuse idiopathic skeletal hyperostosis

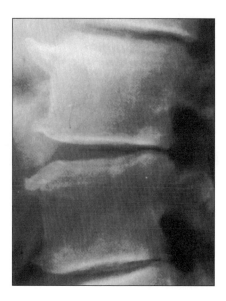

FIGURE 1 Radiograph shows the typical changes of severe osteoarthritis of the lumbar spine, including disk space loss, osteophyte formation, the vacuum phenomenon, and bony sclerosis. (*From* Chandnani and Resnick [14]; with permission.)

and sometimes may be confused with ankylosing spondylitis (Fig. 3). Pain may develop from the hyperostotic process itself, and nerve root impingement from the massive bony overgrowth along the spine may occur. The cause of diffuse idiopathic skeletal hyperostosis is unknown.

DIAGNOSTIC STUDIES

There are no serologic tests or other specific assays for the diagnosis of osteoarthritis. The diagnosis is usually based on the clinical presentation and on findings in selected radiographs (Table 2). Radiographs typically reveal joint space narrowing with some subchondral bony sclerosis and characteristic osteophytes at the joint margins (Fig. 4) [4,5•]. The distribution of joint involvement, as well as the presence of osteophytes and bony sclerosis, serves to differentiate this disease from rheumatoid arthritis. Several other procedures, such as magnetic resonance imaging, are used but are seldom helpful.

Much effort has been devoted to identifying potential serologic markers. These markers could allow the detection of early osteoarthritis and be used to monitor the disease response to various agents that have been proposed as curative or remittive [6,7].

The most commonly used invasive procedure for the diagnosis of osteoarthritis is arthrocentesis. Typically, in osteoarthritic joint fluid, the cell count is below 1000 cells/mm^3, no crystals are seen, the glucose level is normal, and the fluid viscosity is normal.

An invasive procedure that can be useful, but is rarely necessary for the diagnosis of osteoarthritis, is arthroscopy. An arthroscope is inserted into the joint, again most often the knee, and the joint surface is visualized and photographed. This procedure is usually reserved for patients who are suspected of having mechanical abnormalities, such as meniscal tears or ligamentous lesions, or for young individuals with chronic unexplained knee pain, but it is rarely necessary for the diagnosis of osteoarthritis. This technique has improved dramatically in recent years and is now performed with minimal trauma through a very small incision [8]. Patients are usually ambulatory immediately after surgery. Thus, in the future, arthroscopy may become a reasonable method for monitoring osteoarthritis.

MANAGEMENT

No medical cures for osteoarthritis exist. The major medications used in its treatment are analgesics and nonsteroidal antiinflammatory drugs (NSAIDs) (Table 3). An analgesic, such as acetaminophen, is probably the best and safest treatment for osteoarthritis [9••]. Many physicians use NSAIDs to treat osteoarthritis, but the benefits of these agents most likely result from their analgesic effect because relatively little

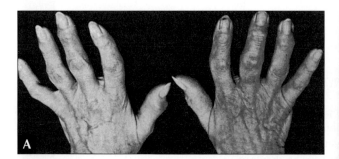

FIGURE 2 **A**, The hands of a patient with osteoarthritis demonstrate Heberden's and Bouchard's nodes. **B**, The corresponding radiograph shows severe joint space narrowing, osteophyte formation, and bony sclerosis of the distal and proximal interphalangeal joints. (*From* McCarty [15]; with permission.)

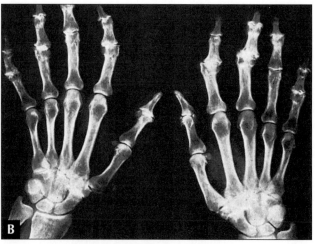

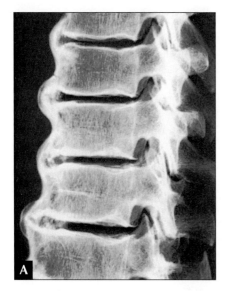

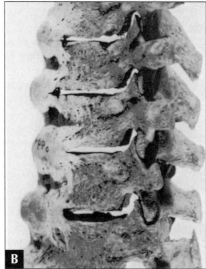

FIGURE 3 **A**, Radiograph and **B**, corresponding pathologic specimen of the lumbar spine from a patient with diffuse idiopathic skeletal hyperostosis demonstrate anterior ossification. (*From* Chandnani and Resnick [14]; with permission.)

TABLE 2 DIAGNOSTIC EVALUATION OF PATIENTS WITH OSTEOARTHRITIS
Imaging
Radiography
Magnetic resonance imaging
Ultrasonography
Markers
Glycosaminoglycans
Proteoglycan fragments
Collagen
Glycoproteins
Invasive procedures
Arthrocentesis with synovial fluid analysis
Arthroscopy

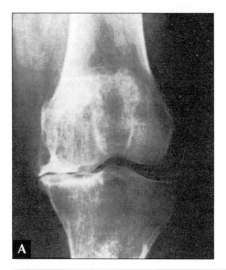

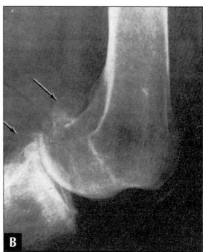

FIGURE 4 Radiographs of **A**, the anteroposterior and **B**, the lateral views of an osteoarthritic knee demonstrate joint space narrowing, osteophyte formation (*arrows*), and bony sclerosis. (*From* McCarty [15]; with permission.)

inflammation is usually present. NSAIDs are more toxic than acetaminophen, especially in the elderly, because of the risk of peptic ulcer disease and renal and liver abnormalities. Acetaminophen should, therefore, be used first in most patients with osteoarthritis.

Physical and occupational therapy are among the mainstays of treatment of osteoarthritis [10]. Educating the patient in exercises to strengthen muscles and maintain joint range of motion is very important and should begin as early as possible. Occupational therapists can provide patients with numerous tools that help make the activities of daily living easier, especially for patients who have problems with their hands. Local heat and ultrasound often help alleviate the painful muscle spasms that can accompany osteoarthritis. Obviously, if weight-bearing joints are affected and the patient is obese, weight reduction and moderate exercise that does not stress the joints (*eg*, swimming, water exercises, and muscle strengthening) are often beneficial.

Surgical intervention can effectively cure osteoarthritis in certain joints [11]. The best procedures are arthroplasty of the knee or hip. These procedures are well developed and have very good success rates. Total joint replacement provides virtually complete relief of pain and remarkable improvement in ambulation. The recovery period from such surgery has diminished greatly, and patients are often functional within a matter of weeks. Lesser procedures include osteotomy and appropriate repair of torn ligaments or menisci. Some of these latter procedures can be performed through the arthroscope, greatly diminishing the surgical risk.

The question of when to refer a patient for a total hip or knee arthroplasty often arises. Patients should be referred if they have severe physical impairment, including decreased range of motion of the involved joint, pain with motion of the joint, nocturnal pain, and progressive difficulty in ambulating; severe or intractable pain with radiographic evidence of significant osteoarthritis of the involved joint; or severe impairment

TABLE 3 MANAGEMENT OF OSTEOARTHRITIS

Medical
Acetaminophen
Nonsteroidal anti-inflammatory drugs

Rehabilitative
Physical therapy
Occupational therapy
Weight reduction

Surgical
Osteotomies
Arthroplasties

Experimental
Joint lavage
Drugs

of ambulation with radiographic evidence of significant osteoarthritis of the involved joint.

A recent innovation in the management of osteoarthritis is joint lavage, which can be performed through a needle or an arthroscope [12]. This technique is undertaken most commonly for the knee. Some studies have suggested that at least short-term relief of pain may result. This procedure remains experimental.

Many agents have been studied for their potential therapeutic use in osteoarthritis. The list is lengthy and includes hyaluronic acid, linseed oil, rhubarb, and extracts of bone or cartilage. Some of these modalities need further testing, and others have been excluded as not beneficial [13].

FUTURE TREATMENT

Future osteoarthritis treatment research will include further attempts to develop curative agents. However, the more we learn about the cause of this common condition, the more successfully we should be able to target its treatment. The number of laboratories that are diligently working on osteoarthritis around the world leads one to hope that we will eventually develop effective curative medical treatment for this often debilitating disease.

REFERENCES AND RECOMMENDED READING

Recently published papers of particular interest have been highlighted as:
• Of interest
•• Of outstanding interest

1.• Peyron JG, Altman RD: The epidemiology of osteoarthritis. In *Osteoarthritis: Diagnosis and Medical/Surgical Management*, edn 2. Edited by Moskowitz RW, Howell DS, Goldberg VM, *et al*. Philadelphia: WB Saunders; 1992:15–37.

2. Kellgren JH, Moore R: Generalized osteoarthritis and Heberden's nodes. *Br Med J* 1952, 1:181–187.

3. Forestier J, Rotes-Querol J: Senile ankylosing hyperostosis of the spine. *Ann Rheum Dis* 1950, 9:321–330.

4. Kellgren JH, Lawrence JS: Radiographic assessment of osteoarthritis. *Ann Rheum Dis* 1957, 16:494–502.

5.• Fife RS, Brandt KD, Braunstein EM,*et al*.: Relationship between arthroscopic evidence of cartilage damage and radiographic evidence of joint space narrowing in early osteoarthritis of the knee. *Arthritis Rheum* 1991, 34:377–382.

6. Fife RS: Imaging, arthroscopy, and "markers" in osteoarthritis. *Curr Opin Rheumatol* 1992, 4:560–565.

7. Ratcliffe A, Shurety W, Caterson B: The quantitation of a native chondroitin sulfate epitope in synovial fluid lavages and articular cartilage from canine experimental osteoarthritis and disuse atrophy. *Arthritis Rheum* 1993, 36:543–551.

8. Ike RW, O'Rourke KS: Detection of intraarticular abnormalities in osteoarthritis of the knee: a pilot study comparing needle arthroscopy with standard arthroscopy. *Arthritis Rheum* 1993, 36:1353–1363.

9.•• Bradley JD, Brandt KD, Katz BP, *et al*.: Comparison of an anti-inflammatory dose of ibuprofen, an analgesic dose of ibuprofen, and acetaminophen in the treatment of patients with osteoarthritis of the knee. *N Engl J Med* 1991, 325:87–91.

10. Hicks JE, Gerber LH: Rehabilitation in the management of patients with osteoarthritis. In *Osteoarthritis: Diagnosis and Medical/Surgical Management*, edn 2. Edited by Moskowitz RW, Howell DS, Goldberg VM, *et al*. Philadelphia: WB Saunders; 1992:427–464.

11. Goldberg VM: Surgery in osteoarthritis: general considerations. In *Osteoarthritis: Diagnosis and Medical/Surgical Management*, edn 2. Edited by Moskowitz RW, Howell DS, Goldberg VM, *et al*. Philadelphia: WB Saunders; 1992:535–544.

12. Chang RW, Falconer J, Stulberg SD, *et al*.: A randomized, controlled trial of arthroscopic surgery versus closed-needle joint lavage for patients with osteoarthritis of the knee. *Arthritis Rheum* 1993, 36:289–296.

13. Fife RS, Brandt KD: Other approaches to therapy. In *Osteoarthritis: Diagnosis and Medical/Surgical Management*, edn 2. Edited by Moskowitz RW, Howell DS, Goldberg VM, *et al*. Philadelphia: WB Saunders; 1992:511–526.

14. Chandnani V, Resnick D: Roentgenologic diagnosis. In *Osteoarthritis: Diagnosis and Medical/Surgical Management*, edn 2. Edited by Moskowitz RW, Howell DS, Goldberg VM, *et al*. Philadelphia: WB Saunders; 1992:263–311.

15. McCarty DJ: *Arthritis and Allied Conditions*, edn 11. Philadelphia: Lea & Febiger; 1989.

SELECT BIBLIOGRAPHY

Altman R, Asch E, Bloch D: Development of criteria for the classification and reporting of osteoarthritis: classification of osteoarthritis of the knee. *Arthritis Rheum* 1986, 29:1039–1049.

Kuettner KE, Schleyerbach R, Hascall VC, eds.: *Articular Cartilage Biochemistry*. New York: Raven Press; 1986.

Muir IHM: The chemistry of the ground substance of joint cartilage. In *The Joints and Synovial Fluid*, vol 2. Edited by Sokoloff L. New York: Academic Press; 1980:27–94.

Resnick D, Niwayama G: *Diagnosis of Bone and Joint Diseases*. Philadelphia: WB Saunders; 1988.

Williams HJ, Ward JR, Egger MJ: Comparison of naproxen and acetaminophen in a 2-year study of treatment of osteoarthritis of the knee. *Arthritis Rheum* 1993, 36:1196–1206.

Regional Pain Syndromes

16

Nortin M. Hadler

Key Points

- Excluding systemic disease as a cause of localized musculoskeletal symptoms remains the top priority.
- Pathology about the shoulder, knee, and foot is common in the asymptomatic person and therefore often nonspecific in the symptomatic.
- Most regional musculoskeletal disorders are spontaneously remittent. Therefore, only the most conservative management is defensible until alternatives are supported by the results of systematic investigation.
- Idiopathic carpal tunnel syndrome has a prevalence approaching 1/1000/year, is not associated with use, and can be diagnosed by tests with known positive and negative predictive values.

There are two general categories of spontaneous localized musculoskeletal pain syndromes. Some are manifestations of a local musculoskeletal disorder in a person who is otherwise well (the regional musculoskeletal disorders) [1••]; others reflect underlying systemic illness. Both are common and familiar to clinicians. For example, shoulder pain and knee pain afflict more than 10% of the population for 1 month each year. Examples of localized musculoskeletal manifestations of (systemic) disease are the pain in the arm that is angina and the pain in the leg that is claudication or pseudoclaudication. This chapter considers three examples of regional musculoskeletal disorders, an example of a focal syndrome that reflects systemic disease, and the entrapment neuropathies, which can be manifestations of regional or systemic illness.

SHOULDER PAIN

Referred shoulder pain seldom interferes with the range of motion of the joint. If the patient can place both palms on the occiput without discomfort, an etiology distant from the shoulder should be sought. This differential diagnosis will test the acumen of any clinician because it runs a gamut of (systemic) illness from angina to bone pain and diaphragmatic irritation. It also includes one common regional musculoskeletal pain syndrome; regional neck pain often presents with discomfort radiating into the trapezius and, if there is an element of C_5 radiculopathy, to the shoulder region itself.

The person with shoulder pain that restricts pectoral girdle motion demands as much attention. The first order of business is to determine whether there is intraarticular pathology. There are three relevant diarthrodial joints: sternoclavicular, acromioclavicular, and glenohumeral. The first two are subcutaneous, therefore erythema, synovitis, and focal tenderness are sensitive signs (Fig. 1). Monarthritis of either of these joints is a critical observation; infection and rheumatoid variants are the likeliest causes.

Arthritis of the glenohumeral joint is another critical finding. This joint lies deep to the deltoid and rotator cuff, rendering signs of inflammation insensitive. However, range of motion is exquisitely sensitive to intraarticular inflammation, and one arc (internal rotation) is specific (Fig. 2). Restriction in this arc of rotation indicates disease of the glenohumeral joint,

which is never a regional musculoskeletal illness. Infection, rheumatoid arthritis and its variants, and reflex sympathetic dystrophy (*vide infra*) are leading etiologies. Whenever infection is a possibility, diagnostic arthrocentesis is mandatory.

The most common cause of regional shoulder pain is a periarthritis. Usually, there is no overt inflammation, only impressive and often focal tenderness about the joint, typically deep to the belly of the deltoid. Many patients experience maximum discomfort in abduction, particularly with external rotation. This posture compresses subdeltoid structures onto the acromion, hence it is an impingement syndrome. However, it is not clear from existing data that further definition of the pathophysiology is possible even with imaging techniques. Dissolution of the rotator cuff has age-dependent prevalence, becoming ubiquitous in later decades; demonstrating such abnormalities in the setting of periarthritis has little value. Abnormalities in tendon hydration, subperiosteal cysts and irregularities, and periarticular calcification are similarly nonspecific. There are no data to establish the reliability, sensitivity, or specificity of the putative hallmarks of bicipital tendonitis, including signs such as tenderness in the bicipital groove and Yergason's sign (pain in the shoulder when the forearm is supinated against resistance with the elbow flexed, thereby stressing the long head of the biceps and its tendon).

Shoulder periarthritis is always a self-limited disease; there is no evidence that these patients are at risk of a frozen shoulder, part of the reflex sympathetic dystrophy syndrome. For nearly all patients, the time to remission is measurable in weeks, occasionally in months. Clinical trials support the use of some forms of physical therapy, of a steroid injection into the region of the subdeltoid bursa (Fig. 3), particularly if there is a point of maximal tenderness, and of NSAIDs [2]. Demonstrating the benefit of acupuncture and ultrasound has proven elusive. There is little convincing evidence that various surgical interventions for periarthritis are of any benefit.

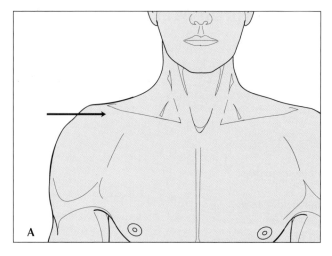

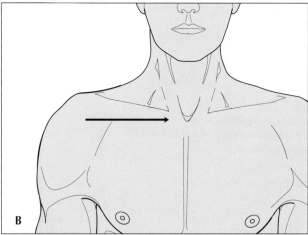

FIGURE 1 **A**, The acromioclavicular and **B**, the sternoclavicular joints are subcutaneous and readily palpable.

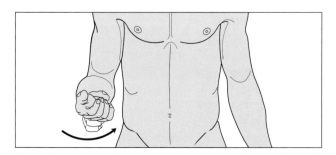

FIGURE 2 Internal rotation from the neutral position with the elbow bent isolates the glenohumeral joint. Restricted motion or pain in this arc is a sign of intra-articular disease.

KNEE PAIN

Knee pain is remarkably common. The frequency increases as we age, from 6% of persons in the third decade of life to 18%

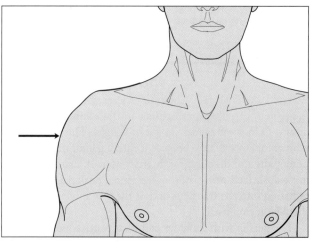

FIGURE 3 Focal tenderness in the region of the subdeltoid bursa as in periarthritis of the shoulder.

in the seventh. Knee pain is highly discordant from radiographic abnormalities of the knee [3••]. This fact holds even in the seventh decade of life, in which radiographic osteoarthritis is apparent in only 1.8% of women and 0.58% of men. Of those afflicted with radiographic osteoarthritis, even if severe, discordance with symptoms is the rule. The inescapable conclusion is that the cause of regional knee pain is unknown; most pathogenetic inferences are unfounded, and most aggressive therapies are unwarranted and unsupported by scientific studies. Certainly there is an end-stage knee readily recognizable by gross loss of cartilage, by severe instability, and by osteophytosis and other bony responses. For the end-stage knee, reconstructive surgery is an option. However, neither physician nor patient should assume that all knee pain is a forme fruste of the end-stage knee so that anxious patients submit to unproven remedies, including the amazing array of unproven arthroscopic procedures that are purveyed.

Most regional knee pain is mechanical; it increases with weight bearing and is relieved with rest. Descending stairs is more difficult than ascending them because of the need to set the knee against considerable shear. However, there are two variations of knee pain that are distinctive both in quality and in indications for therapy (Table 1).

Patients and physicians have been inventive over the decades in their zeal to ascribe knee pain to something special about the joint when there are no osteophytes to blame. Several of these assertions can be put to rest:

1. Joint noise is totally nonspecific. True, palpable crepitation is a feature of the end-stage joint, but popping sounds are a feature of the normal knee.

2. Plicae are folds of synovium that are remnants of the embryologic development of the synovial sac. Cadaveric studies demonstrate plicae in 50% of knees. Plicae have been recognized for generations and were long held to be individual differences to which no symptoms were ascribable. This notion has changed with the use of arthroscopy in the United States to evaluate unexplained knee pain. Visualizing the cause of knee pain in many younger patients is an exercise in inferential leaping. Only the medial plica remains culpable in the minds of some arthroscopists. During flexion, the medial plica crosses the femoral condyle. It is thought that trauma, including the trauma of repetitive motion, perhaps in the setting of subtle malalignment, is a stressor that elicits inflammation. The symptoms ascribed to this process are those of the patellofemoral pain syndrome, with the addition of a sensation of medial snapping or popping. Arthroscopic excision is performed in the absence of a controlled trial.

3. Not all torn or frayed menisci are bad. After all, this finding is common in the later decades of life without associated symptomatology. It is clear the menisci and other intraarticular fibrous structures are relevant to joint biology. For stability, the knee is totally dependent on extra- and intraarticular ligaments. These structures are best viewed as an integrated restraining continuum; perturbing one of them has considerable impact on more global knee function. Menisci serve major functions in knee joint biology (Table 2).

Because not all torn menisci are bad and because menisci are important for normal function, how good are we at defining the meniscal pathology responsible for the syndrome of internal derangement outlined in Table 1? The symptoms and the various orthopedic signs used to detect internal derangements have severely limited sensitivity and specificity; one study documented a 22% false-negative rate and a 33% false-positive rate for the clinical assessment of medial meniscal tears. Furthermore, even in the orthopedic setting with its overt accrual bias, 20% of patients diagnosed with "a probable meniscal tear" experience spontaneous remission of their symptoms. If these data are not enough cause for diagnostic and therapeutic circumspection, the experience with open surgical meniscectomy is further daunting. One decade after the procedure, 70% of the surgically treated knees remain symptomatic, and by two decades, 40% manifest degenerative joint disease. Of course, these results may reflect primary

Feature	Patellofemoral pain syndrome	Internal derangements
Age	Earlier decades, particularly in women Echoed late in life	Earlier decades, particularly in men
Symptoms	Discomfort climbing stairs and sitting for a prolonged period, particularly in the anterior knee	Catching, locking, and giving away
Signs	Tenderness on patella compression	Pain at the joint margin and with maneuvers that compress the menisci
Pathogenesis	Unknown Chondromalacia patellae is nonspecific Patella tracking differences are either insensitive or nonspecific	Anatomical derangement of the menisci occurs with age-dependent frequency Nonetheless, such anatomical derangement seems to underlie this presentation Plicae, on the other hand, are normal variants
Management	Reassurance and conservative measures Surgery is not indicated	Arthroscopic meniscal débridement seems to abrogate symptoms but not long-term risk for osteoarthritis

TABLE 1 DISCRETE REGIONAL KNEE PAIN SYNDROMES

cartilage damage that occurred coincident with the meniscal damage and that would have progressed without the meniscectomy. However, there are no data supporting such an assertion. The contemporary arthroscopic meniscectomy is a major advance in surgical technology in terms of operative and perioperative morbidity, but long-term results must await long-term follow-up.

Given all of these considerations, conservative management becomes the better part of valor if not wisdom. There are several components of conservative management that have withstood scientific testing (Table 3). What remains is to inform the patient and the public.

FOOT PAIN

When we run, each foot distributes approximately six times our body weight in a gliding and stable fashion with each step, seldom with symptoms. To accomplish this activity, an intact and healthy integument is necessary, as is an integrated spring-like musculoskeletal array. There are many disorders of the integument and many systemic diseases that can present as foot pain or compromise this function. The musculoskeletal array and its derangements underlie most regional foot pain.

The midfoot is a longitudinal arch running along the medial border from the first metatarsophalangeal joint to the tuberosity of the os calcis. The forefoot is a transverse arch between the first and fifth metatarsophalangeal joints that transects the necks of the central metatarsal. Gait involves first heel strike, then planting and stabilizing or stance on the first and fifth metatarsal heads, and push off from the first metatarsophalangeal joint and hallux. The arches are the springs that dissipate the force. Close observation of a patient's gait can greatly enhance diagnostic inferences regarding disorders of the feet.

There are many individual differences in the normal foot; the most common is pes planus. It is remarkable how seldom such individuals suffer foot pain. Those who do are greeted with a wealth of empirical orthotic devices attempting to adjust gait. Likewise, lifting devices are prescribed for the common finding of leg-length discrepancy when even an inch of discrepancy does not correlate with symptoms in most systematic studies.

Heel Pain

Many causes of heel pain are obvious on examination: plantaris rupture, retrocalcaneal bursitis, "pump bumps" (granulomas at the site of chronic irritation from foot wear, usually at the distal Achilles tendon). When the discomfort is with heel strike, the examination is usually unremarkable except for tenderness localizing to the tuberosity of the os calcaneus. There is no reason to radiograph such a patient; the finding of an exostosis (a spur) is nonspecific. Furthermore, injection therapy with an anesthetic or corticosteroid is counterintuitive and unsupported by trial. The intuitively appealing intervention is to unload the heel by using orthotics that disperse the pain until the process heals.

Metatarsalgia

Metatarsalgia is pain in some part of the transverse arch. Often there is nothing on examination but diffuse tenderness. In this case, palliation by gait adjustment with footwear or a metatarsal bar is a reasonable empirical trial. Focal tenderness in the sesamoid bones associated with the first metatarsophalangeal joint or in the neck of a metatarsal (often the fourth) may indicate an insufficiency (a stress or march) fracture. Such fractures may be subradiographic when acute, requiring scintiscanning for confirmation. Because treatment provides reassurance and advice as to gait adjustment, there is little need to make the diagnosis with certainty.

TABLE 3 SCIENTIFICALLY SUPPORTED CORNERSTONES OF CONSERVATIVE THERAPY FOR REGIONAL KNEE PAIN

Type of management	Study
Palliation with acetaminophen	Bradley *et al.* [11]
Avoidance of nonsteroidal anti-inflammatory agents	Hadler [12]
Exercise, even in the setting of osteoarthritis	Kovar *et al.* [13]
Weight reduction	Felson *et al.* [14]

TABLE 4	FEATURES THAT ARE COMMON TO ALL ENTRAPMENT NEUROPATHIES UPON CLINICAL PRESENTATION

Dysesthesias characteristically localized to the sensory distribution of the nerve
Discomfort and paresthesia more prominent at rest than with usage
Greater susceptibility of sensory fibers than of motor fibers to the insult
A Tinel's sign (percussion of the nerve at the site of entrapment elicits dysesthesias in the sensory distribution of the nerve)
An electrodiagnostic gold standard (the standard is more reliable and sensitive for some than for others)

Morton's neuroma is a neurofibroma or angioneurofibroma involving the large superficial branch of the external plantar nerve as it courses between metatarsal heads, usually in the more lateral web spaces. It presents with parathesias or cramp-like pain usually near the fourth metatarsal head, and it is usually exacerbated when shoes are worn. Hypesthesias are present in the involved web space. The management is gait adjustment attempting to reduce impingement. Surgical exploration is an option if symptoms persist.

Hallux Rigidus

Hallux rigidus and hallux valgus are deformities that usually occur as a consequence of degenerative disease of the first metatarsophalangeal joint. The latter is part of the bunion complex, usually seen in the later decades of life. Both conditions impede gait by interfering with push off. Furthermore, both are associated with osteophytosis. The range of interventions commences with adaptive footwear and moves on to a menu of inventive surgical empiricisms.

ENTRAPMENT NEUROPATHIES

The major peripheral nerves of the upper and lower extremities are at risk for compression and consequent physiologic compromise at particular sites in their course. Most of these entrapment neuropathies are idiopathic. Several features of the

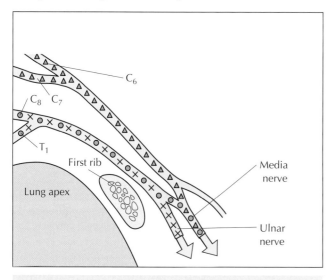

FIGURE 4 Distribution of median and ulnar fibers to the hand as they run in the brachial plexus at the root of the neck. *Crosses* represent ulnar motor and sensory fibers; *closed circles* represent median motor fibers; and *closed triangles* represent median sensory fibers.

clinical presentation are common to all entrapment neuropathies (Table 4).

Thoracic Outlet Syndrome

Almost every imaginable form of pectoral girdle pain has been ascribed to thoracic outlet syndrome despite the overt lack of specificity. Nonetheless, there is such an entity. The diagnosis should be reserved for two presentations: vasculopathic and axonopathic. In the former, often associated with the extremes of usage (as would be the case of a professional baseball pitcher), there is occlusion of the brachial artery or vein, resulting in ischemic symptoms. In the latter, the entrapment is manifest by a painful extremity, notable for the stigmata of axonal degeneration. Given the anatomy at risk (Fig. 4), the presentation reflects compression of the lowest part of the brachial plexus, leading to motor compromise and atrophy first in the thenar eminence (median nerve) and then in the muscles innervated by the ulnar nerve. Reflexes are spared. There is ulnar sensory loss with median sparing (Fig. 5). Documenting this pathophysiology with electrodiagnostic testing is straightforward, as is recourse to the judgment of a surgeon. Short of these two dramatic presentations, thoracic outlet syndrome is a tenuous diagnosis at best.

Ulnar Entrapments

The ulnar nerve is at risk for entrapment at two sites distal to the shoulder: elbow and wrist. In the former, it is superficial at the condylar groove and further at risk as it passes around the ulna, deep to the flexor carpi ulnaris in the cubital tunnel. At the wrist, it is superficial to the flexor retinaculum between the pisiform and the hook of the hamate, deep to the superficial volar carpal ligament in a conduit called Guyon's canal. The clinical presentation of ulnar nerve entrapment is notoriously

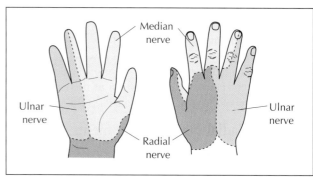

FIGURE 5 Sensory innervation of the hand.

variable. Insidiously progressive atrophy can occur with little discomfort and even little sensory loss (so-called tardy ulnar palsy). More typically, there is neuritic discomfort. However, the sensitivity and specificity of electrodiagnostic testing particularly at the elbow are such that diagnostic certainty is often elusive.

Median Nerve Entrapments

The median nerve is susceptible to entrapment as it enters the forearm lying between the two heads of the pronator teres. The diagnosis is suspected when symptoms suggest the carpal tunnel syndrome, yet Tinel's sign localizes proximally, and late in the course, there is compromise in the power of the long finger flexors. The diagnosis is confirmed electrodiagnostically. Treatment is to restrain forceful pronation so that the pronator muscle involutes.

The median nerve is even more susceptible to entrapment because it traverses the wrist deep to the flexor retinaculum. In fact, the carpal tunnel syndrome is the most frequently encountered entrapment neuropathy. Its prevalence approximates 99 per 100,000 person-years [4], although half of these patients have predisposing medical conditions. Idiopathic carpal tunnel syndrome is not increased in prevalence as a function of upper extremity usage as long as the elements of usage are comfortable and customary [5,6]. In idiopathic carpal tunnel syndrome, impedance to nerve conduction is associated with dramatic increases in the hydrostatic pressure measurable in the carpal tunnel [7].

The clinical presentation is the prototype for an entrapment neuropathy. However, the prototype was generated with the benefit of accrual bias on the part of the publishing surgeons. The prototype performs poorly in screening other populations. If one takes electrodiagnostic abnormalities as the gold standard for diagnostic confirmation, only Tinel's sign and drawings by the patient of the distribution of pain in the hand have sufficient sensitivity and specificity to be diagnostically informative—and then only in a referral population with a high (40%) likelihood of actually having carpal tunnel syndrome [8]. For screening in other populations, even these signs are unreliable and invalid.

Idiopathic carpal tunnel syndrome is bilateral in nearly 50% of patients. Carpal tunnel syndrome is well described as a complication of late pregnancy, hypothyroidism, rheumatoid arthritis, amyloidosis, and acromegaly. The nerve can be impinged on with fractures of the wrist or with intraarticular inflammatory processes, such as tuberculosis. The peripheral neuropathies associated with diabetes and renal failure have some predilection for the median nerve in the tunnel.

The majority of patients respond to conservative management, including splinting and corticosteroid injections [9]. With persistent pain or any indication of thenar atrophy, surgical division of the volar carpal ligament is reasonable.

Radial Nerve Entrapments

The radial nerve is remarkably buffered from compression. It is at risk as it courses around the humerus, usually because of prolonged improper positioning during the administration of anesthesia or because of sleeping on the arm, particularly when inebriated (Saturday night palsy). The result is wrist-drop; sensory impairment is variable.

At the elbow, the radial nerve divides into two branches. The deep branch, the posterior interosseous nerve, passes into the supinator muscle through the arcade of Frohse and courses within the muscle in the supinator canal. Near the elbow, the posterior interosseous nerve is at risk of entrapment, particularly by the synovial proliferation of rheumatoid arthritis.

Lower Extremity Entrapments

Entrapment of peripheral nerves in the lower extremity is far less frequent than that in the upper extremity. For example, both the femoral nerve and its extension in the leg, the saphenous nerve, are rarely compromised in the absence of trauma or hematomas.

The lateral cutaneous nerve of the thigh exits the pelvis through or beneath the inguinal ligament, which is a purely sensory nerve. Compression causes hyperpathia and paresthesia in the lateral thigh, Bernhardt's disease, or meralgia paresthetica (Fig. 6). The symptoms are worsened by abduction of the leg or prolonged standing. The pathogenesis has been ascribed to entrapment either at the inguinal ligament or as the nerve pierces the fascia to reach the skin. Electrodiagnostic confirmation is usually elusive. The differential diagnosis includes L_3 radiculopathy. Treatment is aimed at relieving any pressure of garments to the course of the nerve.

The sciatic nerve is well cushioned throughout its course. It may be at some risk in the pyriform fossa, particularly with prolonged sitting, but this assertion is difficult to establish in the face of the high prevalence of sciatica. In the popliteal fossa, the sciatic nerve divides into the common peroneal nerve and the tibial nerve. The common peroneal nerve courses around the lateral aspect of the proximal fibula to pass through the superficial head of the peroneus longus muscle in the fibular tunnel. In this portion of its course, it is particularly susceptible to external compression, resulting in footdrop and some sensory compromise. The common peroneal nerve divides on emerging from the fibular tunnel into the deep and superficial peroneal nerves. The latter runs in the anterior compartment of the leg. With trauma or even excessive exercise, this compartment can become inflamed to the point of tissue compromise, provoking a surgical emergency.

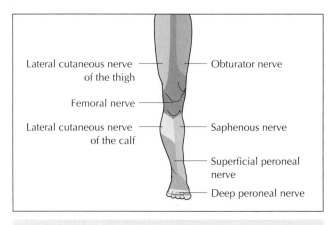

Lateral cutaneous nerve of the thigh

Obturator nerve

Femoral nerve

Lateral cutaneous nerve of the calf

Saphenous nerve

Superficial peroneal nerve

Deep peroneal nerve

FIGURE 6 Sensory innervation of the leg.

The tibial nerve gives off the sural nerve in the popliteal fossa and continues on into the leg, deep to the gastrocnemius. It emerges at the medial aspect of the Achilles tendon and then passes deep to the flexor retinaculum at the medial malleolus to enter the sole, thus serving sensation as the medial plantar nerve (Fig. 7). This retinaculum forms the roof of the tarsal tunnel. Tarsal tunnel syndrome is analogous to carpal tunnel syndrome except that symptoms are even more variable, and electrodiagnostic standards, less definitive.

REFLEX SYMPATHETIC DYSTROPHY

Patients with reflex sympathetic dystrophy (RSD) suffer a global and pervasive neurovascular disorder classically of one upper extremity but often of both. Occasionally, the lower extremity is subjected to a similar process. When the shoulder alone is afflicted, the term *frozen shoulder* pertains. When it is the hip, *regional osteopenia* pertains.

The illness can follow discrete traumatic events. More commonly, the onset is insidious with pain, which can vary from lancinating to burning, and is accompanied by hyperhydrosis, vascular lability, and dysesthesias of the hand. The coincidence of shoulder aching and restriction in motion of the glenohumeral joint (Fig. 2) and hand disease is the reason some label this condition *shoulder-hand syndrome*. Others are struck by the painful neurovascular component and label the condition *causalgia*, whereas others focus on the tender,

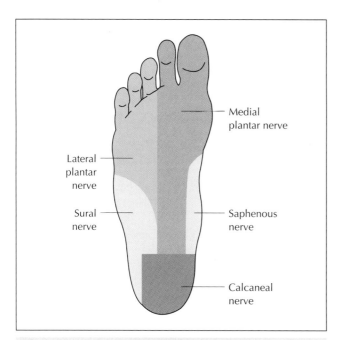

FIGURE 7 Sensory innervation of the sole.

doughy hand with accompanying skin atrophy, calling it *algodystrophy* [10]. Over time, radiographs document patchy osteopenia or Sudeck's atrophy. Scintigrams demonstrate increased vascularity in the early lesion.

For most patients, the illness follows a predictable course to full remission, which may unfortunately take years. Physical therapy is traditionally proscribed. There are advocates for stellate ganglion blocks, distal infusions of reserpine or guanethidine, or even enteral steroids. All of these trials are empirical. More aggressive proclivities should be tempered by the excellent long-term prognosis.

REFERENCES AND RECOMMENDED READING

Recently published papers of particular interest have been highlighted as:
• Of interest
•• Of outstanding interest

1.•• Hadler NM: *Occupational Musculoskeletal Disorders.* New York, NY: Raven Press; 1993:1–273.

2. Petri M, Dobrow R, Neiman R, *et al.*: Randomized, double-blind placebo-controlled study of the treatment of the painful shoulder. *Arthritis Rheum* 1987, 30:1040–1045.

3.•• Hadler NM: Knee pain is the malady: not osteoarthritis. *Ann Intern Med* 1992, 116:598–599.

4. Stevens JC, Sun S, Beard CM, *et al.*: Carpal tunnel syndrome in Rochester, Minnesota: 1961–1980. *Neurology* 1988, 38:134–138.

5. Hadler NM: Cumulative trauma disorders: an iatrogenic concept. *J Occup Med* 1990, 32:38–41.

6. Hadler NM: Arm pain in the workplace: a small area analysis. *J Occup Med* 1992, 34:113–119.

7. Gelberman RH, Rydevik BL, Pess GM, *et al.*: Carpal tunnel syndrome: a scientific basis for clinical care. *Orthop Clin North Am* 1988, 19:115–124.

8. Katz JN, Larson MG, Sabra A, *et al.*: The carpal tunnel syndrome: diagnostic utility of the history and physical examination findings. *Ann Intern Med* 1990, 112:321–327.

9. Gelberman RH, Aronson D, Weisman MH: Carpal tunnel syndrome: results of a prospective trial of steroid injection and splinting. *J Bone Joint Surg Am* 1980, 62A:1181–1184.

10. Chard MD: Diagnosis and management of algodystrophy. *Ann Rheum Dis* 1991, 50:727–730.

11. Bradley JD, Brandt KD, Katz BP, *et al.*: Comparison of an anti-inflammatory dose of ibuprofen, an analgesic dose of ibuprofen, and acetaminophen in the treatment of patients with osteoarthritis of the knee. *N Engl J Med* 1991, 325:87–91.

12. Hadler NM: There's the forest: the object lesson of NSAID "gastropathy." *J Rheumatology* 1990, 17:280–282.

13. Kovar PA, Allegrante JP, MacKenzie CR, *et al.*: Supervised fitness walking in patients with osteoarthritis of the knee: a randomized, controlled trial. *Ann Intern Med* 1992, 116:529–534.

14. Felson DT, Zhang Y, Anthony JM, *et al.*: Weight loss reduces the risk for symptomatic knee osteoarthritis in women: the Framingham study. *Ann Intern Med* 1992, 116:535–539.

Arthritis Associated with Hematologic Disease, Sarcoidosis, or Storage Disorders

17

Juan J. Canoso

Key Points

- Rheumatic complaints, from a variety of mechanisms, occur commonly in the leukemias, lymphomas, and plasma cell dyscrasias.
- Bone ischemia and marrow necrosis explain the painful crises of sickle cell disease.
- In hemophiliacs, recurrent hemarthroses destroy joints.
- Acute ankle periarthritis is a well-known feature of sarcoidosis, but chronic tenosynvoial or articular lesions are often misdiagnosed.
- Hypercholesterolemia should be suspected in patients with Achilles tendon nodules.
- The rare multicentric reticulohistiocytosis is a member of the seronegative nodular rheumatoid arthritis group.
- Bone findings, including ischemic pain and aseptic necrosis, are prominent in Gaucher's disease.

Patients with myeloproliferative diseases, hemoglobinopathies, bleeding disorders, sarcoidosis, or storage diseases may present or develop musculoskeletal disorders that pose diagnostic or treatment problems. Because many of these conditions are rare, concurrent consultant's care is highly desirable. In sickle cell disease, the primary physician should be aware of the serious implications of rheumatic complaints (vasoocclusive crises, bone necrosis, osteomyelitis) so that appropriate study and consultation can be focused on the problem.

HEMATOLOGIC DISEASE

Leukemia

Rheumatic complaints are frequent in patients with leukemia. They may result from tissue infiltration or bone marrow expansion (arthritis, bone pain) [1,2], immunologic mechanisms (arthritis, vasculitis, lupus-like illness), increased cell breakdown and purine catabolism (gout), thrombocytopenia and hemorrhagic diathesis (hemarthrosis), immunosuppression (septic arthritis), and iatrogenesis (aseptic necrosis of bone, vasculitis). Chest pain from sternal and rib marrow expansion, mimicking pleuritic pain, in a context of arthritis, anemia, and thrombocytopenia, may initially suggest systemic lupus erythematosus. Finally, juxtaarticular bony leukemic infiltrates may result in pain and limitation of motion with noninflammatory findings in the joint fluid [1,2]. Bone tenderness is often a helpful diagnostic clue in leukemic (or metastatic) synovitis (Table 1). Both leukemic synovitis and bone pain respond rapidly to antileukemic therapy.

TABLE 1 LEUKEMIC SYNOVITIS

Manifestation	Characteristics	It may be mistaken for	Diagnostic clues
Acute leukemia	A frequent manifestation, particularly in children	Juvenile rheumatoid arthritis or systemic lupus erythematosus (pseudopleuritis from rib infiltration, cytopenias)	Bone tenderness Severe anemia or thrombocytopenia
	Monoarthritis, oligoarthritis, or polyarthritis; acute or subacute		
	Synovial fluid leukocyte counts, 50–50,000 cells/mm^3; neutrophils may predominate		
	Rapid improvement with antileukemic therapy		
Chronic leukemia	An unusual manisfestation in lymphoid, T-cell, or hairy cell leukemia	Rheumatoid arthritis	Adenopathy, splenomegaly, negative rheumatoid factor
	Mono-, oligo-, or polyarticular chronic arthritis caused by leukemic synovial infiltration		

Additional rheumatic conditions may occur in leukemia patients [3••]. Vasculitis usually occurs late in the course of malignant disease (Table 2). Hairy cell leukemia may be preceded by an antinuclear antibody–positive lupus-like illness [4]. In myelodysplasia, in which ineffective hematopoiesis may be followed by acute leukemia, seronegative polyarthritis, small vessel vasculitis, systemic lupus erythematosus, and Sjögren's syndrome have all been described [3••,4,5]. Acute arthritis in leukemia patients may result from gout (chronic myelogenous leukemia, polycythemia vera), hemarthrosis, and septic arthritis. Synovial aspiration is essential for diagnosis and may require antecedent platelet transfusion. Finally, aseptic necrosis of bone should be suspected in corticosteroid-treated patients who develop joint pain (usually in the hip) on weight bearing with a relatively preserved range of motion. It is often difficult to determine whether one is dealing with a rheumatologic complication of leukemia or a coincidental rheumatic disease.

Lymphoma

Rheumatic manifestations of lymphoma include:

Tissue infiltration: rheumatoid-like arthritis (synovial infiltration in B-cell and T-cell lymphoma and angioimmunoblastic lymphadenopathy) and bone pain or midlumbar plexopathy (bone infiltration or neural compression in B-cell and T-cell lymphoma and Hodgkin's disease)

Immunologic manifestations: vasculitis and erythema nodosum

Lymphoma developing in rheumatic disease: B-cell lymphoma in Sjögren's syndrome (rare), B-cell lymphoma in rheumatoid arthritis (very rare), and iatrogenic manifestations, including B-cell lymphomas in immunosuppressive treatment

These manifestations may be due to synovial infiltration [6,7], bone infiltration, epidural space invasion [8], and compressive adenopathies. Fever, adenopathy, and splenomegaly are help-

TABLE 2 VASCULITIS IN MALIGNANT DISEASE

Disease	Type of vasculitis
Hairy cell leukemia	Polyarteritis nodosa
	Cutaneous vasculitis
Myelodysplastic syndromes	Cutaneous vasculitis
Lymphoma	Cutaneous vasculitis
Plasma cell dyscrasias	Cutaneous vasculitis
	Cryoglobulinemia
	λ Light chain vasculopathy (limb and visceral necrosis)
Solid tumors	Cutaneous vasculitis
	Polyarteritis nodosa (rare)
Complication of chemotherapy or bone marrow transplantation	Usually cutaneous vasculitis

ful diagnostic clues. Lymphoma and other malignant processes involving the retroperitoneum should be suspected when femoral neuropathy develops in patients without diabetes, particularly when the erythrocyte sedimentation rate and the serum lactic dehydrogenase levels are elevated. An abdominal computed tomography scan with attention to the retroperitoneum should be obtained when evaluating these patients. Rare manifestations of lymphoma include small vessel vasculitis and erythema nodosum. On the other hand, B-cell lymphoma may complicate Sjögren's syndrome, particularly in patients with lymphadenopathy, splenomegaly, and previous radiography or cytotoxic treatment, and it may develop in rheumatoid arthritis patients treated with immunosuppressive agents, particularly azathioprine.

Plasma Cell Dyscrasias

In the plasma cell dyscrasias, rheumatic manifestations in the form of infiltrative lesions may include bone pain, bone tumor (plasmocytoma), osteolytic lesions, osteopenia, and osteosclerosis (osteosclerotic myeloma). Scleredema, scleromyxedema, L-amyloidosis, erosive arthritis, vasculitis, cryoglobulinemia, light chain occlusive vasculopathy, peripheral neuropathy, and the POEMS syndrome (Table 3) are rheumatic manifestations of a paraneoplastic nature. Scleredema, an indurated nonpitting edema of the posterior neck that spreads to face, shoulders, upper arms, abdomen, and thighs, may be confused with eosinophilic fasciitis. Scleromyxedema is a superficial, pebbled lesion in which the skin is freely movable over the subcutaneous tissues. Although some cases resemble scleroderma, Raynaud's phenomenon is typically absent. A neutrophilic dermatosis, Sweet's syndrome, also may occur [3••]. L-amyloidosis [9] causes an array of clinical manifestations, such as skin fragility, macroglossia, hepatomegaly, proteinuria, cardiomyopathy, carpal tunnel syndrome, peripheral neuropathy, the "shoulder pad" sign, arthritis resembling rheumatoid arthritis, including subcutaneous nodules, and bone masses (amyloidomas). Amyloidosis, as well as other mimickers, should be suspected in rheumatoid factor–negative, nodular rheumatoid arthritis. Full-blown amyloidosis is unmistakable, but a high index of suspicion is required to diagnose initial or incomplete cases. An atypical erosive arthritis, with or without amyloid deposition, also has been described in plasma cell dyscrasias [10]. Cryoglobulinemia may lead to purpuric lesions and nephritis. A dramatic and fatal vasculopathy resembling necrotizing vasculitis may occur in patients with monoclonal

gammopathy [11]. Finally, peripheral neuropathy may occur in isolation or in the context of osteosclerotic myeloma or the POEMS syndrome [12]. Osteosclerotic lesions are noted on radiographs in most patients; prognosis (both in POEMS and in osteosclerotic myeloma) is far better than that in nonneuropathic multiple myeloma [12].

Sickle Cell Disease and Other Hemoglobinopathies

Musculoskeletal complaints are extremely common in the hemoglobinopathies, particularly in sickle cell disease (Table 4). Soft tissue, bone, and articular findings as a result of microvascular occlusion leading to tissue infarction represent a major cause of disability in sickle cell disease. Bone marrow expansion results in a weakened bone that is prone to fractures and is a suboptimal environment for a femoral prosthesis, which is eventually required in many of the patients. Hyperuricemia secondary to increased purine catabolism and renal disease occurs in 40% of patients, but gout is rare. Finally, as in thalassemia, hemochromatotic arthropathy may rarely complicate sickle cell disease.

The hand-foot syndrome (self-limited diffuse swelling and pain of abrupt onset) is caused by bone and soft tissue ischemia and occurs in children aged 6 months to 2 years. Bone ischemia also results in the characteristic, excruciatingly painful but self-limited vasoocclusive crises and leads to irreversible avascular necrosis of bone. A correlation between the frequency of vasoocclusive crises and osteonecrosis has been noted. Osteonecrosis, affecting the femoral head unilaterally or bilaterally (Fig. 1), eventually occurs in 10% to 40% of patients. Concurrent care with an experienced orthopedist is essential for these patients. Patients with the SS genotype plus homozygous α-thalassemia are at the highest risk for osteonecrosis [13••].

TABLE 3 THE POEMS SYNDROME

Polyneuropathy
Organomegaly (hepatomegaly, splenomegaly, lymphadenopathy)
Endocrinopathy (gonadal failure, gynecomastia, hypothyroidism, diabetes)
M component (usually with lambda light chains)
Skin changes (hyperpigmentation, hypertrichosis, coarse dark hair, skin thickening)

TABLE 4 MUSCULOSKELETAL MANIFESTATIONS OF SICKLE CELL DISEASE

Ischemia (microcirculatory vaso-occlusion)
Hand-foot syndrome
Sickle cell crises (with or without synovial effusions: noninflammatory, inflammatory, hemarthrosis); indurated, tender muscle may occur
Osteonecrosis
Joint and bone infections
Leg ulcers

Bone marrow expansion
Coarse bone trabeculation
Osteopenia
Bone fractures; failures of femoral prostheses
"Hair on end" trabeculae in the skull
Vertebral indentations

Chronic hemolysis, renal disease
Hyperuricemia
Gout
Hemochromatosis

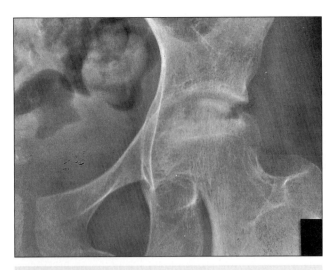

FIGURE 1 Aseptic necrosis of the left femoral head in a 17-year-old boy with sickle cell disease. The contralateral side became involved as well. Bilateral total hip replacement was eventually required.

years. The results of hip arthroplasty are poor, with a 30% chance of revision within 4.5 years [13••,14]. Synovial effusions may occur during painful crises and range from noninflammatory to inflammatory. Areas of indurated, tender muscle also may occur during the vasoocclusive crises. Magnetic resonance studies may help to distinguish this condition from intramuscular abscesses. The treatment of painful crises consists largely of hydration and the use of narcotic agents. Methylprednisolone administered as large intravenous boluses on admission and 24 hours later was shown to reduce significantly the use of analgesics. Whether or not this treatment alters the rate of osteonecrosis remains to be shown. Ischemic leg ulcers are another complication of the disease that may require extensive grafting. Finally, patients with sickle cell disease are prone to bone infection; *Staphylococcus aureus* and *Salmonella* are the usual pathogens. Treatment requires bone débridement and prolonged antibiotic therapy (Table 5) [15••]. It may be difficult to distinguish vasoocclusive crises from osteomyelitis; the latter is suggested by fever, malaise, focal bone tenderness, swelling and tenderness at the involved sites, leukocytosis, and an increased erythrocyte sedimentation rate.

Hemophilia

Hemarthrosis represents the most frequent and disabling complication of hemophilia (Table 6) [16]. Hemophilia A

Femoral head osteonecrosis may be a radiographic finding in an asymptomatic patient, but pain eventually develops in all patients. With an average onset of symptoms at 25 years of age, bilateral hip arthroplasty is usually required by the age of 30

TABLE 5 MANAGEMENT OF SUSPECTED BONE INFECTION IN SICKLE CELL DISEASE

Admit patient to hospital

Obtain complete blood cell count and erythrocyte sedimentation rate (ESR); if leukocyte count and ESR are elevated, osteomyelitis must be considered

Obtain blood cultures

Determine febrile agglutinins and culture stools for *Salmonella* species

Consult hematologist and infectious diseases specialist

Obtain plain bone radiographs; repeat in 10–14 d if initial findings are negative

Obtain technetium or gallium scintigram; these tests do not distinguish osteomyelitis from bone infarction, but they serve to detect multiple sites of infection and osteomyelitis involving the pelvis and spine

Any bone thought to be infected should be aspirated for culture

From Epps Jr. and coworkers [15••]; with permission.

TABLE 6 MUSCULOSKELETAL MANIFESTATIONS OF HEMOPHILIA

Arthritis

Most frequently involved joints: knees, elbows, ankles, hips

In a given patient the same set of joints tends to be affected in recurrent attacks

    Acute (hemarthrosis)

    Chronic synovitis (proliferative)

    Osteoarthritis (early osteoarthritis with prominent cyst formation)

Soft tissue hematomas

Joint contractures, nerve compressions, and others

Bone hematomas

May produce massive expansion of bone, such as the ilium

(classic hemophilia) is due to a deficiency of Factor VIII, and hemophilia B (Christmas disease) is due to a deficiency of Factor IX. Because both genes are in the X chromosome, the disease is usually restricted to men, except in extensively inbred kindreds. In the evaluation of a patient with unexplained hemarthrosis or soft tissue hematoma, a prolonged partial thromboplastin time and a normal prothrombin time indicate a defect in the intrinsic limb of the coagulation cascade, and hematology consultation must be sought. In hemophilia, spontaneous bleeding occurs in patients with less than 1% of Factor VIII activity, requires some degree of trauma with concentrations of 1% to 5% percent, and complicates major trauma or surgery in patients with concentrations of 5% to 50%. Mechanical and biochemical factors contribute to joint damage in hemophilia; the involved joint adopts a position, specific for each joint, in which intra-articular pressures are lowest (semiflexion in knees and elbows). Altered mechanics result in degenerative joint changes with prominent cyst formation (Fig. 2) [17]. Unfortunately, because more than 90% of patients with severe hemophilia are now infected with the HIV virus, bacterial infection of damaged and prosthetic joints is not uncommon. Although the preceding scenario is indeed a grim one, a revolution in biotechnology (recombinant Factor VIII, new processing methods of Factor VIII concentrates that eliminate virus transmission) and advances in orthopedic surgery (arthroscopic surgery, improved prostheses) and physical medicine (preventive muscle conditioning, early mobilization) should improve the quality of life of patients with hemophilia.

SARCOIDOSIS

Sarcoidosis, both in its acute and chronic forms, may have rheumatologic manifestations (Table 7) [18]. In acute sarcoidosis, in particular Löfgren's syndrome (fever, erythema nodosum, tender distal edema, ankle arthritis, hilar adenopathy), clinical and radiographic findings are so characteristic (Fig. 3) that biopsy is usually withheld and the patient watched while awaiting spontaneous resolution. Aspirin or other nonsteroidal antiinflammatory drugs provide symptomatic relief in this form of sarcoidosis. In chronic sarcoidosis, prominent skin, joint, muscle, bone, or central nervous system

TABLE 7   RHEUMATIC MANIFESTATIONS OF SARCOIDOSIS
Acute (with hilar adenopathy on chest radiography)*
Erythema nodosum
Swollen, tender lower extremities
Acute ankle arthritis
Chronic (with interstitial and nodular changes on chest radiography)
Proliferative tenosynovitis
Rheumatoid-like arthritis
Skin nodules (hard, superficial)
Bone cysts (rarely widespread), usually affecting metacarpals, metatarsal, and phalanxes
Myositis (proximal weakness, nodules)†
Eye manifestations (episcleritis, granulomatous uveitis, and others)
Peripheral neuropathy (facial nerve and others)
Central nervous system manifestations (meningitis, granulomas)
Renal disease
*Computed tomography may reveal nodes in patients with negative chest radiographs.
†Subclinical muscle granulomas are common in both acute and chronic sarcoidosis.

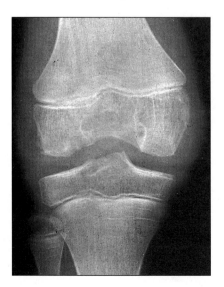

FIGURE 2
Epiphyseal expansion, coarse trabeculae, and widened intercondylar notch with cyst formation in a 14-year-old boy with chronic hemophilic arthropathy involving both knees.

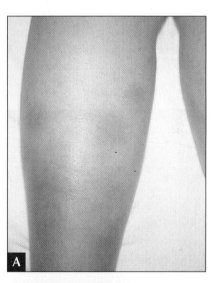

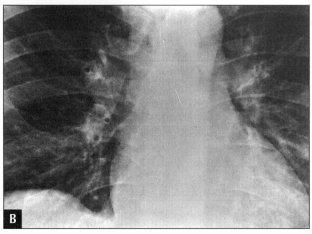

FIGURE 3
A, A 22-year-old nurse developed fever, malaise, and tender leg lesions of erythema nodosum. **B**, Bilateral hilar adenopathy and a right paratracheal node strongly suggested Löfgren's syndrome in this patient.

findings due to granulomatous infiltration require biopsy to exclude lymphoma, mycobacterial infection, and other processes. Treatment of chronic sarcoidosis includes the use of prednisone plus, in refractory cases or as steroid-sparing agents, hydroxychloroquine, methotrexate, or other immuno-suppressant drugs.

STORAGE DISORDERS

Hyperlipidemia

Tendon xanthomas affecting predominantly the Achilles tendon (Fig. 4), Achilles tendon tendinitis, and oligoarthritis are the typical manifestations of adult familial hypercholes-terolemia (Frederickson type IIa) and mixed hyperlipidemia [19••]. Cholesterol levels tend to be higher in patients with tendon findings than in those without, and the use of choles-terol-lowering agents is followed by improvement in most cases. Other possible associations of hyperlipidemia include gout and arthralgias.

Multicentric Reticulohistiocytosis

This rare condition of unknown origin is characterized by skin nodules (various sizes and locations; periungual "beading" is characteristic) and erosive rheumatoid-like arthritis with pseudo-widening of the distal interphalangeal joints. The arthropathy may progress to osteolysis and extreme deformity (arthritis mutilans). An association with neoplasm has been noted in approximately 20% of cases [20]. Although the process may be self-limited, immunosuppressive agents such as cyclophosphamide and methotrexate are successful in arresting disease activity [21].

Gaucher's Disease

Gaucher's disease is an autosomal recessive disorder caused by a deficiency of glucocerebrosidase (glucosylceramidase), an enzyme required in the lysosomal degradation of glycolipids [22]. Lipid-engorged macrophages crowd the liver, the spleen, the bone marrow, the adventitia and inner walls of blood vessels, and the Virchow-Robin space of the brain. Gaucher's disease is diagnosed by determination of leukocyte β-glucosi-dase activity or by the finding of Gaucher's cells (20 to 100 μm cells with an eccentric nucleus and a "wrinkled tissue paper" appearance of their cytoplasm) on bone marrow examination. Serum levels of acid phosphatase and angiotensin-converting enzyme are increased. The clinical subtypes of Gaucher's disease are recognized based on the presence or absence of neurologic involvement and the time course of the disease [22,23]. Of these subtypes, the most common form is (more than 99% of cases) Type 1 (chronic nonneuronopathic), which may present when symptoms secondary to bone marrow engorgement with Gaucher's cells develop. This form, which is seen predominantly in Ashkenazi Jews and is usually diagnosed in patients aged in their early 30s, is suggested by splenomegaly with variable cytopenias (usually thrombocytopenia) or bone disease. Bone disease is characterized by a flaring of the distal femur (Erlenmeyer flask deformity) on radiographs (Fig. 5); aseptic necrosis of the femoral heads; bone crises (pain, swelling, sometimes fever) with decreased uptake on bone scan [24•]; and long-bone pathologic fractures. The sacroiliac joints may be secondarily involved from bone infarction in the adja-cent ilium. Treatment of Gaucher's disease includes pain management; partial or total splenectomy for the treatment of thrombocytopenia, hypersplenism, and painful splenic infarc-tion; orthopedic measures; genetic counseling; and attempts at

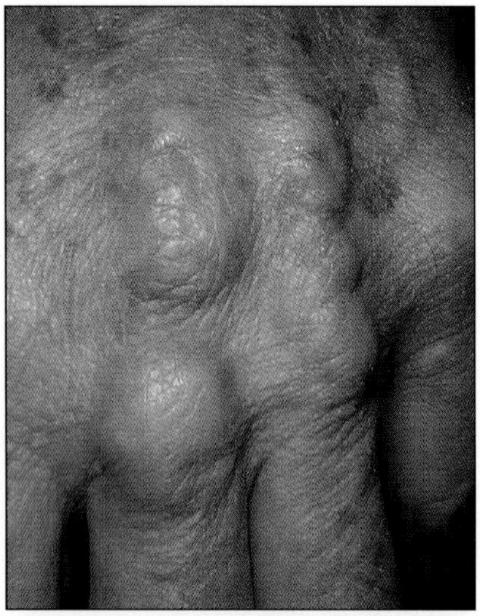

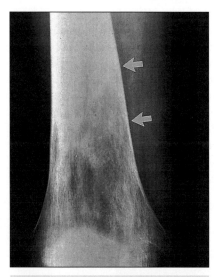

FIGURE 4 Extensor tendon xanthomas in the hand of a 47-year-old man with type IIa hypercholesterolemia. Recur-rent, very painful attacks of Achilles tendinitis and ankle arthritis (with microspherules that casted a Maltese cross on polarizing microscopy) ceased with the successful treatment of the hypercholesterolemia.

FIGURE 5 Type 1 Gaucher's disease. The normal concavity of the bone near the epiphysis is replaced by a convexity (*arrows*), the Erlenmeyer flask deformity of distal femur.

restoring the glucocerebrosidase depletion by bone marrow transplantation or enzyme replacement [24•].

Fabry's Disease

Fabry's disease is an X-linked disorder resulting from deficient lysosomal hydroxylase α-D-galactosidase A activity [25]. As a result, there is a systemic deposition of glycosphingolipids. Vascular deposits are responsible for the major manifestations of the disease (Fig. 6). Musculoskeletal, neurologic, and other systemic manifestations may be prominent, and fever and leukocytosis may be present, thus leading to confusion with connective tissue disease (Table 8). Male hemizygotes show full-blown disease, whereas female carriers either show mild disease (corneal dystrophy, angiokeratoma, acroparesthesias) or are asymptomatic.

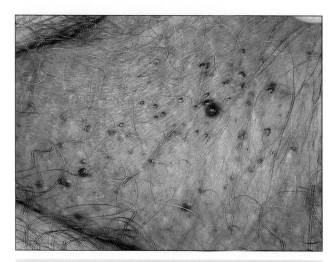

FIGURE 6 A typical angiokeratoma corporis diffusum lesion consisting of 2 to 4 mm in diameter dark red nodules (they can be darker) in the scrotum of a 34-year-old man with Fabry's disease.

ACKNOWLEDGMENT

The author is grateful to Roy G.K. McCauley, MD, for radiographs.

TABLE 8 MANIFESTATIONS OF FABRY'S DISEASE

Skin

Angiokeratoma corporis diffusum (clusters of dark-red or blue angiectases that do not blanch on pressure) between the umbilicus and the knees (hidden lesions should be looked for at the scrotum and the umbilicus)

Heart

Cardiomegaly, mitral insufficiency, conduction abnormalities

Central nervous system

Cerebrovascular lesions range from transient ischemic attacks to stroke; personality changes are common in older patients

Kidney

Nephrotic syndrome; progressive renal insufficiency is a leading cause of death

Musculoskeleton

Distal interphalangeal joint changes, enthesial ossification, intra- and extra-articular erosions, aseptic necrosis of the bone

Eyes

Corneal opacities similar to those observed during hydroxychloroquine therapy

Chronic pain

Episodic (crises) or chronic; it may affect palms and soles, diffusely the extremities, or the abdomen. Pain is intensified by fever and exercise. Raynaud's phenomenon may be an association

Autonomic dysfunction

Impaired sweating, decreased saliva and tear production, impaired constriction of the pupil, abnormal bowel motility

REFERENCES AND RECOMMENDED READING

Recently published papers of particular interest have been highlighted as:
• Of interest
•• Of outstanding interest

1. Eguchi K, Aoyagi I, Nakashima M, *et al.*: A case of adult T cell leukemia complicated by proliferative synovitis. *J Rheumatol* 1991, 18:297–299.

2. Fort JG, Fernandez C, Jacobs SR, Abruzzo J: B cell surface marker analysis of synovial fluid cells in a patient with monarthritis and chronic lymphocytic leukemia. *J Rheumatol* 1991, 19:481–488.

3.•• Mertz LE, Conn DL: Vasculitis associated with malignancy. *Curr Opin Rheumatol* 1992, 4:39–46.

4. Strickland RW, Limmani A, Wall JG, Krishnan J: Hairy cell leukemia presenting as a lupus-like illness. *Arthritis Rheum* 1988, 31:566–568.

5. George SW, Newman ED: Seronegative inflammatory arthritis in the myelodysplastic syndrome. *Semin Arthritis Rheum* 1992, 21:345–354.

6. Dorfman HD, Siegel HL, Perry MC, Oxenhandler R: Non-Hodgkin's lymphoma of the synovium simulating rheumatoid arthritis. *Arthritis Rheum* 1987, 30:155–161.

7. Boumpas DT, Wheby MS, Jaffe ES, *et al.*: Synovitis in angioimmunoblastic lymphadenopathy with dysproteinemia simulating rheumatoid arthritis. *Arthritis Rheum* 1990, 33:578–582.

8. Gaudin P, Juvin R, Rozand Y, *et al.*: Skeletal involvement as the initial disease manifestation in Hodgkin's disease: a review of 6 cases. *J Rheumatol* 1992, 19:146–152.

9. Cohen AS: Amyloidosis. In *Arthritis and Allied Conditions*, edn 12. Edited by McCarty DJ, Koopman WJ. Philadelphia: Lea & Febiger; 1993:1427–1447.

10. Vitali C, Baglioni P, Vivaldi I, *et al.*: Erosive arthritis in monoclonal gammopathy of uncertain significance: report of four cases. *Arthritis Rheum* 1991, 34:1600–1605.

11. Stone GC, Wall BA, Oppliger IR, *et al.*: A vasculopathy with deposition of lambda light chain crystals. *Ann Intern Med* 1989, 110:275–278.

12. Miralles GD, O'Fallon JR, Talley NJ: Plasma-cell dyscrasia with polyneuropathy: the spectrum of POEMS syndrome. *N Engl J Med* 1992, 327:1919–1923.

13.•• Milner PF, Kraus AP, Sebes JI, *et al.*: Sickle cell disease as a cause of osteonecrosis of the femoral head. *N Engl J Med* 1991, 325:1476–1481.

14. Acurio MT, Friedman RJ: Hip arthroplasty in patients with sickle-cell haemoglobinopathy. *J Bone Joint Surg Br* 1992, 74:367–371.

15.•• Epps CH Jr., Bryant DD III, Coles MJ, Castro O: Osteomyelitis in patients who have sickle-cell disease: diagnosis and management. *J Bone Joint Surg Am* 1991, 73:1281–1294.

16. Madhok R, York J, Sturrock RD: Hemophilic arthritis. *Ann Rheum Dis* 1991, 50:588–591.

17. Herman G, Gilbert MS, Abdelwahab IF: Hemophilia: evaluation of musculoskeletal involvement with CT, sonography, and MR imaging. *AJR Am J Roentgenol* 1992, 158:119–123.

18. Schumacher HR Jr.: Sarcoidosis. In *Arthritis and Allied Conditions*, edn 12. Edited by McCarty DJ, Koopman WJ. Philadelphia: Lea & Febiger; 1993:1449–1455.

19.•• Klemp P, Halland AM, Majoos FL, Steyn K: Musculoskeletal manifestations in hyperlipidaemia: a controlled study. *Ann Rheum Dis* 1993, 52:44–48.

20. Janssen B, Kencian J, Brooks PM: Close temporal and anatomic relationship between multicentric reticulohistiocytosis and carcinoma of the breast. *J Rheumatol* 1992, 19:322–324.

21. Ginsburg WW, O'Duffy D, Morris JL, Huston KA: Multicentric reticulohistiocytosis: response to alkylating agents in six patients. *Ann Intern Med* 1989, 111:384–388.

22. Beutler E: Gaucher's disease. *N Engl J Med* 1991, 325:1354–1360.

23. Sidranski E, Ginns EI: Clinical heterogeneity among patients with Gaucher's disease. *JAMA* 1993, 269:1154–1157.

24.• Katz K, Mechlis-Frish S, Cohen IJ, *et al.*: Bone scans in the diagnosis of bone crisis in patients who have Gaucher's disease. *J Bone Joint Surg Am* 1991, 73:513–517.

25. Desnick RJ, Bishop DF: Fabry disease: α-galactosidase deficiency and Schindler disease. Alpha-N-Acetylgalactosaminidase deficiency. In *The Metabolic Basis of Inherited Disease.*. Edited by Scriver CR, Beaudet AL, Sly WS, Valle D. New York: McGraw Hill; 1989:1751–1796.

SELECT BIBLIOGRAPHY

Careless DJ, Cohen MG: Rheumatic manifestations of hyperlipidemia and antilipidemia drug therapy. *Semin Arthritis Rheum* 1993, 23:90–98.

Griffin TC, McIntire D, Buchanan GR: High-dose intravenous methylprednisolone therapy for pain in children and adolescents with sickle cell disease. *N Engl J Med* 1994, 330:733–737.

Weisman MH: Arthritis associated with hematologic disorders, storage diseases, disorders of lipid metabolism, and dysproteinemias. In *Arthritis and Allied Conditions*, edn 12. Edited by McCarty DJ, Koopman WJ. Philadelphia: Lea & Febiger; 1993:1457–1482.

Miscellaneous Arthritic Syndromes 18
David E. Trentham

Key Points
- Palindromic rheumatism and intermittent hydrarthrosis are best viewed as rare variants of rheumatoid arthritis.
- Familial Mediterranean fever is an autosomal recessive disorder causing recurrent polyserositis.
- Relapsing polychondritis can inflame and even destroy cartilage at any site in the body.
- Painful but benign knee effusions can accompany adrenocorticosteroid withdrawal.
- Hypertrophic osteoarthropathy can cause polyarthritis and be associated with neoplasia.
- Joint tumors can cause pain and swelling.

The arthritic conditions described in this chapter are important to recognize early because most respond well to appropriate therapy, and incorrect diagnosis makes their subsequent management more difficult. Because of the relative rarity of these diseases, much of the relevant literature has consisted of recapitulations of earlier treatises. This chapter provides a fresh description of the clinical features of arthritic conditions and their appropriate management. The grouping of these entities reflects their propensity to follow markedly rhythmic courses.

Gout, pseudogout, palindromic rheumatism, Reiter's syndrome, and peripheral arthropathies associated with inflammatory bowel disease are the most common rheumatic syndromes that possess intermittent patterns of activity. The diagnosis of palindromic rheumatism and that of a rare disease called intermittent hydrarthrosis depend on recognition of their prototypic features. When the diagnosis is in doubt, the advice of an experienced rheumatologist is often useful.

PALINDROMIC RHEUMATISM

Palindromic rheumatism is probably best viewed as a variant of rheumatoid arthritis. Patients begin to experience, at markedly irregular intervals, the sudden onset of periarticular or paraarticular pain that often begins in the late afternoon, reaches peak intensity within a few hours, and fully resolves spontaneously within a few hours, up to 3 to 4 days later, or rarely, 2 or more weeks later. True synovitis is unusual. There is no sex predilection for the disorder. Incipient episodes are typically localized to a single region, most commonly involving tissues about a knee, wrist, metacarpophalangeal–proximal interphalangeal joint, or a shoulder. Later attacks can involve more areas. Between attacks, no signs or symptoms are present. This characteristic picture led Philip K. Hench to use the term *palindromic* (eg,

"Madam I'm Adam.")—the patient's condition looks the same before the onset and after the recovery.

Although the severity of pain is variable, some objective evidence of inflammation, such as localized swelling, tenderness, or skin redness, is evident. Swelling of the finger pads, heels, or tendons of the hands or feet may occur. Small transitory rheumatoid nodules can also develop. Systemic features and laboratory abnormalities are generally absent, although fever accompanies the episodes in some patients [1–3].

Palindromic rheumatism closely simulates crystal-induced synovitis, and if a joint is swollen, aspiration should be performed to exclude the presence of calcium pyrophosphate or sodium urate crystals. Unlike the inflammatory synovial fluid found in gout or pseudogout attacks, a benign fluid with a low leukocyte count is almost invariably encountered in patients with palindromic rheumatism. Perhaps as many as 50% of patients with periodic attacks diagnosed originally with palindromic rheumatism eventually display features more characteristic of seropositive rheumatoid arthritis. Early in this disease, no differentiating laboratory parameters exist because rheumatoid factor is usually absent; the erythrocyte sedimentation rate is, at most, minimally elevated but only during attacks. When rheumatoid arthritis supervenes, a pattern of fixed symmetrical arthritis is noted. Usually, the palindromic attacks stop, but they may continue, superimposed on rheumatoid arthritis. Palindromic attacks may continue for years in other patients, never evolving into rheumatoid arthritis. In still others, the attacks may spontaneously stop. Approximately 20% of patients with rheumatoid arthritis have a palindromic onset. In palindromic rheumatism, biopsy of the paraarticular lesion (often a bursa) reveals fibrin deposition.

Therapy should focus on prophylaxis because the temporally compressed nature of the attacks otherwise leads to nonresponsiveness to nonsteroidal antiinflammatory drugs (NSAIDs). Oral corticosteroids may be needed for painful attacks not responding to an NSAID. Although the variable nature of palindromic rheumatism makes judgments regarding the efficacy of most drug therapy difficult, treatment programs similar to those used for rheumatoid arthritis are probably the best approach, particularly if prophylactic colchicine (0.6 mg twice per day) fails to control the problem. In individual patients, NSAIDs with long half-lives, such as piroxicam (20 mg/d), naproxen (500 mg twice per day), or hydroxychloroquine (200 mg twice per day), may be effective. In patients with frequent and severe attacks, injectable gold, methotrexate, or penicillamine administration is probably indicated.

INTERMITTENT HYDRARTHROSIS

Like palindromic rheumatism, another intermittent disorder that may culminate in rheumatoid arthritis in many patients is intermittent hydrarthrosis. This syndrome is truly rare, is generally considered to be fairly benign, and as stated in the literature, is refractory to treatment.

Features necessary for the diagnosis of intermittent hydrarthrosis are presented in Table 1. Intermittent hydrarthrosis generally persists for decades, although spontaneous resolution can occur. Some patients with this disorder have concomitant rheumatoid arthritis, typically of a mild degree.

Therapy, even synovectomy, is ineffective, with the possible exception, based on anecdotal reports, of a prophylactic effect of intraarticular glucocorticoid crystal instillation. For this reason, a determination of the effect of joint injection in individual patients should be systematically appraised.

FAMILIAL MEDITERRANEAN FEVER

Familial Mediterranean fever is an autosomal recessive disorder that primarily occurs in people of Mediterranean origins (Arabs, Jews, Turks, and Armenians). Perhaps *recurrent polyserositis* is a more descriptive term for this disease. Beginning in childhood or adolescence, patients begin to experience attacks at irregular intervals that consist of fever and severe pain in the abdomen, chest, or joints [4]. Familial Mediterranean fever must be accurately diagnosed as early as possible because prophylactic colchicine therapy is effective in stopping the attacks and eventual amyloidosis. In the absence of such therapy, death from amyloidosis is common [5•].

Episodes begin precipitously, are accompanied by varying levels of fever, and usually resolve within 24 hours, or more rarely, in 3 to 4 days. Abdominal pain mimics acute diffuse peritonitis, whereas chest pain is generally limited to a hemithorax. Transitory, small pleural, or pericardial effusions may occur during an event, as may an elevated erythrocyte sedimentation rate. Infrequently, recurrent aseptic meningitis is a feature of familial Mediterranean fever.

Joint involvement, typically in a knee, ankle, hip, shoulder, elbow, wrist, or hand, is a common initial presentation. Less commonly, pain occurs in several joints, often in an asymmetric distribution. Pain is severe and accompanied by periarticular spasm, but little swelling or redness of overlying skin occurs—an observation that should suggest the diagnosis. Articular attacks are more long-lived than are abdominal or

TABLE 1 FEATURES NECESSARY FOR THE DIAGNOSIS OF INTERMITTENT HYDRARTHROSIS
Intermittent attacks cause an acute, readily detectable knee effusion that is relatively painless, superimposed on a background of complete normalcy
Recurrences involve the same joint, usually the knee. On rare occasions, bilateral knee involvement has been reported
Local, systemic, or joint fluid evidence of inflammation should not be apparent
Effusion has an abrupt onset with a maximal swelling within 4 h premorbid state is reestablished in less than 1 wk
A completely predictable periodicity occurs, often in striking parallel to the menstrual cycle in female patients

chest crises, lasting days or even weeks. Splenomegaly may be observed, and low levels of proteinuria generally signify the onset of secondary amyloidosis resulting from amyloid A protein, an acute-phase reactant made in response to persistent inflammatory stimulus. Continuous prophylactic use of colchicine at a dosage of 1.2 to 1.8 mg/d aborts attacks and prevents amyloidosis. If amyloidosis develops, hemodialysis or kidney transplantation can prolong survival.

RELAPSING POLYCHONDRITIS

Relapsing polychondritis inflames and eventually destroys cartilage at virtually any site within the body (Table 2). With time, it generally assumes an intermittent or fluctuating pattern. Additional problems are caused by coexisting cutaneous or systemic vasculitis and inflammation of proteoglycan-rich tissues, such as those in the aortic valve or eye [6].

Anatomic factors account for the pathophysiology of polychondritis. The soft inferior lobe of the external ear lacks cartilage, which explains why only the superior cartilaginous part becomes inflamed (Fig. 1). The septum of the nose consists of a bony and more distal cartilaginous segment, accounting for the preservation of the proximal region of the nose as the cartilage-supported area collapses into the hallmark saddle-nose deformity (Fig. 2). An abundance of cartilage is present in the larynx, and hoarseness is common in patients with polychondritis. Hearing can be impaired mechanically or by inflammation if the thick cartilage sheaths swell and occlude the lumens of either the external auditory canal or the eustachian tube. In addition to this conductive hearing loss, a sensorineural hearing deficit, accompanied by vestibular symptoms, can occur, probably as a result of vasculitis.

Ocular involvement can be complex, representing an overlap of forms of inflammation found in either adult or juvenile rheumatoid arthritis or ankylosing spondylitis. As in adult rheumatoid arthritis, conjunctivitis or episcleritis can occur; as in juvenile rheumatoid arthritis or ankylosing spondylitis damage of the ascending portion of the aorta or aortic valve can develop.

Polychondritis is commonly misdiagnosed as an infectious perichondritis of the ear, but during an infection, the entire ear is inflamed. Another serious disease that can present with a polychondritis-like picture is Wegener's granulomatosis, but unlike polychondritis, the latter disorder destroys non–cartilage-containing tissues as well. It can be differentiated by the presence of granulomas on a biopsy specimen and by the detection of cytoplasmic antineutrophil cytoplasmic antibodies in the serum. Polychondritis can develop in patients with a preexisting autoimmune disease, such as rheumatoid arthritis, systemic lupus erythematosus, Hashimoto's thyroiditis, ankylosing spondylitis, Reiter's disease, primary biliary cirrhosis, or vasculitis.

Life expectancy is shortened in patients with polychondritis. In a retrospective review [7], the overall survival was 74% and 55% at 5 and 10 years, respectively. Most deaths related to the disease were caused by bacterial pneumonia following airway collapse or aortic insufficiency. Side effects from immunosuppressive regimens or organ damage from vasculitis led to other fatalities. Although decreased survival is difficult to predict in individual patients, in the retrospective study, potential markers for decreased survival included, in patients younger than 50 years of age, anemia, saddle-nose deformity, or systemic vasculitis. In older patients, only anemia correlated with decreased survival. The use of glucocorticoid therapy did not influence survival in either age group.

Treatment of polychondritis is frequently suboptimal and creates additional morbidity; however, prolonged administra-

TABLE 2 SITES OF INFLAMMATION AND CARTILAGE DESTRUCTION IN RELAPSING POLYCHONDRITIS

Tissue	Site of inflammation
Elastic cartilage	External ear (pinna)
	Nose (distal)
Hyaline cartilage	Peripheral joints
Fibrocartilage	Axial sites, *eg*, symphysis pubis
Other (proteoglycan-rich) cartilage	Aorta
	Bronchotracheal tree

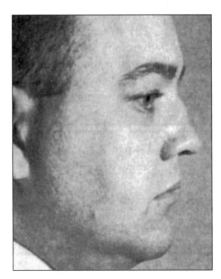

FIGURE 1 Inflammation of the superior (cartilage-containing) portion of the ear in relapsing polychondritis. (*From* McCarty and Koopman [6]; with permission.)

FIGURE 2 Collapse of the distal (cartilage-containing) region of the nose in relapsing polychondritis. (*From* McCarty and Koopman [6]; with permission.)

Adult-Onset Still's Disease 19

James T. Cassidy

> **Key Points**
> - Early diagnosis of adult-onset Still's disease is difficult and demands a high degree of suspicion.
> - Long-term prognosis is related to extent of joint disease.
> - Treatment should be approached cautiously, especially early in course.

Adult-onset Still's disease (AOSD) has become an increasingly frequent consideration in the differential diagnosis of febrile disorders in adults, characterized by rash and clinical manifestations of visceral disease [1,2]. Because objective arthritis is often absent during the initial course of the syndrome and AOSD almost always lacks other specific clinical, laboratory, or histologic features, a definite diagnosis is often difficult to make early, and patients are subjected to unnecessary and potentially dangerous diagnostic procedures [3]. Approximately half of the patients who present with this syndrome represent the *de novo* onset of disease as adults, whereas the other half are experiencing exacerbations of long quiescent systemic-onset juvenile rheumatoid arthritis (JRA) [2]. An accurate history of the latter or the detection on physical examination of evidence for JRA can often be an important clue to early diagnosis of AOSD.

EPIDEMIOLOGY

The frequency of AOSD is unknown. The prevalence of rheumatoid arthritis has been variously cited as 0.3% to slightly more than 1% of the adult North American population, a frequency influenced by the mean age of the population in question. It can be estimated that AOSD represents no more than 1% of new cases, a rarity that leads to unfamiliarity with its features by primary care physicians, thereby confounding or delaying appropriate diagnosis (Table 1) [1,2]. It is slightly more frequent in women [1] and has onset in the third or fourth decade of life in a pattern similar, if not identical, to that of systemic onset JRA [4•]. Its frequency in populations of varying ethnic background is basically unknown, although there have been publications from Japan [4–6] and India [7,8], as well as from North American and Europe [9–15]. In one report [5••], patients with AOSD represented 2.9% of the total rheumatology clinic population. In another, patients with AOSD constituted 5% of adults presenting with fever of unknown origin.

TABLE 1 CLINICAL CHARACTERISTICS OF ADULT-ONSET STILL'S DISEASE

Women
Quotidian fever
Rheumatoid rash
Serositis
Poly- and oligoarthritis
Seronegativity, no subcutaneous nodules
Age of onset
    Mean, 27.5 y
    Range, 17–35 y
Small and large joint involvement
    Erosions and ankylosis
    Cervical spine disease

From Bywaters [1]; with permission.

ETIOLOGY AND GENETIC PREDISPOSITION

The etiology of AOSD is unknown. Because of its presentation, it resembles an acute febrile infectious disease, but no specific organism has been isolated. An immunogenetic predisposition to this syndrome has also eluded geneticists, although there has been evidence for an increase in the frequency of HLA-B35 in children with systemic-onset JRA [3].

CLINICAL MANIFESTATIONS

Adult-onset Still's disease generally presents as an acute illness with marked constitutional signs and an intermittent fever (Table 2) [1,4•,13,15]. Its presentation closely resembles that of systemic-onset JRA [2,3,6,12,13,16]. The fever is most often quotidian, that is, there is a single febrile peak per day of 102°F to 105°F (Fig. 1). This peak is repeated daily and generally occurs at the same time, often in late afternoon or

TABLE 2 CLINICAL PRESENTATION OF ADULT-ONSET STILL'S DISEASE

Manifestation	Patients, *n/10*
Fever (> 105°F)	9
Rheumatoid rash	7
Adenopathy	7
Splenomegaly	6
Pneumonitis	6
Pericarditis	3
Abdominal pain	3
Arthritis	5

Adapted from Aptekar and coworkers [2]; with permission.

early evening; however, it may occur at any time of day or night. The temperature after each peak often decreases to below normal before returning to baseline. When the patient is febrile, there are usually marked signs of anorexia, extreme fatigue, and malaise. In contrast to other causes of unknown origin, including sepsis, the patient when afebrile often feels much better than the overall course of the disease would suggest. These episodes may last a few weeks or months and then not appear again for some time. In this matter, AOSD resembles early descriptions of periodic diseases (other than familial Mediterranean fever).

Each febrile peak is almost always accompanied by a characteristic rash (Fig. 2). This rash is macular and may be limited to small areas of the torso, extensor surfaces of the extremities, or the face, or it may be more generalized. It is not urticarial, pruritic, or vesicular. Its most characteristic feature is the fact that any lesion or group of lesions tends to be quite transient over 1 or 2 hours, although other lesions continue to appear elsewhere, giving the false impression of a more chronic dermatitis. The rash fades with central clearing, but coalescent areas may be present. Because this rash tends to be associated with the febrile peaks and is often limited in distribution on the body, a physician may be unaware that the patient has a rash unless that patient is examined at the time of the fever. The rash is also characterized by the isomorphic (Koebner) response and can often be precipitated by trauma to the skin or by a hot shower.

Objective arthritis may not be present at onset of the disease [1,2,4•,15] or for days, weeks, or months thereafter. Rarely, arthritis may not become evident until years after the initial febrile episode. The arthritis may be polyarticular, involving many joints, or oligoarticular, involving just a few or, indeed, only one joint [9••,10•]. If oligoarticular, the large joints, such as the wrists, knees, and ankles, tend to be involved; if polyarticular, small joint disease may also be present. Axial joints, such as the hips or shoulders, tend not to be involved at onset. Subcutaneous nodules are quite rare in patients with AOSD [1].

Over time, the systemic features of the illness tend to fade gradually into the background, and the articular component becomes more prominent. It, too, may adopt a pattern of repeated exacerbations and remissions. However, if chronic, the arthritis tends to establish itself as distinctly polyarticular or oligoarticular [10•]. This articular pattern of disease is important relative to prognosis.

Evidence of visceral involvement is usually quite prominent at onset of AOSD. The patient is often thought to have an acute infectious process, malignancy, leukemia, or lymphoma. The most characteristic manifestations are hepatomegaly, splenomegaly, and lymphadenopathy, know as the Still's triad; however, pericarditis with effusion, and pleuritis and effusion are common. Disease involving the central nervous system, gastrointestinal tract, or kidneys is rare in contrast to the other acute rheumatic diseases that may at onset be confused with AOSD. Patients have been described with this type of more extensive involvement [4•,11•].

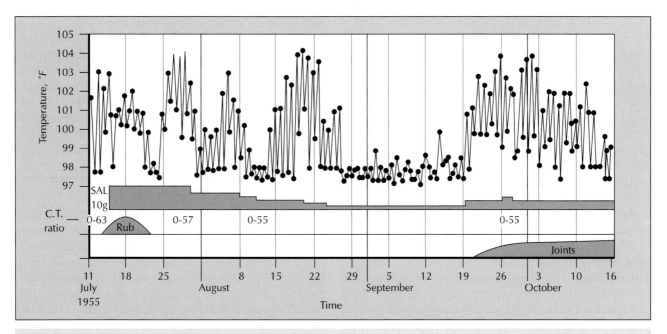

FIGURE 1 A single febrile peak of adult-onset Still's disease. CT–cardiothoracic. (*From* Bywaters [1]; with permission.)

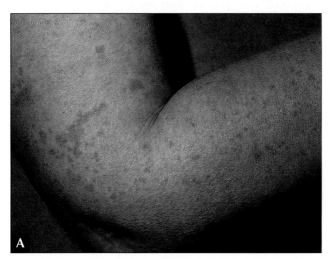

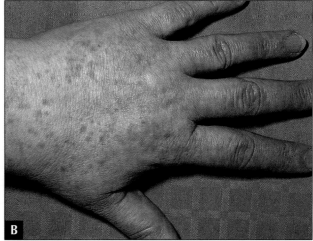

FIGURE 2 The rash of adult-onset Still's disease (AOSD) on **A**, the forearm and **B**, the dorsum of hand. The rash of AOSD is identical to that which occurs in systemic-onset juvenile rheumatoid arthritis. It is macular and pink, and individual lesions tend to occur in linear or coalescent groups. Each lesion is transient, lasting 0.5 to 2 hours, although new areas continue to appear.

PATHOLOGY AND LABORATORY EXAMINATION

There are relatively few objective measures that will confirm a diagnosis of AOSD. The most distinctive pathologic lesion involves features of the rash on histopathologic examination [1,9••]. It tends to be a neutrophilic perivasculitis rather than a necrotizing lesion with only minimal diapedesis of erythrocytes into the surrounding tissues. Perhaps most important, more specific evidence of other forms of idiopathic vasculitis is absent, and the lupus band test is negative. There are few reports of additional histologic studies in AOSD. The lymphadenopathy is characterized by a nonspecific reactive

hyperplasia that may resemble a lymphoma closely enough to cause diagnostic confusion [14]. The pericardial and pleural surfaces are affected by nonspecific inflammation, as well, that seldom progresses to fibrosis.

There are no specific laboratory findings. The patients almost always have a neutrophilic leukocytosis that may reach levels of 40,000 to 60,000 cells/mm^3 [4•,5,9••,15]. The cells on examination appear normal, although there may be toxic granulation of the neutrophils. Eosinophilia is not characteristic, although it has been described (as in adult rheumatoid arthritis). Bone marrow examination reflects a reactive hyperplasia of the granulocytic elements. Thrombocytosis of 450,000 to 750,000 platelets/mm^3 is also characteristic of the acute febrile phase of this disease, the platelets responding as acute-phase reactants. A normocytic, normochromic anemia is also found in these patients at onset or during the course of the disease and has the characteristics of the anemia of chronic inflammation with markedly depressed serum iron levels and moderately low total iron-binding capacity. The serum ferritin concentration may be misleading, however, because it is often elevated as an acute phase response. In fact, hyperferritinemia has been proposed as a helpful diagnostic clue for AOSD [17,18]. The erythrocyte sedimentation rate (ESR), the C-reactive protein concentration, and immunoglobulin levels are almost always elevated in patients with AOSD. At onset, this information may be useful diagnostically because serum sickness is usually associated with a normal ESR.

The rheumatoid factor test as performed on IgG-coated latex beads (Singer-Plotz tube dilution test) is negative. However, the slide latex agglutination is not a reliable measure of rheumatoid factor seropositivity and should not be used. Antinuclear antibodies are almost always absent in these patients when assayed on HEp-2 cell substrate. However, the background frequency of antinuclear antibody seropositivity increases markedly with the age of the patient after childhood; therefore, a positive result on antinuclear antibody testing, unless a distinctive pattern and high titer are present, may be misleading [3].

RADIOLOGIC CHANGES

The most prominent radiologic changes are in joints that are characteristically involved in this disease: knees, wrists, small joints of the hands, and cervical spine. Bony erosions, at least

early in the disease, are unusual, which also is often characteristic of children with systemic-onset JRA. A distinctive finding has been noted in the carpometacarpal joints with narrowing or ankylosis, especially at the second and third metacarpal bases [1,10•]. The intercarpal joints are also involved in AOSD patients. Loss of neck motion may be striking, and cervical spine disease, if present radiologically, preferentially begins at the C_2-C_3 apophyseal joint [1]. Cervical involvement may progress to atlantoaxial subluxation.

DIAGNOSIS

The diagnosis of AOSD is often delayed for months or occasionally years. In one report, the mean delay was 16 months [12]. Recently, preliminary criteria for the classification of AOSD were proposed in a study of Japanese patients to aid in its early recognition [5]. In this report, 90 patients were compared with 267 control subjects, and the criteria were divided into major and minor categories (Table 3). Definitions of these criteria were reminiscent of the pediatric criteria for JRA. Thirteen control subjects satisfied the proposed criteria, including two patients with polyarteritis nodosa, two with rheumatoid vasculitis, one with sepsis, and eight with fever of unknown origin. Five of these latter patients were eventually diagnosed with viral meningitis, an HIV-associated complex, Takayasu's arteritis, hypersensitivity angiitis, and sarcoidosis in one patient each. These authors also compared their criteria with those of four previously published studies for sensitivity and specificity. The Japanese criteria, because of their specificity, performed least well in the likelihood ratio in comparison with those of the other studies.

TABLE 3 PRELIMINARY CRITERIA FOR CLASSIFICATION OF ADULT-ONSET STILL'S DISEASE*
Major criteria Fever of 102°F (39°C) or higher lasting 1 wk or longer Arthralgia lasting 2 wk or longer Typical rash Leukocytosis ($\geq$ 10,000 cells/mm³), including granulocytes ($\geq$ 80%) **Minor criteria** Sore throat Lymphadenopathy or splenomegaly Liver dysfunction† Negative rheumatoid factor and negative antinuclear antibody **Exclusions** Infections (especially sepsis and infectious mononucleosis) Malignancies (especially lymphoma) Rheumatic diseases (especially polyarteritis nodosa and rheumatoid vasculitis with extra-articular features) *Classification of adult-onset Still's disease requires five or more criteria, including two or more major criteria. † Defined as abnormally elevated levels of transaminases or lactate dehydrogenase, which are attributed to liver damage associated with this disease but not with drug allergy, toxicity, or other causes. *Adapted from* Yamaguchi and coworkers [5]; with permission.

MANAGEMENT

The key to appropriate treatment is early diagnosis. The varying clinical manifestations of AOSD are managed consistent with their treatment in more typical rheumatoid arthritis. Nonsteroidal antiinflammatory drugs often provide considerable relief of joint pain or stiffness and constitutional symptoms. At onset, they may not have a dramatic impact upon the fever or rash, however. Indomethacin may be more effective as an antipyretic agent. Glucocorticoids occasionally have to be used to control visceral disease or very high fevers unresponsive to other treatment. Steroids should be avoided if at all possible; if not, they should be given as a single morning dose. It is not known whether patients with AOSD may be at risk for the same adverse reactions to disease-modifying antirheumatic drugs, as described in children with systemic-onset JRA [3]. Such reactions have often been serious, involving diffuse intravascular coagulation and even death. Caution should be observed when any of these agents are given to patients with AOSD early after onset during the acute febrile phase.

COURSE OF THE DISEASE AND PROGNOSIS

The febrile phase of the disease tends to be self-limited after some months to a few years [2,8,11•,12,16]. Thereafter, these patients pursue a pattern of chronic arthritis of either the polyarticular or the oligoarticular type [9••,10•] or they continue to have exacerbations and remissions of the febrile syndrome (Table 4) [2]. Patients with oligoarticular disease tend to do somewhat better than do those with more widespread joint involvement [10•]. Bywaters [1] published the results from a series of 14 young women with characteristic features of Still's disease, including fever, rash, polyarthritis, and an elevated ESR (Table 1). In a study from the National Institutes of Health, however, all of the patients were men, half of whom were experiencing an exacerbation of arthritis after a long remission of systemic-onset disease that began in childhood (Tables 2 and 4) [2]. In a report by Elkon and coworkers [9] of 11 white women with AOSD followed for a mean of 20 years, 10 had a polycyclic pattern characterized by remissions and exacerbations; there was a tendency for each exacerbation, although similar to the one before, to be progressively less severe (Table 5). Loss of wrist extension with carpal ankylosis was the most common chronic joint abnormality in these patients, although five developed involvement of the distal interphalangeal joints (again characteristic of childhood-onset disease). In another series of 21 patients by Cush and coworkers [10], four patterns of disease emerged: 1) monocyclic-systemic, 2) polycyclic-systemic, 3) chronic monocyclic-systemic, and 4) chronic polyarticular-systemic. The first two groups (good-prognosis AOSD) had articular disease only during exacerbations of the syndrome, whereas the latter two (poor-prognosis AOSD) developed significant long-term disability. One fifth of the patients had severe enough erosive disease that functional deterioration to a Steinbocker classification of III or IV developed, often related to involvement of the hips.

The recurring nature of AOSD was also documented in a Japanese study in which 55% of 90 patients had repeated exacerbations and remissions [4,5]. This report estimated the frequency of development of secondary amyloidosis to be as high as 30% after 10 years of illness. It is assumed that North American patients with AOSD probably do not develop a similar frequency of this complication because amyloidosis is exceedingly rare in children with JRA on this continent.

TABLE 4 EXACERBATIONS AND REMISSIONS OF ADULT-ONSET STILL'S DISEASE

Age of onset, y	Asymptomatic interval, y	Current age, y
6	10	31
6	6,4,4	19
7	3	28
7	6,10	29
8	10,13	26
17	2	20
17	11,8	40
22	3	25
23	0.5	25
29	0	31

From Aptekar and coworkers [2]; with permission.

TABLE 5 PROGNOSIS OF ADULT-ONSET STILL'S DISEASE

White women–11
Quotidian fever and rheumatoid rash–11
Polycyclic clinical pattern, mnemic, decreasing severity–11
Carpal ankylosis–10
Distal interphalangeal joint arthritis–5

From Elkon and coworkers [9••]; with permission.

REFERENCES AND RECOMMENDED READING

Recently published papers of particular interest have been highlighted as:

• Of interest
•• Of outstanding interest

1. Bywaters EGL: Still's disease in the adult. *Ann Rheum Dis* 1971, 30:121–133.
2. Aptekar RG, Decker JL, Bujak JS, Wolff SM: Adult onset juvenile rheumatoid arthritis. *Arthritis Rheum* 1973, 16:715–718.
3. Cassidy JT, Petty RE: *Textbook of Pediatric Rheumatology*, edn 3. Philadelphia: WB Saunders; 1994.
4.• Ohta A, Yamaguchi M, Tsunematsu T, *et al.*: Adult Still's disease: a multicenter survey of Japanese patients. *J Rheumatol* 1990, 17:1058–1063.
5.•• Yamaguchi M, Ohta A, Tsunematsu T, *et al.*: Preliminary criteria for classification of adult Still's disease. *J Rheumatol* 1992, 19:424–430.

6. Tanaka S, Matsumoto Y, Ohnishi H, *et al*.: Comparison of clinical features of childhood and adult onset Still's disease. *Ryumachi* 1991, 31:511–518.

7. Singh YN, Adya CM, Kumar A, Malviya AN: Adult-onset Still's disease in India. *Br J Rheum* 1992, 31:417–419.

8. Bambery P, Thomas RJ, Malhotra HS, *et al*.: Adult-onset Still's disease: clinical experience with 18 patients over 15 years in northern India. *Ann Rheum Dis* 1992, 51:529–532.

9.•• Elkon KB, Hughes GRV, Bywaters EGL, *et al*.: Adult-onset Still's disease: twenty-year followup and further studies of patients with active disease. *Arthritis Rheum* 1982, 25:647–654.

10.• Cush JJ, Medsger TA Jr., Christy WC, *et al*.: Adult-onset Still's disease: clinical course and outcome. *Arthritis Rheum* 1987, 30:186–194.

11.• Reginato AJ, Schumacher HR, Baker DG, *et al*.: Adult onset Still's disease: experience in 23 patients and literature review with emphasis on organ failure. *Semin Arthritis Rheum* 1987, 17:39–57.

12. Sanchez Loria DM, Moreno Alvarez MJ, Maldonado Cocco JA, *et al*.: Adult onset Still's disease: clinical features and course. *Clin Rheumatol* 1992, 11:516–520.

13. Neve P, Decaux G: Still's disease in adults. *Rev Med Brux* 1991, 12:399–401.

14. Quaini F, Manganelli P, Pileri S, *et al*.: Immunohistological characterization of lymph nodes in two cases of adult onset Still's disease. *J Rheumatol* 1991, 18:1418–1423.

15.• van de Putte LB, Wouters JM: Adult onset Still's disease. *Baillieres Clin Rheumatol* 1991, 5:263–275.

16.•• Cabane J, Michon A, Ziza JM, *et al*.: Comparison of long term evolution of adult onset and juvenile onset Still's disease, both followed up for more than 10 years. *Ann Rheum Dis* 1990, 49:283–285.

17. Coffernils M, Soupart A, Pradier O, *et al*.: Hyperferritinemia in adult onset Still's disease and the hemophagocytic syndrome. *J Rheumatol* 1992, 19:1425–1427.

18. Schwarz-Eywill M, Heilig B, Bauer H, *et al*.: Evaluation of serum ferritin as a marker for adult Still's disease activity. *Ann Rheum Dis* 1992, 51:683–685.

Metabolic Bone Diseases 20

Catherine Cormier
Charles J. Menkes

Key Points

- Bone densitometry has considerably improved the management of osteoporosis and the evaluation of fracture risk.

- Management of glucocorticoid-induced osteopenia is based on baseline bone densitometry and rate of bone loss.

- The distinction between parathyroid and nonparathyroid-mediated causes of hypercalcemia is best made with the two-site type of assay that measures intact parathyroid hormone.

- Hypocalcemic disorders can be divided into hypoparathyroidism and hypocalcemia due to target organ malfunction.

- Osteomalacia is difficult to recognize in adults; bone biopsy may be necessary.

- The skeletal disorders of renal osteodystrophy are classified as high or low turnover lesions.

- Indications for therapy in Paget's disease include bone pain, rapid deformity, and risk of complications; bisphosphonates are now currently used for the treatment.

Osteoporosis decreases bone mass, causing bones to become more susceptible to fracture. The bone density of elderly people appears to depend on their peak bone mass during adolescence. Genetic factors strongly influence adult peak bone mass (responsible for 80% of total variance in bone density), but the importance of genetic effects diminishes with aging, owing to the cumulative effects of environmental factors [1]. Of the environmental factors, calcium and physical activity may play critical roles in skeletal development and maintenance of bone mass, and the two factors are interrelated. Estrogen also is involved and is the major determinant of postmenopausal osteoporosis. Sex steroid deficiency and calciotropic hormone disturbances are the most likely contributors to aging-associated bone loss.

Because bone loss can be the result of any of a diverse group of diseases, its etiology must be determined before therapy begins. Table 1 shows a classification of the causes of osteoporosis.

PRIMARY OSTEOPOROSIS

Clinical Presentation

Osteoporosis is associated with back pain, loss of height, spinal deformity, and fractures of the vertebrae, hips, and wrists. Vertebral compression fractures affecting the lower thoracic and lumbar vertebrae (fracture of trabecular-rich bones in type 1 or postmenopausal osteoporosis) can occur as a result of minimal trauma. Pain is

TABLE 1 CLASSIFICATION OF OSTEOPOROSIS

Primary osteoporosis
Juvenile
Type 1 (postmenopausal)
Type 2 (senile)

Secondary osteoporosis
Endocrine diseases
  Hypogonadism, hyperparathyroidism, hyperthyroidism, cushing's syndrome, diabetes mellitus (?)
Gastrointestinal diseases
  Gastrectomy, malabsorption, chronic liver disease, alcoholism
Bone marrow disorders
  Multiple myeloma, lymphoma, leukemia, disseminated carcinoma, systemic mastocytosis
Genetic skeletal disorders
  Osteogenesis imperfecta, hypophosphatasia, homocystinuria, Ehlers-Danlos and Marfan syndromes
Acquired osteoporosis
  Immobilization, chronic obstructive pulmonary disease, rheumatoid arthritis
Drug addictions
  Glucocorticoids, anticonvulsants, heparin

usually severe, and acute pain generally subsides within 6 to 8 weeks. With repeated fractures, the rib cage comes to rest on the pelvic rim. Many radiologically documented vertebral deformities are asymptomatic. Proximal femur subcapital and trochanteric fractures (type 2 or senile osteoporosis associated with vertebral fractures) are a significant health problem.

Diagnostic Methods
Bone densitometry
Techniques enabling safe and precise measurements of bone mineral density have considerably improved the management of osteoporosis in terms of diagnosing patients with vertebral abnormalities or roentgenographic osteopenia and of monitoring treatment. Such measurements can be used to classify patients according to fracture risk [2]. The technique of choice (simply because of its lower radiation dose) is dual photon absorptiometry or its roentgenographic equivalent, dual energy roentgenogram absorptiometry (Fig. 1).

Biochemical investigations
The most sensitive markers of bone formation (serum alkaline phosphatase, osteocalcin, and type 1 collagen peptide) and resorption (fasting urinary calcium, hydroxyproline, and urinary pyridinoline and deoxypyridinoline) can be used together to determine the rate of bone turnover in patients with vertebral osteoporosis. Which menopausal women have the highest risk of developing osteoporosis also can be determined by bone mass measurements [3].

Vertebral roentgenograms
The vertebral fracture rate assessed by vertebral roentgenograms has been the most objective indicator of osteoporosis in therapeutic trials. Defining vertebral deformities requires further studies to assess the relationship between them and symptomatic osteoporosis (Fig. 2).

Bone biopsy
Bone biopsy may be valuable for managing fractures that have occurred at sites other than those commonly associated with postmenopausal osteoporosis; for treating patients with nontraumatic fractures but normal vertebral bone mass; and for

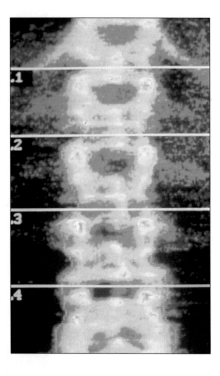

FIGURE 1
Dual energy roentgenographic absorptiometry showing osteoporosis in the spine.

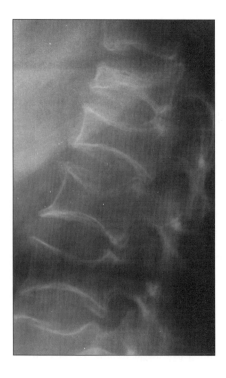

FIGURE 2
Multiple compression fractures of osteoporosis.

assessing, in treatment trials, whether patients with different remodeling characteristics respond differently to treatment.

Management

Prevention

Optimizing peak adult bone mass, stabilizing bone mass, and preventing falls are of paramount importance to prevention [4•]. The calcium content of diet should be increased to 1200 mg/d starting in adolescence, and physical exercise should be encouraged. Estrogen therapy is effective for preserving bone mass in postmenopausal and elderly women and for decreasing the number of osteoporotic fractures. Bone densitometry appears to influence patients' decisions and may improve compliance with estrogen therapy. Estrogen therapy decreases the risks of coronary heart disease and hip fracture; however, long-term therapy increases the risk of endometrial cancer and may be associated with a small increase in the risk of breast cancer. The effect of combination hormones (estrogen-progestin) on risks or benefits requires further study. Calcium may exert an effect by suppressing parathyroid hormone secretion, thus reducing bone loss. The absorption of calcium can be improved by adding 400 to 1000 units of vitamin D to the diet. Women who cannot take estrogens can use calcitonin (subcutaneous or nasal spray); however, it is not yet known whether calcitonin is effective for preventing fractures. Exercise and maintaining an adequate calcium intake help prevent bone loss.

Therapy

For symptomatic therapy of established osteoporosis, strong analgesics and muscle relaxants may be necessary initially. After the acute pain subsides, physical therapy is useful.

Drugs that decrease bone resorption include estrogens. Estrogen replacement therapy reduces the incidence of fractures among older osteoporotic women [5•]. Calcitonin increases lumbar spine bone density, but it is unclear whether the rate of new vertebral fracture is reduced. With both intermittent and low-dose continuous administration of bisphosphonates [6], lumbar spine mineral density increases and not at the expense of cortical bone; controlled studies of the effect of bisphosphonates on rates of new vertebral fractures are now necessary to confirm that they protect skeletal integrity. Calcium and vitamin D supplementation for residents of homes for elderly persons lowered hip fracture incidence [7•], but calcium had no demonstrated effect on vertebral fracture rate. Almost all medical treatments of established osteoporosis include calcium as an obligatory adjuvant.

Drugs that stimulate bone formation include fluoride, which directly stimulates osteoblasts. The drug is effective for increasing trabecular bone volume, but posology should be adapted [8]; a dosage of 15 to 25 mg/d is recommended. The results of trials with calcitriol (vitamin D) are conflicting. Trials with human synthetic 1-34 parathyroid hormone fragments are ongoing. Anabolic steroids may be indicated in osteoporosis, but they have the great disadvantage of inducing virilization effects.

SECONDARY OSTEOPOROSIS

Glucocorticoid-induced osteopenia results from direct glucocorticoid suppression of osteoblast activity and increased osteoclastic activity caused by increased parathyroid hormone secretion. Bone loss is more severe in regions of the skeleton with high trabecular bone content (ribs, vertebrae). The reported incidence of bone fractures among steroid-treated patients ranges from 8% to 18%. Steroid-induced osteopenia is diagnosed on the basis of the clinical situation and the exclusion of other causes of osteopenia. There is evidence of increased bone formation in patients with Cushing's disease after adrenalectomy. A direct relationship has been established between a cumulative dose of glucocorticoids and osteopenia. Osteopenia has been observed in patients treated chronically with daily doses of prednisone as low as 7.5 to 10 mg. Treatment regimens for steroid-induced osteopenia are directed toward reversing the disordered osteoblastic and osteoclastic activity (Table 2).

HYPERCALCEMIA

Hypercalcemia is an abnormal elevation in the serum concentration of ionized calcium (total calcium is influenced by serum

---

TABLE 2 MANAGEMENT OF GLUCOCORTICOID-INDUCED OSTEOPENIA

Initiation of glucocorticoid therapy
    Maintain lowest possible glucocorticoid dose
    Identify osteoporosis risk factors and intervene with general measures
    Regular program of weight-bearing physical activity
    Adequate calcium intake
    Estrogen therapy for postmenopausal women
    Measure baseline bone densitometry
Prophylaxis
    If 24-h urine calcium ≥ 4 mg/kg/d, use thiazide
    If 24-h urine calcium ≤ 3.5 mg/kg/d, treat with vitamin D and calcium, with or without thiazide
    Measure bone densitometry to evaluate rate of bone loss and adjust therapy
        Add sodium fluoride? Add bisphosphonate?
        Add nandrolone therapy?
    Treat fractures during glucocorticoid therapy with sodium fluoride, nandrolone therapy, or antiresorptive agents

TABLE 3 HYPERCALCEMIA

Clinical manifestations	Causes
Neuromuscular	Parathyroid-related
Altered states of consciousness: impaired ability to concentrate, confusion, stupor, coma	Primary hyperparathyroidism: adenoma, hyperplasia, carcinoma, familial multiple endocrine neoplasia types 1 and 2
Muscle weakness, hyporeflexia, paralysis	Familial hypocalciuric hypercalcemia
Headache	Secondary hyperparathyroidism
Depression	Ectopic secretion of parathyroid hormone by tumors
Gastrointestinal	Lithium
Anorexia, constipation	Non–parathyroid-related
Nausea, vomiting, peptic ulcer, acute pancreatitis	Malignancy: local osteolytic hypercalcemia, humoral hypercalcemia (secretion of parathyroid hormone–related peptide)
Renal	Vitamin D–related: vitamin D intoxication, excessive production of $1,25(OH)_2 D_3$ (granulomatous disorders)
Polyuria, polydipsia	Increased bone turnover: hyperthyroidism, immobilization with increased base turnover (*eg*, Paget's disease, children), vitamin A intoxication
Impaired renal function	Decreased bone mineralization: aluminum, iron intoxication
Nephrolithiasis, nephrocalcinosis	Endocrinopathies: hypoadrenalism, pheochromocytoma, pancreatic VIP syndrome
Cardiovascular	Calcium carbonate ingestion: milk-alkali syndrome
Hypertension	**Pharmaceutical**
Reduced QT interval, bradycardia, first-degree arteriovenous block	Vitamin D, vitamin A intoxication
Miscellaneous	Estrogen and antiestrogen in breast cancer
Dehydration	Lithium (dependent or independent of parathyroid function)
Deposition of calcium in soft tissue, often associated with hyperphosphatemia	Thiazide diuretics
	Aminophylline

albumin concentration and acid-base status). Clinical manifestations and causes are listed in Table 3. In more than 90% of patients with hypercalcemia, either primary hyperparathyroidism or malignancy will prove to be the cause. The distinction between parathyroid- and non–parathyroid-mediated causes of hypercalcemia is best made with the two-site type of assay that measures intact parathyroid hormone. If the intact parathyroid hormone level is elevated, primary hyperparathyroidism is the most likely diagnosis. Family history should be checked to distinguish sporadic from familial disease. Urine calcium should be measured to exclude familial hypocalciuric hypercalcemia. If the parathyroid hormone level is low or undetectable, increased urinary cyclic AMP excretion suggests tumor secretion of parathyroid hormone–related peptide (PTHrp), and increased serum 1,25 dihydroxyvitamin D suggests granulomatous diseases, such as sarcoidosis. The definitive treatment of hypercalcemia is removal of the cause, but initial treatment can and should be instituted without specific diagnosis. General management of hypercalcemia includes hydration, saline diuresis, diuretics, dialysis, and mobilization, whereas specific treatment can include calcitonin, bisphosphonates, corticosteroids, mithramycin, phosphate, and therapy for the underlying etiology.

HYPOCALCEMIA

Hypocalcemia is an abnormally low serum ionized calcium concentration. Hypocalcemic disorders can be divided into two categories: primary hypoparathyroidism and hypocalcemia due to target organ malfunction with normal or even increased parathyroid hormone secretion (Table 4). Clinical manifestations of hypocalcemia include increased neuromuscular excitability, paresthesia, muscle cramping, carpopedal spasm, Chvostek's sign (twitching of the circumoral muscles in response to gently tapping the skin over the facial nerve just anterior to the ear), laryngeal stridor, and convulsions.

The decision to treat a hypocalcemic patient is based on both the degree of hypocalcemia and the rate at which the condition developed. Serum calcium levels of less than 7.5 mg/dL—or any level in patients with symptoms—should be treated (Table 4).

OSTEOMALACIA AND RICKETS

In children, clinical features of osteomalacia and rickets include hypotonia, proximal weakness, skeletal deformities, and fractures. In adults with symptoms, diffuse skeletal pain and generalized muscular weakness may dominate [9]. The various forms are listed in Table 5. Radiographic abnormalities, like the clinical presentation, are not precise. A more specific abnormality is Looser's zones, ribbon-like zones of rarefaction ranging from a few millimeters to several centimeters in length and usually oriented perpendicular to the bone surface, near the femoral heads in the metatarsals or in the pelvis. Common laboratory findings are listed in Table 6.

TABLE 4 HYPOCALCEMIA

Causes

Hypoparathyroidism
  Idiopathic
  Autoimmune
  Acquired: infiltrative (hemachromatosis, Wilson's disease, thalassemia, metastatic carcinoma, Di George's syndrome), surgical, postirradiation
  Functional: hypomagnesemia, transient neonatal and postoperative
Deficient parathyroid action (hormone resistance)
  Pseudohypoparathyroidism
Deficiency of vitamin D and abnormalities of vitamin D metabolism
  Vitamin D deficiency: decreased precursors, insufficient exposure to sunlight, dietary insufficiency, malabsorption, liver disease, abnormal enterohepatic circulation, drugs (phenobarbital, phenytoin), nephrotic syndrome
  Decreased production of active metabolite: vitamin D–dependent rickets type 1, renal disease
Resistance to vitamin D
  Vitamin D–dependent rickets type II
  Altered bone remodeling
  Increased osteoblastic activity: "Hungry bone" syndrome (postparathyroidectomy)
  Drug-decreased bone resorption: calcitonin, mithramycin
  Osteoblastic metastases
Phosphate excess
  Exogenous, rhabdomyolysis
Miscellaneous
  Acute pancreatitis
  Multiple citrated blood transfusions

Management

Acute
  An ampule of 10% calcium gluconate (90 mg of elemental calcium) infused over 5–10 min
Less acute
  Calcium solution diluted in dextrose, 15 mg/kg of calcium over 4–6 h
Chronic
  Treatment of specific cause, *eg*, hypoparathyroidism, with 1 g/d calcium; $1,25(OH)_2 D_3$, with 0.25–2 µg/d; or 25-OH D_3, with 25–200 µg/d
  Correction of vitamin D status

TABLE 5 ETIOLOGY OF RICKETS AND OSTEOMALACIA

Vitamin D disorders

Vitamin D deficiency
  Insufficient exposure to sunlight
  Dietary deprivation
  Loss of vitamin D metabolites: nephrotic syndrome and peritoneal dialysis
Vitamin D malabsorption
  Gastrointestinal disorder: gastrectomy, sprue, regional enteritis, jejunoileal bypass
  Pancreatic insufficiency
  Hepatobiliary disease: biliary atresia and obstruction, cirrhosis
Disorders of vitamin D metabolism
  Impaired 25-hydroxylation: liver disease, anticonvulsant agents
  Impaired 1-hydroxylation: chronic renal failure, hereditary vitamin D–dependent rickets type 1, hypoparathyroidism
Abnormal target tissue response
  Hereditary vitamin D–dependent rickets type 2
Metabolic acidosis

Phosphate disorders

Decreased intestinal malabsorption: malnutrition, malabsorption, ingestion of phosphate-binding factors or acids
Increased renal loss
  Hereditary: X-linked hypophosphatemic rickets, De Toni-Debré-Fanconi (phosphaturia, aminoaciduria, glycosuria, bicarbonaturia), cystinosis, Wilson's disease, tyrosinemia
  Acquired: tumoral hypophosphatemia osteomalacia, sporadic hypophosphatemia osteomalacia, fibrosis dysplasia, multiple myeloma
  Drug-induced: cadmium, tetracycline outdated
Calcium deficiency
Primary disorders of bone matrix
  Hypophosphatasia
  Fibrogenesis imperfecta ossium
Inhibitors of mineralization
  Aluminum
  Etidronate

TABLE 6 LABORATORY FINDINGS IN RICKETS OR OSTEOMALACIA

	Calcipenic form	Phosphopenic form
Calcium	↓	↓ or N
Phosphate	↓	↓↓
25-OH D	↓ < 3 ng/mL	N
1,25(OH)$_2$ D	↓ or N	N unadapted
Parathyroid hormone	↑ or N	N

↓—decreased; ↑—increased; N—normal.

Osteomalacia is difficult to diagnose in adults; bone biopsy may be necessary. In osteomalacia, bone is poorly and slowly mineralized, resulting in wide osteoid seams and a large fraction of bone covered by unmineralized osteoid. The mineralization lag time is determined by the fluorescence of previously ingested tetracycline.

The goal of treatment is to normalize the clinical, biochemical, and radiologic abnormalities without producing hypercalcemia, hyperphosphatemia, hypercalciuria, nephrolithiasis, or ectopic calcification. Table 7 lists the available vitamin D metabolites and clinical applications.

RENAL OSTEODYSTROPHY

The skeletal disorders of renal osteodystrophy are classified as either high turnover lesions related to persistently elevated serum levels of parathyroid hormone or low turnover lesions related predominantly to excess bone aluminum accumulation (Table 8).

Clinical manifestations are bone pain (generally not localized), progressive muscular weakness, vascular calcification, and skeletal deformities. Circulating parathyroid hormone levels are elevated early during the course of the disease, and hypocalcemia and low levels of calcitriol appear later [10]. Hypercalcemia may be observed in patients with severe secondary hyperparathyroidism, ingestion of large amounts of calcium and vitamin D, sarcoidosis, malignancies, or osteomalacia secondary to aluminum retention. Long-term hemodialysis patients frequently develop amyloid deposits that produce cysts adjacent to large joints. In cases of renal failure, low 1,25(OH)$_2$ D$_3$ levels precede calcium, phosphorus, and parathyroid hormone level changes.

TABLE 7 VITAMIN D METABOLITES AND CLINICAL APPLICATIONS

Application	Ergocalciferol D$_2$	Calcifediol 25-OH D$_3$	Calcitriol 1,25(OH)$_2$ D$_3$ 1α-hydroxycholecalciferol
Physiologic dose	2.5–10 μg (10 μg = 400 UI)	1–5 μg	0.25–0.5 μg
Pharmacologic dose	0.625–5 mg	20–200 μg	0.5–2 μg 0.5–5 μg
Half-life	4–5 d	10–20 d	5–18 h
Clinical dose	Vitamin D deficiency	Vitamin D deficiency	Chronic renal failure
	Hypophosphatemic rickets	Chronic renal failure	Hypoparathyroidism
	Anticonvulsant		Hypophosphatemic rickets
	Chronic renal failure		Acute hereditary hypocalcemia
			Vitamin D–dependent rickets types 1 and 2
			Osteoporosis

TABLE 8 RENAL OSTEODYSTROPHY

Pathogenesis	Roentgenography
High turnover bone disease: uremic hyperparathyroidism	
Hyperphosphatemia	Subperiosteal erosion of digital phalanges and distal ends of clavicles
Decreased 1α-hydroxylase	Brown tumors
Decreased calcium intake and absorption	Soft tissue calcification
Skeletal resistance to calcemic action of parathyroid hormone	
Parathyroid gland insensitivity to suppressive effects of calcium	
Low turnover base disease: adynamic bone diseases	
Osteomalacia	Pseudofracture
Vitamin D deficiency	Fractures of the ribs and hips and vertebrae fractures
Persistent hypocalcemia or hypophosphatemia, or both	Rickets-like lesions
Aluminum accumulation	Spontaneous fractures
Iron	

Successful management of renal osteodystrophy includes interventions to correct or counteract the major pathogenic factors responsible for the bone disease (Table 9).

PAGET'S DISEASE OF BONE

The clinical presentation of Paget's disease is variable: with or without symptoms, monostotic or polyostotic. The most common features are skeletal deformity and musculoskeletal pain [11•]. The complications of Paget's disease include

Fractures, including fissures, complete fracture, vertebral fractures

Compression of neural structures, including various cranial nerves, spine

Degenerative joint disease of the hip and knee

Hypercalciuria, hypercalcemia, nephrolithiasis

High-output cardiac failure

Sarcoma in 1% of the diseased population

Another family member is affected in 1% to 5% of cases, and 3% to 4% of the population older than 40 years of age are afflicted. Considerable evidence now suggests that Paget's disease is caused by infection with a virus with a prolonged latent period.

The diagnosis is based on radiologic findings. Osteolytic lesions include osteoporosis circumscripta (Fig. 3), well-demarcated areas of decalcification in frontal and occipital regions, and V-shaped lytic edges in long bones (Fig. 4). The radiographic manifestations of osteoblastic activity are sclerosis in long bones and in the vertebral column with enlargement (Fig. 5) and the classic cotton-wool lesions of exuberant chaotic bone formation (Fig. 6). Computed tomography is the most useful imaging technique for diagnosing sarcoma, and magnetic resonance imaging combined with computed tomography is particularly helpful in cases of neurologic complications. Bone scans are the most sensitive means of detecting active lesions that are discernible by roentgenography [12].

A major histologic feature is the increased number of multinucleated osteoclasts with an increased rate of bone remodeling. Markers of matrix synthesis or osteoblastic activity (plasma alkaline phosphatase and osteocalcin) and markers of bone resorption (urinary hydroxyproline) are often elevated. There is a significant correlation between the severity of Paget's disease and the plasma concentration of alkaline phosphatase.

Patients are frequently asymptomatic and thus do not require therapy. Indications for therapy include severe bone pain corresponding to areas of Paget's disease, rapid deformity, and complications. Subcutaneous injections of 50 to 100 MRC units of calcitonin per day or per every 2 days improve many manifestations of the disease and produce a 50% decrease in biochemical markers. Given the problems with parenteral administration, nasal calcitonin may be preferable.

Bisphosphonates are now well established in treating Paget's disease. Etidronate (5 mg/kg/d for 6 months) produces benefits similar to those of calcitonin, but calcitonin or another bisphosphonate should be used for treating osteolytic lesions. Pamidronate is considered superior in terms of symptomatic and biochemical response. Predicting the dose required for any given patient remains problematic. Unfortunately, this drug is not available in the United States.

Orthopedic procedures such as total hip replacement and tibial osteotomy also have a role in the treatment of selected patients. Adjuvant medical therapy should be administered before surgery to reduce intraoperative and postoperative bleeding and to prevent immobilization hypercalcemia.

TABLE 9 TREATMENT OF RENAL OSTEODYSTROPHY

Control serum phosphate

Phosphorus intake in diet should be restricted to 600–800 mg/d to reduce serum parathyroid hormone levels in patients with moderate renal failure

Phosphate-binding agents: acceptable doses of aluminum hydroxide

Calcium carbonate improves calcium balance when phosphate is controlled

Use of vitamin D sterols

25-OH D$_3$, 1alpha-dihydroxycholecalciferol

1,25(OH)$_2$ D$_3$, 0.25–1.5 µg/d

1,25(OH)$_2$ D$_3$ intravenously

Parathyroidectomy indications

Persistent hypercalcemia: serum calcium, > 11.5–12 mg/dL

Intractable pruritus

Progressive extraskeletal calcifications and persistent hyperphosphatemia despite appropriate phosphate restriction

Severe skeletal pain or fractures

Calciphylaxis: ischemic ulcers and necrosis

(Aluminum-related bone disease must be excluded)

Postparathyroidectomy

Only calcium carbonate should be used as the phosphate-binding agent

Management of aluminum intoxication

Deferoxamine only for patients with symptomatic intoxication

In asymptomatic patients: withdrawal of aluminum-containing agents and substitution of calcium carbonate

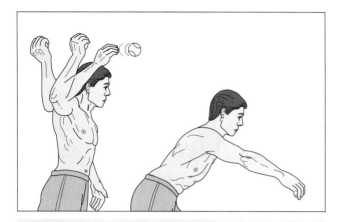

FIGURE 1 Biomechanics of the throwing motion: cocking, acceleration, and follow-through phases.

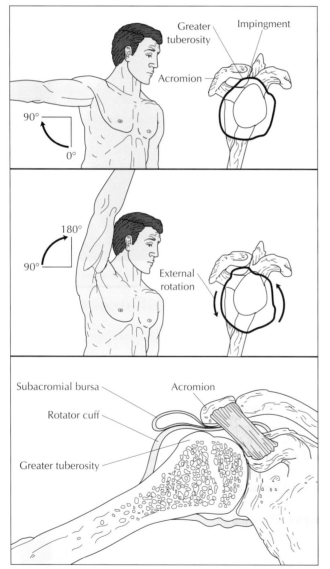

FIGURE 2 The impingement syndrome of the shoulder, involving compression of the rotator cuff muscles between the greater tuberosity of the humerus head and the acromion and soft tissues on the shoulder roof.

The supraspinatus muscle can be isolated by having the patient hold the hands outstretched in the thumbs-down position, with the wrists brought 30° forward from neutral in the abducted position. With the wrists held approximately 45° to 60° away from the body, resistance is applied against the wrist, and the patient is asked to press upward. Pain or weakness with this motion is often associated with tendinitis or a tear to the supraspinatus muscle. The infraspinatus muscle is best assessed by asking the patient to externally rotate the shoulder against resistance with the elbow held at 90° and the arms abducted against the body. The subscapularis muscle is assessed with the arm held in a similar position but with resistance placed against internal rotation (Fig. 3). The teres minor muscle is very difficult to isolate and individually assess.

Glenohumeral dislocation is evaluated by several methods. The most common is the apprehension test, in which the arm is held at a 90° angle in an abducted, externally rotated position. Posterior forces are applied against the glenohumeral joint, and the patient is asked to press the hand forward against resistance. The sensation of instability or apprehension is highly suggestive of subluxation (dislocation) of the shoulder (Fig. 4).

Injuries to the rotator cuff also can occur in sports such as swimming and gymnastics, which involve a forceful arc of the shoulder girdle. The throwing motion does not necessarily have to be involved.

Treatment

Management of rotator cuff injuries depends on their severity. Using the Neer classification of rotator cuff tears, the following treatment schedules apply [4]. Grade I rotator cuff injuries involve pain with normal range of motion and mild

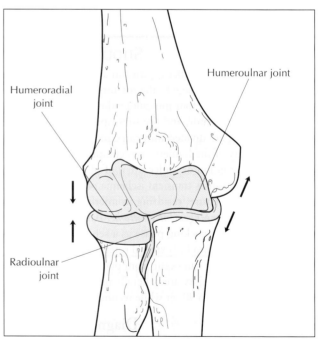

FIGURE 3 Valgus and varus stresses to the elbow associated with the throwing motion.

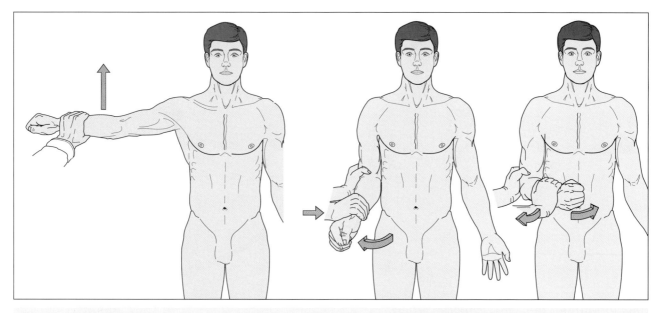

FIGURE 4 Strength testing the rotator cuffs: supraspinatus, infraspinatus, and subscapularis muscles.

pain with strength testing for each rotator cuff muscle but no weakness whatsoever; these injuries can be managed conservatively with rest, the use of nonsteroidal antiinflammatory drugs (NSAIDs), and physical therapy. Grade II rotator cuff tears demonstrate weakness but with a capacity to produce significant power upon rotator cuff muscle strength testing; these injuries must be observed closely, with rest, physical therapy, NSAIDs, and vigilance for progression of weakness. Grade III tears involve significant weakness and the classical drop arm test associated with strength testing: with the arm held above 90°, the deltoid muscle supports the shoulder; as the arm is lowered to below 90°, it drops because stability depends on rotator cuff strength (Fig. 5). For all grades of rotator cuff injury, a radiographic assessment of the shoulder is indicated to determine instability, calcific tendinitis, or osteoarthritis.

When to Refer

Generally, grade III rotator cuff tears and progressively weakening grade II rotator cuff injuries should be referred to an orthopedic surgeon for evaluation.

ELBOW

During the acceleration phase of throwing, the elbow is held in a position of extreme valgus strain, which can result in two major injuries (Fig. 6). These biomechanical stresses from the throwing motion in young pitchers, whose growth plates have not yet closed, is commonly referred to as *Little Leaguer's elbow* [5].

Diagnosis

A symptom of Little Leaguer's elbow is pain associated with throwing.

Valgus strain to the elbow can be assessed using several methods. A normal range of motion can be ascertained by measuring full flexion and extension of the elbow, pronation, and supination. The medial collateral ligament can be stressed by holding the elbow bent at 10° and placing a valgus stress across the elbow, checking for an end point of laxity. An injury to the radial head or to the distal humerus can be assessed by palpating the radial head with the elbow flexed at 90°, then pronating and supinating the forearm. Positive findings with this examination include pain or swelling.

Treatment

Managing Little Leaguer's elbow requires rest and a radiographic evaluation of the elbow. Physical therapy with ice, electrical stimulation, and ultrasound can be useful.

When to Refer

Generally, growth plate abnormalities evident on roentgenogram, osteochondritis dissecans, radial head compression fracture, or tear of the ulnar collateral ligament of the elbow require referral to an orthopedic surgeon.

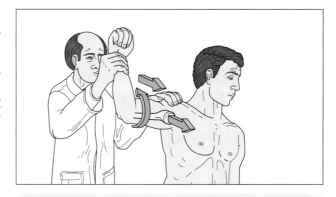

FIGURE 5 The apprehension test for glenohumeral instability of the shoulder.

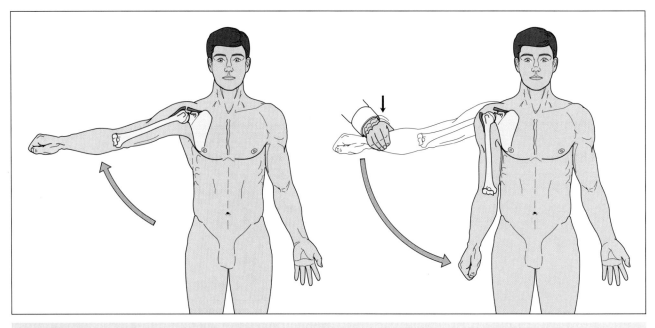

FIGURE 6 The drop arm test for grade III (complete) tear of the rotator cuff.

SPINE

Significant injuries to the spine in collision sports, such as football and rugby, may be associated with cervical spinal stenosis [6•]. Patients may have pain, weakness, or numbness in an upper extremity, usually in a cervical nerve root distribution area.

Diagnosis

The diagnosis of cervical spinal stenosis has been confusing [7–9]. Both anatomic and functional definitions have been proposed. The problem with the anatomic definition is its lack of sensitivity and specificity for predicting future significant injury. Patients with cervical spinal stenosis often come for medical attention because of neurologic symptoms, such as hand numbness or weakness, associated with an injury to the neck while playing a collision sport. Spinal stenosis also can be defined functionally by loss of fluid around the cervical spinal cord or, in more extreme cases, deformation of the spinal cord documented by magnetic resonance imaging, contrast computed tomography scan, or myelography [6•].

KNEE AND LOWER EXTREMITY

Anterior Cruciate Ligament Injury

One of the most devastating injuries in collision and contact sports, such as football, soccer, and basketball, is a tear of the anterior cruciate ligament of the knee (Fig. 7) [10]. Classically, with an acute tear, a knee effusion occurs within the first 1 to 2 hours, with or without ecchymoses, accompanied by severe pain about the knee.

Diagnosis

An anterior cruciate ligament injury can be classified into first-, second-, or third-degree sprains (a stretch, a partial tear, and a complete rupture, respectively). Physical examination of the knee for anterior cruciate ligament integrity can be performed using two basic tests. The Lachman test is performed while holding the knee at approximately 10° flexion and placing an anterior stress over the tibia and fibula while holding the femur stable (Fig. 8). Anterior slippage of the tibia and fibula

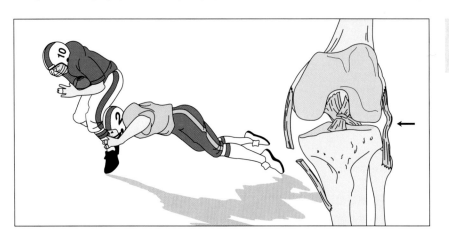

FIGURE 7 Direct lateral blow to the knee resulting in a torn anterior cruciate ligament.

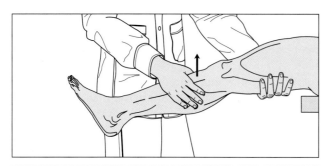

FIGURE 8 Lachman test of the knee to determine stability of the anterior cruciate ligament.

across the femoral condyles is a positive test, indicating at least partial loss of the integrity of the ligament.

Another test is the anterior drawer test, which is performed while holding the knee at 80° to 90° flexion with weight placed on the patient's foot to stabilize the leg. After placing the hands at the proximal calf with the thumbs at the anterior joint line of the knee, the knee is pulled forward; anterior slippage of the tibia suggests a positive test (Fig. 9). Assessing an acute anterior cruciate ligament tear should always include a radiographic examination to rule out an avulsion fracture of the distal portion of the anterior cruciate ligament from the tibial eminence; this lesion is easily corrected surgically by replacing the bony avulsed fragment, and it does not require the more complex reconstruction of the anterior cruciate ligament as most tears do. In addition to radiographic analysis after an acute injury, arthrocentesis can be performed for diagnostic purposes. A bloody tap is highly suggestive of an anterior cruciate ligament tear; fat in bloody joint fluid is highly suggestive of a tibial plateau fracture, with release of fat from the bone marrow.

Treatment

Managing an acutely torn anterior cruciate ligament requires immobilization of the knee, crutches to prevent weight bearing, and follow-up evaluation by an orthopedic surgeon. Nonsurgical management of such a tear is possible, particularly for sedentary people who do not place significant stresses on the knee. Surgical reconstruction of the ligament must be followed by a rigorous physical therapy program, initially involving isometric exercises, followed by dynamic quadriceps- and hamstring-strengthening exercises. Whether surgical management is chosen or not, the strength of the quadriceps and hamstring muscles must be optimized to prevent instability of the knee. Repetitive injury to a knee with a deficient anterior cruciate ligament can lead to the accelerated development of osteoarthritis.

When to Refer

All acute anterior cruciate ligament tears should be referred to an orthopedic surgeon, who will generally recommend reconstructive repair for physically active individuals. Chronic injuries with recurrent effusions also should be referred.

Patellofemoral Pain Syndrome

The patellofemoral pain syndrome (formerly called chondromalacia patellae), is a softening of the patellar articular cartilage [11]. The syndrome encompasses patellofemoral cartilage damage, malalignment of the patellofemoral joint, and overuse. Malalignment of the patellofemoral joint is typically associated with an increased tubercle-sulcus angle (the quadriceps, or Q angle) across the knee (Fig. 10). With knee flexion, a lateral force vector is applied to the misaligned patellae. As the patella is forced laterally, the medial retinaculum may be stretched or torn. The persistent lateral tracking of the patella can be associated with thickening of the lateral structures of the knee, stretching of the medial structures of the knee, and pain and tenderness posterior to the patella. Patellofemoral pain also can occur with normal alignment and is associated with overtraining.

Diagnosis

A patient with patellofemoral pain syndrome will often have an initial complaint of a dull ache in the anterior knee, generally underneath the kneecap. The pain is often exacerbated by climbing or descending stairs, and it worsens after prolonged sitting. During the physical examination, three tests are considered diagnostic. The patellar shrug test is performed by gently anchoring the superior portion of the patella with the hands and then having the patient contract the quadriceps muscle. The patellar compression test is performed by placing the hand directly over the patella and having the patient flex and extend the knee from approximately 30° flexion to

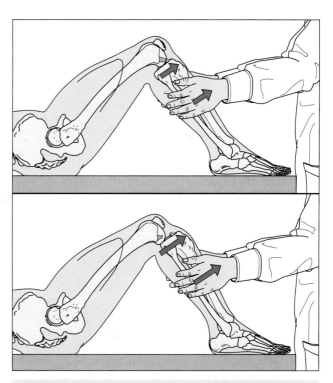

FIGURE 9 Anterior drawer test of the knee to determine stability of the anterior cruciate ligament.

complete extension. The patellar apprehension test is performed by placing a lateral and medial stress across the patella with the patient's leg held in full extension (Fig. 11). All of these maneuvers cause pain in patients with patellofemoral pain syndrome.

Treatment

Treatment consists of rest, either by resting complete or by reducing physical activity by one half to three quarters. The judicious use of NSAIDs, generally for 2 to 3 weeks, and applying ice and occasionally electrical stimulation to the affected area are effective. Specific exercises should include isometric strengthening of the quadriceps muscles. Dynamic knee-extension exercises from 90° flexion to full extension and against heavy resistance should be avoided. If an anatomic abnormality, such as malalignment, exists, correction should be attempted by means of an orthotic device.

When to Refer

When patellofemoral pain is associated with subluxation or dislocation, referral to an orthopedic surgeon is recommended.

EXERCISE GUIDELINES FOR PATIENTS WITH RHEUMATOLOGIC CONDITIONS

It is prudent for physicians to advise their patients strongly about a healthful program of physical exercise. By taking a common sense approach, a physical exercise program for a patient with musculoskeletal injury or arthritic condition can be devised. If the injury involves the upper extremity, such as a rotator cuff tear of the shoulder, walking, running, or bicycling—predominately lower-extremity activities—can be advised. Similarly, if an injury to the spine precludes involvement in sports that would place compressive forces across the spine, an activity such as swimming may be indicated.

The US Centers for Disease Control and Prevention recommends 20 to 30 minutes of aerobic exercise three to four times per week as the minimum physical activity necessary to benefit health. These guidelines do not include specific recommendations for the intensity of such exercise. It is thought that the quantity of exercise, rather than its intensity, is most important [12].

In 1990, the American College of Sports Medicine updated its exercise recommendations to include 20 to 60 minutes of physical, aerobic exercise performed three to five times per week at sufficient intensity to induce 60% to 90% of the predicted maximal heart rate (PMHR) [13•], which can be determined using the equation: PMHR = 220 less the patient's age. This recommendation reinforces the contention of the US Centers for Disease Control and Prevention that exercise of lesser intensity has significant benefit for many patients and may lead to greater compliance with an exercise program.

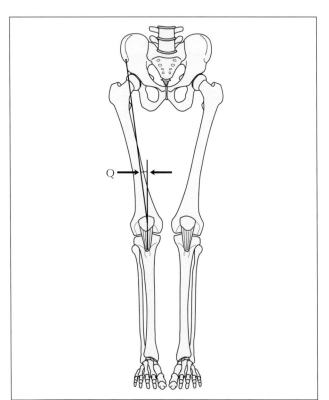

FIGURE 10 Quadriceps (Q) angle of the knee used to predict lateral stresses to the knee.

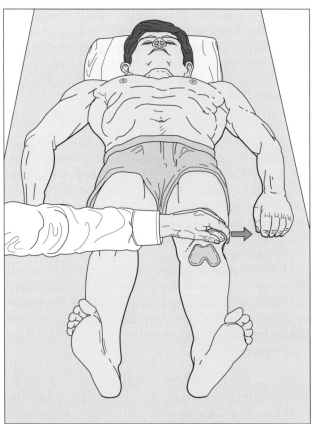

FIGURE 11 The patellar apprehension test for the patellofemoral pain syndrome.

References and Recommended Reading

Recently published papers of particular interest have been highlighted as:
- • Of interest
- •• Of outstanding interest

1.• McKeag DB, Hough DO: The shoulder. In *Primary Care Sports Medicine*, edn 1. Dubuque, IA: Wm C. Brown; 1993:281–301.

2. Tullos HS, King JW: Throwing mechanism in sports. *Orthop Clin North Am* 1973, 4:709–720.

3. Julin MJ, Mathews M: Shoulder injuries. In *The Team Physician's Handbook*, edn 1. Edited by Mellion MB. Philadelphia: Hanley and Belfus; 1990:313–333.

4. Neer CS: Anterior acromioplasty for the chronic impingement syndrome of the shoulder. *J Bone Joint Surg* 1972, 54A:41–50.

5. Barnes DA, Tullos HS: An analysis of 100 symptomatic baseball players. *Am J Sports Med* 1978, 6:62–67.

6.• Cantu RC: Functional cervical spinal stenosis: a contraindication to participation in contact sports. *Med Sci Sports Exerc* 1993, 25:316–317.

7. Torg JS, Pavlov H, Genuano SE, *et al.*: Neuropraxia of the cervical spinal cord with transient quadriplegia. *J Bone Joint Surg* 1986, 68A:1354–1370.

8. Pavlov H, Torg JS, Robie B, *et al.*: Cervical spinal stenosis: determination with vertebral body ratio method. *Radiology* 1987, 164:771–775.

9. Herzog RJ, Wiens JJ, Dillingham MF, Sontag MJ: Normal cervical spine morphometry and cervical spinal stenosis in asymptomatic professional football players. *Spine* 1991, 16:178–186.

10. Cross MJ, Wootton JR, Bokor DJ, Sorrenti SJ: Acute repair of injury to the anterior cruciate ligament. *Am J Sports Med* 1993, 21:128–131.

11. Grabiner MD, Koh TJ, Draganich LF: Neuromechanics of the patellofemoral joint. *Med Sci Sports Exerc* 1994, 26:10–21.

12. Caspersen CJ, Christensen GM, Pollard RA: Status of the 1990 physical fitness and exercise objectives: evidence from NHIS 1985. *Pub Health Rep* 1986, 101:587–592.

13.•• American College of Sports Medicine: Position statement on the recommended quantity and quality of exercise for developing and maintaining fitness in healthy adults. *Med Sci Sports Exerc* 1990, 22:265–274.

Select Bibliography

American College of Sports Medicine: Physical activity, physical fitness and hypertension: position stand. *Med Sci Sports Exerc* 1993, 25:i–x.

Glasgow SG, Gabriel JP, Sapega AA, *et al.*: The effect of early v. late return to vigorous activities on the outcome of ACL reconstruction. *Am J Sports Med* 1993, 21:243–248.

Reid DC: The myth, mystique, and frustration of anterior knee pain. *Clin J Sport Med* 1993, 3:139–143.

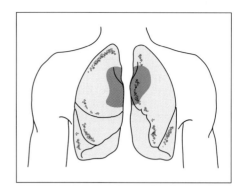

ALLERGY

AND IMMUNOLOGY

VII

Section Editor

Phillip L. Lieberman

The Allergy and Immunology section of *Current Practice of Medicine* reflects the broad-based character of the specialty. Chapters detail approaches to organ-related illnesses (*eg*, rhinitis, asthma, and urticaria), and those conditions that are not organ limited (*eg*, complement deficiency syndromes, immune deficiencies, and immunomodulation).

Several sections of text highlight the immunologic disorders most commonly seen in the practice of medicine, the atopic diseases. Chapters cover the management of chronic asthma, rhinitis, urticaria, angioedema, allergic disorders of the eye, anaphylaxis, and reactions to insect stings and bites. In this regard, the intent is to offer a practical guideline for therapy and management of these disorders to the practicing internist.

Immunology, however, extends far beyond the atopic diseases. Therefore, this section includes discussions of complement deficiency, vasculitis, immune deficiencies, AIDS, immunotherapy, and immunomodulation as well. These chapters are designed to assist the internist in the practical steps of diagnosis and management, while simplifying the scientific rationale for the approach to the patient who has an immunologic disorder.

The field of allergy and immunology is expanding exponentially. As this volume was being prepared, new advances in molecular biology, the identification of cytokines, and the genetics of atopic disease were beginning to revolutionize the practice of this discipline. We look forward to a rapid update of this volume in keeping with these changes. This feature, the ability to maintain current and salient updates and to translate them for the practicing internist, is our primary goal in the presentation of this volume.

Management of Chronic Asthmatic Symptoms

Sheldon L. Spector

Key Points

- Allergic, irritant, and occupational triggers may play an important role in initiating or perpetuating asthma.

- Nonpharmacologic treatment should emphasize avoidance of such triggers as pollens, house dust mites, cockroaches, and pets.

- Filtering devices, such as high-efficiency particulate filters, can diminish the allergen load.

- Pharmacologic management should address upper and lower airway therapy.

- A stepwise approach to asthma therapy can be useful, depending on the severity of the asthma.

- Agents such as cromolyn, nedocromil, and anticholinergics may also be useful.

- Immunotherapy (allergy injections) and allergen avoidance may be indicated, and pharmacologic therapy is inadequate or is associated with significant side effects.

This chapter discusses the long-term management of bronchial asthma. The prevalence of asthma varies somewhat with age, most cases occurring in patients less than 18 years of age (Fig. 1). Because more than 4000 deaths occur in the United States each year from acute asthma, there is room for improvement in the management of chronic asthmatic symptoms so that severe asthma never develops [1]. In most countries there has been an increased asthma mortality; in the United States, asthma mortality is more prevalent in black than in white patients (Fig. 2). Many patients with asthma show early signs of deterioration that are not recognized by the patient, the physician, or both.

Asthma is a potentially life-threatening disease that by its chronic nature can be frustrating and disruptive to a patient's lifestyle and budget. When properly controlled, asthma can cause little danger or discomfort. From a physician's point of view, asthma is a heterogeneous disease process with multiple triggering factors, including irritants and allergens. Although its hallmark is reversible airway obstruction, it also involves an inflammatory process characterized by epithelial damage, mucosal edema, increased vascular permeability, excess mucus production, and an infiltrate of eosinophils, neutrophils, monocytes, and T lymphocytes.

RECOGNITION OF POSSIBLE TRIGGERS

Allergic factors often play an important role in initiating or perpetuating asthma. Airborne pollens, molds, dust, or even food allergens or additives might trigger asthmatic problems. One of the most prominent allergens to cause symptoms is the dust mite, which is the most important component of house dust [2]. Many modern practices, such as maintaining high indoor humidity with a humidifier or swamp coolers, nurture the house dust mite. Cockroach allergen may also represent

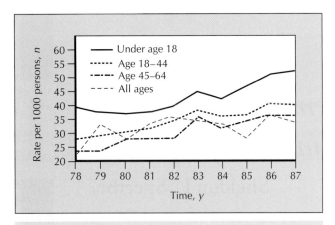

FIGURE 1 Trends in asthma prevalence.

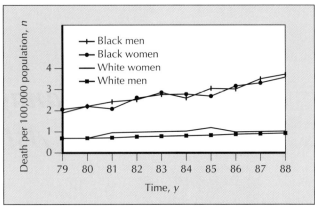

FIGURE 2 Trends in asthma mortality: United States age-adjusted death rates 1979–1988.

a major allergic trigger in certain communities [3]. Alcoholic beverages can cause symptoms by direct histamine release or secondary to components within the alcohol, such as metabisulfite, which is used to stop the fermentation of wines. Aspirin might result in bronchoconstriction in up to 20% of asthmatic individuals [4]. Such individuals generally cannot tolerate nonsteroidal anti-inflammatory agents, but can usually ingest acetaminophen and salicylate without provoking asthma. Occupational triggers, such as chemicals, gases, and organic substances, can cause asthma through immunologic, pharmacologic, or irritant mechanisms. Sinusitis can occur as a result of an allergic or infectious trigger, or it can exist as an important component of aspirin idiosyncrasy. Rhinitis and sinusitis often occur concomitantly with asthma, and treatment of either one often helps the asthma [5]. In some cases, if medical therapy is insufficient for the treatment of sinus infection, surgery provides effective management of the asthma. Viral infections can be potent triggers for a severe asthmatic attack. They cause an increase in bronchial reactivity that can last for days or weeks. Some people feel that they are the initiating factor for chronic asthma. An association exists between gastroesophageal reflux and asthma; reflux is often worsened with the use of bronchodilators because they relax the gastroesophageal sphincter. Hormonal factors also seem to play a role in exacerbating asthma, but the causative mechanism is unclear. Certain patients with hyperthyroidism have intractable asthma, and asthma typically gets worse before menstrual periods in women. Although asthma is not a psychogenic illness, as with any chronic illness certain individuals cope poorly with their disorder and can augment its consequences. Asthma is typically worse at night for many reasons, including recumbency itself, reduced mucociliary clearance, cooling of the airways, altered metabolism of medications, and various circadian rhythms within the body, such as endogenous epinephrine and cortisol secretion.

SIGNS AND SYMPTOMS OF ASTHMA

The signs and symptoms of asthma differ, depending on the severity of the disorder. Some individuals with exercise-induced asthma predominately describe being winded, tired, or dizzy after exercising and may even experience a stomach ache. These patients may describe their chest as being too small for their lungs; they might also experience cough, chest pain, or tightness. Worsening of these symptoms at night strongly suggests asthma. Although wheezing is more commonly a doctor's description of the symptoms, this may be a pertinent part of the history. Often, a patient historically has been treated for asthma or has been given a bronchodilator and had a beneficial response. A persistent cough that does not respond to cough suppressants and is made worse by cold air or exercise is typical of cough-variant asthma. The presence of associated conditions or family history of rhinitis, sinusitis, eczema, or migraine headaches also suggest asthma.

Symptoms may be seasonal or perennial, continuous or paroxysmal, or they may result from an allergen, irritant, or occupational trigger. Many allergic conditions, including asthma, are worsened before or during menstruation, sometimes because of aspirin or nonsteroidal anti-inflammatory agents taken at the time of the period itself.

Findings on the physical examination depend on the severity of the asthma. In severely compromised patients, cyanosis may be present, along with the use of accessory muscles and pulsus paradoxus. The patient may be unable to speak in complete sentences. A hyperinflated chest or increased anteroposterior diameter is more commonly recognized in a child, and wheezing and rhonchi may also be present. With severe obstruction, a silent chest may be more characteristic.

CONFIRMING DIAGNOSIS

Although history taking and physical examination are helpful, some historical data may be misleading. For example, designations other than asthma may have been used for asthmatic patients, such as chronic bronchitis, bronchiolitis, or even a "wheezy cold." Although an anteroposterior lateral chest radiograph is indicated during the initial evaluation of a patient with asthma, a radiograph *per se* is usually not very helpful in diagnosing asthma. Radiographic signs of air trapping include flattening of the diaphragm, increased anteroposterior diame-

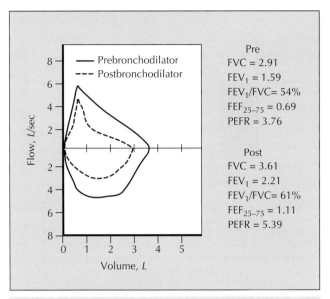

FIGURE 3 Pre- and postbronchodilator flow volume loops. FVC—forced vital capacity; FEV$_1$—forced expiratory volume in one second; FEF$_{25-75}$—forced expiratory flow during the middle half of the forced vital capacity; PEFR—peak expiratory flow rate.

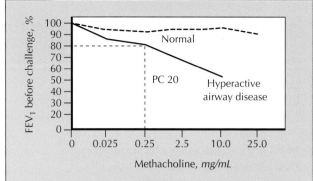

FIGURE 4 Asthmatic response to methacholine (or histamine) challenge. FEV$_1$—forced expiratory volume in one second; PC 20— provocative concentration causing a 20% decrease in FEV$_1$.

Histologic evaluations of the nasal secretions might help establish the diagnosis of allergic rhinitis or sinusitis. A radioallergosorbent test (RAST) or other *in vitro* testing for specific IgE antibodies is slightly less sensitive than skin testing, but both of these tests help evaluate the role of IgE in the allergic state.

Classification of Asthma by Severity

The National Heart, Lung, and Blood Institute (NHLBI) Guidelines clarify asthma severity by such criteria as symptom frequency, activity, tolerance, nocturnal symptoms, interference with work/school and pulmonary function [6]. Although this classification lends itself to an overview of pharmacologic therapy based on severity (Fig. 6), in reality, many patients cross categories and don't quite fit such a rigid categorization [7]. Thus, one patient may appear mild by most criteria, yet develops severe life-threatening asthma secondary to an upper respiratory infection. Certain patients also fall into high-risk categories (Table 1). A peak flow meter or forced expiratory volume in one second (FEV$_1$) determination (Fig. 7) can also assess exercise-induced asthma with the characteristic worsening 5 to 15 minutes after exercise.

ter, hyperlucency, and horizontal positioning of the ribs. Increased lung markings or even atelectasis may also be present. The results of pulmonary function testing incorporating spirometry alone, with and without a bronchodilator, often suggest the diagnosis (Fig. 3). Even with normal spirometry, a positive response to histamine or methacholine has been a useful tool to establish the diagnosis of asthma and may be slightly more sensitive than a controlled exercise challenge (Fig. 4). Most laboratory evaluations do not differentiate asthma from other allergic or even nonallergic diseases (Fig. 5). The presence of eosinophilia in a blood specimen or even sputum sample suggests an allergic condition such as asthma.

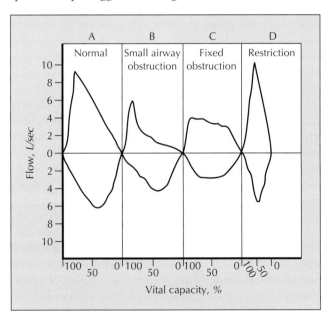

FIGURE 5 Flow-volume curve of certain lung conditions.

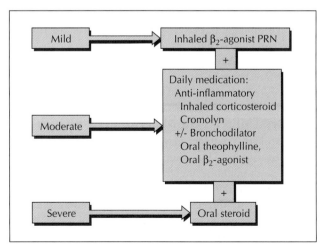

FIGURE 6 Overview of pharmacologic therapy for asthma.

TABLE 1 CHARACTERISTICS IDENTIFYING PATIENTS AT PARTICULAR RISK FOR LIFE-THREATENING DETERIORATIONS

Infants < 1 year of age

Prior history of life-threatening exacerbations

Less than 10% improvement in PEFR in the emergency department

PEFR or FEV, < 25% of predicted value

$PCO_2 \geq 40$ mm Hg

Wide daily fluctuations in PEFR

Patient cannot recognize airflow obstruction

FEV—forced expiratory volume; PEFR—peak expiratory flow rate; PCO_2—partial pressure of carbon dioxide.

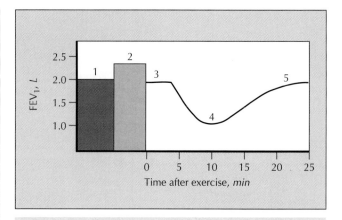

FIGURE 7 Course of exercise-induced bronchospasm. 1 = baseline lung function; 2 = exercise; 3 = striking decrease in forced expiratory volume in one second (FEV_1) beginning a few minutes after cessation of exercise; 4 = decline reaches its lowest point 5 to 10 minutes after cessation of exercise; 5 = after 20 minutes, FEV_1 has greatly improved.

AVOIDANCE OF SUSPECTED TRIGGERS

Avoidance of airborne pollens or other allergens or irritants is often impractical, if not impossible [1]. Vacuuming alone usually does not effectively remove house dust mites from upholstered furniture or carpeting. However, washing bed linens in hot water, employing special bed covers, and minimizing carpets in favor of hardwood floors may help minimize dust exposure. Acaricides, *ie*, special chemicals used to kill mites, are presently being studied for their effectiveness and safety. Removal of cockroaches requires vigorous and often repeated extermination procedures. For apartment dwellers, the whole complex ideally must be treated rather than one apartment alone. Cat lovers rarely get rid of their cats; however, exposure can be minimized by keeping the cat out of the bedroom, washing it at least once per week, and using air-filtering devices, such as a high-efficiency particulate filter to reduce the allergen load. With children in the house, a constant reservoir of viral infections spreads through the environment. Such infections can lead to sinusitis and exacerbations of asthma. These viral triggers are very difficult to avoid. Ideally, a recognized occupational trigger can be avoided by changing the job or exposure level. Workers are often unable to change their immediate environment for fear that they will lose their job and may have to resort to specific treatments, such as cromolyn sodium, atropine sulfate, or even round-the-clock bronchodilators or specific anti-inflammatory medications, before exposure.

TREATMENT FOR SUSPECTED TRIGGERS

Pharmacologic treatment may be specifically directed toward suspected triggers. Thus, antibiotics, nasal decongestants, and nasal steroids might be used for episodes of recurrent sinusitis. Cromolyn sodium or aerosolized corticosteroids might serve as a substitute for theophylline or an oral β-agonist if the latter agents are thought to contribute to esophageal reflux. Additional treatment might include H_2-blockers and specific mucosal protectants, or in patients with severe, intractable reflux, surgical correction. Hyperthyroidism can be treated

with appropriate medications. Hormone therapy might even be considered in women who have an exacerbation of asthma before menstruation. A better understanding of the interplay of psychological factors contributing to asthma allows for tailored approaches to the treatment of individual patients. Relaxation procedures and techniques to improve patient compliance may be particularly useful in noncompliant or suggestible patients. Eye drops containing β-blockers or anti-hypertensive agents that produce cough and wheezing might have to be discontinued if they are suspected of causing the adverse effects.

PHARMACOLOGIC TREATMENT OF ASTHMA

β-Adrenergic Agonists

It is preferable to use the relatively selective β_2-agonists, such as albuterol, terbutaline, bitolterol, or pirbuterol, rather than the relatively nonselective β_1-agonists, such as isoproterenol, because β_2-agonists have a longer duration of action and are less likely to produce cardiovascular side effects. The route of delivery is probably even more important than receptor specificity in reducing cardiovascular and peripheral effects. Thus, inhaled β_2-agonists are preferable to oral medications. Marked individuality of response to all of these agents exists. There is controversy over the proper aerosol dose and the frequency of delivery of the selective β_2-agonists. In some studies, a progressive bronchodilatation occurs with increasing doses [8]. In addition, the inhaled β_2-agonist may be more effective when administered on an as-needed basis rather than on a regular basis. If more than six to eight inhalations per day (or approximately one canister per month) are needed, the addition or substitution of other medication, such as cromolyn or inhaled corticosteroids, should be strongly considered [6]. If patients fail to use their inhaler devices correctly, spacers should be given to maximize their effectiveness. Inhaled β-agonists given 15 to 30 minutes before exercise are considered the ideal treatment for prevention of exercise-induced bronchospasm [9].

Adverse effects

Although oral preparations produce more unwanted adrenergic effects than aerosols, tachycardia, increased blood pressure, and potential arrythmias can occur, especially in individuals with pre-existing heart disease. Tremor and central nervous system side effects can be minimized when selective β_2-agonists are administered by the inhaled route. In a small subgroup of asthmatic patients, inhalation of β-agonists, especially those with both α- and β-adrenergic effects, such as epinephrine, can produce a paradoxical increase in airway obstruction. This adverse effect is reportedly commoner with solutions, sulfites, or even benzalkonium.

Occasionally, a paradoxical bronchospasm occurs during the first use of a new canister or bottle of a metered dose inhaler even in patients who have used the same product without difficulty. Hypoxemia can occur after the use of such products as isoproterenol as a result of ventilation-perfusion abnormalities, despite improvement in airway obstruction. Concomitant administration of oxygen can usually take care of the relatively small decrease in PO_2 described after β-agonist or aminophylline therapy. Tachyphylaxis, also called drug tolerance or subsensitivity, has been described after both oral and aerosolized β-agonists and results in a decrease in peak or duration of bronchodilatation. The clinical significance of the development of tolerance is unclear; however, concern exists that tolerance can lead to overuse of inhaled β-agonists, a development considered by some to be associated with

---

TABLE 2 MEDICATIONS AND CONDITIONS THAT MIGHT PROMPT A CHANGE IN THEOPHYLLINE DOSAGE

Increase in dose
Phenobarbital
Phenytoin
Carbamazepine
Aminoglutethimide
Low-carbohydrate, high-protein diet
Charcoal-broiled beef consumption
Cigarette smoking

Decrease in dose
Antibiotic, *eg*, troleandomycin or erythromycin
Oral contraceptives
Allopurinol
Cimetidine
High-carbohydrate, low-protein diet
Liver failure or heart failure
Influenza A vaccine
Prolonged fever
Intravenous isoproterenol
Ciprofloxacin

---

increased asthma mortality. It is unclear whether this tolerance to β-adrenergic agents is associated with an increase in bronchial reactivity, especially after routine rather than as-needed use of β-agonists. Overuse has also been also been associated with hypokalemia, which can lead to cardiac arrhythmias. B-agonists, as well as other bronchodilators, theoretically can allow an increased allergen deposition onto the lower respiratory tract, which can change an individual's response to allergens and increase the likelihood of a late-phase reaction. Longer-acting β-agonists not presently available in the United States are formoterol and salmeterol. These agents may produce effective bronchodilatation for 12 to 18 hours and have some antiinflammatory properties.

Theophylline

Although its popularity has diminished, theophylline remains one of the most widely used bronchodilators in the United States. By contrast, popularity of corticosteroid aerosols and cromolyn has increased. Although theophylline is less effective than inhaled or injected β-agonists for the treatment of acute asthma, it is effective in reducing the frequency and severity of the symptoms of chronic asthma. Many studies have reported it to be as useful as cromolyn or β_2-agonists for long-term management [10], and once-daily formulations have contributed to its popularity, especially for the treatment of nocturnal asthma [11]. Once-daily dosing in particular results in improved patient compliance. The rate and extent of absorption varies between formulation, between individuals, and possibly within the same individual from time to time. Food ingestion may alter the rate of absorption, depending on the specific formulation administered [12]. The therapeutic range is approximately 8 to 15 μg/mL. Lower doses have the advantage of minimal side effects. Although certain patients derive additional benefit from serum concentrations higher than 20 mg/mL, the frequency and severity of adverse affects increases progressively with increasing serum levels.

Adverse effects

Slowly increasing the dosage of theophylline over a period of days can circumvent transient caffeine-like side effects, such as nausea, headache, nervousness, and insomnia. Many factors affect theophylline clearance. Children typically eliminate theophylline faster than adults, and elimination is prolonged in patients with liver or cardiac decompensation. Selected medications, or conditions that might prompt a change in theophylline dosage are listed in Table 2. Theophylline toxicity can be treated with ipecac, to remove theophylline from the stomach, and orally administered activated charcoal, which inhibits further absorption. Intravenous phenobarbital has been used to prevent seizures and speed theophylline clearance, but diazepam rather than phenytoin should be used to terminate seizures. Most intravenous preparations include ethylenediamine which has rarely been associated with allergic reactions.

Cromolyn Sodium

Cromolyn sodium is frequently prescribed prophylactically to prevent such asthma triggers as allergen and exercise [13]. It blocks both the immediate and late-phase asthmatic responses after allergen exposure and prevents experimentally induced asthma provoked by exercise; irritants, such as sulfur dioxide and aspirin; and even occupational triggers [13]. Its efficacy is difficult to predict, and often a trial of 4 to 6 weeks is necessary for such a determination. It is available in three forms: the original Spinhaler powder formulation, a metered dose inhaler, and a nebulized aqueous solution. The effectiveness of any form is usually equivalent.

Adverse effects

Cromolyn is one of the safest medications used in the treatment of asthma. Occasionally, it is irritating to the throat or tracheobronchial tree, and rarely hypersensitivity reactions can occur.

Corticosteroid Aerosols

Because of the renewed awareness of the importance of airway inflammation in the pathogenesis of asthma, inhaled corticosteroids have gained in popularity and should even be considered the primary therapy in patients with moderate and severe chronic asthma [6]. They block late-phase allergic reactions and are probably the most effective agents in decreasing bronchial reactivity, as measured by methacholine. Three inhaled corticosteroid preparations are presently available in the United States: beclomethasone dipropionate (Vanceril Schering; Beclovent Allen and Hanburys, Research Triangle Park, NC), flunisolide (AeroBid, Forest, Maryland Heights, MO), and triamcinolone acetonide (Azmacort, Rhone-Poulenc Rorer, Fort Washington, PA). Some patients respond to corticosteroid aerosols when the agents are administered in greater than the recommended doses or to highly topical preparations, such as budesonide, rather than those given in standard doses.

Adverse effects

The commonest side effect is oral candidiasis (thrush), and increased risk for its development occurs with concomitant antibiotic or oral corticosteroid use, diabetes, or poor oral hygiene. The risk of thrush can be minimized if the patient is instructed to rinse the mouth after each treatment. With persistence, an antifungal mouthwash, such as nystatin, may be used, but occasionally, the dose of steroid aerosol may have to be reduced and a spacer device employed to minimize impaction on the pharynx. Other side effects include dysphonia, coughing, and wheezing. Another concern has been the effect of these aerosols on the hypothalamic-pituitary-adrenal axis, and suppression is the commonest effect at the higher-than-recommended doses. Recent studies have implicated two other side effects: osteoporosis (loss of bone mass) [14] and growth retardation in children [15]. The latter side effect in particular must be substantiated by further studies.

Nedocromil Sodium

Nedocromil sodium is structurally related to cromolyn sodium and is marketed in the United States as Tilade (Fisons, Rochester, NY). Like cromolyn, it blocks immediate and late-phase allergen reaction as well as reaction provoked by exercise and has been proved effective as an aerosol given twice daily

[16]. The commonest adverse effects have been nausea, headache, and unpleasant taste.

Anticholinergic Agents

Atropine sulfate, a tertiary compound, and ipratropium bromide, a quaternary compound, are effective in a subgroup of asthmatic patients, especially those with a bronchitic component. In fact, they have equal efficacy to β-agonists in patients with chronic bronchitis. The quaternary compounds are not as well absorbed from the gastrointestinal tract and are less capable of crossing the blood-brain barrier than other agents. Many anticholinergic agents are useful when inhaled β-agonists or theophylline are ineffective. They can prolong the effectiveness of a β-agonist when given concomitantly and are often useful in cough-variant asthma. Ipratropium bromide is available as a metered dose inhaler (Atrovent, Boehringer Ingelheim, Ridgefield, CT), which delivers 18 mcg per actuation. The usual dose is one to four inhalations four times per day. The maximum effect occurs after 1 1/2 to 2 hours, and the duration of action is 4 to 6 hours.

Adverse effects

Although ipratropium bromide theoretically causes drying, clinically this does not seem to be much of a problem. It also does not show much cardiac effect, although it can cause slowing of the heart rate.

H_1 Receptor Antagonists

In the past, it was feared that the usual oral H_1-antihistamines were associated with worsening of bronchial asthma, and such a warning is printed on the package inserts of the classic antihistamines. Recent studies have shown that asthmatics can derive benefit from the use of the nonsedating antihistamines, which serve as mild bronchodilators in many individuals [17].

Adverse effects

Recently, warnings have appeared about the interaction of the nonsedating antihistamines, such as terfenadine or astemizole, with medications such as ketoconazole and erythromycin [18]. These agents should also not be given to patients with severe liver disease, congenital heart disease, conditions that prolong the QT interval, and hypokalemia. Although such side effects have been attributed to the nonsedating antihistamines, they are also present, possibly to a greater degree, in patients taking sedating antihistamines.

Oral Corticosteroids

When the previously mentioned medications fail, resorting to oral corticosteroids may be necessary. They are also given for the management of acute asthma when the patient does not respond readily to bronchodilators. They are generally the last medications to be added to an asthmatic program and the first to be removed because of the risk of side effects, especially when given on a daily basis in large doses [1,19]. Prednisone, prednisolone, and methylprednisolone are the three agents of choice because of their short-acting effects and minimal salt-retaining properties. Oral steroids often have the advantage of controlling other problems that may have contributed to the asthma, such as sinusitis, rhinitis, and nasal polyps. They are thought to restore the responsiveness of leukocytes and bronchial smooth muscle to the effects of β-adrenergic medications.

Adverse effects

Some of the common adverse effects of oral corticosteroids are shown in Table 3. Side effects of oral corticosteroids can virtually be avoided if they are taken on an alternate day basis. Side effects are generally influenced by the type of steroid, route of administration, frequency and duration of administration, and the preexisting disease state. Patients with esophagitis, gastritis, and peptic ulcer may also be at increased risk for side effects in the organs mentioned. In children, growth retardation is always a concern, and in certain individuals, hypertension and osteoporosis may be a significant complication. Live viral vaccines are contraindicated in patients taking oral steroids. A 3- or 4-day course of oral corticosteroids, for example, during an upper respiratory infection, in which the agent is given multiple times per day can be rapidly tapered or even abruptly discontinued with virtually no side effects in most patients. Other individuals, particularly the elderly, might develop aching of muscles and joints, fatigue, poor appetite, and even fever, the so-called steroid withdrawal syndrome.

SPACER DEVICES

Use of various spacer devices is helpful for patients who are unable to properly coordinate the metered dose inhaler. These spacers, or holding chambers, vary in size and design and provide a reservoir in which the drug is delivered from the metered dose inhaler. Because the aerosol remains suspended in the chamber for approximately 5 seconds, it permits the patient to inhale within that period of time. Examples of such tube spacer devices include the Monaghan AeroChamber (Forest, Maryland Heights, MO) and the collapsible, accordion-like InspirEase (Schering Corp., Kenilworth, NJ). An alternative is inhalation of a dried powder preparation through a flow-activated device.

IMMUNOTHERAPY

Allergy injection therapy (immunotherapy, hyposensitization) is a well-accepted treatment for allergies, but only recently has it been appreciated for its value in asthma in which allergic triggers are playing a significant role [20]. It is indicated when allergen avoidance and pharmacologic therapy has proved to be inadequate or associated with significant side effects. Maintenance immunotherapy has a proven safety record in pregnancy (Table 4). Experimentally, it is an antiinflammatory therapy inasmuch as it blocks late-phase allergic reactions as well as the ensuing hyperreactivity in many circumstances.

Adverse effects

Local effects include swelling and itching at the site of injection. However, generalized reactions can uncommonly occur, including generalized itching, hives, shortness of breath, and tightness of the chest. Death has been reported, especially when injections have not been given by experienced physicians or when adequate resuscitative equipment has not been available.

UNCOMMON TREATMENTS FOR ASTHMA

Agents such as troleandomycin, ketotifen, methotrexate, gold, intravenous gamma globulin, and antileukotrienes are presently being studied more extensively for their possible role in the treatment of asthma [1].

Other agents, such as potassium channel blockers, diuretics, and cyclosporine, are in the early stages of development for the treatment of asthma. The medical community is enthusiastic about their potential benefit in asthmatic patients.

OBJECTIVES OF MANAGEMENT

One main goal of treatment is to obtain sufficient control so that no severe exacerbations occur and the symptoms are not

TABLE 3 SIDE EFFECTS OF ORAL CORTICOSTEROIDS*
Skin changes: acne, thinning of the skin
Easy bruising of skin
Eye changes: cataracts, glaucoma
Fullness of the face
Hair growth (especially on the cheeks of females)
Weight gain
Change in fat distribution ("buffalo hump")
High blood pressure
Increased blood glucose level
Osteoporosis
Altered growth (in children)
Muscle weakness
Mood changes
Increased wakefulness at night (from large doses)
Decreased resistance to infection
Suppression of normal steroid production
Increased risk for ulcer or pancreatitis
*These side effects are almost invariably avoided with alternate-day morning dosage.

TABLE 4 MEDICATIONS TO BE AVOIDED DURING PREGNANCY
Decongestants
Antibiotics: tetracycline, aminoglycosides, sulfonamides, ciprofloxacin
Vaccines: live virus
Immunotherapy: do not start, do not increase dose if continuing
Iodides: liquid or tablet expectorants
α-adrenergic compounds, epinephrine, phenyl-propanolamine, phenylephrine, brompheniramine

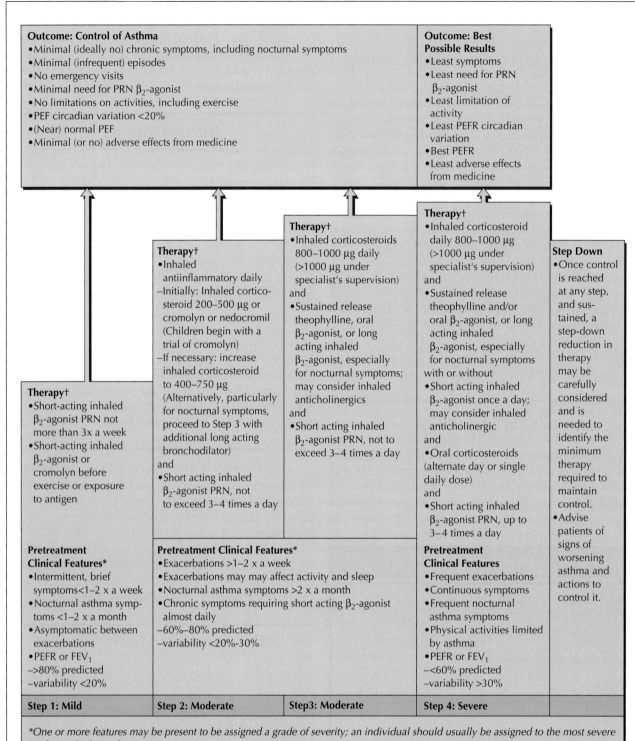

Outcome: Control of Asthma
- Minimal (ideally no) chronic symptoms, including nocturnal symptoms
- Minimal (infrequent) episodes
- No emergency visits
- Minimal need for PRN β_2-agonist
- No limitations on activities, including exercise
- PEF circadian variation <20%
- (Near) normal PEF
- Minimal (or no) adverse effects from medicine

Outcome: Best Possible Results
- Least symptoms
- Least need for PRN β_2-agonist
- Least limitation of activity
- Least PEFR circadian variation
- Best PEFR
- Least adverse effects from medicine

Therapy†
- Inhaled corticosteroid daily 800–1000 µg (>1000 µg under specialist's supervision) and
- Sustained release theophylline and/or oral β_2-agonist, or long acting inhaled β_2-agonist, especially for nocturnal symptoms with or without
- Short acting inhaled β_2-agonist once a day; may consider inhaled anticholinergic and
- Oral corticosteroids (alternate day or single daily dose) and
- Short acting inhaled β_2-agonist PRN, up to 3–4 times a day

Therapy†
- Inhaled corticosteroids 800–1000 µg daily (>1000 µg under specialist's supervision) and
- Sustained release theophylline, oral β_2-agonist, or long acting inhaled β_2-agonist, especially for nocturnal symptoms; may consider inhaled anticholinergics and
- Short acting inhaled β_2-agonist PRN, not to exceed 3–4 times a day

Therapy†
- Inhaled antiinflammatory daily
  - Initially: Inhaled corticosteroid 200–500 µg or cromolyn or nedocromil (Children begin with a trial of cromolyn)
  - If necessary: increase inhaled corticosteroid to 400–750 µg (Alternatively, particularly for nocturnal symptoms, proceed to Step 3 with additional long acting bronchodilator) and
- Short acting inhaled β_2-agonist PRN, not to exceed 3–4 times a day

Therapy†
- Short-acting inhaled β_2-agonist PRN not more than 3x a week
- Short-acting inhaled β_2-agonist or cromolyn before exercise or exposure to antigen

Step Down
- Once control is reached at any step, and sustained, a step-down reduction in therapy may be carefully considered and is needed to identify the minimum therapy required to maintain control.
- Advise patients of signs of worsening asthma and actions to control it.

Pretreatment Clinical Features*
- Intermittent, brief symptoms<1–2 x a week
- Nocturnal asthma symptoms <1–2 x a month
- Asymptomatic between exacerbations
- PEFR or FEV_1
  - >80% predicted
  - variability <20%

Pretreatment Clinical Features*
- Exacerbations >1–2 x a week
- Exacerbations may may affect activity and sleep
- Nocturnal asthma symptoms >2 x a month
- Chronic symptoms requiring short acting β_2-agonist almost daily
  - 60%–80% predicted
  - variability <20%-30%

Pretreatment Clinical Features
- Frequent exacerbations
- Continuous symptoms
- Frequent nocturnal asthma symptoms
- Physical activities limited by asthma
- PEFR or FEV_1
  - <60% predicted
  - variability >30%

| Step 1: Mild | Step 2: Moderate | Step3: Moderate | Step 4: Severe | |

*One or more features may be present to be assigned a grade of severity; an individual should usually be assigned to the most severe grade in which any feature occurs.
†All therapy must include patient education about prevention (including environmental control where appropriate) as well as control of symptoms.

FIGURE 8 A stepwise approach to the management of chronic asthma.

so bothersome as to disallow normal activity. This control should be realized with a minimum amount of medications, selected to minimize or avoid side effects. For example, overuse of β-agonists should be avoided as should toxic doses of theophylline. Results of pulmonary function tests ideally should not vary excessively throughout the day and should be as normal for a given individual as possible, even though they may not always reach predicted values. Sometimes the physician must make a conscious decision not to overmedicate to reach normal pulmonary function, especially if the patient is leading a rather sedentary life and if additional medications might lead to uncomfortable side effects. In this respect, environmental control rather than pharmacotherapy should be stressed whenever possible.

STEPWISE APPROACH TO THE MANAGEMENT OF CHRONIC ASTHMA

A stepwise approach to the long-term management of asthma has been suggested by various groups, such as the National Heart, Lung, and Blood Institute [21], the American Academy and College of Asthma [22], and an international consensus panel of experts [23]. The suggestion of the international consensus is included in Figure 8. The consensus recommendations include short-acting inhaled β-agonists, administered as needed for mild asthmatic subjects, cromolyn, taken before exercise, or both. It also suggests high doses of inhaled corticosteroids, sustained-release theophylline, short-acting inhaled β-agonists, and oral corticosteroids, if necessary in more severe cases. Once control is reached, a step-down reduction is also advised. A special note is made of patient education in environmental control as part of the overall therapy.

REFERENCES AND RECOMMENDED READING

Recently published papers of particular interest have been highlighted as:
• Of interest
•• Of outstanding interest

1. Spector SL: Asthma and chronic obstructive lung disease: A pharmacologic approach. *Dis Mon* 1991, 37.
2. Platts-Mills TAE, Chapman MD: Dust mites: Immunology, allergic disease, and environmental control. *J Allergy Clin Immunol* 1987, 80:755–777.
3. Kang B, Vellody D, Homburger H, *et al*.: Cockroach cause of allergic asthma: Its specificity and immunologic profile. *J Allergy Clin Immunol* 1979, 63:80.
4. Spector SL: What you should know about aspirin idiosyncrasy. *Mod Med* 1981, 49:97–104.
5. Slavin RG: Relationship of nasal disease and sinusitis to bronchial asthma. *Ann Allergy* 1982, 49:76–80.
6. *Guidelines for the Diagnosis and Management of Asthma*. National Asthma Education Program, Expert Panel Report, 1991, Publication no. 91–3042.
7. Spector SL, et al: Practice parameters for the diagnosis and treatment of asthma. March 1993. Library of Congress Catalogue Card #93-72193.
8. Nelson HS, Spector SL, Whitsett TL, *et al*.: The bronchodilator response to inhalation of increasing doses of aerosolized albuterol. *J Allergy Clin Immunol* 1983, 72:371–375.
9. Rohr AS, Siegel SC, Katz RM, *et al*.: A comparison of inhaled albuterol and cromolyn in the prophylaxis of exercise-induced bronchospasm. *Ann Allergy* 1987, 59:107–109.
10. Weinberger M: Pharmacology and therapeutic use of theophylline. *J Allergy Clin Immunol* 1984, 73:525–540.
11. Arkinstall WW, Atkins ME, Harrison D, *et al*.: Once-daily sustained-release theophylline reduces diurnal variation in spirometry and symptomatology in adult asthmatics. *Am Rev Respir Dis* 1987, 135:316–321.
12. Spector SL: Advantages and disadvantages of 24-hour theophylline. *J Allergy Clin Immunol* 1985, 76:302–311.
13. Spector SL: Allergen inhalation challenge procedures. In *Provocative Challenge Procedures: Background and Methodology*. Edited by Spector SL. Mount Kisco, NY: Futura Publishing Company; 1989:293–339.
14. Toogood JH, Hodsman AB: Effects of inhaled oral corticosteroids on bone. *Ann Allergy* 1991, 67:87–88.
15. Wolthers OD, Pedersen S: Controlled study of linear growth in asthmatic children during treatment with inhaled glucocorticosteroids. *Pediatrics* 1992, 89:839–842.
16. Holgate ST: Clinical evaluation of nedocromil sodium in asthma. *Eur J Respir Dis* 1986, 69(suppl 147):149–159.
17. Spector SL, Lee N, McNutt B, *et al*.: Effect of terfenadine in asthmatic patients. *Ann Allergy* 1992, 69:212–216.
18. Casillas AM, Spector SL: Nonsedating antihistamines, an overview. *Phys Assist J* 1993, 17:48–54.
19. Spector SL: Outpatient treatment of asthma. *Ann Allergy* 1989, 63:1–7.
20. Greenberger P: Immunotherapy of IgE-mediated disorders. *Immunol Allergy Clin North Am* 1992, 12.
21. *Guidelines for the Diagnosis and Management of Asthma*. US Department of Health and Human Services, Public Health Service, National Institutes of Health, Publication no. 91–3042, August 1991.
22. American Academy and College of Allergy and Immunology: Practice Parameters for the Diagnosis and Treatment of Asthma, American Academy of Allergy and Immunology, American College of Allergy and Immunology, March 1993.
23. *International Consensus Report on Diagnosis and Management of Asthma*. US Department of Health and Human Services, Public Health Service National Institutes of Health, Publication no. 92–391, June 1992.

SELECT BIBLIOGRAPHY

Corren J, Adinoff AD, Buchmeier AD, Irvin CG: Nasal beclomethasone prevents the seasonal increase in bronchial responsiveness in patients with allergic rhinitis and asthma. *J Allergy Clin Immunol* 1992, 90:250–256.

Enberg RN, Shamie SM, McCullough J, Ownby DR: Ubiquitous presence of cat allergen in cat-free buildings: probable dispersal from human clothing. *Ann Allergy* 1993, 70:471–474.

Kang BC, Johnson JJ, Veres-Thorner C: Atopic profile of inner-city asthma with a comparative analysis on the cockroach-sensitive and ragweed-sensitive subgroups. *J Allergy Clin Immunol* 1993, 92:802–811.

Linter TJ, Brame KA: The effects of season, climate, and air-conditioning on the prevalence of *Dermatophagoides* mite allergens in household dust. *J Allergy Clin Immunol* 1993, 91:862–867.

O'Hollaren MT, Yunginger JW, Offord KP, *et al*.: Exposure to an aeroallergen as a possible precipitating factor in respiratory arrest in young patients with asthma. *New Engl J Med* 1991, 324:359–363.

Occupational Respiratory Allergy

Emil J. Bardana, Jr.

2

Key Points

- After the skin, the respiratory tract is the most commonly affected organ system in the workplace.
- Occupational allergy is caused by one of two basic mechanisms: immunologically mediated inflammation, or several variants of irritant-induced inflammation.
- Many industrial reactants cause occupational allergy by more than a single mechanism, and several mechanisms may be operative in any given patient.
- Diagnosis of immunologic occupational allergy depends on the demonstration of variable airway obstruction on exposure to subirritant doses of the putative asthmogenic agent.
- There should be improvement of symptoms with timely diagnosis and removal from the incriminated agent.

The rapid proliferation of complex plastic polymers and other chemicals in industry is felt to be associated with the increased incidence of allergic work-related respiratory disorders. After the skin, the respiratory tract is the most commonly affected organ system in the workplace. This relates to the lung's role as the final common pathway for a variety of potentially annoying, irritating, sensitizing, and intoxicating agents. In considering occupational respiratory allergies, the clinician must possess a balanced perspective so that common, nonoccupational causes of symptoms can be carefully considered before implicating a potential industrial agent. This exercise in differential diagnosis demands a comprehensive grasp of the possible causes and mechanisms of work-related allergies.

Despite the many advances in our knowledge of occupational asthma, most of the data on which we rely for its prevalence are retrospective in nature. It is not possible to be certain that preexisting bronchial hyperreactivity was not present before the diagnosis of occupational asthma based on genetic or other nonindustrial factors. Current estimates of occupational asthma range between 2% and 15% of cases of adult asthma in men [1]. Many investigators believe that this prevalence is underestimated and would argue for the higher figure [2•]. They believe many workers become ill and leave the industry without reporting their illness, creating a resistant "survivor population." There are few data to support this concept in our modern era of workers' compensation. It is also thought that other workers remain at their posts but fail to report their disease for fear of losing their job and seniority. Other affected workers are said to be misdiagnosed. These arguments must be balanced by equally cogent observations that, in a medical system where many people lack adequate medical insurance, involving occupational illness is a tempting strategy to assure reimbursement from the workers' compensation system. In addition, there are the occasional workers who abuse the system for secondary gain [3].

Definitions

A variety of respiratory occupational syndromes occur at work. Many have immunologic components as part of their pathogenesis. The principal focus of this chapter is occupational rhinitis and asthma.

Occupational asthma is defined as a condition, characterized by reversible obstruction of the airways, originating in the inhalation of ambient dusts, vapors, gases, or fumes manufactured or used by the worker or incidentally present at the workplace [4]. Diagnostic criteria for the diagnosis of occupational asthma have been established (Table 1). Causative agents can be divided into major categories including plastics/chemicals, wood/vegetable dusts, pharmacologic agents, and substances of animal origin (Table 2). True asthma, regardless of origin, incorporates bronchial inflammation. Many cases of occupational asthma occur in association with chronic bronchitis and varying degrees of irreversible obstructive airway disease (emphysema).

In evaluating any patient for work-related asthma, it is critical to consider the diagnosis in the context of the entire medical history. Any preexisting lung condition should be considered as a potential contributor to the suspected occupational asthma. Disorders that may mimic asthma include chronic bronchitis, emphysema, vocal cord dysfunction syndrome, and hypersensitivity pneumonitis, among others. *Chronic bronchitis* has been defined as productive cough for 3 months of the year for 2 consecutive years. Although it is defined in symptomatic terms, it also connotes an inflammatory process in the bronchi [5]. *Emphysema* is defined in pathologic terms as destruction of the alveoli.

Occupational rhinitis has been defined as the episodic work-related occurrence of sneezing, nasal discharge, and nasal obstruction [6•]. It often coexists with occupational asthma. The incidence of occupational rhinitis is unknown, but in a survey of laboratory animal workers in whom allergic symptoms were studied, all the affected workers had rhinoconjunctivitis and only 70% had allergic asthma.

Hypersensitivity pneumonitis or extrinsic allergic alveolitis is a granulomatous inflammatory reaction in the terminal airways, alveoli, and surrounding interstitium caused by inhaled organic dusts or by volatile low-molecular-weight organic compounds that react with tissue proteins [7]. This subject is covered in detail in Chapter 4.

Predisposing Factors for Occupational Asthma

Epidemiologic studies have examined a variety of industrial, climatic, personal, social, and medical factors associated with the development of occupational asthma (Table 3). A variety of workplace issues influence the development of workplace asthma. Chief among these are the nature of chemicals employed and the concentration in which they are likely to be encountered. This is also influenced by employer/employee attitude toward work safety, for example, availability of material data safety sheets (MSDS) (Fig. 1). Adequate worker protective devices, such as hard hats, earplugs, goggles, and face masks (Fig. 2) as well as the institution and enforcement of effective industrial hygiene measures (Fig. 3) are also important in this regard.

A variety of climatic factors prevalent in a specific area may also play a role in the development of work-related asthma. Environmental contamination has been incriminated in a number of asthma epidemics [8]. Epidemics of emergency

---

TABLE 2 SELECTED CAUSATIVE AGENTS OF OCCUPATIONAL ASTHMA

Category/agent	Industrial exposure
Plastics/chemicals	
Acid anhydrides (phthalic and trimellitic)	Amine-based epoxy resins Adhesives, plastics
Diisocyanates (toluene, hexamethylene, and diphenylmethaline)	Polyurethanes, catalyzed Paints, adhesives
Formaldehyde	Lamination, plywood
Complex platinum salts	Photography, refining
Cobalt, vanadium	Hard metal industry
Nickel salts	Metal plating
Reactive azo dyes	Textile
Wood/vegetable dusts	
Flour	Bakers, grain handlers
Green coffee bean	Food processing
Castor bean	Oil industry
Soybean	Food industry
Vegetable gums	Printing, chewing gum
Colophony	Electronic
Cotton, flax, hemp	Textile
Pharmaceutical/biological agents	
Antibiotics, *eg*, penicillin	Pharmaceutical
Pancreatic enzymes	Pharmacists
Piperazine	Veterinary practice
Enflurane	Anesthesiologists
Papain	Packaging
Tryspin	Plastics
Bacillus subtilis (alcalase)	Detergent
Animal origin	
Insects	Bait, laboratory workers
Hair dander, mites, molds	Animal handlers
Birds	Breeders, fanciers

TABLE 1 DIAGNOSTIC CRITERIA FOR OCCUPATIONAL ASTHMA

Symptoms related temporally to the workplace

Established industrial asthmogenic agent

Persistent variable airway obstruction

Demonstration of variable airway obstruction to the putative work-related agent

Bronchial provocation with a controlled, subirritant dose of suspected agent

Improvement in symptoms with timely diagnosis and removal of putative agent

TABLE 3 PREDISPOSING FACTORS INFLUENCING THE DEVELOPMENT OF OCCUPATIONAL ASTHMA

Workplace factors
   Sources of chemicals and their concentration
   Industrial hygiene practice
   Job description
Climatic factors
   Presence of oxidizing pollutants
   Incidence of temperature inversions
   Wind conditions
   Proximity of other allergens or irritants
Atopic background
Tobacco abuse
Recreational drug use
Viral upper respiratory infections
Bronchial hyperreactivity
Miscellaneous medical factors
   Aspirin idiosyncrasy syndrome
   Pharmacologic influences, *eg*, β-blocking drugs
   Gastrointestinal reflux
   Stress/hyperventilation

room admissions for asthma occurring in Barcelona between 1981 and 1987 were caused by soybean dust. In addition to the prevailing wind and weather conditions, atopy and cigarette smoking played an important synergistic role. As well, exposure to ozone has been found to cause increased airway responsiveness and has been associated with an influx of mucosal neutrophils. Other oxidizing pollutants may also play a facilitory role in the generation of work-related asthma.

A personal or family history of atopic disease predisposes patients to allergic sensitization. This is well established for industrial agents of higher molecular weight, that is, greater than 1000 d [9] (Table 4).

In addition to atopy, the habit of smoking tobacco products is both a predisposing and an aggravating factor in the development of work-related asthma. There is a clear relationship between smoking, the development of chronic obstructive pulmonary disease, and the presence of bronchial hyperreactivity. Chronic tobacco abuse is associated with higher levels of serum IgE and a higher incidence of respiratory infections, which, in turn, are associated with the development of asthma [10•]. However, smoking has never been causally linked to the development of bronchial asthma. In addition to tobacco products, recreational drug use may also have profound

MATERIAL SAFETY DATA SHEET

I PRODUCT IDENTIFICATION

MANUFACTURER'S NAME	REGULAR TELEPHONE NO EMERGENCY TELEPHONE NO
ADDRESS	
TRADE NAME	
SYNONYMS	

II HAZARDOUS INGREDIENTS

MATERIAL OR COMPONENT	HAZARD DATA

III PHYSICAL DATA

BOILING POINT 760 MM HG		MELTING POINT	
SPECIFIC GRAVITY (H$_2$0•1)		VAPOR PRESSURE	
VAPOR DENSITY (AIR•1)		SOLUBILITY IN H$_2$0 % BY WT	
% VOLATILES BY VOL		EVAPORATION RATE IBUTYL ACETATE II	
APPEARANCE AND ODOR			

FIGURE 1 Format of Material Safety Data Sheet (MSDS). Daytime and emergency telephone numbers are usually located in the upper-right-hand corner. (*From* O'Hollaren [26•]; with permission.)

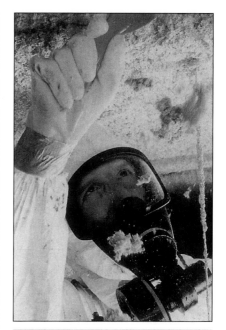

FIGURE 2 Certain highly toxic exposures (asbestos, isocyanate vapors) require full-face, enclosed respirators or air-supply respirators.

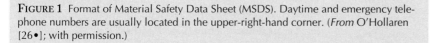

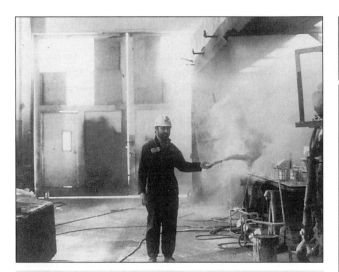

FIGURE 3 Inspection of a waterfall exhaust system proximal to a spray-pain work area. Smoke bomb provides visual assurance of effective performance.

adverse effects on the lung. There are data suggesting that the combined use of marijuana and tobacco may be more harmful than either used alone [11].

Viral infections of the respiratory tract are frequently noted to be the initial precipitating event in the onset of bronchial asthma [12]. It has also been noted that *Chlamydia pneumoniae* infection increases the likelihood of asthma [13]. The association of viral infection and asthma is based on a number of specific pathogenic events including epithelial injury, development of viral-specific IgE, leukocyte-dependent inflammation, and enhanced mediator release (Table 5).

Individuals with nonspecific airway hyperresponsiveness may have an exaggerated response to airway irritants. It is a finding in work-related asthma, but is also present in individuals without this diagnosis. There is evidence suggesting a role for genetic factors influencing the development of allergy, bronchial hyperresponsiveness, and symptomatic asthma [14]. However, it should be noted that the prevalence of bronchial hyperreactivity in the general population is much greater than previously thought: 30% of subjects challenged in a normative aging study had a positive methacholine challenge (23% of the group had never smoked) [15]. Because most of what we know in occupational asthma is the result of retrospective study, it is not possible to state whether a variety of genetic proclivities dictate the manner by which any exposure will precipitate overt asthma.

Finally, there are various miscellaneous factors which may affect the development of work-related asthma. Among these are the use of aspirin and related compounds in patients with aspirin idiosyncrasy syndrome. Some prescription medications may exacerbate asthma or trigger its initial appearance, for example, beta-adrenergic blocking drugs and angiotensin converting enzyme inhibitors [10•]. Other factors include exercise, exposure to cold air, stress, and gastroesophageal reflux.

TABLE 4 SELECTED HIGH-MOLECULAR-WEIGHT ALLERGENS IMPLICATED IN THE CAUSATION OF OCCUPATIONAL ASTHMA

Animal proteins
Urine, salivary, and pelt-derived protein from virtually any mammalian species
Insect proteins
Bee moths, lake flies, midges, screwworm flies, sewer flies, mealworms, locusts, etc.
Plant proteins
Green coffee-bean dust
Castor-bean dust
Gum arabinocytidine
Gum acacia
Hardwood/exotic wood dusts
Grains and flour
Foods and enzymes
Pepsin, flourastase, papain
Penicillin
Cephalosporins
Spiromycin
Garlic powder
Egg powder
Sea squirts, crabs, prawns

TABLE 5 RATIONALE FOR INFECTIOUS EVENTS PREDISPOSING TO THE DEVELOPMENT OF OCCUPATIONAL ASTHMA

Viral infections frequently precipitate initial asthmatic episode
Viral infections are commonly associated with exacerbations of asthma
Viral infections damage irritant receptors in the lung
Viral-specific IgE could result in release of vasoactive amines from mast cells
Viral infections may depress cellular immunity
Chlamydia pneumoniae infection is associated with development of asthma
Chronic pyogenic sinusitis may be associated with intensification of bronchial asthma

CLINICAL AND PATHOGENETIC FEATURES OF OCCUPATIONAL ASTHMA

Occupational asthma can be divided into two broad categories, based on whether immunologic sensitization is believed to play a role in its development. Nonimmunologic occupational asthma can be further subdivided into several subsets depending on the major pathogenetic mechanism: acute inflammatory bronchoconstriction, reflex bronchoconstriction, or pharmacologic bronchoconstriction (Fig. 4) [16••].

Allergic occupational asthma results from exposure and sensitization to a high-molecular-weight protein agent present at the work site (Table 4). Most of these patients report preceding or concomitant upper airway and ocular symptoms of work-related sneezing, nasal discharge, tearing, and nasal obstruction [17]. There is usually a latent period of months or years before upper and lower respiratory symptoms develop. Patients note work-related airflow obstruction characterized by chest tightness, cough, and dyspnea, which may intensify as the work week goes on. Onset of symptoms with work exposures may be immediate, delayed, or biphasic (dual), consistent with early- and late-phase allergic responses. In conceptualizing the development of bronchial asthma, Cock-croft [18] divided potential triggers into those agents inducing a symptomatic expression of asthma (*ie*, a bronchospastic response) and those likely to produce bronchial mucosal injury and inflammation.

There are a number of low-molecular-weight agents that also mediate a spectrum of specific immune responses believed to play a role in the development of work-related asthma. The complex salts of platinum, nickel, and chromium have the capacity to react as haptens and result in an IgE-specific reaction. Other low-molecular-weight compounds appear to act as copolymerizing agents and may produce limited immunologic responses. These include polyurethane, polystyrene, polyvinyl, and others. The acid anhydrides are a group of chemicals

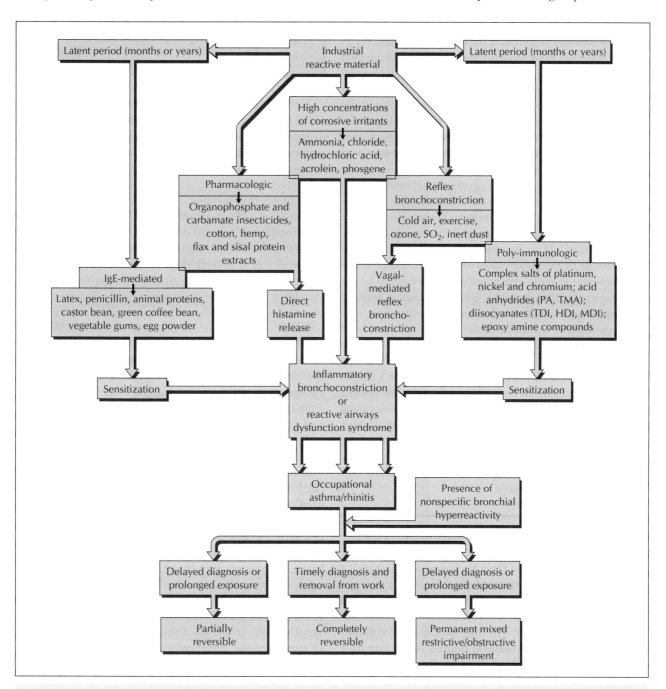

Figure 4 Schematic conceptualization of overlapping pathogenetic mechanisms operative in occupational asthma. HDI—hexamethylene diidocyanate; MDI—methylene diphenyl-diisocyanate; PA—phthalic anhydride; TDI—toluene diisocyanate; TMA—trimellitic anhydride. (*Adapted from* Bardana [16••]; with permission.)

TABLE 1 PULMONARY INFILTRATES WITH EOSINOPHILIA SYNDROME

Diagnosis	Asthma	IgE	Etiology	Characteristics
Löffler's syndrome	No	Normal	Unknown	Transient pulmonary infiltrates with eosinophilia
Eosinophilic pneumonia	No	Variable	Infectious	Treat infection
			Drug reaction	Corticosteroids
Tropical eosinophilia	Yes	++	Filariasis	Coughing, wheezing, and dyspnea: treat with diethylcarbamazine
Allergic bronchopulmonary aspergillosis	Yes	+++	*Aspergillus fumigatus*	Asthma with constitutional symptoms
Churg-Strauss syndrome (allergic granulomatosis with angiitis)	Yes	++	Vasculitis	Multisystem involvement
Hypereosinophilic syndrome	No	Normal	Unknown	Highest eosinophilia; multiple organs are involved, particularly the heart and brain

nia, an indolent, cavitating disease reported in diabetics and alcohol abusers; and allergic aspergillus sinusitis, which is caused by a hypersensitivity reaction to *Aspergillus* species that can aggravate concomitant asthma or ABPA.

DIAGNOSIS

It is important to remember that ABPA is not an invasive infectious disease, and it does not require or respond to anti-fungal therapy. Instead, it is a hypersensitivity state caused by aberrant type-I (IgE) mechanisms directed against *A. fumigatus* antigens. Other immune mechanisms may be responsible for the extensive pulmonary damage that may occur [6]. Precipitating (IgG) antibodies to *A. fumigatus* are commonly found in these patients [7], but no definitive pathologic role for type-II or type-III hypersensitivity has yet been identified.

Diagnostic Criteria

There are eight major criteria characteristic of ABPA (Table 2).

If all eight criteria are met, the diagnosis is obvious. These patients' conditions are classified as ABPA with central

TABLE 2 MAJOR CRITERIA OF ALLERGIC BRONCHOPULMONARY ASPERGILLOSIS

Asthma
Pulmonary infiltration seen on chest radiography (although they may not be present if the patient has received systemic corticosteroids)
Peripheral blood eosinophilia (may also be affected by systemic corticosteroids)
Elevated serum IgE levels (usually highly elevated on an order of > 1000 ng/mL)
Immediate cutaneous reactivity to *Apsergillus fumigatus* antigen
Precipitating antibodies (precipitins) to *A. fumigatus*
Elevated titers of IgE and IgG specific for *A. fumigatus* and
Central bronchiectasis with normal tapering of distal bronchi

bronchiectasis (ABPA-CB). A recent variant demonstrates a subgroup of patients with APBA without evidence of central bronchiectasis, who are hence designated as being ABPA seropositive (ABPA-S). Current thinking suggests that patients with ABPA-S have an early stage of disease compared with patients with ABPA-CB [8•]. The most common findings in ABPA are central bronchiectasis and elevated serum levels of IgE and IgG specific for *A. fumigatus*; but the absence of either of these findings does not exclude the diagnosis if other criteria are met. Most patients with ABPA have a positive immediate skin test response to *A. fumigatus*. Family history is important because familial occurrences have been reported. Once a definitive diagnosis has been made, ABPA should be excluded in family members with asthma. Thus, the definitive work-up, once initiated, must be methodical and thorough.

Differential Diagnosis

Of the PIE syndromes, ABPA most commonly presents with asthma (Table 1). Patients with Löffler's syndrome and eosinophilic pneumonia do not usually present with bronchospasm. Löffler's syndrome is typically transient and produces no significant symptomatology of its own, whereas eosinophilic pneumonia causes constitutional symptoms such as fever and sputum production. Tropical eosinophilia should be suspected with a travel history to locations endemic for filaria (*Wuchereria bancrofti*). In a wheezing patient with eosinophilia and other systemic involvement (*ie*, renal, hepatic, or cutaneous), Churg-Strauss vasculitis should be considered. Clinical and laboratory findings typical of vasculitis (*eg*, extreme complement consumption) are commonly found.

If a patient presents with wheezing, diagnoses other than ABPA are more often considered. If evidence of purulent sputum, the need for recurrent systemic corticosteroids, or both are present, ABPA must be considered. In children, cystic fibrosis may present with wheezing, sputum production, and bronchiectasis. Asthmatic bronchitis, sarcoidosis, pneumonia, chronic obstructive pulmonary disease, and congestive heart failure can all present with various combinations of the previously mentioned symptoms. Other diseases that present with eosinophilia (hypoadrenalism, collagen vascular diseases, neoplasms, and parasitism), highly elevated IgE levels (Job's syndrome and atopic dermatitis), or both must be considered.

The clinical picture associated with ABPA can also be caused by other allergic bronchopulmonary mycoses [9], such as those caused by *Alternaria*, *Candida*, *Curvularia*, and *Dreschlera* species. This fact is important because test results for IgE and IgG specific for *A. fumigatus* would probably be negative. The proper diagnosis might be made if evidence of specific fungi can be recovered in sputum from affected patients.

CLINICAL COURSE

Clinical Presentation

The acute form of ABPA can be difficult to distinguish from an asthma exacerbation. On presentation, the patient may experience wheezing, dyspnea, and cough. Because chest radiographs and hemograms are not routinely ordered for simple asthma exacerbations, other signs should be sought. They may include significant malaise, often with fever, and cough with sputum production (including brown mucous plugs). Subsequent chest radiography may show hyperinflation with alveolar infiltrates and eosinophil-containing sputum, as well as marked peripheral blood eosinophilia. A subsequent work-up of the PIE can then be initiated for definitive diagnosis.

Chronic ABPA can be mistaken for chronic obstructive pulmonary disease, particularly in an older patient with a history of smoking. However, acute symptoms occur in addition to the chronic productive cough. Pulmonary function testing can reveal a mixed obstructive-restrictive pattern, particularly if fibrosis is present. Once again, a high index of suspicion regarding possible *A. fumigatus* sensitivity must be present to initiate the appropriate diagnostic work-up.

Staging

The staging of ABPA is important for prognostic and therapeutic strategies (Fig. 1). The basic assumptions are that chronic disease follows uncontrolled acute episodes and that irreversible pulmonary damage can be prevented by corticosteroid therapy.

Stage I is the acute phase, with little or no permanent damage. This stage is most likely to have all of the diagnostic criteria. Pulmonary infiltrates are very commonly observed, as is significant peripheral blood eosinophilia. This stage is typically most responsive to short-term high-dose corticosteroid therapy.

Stage II is remission, defined as no subsequent chest infiltration after corticosteroids have been tapered and discontinued for at least 6 months. Total serum IgE levels often decrease substantially (although not always to normal) and remain low while the disease is in remission. Remission can be permanent, although exacerbations up to 7 years later have been reported.

Stage III is exacerbation, which is characterized by new pulmonary infiltration unexplainable from other diagnoses and by a marked elevation in serum IgE levels (at least double, and typically three- to tenfold). The clinical picture is exacerbation

of asthma symptoms with or without constitutional symptoms such as malaise, fever (usually a temperature of <38.5°C), myalgias, and sputum production.

Stage IV is steroid-dependent asthma from APBA and is recognized by exacerbations (asthma, new chest infiltrates, or an elevation in IgE levels) from either stage I or III disease when repeated attempts to taper systemic corticosteroids fail. Although IgE levels may remain low, *A. fumigatus*–specific IgE and IgG levels are typically elevated.

Stage V is end-stage fibrotic lung disease from repeated inflammatory episodes of ABPA. These patients have defined ABPA as well as an irreversible obstructive-restrictive clinical picture. They are steroid-dependent asthmatics. With end-stage lung disease that worsens despite corticosteroid therapy, patients typically die from acute respiratory failure (*eg*, superimposed pneumonia) or cor pulmonale.

LABORATORY PRESENTATION

Radiographic Findings

The most characteristic radiologic findings in patients with ABPA are pulmonary infiltrates and central bronchiectasis. ABPA without central bronchiectasis (ABPA-S) may represent early disease that has not yet progressed to bronchiectasis, or it may truly be a disease variant. Central bronchiectasis is most commonly found by hilar tomography. Computed tomography may be useful but, because of its axial orientation, can miss central bronchiectasis. The utility of chest magnetic resonance imaging for this indication is currently under study.

Plain films of the chest can be most useful, from the initial infiltrate recognition to a baseline study to distinguish the development of fibrosis. Other findings, such as mucoid impactions or new infiltrates, can be a monitor of disease exacerbation or progression. A characteristic finding in ABPA is the development of ring shadows, typically 1 to 2 cm in diameter, which reflect ectatic central bronchi with peribronchial thickening seen en face. If seen tangentially, the dilated bronchus is called a parallel-line shadow. These findings are most common in the posterior segments of the upper lobe.

Other radiographic findings seen in ABPA include perihilar infiltrates, tramlines (representing bronchial wall edema), and occasionally, significant consolidation. Although none of these latter findings is specific for ABPA, their presence is associated with disease activity, and they may be useful markers of the response to therapy.

Pulmonary Function Test Findings

Asthma is an obstructive disease, and patients with asthma typically present with a decreased forced expiratory volume in 1 second (FEV_1) level. However, during acute exacerbations of ABPA, a decrease in total lung capacity and diffusing capacity occurs [10]. If the changes become chronic (*ie*, unresponsive to corticosteroids), lung fibrosis has probably occurred (or at least begun). Thus, even normal pulmonary function in a clinical exacerbation of ABPA should not preclude aggressive corticosteroid therapy. Fortunately, not all patients with ABPA will have progression to irreversible

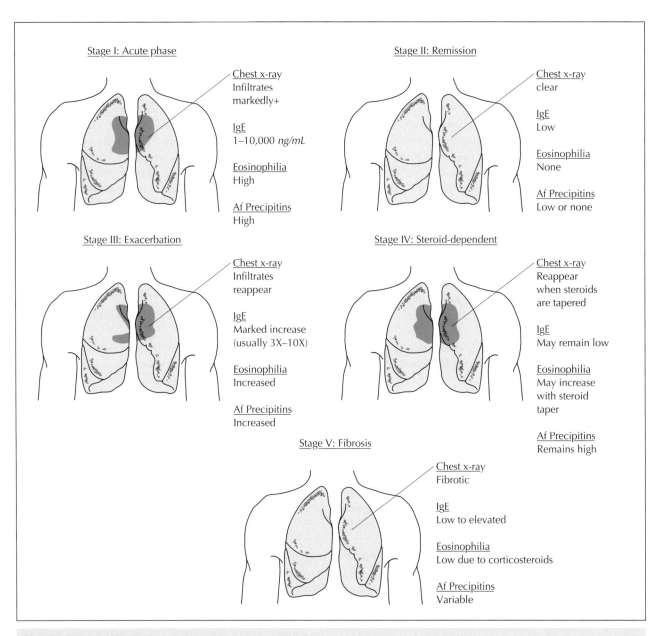

FIGURE 1 Staging of allergic bronchopulmonary aspergillosis.

obstructive-restrictive disease, despite multiple exacerbations. This may be due to the aggressiveness with which the exacerbations are treated [11].

Serologic Findings

Virtually all patients with ABPA have a positive percutaneous immediate reaction to *A. fumigatus*, unless they have been taking antihistamines or other medications that interfere with mast cell degranulation (*eg*, long-term high-dose corticosteroids). Occasionally, intradermal testing is necessary to demonstrate a positive skin test response. In as many as one third of ABPA patients, a dual skin reaction at 20 minutes and at 6 hours can be demonstrated. No correlation has yet been established with prognosis or response to therapy.

Serologic tests are still the most useful in confirming or excluding ABPA. They can also be useful in staging of the disease. Precipitins to *A. fumigatus* are commonly found in

stages I and III, and are less commonly seen in other stages. They can also be useful in differentiating ABPA caused by non–*A. fumigatus* species.

Many asthmatics who do not have ABPA may have a positive skin test response to *A. fumigatus*. However, serum from patients with ABPA has a highly elevated level of *A. fumigatus*–specific IgE and IgG compared with levels in mold-sensitive asthmatics without ABPA [12]. Unfortunately, the *A. fumigatus*–IgG serology is not commonly available in many diagnostic laboratories.

Serum IgE levels are typically highly elevated in patients with ABPA, particularly in stage I and III disease. The levels are usually in the range of 1000 to 10,000 ng/mL or higher, and they often decrease with remission. Even in stage II disease, serum IgE levels are typically in the range of 500 to 1000 ng/mL. These values are far in excess of those in other allergic diseases (rhinitis and asthma), except atopic dermatitis. Only conditions such as hyper-IgE (Job's) syndrome or IgE myeloma (extremely rare) have higher levels of serum IgE.

THERAPY

The specific therapeutic regimen for patients with ABPA depends primarily on the stage of disease. Specific therapeutic goals should be set for each patient (Table 3). These include 1) the rapid detection and treatment of pulmonary infiltrates because these are believed to be the sites most at risk for the development of bronchiectasis; 2) the management of associated lung diseases (asthma and fibrosis); and 3) the search for environmental sources of the fungus that can be controlled. In addition, ABPA should be excluded in at least first-degree family members with asthma. It can be screened for with immediate skin testing to *A. fumigatus*. A negative percutaneous and intradermal test result excludes the diagnosis (assuming adequate expertise of the tester).

In 60% to 70% of patients with ABPA, asthma is the most persistent symptom. Thus, proper control of asthma symptoms is a major consideration for long-term control. In stages I and III, systemic corticosteroids are usually necessary. They should be given in relatively large amounts (0.5 mg/kg of prednisone, up to 40 mg) daily for at least 2 weeks and should be converted to alternate-day regimens for at least 2 to 3 months. Serum IgE levels typically decrease as remission is achieved. Thus, monthly monitoring of IgE levels for the first year is useful because pulmonary infiltration may worsen in up to 30% of ABPA patients with few or no pulmonary symptoms. Sharp increases in IgE levels (at least doubling) are often associated with the appearance of new pulmonary infiltrates long before the development of clinical symptoms. After a 3-month trial, tapering and discontinuation of corticosteroids can be attempted, dictated by clinical symptomatology, IgE levels, and chest radiographic findings. The patient may remain in stage II (remission) indefinitely, but should be followed up at frequent intervals for the first year with IgE determinations and clinical assessment.

Antifungal agents (amphotericin B, ketoconazole, and itraconazole) have been suggested or tried in ABPA patients, but little success has been reported [13]. This result is to be expected, because ABPA is a hypersensitivity disease, and is not a condition associated with invasive organisms. Because the source of mold spore inhalation can be essentially ubiquitous, sterilization of the airways is not feasible.

When exacerbation occurs (stage III), repeated therapy as outlined previously can be attempted. If the patient has progression to stage IV, alternate-day administration of corticosteroids should be attempted repeatedly. Even in a stable stage IV patient receiving prednisone, exacerbations occur. If symptoms are primarily asthmatic and no new chest infiltration or sharp increases in serum IgE levels have occurred, other medications, such as bronchodilators, cromolyn, and even anticholinergics, can be used.

Patients with stage V disease have a poorer prognosis. An initial FEV_1 level of 0.8 L or less is a very poor prognostic indicator. Daily corticosteroids are usually indicated. The conditions of some patients with stage V disease remain stable with daily corticosteroid use. However, most such conditions progress to parenchymal destruction with the development of fibrosis, cor pulmonale, and pulmonary hypertension. These complications are managed until the patient finally dies.

ROLE OF THE GENERALIST

With ABPA, as with many other diseases, successful diagnosis depends on an index of suspicion. Asthmatic patients with constitutional symptoms, chronic brown sputum production, and historical exacerbations in areas expected to harbor *A. fumigates* spores (*eg*, damp areas and moldy hay) should be evaluated for ABPA. Although basic screening is easily performed in a primary care setting, determining the definitive diagnosis and deciding on a specific treatment protocol should involve specialists who have experience with ABPA patients (*eg*, allergist-immunologists).

Careful monitoring of a diagnosed patient is often best accomplished in a primary care setting, with periodic specialist follow-ups. This practice allows detection of early clinical changes that could trigger more prompt therapeutic intervention and hopefully lessen progression.

FUTURE DIRECTIONS

Learning more about the aberrant immune mechanisms responsible for the aggressive hypersensitivity response to *A. fumigatus* may lead to new treatments involving the use of immunotherapies. Controlling the inflammatory mechanisms with agents such as cytokines may allow nonsteroidal control of asthma in general and of ABPA in particular. Fibrocyte production of collagen, and thus, fibrosis, is also influenced by inflammatory factors, including cytokines. Such studies are ongoing, offering hope for management of the long-term effects of the disease, as well as its therapy.

TABLE 3 THERAPEUTIC GOALS FOR ALLERGIC BRONCHOPULMONARY ASPERGILLOSIS
Rapidly detect pulmonary infiltrates
Aggressively treat pulmonary infiltrates with corticosteroids
Manage associated lung diseases
Asthma (stages I, III, and IV)
Fibrosis (stage V)
Search for environmental exposure to *Aspergillus fumigatus* spores
Rule out ABPA in family members with asthma
ABPA—allergic bronchopulmonary aspergillosis.

REFERENCES AND RECOMMENDED READING

Recently published papers of particular interest have been highlighted as:
• Of interest
•• Of outstanding interest

1.•• Greenberger PA: Allergic bronchopulmonary aspergillosis. In *Allergy Principles and Practice*, edn 4. Edited by Middleton E, Reed CE, Ellis EF, *et al.* St. Louis: CV Mosby; 1993:1395–1414.

2.• Hinson KFW, Moon AJ, Plummer NS: Bronchopulmonary aspergillosis. *Thorax* 1952; 7:317–333.

3. Patterson R: Pulmonary infiltrates and eosinophilia. *Masters Allergy* 1989, 1:4–6.

4.• Wardlaw A, Geddes DM: Allergic bronchopulmonary aspergillosis: a review. *J R Soc Med* 1992, 85:747–751.

5. Radin RC, Greenberger PA, Patterson R, Ghory A: Mold counts and exacerbations of allergic bronchopulmonary aspergillosis. *Clin Allergy* 1983, 13:271–278.

6. Slavin RG, Bedrossian CW, Hutchison PS, *et al.*: A pathologic study of allergic bronchopulmonary aspergillosis. *J Allergy Clin Immunol* 1988, 81:718–725.

7. Moser M, Cramer R, Brust E, *et al.*: Diagnostic value of recombinant *Aspergillus fumigatus* allergen 1/a for skin testing and serology. *J Allergy Clin Immunol* 1994, 93:1–11.

8.• Greenberger PA, Miller TP, Roberts M, Smith LL: Allergic bronchopulmonary aspergillosis in patients with and without evidence of bronchiectasis. *Ann Allergy* 1993, 70:333–338.

9. Miller MA, Greenberger PA, Amerian R, *et al.*: Allergic bronchopulmonary mycosis caused by *Pseudoallerescheria boydii*. *Am Rev Respir Dis* 1993, 148:810–812.

10. Nichols D, Dopico GA, Braun S, *et al.*: Acute and chronic pulmonary function changes in allergic bronchopulmonary aspergillosis. *Am J Med* 1979, 677:631–640.

11. Lee TM, Greenberger PA, Patterson R: Stage V (fibrotic) allergic bronchopulmonary aspergillosis: a review of 17 cases followed from diagnosis. *Arch Intern Med* 1987, 147:139–145.

12. Wang JLF, Patterson R, Rosenberg M, *et al.*: Serum IgE and IgG antibody activity against *Aspergillus fumigatus* as a diagnostic aid in allergic bronchopulmonary aspergillosis. *Am Rev Respir Dis* 1978, 117:917–926.

13. Denning DW, Van Wye JE, Lewiston NJ, Steven DA: Adjunctive therapy of allergic bronchopulmonary aspergillosis with itraconazole. Chest 1993, 100:813–819.

Hypersensitivity Pneumonitis

Jordan N. Fink

4

Key Points

- Hypersensitivity pneumonitis is an immunologic inflammatory lung disease that differs from asthma and is caused by the interaction of environmental organic dusts and the immune system.
- Recurrent chills, fever, cough, dyspnea, and arthralgia reminiscent of influenza are characteristic of the disorder.
- Characteristic pulmonary function, chest x-ray, and immunologic features can be demonstrated.
- The episodes can be reproduced by purposeful inhalation challenge with the offending organic dust.
- Avoidance of exposure results in complete recovery in most cases.

Hypersensitivity pneumonitis, or extrinsic allergic alveolitis, is a nonimmunoglobulin immunologic-mediated, inflammatory, interstitial, and alveolar pulmonary disease occurring after repeated exposure to any of a number of organic dusts present in work, home, or hobby environments (Table 1). The clinical, immunologic, and pathophysiologic features of the disease are similar in susceptible individuals despite the multiple antigens [1–3••].

The major clinical features of the disease include peripheral airway dysfunction with constitutional symptoms but without systemic organ involvement. The interstitial lung infiltrates are characterized by lymphocytosis with increased suppressor T cells (CD8 cells), activated macrophages, and natural killer (NK) cells as well as granuloma formation. Serum immunoglobulins are broadly elevated and specific antibodies against the offending agent can be detected in the peripheral blood and lung lavage [1••].

CLINICAL FEATURES

Hypersensitivity pneumonitis is a syndrome with a broad spectrum of signs and symptoms (Table 2). The clinical features may be divided into acute and chronic forms. The type of organic dust inhaled is less important than the nature, intensity, and frequency of inhalation of the dust or the immune response of the host. Sensitization of susceptible individuals occurs after exposure to offending agents. After a variable latent period, the symptoms occur acutely or insidiously following further exposure [1–3••].

ACUTE FORM

In the acute form, explosive flulike symptoms of fever up to 40°C, chills, headache, malaise, myalgia, minimally productive cough, and dyspnea may occur approximately 4 to 6 hours after inhalation of the offending agent. The symptoms may persist for up to 24 hours, and spontaneous recovery follows (Fig. 1). The attacks may recur repeatedly following subsequent exposure and patients often recognize the episodes as a part of their life. The physical examination during an episode reveals an acutely ill patient with dyspnea. Bibasilar end-inspiratory crepitant rales are prominent and

TABLE 1 SOME CAUSATIVE AGENTS OF HYPERSENSITIVITY PNEUMONITIS

Antigen	Source	Disease
Bacteria		
Thermophilic actinomycetes		
Micropolyspora faeni	Moldy hay, grain, or compost	Farmer's lung
Thermoactinomyces vulgaris	Moldy hay, grain, or compost	Farmer's lung
T. sacchari	Moldy sugarcane	Bagassosis
T. candidus	Humidifier or air conditioner	Ventilation pneumonitis
T. viridis	Mushroom compost	Mushroom worker's lung
Fungi		
Aspergillus species	Moldy malt dust	Malt worker's lung
Alternaria species	Moldy wood dust	Woodworker's lung
Penicillium caseii	Cheese mold	Cheese worker's lung
Cryptostroma corticale	Wet maple bark	Maple bark stripper's disease
Penicillium frequentans	Moldy cork dust	Suberosis
Pullularia species	Moldy redwood dust	Sequoiosis
Trichosporum cutaneum	Japanese house mold	Summer type
Animal proteins		
Avian serum proteins	Avian dust	Bird breeder's disease
Bovine and porcine protein	Pituitary snuff	Pituitary-snuff user's lung
Rat urinary protein	Rat urine	Laboratory worker's lung
Oyster or mollusk shell protein	Shell dust	Oyster shell lung
Insect proteins		
Sitophilus granarius	Infested wheat flour	Wheat weevil disease
Silkworm larvae	Cocoon fluff	Sericulturist's lung disease
Amoebae		
Naegleria gruberi	Contaminated ventilation system	Ventilation pneumonitis
Acanthamoeba castellani	Contaminated ventilation system	Ventilation pneumonitis
Medication		
Amiodarone, gold, and procarbazine	Drugs	Drug-induced
Chemicals		
Toluene diisocyanate	Paint catalyst	Paint refinisher's disease
Diphenylmethane diisocyanate	Paint catalyst	Bathtub refinisher's lung
Phthalic anhydride	Epoxy resin	Epoxy resin worker's lung
Trimellitic anhydride	Plastics industry	Plastic worker's lung

TABLE 2 CHARACTERISTICS OF HYPERSENSITIVITY PNEUMONITIS

	Acute form	Chronic form
Symptoms	Constitutional and respiratory	Respiratory
Examination	Bibasilar rales	Dry crackles
Laboratory	Elevated leukocytes, eosinophils, immunoglobulins (except IgE)	Elevated leukocytes, eosinophils, immunoglobulins (except IgE)
Chest radiographs	Diffuse nodular to normal	Fibrosis
Pulmonary function	Restrictive defect	Restrictive or obstructive defect
	Decrease gas transfer	Decrease gas transfer
Reversibility	Good	Poor

may persist for weeks after cessation of exposure. Wheezing is not prominent.

Pulmonary function abnormalities include a restrictive pattern with a decrease in the forced vital capacity (FVC), forced expiratory volume in 1 second (FEV_1), diffusing lung capacity for carbon monoxide, and decrease in oxygen saturation (PaO_2). The expiratory flow rates and the FEV_1 and FVC are usually normal. If sufficient pulmonary damage has occurred as a result of the inflammatory process, decreases in volume and flow may occur and persist after the acute episode subsides [3••]. The pulmonary function may return to normal between episodes or there may be a subtle persistent decrease in PaO_2 demonstrable only on exercise. During an acute episode, the chest radiograph reveals diffuse, bilateral, soft, patchy, parenchymal densities that tend to coalesce. The radiograph results may appear normal between episodes or may show reticulations and fine sharp nodulations with coarsening of the bronchovascular markings (Fig. 2) [2••].

Routine laboratory test results are usually normal between attacks, but during acute episodes a moderate leukocytosis with a marked left shift and on occasion eosinophilia may be detected in up to 10% of patients. Except for IgE, all immunoglobulin isotypes are usually elevated. Specific precipitating antibodies are detectable in the serum and rheumatoid factor may be elevated, reflecting a nonspecific pulmonary inflammatory response (Table 3) [4•].

Bronchoalveolar lavage reveals elevated total protein, immunoglobulin level–specific IgG and IgA antibody, albumin, and adhesive glycoproteins such as vitronectin and fibronectin. The increased cellular constituents of the lavage include neutrophils. T lymphocytes expressing CD8 and the NK cell markers CD56 and CD57, and reversal of the normal CD4 to CD8 ratio, large foamy macrophages, mast cells, and eosinophils are present. Lung biopsy specimens demonstrate lymphocytic infiltration of the alveolar walls with plasma cells and macrophages occluding the alveolar spaces [5•]. Early gran-

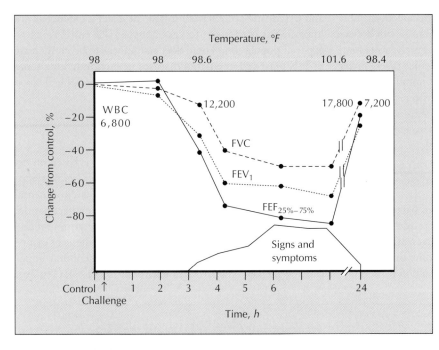

FIGURE 1 Pulmonary function and other clinical abnormalities induced in a sensitized pigeon breeder following exposure to pigeons. WBC—white blood cell count; FVC—forced vital capacity; FEV_1—forced expiratory volume in 1 second; $FEF_{25\%-75\%}$—forced expiratory flow during the middle half of the forced vital capacity.

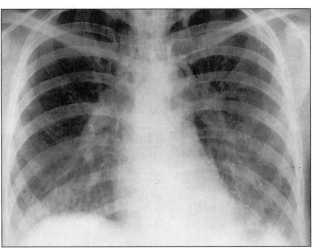

FIGURE 2 Chest radiograph of pigeon breeder with hypersensitivity pneumonitis demonstrating diffuse soft infiltrations.

TABLE 3 IMMUNOLOGIC FEATURES OF HYPERSENSITIVITY PNEUMONITIS
Serum
Precipitating antibodies to offending antigen
Normal complement levels
Elevated immunoglobulins
Antibodies of IgG, IgA, IgM class bronchoalveolar lavage
Cells
Peripheral blood studies normal
Lymphocytosis cells of lavage fluid
Elevated CD8 (suppressor) over CD4 (helper) cells
Activated macrophages

ulomas may be detected. As the disease progresses, the alveolar spaces become obliterated and interstitial infiltration with fibroblasts occurs. Some investigators believe that the histiocytes with foamy cytoplasm surrounded by activated macrophages may be unique to hypersensitivity pneumonitis [1–3••].

CHRONIC FORM

In the chronic form of hypersensitivity pneumonitis, antigen exposure is less often intense but may be continuous. An intense inflammatory reaction occurs in the lung, usually progressing to irreversible pulmonary parenchymal damage. Acute episodes are not usual in this form. The symptoms of the chronic form are largely respiratory with progressive dyspnea, with cyanosis on exertion. Cough, weakness, malaise, and anorexia with occasional weight loss and often without fever may also be present. The physical examination may reveal fine bibasilar rales and clubbing of the fingers. Pulmonary function tests demonstrate a predominantly restrictive ventilatory defect with a decreased diffusing capacity. Chest radiographs demonstrate a reticulonodular infiltrate; in advanced disease, diffuse infiltrative fibrosis with honeycombing is seen. Laboratory features are similar to the acute form of hypersensitivity pneumonitis. Lavage studies reveal lower percentages of lymphocytes, less protein and immunoglobulin, and fewer neutrophils. Lung biopsy demonstrates interstitial fibrosis of varying degrees, lymphocytic alveolitis with alveolar septal wall thickening and plasma cell infiltration, and intraalveolar foamy macrophages and granulomas [4•, 5•].

ETIOLOGY

A number of organic antigens derived from bacteria, fungi, protozoa, or plant and animal proteins of approximately 5 μm or smaller have been shown to cause hypersensitivity pneumonitis (Table 1). Volatile chemicals including diisocyanates and anhydrides used in the plastics industry and in paint refin-ishing have also been implicated. Drugs such as amiodarone, gold, procarbazine, and hydrochlorothiazide have also been associated with lung diseases resembling hypersensitivity pneumonitis [6•].

The most common form of hypersensitivity pneumonitis is associated with repeated inhalation of thermophilic actinomycetes, a common compost organism, either at home or work. The bacteria may also contaminate stagnant water in air conditioning, humidification, and forced-air heating systems. Actinomycetes are ubiquitous and thrive at 60°C in soil, manure, grain, compost, and hay; inhalation exposure is thus likely from many sources [1–3••, 4•].

A second common form of hypersensitivity pneumonitis occurs in bird breeders, particularly pigeon breeders, in which susceptible individuals develop symptoms after repeated inhalation of avian proteins in serum, bird dander, feathers, or excrement. Disease has been described in wives and children of pigeon breeders exposed to antigens on the breeder's clothes.

Hypersensitivity pneumonitis occurs relatively infrequently and diagnostic accuracy is limited. Its exact incidence is not known, but is thought to vary between 5% and 15% in an exposed population. There does not appear to be an increase in IgE mast cell–mediated diseases in such individuals and serum levels of IgE in pulmonary lavage and peripheral blood are usually normal [1–3••, 4•].

DIAGNOSIS

The diagnosis of hypersensitivity pneumonitis is based on the clinical history of intermittent pulmonary and systemic symptoms temporally associated with a particular environmental exposure (Fig. 3). A detailed history regarding occupation, medication, hobbies, exposure to forced air equipment and ventilation systems may be helpful. Improvement of symptoms after avoidance of the suspected environment may implicate the allergen or a particular environment (Fig. 4) [1••, 2••].

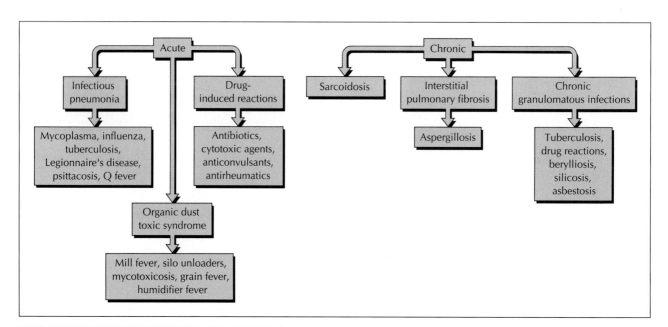

FIGURE 3 Differential diagnosis of hypersensitivity pneumonitis.

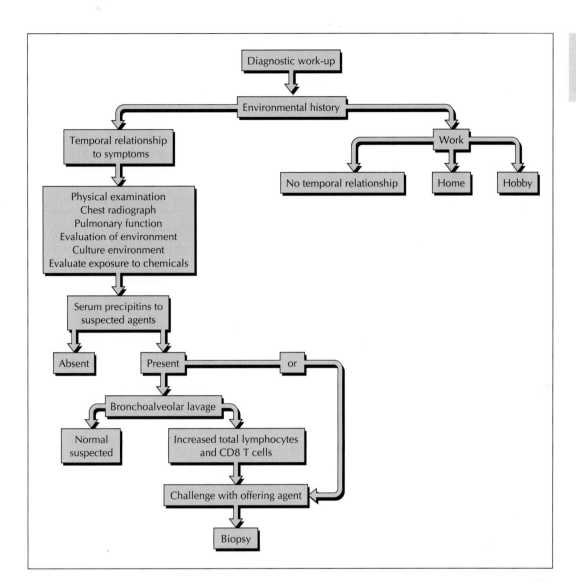

FIGURE 4
Diagnosis of hypersensitivity pneumonitis.

In asymptomatic individuals who may be in-between episodes, routine laboratory tests are frequently nonspecific. The demonstration of serum precipitating antibodies against the suspected antigen supports the diagnosis; however, this reaction indicates exposure and not necessarily disease. The presence of antibodies must, therefore, be correlated with the clinical features. Skin testing is not helpful in the diagnosis. Intradermal skin testing is limited as standardized extracts are not available and crude extracts tend to irritate. Skin testing with avian serum in pigeon breeder's disease may detect an immediate wheal-and-flare reaction followed by a late erythema and edema 4 to 8 hours from time of testing. Pulmonary function testing and chest radiography may be helpful immediately after an acute exposure or in the chronic phase of the disease, but may be normal if obtained during an asymptomatic period [1–3••, 4•].

If further evidence is needed to support the diagnosis, bronchial inhalation challenge may be carried out with suspected antigenic material. Repeated pulmonary function studies, leukocyte counts, and temperature measurement follow a characteristic course that normalizes within 24 hours (Fig. 1).

Lung biopsy may reveal characteristic histopathologic features in patients with chronic or subacute disease, or the features may be nonspecific or may aid in diagnosis by eliminating other possibilities [5•].

DIFFERENTIAL DIAGNOSIS

The differential diagnosis of hypersensitivity pneumonitis includes a number of interstitial pulmonary disorders of both known and unknown etiologies (Fig. 4) [1–3••, 4•]. These diseases may progress with time and may present with constitutional symptoms as well. The acute form may be mistaken for community-acquired infectious diseases, usually mycoplasma or influenza, but also disseminated tuberculosis, psittacosis, and Q-fever, as well as building-related infections such as Legionnaire's disease. Microbial pneumonias cause single attacks of severe illness and lack recurrent episodes after exposure to an offending antigen or organic dust. The lack of specific serum precipitins in such cases also suggests the need for an alternative diagnosis. Reactions that involve the lung parenchyma have been described with antibiotics, cytotoxic agents, anticonvulsants, and antirheumatic drugs. Antibiotics most commonly implicated are nitrofurantoin and sulfonamides. Generally these reactions involve other organ systems and show peripheral eosinophilia and elevated levels of serum

IgE. The organic dust toxic syndrome may be difficult to distinguish clinically from hypersensitivity pneumonitis. This acute febrile noninfectious illness with pulmonary and systemic symptoms occurs 2 to 12 hours after exposure to high levels of organic dust contaminated with bacteria and fungi and occurs associated with agricultural exposure such as Mill fever, Silo filler disease, pulmonary mycotoxicosis, and Grain fever. Contaminated humidification and ventilation systems may also cause a similar disorder, probably related to bacterial endotoxin. Other characteristics of these disorders include a high attack rate, the absence of a sensitizing exposure or symptoms on repeated low-dose exposure, less frequent radiographic and pulmonary function abnormalities, lack of relevant precipitins, and a rapidly reversible reaction without permanent damage. Exposure to sulfur dioxide or nitrogen dioxide can occur in a variety of occupational and industrial settings, resulting in bronchiolitis characterized by an increased number of neutrophils rather than lymphocytes in the alveolar lavage fluid. Silo filler's disease is acute pulmonary edema caused by the inhalation of nitrogen oxides generated by fresh silage [1–3••, 4•, 6•].

Chronic hypersensitivity pneumonitis should be differentiated from other causes of progressive dyspnea with interstitial pulmonary fibrosis. Chronic aspergillosis, sarcoidosis, chronic granulomatous infections, chronic bronchitis, drug reactions, collagen vascular diseases, building-related illnesses, and inorganic respiratory dust syndromes including berylliosis, silicosis, and asbestosis should be considered [1–3••, 4•].

The diagnosis of pneumoconioses or inorganic dust respiratory disorders is usually established by a careful environmental history (Fig. 3). Nonpulmonary manifestations distinguish the collagen vascular diseases. Sarcoidosis may present with pulmonary symptoms, but is differentiated from hypersensitivity pneumonitis by bilateral hilar adenopathy, lack of exposure to known inciting agents, presence of several affected organ systems, and CD4 helper T lymphocytes

predominating in the lavage fluid. Sick building syndrome, which manifests as irritative ocular and respiratory symptoms in exposed individuals, is likely due to increased concentrations of fungal spores, carbon monoxide, and formaldehyde after energy-conserving practices are instituted. The problem is usually resolved with adequate ventilatory exchanges. Idiopathic pulmonary fibrosis has clinical features similar to chronic hypersensitivity pneumonitis but is a diagnosis of exclusion. A biopsy may be necessary in some cases to solidify the diagnosis [6•].

THERAPY

Removal or avoidance of the offending antigen is as effective as it is in other allergic disorders (Table 4). Patients with the acute form will spontaneously improve after avoidance measures are implemented. After identification of the antigen, avoidance techniques may include air-filtering systems, personal protective masks, or changes in cooling and forced-air systems. A change of habit, hobby, or occupation may be necessary for some. Elevated levels of bird antigen may be detectable for months in the home environment even after removal of the birds and environmental clean-up [1–3••, 4•].

Oral corticosteroids can dramatically improve acute disease. Single-morning dosing should be used with a gradual daily tapering regimen as pulmonary functions stabilize. When long-term therapy is needed, alternate-day dosing should be used and careful environmental investigations should be repeated to totally eliminate antigen exposure. Cromolyn sodium and inhaled corticosteroids have been tried, but are usually of little benefit [1••].

PROGNOSIS

The prognosis in hypersensitivity pneumonitis is related to the reversibility of the disease, which depends on the degree

TABLE 4 THERAPY OF HYPERSENSITIVITY PNEUMONITIS
Therapy
Environmental control
Avoidance of antigen
Removal of antigen when identified
Removal of patient
Environmental modification
Respirators
Improve ventilation
Use of alternative agents
Pharmacotherapy
Corticosteroids
To be used with avoidance
Inhaled form–poor response
Oral form: start prednisone 0.5 mg/kg for 2–4 wk
and taper as improvement progresses
Antihistamines, β-agonists and cromolyn of little help

TABLE 5 FOLLOW-UP EVALUATION OF HYPERSENSITIVITY PNEUMONITIS AT INTERVALS
History
Avoidance measures instituted
Absence of symptoms
Physical examination
No evidence of interstitial pulmonary disease unless recent exposure
Serologic studies
Normal leukocyte count
Precipitating antibody titers wane over time as avoidance continues
Lung lavage may continue to demonstrate lymphocytosis
Chest radiograph
Returns to normal over time
Pulmonary function
Spirometry returns to normal decrease in PaO$_2$ with exercise may persist

of permanent respiratory impairment, the ability of the patient to avoid re-exposure, and the patient's age (Table 5). More than four episodes of recurrent acute symptoms or low-grade exposure may result in progressive pulmonary disease with irreversible pulmonary fibrosis and, rarely, early death. Digital clubbing, which is associated with fibrosing interstitial lung disorders, has been proposed as a prognostic tool. Chest radiographs and pulmonary functions should be monitored carefully. A reduced diffusing capacity appears to be the most sensitive index of impaired lung function, but any abnormalities persisting for at least 6 months are suggestive of the chronic stage of hypersensitivity pneumonitis [1••].

REFERENCES AND RECOMMENDED READING

Recently published papers of particular interest have been highlighted as:
• Of interest
•• Of outstanding interest

1.•• Salvaggio JE: Recent advances in pathogenesis of allergic alveolitis. *Clin Exp Allergy* 1990, 20:137–144.
2.•• Fink JN: Hypersensitivity pneumonitis. *Clin Chest Med* 1992, 13:303–309.
3.•• Fink JN: Hypersensitivity pneumonitis. In *Allergy Principles and Practice.* Edited by Middleton RJ, Reed CE, Ellis EF, *et al.* St. Louis: CV Mosby Co., 1993:1415–1431.
4.• Parker JE, Petsonk EL, Weber SL: Hypersensitivity pneumonitis and organic dust toxic syndrome. *Immunol Allergy Clin North Am* 1992, 12:279–290.
5.• Kawanami O, Basset F, Barrios R, *et al.*: Hypersensitivity pneumonitis in man. Light and electron microscope studies of 18 lung biopsies. *Am J Pathol* 1983, 110:275–289.
6.• Pitcher WD: Southern Internal Medicine Conference: Hypersensitivity pneumonitis. *Am J Med Sci* 1990, 300:251–266.

SELECT BIBLIOGRAPHY

Fink JN, Kelly KJ: Immunologic aspects of granulomatous and interstitial lung diseases and cystic fibrosis. *JAMA* 1992, 268:2874–2881.

Kaltreider HB: Hypersensitivity pneumonitis. West J Med 1993, 159:570–578.

Semenzato G: Immunology of interstitial lung diseases: cellular events taking place in the lung of sarcoidosis, hypersensitivity pneumonitis and HIV injection. *Eur Resp J* 1991, 4:94–102.

Salvaggio JE: Pathogenetic mechanisms in occupational lung disease. In *Advances in Allergology and Clinical Immunology.* Edited by Goddard PH, Bosquet J, Michel FB. Pearl River, NY: Parthenon Publishing Group; 1992:435–456.

Salvaggio JE: Recent advances in pathogenesis of allergic alveolitis. *Clin Exp Allergy* 1990, 20:137–144.

Rhinitis 5

Phillip Lieberman

> ### *Key Points*
> - Rhinitis is an important health problem in the United States today and accounts for significant numbers of lost work and school days.
> - The approach to the patient with rhinitis should emphasize a differential diagnosis.
> - Patient history is the most important diagnostic tool to establish the diagnosis.
> - Only approximately 50% of adults have an allergic component to their rhinitis.
> - Therapy should include pharmacologic measures, and when appropriate, environmental control and allergen immunotherapy.

DIAGNOSIS

Rhinitis is arguably the most common illness seen in the outpatient practice of medicine (Table 1). The mean age of onset of nonseasonal allergic rhinitis is 9.1 years and of seasonal allergic rhinitis 10.6 years [1]. Prevalence decreases with age (Fig. 1). However, the disease can begin in young adults, with 3.1% of asymptomatic college freshmen developing symptoms by the time of their senior year [1] (Figs. 2 and 3). Occasionally allergic rhinitis can begin in the middle and older years [2,3]. Sixty-four percent of patients have a history of allergy in first-degree relatives [1]. There is an equal incidence in males and females and no known racial or ethnic difference in incidence [2]. The illness is clearly an important health problem in the United States, exacting a prominent toll on the workplace, and resulting in over 3.5 million lost workdays. This does not take into consideration loss in efficiency while workers are impaired by the illness itself or drugs used to treat it.

Many patients refer to nasal symptoms, regardless of cause, as "allergies," but only 50% of adults have allergies contributing to their rhinitis. All nasal disease produces the same symptoms of congestion, drainage, rhinorrhea, sneezing, and loss of olfaction. The causes of these symptoms are numerous (Table 1).

The patient's history is by far the most important tool used to establish etiology (Table 2). A physical examination is done to detect mechanical or anatomic abnormalities (Fig. 4). Anterior rhinoscopy is preferably performed with a strong light source and a nasal speculum. Fiberoptic rhinoscopy is an optimal means of examination but need not be used in every patient.

The symptoms of allergic rhinitis are produced by mediators released from mast cells and basophils. The allergic reaction occurs in two phases. Acute symptoms (early-phase reaction) begin 5 to 10 minutes after allergen exposure and abate within 1 hour. Symptoms often recur 2 to 4 hours later. This return of symptoms is called the late-phase reaction. The late-phase reaction produces a state of hyperirritability of the turbinates, making them more sensitive to exacerbants of rhinitis, including aeroallergens as well as irritants [4••].

TABLE 1 DIFFERENTIAL DIAGNOSIS OF RHINITIS

Allergic
Seasonal
Perennial

Chronic idiopathic nonallergic
Nonallergic rhinitis with eosinophilia
Neurogenic (vasomotor)

Mechanical/anatomic obstruction
Tumors
Granulomas
Sarcoid
Wegener's
Septal deviation
Septal perforation
Foreign bodies

Drug-induced (rhinitis medicamentosa)
Topical agents
  α-adrenergic vasoconstrictors
  Cocaine
Oral agents
  Antihypertensives
  Birth control pills
  Phenothiazines

Endocrinologic
Pregnancy
Hypothyroidism
Acromegaly

Acute cholinergic-induced rhinitis
Gustatory
Skier's-jogger's nose

Cerebrospinal leakage

Atrophic

Infectious

The pathogenesis of chronic nonallergic rhinitis is unknown, and indeed this disorder is not one entity but rather a diagnosis of exclusion. That is, when symptoms are chronic and no specific cause for the rhinitis can be determined, the diagnosis of chronic nonallergic rhinitis is made. Approximately 15% to 20% of patients with this syndrome have an increase in nasal eosinophils. The term *nonallergic rhinitis with eosinophilia* (NARES) has been coined to describe these patients. Patients with NARES respond to topical corticosteroid treatment more readily than some other patients with chronic nonallergic rhinitis. Since most patients with chronic rhinitis will have either allergic or chronic nonallergic rhinitis, it is important to be familiar with the features distinguishing these two entities. They are summarized in Table 3.

Although allergic and chronic nonallergic rhinitis are the most common entities seen in practice, one must have a high index of suspicion regarding the presence of other causes. When obstruction is unilateral, a tumor, foreign body, synechia, or nasal septal deviation is to be expected. The presence of unilateral obstruction due to a tumor or foreign body

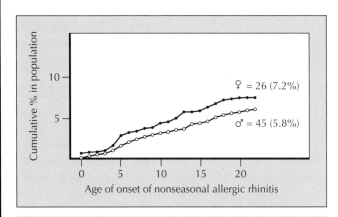

FIGURE 2 The cumulative incidence of nonseasonal allergic rhinitis.

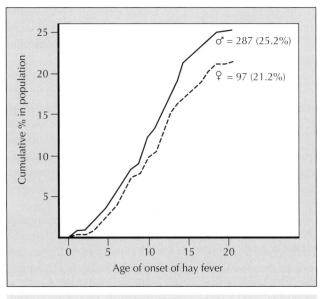

FIGURE 3 The cumulative incidence of seasonal allergic rhinitis.

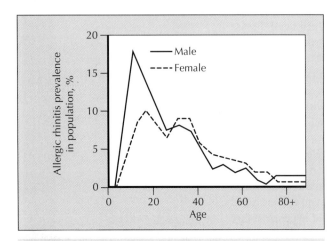

FIGURE 1 The prevalence of allergic rhinitis.

is often accompanied by purulence or a unilateral maxillary or ethmoid sinusitis.

Nasal polyps are usually bilateral. They are distinguished from nasal turbinates by their pale color and the fact that gentle pressure sufficient to cause movement of the polyp fails to produce pain, whereas turbinates are relatively immobile and pain is produced by such pressure (*see* Chapter 6).

The use of topical vasoconstrictors, birth control pills, antihypertensives, or phenothiazines suggests rhinitis medicamentosa. Topical vasoconstrictors account for most

TABLE 2 IMPORTANT ELEMENTS OF THE HISTORY NECESSARY TO ESTABLISH THE CAUSE OF RHINITIS

Age of onset

Chronological variations in symptoms
Perennial without seasonal variation
Perennial with seasonal variation
Seasonal
    If seasonal or with seasonal variation, denote specific months

Exacerbating factors
Allergens
    Fresh cut grass, animal exposure, house dust, hay
Irritants
    Cigarette smoke, odors, perfumes, detergents, soap powder
    Particulate dust
    Automobile exhaust fumes
Weather conditions
    Weather fronts
    Changes in humidity temperature
    Damp humid weather
    Cold air
Ingestants
    Alcohol
    Spicy foods
    Other
Nature of symptoms
    Sneezing
    Congestion
    Postnasal drainage
    Pruritus
    Anterior rhinorrhea
    Unilateral versus bilateral

Environmental exposures
Workplace
Home
Pets
Feathers
Air-conditioning, heating

Hobbies/activities

Medications used to treat rhinitis, response to same
Topical
Oral

Medications used for other conditions
Topical
Oral
    Antihypertensives
    Birth control pills
    Tranquilizers

Family history of atopy

Other personal manifestations of atopy
Asthma
Atopic dermatitis
Allergic conjunctivitis

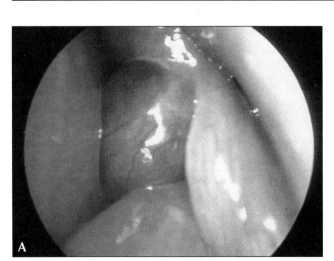

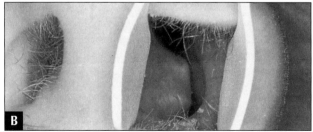

FIGURE 4 Mechanical obstruction of the nose. **A**, Nasal polyps. The color of the polyp distinguishes it from normal turbinates. Polyps are pale and have a gunmetal-gray or bluish-gray tint (*courtesy of* Dr. Sylvan Stool, Pittsburgh, PA). **B**, Nasal septal deviation. A spur of septal cartilage occludes the inferior nasal meatus on the left (*see* Color Plates). (*continued*)

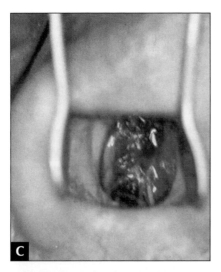

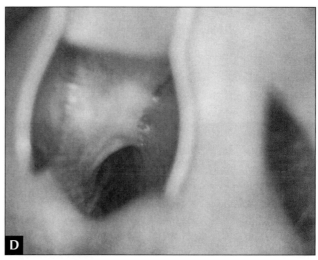

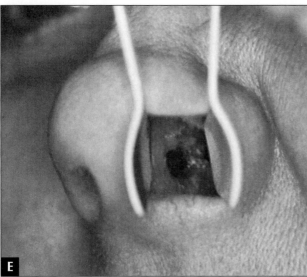

FIGURE 4 (*continued*) **C**, Nasal tumor. Pigmentation of a polypoid structure or a polyp that bleeds should arouse suspicion of a nasal carcinoma or malignant granuloma. **D**, Synechia connecting the turbinates with the septum following nasal trauma. They can occur after surgery. **E**, A nasal septal perforation, because it produces alterations in nasal air flow, can produce symptoms of nasal obstruction (*see* Color Plates). (**B–E**, *From* Bull [11]; with permission.)

drug-induced rhinitis. They induce a rebound nasal congestion that encourages an escalating frequency of use. Cocaine causes a similar problem.

Rhinitis of pregnancy is characterized mainly by congestion. The nasal capacitance vessels have receptors for estrogen which cause vasodilatation. This effect is magnified by the increased blood volume during pregnancy. Endocrine-related rhinitis is also seen in hypothyroidism and in acromegaly.

Gustatory rhinitis and "skier's-jogger's nose" have a similar pathogenesis—excessive cholinergic activity. These conditions are due to exogenously triggered parasympathetic discharge. They are characterized by a clear, copious rhinorrhea beginning shortly after eating or exposure to cold air, as occurs in jogging and skiing.

Atrophic rhinitis is usually a disease of the elderly produced by withering of the turbinates. It can occur in younger age groups as well.

Rhinitis due to leakage of cerebrospinal fluid is characterized by a clear, watery, unilateral or bilateral rhinorrhea that becomes more profuse when the head is tilted forward [1]. The flow is usually sufficient to allow collection in a beaker. Cerebrospinal fluid can be distinguished from nasal secretions because it contains glucose. A dipstick analysis will suffice to detect the presence of glucose in cerebrospinal fluid.

In the evaluation of a patient with rhinitis, ancillary testing, with the exception of allergy tests, plays a lesser role than does history and physical examination. Allergy tests are the definitive tool for distinguishing allergic from nonallergic rhinitis. The test of choice is clearly the allergy skin test. In vitro tests, because of their expense and relative lack of sensitivity [2], should be reserved for patients in whom skin testing is not possible for reasons such as generalized dermatitis. Nasal eosinophil smears are useful in strengthening the case for allergic rhinitis or determining whether a patient with chronic nonallergic rhinitis has NARES. Total IgE levels are not indicated because of the overlap existing between allergic and nonallergic individuals [3]. Sinus roentgenograms and CT scans are obtained when a complicating sinusitis is suspected.

THERAPY

Pharmacologic management is the mainstay of therapy for rhinitis. When the patient is atopic, environmental control

Manifestation	Allergic rhinitis	Chronic nonallergic rhinitis
Age of onset	Usually before 20	Usually after 30
Seasonality	Usually with seasonal variation; spring, fall	Usually perennial but not infrequently worse during weather changes such as occur during fall and early spring
Exacerbating factors	Allergen exposure	Irritant exposure, weather conditions
Nature of symptoms		
Pruritus	Common	Rare
Congestion	Common	Common
Sneezing	Prominent	Usually not prominent but can be dominant in some cases
Postnasal drainage	Not prominent	Prominent
Other related manifestations (eg, allergic conjunctivitis, atopic dermatitis)	Often present	Absent
Family history	Usually present	Usually absent
Physical appearance	Variable, classically described as pale, boggy, swollen—may appear normal	Variable, erythematous
Ancillary studies	Allergy skin tests always positive	Allergy skin tests negative
Nasal eosinophilia	Usually present	Present 15%–20% of the time (nonallergic rhinitis with eosinophilia)
Peripheral eosinophilia	Often present, especially during allergy season	Absent

and allergen immunotherapy may also be indicated. The drugs employed are H_1 antagonists (antihistamines), decongestants, anticholinergics, cromolyn sodium, and corticosteroids.

Antihistamines

H_1 antagonists are competitive inhibitors of histamine at the H_1 level. They are classified as first- and second-generation drugs. First-generation drugs are further divided on the basis of their structure into six groups, each of which is said to have individual characteristics that bestow certain therapeutic qualities (Table 4). Three second-generation, nonsedating antihistamines are available in the United States. They are terfenadine, astemizole, and loratadine.

Antihistamines have other actions that may enhance their therapeutic activity or cause side effects. First-generation antihistamines, but not second-generation drugs, have anticholinergic activity. This can be useful in the control of symptoms due to cholinergic discharge (rhinorrhea and sneezing) but can also cause side effects. Some antihistamines also have antiserotonergic effects and inhibit histamine release from mast cells and basophils.

All presently available antihistamines are rapidly absorbed from the gastrointestinal tract and are metabolized in the liver via the cytochrome P-450 system. Thus hepatic dysfunction or drugs which interfere with cytochrome P-450 activity can prolong the half-life of these drugs. Most antihistamines have tissue effects extending beyond detectable serum levels. However, the tissue effect is delayed relative to peak serum concentrations. This is perhaps one reason why clinical results

appear to be better when these drugs are administered prior to exposure to allergen. The pharmacokinetic and pharmacodynamic characteristics of selected first-generation H_1 antagonists are seen in Table 5.

Antihistamines are effective for the treatment of sneezing, rhinorrhea, and pruritus. They are less useful for therapy of postnasal drainage and fairly ineffective for nasal congestion. Thus they are usually more useful in acute, seasonal allergic rhinitis than in chronic perennial allergic rhinitis, in which congestion is likely to be more pronounced. They are more effective in allergic than in chronic nonallergic rhinitis.

The most common side effect due to first-generation antihistamine administration is drowsiness. Approximately one third of patients taking first-generation antihistamines complain of this effect. It is important to note that reaction time, ability to concentrate, and other cognitive functions can be impaired without the patient sensing drowsiness [5]. This is noteworthy, as it means that patients may not notice drowsiness but yet may be at risk if operating machinery, or driving, for example. Drowsiness can be overcome by the exertion of will, but impairment of function persists until the effect of the drug abates [6]. Thus airline pilots are prohibited from taking first-generation antihistamines while flying [7].

The next most frequent side effects of first-generation agents are those produced by their antimuscarinic action. These include dryness of the mouth; urinary retention and dysuria; blurring of vision; and constipation.

TABLE 4 CHARACTERISTICS OF REPRESENTATIVE FIRST-GENERATION H₁ ANTAGONISTS BASED ON CHEMICAL CLASSIFICATION

Chemical class	Examples	Comments
Ethanolamines	Diphenhydramine Clemastine Carbinoxamine	Significant antimuscarinic effects. Can be potent sedatives, but sedative potential varies, with clemastine producing the least amount. Can have some anti–motion-sickness activity
Alkylamines	Chlorpheniramine Brompheniramine Dexchlorpheniramine Tripolidine	Relatively moderate incidence of drowsiness. Moderate anticholinergic effect. No anti-emetic or anti–motion-sickness activity. Few gastrointestinal side effects
Ethylenediamines	Tripelennamine Pyrilamine Antazoline	Mild to moderate sedation. Slight anticholinergic effect. Some local anesthetic effect. As a group said to have frequent gastrointestinal side effects
Piperazines	Hydroxyzine Meclizine Cyclizine	Meclizine and cyclizine relatively low sedative activity with main use being for vertigo, anti-motion sickness, and antiemetic activity. Hydroxyzine has significant anticholinergic activity
Piperadines	Cyproheptadine Azatadine Phenindamine	Mild to moderate sedation. Little anticholinergic activity, antiemetic activity, and anti–motion sickness activity. Cyproheptadine has a potent antiserotonin effect.
Phenothiazines	Methdilazine Promethazine Trimeprazine	Usually highly sedating. Main clinical use is as antiemetic

TABLE 5 COMPARISON OF PHARMACODYNAMIC CHARACTERISTICS OF SELECTED FIRST-GENERATION H₁ ANTAGONISTS

Drug	Approximate time at which peak serum concentration is reached after oral dose, h	Approximate half-life, h	Approximate duration of biological activity, suppression wheal and flare, h	Route of metabolism
Diphenhydramine	.75–2.5	8–9	6–10	Liver
Chlorpheniramine	1.5–2.5	20–24	24	Liver
Hydroxyzine	1–2.5	20	36	Liver
Brompheniramine	2–3	24	9	Liver
Tripolidine	1–2	2.1	—	Liver

Second-generation, nonsedating antihistamines cause neither drowsiness nor anticholinergic side effects. However, both terfenadine and astemizole can cause adverse cardiovascular events, specifically arrhythmias, and most notably torsades de pointes. These events have usually been due to an increased serum level of the drug secondary to overdose or decreased catabolism because of hepatic dysfunction or the simultaneous administration of another drug also metabolized by the cytochrome P-450 system. Adverse cardiovascular events are thought to be caused by interference with the functioning of the delayed potassium rectifier channel [8•].

Nonetheless, both terfenadine and astemizole appear to be safe when administered in the recommended dosage without drugs that retard their metabolism, specifically keta-conazole, itraconazole, and erythromycin. It would be reasonable to assume, however, that some caution would be advisable in regard to the simultaneous administration of these antihistamines with other drugs metabolized via the cytochrome P-450 system. Other risk factors include liver disease, hypokalemia, hypocalcemia, and congenital prolongation of the QT interval.

Terfenadine and astemizole are not equivalent drugs. The onset of action of astemizole is somewhat delayed and the drug has an extremely long half-life. Thus, there is question as to whether astemizole is appropriate for "as needed" use or in women of childbearing age, since it persists in tissues several weeks after cessation of therapy. Loratadine administration has not been associated with ventricular arrhythmias.

Decongestants

All nasal decongestants are alpha-adrenergic agents that contract the sphincters controlling the blood supply to the venous plexuses in the turbinates. As implied by their name, decongestants are effective only for turbinate swelling and exert little if any effect on other manifestations of rhinitis. Topical application is far more effective and rapid in onset than oral administration. However, topical use can cause rhinitis medicamentosa and therefore use should be limited to 1 week. Topical decongestants do have a role in the therapy of sinusitis, upper respiratory tract infections, and the prevention of barotrauma and otitis due to air travel.

The number of decongestants available for use is quite limited (Table 6). There is no clear-cut choice as far as an oral decongestant is concerned. The long-acting topical drugs, oxymetazoline and xylometazoline, are probably superior to the shorter-acting topical agents if for no other reason than convenience.

Side effects of oral decongestants include insomnia, nervousness, and stranguria, especially in patients with prostatism. Other side effects are infrequent. Although there is a well-known admonition not to prescribe these drugs to patients with hypertension, they appear to be safe in patients with stable hypertension [9].

Anticholinergics

Anticholinergics are used primarily for the treatment of anterior watery rhinorrhea. They are therefore recommended for controlling gustatory rhinitis and skier's-jogger's nose. They can also alleviate the anterior rhinorrhea associated with acute upper respiratory tract infections.

Ipratroprium bromide, which is used for rhinitis in Europe, is available in the United States in the form of a metered-dose inhaler for pulmonary disease. These inhalers can be converted for topical nasal use with a baby-bottle nipple. The nipple is fitted over the mouthpiece of the inhaler and its end truncated halfway down the stem. For gustatory rhinitis or skier's-jogger's nose, the dose is 1 to 2

TABLE 6 DECONGESTANTS
Oral
Pseudoephedrine
Phenylpropanolamine
Phenylephrine
Topical long-acting (8–12 *h*)
Oxymetazoline
Xylometazoline
Topical short-acting (3–8 *h*)
Tetrahydrozoline
Naphazoline
Phenylephrine

puffs before eating or exposure to cold, respectively. Side effects of dryness and nasal irritation rarely occur. Care must be taken to avoid spraying the drug into the eye.

In addition to topical use of anticholinergics, some antihistamine-decongestant combinations contain anticholinergic drugs in the form of belladonna alkaloids.

Antihistamines, decongestants, and anticholinergics are often administered orally in the form of combination medications (Table 7).

Cromolyn Sodium

Cromolyn sodium can be an extremely effective drug for the therapy of allergic rhinitis, especially seasonal allergic rhinitis. It is also useful in preventing symptoms due to isolated exposure to allergens. For example, it can be used prior to cutting the lawn or visiting someone who has a pet.

This drug blocks both early- and late-phase allergic reactions. Although the mechanism of action is not understood, it does prevent mast cell degranulation and the resultant release of mediators.

TABLE 7 SELECTED COMBINATION ANTIHISTAMINE, DECONGESTANT, AND ANTICHOLINERGIC AGENTS			
Trade name	**Antihistamine**	**Decongestant**	**Anticholinergic**
Seldane-D (Marion Merrell Dow, Kansas City, MO)	Terfenadine	Pseudoephedrine	—
Trinalin (Schering-Plough, Kenilworth, NJ)	Azatadine maleate	Pseudoephedrine	—
Bromfed (Muro, Tewksbury, MA)	Brompheniramine maleate	Pseudoephedrine	—
Poly-Histine-D (Bock, St. Louis, MO)	Phenyltoxolamine citrate Pyrilamine maleate Pheniramine maleate	Phenylpropanolamine	—
Atrohist Plus (Adams, Ft. Worth, TX)	Chlorpheniramine maleate	Phenylephrine Phenylpropanolamine	Hyoscyamine sulfate Atropine sulfate Scopolamine hydrobromide
Extendryl S (Fleming, Fenton, MO)	Chlorpheniramine maleate	Phenylephrine	Methscopolamine nitrate

Cromolyn sodium must be administered before exposure. In treating seasonal allergic rhinitis, it should be started a week prior to the allergy season; when used to prevent symptoms due to isolated exposure, it can be given immediately before such exposure. Cromolyn sodium is not effective in the therapy of chronic nonallergic rhinitis. It is almost totally devoid of side effects.

Corticosteroids

Corticosteroids are the most effective drugs for the therapy of both allergic and nonallergic rhinitis. Oral therapy is more effective and more rapid in onset than topical therapy. A 10-day tapering curse of prednisone beginning at 40 to 50 mg/day is almost universally effective in controlling all symptoms of chronic rhinitis, regardless of cause. This regimen is recommended prior to the initiation of topical therapy with either cromolyn sodium or corticosteroids. Pretreatment in this way reduces the exacerbation of symptoms that can occur when topical treatment is applied to an inflamed nasal mucosa. Five drugs are available for topical use (Table 8).

Topical dexamethasone may be the most potent agent. However, because this drug is absorbed in its active form, it can exert detectable albeit modest systemic effects. This limits its usage. Nonetheless, it is appropriate for therapy of seasonal rhinitis lasting no longer than 6 weeks. The other topical corticosteroid preparations have high topical/systemic ratios of activity and are catabolized rapidly. Thus they exert no detectable systemic effect in recommended doses. In addition, topical side effects, even after long-term use, are minimal. Nasal irritation is probably the most common side effect. Nasal bleeding, especially when blowing the nose, occurs with significant frequency, especially during the winter months. Unprovoked nasal bleeding can also occur and should prompt discontinuation of the medication. Nasal septal perforation has been reported, and patients should be monitored for this side effect. Because of the possibility of nasal septal perforation, patients should be told to avoid pointing the spray toward the septum and instructed to point it toward the ear on the side they are spraying.

Exactly how long corticosteroids can be used with safety has not been established, but it is clear that they (with the exception of dexamethasone) can be used for at least several months. Nasal biopsy specimens obtained from patients using beclomethasone continuously for several years have shown no significant mucosal atrophy [10]. Nonetheless, patients on long-term therapy should be monitored.

Application of Individual Medications

Mild seasonal allergic rhinitis can be controlled with antihistamines or antihistamine-decongestant combinations. If sedation occurs, a nonsedating antihistamine can be employed. For more severe symptoms, a topical corticosteroid or cromolyn sodium can be added.

Both allergic and nonallergic perennial rhinitis forms usually require long-term therapy with topical corticosteroids. Dexamethasone should not be used in this setting, but beclomethasone, flunisolide, budesonide, and triamcinolone acetonide can be safely administered for several months. Antihistamine-decongestants can be used as needed. Occasionally anticholinergics are helpful. Intermittent 7- to 10-day courses of corticosteroids are occasionally needed.

Rhinitis medicamentosa is treated with an oral corticosteroid in a tapering dose administered over a 10-day period.

TABLE 8 TOPICAL CORTICOSTEROID PREPARATIONS USED TO TREAT RHINITIS				
Drug	Trade name	Type of delivery	Dose	Sprays per container
Beclomethasone	Beconase (Allen & Hanburys, Research Triangle Park, NC)	Fluorocarbon aerosol	1 spray = 42µg 1–2 sprays each nostril bid to tid	200
	Beconase AQ (Allen & Hanburys)	Liquid spray		
	Vancenase (Schering-Plough, Kenilworth, NJ)	Fluorocarbon aerosol		
	Vancenase AQ (Schering-Plough)	Liquid spray		
Triamcinolone	Nasacort (Rhone-Poulenc Rorer, Ft. Washington, PA)	Fluorocarbon aerosol	1 spray = 55µg 1–2 sprays each nostril qd to bid	100
Flunisolide	Nasalide (Syntex, Palo Alto, CA)	Liquid spray	1 spray = 25µg 1 to 2 sprays each nostril bid	200
Dexamathasone	Decadron Turbinaire (Merck Sharpe & Dohme, West Point, PA)	Fluorocarbon aerosol	1 spray = 0.084 mg 1–2 sprays each nostril bid to tid	170
Budesonide	Rhinocort	Fluorocarbon aerosol	1 spray = 32µg 4 sprays each nostril qd	200

AQ—aqueous; bid—twice daily; qd—daily; tid—three times daily.

TABLE 9 ENVIRONMENTAL CONTROL MEASURES USED TO REDUCE ALLERGEN EXPOSURE

House dust mite
Enclose mattress, box springs, pillows in allergen-proof casings
Wash bed linen on ``hot cycle,'' 130° F
Reduce indoor humidity<50%
Consider use of benzyl benzoate (acaricide) or tannic acid (to denature antigen)

Pollens
Avoid fresh-cut grass, do not mow lawn
Utilize air conditioning

Pets
Should be removed from home whenever possible
Cat allergen can be reduced by frequent bathing of cat (every 2 weeks)
Use of HEPA filter may be helpful

On the third day of administration, a topical corticosteroid is also given. The topical corticosteroid should be used for at least 1 month. The patient should discontinue the topical decongestant. To avoid discomfort, this need not be done precipitously but can be tapered off gradually over a period of 1 week. Oral decongestants can be used as needed.

Gustatory rhinitis and skier's-jogger's nose, as mentioned, usually respond to ipratropium bromide administered 30 minutes to an hour prior to eating or exposure to cold.

Rhinitis of pregnancy is a particularly difficult therapeutic problem because of the admonition not to use drugs, especially during the first trimester. It usually responds only to corticosteroids. The decision to initiate oral or topical corticosteroid therapy should be taken in conjunction with the obstetrician. This condition usually worsens as the pregnancy proceeds but subsides spontaneously shortly after parturition.

Nonpharmacologic Measures

An environmental control regimen can be helpful (Table 9). In some instances, the removal of a pet from the home totally resolves the problem. Allergen immunotherapy alleviates the symptoms of allergic rhinitis caused by pollens and dust mites. The exact mechanism of action of immunotherapy has not been established but is attributable to a number of immunologic events occurring during administration (see Chapter 17). Relief can persist permanently after cessation of therapy. The duration of immunotherapy is usually 3 to 5 years.

Complications

A number of abnormalities in facial development can occur in severe perennial rhinitis due to obligate mouth breathing. It is therefore essential to treat adolescents and children with chronic rhinitis aggressively. Otitis media and sinusitis are a result of obstruction of the eustachian tubes and sinus ostia, respectively. Correction of nasal obstruction is necessary in the therapy of both disorders. There is significant evidence that nasal obstruction can predispose to bronchoconstriction through the activation of nasal reflexes. Thus, control of rhini-

tis is considered helpful in the treatment of asthma. Finally, rhinitis can produce sleep disturbances and contribute to sleep apnea. Correction of the rhinitis exerts a salutary effect on sleep apnea.

References and Recommended Reading

Recently published papers of particular interest have been highlighted as:
• Of interest
•• Of outstanding interest

1. Schiano CM: Non traumatic cerebrospinal fluid rhinorrhea. *Immunol Allerg Prac* 1990, 12:336–338.
2. Bousquet J, Francois-Bernard M: Diagnostic tests. In *Allergy Theory and Practice*, edn 2. edited by Kornblatt P, Wedneser HJ. Philadelphia: WB Saunders; 1992:143–163.
3. Owenby DR: Clinical significance of IgE. In *Allergy Principles and Practice*, vol 2, edn 4. Edited by Middleton E Jr, Reed CE, Ellis EF, *et al.* St Louis: Mosby; 1993:1059–1076.
4.•• Naclerio RM: Allergic rhinitis. *N Engl J Med* 1991, 325:869.
5. Druce H: Impairment of function by antihistamines. *Ann Allerg* 1990, 64:403–405.
6. Gengo FM, Gabos C: Antihistamines, drowsiness, and psychomotor impairment: central nervous system effect of cetirizine. [Proceedings of a symposium—Cetirizine, a recent advance in selective antihistamine therapy—supplement.] *Ann Allerg* 1987, 59(part II):53–57.
7. Kaliner MA, Check WA: Nonsedating antihistamines. *Allerg Proc* 1988, 9:649–663.
8.• Kemp JP: Antihistamines: is there anything safe to prescribe? *Ann Allerg* 1992, 69:276–280.
9. Kroenke K, Omori D, Simmons J, Wood D, Meier N: The safety of phenylpropanolamine in patients with stable hypertension. *Ann Intern Med* 1989, 3:1043–1044.
10. Mygand N, Sorensen H, Peterson CB: The nasal mucosa during long term treatment with beclomethasone dipropionate aerosol: a light and scanning electron microscopic study of nasal polyps. *Acta Otolaryngol* 1978, 85:437.
11. Bull TR, ed.: *A Colour Atlas of ENT Diagnosis*, edn. 2. London: Wolfe Medical Publications; 1987:123—155.

etiology of nasal polyps [2], and the routine referral of nasal polyp patients for allergy evaluation is not indicated [3–7].

Management

The management of nasal polyps may include both medical and surgical approaches. Antihistamines, decongestants, and cromolyn sodium are of little benefit. In the case of superimposed bacterial infection, appropriate antibiotics should be administered. Corticosteroids are extremely effective in reducing polyp size. Well-controlled studies have revealed a variety of intranasal preparations of corticosteroids to be effective in managing nasal polyps. With treatment, significant improvement in 80% of patients with moderate-to-severe polyposis occurs. In addition to decreasing polyp size and increasing airway conductance, there is also a decrease in eosinophils in the nasal smear with a decrease in albumin, IgG, and IgE in the secretions.

A fundamental effect of corticosteroids in inhibiting protein synthesis at the cellular level has led to fears that protracted use of intranasal steroids might lead to atrophic changes. Examination of nasal polyp biopsy specimens after 5 years of local beclomethasone treatment demonstrated no change from pseudostratified to squamous metaplasia of surface epithelium that would be indicative of atrophic rhinitis. This is probably because of the rapid removal of beclomethasone from mucous membranes. The mucous membrane half-life of beclomethasone is 30 minutes compared with 6 to 8 hours in the skin [8].

One method for corticosteroid administration in treating nasal polyps is direct injection into the polyp. Although the technique is widely used, there are well-documented studies of unilateral visual loss after intranasal steroid injection. This has prompted the US Food and Drug Administration not to approve the use of steroids for this procedure.

Nasal polypectomy alone is associated with an extraordinary recurrence rate of polyps after surgery [9]. In a past study, surgical removal of nasal polyps was compared with the use of systemic steroids. After initial treatment with either surgery or systemic steroids, both groups of patients were administered topical steroids and their progress followed for 1 year. Both

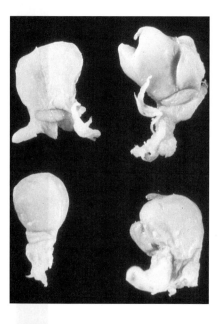

FIGURE 1 Four nasal polyps removed from same individual.

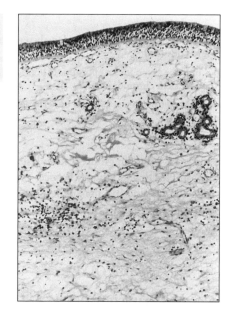

FIGURE 2 Photomicrograph of nasal polyps showing edema fluid, pseudostratified epithelium, and inflammatory cell infiltrate.

TABLE 1 FREQUENCY OF NASAL POLYPS IN VARIOUS CONDITIONS

Diagnosis	Frequency, %
Aspirin intolerance	36.0
Adult asthma	7.0
Intrinsic	13.0
Atopic	5.0
Chronic rhinitis	2.0
Nonallergic	5.0
Allergic	1.5
Childhood asthma/ rhinitis	0.1
Cystic fibrosis	20.0

From Settipane [1]; with permission.

TABLE 2 MECHANISMS IMPLICATED IN THE FORMATION OF NASAL POLYPS

Allergy
Infection
Autonomic imbalance
Mucopolysaccharide abnormality
Enzyme abnormality
Drug sensitivity
Mechanical obstruction
Histamine
Proto-oncogene

TABLE 3 MANAGEMENT OF NASAL POLYPS

A 12-day tapering course of oral prednisone beginning with 20 mg three times a day and decreasing by 5 mg each day

On the third day, begin administering a topical nasal corticosteroid

Reserve polypectomy for medically resistant cases

groups experienced similar increase in nasal expiratory peak flow and sense of smell with a statistically significant increase in benefit from medication. The two major conclusions of the authors, who were otolaryngologists, were: 1) the continued postoperative use of topical steroids postpones or prevents recurrence of nasal polyps, and 2) surgical removal should be reserved for those few cases in which the presence of residual or recurrent polyps justifies the inherent risks and discomfort for the patient [10].

Based on these and other studies, it would appear that a reasonable medical approach to management of nasal polyps would be a 10- to 14-day course of oral prednisone followed by intranasal beclomethasone, flunisolide, triamcinolone, budesonide, or fluticasone (Table 3).

SINUSITIS

Pathophysiology

Protection against infection of the paranasal sinuses is largely provided by the mucociliary apparatus. Microorganisms, pollutants, irritants, and other foreign particles that escape the filtering apparatus of the nose are trapped in the mucus of the sinuses, then removed through the draining ostia by constant movement of the mucus blanket propelled by the underlying cilia. When this self-cleansing mechanism is impaired, bacterial infection occurs.

Several factors may result in retention of secretions in the paranasal sinuses: 1) swelling of the mucus membrane leading to reduced patency of ostia; 2) reduced transport capacity related to abnormalities of the cilia including quantitative reduction, retardation of movement, and insufficient coordination of movement; and 3) overproduction of secretions.

Of these three factors, patency of the ostia is the most important in the development of sinusitis. The ostia functions primarily for drainage of secretions and for gas exchange. Obstruction of the ostium leads to retention of secretions and a low oxygen content in the sinuses, both of which favor increased bacterial growth and purulence. Mucociliary activity of the sinuses is of extreme importance in protection against sinusitis because spontaneous drainage of the maxillary sinus is nearly impossible for two reasons. First, the maxillary ostium is not simply an opening of 1 to 3 mm in diameter, but rather a circuitous channel 6 mm in length that connects the maxillary antrum to the middle meatus. This is referred to as the *ostiomeatal complex*. Second, the maxillary ostium is located in the superior portion of the maxillary antrum. Therefore, for spontaneous drainage to occur into the nose in the upright position, the antrum must be completely filled before the contents can spill over or ciliary action must move secretions in a cephalad direction against the force of gravity. For these reasons, the maxillary sinus is by far the most common site of sinusitis, followed in decreasing order of incidence by the ethmoid, frontal, and sphenoid sinuses. With this information on pathophysiology we can now logically turn to Table 4, showing the factors that predispose to the development of sinusitis.

While systemic factors, particularly hypogammaglobulinemia, may play some role, far and away the most common factors predisposing to sinusitis are local. Heading the list are viral upper respiratory infections and allergic rhinitis in which the mechanism for the development of sinusitis would appear to be similar. Acute rhinitis of either infectious or allergic etiology results in edematous obstruction of the nasal ostia, decreased paranasal sinus ciliary action, and increased mucus production. With the subsequent accumulation of mucus in the sinus, the stage is set for secondary bacterial infection and the conversion of mucus to mucopus. Mucopus further impairs ciliary function and increases swelling around ostia when it discharges into the nose, creating a vicious cycle.

Diagnosis
History and physical examination
Table 5 shows the ways in which the diagnosis of sinusitis can be made. The most important clinical clue to the diagnosis of acute sinusitis is the continuation of symptoms after a typical cold has subsided. The previously clear nasal discharge becomes yellow or green. Fever persists, and chills may develop. Pain that is felt in the forehead may be associated with maxillary sinusitis. The patient's discomfort often worsens when bending or straining.

On physical examination, the patient will have thick, purulent, green or deep yellow secretions in the nose on the side of the diseased sinus. Because the maxillary sinus is most frequently involved, purulent secretions will be seen most often in the middle meatus, which is the drainage site of the maxillary sinus.

In chronic sinusitis, the general lack of pain or systemic symptoms makes this condition difficult to diagnose based on history alone. There is usually a poor correlation between clinical characteristics and evidence obtained from an antral puncture. Patients with chronic sinusitis generally do not complain of headache, facial pain, fullness in the face, pain in the teeth, or discomfort when they bend over. Rather, nasal obstruction that is sometimes unilateral, purulent postnasal drainage,

TABLE 4 FACTORS PREDISPOSING TO SINUSITIS	
Local	**Systemic**
Upper respiratory infection	Immune deficiency
Allergic rhinitis	Bronchiectasis
Overuse of topical decongestants	Immotile cilia syndrome
Hypertrophied adenoids	
Deviated nasal septum	
Bone spurs	
Nasal polyps	
Tumors	
Foreign bodies	
Swimming and diving	
Cigarette smoke	
Barotrauma	
Dental extraction/injections	

TABLE 5 DIAGNOSIS OF SINUSITIS
History Physical examination Nasal secretions Fiberoptic nasopharyngoscopy Ultrasonography Radiography Computed tomography

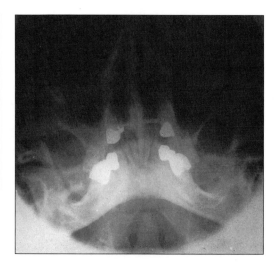

FIGURE 3 Sinus radiograph showing haziness of left maxillary antrum with bilateral maxillary mucoperiosteal thickening.

chronic cough, hyposmia, sore throat, and unpleasant breath are the most common presenting signs. Physical examination of the patient with chronic sinusitis will reveal an edematous nasal mucosa bathed in mucopus.

Although a nasal culture does not give an appropriate picture of the organisms responsible for sinusitis, a microscopic examination of nasal secretions will demonstrate sheets of polymorphonuclear neutrophils and bacteria. The recently introduced technique of fiberoptic nasopharyngoscopy affords a splendid opportunity for better visualization of the draining ostia of infected sinuses and for obtaining specimens for culture.

Radiography and other diagnostic techniques

Evidence from sinus roentgenograms is the most common means of establishing a clinical diagnosis of sinusitis. The occipitomental or Waters view best demonstrates the maxillary sinuses. The head is tilted back so the dense petrous bone does not occlude the lower part of the maxillary antra. The occipitofrontal or Caldwell view demonstrates both the ethmoid and frontal sinuses. The sphenoid sinus is seen on a lateral view. Correlation between antral puncture and radi-

ographic appearance [11] reveals that true sinusitis is associated with either mucosal thickening of 6 mm or greater (Fig. 3), an air-fluid level (Fig. 4), or opacification (Fig. 5).

Transillumination has been shown to be of very limited usefulness in the diagnosis of sinusitis, particularly with maxillary involvement [12]. Ultrasonography consists of transmitting low-power pulsed ultrasound into the selected sinus cavity by direct contact of the transducer on the patient's face. At the frequency used, ultrasound does not propagate through air. When the sinus is healthy and filled with air, no echo appears from the back wall. If fluid is present, a strong echo will be reflected by the back wall of the sinus. Advantages of ultrasonography are that it is noninvasive, nonionizing, and painless. However, to date no consensus has been reached as to the diagnostic accuracy and validity of ultrasonography. More studies and improvement in technology will be necessary before this technique can be recommended for general use.

A major development in the diagnosis of sinusitis is the application of computed tomographic (CT) scans. There is no question that disease of the sinuses, particularly of the ethmoids, may be missed on ordinary roentgenography

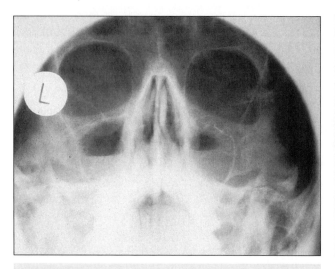

FIGURE 4 Sinus radiograph showing bilateral maxillary air-fluid levels.

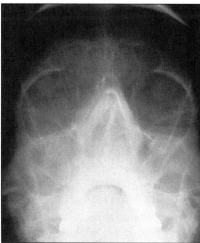

FIGURE 5 Sinus radiograph showing bilateral maxillary opacification.

(Fig. 6). CT scans will demonstrate the ostiomeatal complex and will detect subtle disease not demonstrated on sinus radiographs. A major problem in the past has been the rather prohibitive cost of CT scans. Through improvement in technology and the utilization of limited scans, the price of the technique has diminished to a much more reasonable level and in some centers is quite close to that of ordinary sinus radiographs. A recent study demonstrated a strong correlation between extensive disease of the sinuses and asthma, specific IgE antibodies, and eosinophilia in particular, with 87% of patients with peripheral blood eosinophilia having extensive sinus disease [13•].

Management
Medical

Sinusitis should be thought of as an abscess (*ie*, an infection within a closed anatomic space). The medical approach to managing infectious sinusitis is shown in Table 6 and Figure 7. Saline nasal spray or douches are useful to liquefy secretions and also decrease blood flow to the nose with a resultant decongestant effect. It is vital to increase the diameter of the maxillary ostium and promote mucociliary activity. In this way, purulent secretions are removed with an associated increase in sinus PaO_2, a decrease in sinus PCO_2, a decrease in lactate content, an increase in ciliary movement, and a decrease in proteolytic enzymes. When administered orally, phenylpropanolamine has been shown to increase the functional diameter of the maxillary sinus. There would also

appear to be benefit in reducing mucosal inflammation, allowing host clearance mechanisms to recover. One controlled study [14•] showed that a nasal spray incorporating flunisolide was more effective than a placebo in treating sinusitis. There is no controlled study demonstrating the efficacy of mucoevacuants in treating sinusitis. However, based on the discussion here, it seems reasonable that thinning of sinus secretions would increase drainage and promote the recovery of host clearance mechanisms.

The bacteria responsible for acute sinusitis are largely aerobic. *Streptococcus pneumoniae*, *Moraxella catarrhalis*, and *Haemophilus influenzae* are the most common. Anaerobic bacteria are largely responsible for chronic sinusitis. Common pathogens include alpha streptococci and species of *Bacteroides*, *Veillonella*, and *Corynebacterium*.

Fungal infection of the paranasal sinuses may occur in both immunocompromised and immunocompetent individuals. *Aspergillus fumigatus* is the most common fungus responsible for sinusitis [15]. Other fungi causing sinusitis include actinomycetes, *Nocardia* and *Mucor* species, *Sporothrix schenckii*, and bipolaris. Mucormycosis is particularly associated with diabetes mellitus. Fungal sinusitis should be suspected in any case of antibiotic-resistant sinusitis. The sinus exudate is generally thick, of a peanut butter–like consistency. The management of invasive fungal sinusitis includes extensive debridement and parenteral antifungal drugs.

The antibiotic of choice in managing acute or chronic bacterial sinusitis is ampicillin or amoxicillin. The responsible

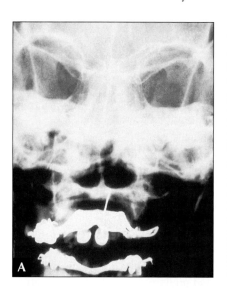

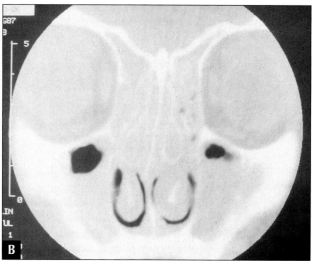

FIGURE 6 A, Sinus radiograph showing normal ethmoid sinuses. B, computed tomographic scan of same patient revealing opacified ethmoid sinuses.

TABLE 6 MEDICAL TREATMENT OF SINUSITIS

Analgesics	Corticosteroids	Antibiotics
Steam and saline	Topical: beclomethasone, flunisolide, triamcinolone, budesonide, fluticasone	Ampicillin or amoxicillin
Decongestants	Oral: prednisone	Trimethoprim with sulfamethoxazole (in case of penicillin sensitivity)
Topical: oxymetazoline, phenylephrine	**Mucoevacuants**	Cefprozil
Oral: pseudoephedrine, phenylpropanolamine	Guaifenesin	Amoxicillin-clavulanate
		Cefuroxime

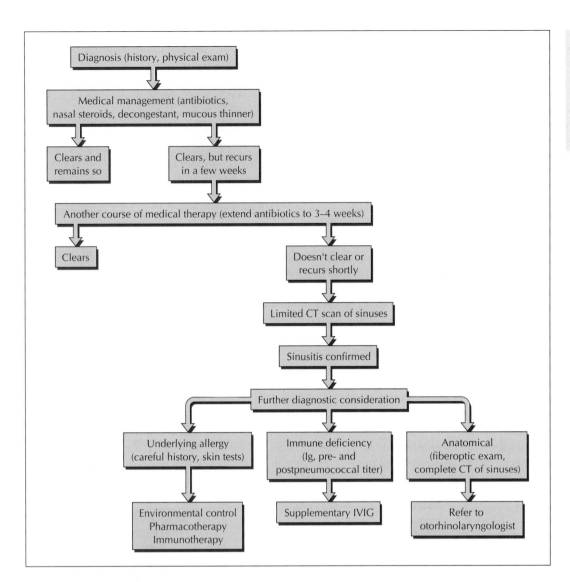

FIGURE 7
Management of sinusitis. CT—computed tomography; IVIG—intravenous immunoglobulin.

organisms are generally sensitive to these antibiotics, and adequate mucosal and sinus fluid concentrations of these antibiotics are obtained. For patients who are sensitive to penicillin, an adequate alternative is trimethoprim–sulfamethoxazole.

It is estimated that approximately 20% of bacteria responsible for sinusitis have become resistant to penicillin and to cephalosporins by producing β-lactamase enzymes that destroy the β-lactam nucleus of these antibiotics. Clavulinic acid, an inhibitor of the β-lactamases, has been introduced in combination with some penicillins, and these drugs have proven to be useful in patients with β-lactamase–producing organisms. Other antibiotics useful in such instances are Cefprozil and Ceftin (Glaxo, Research Triangle Park, NC).

The duration of treatment is as important as the choice of antibiotics. Two weeks of antibiotic therapy is generally adequate for acute sinusitis, with chronic sinusitis requiring 3 to 4 weeks or longer.

Surgical

If there is no significant clinical or roentgenographic improvement after 1 month of antibiotic therapy, or if the patient's sinusitis recurs on a regular basis, then the advice of an otolaryngologist should be sought. The tasks of the otolaryn-gologist consist basically of removing diseased tissue, relieving obstruction, and providing a nasal airway with drainage for all nasal and sinus compartments.

The technique of functional endoscopic sinus surgery is gaining increasing acceptance for treatment of medically resistant sinus disease. Reestablishment of ventilation and mucociliary clearance of the sinuses is accomplished by the endoscopic removal of diseased tissue from the key areas of the anterior ethmoid sinus, middle turbinate, and middle meatus. The objective is to remove, in a limited resection, the inflammatory and anatomic defects that interfere with normal mucociliary clearance and produce the resistant inflammation. Advantages are minimal trauma to normal nasal and sinus structures and conservative removal of diseased tissue. A return to the natural physiology and mucociliary clearance and function of the sinuses are thus made possible [16].

Relationship with Asthma

The frequent association of nasal and paranasal sinus disease with bronchial asthma is being increasingly appreciated. There are a number of studies that strongly suggest that appropriate medical or surgical management of underlying sinusitis will frequently result in an improvement of the associated asthmatic state. Rachelefsky *et al.* [17] demonstrated that children

TABLE 7 DISEASE CHARACTERISTICS BEFORE AND AFTER TREATMENT OF SINUSITIS IN 48 CHILDREN WITH ASTHMA

Characteristic	Before treatment, %	After treatment, %
Cough	100	29
Wheeze	100	15
Normal pulmonary function tests	0	67
Bronchodilator treatment	100	21

with combined sinusitis and lower airway hyperreactivity show significant improvement of the asthmatic state when they receive appropriate medical treatment of their sinusitis. In Table 7, we see disease characteristics before and after treatment for sinusitis in 48 children with hyperreactive airway disease. Seventy-nine percent of these children were able to discontinue bronchodilators with resolution of their sinusitis. In our own series of medically resistant adults with nasal polyps, sinusitis, and asthma, definitive nasosinus surgery resulted in significant subjective improvement in the asthmatic state in 66% of patients. Two thirds were able to decrease the corticosteroid dose significantly, with one third eliminating steroids entirely. In a 5-year follow-up of patients with chronic sinusitis and asthma who underwent bilateral intranasal sphenoethmoidectomy, the improvement noted within 2 years continued, for the most part, for 5 years [18].

REFERENCES AND RECOMMENDED READING

Recently published papers of particular interest have been highlighted as:
• Of interest
•• Of outstanding interest

1. Settipane GA: Nasal polyps. *Immunol Allergy Clin North Am* 1987, 7:105–107.

2. Slavin RG: Allergy is not a significant cause of nasal polyps. *Arch Otolaryngol Head Neck Surg* 1992, 118:771–773.

3. Caplan I, Haynes TJ, Spahn J: Are nasal polyps an allergic phenomenon? *Ann Allergy* 1971, 29:631–634.

4. Settipane GA, Chafee FH: Nasal polyps in asthma with rhinitis: a review of 6,037 patients. *J Allergy Clin Immunol* 1977, 59:17–21.

5. Drake-Lee AB, Lowe D, Swanson A, Grace A: Clinical profile and recurrence of nasal polyps. *J Laryngol Otol* 1984, 98:783–787.

6. Drake-Lee AB, Pitcher-Wilmott RW: The clinical and laboratory correlates of nasal polyps in cystic fibrosis. *Int J Pediatr Otorhinolaryngol* 1982, 4:209–220.

7. Wong D, Jordana G, Denburg J, Dolovich J: Blood eosinophilia and nasal polyps. *Am J Rhinol* 1992, 6:195–198.

8. Mygind N, Prytz S, Sorenson H, Pederson CB: Long-term treatment of nasal polyps with beclomethasone dipropionate aerosol. I. Treatment and rationale. *Acta Otolaryngol* 1976, 82:252–259.

9. Settipane GA: Nasal polyps. In *Rhinitis*, edn 1. Edited by Settipane GA. Providence, RI: Brown University; 1984:133–140.

10. Lildholdt T, Fogstrip J, Gamelgoord N, *et al.*: Surgical versus medical treatment of nasal polyps. *Acta Otolaryngol* 1988, 105:14–143.

11. Evans FO Jr, Sydnor VB, Moore WE, *et al.*: Sinusitis of maxillary antrum. *N Engl J Med* 1975, 293:735–739.

12. Spector SL, Loton A, English G, Philpot L: Comparison between transillumination and the roentgenogram in diagnosing paranasal sinus disease. *J Allergy Clin Immunol* 1981, 67:22–26.

13.• Newman LV, Platts-Mills TAE, Phillips CD, *et al.*: Chronic sinusitis: relationship of computed tomographic findings to allergy, asthma, and eosinophils. *JAMA* 1994, 271:363–367.

14.• Meltzer EO, Orgel HA, Bockhaus JW: Intranasal flunisolode spray as an adjunct to oral antibiotic therapy for sinusitis. *J Allergy Clin Immunol* 1993, 92:812–823.

15. Morgan MA, Wilson WR, Neel HB III, Robert GD: Fungal sinusitis in health and immunocompromised individuals. *Am J Clin Pathol* 1984, 82:597–601.

16. Kennedy DW: Functional endoscopic sinus surgery technique. *Arch Otolaryngol* 1985, 3:643–649.

17. Rachelefsky GS, Katz RM, Siegel SC: Chronic sinus disease with associated reactive airway disease in children. *Pediatrics* 1984, 783:526–529.

18. Mings R, Friedman WH, Linford P, Slavin RG: Five year follow-up of the effects of bilateral intranasal sphenoethmoidectomy in patients with sinusitis and asthma. *Am J Rhinol* 1988, 71:123–132.

SELECT BIBLIOGRAPHY

Slavin RG: Management of sinusitis. *J Am Geriatr Soc* 1991, 39:212–217.

Slavin RG: Medical management of nasal polyps and sinusitis. *J Allergy Clin Immunol* 1991, 88:141–146.

Slavin RG: Nasal polyps and sinusitis. In *Allergy: Principles and Practice*, edn 4. Edited by Middleton EJ, Reed CE, Ellis EF, *et al.* St. Louis: Mosby-Year Book; 1993:1455–1470.

Slavin RG: Sinusitis. In *Atlas of Allergies*. Edited by Fireman P, Slavin RG. Philadelphia: J.B. Lippincott; 1991:102–110.

Slavin RG: Sinusitis and asthma. In *Pediatric Sinusitis*. Edited by Lusk RP. New York: Raven Press; 1992:59–64.

Allergic Disorders of the Eye

7

Leonard Bielory

Key Points

- Mast cell activation is the primary event associated with acute allergic ocular disorders.

- Eosinophils and lymphocytes are involved in the more chronic allergic ocular disorders.

- A multidisciplinary management assessment (allergist/immunologist and ophthalmologist) should be considered in more persistent and recurrent forms.

- Management involves the use of topical application of lubricants and antihistamines/vasoconstrictors, as well as systemic antihistamines. Immunotherapy has been shown to be an excellent adjunctive therapy that can improve and control acute allergic ocular disorders.

Immunologic hypersensitivity reactions involving the eye include mast cell, cytotoxic antibody, circulating immune complexes, and cell-mediated reactions [1,2,3•] (Table 1). Like our other sensory organs, the eye instantly alerts us to any dysfunction. The eye allows for direct visualization of the active immunologic processes such as corneal immune rings reflecting immune complex deposition, which are analogous to precipitins in Ouchterlony plates, and *floating* lymphocytes (floaters) in the anterior chamber, which may be compared to cells migrating into a Boyden chamber.

Allergic diseases affecting the eye are very common, affecting approximately 25% of the general population. In one study of 5000 allergic children, 32% had ocular disease as the single manifestation of their allergies [4]. Ocular allergies are thought to comprise 10% of the ophthalmologist's practice, 25% of the allergist/clinical immunologist's practice, and 5% of the general pediatric and internist's practice. However, the varying definitions and treatment regimens make allergic diseases of the eye difficult to diagnose, and sometimes, frustrating to treat.

CLINICAL EXAMINATION

The eyelids are carefully examined for evidence of blepharitis, dermatitis, swelling, discoloration, blepharospasm, or ptosis (Fig. 1). The conjunctivae are examined for evidence of chemosis, hyperemia, palpebral and bulbar papillae, and cicatrization (Fig. 2). Increased or abnormal secretions are noted. A funduscopic examination will reveal uveitis, sometimes associated with autoimmune disorders, and cataracts, which may be associated with atopic disorders and chronic steroid use.

A fundamental principle of the ocular examination is determining whether conjunctival inflammation is nonspecific or punctuated by the presence of follicles or papillae involving the bulbar and tarsal conjunctivae. Follicles appear as grayish, clear, or yellow bumps varying in size from pinpoint to 2 mm in diameter with conjunctival vessels on their surface; these are generally distinguishable from papillae, which contain a centrally located tuft of vessels. For a clinician to determine an acceptable (nonpathologic) level of follicular and papillary reactivity, the upper and lower tarsal plates and bulbar conjunctivae should be examined on a routine basis (Fig. 3).

The cornea is best examined by an ophthalmologist, using a slit-lamp biomicroscope, although many important clinical features can be seen with the naked eye or with the use of a hand-held direct ophthalmoscope. The cornea should be perfectly smooth and transparent. Dusting of the cornea may indicate punctate epithelial keratitis. A localized corneal defect may develop into a localized erosion or a larger ulcer. A corneal plaque may be present if the surface is dry and white or yellow in appearance. Mucus adhering to the corneal or conjunctival surface is considered pathologic. The limbus is the zone immediately surrounding the cornea and is normally

TABLE 1 CATEGORIES OF OCULAR INFLAMMATION					
Category	**Recognition component**	**Soluble mediators**	**Time course**	**Cellular response**	**Clinical example**
IgE/mast cell	IgE	Leukotrienes, arachadonates, histamine	*s, min*	Eosinophils, neutrophils, basophils	Allergic conjunctivitis, anaphylaxis, atopic keratoconjunctivitis, vernal keratoconjunctivitis
Cytotoxic antibody	IgG, IgM	Complement	*h, d*	Neutrophils, macrophages	Mooren's ulcer, pemphigus, pemphigoid
Immune complex	IgG, IgM	Complement	*h, d*	Neutrophils, eosinophils, lymphocytes	Serum sickness uveitis, corneal immune rings, lens-induced uveitis, Behçet's syndrome, vasculitis
Delayed hypersensitivity	T-lymphocytes, monocytes	Lymphokines, monokines	*d, wk*	Lymphocytes, monocytes, eosinophils, basophils	Corneal allograft rejection, sympathetic ophthalmia, sarcoid-induced uveitis, Vogt-Koyanagi-Hirada syndrome

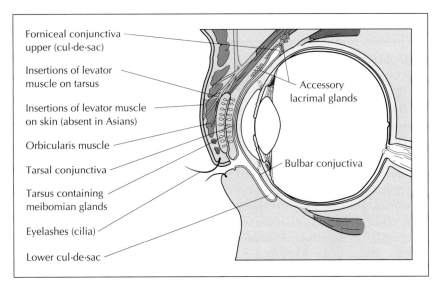

FIGURE 1 The position of the eyelid is important in the examination of the eye. The upper eyelid commonly rests on the top portion of the iris. **A,** normal; **B,** exophthalmos; **C,** ptosis.

A   B   C

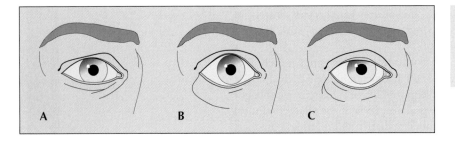

Forniceal conjunctiva upper (cul·de·sac)

Insertions of levator muscle on tarsus

Insertions of levator muscle on skin (absent in Asians)

Orbicularis muscle

Tarsal conjunctiva

Tarsus containing meibomian glands

Eyelashes (cilia)

Lower cul·de·sac

Accessory lacrimal glands

Bulbar conjunctiva

FIGURE 2 Cross-section of parts of the eye commonly involved in allergic reactions.

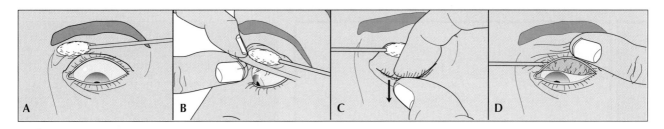

FIGURE 3 Proper examination of the conjunctival surfaces involves eversion of the upper eyelid, which can be done by **A**, placing a cotton-tipped swap above the eyelid; **B**, asking the patient to look down while gently grasping onto the upper eyelashes; **C**, pulling the eyelid down while placing pressure with the cotton swab; and **D**, lifting the eyelid up and over the cotton swab.

invisible to the naked eye; however, when inflamed, this area becomes visible as a pale or pink swelling. Discrete swellings with small white dots (Trantas–Horner's dots) are indicative of degenerating cellular debris, which is commonly seen in chronic forms of conjunctivitis (Table 2).

Allergic Conjunctivitis

Mast cell and IgE-mediated reactions are the most common hypersensitivity responses of the eye (Table 3). Allergic conjunctivitis is caused by direct exposure of the ocular mucosal surfaces to environmental allergens.

Allergic conjunctivitis is more notable for its frequency than for its severity. Prevalence ranges from 5% to 22% of the population depending on the area studied [5]. Unlike several other ocular diseases, it is seldom followed by permanent visual impairment. The most prevalent forms of ocular allergy are seasonal and perennial allergic conjunctivitis; the former, which is due to grass pollen, is the most common. IgE sensitization to papain enzyme in contact-lens cleaning solutions has been reported, with serum-specific IgE via skin tests to papain and chymopapain detected [6]. Symptoms of conjunctivitis include itching, tearing, and burning. There may also be corneal symptoms of photophobia and blurring of vision. Clinical signs include milky or pale pink conjunctivae with vascular congestion, which may progress to conjunctival swelling (chemosis). A white exudate may form during the acute state, which becomes stringy in the chronic form. Tear fluid has been found to contain a small quantity of eosinophils and histamine.

Vernal Conjunctivitis

Vernal conjunctivitis (VC) is a chronic inflammatory disorder of the conjunctiva that primarily affects young men. It usually begins in the spring with symptoms that include intense pruritus exacerbated by time, exposure to wind, dust, bright light, hot weather, or physical exertion associated with sweating. Associated symptoms involving the cornea include photophobia, foreign body sensation, intense pruritus, and lacrimation. Signs include conjunctival hyperemia with papillary hypertrophy (*cobblestoning*) of the upper tarsal plate reaching 7 to 8 mm in diameter (Fig. 4); a thin, copious, milk-white fibrinous secretion; limbal or conjunctival "yellowish-white points" (Horner's points and Trantas' dots; Fig. 5); an extra lower eyelid crease (Dennie's line); corneal ulcers; or pseudomembrane formation of the upper eyelid when everted and exposed to heat (Maxwell-Lyon's sign). Although VC is a bilateral disease, it may affect one eye more than the other. Vernal conjunctivitis is a childhood disease, appearing more often in boys than in girls before pubescence, after which it is equally distributed between the sexes and, by the third decade of life (4 to 10 years after onset), it will commonly attenuate and finally disappear.

Unlike VC, atopic keratoconjunctivitis is a chronic inflammatory disorder of the conjunctivae that affects persons well beyond their teenage years. A familial history for atopy and its association with atopic dermatitis is common. Ocular complications include blepharoconjunctivitis, cataract, keratoconus, and ocular herpes simplex. Symptoms commonly include itching, burning, and tearing. Signs include involvement of the conjunctiva (primarily upper) in the form of a papillary conjunctivitis. The corneal epithelium reveals mild to moderate inflammatory changes that can result in scarring and neovascularization leading to blindness. Limbal infiltrates of cellular debris are known as Horner's points or Trantas' dots (Fig. 3). Many patients may develop secondary staphylococcal blepharitis.

TABLE 2 COMMON CLINICAL SIGNS AND SYMPTOMS OF OCULAR INFLAMMATION

Trichiasis—inturned eyelashes

Epiphora—excessive tearing

Blepharospasm—spasm of the obicularis oculi muscles

Subconjunctival hemorrhages—benign lesions occurring spontaneously, but may follow vigorous rubbing of the eye, vomiting, coughing or Valsalva's maneuvers

Blepharitis—inflammation of the eyelids

Madarosis—loss of eyelashes

Chalazion—inflammation of the meibomian gland

Hordeolum—a sty

Cicatrization—shrinkage and scarring of the conjunctival surface

Episcleritis—benign self-limiting sometimes bilateral inflammatory process of the tunic that surrounds the ocular globe

Scleritis—an inflammatory process of the outer tunic surrounding the globe associated with autoimmune disorders (*eg*, systemic lupus erythematosus, rheumatoid arthritis)

TABLE 3 DIFFERENTIAL DIAGNOSIS OF CONJUNCTIVAL INFLAMMATORY DISORDERS

	AC	VC	AKC	GPC	Contact	Bacterial	Viral	Chlamydial	KCS	BC
SIGNS										
Predominant cell type	Mast cell EOS	Lymph EOS	Lymph EOS	Lymph EOS	Lymph	PMN	PMN mono lymph	Mono lymph	Lymph mono	Mono lymph
Chemosis	+	±	±	±	–	±	±	±	–	±
Lymph node	–	–	–	–	–	+	++	±	–	–
Cobblestoning	–	++	++	++				+	–	–
Discharge	Clear mucoid	Stringy mucoid	Stringy mucoid	Clear white	+–	++ Mucopurulent	– Clear mucoid	++ Mucopurulent	± Mucoid	++ Mucopurulent
Eyelid involvement	–	+	+	–	++	–	–	–	–	++
SYMPTOMS										
Pruritus	+	++	++	++	+	–	–	–	–	+
Gritty sensation	±	±	±	+	–	+	+	+	+++	++
Seasonal variation	+	+	±	±	–	±	±	±	–	–

AC—allergic conjunctivitis; AKC—atopic keratoconjunctivitis; BC—blepharoconjunctivitis; EOS—Eosinophil; GPC—Giant papillary conjunctivitis; KCS—keratoconjunctivitis sicca; Lymph—lymphocyte; Mono—monocyte; PMN—polymorphonuclear cells; VC—vernal conjunctivitis; +—present; — —not present; ±—may or may not be present.

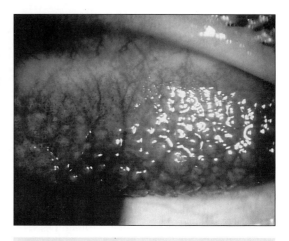

FIGURE 4 In vernal conjunctivitis, the conjunctival changes are primarily found on the upper tarsal plate, which include giant papilla typically described as "cobblestoning." These cobblestones persist during the quiescent phase of the disease, but become extremely swollen during the active phase, commonly in the spring (*ie*, vernal season). This figure also reveals mucus threads lying in the crypts of the papilla.

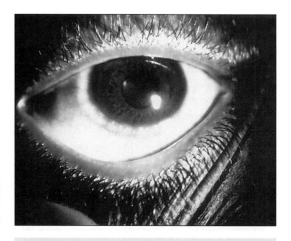

FIGURE 5 Vernal conjunctivitis may also present as a limbal infiltration of inflammatory cells commonly in the upper limbus. The blood vessels are not prominent and there is no mucus. Trantas' dots may be present and appear as small grayish-white epithelial collections of cellular debris (including eosinophil cationic protein) at the upper limbus.

Giant papillary conjunctivitis (GPC) is a mixed mast cell and lymphocyte-mediated process that has been directly linked to the continued use of contact lenses or other ocular prostheses. Symptoms include itching. Signs include a white or clear exudate on awakening, which chronically becomes thick and stringy, and the patient may develop Trantas' dots, limbal infiltration, and bulbar conjunctival hyperemia and edema. Upper tarsal papillary hypertrophy (*cobblestoning*; Fig. 4) has been described in 5% to 10% of soft and 3% to 4% of hard contact lens wearers.

Contact dermatitis involving the eyelids frequently causes the patient to seek medical attention because of the cutaneous reaction that elsewhere on the skin would be of less concern. The eyelid skin being soft, pliable, and thin increases its susceptibility to contact dermatitis. The eyelid skin is capable of developing significant swelling and redness with minor degrees of inflammation. Preservatives such as thimerosal, which is found in contact lens cleaning solutions, have been shown by patch tests to be one of the major culprits. Besides avoidance of the suspected allergen, topical steroids (1% creams) are used to resolve the inflammatory process.

MANAGEMENT

The treatment of ocular allergic disorders begins with nonpharmacologic interventions. These include avoidance of allergens; use of cold compresses, which provide symptomatic relief from ocular pruritus; and lubrication, which assists in the direct removal and dilution of allergens.

Decongestants are effective in reducing erythema and are widely used in combination with topical antihistamines [7] (Table 4). Antihistamines for ocular use include pheniramine maleate, pyrilamine maleate, and antazoline phosphate and levocabastine. Sodium cromoglycate is used to treat allergic conjunctivitis, and has an excellent safety record, though the original studies reflecting its clinical efficacy were marginal [8]. Topical sodium cromoglycate and lodoxamide have greater efficacy in the treatment of vernal conjunctivitis. Both solutions are applied four times a day, the dose being decreased to twice a day as symptoms permit.

Topical nonsteroidal anti-inflammatory drugs (NSAIDs) decrease conjunctival, ciliary, and episcleral hyperemia and ocular pruritus when compared with controls (vehicle-treated eyes) [9•]. Ketorolac tromethamine, an NSAID, significantly diminishes the ocular itching and conjunctival hyperemia associated with seasonal antigen-induced and allergic conjunctivitis. Unlike topical corticosteroids, NSAIDs do not mask ocular infections, affect wound healing, increase intraocular pressure, or contribute to cataract formation.

Topical corticosteroids are highly effective in the treatment of acute and chronic forms of allergic conjunctivitis and ocular hypersensitivity reactions. However, local administration of these medications is associated with increased intraocular pressure (glaucoma), viral infections, and cataract formation and should be prescribed in consultation with an ophthalmologist (Table 5). The efficacy of immunotherapy (*allergy desensitization*) is well established. It requires fewer medications, and higher concentrations of allergen are needed to induce a similar intensity of allergic symptoms of redness, pruritus, and swelling [10].

DIFFERENTIAL DIAGNOSIS

The differential diagnosis of ocular allergic disorders includes infectious causes (*eg*, chlamydial disease, molluscum contagiosum, Parinaud's oculoglandular syndrome); chronic forms of conjunctivitis (*eg*, giant papillary conjunctivitis, vernal conjunctivitis, atopic keratoconjunctivitis, superior limbic conjunctivitis, follicular conjunctivitis), and miscellaneous disorders including keratoconjunctivitis sicca, acne rosacea, ocular pemphigoid, and blepharoconjunctivitis.

Keratoconjunctivitis sicca is the most common entity confused with ocular allergic disorders. It is a dry eye syndrome that is commonly associated with an underlying systemic autoimmune disorder such as Sjogren's syndrome or rheumatoid arthritis. Clinically it occurs more commonly in postmenopausal women and in patients with AIDS. It is characterized by an insidious and progressive dysfunction of the lacrimal glands. Patients initially complain of a mildly irritated eye with excessive mucus production. Symptoms include a gritty, sandy sensation in the eye compared with the itching and burning many patients complain of with histamine release into the eye. Symptoms worsen throughout the day as the limited portion of the aqueous tear film evaporates. Exacerbation of symptoms also occurs in the winter months when heating systems decrease the relative humidity in the household to less than 24%. Schirmer's test demonstrates decreased tearing generally with 0 to 1 mm (normal > 4 mm) of wetting at 1 min and 2 to 3 mm (normal > 10 mm) at 5 min (Fig. 6). Rose bengal stain, providing a distinct staining pattern over the central portion of the eye, also assists in identifying the defect in tear film production. Biopsy of the lacrimal or minor salivary gland reveals an abnormal infiltration of lymphocytes. Treatment has primarily focused on the replacing tear fluid constituents with a variety of lubricants and artificial tears.

UVEITIS

Commonly, a red eye presenting to the generalist may also point to disorders affecting the internal uveal portion (iris, ciliary body, or choroid). However, these disorders would require the assistance of an ophthalmologist to better define the extent of ocular involvement.

Signs include diminished or hazy vision, black floating spots, severe pain, photophobia, blurred vision, and pupillary miosis. A ciliary/perilimbal flush can be easily confused with "conjunctivitis." The differential diagnosis of uveitic syndromes will often involve the assistance of an astute generalist, as they are commonly associated with a systemic autoimmune disorder, in approximately 50% of the cases with HLA-B27 spondyloarthropathy (such as ankylosing

TABLE 4 TREATMENT OF OCULAR ALLERGIES

Identification and avoidance of allergens
SAC
  Seasonal allergens
PAC
  Dust mites, animal dander

Cold compresses for ocular pruritus
Provision of all ocular medications in refrigerated form provides additional relief

Lubrication (artificial tears) applied topically PRN 2–4 times a day
Preservatives
  Most artificial tears use benzalkonium chloride, thimerosal, parabens, chlorobutanol, or sorbic acid
Preservative free
  Carboxymethylcellulose (0.5% or 1.0%) (Cellufresh, Celluvisc, Allergan, Irvine, CA)
  Hydroxypropyl cellulose (Lacrisert, Merck, West Point, PA)
  Hydroxypropyl methylcellulose (Tears Naturale Free, Alcon, Ft. Worth, TX)
  Polyvinyl alcohol + povidone (Refresh, Allergan)

Decongestants (vasoconstrictors)
Naphazoline hydrochloride, phenylephrine hydrocloride, tetrahydrozoline hydrochloride
  (applied topically PRN 2–4 times a day)

Antihistamines
Topical
  Levocabastine applied 4 times a day for 2 weeks
Oral
  When nonocular symptoms prevail

Mast cell stabilizing agents
Cromolyn sodium indicated in VC
Lodoxamide indicated in VC applied 4 times a day for 3 months

Nonsteroidal antiinflammatory agents
Topical
  Ketorolac applied 4 times a day for 1 week
Oral
  Aspirin in forms of VC

Steroids
Topical
Mild formulations (predinisolone acetate suspensions and prednisolone phosphate solutions)

Immunotherapy
Efficacy shown in SAC and PAC

Experimental
Topical immunophilins
  Cyclosporine A in VC, AKC
Cetirizine

SAC—seasonal allergic conjunctivitis; PAC—perennial allergic conjunctivitis; VC—vernal conjunctivitis; AKC—atopic keratoconjunctivitis.

TABLE 5 PATIENTS REQUIRING OPHTHALMOLOGIC CONSULTATION
Any patient using ocular steroids for more than 2 weeks for the presence of cataracts and level of intraocular pressure
Those with persistent qualities of any ocular complaint
The consideration of strong topical steroids or systemic steroids
With the presence of ciliary blush suggesting uveitis

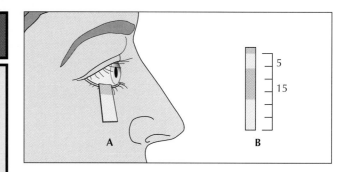

FIGURE 6 Tear secretion is clinically measured with Schirmer test paper. **A**, a piece of filter paper is placed in the inferior cul-de-sac of an unanesthetized eye at the junction of the lateral one-third and the medial two thirds of the eyelid. **B**, normal tear secretion wets more than 10 mm of filter paper at 5 minutes. Wetting of the test paper can be easily discerned by using paper that changes color on contact with tears (Eagle Vision, Memphis, TN).

spondylitis or Reiter's syndrome), or inflammatory bowel disease such as Crohn's disease; infections such as toxoplasmosis, syphilis, toxocariasis, tuberculosis, histoplasmosis, and AIDS; or sarcoid. Treatment requires the assistance of an ophthalmologist and includes the local use of corticosteroids (periocular or systemic drops), mydriatic/cycloplegic drops, as well as systemic immunomodulation or antibiotics.

REFERENCES AND RECOMMENDED READING

Recently published papers of particular interest have been highlighted as:

- Of interest

1. Allansmith MR, Ross RN: Ocular allergy. *Clin Allergy* 1988, 18:1–13.

2. Friedlaender M: Immunologic aspects of disease of the eye. *JAMA* 1992, 268:2869–2873.

3.• Bielory L, Frohman L: Allergic and immunologic disorders of the eye. *J Allergy Clin Immunol* 1992, 86:1–20.

4. Marrache F, Brunet D, Frandeboeuf J, et al.: The role of ocular manifestations in childhood allergy syndromes. *Rev Fr Allergol Immunol Clin* 1978, 18:151–155.

5. Weeke ER: Epidemiology of hay fever and perennial allergic rhinitis. *Monographs in Allergy* 1987, 21:1–20.

6. Bernstein DI, Gallagher JS, Grad M, Bernstein IL: Local ocular anaphylaxis to papain enzyme contained in a contact lens cleaning solution. *J Allergy Clin Immunol* 1984, 74:258–260.

7. Abelson MB, Paradis A, George MA, et al.: The effects of Vasocon-A in the allergen challenge model of acute conjunctivitis. *Arch Ophthalmol* 1990, 108:520–524.

8. Sorkin EM, Ward A: Ocular sodium cromoglycate: an overview of its therapeutic efficacy in allergic eye disease. *Drugs* 1986, 31:131–148.

9.• Bishop K, Abelson M, Cheetham J: Evaluation of flurbiprofen in the treatment of antigen-induced allergic conjunctivitis (abstract). *Invest Ophthalmol Vis Sci* 1990, 31:487.

10. Dreborg S, Agrell B, Foucard T, et al.: A double blind, multicenter immunotherapy trial in children, using a purified and standardized Cladosporium herbarum preparation. I. Clinical results. *Allergy* 1986, 41:131–140.

SELECT BIBLIOGRAPHY

Bielory L, Frohman L: Allergic and immunologic disorders of the eye. *J Allergy Clin Immunol* 1992, 86:1–20.

Bonini S, Bonini S, Bucci MG: Allergen dose response and late symptoms in a human model of ocular allergy. *J Allergy Clin Immunol* 1990, 86:869–876.

Friedleander MH: Current concepts in ocular allergy. *Ann Allergy* 1991, 67:5–13.

Urticaria and Angioedema 8

Roger W. Fox

Key Points

- Urticaria and angioedema occur in approximately 20% of the population.
- Chronic urticaria and angioedema are idiopathic in most cases.
- The differential diagnosis of urticaria and angioedema is extensive, and includes allergic, immunologic, and nonimmunologic etiologies. The laboratory evaluation must be directed by the history and physical exam, and only appropriate, cost-effective studies should be ordered.
- Antihistimines are the mainstay of treatment for acute and chronic urticaria and angioedema. Both classical and new generation antihistimines are effective in controlling some or all symptoms.
- Corticosteroids are often used in management of urticaria and angioedema, but the risk-benefit ratio must be strongly considered in the cases of chronic idiopathic urticaria and angioedema.

URTICARIA

Urticarial reactions are characterized by pale, localized swellings of the skin with a surrounding border of erythema. These pruritic lesions range from 1 or 2 mm (cholinergic urticaria; Fig. 1) to several centimeters (giant urticaria; Fig. 2) in diameter, and each may be round to serpiginous in configuration (Fig. 3). A single hive or a generalized outbreak (Fig. 4) may occur in an individual patient. Urticaria is typified by the wheal and flare reaction induced by injection of histamine into the superficial dermis, or by cutaneous mast cell degranulation. The individual lesions of urticaria arise suddenly, and persist for a brief period, usually less than 24 hours. The hives can recur in episodes, or continuous outbreaks of groupings of urticaria can develop until treatment intervenes or spontaneous remission occurs. With a few exceptions, such as physical urticaria and urticaria pigmentosa, the cause of urticaria cannot be identified by its physical appearance.

ANGIOEDEMA

Angioedema, in most cases, is a manifestation of the same pathogenetic process as urticaria, although angioedema is characterized by well-demarcated swelling of deeper cutaneous tissues. The sites of predilection are the palms, soles, face (Fig. 5), and oral area. The overlying skin appears to be erythematous, and the lesion is nonpruritic. The associated discomfort is described as a burning or pins-and-needles sensation. Angioedema persists longer than urticaria, because the quantity of accumulated tissue fluid is greater in angioedema. Urticaria and angioedema may coexist, or each may appear alone. The cumulative prevalence rate of these cutaneous manifestations in the general population is approximately 15% to 20%, and all ages are affected [1].

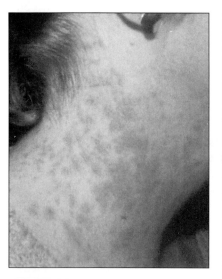

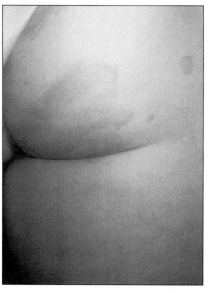

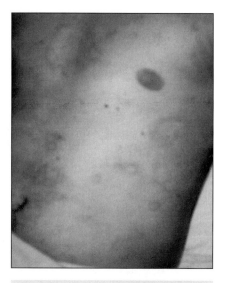

FIGURE 1 Cholinergic urticaria (heat-induced). Note the small punctate wheals with flare.

FIGURE 2 Giant urticaria.

FIGURE 3 Large urticaria with serpiginous border caused by drug-induced serum sickness.

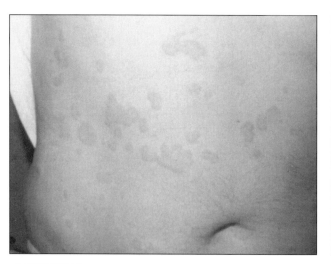

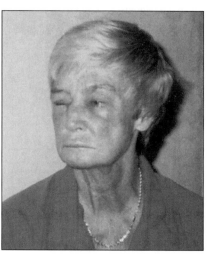

FIGURE 4 Generalized urticaria.

FIGURE 5 Facial angioedema.

CLASSIFICATION

Urticaria and angioedema are classified as acute or chronic, based on whether the episodes persist for more or less than 6 to 8 weeks. Acute urticaria and angioedema are short-lived, and are generally associated with allergic reactions to foods, Hymenoptera venom, or medications such as penicillin. Acute urticaria and angioedema occur more frequently in children and young adults, and represent the most common types of hives. In addition to the immediate, IgE-mediated hypersensitivity reaction, urticaria and angioedema are clinical manifestations of other immunologic and nonimmunologic etiologies, and each is categorized by a causative mechanism (Table 1) [2•]. Immunologic urticaria and angioedema include the classic allergic reaction, physical urticaria and complement-mediated urticaria and angioedema, and urticarial vasculitis. An IgE mechanism has been implicated in several of the physical

urticarias (Table 2), including dermatographism (Fig. 6), cold (Fig. 7) and solar urticaria [3]. These types of urticaria can be passively transferred to a normal skin site of a volunteer by injecting a serum sample from an affected patient. But not all physical urticarias are IgE-mediated and passively transferred with serum, for example, delayed-pressure urticaria, cholinergic urticaria, and four of six types of solar urticaria (Table 2).

Signs and Symptoms

The skin disorders listed in Table 1 that result from the activation of the complement cascade and subsequent generation of anaphylotoxins—C3a, C4a, and C5a—and other mediators, such as bradykinin, are a diverse group [4•,5]. Autoantibodies associated with systemic lupus erythematosus and thyroiditis, and immune complex formation associated with serum sickness, hepatitis B, and transfusion reactions result in urticaria and cutaneous vasculitis. In some patients, cutaneous leukocytoclastic vasculitis is a rare cause of chronic urticaria. Unlike the typical hive, the individual lesions of urticarial vasculitis may persist for 1 to 3 days. Some of the cutaneous vasculitis lesions are described as palpable purpura which are more often localized on the lower extremities. Constitutional symptoms associated with cutaneous vasculitis include myalgias, arthralgias, fever along with the laboratory findings of a leukocytosis, elevated erythrocyte sedimentation rate, and low total complement level (CH_{50}). A skin biopsy can be used to confirm the diagnosis. Hypocomplementemic urticarial vasculitis syndrome (HUVS) is associated with low complement levels and a low molecular weight precipitin (monomeric IgG), which binds to C1q. Other systemic symptoms and organ involvement (eg, lung, joints, and kidneys) are described in Table 1.

Hereditary and acquired C1 esterase inhibitor (C1INH) deficiencies are characterized clinically by recurrent attacks of angioedema involving the extremities, upper airway, or

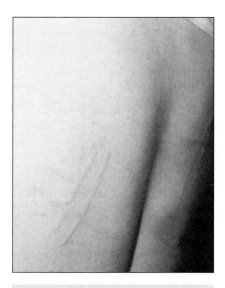

FIGURE 6 Dermatographism after stroking the back.

FIGURE 7 Cold-induced urticaria, after a positive ice cube test on forearm.

TABLE 1 CLASSIFICATION OF URTICARIA AND ANGIOEDEMA	
Immunologic mechanisms	**Nonimmunologic mechanisms**
IgE-mediated	Direct mast cell-releasing agents
Allergic reactions	Opiates and muscle relaxants
Foods	Radiocontrast media
Drugs	Others
Hymenoptera venom	Alteration of arachidonic acid metabolism (aspirin and other nonsteroidal antiinflammatory drugs)
Physical urticaria	Acute urticaria
Cholinergic urticaria	Chronic idiopathic urticaria exacerbations
Cold-dependent urticaria	Systemic diseases manifesting with urticaria/angioedema
Delayed pressure urticaria and angioedema	Urticaria pigmentosa/systemic mastocytosis
Solar urticaria	Angioedema associated with eosinophilia
Dermatographism	Chronic idiopathic urticaria
Aquagenic urticaria	
Vibratory angioedema	**Hereditary forms**
Local heat urticaria	Familial cold urticaria
Complement-mediated	Vibratory angioedema
Collagen vascular diseases	C3b inactivator deficiency
Systemic lupus erythematosus	Amyloidosis, deafness, and urticaria
Chronic cutaneous vasculitis	Hereditary angioedema
Hypocomplementemic urticarial vasculitis syndrome	
Thyroiditis	
Transfusion-related reactions	
ABO mismatched reactions	
IgA deficiency (IgG-IgA immune complexes)	
Hereditary angioedema and C1INH deficiencies	
Absent C1INH	
Nonfunctional C1INH	
Acquired C1INH deficiency	
Autoantibodies to C1INH	
Infections	
Hepatitis B	
Mononucleosis	
Other viral infections (mostly in children)	
Parasites	
Malignancies	
Serum sickness	
Paraproteinemias	

From Fox and Russell [2•]; with permission
C1INH—C1 esterase inhibitor.

TABLE 2 PHYSICAL URTICARIA AND/OR ANGIOEDEMA

Type	Diagnostic test	Treatment
Cold dependent	Ice cube test	H$_1$ antihistamines
Idiopathic (cutaneous only, or systemic)		
Associated with abnormal serum proteins	Cryoproteins	Cyproheptadine HCl
Cold agglutinins		Doxepin
Cryoglobulin		
Cryofibrinogen		
Donath-Landsteiner antibody		
Cold-induced cholinergic urticaria		
Cold-dependent dermatographism		
Delayed cold urticaria		
Familial cold urticaria		
Heat-induced disorder	Exercise	H$_1$ antihistamines
Cholinergic	Methacholine skin test	Hydroxyzine
Local heat urticaria		Danazol
Dermatographism	Stroke back	H$_1$ antihistamines
Idiopathic		
Following cutaneous allergic reaction		
Delayed form		
Mastocytosis/urticaria pigmentosa		
Delayed pressure angioedema	15-lb weight for 15 min	Corticosteroids
Idiopathic		
Associated with chronic idiopathic urticaria/angioedema		
Solar urticaria	Phototesting	Sunblock
		Antihistamines
		Antimalarials

Type	Wavelength (nm)
I	290–320 (UVB) passively transferred (IgE)
II	320–400 (UVA)
III	400–700 (visible)
IV	290–900 passively transferred (IgE)
V	280–500
VI	400–500 (protoporphyrin IX)

Differential diagnosis SLE/photoallergic drug reaction
PABA sunscreen blocks 280–320 (UVB)
Window glass blocks <320 (UVB)

Type	Diagnostic test	Treatment
Vibratory	Vortex for 4 min	H$_1$ antihistamines
		Terfenadine
		Diphenhydramine
Aquagenic urticaria	Water compresses	H$_1$ antihistamines
Urticaria pigmentosa	Stroke back	H$_1$ antihistamines
	Darier's sign	PUVA
	"String of pearls"	

UVA—ultraviolet A; UVB—ultraviolet B; SLE—systemic lupus erythematosus; PABA—para-aminobenzoic acid; PUVA—psoralen ultraviolet light.

gastrointestinal tract [6]. Attacks abate spontaneously, lasting up to 24 to 72 hours. Upper airway obstruction may become life-threatening.

Hereditary Versus Acquired Angioedema

Hereditary angioedema is managed with oral, attenuated androgens, stanozolol 1 to 4 mg/day or danazol 50 to 300 mg/day which stimulates the hepatic synthesis of C1INH [7]. Delayed-pressure urticaria/angioedema can be differentiated from the clinical criteria and normal complement studies. Two types of hereditary angioderma exist. Low levels of C1INH or nonfunctional C1INH in normal quantities must be assayed.

Hereditary—type I, type II

Acquired—acquired C1INH deficiency associated with lymphoproliferative disorders or autoantibody to C1INH. Angioedema associated with systemic lupus erythematosus, angioedema associated with eosinophilia, drug-induced (angiotensin-converting enzyme inhibitors), and idiopathic, delayed pressure must be included in the differential diagnosis of angioedema.

Among the nonimmunologic causes are drugs that directly perturbate the mast cell to degranulate. Opiates, some general anesthetics, dextran, and conventional radiocontrast materials are the best examples of medication and diagnostic agents that cause hives by a nonallergic mechanism. The nonsteroidal antiinflammatory drugs apparently alter arachidonic acid metabolism, which generates vasoactive substances such as leukotrienes, causing the formation of urticaria and angioedema in susceptible subjects. These drugs may exacerbate chronic, idiopathic urticaria in some patients.

The hereditary forms of urticaria and angioedema are of academic interest, and each must be excluded along with all other forms before the diagnosis of chronic idiopathic urticaria can be confirmed (Table 1).

Chronic urticaria and angioedema (>6 to 8 weeks' duration) are idiopathic in most cases (70 to 95%) [10,11]. Women are more commonly affected (Fig. 8). The average duration of such hives is 6 months, but some patients continue with persistent or recurring urticaria and angioedema for several years. Chronic hives generally occur daily, with lesions lasting

up to 12 hours. A diurnal pattern is apparent in many subjects with exacerbations of lesions at night and early morning. The typical skin biopsy obtained from a chronic urticarial lesion reveals, unlike vasculitis, non-necrotizing perivascular mononuclear cell infiltrate involving small venules. Activated T lymphocytes, monocytes, mast cells (with a six- to ninefold increase) and variable numbers of neutrophils or eosinophils are identified.

Mastocytosis

Mastocytosis is a spectrum of conditions characterized by mast cell hyperplasia. Clinical manifestations result principally from the reactions of mast cell-derived mediators [8]. Mastocytosis can be divided into presentations in which the skin is the only organ obviously involved (urticaria pigmentosa is one form; Fig. 9) and systemic mastocytosis, either with or without skin involvement. Most patients with systemic mastocytosis experience a chronic, indolent course with episodic exacerbations. Antihistamines are the mainstay of treatment [9]. Psoralen plus ultraviolet light A wavelength photochemotherapy is recommended for urticaria pigmentosa. For systemic mastocytosis, interferon α-2b is being used in clinical trials. Oral cromolyn 100 mg qid is recommended for the treatment of uncontrolled symptoms of urticaria pigmentosa and systemic mastocytosis.

CLINICAL EVALUATION

The possibility of an adverse or allergic reaction to venom, food, or a drug is always considered in the patient presenting with urticaria and angioedema. If a comprehensive clinical evaluation is indeterminate, a cost-effective laboratory work-up is needed (Figs. 10 and 11). Because most episodes of acute urticaria are self-limiting or associated with an obvious allergic reaction, no further evaluation is necessary, with these exceptions: when venom immunotherapy is required and when penicillin desensitization is mandatory. Basic laboratory studies are needed to further evaluate the patient with unrelenting urticaria (Table 3). After a complete cognitive review of the clinical information and laboratory data other immunologic studies may be ordered, although these tests are rarely required

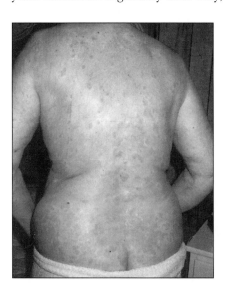

FIGURE 8
Severe, chronic idiopathic urticaria and angioedema (note patches of vitiligo on upper back). In addition, the patient was treated for hyperthyroidism.

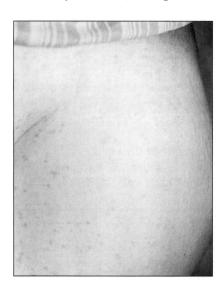

FIGURE 9
Urticaria pigmentosa (cutaneous mastocytosis), displaying numerous brown macules.

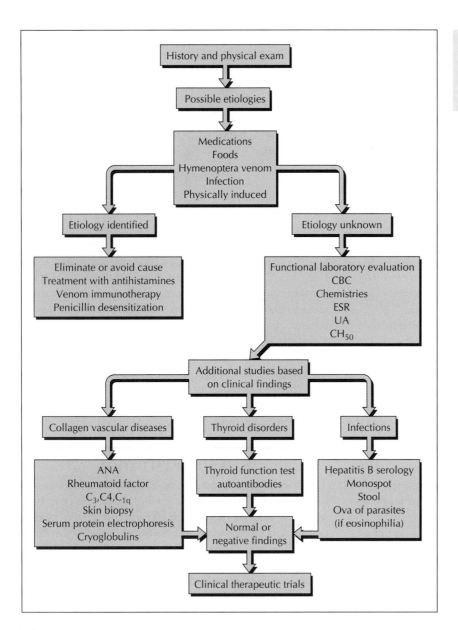

FIGURE 10 Algorithmic approach to the workup of urticaria. CBC—complete blood count; ESR—erythrocyte sedimentation rate; CH_{50}—total hemolytic complement.

in an otherwise healthy individual with only the cutaneous manifestations of urticaria and angioedema (as is the case with chronic idiopathic urticaria and angioedema). An evaluation for an occult malignancy or infection is not appropriate. *Hidden* food and food additive sensitivities are frequently considered as a cause of hives by the patient. A detailed food diary or elimination diet of a specific food or food additive can evaluate such possibilities. A hypoallergenic diet, such as a lamb and rice type diet, is sometimes required to determine if food is contributing. The double-blind, provocative oral challenge with a suspected food or food additive establishes a causal relationship, if one exists.

A skin biopsy is not recommended in the evaluation of most cases of urticaria and angioedema, unless cutaneous vasculitis or neutrophilic urticaria is strongly suspected [12].

TREATMENT

The rational therapy of urticaria is identification and then avoidance of the causative agents such as foods or medica-

tions, or of the specific conditions that induce physical urticarias. However, the precipitating cause is not always recognized immediately, or some other substance or activity is wrongly assigned. In any case, the acute phase requires treatment, which is usually accomplished satisfactorily with the classic H_1 antihistamines. When the urticarial reaction is severe or accompanied by signs or symptoms of anaphylaxis, subcutaneous epinephrine, parenteral antihistamines, both H_1 and H_2 antagonists, and systemic corticosteroids are indicated.

With chronic urticaria and angioedema, avoidance of potentiating factors such as alcoholic beverages, heat, emotional stress, aspirin, and exertion is advocated. The treatment of this condition is generally considered palliative rather than curative [2]. Long-term treatment is the rule for patients with chronic urticaria and angioedema; therefore, careful selection of therapy is mandatory in order to maximize the benefit without resulting in severe drug side effects (Table 4). Because most chronic urticaria is idiopathic, the physician should dispel patients' unrealistic expectations, if any, and

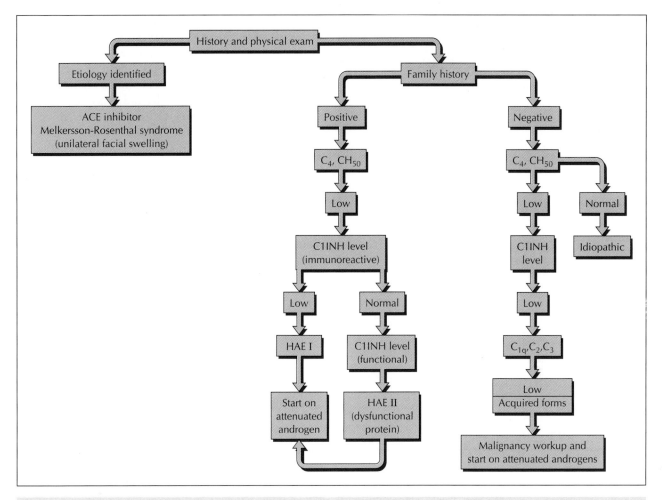

FIGURE 11 Algorithmic approach to the workup of patient with angioedema without associated urticaria. ACE—angiotensin-converting enzyme; CH$_{50}$—total hemolytic complement; C1INH—C1 esterase inhibitor.

TABLE 3 INVESTIGATION OF CHRONIC IDIOPATHIC URTICARIA AND/OR ANGIOEDEMA	
In all patients	**In certain patients**
History and physical exam	Stool for ova and parasites
Provocative challenges for physical urticarias	Antinuclear factor
CBC	Hepatitis B virus surface antigen and antibody
ESR	Allergy skin testing or RAST
Urinalysis	Thyroid autoantibodies
CH$_{50}$	Serum protein electrophoresis
Blood chemistry profile	Cryoproteins
	Skin biopsy

CBC—complete blood count; ESR—erythrocyte sedimentation rate; CH$_{50}$—total hemolytic complement; RAST—radioallergosorbent test.

reassure them that the prognosis is good and spontaneous remission is anticipated.

Antihistamines

H$_1$ antihistamines

Antihistamines are the mainstay of symptomatic management, mainly for pruritus. The diversity of mediators produced and the variety of inflammatory cells involved in urticarial reactions explain why antihistamines do not completely eliminate all the signs and symptoms of chronic urticaria. Sedation is common with most of the classic H$_1$ antagonists. The patient's tolerance for this side effect and others, such as dry mouth, urinary retention, and blurred vision, will dictate the maximum antihistamine dose to be utilized. The limiting nature of the side effects of the classic antihistamines may not allow optimal control of the hives.

TABLE 4 CHRONIC IDIOPATHIC URTICARIA AND ANGIOEDEMA TREATMENT PLAN

Begin daily H₁ antihistamine

Hydroxyline or other classical/new

May use combinations

Incomplete relief with above

Add daily H₂ antihistamine or doxepin

1 month trial

For severe, refractory cases

Add corticosteroid for remission

Alternate day, tapering schedule

Other reported therapies in open clinical trials—limited cases

To steroid-dependent group
  (urticarial vasculitis, neutrophilic urticaria)
  Nifedipine
  Dapsone
  Hydroxychloroagine
  Azulfidine
  Stanozolol
  Methotrexate
  Cyclosporin A

There are six groups of classic H₁ antihistamines (Table 5). The newer category of less sedating antihistamines, terfenadine, astemizole, and loratadine, are not necessarily more effective, but compliance improves when drugs are easy to take (qd and bid) and no symptomatic adverse effects are experienced. The United States Food and Drug Administration has issued a warning that terfenadine and astemizole can cause significant electrocardiogram abnormalities, including prolonged QT interval and ventricular tachyarrhythmia, such as torsades de pointes. The cardiotoxicity caused by these antihistamines is caused by overdose, by drugs that inhibit the hepatic metabolism such as erythromycin and ketoconazole, and by association with cirrhosis and hypokalemia. Otherwise, terfenadine and astemizole are considered safe (Table 5).

In general, when one antihistamine is ineffective or tachyphylaxis develops, select another antihistamine from a separate pharmacologic group. Hydroxyzine is traditionally first-line treatment for chronic idiopathic urticaria, and it remains the standard to which all other antihistamines are compared. When choosing two antihistamines for the patient with the more difficult chronic urticaria, choose from different groups. The combination of hydroxyzine and cyproheptadine is particularly effective [13]. A popular combination is a nonsedating antihistamine in the morning and a sedating antihistamine, such as hydroxyzine, at bedtime. Patients with chronic urticaria should not be managed with *as needed* antihistamines exclusively, as this therapeutic rationale does not approach the problem from a preventive standpoint. Once an effective dose schedule is established with an antihistamine, the total dose can be gradually reduced according to the schedule until the lowest effective dose is found or the drug is withdrawn.

H₂ antihistamines

The patient with inadequate symptomatic control on an H₁ or combination of H₁ antihistamines at the highest tolerated or recommended dose should be prescribed an H₂ antihistamine. Cimetidine, 300 mg four times daily, or ranitidine, 150 mg twice daily can be combined with an H₁ antihistamine. H₂ receptors make up about 10% to 15% of the total number of histamine receptors in the cutaneous vasculature [14]. The H₂ antihistamine should be discontinued after 3 to 4 weeks if there is no definitive clinical benefit.

TABLE 5 CLASSIC H₁ ANTIHISTAMINES EXAMPLES

Class	Generic name	Trade name	Doses (divided daily)
Piperazines	Hydroxyzine	Atarax (Roerig)	40–200 mg
Piperidines	Cyproheptadine	Periactin (Merck)	8–32 mg
	Azatadine	Optimine (Schering)	2–4 mg
Ethanolamines	Diphenhydramine	Benadryl (Parke-Davis)	25–200 mg
	Clemastine	Tavist (Sandoz)	2.6–5.3 mg
Ethylenediamines	Tripelennamine	PBZ (Geigy)	75–200 mg
Propylamines	Chlorpheniramine	Chlor-Trimeton (Schering)	16–64 mg
Phenothialines	Methdilazine	Tacaryl (Westwood Squibb)	8–32 mg
New H₁ antihistamines			
	Terfenadine	Seldane (Marion Merrell Dow)	120 mg
	Astemizole	Hismanal (Janssen)	10 mg
	Loratadine	Claritin (Schering)	10 mg
	*Cetirizine		10 mg

*Not currently available in the United States.

Doxepin

Doxepin, a heterocyclic variant of amitriptyline, is approximately 800 times more potent than diphenhydramine in vitro on a molar basis, and doxepin is six times more potent than cimetidine. Clinical efficacy for doxepin in the management of chronic idiopathic urticaria has been established in doses ranging from 30 to 150 mg/day [15,16]. Doxepin is now considered a first-line treatment for chronic idiopathic urticaria. A concentrated syrup of doxepin allows for flexibility in dosing for the sedated patient.

Corticosteroids

Corticosteroids are very effective in suppressing most signs and symptoms of all categories of urticaria. The physical urticarias (excluding delayed pressure urticaria/angioedema) are the exception. Corticosteroids should be judiciously prescribed only in severe chronic urticaria and for uncontrolled exacerbations of urticaria and angioedema [11]. Their exact pharmacologic action is not completely understood. The patient should be tapered off the corticosteroids, with complete withdrawal of the drug prior to the onset of significant side effects as the desirable objective. An alternate-day regimen of corticosteroids, prednisone 25 to 40 mg or equivalent dose of methylprednisolone, is used in the management of the patient with *steroid-dependent* chronic urticaria to maintain a clinical remission. Several months of therapy may be required. Corticosteroid-sparing agents and alternative drugs have been reported in the management of severe chronic idiopathic urticaria [2•,17•]. Prescribing such treatment without adequate knowledge of side effects and effectiveness places the patient at considerable risk from an unproven drug.

CONCLUSION

Standard treatments for urticaria and angioedema are well established. Further evaluations of unsubstantiated or new treatments are needed before they can be generally accepted, even in the most severe cases of chronic idiopathic urticaria. Future treatments will be guided by scientific discoveries on the molecular and cellular interactions involved in the pathophysiology of chronic idiopathic urticaria and angioedema.

REFERENCES AND RECOMMENDED READING

Recently published papers of particular interest have been highlighted as:

• Of interest

1. Warin RP, Champion RH: Urticaria. London: WB Saunders, 1974.
2.• Fox RW, Russell D: Drug therapy of chronic urticaria and angioedema. In *Pharmacologic Management of the Difficult to Treat Allergic Patient.* Edited by Kemp J. Philadelphia: WB Saunders; 1991:45–63.
3. Casale TB, Sampson HA, Hanifin J, *et al.*: Guide to physical urticarias. *J Allergy Clin Immunol* 1988, 82:758–763.
4.• Kaplan AP: Urticaria and angioedema. In *Allergy: Principles and Practice.* Edited by Middleton E, Reed CE, Ellis F, *et al.*, edn 4. St. Louis: Mosby; 1993:1553–1580.
5. Sanchez NP, Winkleman R, Schroeter AL, *et al.*: The clinical and histopathologic spectrum of urticaria vasculitis: study of 40 cases. *J Am Acad Dermatol* 1982, 7:599–605.
6. Frank MM, Gelfand JA, Atkinson JP: Hereditary angioedema: the clinical syndrome and its management. *Ann Intern Med* 1976, 84:580–507.
7. Sheffer AL, Fearon DT, Austen KF: Clinical and biochemical effects of stanozolol therapy for hereditary angioedema. *J Allergy Clin Immunol* 1981, 68:181–187.
8. Metcalfe DD: Classification and diagnosis of mastocytosis: current status. *J Invest Dermatol* 1991, 96:2S–4S.
9. Metcalfe DD: The treatment of mastocytosis: an overview. *J Invest Dermatol* 1991, 96:55S–59S.
10. Paul E, Greilich KD, Dominante G: Epidemiology of urticaria. *Monogr Allergy* 1987, 21:87–115.
11. Kaplan AP: Urticaria and angioedema. In *Allergy.* Edited by Kaplan AP. New York: Churchill Livingstone, 1985:439–471.
12. Winkleman RK, Reizner GT: Diffuse dermal neutrophilia in urticaria. *Hum Pathol* 1988, 19:389–393.
13. Harvey RP, Wegs J, Schocket AL: A controlled trial of therapy and chronic urticaria. *J Allergy Clin Immunol* 1981, 68:262–266.
14. Harvey RP, Schocket AL: The effect of H1 and H2 blockade on cutaneous histamine response in man. *J Allergy Clin Immunol* 1980, 65:136–139.
15. Goldgobel AB: Efficacy of doxepin in the treatment of chronic idiopathic urticaria. *J Allergy Clin Immunol* 1986, 78:867–871.
16. Greene SL, Reed CE, Schroeter AL: Double-blind crossover study comparing doxepin with diphenhydramine for the treatment of chronic urticaria. *J Am Acad Dermatol* 1985, 12:669–664.
17.• Czarnetzki BM: Chronic Urticaria. In *Current Therapy in Allergy, Immunology, and Rheumatology*, edn 4. Edited by Lichtenstein LM, Fauci AS. St. Louis: Mosby; 1992:49–52.

Anaphylaxis and Anaphylactoid Reactions

Michael S. Blaiss

9

Key Points
- Anaphylaxis and anaphylactoid reactions can be produced by various agents, can affect virtually all organ systems, and can range from mild to fatal symptoms within minutes.
- The most common causes of anaphylaxis in man are medications, stinging insects, and foods.
- Treatment of anaphylaxis requires rapid assessment and management of the patient with the use of epinephrine as the cornerstone of therapy.
- Prevention of anaphylaxis requires identifying the causative agent and educating the patient in avoiding future exposure.
- All patients with a history of anaphylaxis should wear medical identification jewelry and should be equipped and educated regarding the use of an auto-injector of epinephrine.

Anaphylaxis is an immediate hypersensitivity reaction that is unexpected and potentially fatal. It results from the release of potent pharmacologic mediators from tissue mast cells and peripheral blood basophils. Anaphylactoid reactions have the same clinical manifestations as anaphylaxis but do not involve IgE in the pathogenesis. Anaphylaxis and anaphylactoid reactions can be produced by various agents and can affect virtually all organ systems. They can progress from mild symptoms, such as pruritus and urticaria, to life-threatening hypotension and cardiac arrhythmias. The physician must rapidly diagnose these conditions and begin treatment immediately to prevent possible death.

PATHOPHYSIOLOGY OF ANAPHYLAXIS

Anaphylaxis is an IgE-mediated reaction to a foreign antigen such as a protein, polysaccharide, or hapten. In susceptible individuals, initial exposure to an antigen results in the formation of specific IgE antibodies to that antigen. These antibodies attach to receptors on the surface of mast cells and basophils. On re-exposure, the antigen can bind and crosslink the IgE antibodies on these cells. This leads to changes in the cell membrane with degranulation and release of preformed chemical mediators and generation of new potent mediators. It is these mediators that produce the clinical symptoms of anaphylaxis (Fig. 1).

Anaphylactoid reactions can be initiated by several mechanisms: 1) activation of the complement system resulting in the formation of anaphylatoxins $C3_a$ and $C5_a$, which can directly trigger mast cell and basophil degranulation; 2) direct action of certain agents on mast cells and basophils, stimulating the release of mediators; this mechanism is independent of IgE and complement; and 3) situations where the involvement of mast cells and basophils is not apparent. Treatment of classic anaphylaxis and anaphylactoid reactions is identical, because the symptoms in both conditions are caused by the release of chemical mediators.

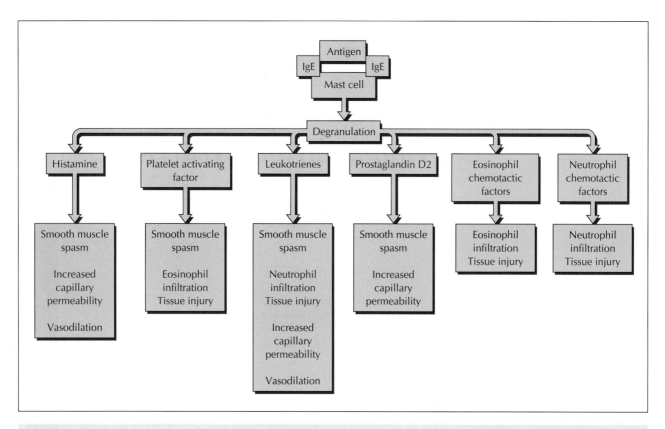

FIGURE 1 Major chemical mediators of anaphylaxis and their actions.

SIGNS AND SYMPTOMS OF ANAPHYLAXIS

Anaphylaxis may present with symptoms ranging from mild to fatal within minutes. The majority of reactions occur within 1 hour after exposure to the provoking agent. However, in some individuals the time course of the symptoms may be delayed for several hours. The onset of symptoms depends on the dose of the inciting agent, the route of administration, and the degree of the host's immunologic responsiveness to the triggering substance. In some patients, a protracted or a biphasic reaction takes place [1]. A biphasic reaction occurs when symptoms reappear several hours after resolution of the immediate anaphylactic manifestations.

Four organ systems are most commonly involved: the skin, gastrointestinal tract, respiratory tract, and cardiovascular system. The common clinical symptoms that may occur in each organ system during anaphylaxis are listed in Figure 2. Usually only the skin is involved in mild cases, whereas in more severe episodes virtually every organ system can be affected. Fatal anaphylaxis usually results from upper airway obstruction or cardiovascular collapse.

When the signs and symptoms of anaphylaxis occur within minutes of exposure to a known causative agent, the diagnosis of anaphylaxis is easy to make. However, if a cause and effect situation is not obvious, the diagnosis could be confused with many other medical emergencies that clinically mimic anaphylaxis (Table 1). The condition most frequently mistaken for anaphylaxis is a vasodepressor or vasovagal reaction. These reactions are usually preceded by a stressful or frightening event and are characterized by syncope and hypotension. These attacks can usually be distinguished from anaphylaxis by the absence of pruritus, tachycardia, urticaria, and bronchospasm. In general, laboratory tests are seldom needed to make the diagnosis of anaphylaxis. An anaphylactic reaction can be verified by measuring a serum mast-cell tryptase level [2]. Unlike plasma histamine, which usually declines within 30 minutes of an anaphylactic reaction, mast-cell tryptase level peaks 60 to 90 minutes after anaphylaxis and then declines with a half-life of approximately 2 hours.

CAUSATIVE AGENTS

Hundreds of agents have been documented as causes of anaphylaxis. Medications comprise one of the largest groups of substances that provoke anaphylaxis (Table 2), with penicillin designated as the major causative agent [3]. Penicillin skin testing (discussed in the chapter on drug reactions) can be performed to confirm allergy in individuals whose history is suggestive of an anaphylactic reaction [4].

Foods are another major source of anaphylaxis. Legumes (peanuts, peas, soybeans, and beans), nuts, fish, shellfish, cow's milk, and eggs are the most common food allergens (Table 3). Recently, several reports have documented that anaphylaxis to foods is a more common cause of fatalities in adults and children than previously recognized [5,6••].

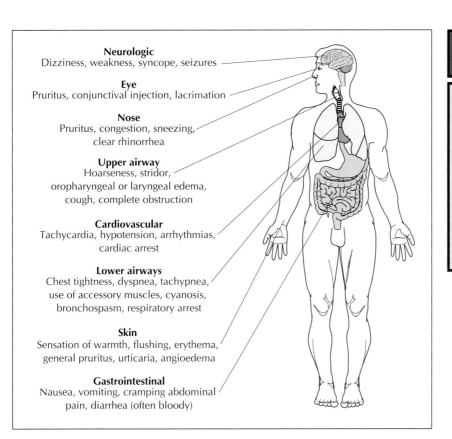

Neurologic
Dizziness, weakness, syncope, seizures

Eye
Pruritus, conjunctival injection, lacrimation

Nose
Pruritus, congestion, sneezing, clear rhinorrhea

Upper airway
Hoarseness, stridor, oropharyngeal or laryngeal edema, cough, complete obstruction

Cardiovascular
Tachycardia, hypotension, arrhythmias, cardiac arrest

Lower airways
Chest tightness, dyspnea, tachypnea, use of accessory muscles, cyanosis, bronchospasm, respiratory arrest

Skin
Sensation of warmth, flushing, erythema, general pruritus, urticaria, angioedema

Gastrointestinal
Nausea, vomiting, cramping abdominal pain, diarrhea (often bloody)

FIGURE 2 Clinical manifestations of anaphylaxis.

TABLE 1 DIFFERENTIAL DIAGNOSIS OF ANAPHYLAXIS

Vasodepressor or vasovagal response
Globus hystericus
Hyperventilation syndrome
Carcinoid
Hereditary angioneurotic edema
Systemic mastocytosis
Foreign-body aspiration
Drug overdose
Severe asthma
Pheochromocytoma

TABLE 2 MEDICINAL AGENTS CAUSING ANAPHYLAXIS

Antibiotics	Chemotherapeutic agents	Miscellaneous
Penicillin and derivatives	Asparaginase	Aspirin
Cephalosporins	Vincristine	Nonsteroidal antiinflammatory agents
Tetracycline	Cyclosporine	Allergy extracts
Chloramphenicol	Methotrexate	Human gamma globulin
Sulfonamides	5-Fluorouracil	Insulin
Ciprofloxacin		Radiocontrast media
Nitrofurantoin		Heparin
Vancomycin		Vaccines (tetanus, measles, influenza, mumps)
		Dextran
		Opiates
		Protamine
		Local anesthetics
		Glucocorticosteroids
		Antithymocyte globulin

TABLE 3 FOODS CAUSING ANAPHYLAXIS

Legumes
 (peanuts, beans, peas, soybeans)
Shellfish
 (shrimp, lobster, crab, crawfish)
Milk
Eggs
Wheat
Fish
Nuts
 (cashews, almonds, pecans, walnuts)
Seeds (sesame, sunflower, poppy, cottonseed)
Spices (cinnamon, nutmeg, mustard, sage)
Fruits (apples, bananas, peaches, oranges, melons)
Chocolate
Potato
Corn

There are numerous other agents known to provoke anaphylaxis in humans (Table 4). Up to 0.5% of the population has had anaphylaxis to insect stings. These insects belong to the order *Hymenoptera* and include fire ants, hornets, yellow jackets, wasps, and honey bees. All patients with anaphylaxis from one of these insects should have venom skin testing to document sensitivity [7].

Rubber or latex products have recently been recognized as an important cause of anaphylactic reactions [8]. Many reports have documented anaphylaxis during surgical and radiologic procedures due to latex objects such as gloves and catheters. Three groups appear to be at high risk for development of anaphylaxis to latex: medical personnel, people with a history of pruritus from exposure to latex objects, and patients with spina bifida. Skin testing and the radioallergosorbent test (RAST) for latex are reliable methods of diagnosing patients with latex allergy. Since there is not a standardized extract in the United States for latex skin testing, the RAST is more useful at this time [9].

Exercise has also been documented as a trigger of severe anaphylactoid reactions [10]. A certain group of patients with exercise-induced anaphylaxis develop symptoms only if they exercise within 2 to 4 hours of eating. This condition is called food-dependent exercise-induced anaphylaxis [11]. Some patients with this condition can develop symptoms if they exercise after any meal, whereas others suffer from exercise-induced anaphylaxis only after eating certain foods such as celery, wheat, shellfish, and oysters. All patients with these conditions should exercise with a companion capable of administering epinephrine. Individuals with food-dependent exercise-induced anaphylaxis should avoid exercise within 2 to 4 hours of eating.

In rare cases, no identifiable precipitant for the patient's anaphylaxis can be found. These individuals are classified as having idiopathic anaphylaxis [12•]. Patients who are victims of frequent and life-threatening episodes of idiopathic anaphylaxis may need prophylactic treatment with oral H_1 antihistamines and prednisone.

TREATMENT OF ANAPHYLAXIS

All physicians should have ready access to equipment to treat anaphylaxis (Table 5). Since anaphylaxis can be a life-threatening event, assessment and management must begin without delay (Table 6). This requires a rapid evaluation of recent events and a medical history including known allergies, present medications, and underlying health problems. The severity of the clinical manifestations, rate of progression of symptoms, evaluation of vital signs, and assessment of the airway should be performed quickly.

Epinephrine is the cornerstone of therapy for anaphylaxis [13]. Many deaths from anaphylaxis could be prevented if epinephrine was given at the first sign of symptoms. Epinephrine has both α- and β-adrenergic properties that reverse the symptoms of anaphylaxis. The α-adrenergic effects elevate diastolic blood pressure and increase systemic vascular resistance, while the β-adrenergic stimulation leads to bronchodilation.

TABLE 4 MISCELLANEOUS CAUSES OF ANAPHYLAXIS
Stinging insects (yellow jackets, white-face hornets, yellow hornets, honeybees, wasps, fire ants)
Physical agents (cold, exercise)
Preservatives (sulfites, benzoates)
Latex (rubber)
Idiopathic

TABLE 5 EQUIPMENT FOR TREATMENT OF ANAPHYLAXIS
Medications
Epinephrine 1:1000 for SC, IM
Epinephrine 1:100,000 for IV
Corticosteroids (methylprednisolone, hydrocortisone)
H_1 antihistamines (diphenhydramine, hydroxyzine)
H_2 antihistamines (cimetidine, ranitidine)
β_2 agonists (albuterol)
Aminophylline
Glucagon
Dopamine
Norepinephrine bitartrate
Oxygen, face mask, nasal cannula
IV fluids (normal saline, albumin)
Airway kit, Ambu bag, laryngoscope, scalp and 11-gauge needle for cricothyroidotomy
Electrocardiogram
Sphygmomanometer and stethoscopes
Tourniquets
SC—subcutaneous; IM—intramuscular; IV—intravenous.

TABLE 6 INITIAL MANAGEMENT OF ANAPHYLAXIS
Place patient in recumbent position with feet elevated
Secure and maintain airway, administer oxygen at 4–6 L/min; if life-threatening airway obstruction occurs, place endotracheal tube; if this is not possible, cricothyroidotomy
Epinephrine 1:1000, 0.01 mL/kg up to 0.30 mL SC, repeat every 15 min if necessary
Tourniquet above injection site and infiltrate site with additional epinephrine 1:1000, 0.01 mL/kg 0.10–0.20 mL SC; release the tourniquet for 5 min every 10 min
Administer H_1 antihistamine (diphenhydramine 1–2 mg/kg IM or IV up to 50 mg every 4–6 h)
Administer corticosteroids (hydrocortisone 5–10 mg/kg up to 500 mg IV every 4–6 h)
Administer H_2 antihistamine (ranitidine 12.5–50 mg IV every 6–8 h)
Monitor vital signs frequently
IM—intramuscular; IV—intravenous; SC—subcutaneous.

Although not effective in the initial management of anaphylaxis, H$_1$ antihistamines, H$_2$ antihistamines, and corticosteroids are commonly used to supplement epinephrine. H$_1$ antihistamines help decrease the pruritus and cutaneous symptoms, whereas H$_2$ antihistamines in conjunction with H$_1$ antihistamines may be beneficial in treating histamine-induced hypotension, flushing, cardiac arrhythmias, and atrioventricular conduction delay [14,15]. Corticosteroids may help reduce or prevent a protracted or late-phase reaction of anaphylaxis.

Further measures may need to be taken if the above intervention does not control the patient's anaphylactic symptoms (Table 7). Treatment with volume expanders is indicated if the patient remains hypotensive after subcutaneous epinephrine administration. Patients having hypotension during anaphylaxis due to stinging insects are found to have elevated levels of endogenous epinephrine, norepinephrine, and angiotensin II [16]. This may explain why some patients with hypotension do not respond to epinephrine and need fluid administration. If volume expanders do not stabilize blood pressure then pressor agents, norepinephrine bitartrate, or dopamine should be administered. Cardiac arrhythmias can result from a combination of chemical mediators, hypoxia, hypotension, and from the epinephrine itself. This condition requires the use of specific antiarrhythmic agents. Resistance to epinephrine may be seen in patients treated with β-blocking agents [17]. In these situations, the use of glucagon can partially overcome this resistance [18]. Bronchospastic symptoms should be managed with β$_2$-agonist aerosols and IV-aminophylline therapy. Patients with severe anaphylaxis should be hospitalized and monitored for at least 24 hours because of the possibility of a protracted or biphasic course.

PREVENTION OF ANAPHYLAXIS

Prevention of recurrence of anaphylaxis is aimed at identifying the etiologic agent and educating the patient on avoidance of this agent (Table 8). In cases where the reaction may have been IgE-mediated such as foods, certain medications, and stinging insects, allergy skin testing can be performed to confirm the diagnosis. IgE sensitivity to certain medications such as insulin and protamine can also be accomplished by RAST. The list of agents that can be evaluated by this method is growing.

Certain pharmaceutical agents should be avoided by patients with a history of anaphylaxis. Patients treated with beta blocking agents who experience anaphylaxis may have profound hypotension and may not respond to epinephrine. In addition, angiotensin-converting enzyme (ACE) inhibitors may potentiate anaphylaxis. This has been described in patients who developed anaphylactoid reactions to high-flux membrane dialysis when treated with ACE inhibitors [19].

In certain cases where avoidance of an anaphylactic agent is not possible, other measures of prevention are available. Venom immunotherapy should be offered to all patients with documented *Hymenoptera* anaphylaxis [20]. It has been shown to be effective in the prevention of anaphylaxis in over 95% of patients who were re-stung by insects. In patients showing

positive skin tests to penicillin to whom penicillin or one of its derivatives must be administered, desensitization protocols are available. These procedures should be done in a setting equipped for treating anaphylaxis by physicians well versed in the procedure.

There are many steps that the physician can take to prevent anaphylaxis (Table 9). A detailed history of drug reactions should be obtained prior to prescribing any medication. Whenever possible, medications should be given orally instead of parenterally, because the incidence of allergic drug reactions is much lower when given by the oral route. When a medication is given by the intramuscular route, the patient should remain in the physician's office for at least 30 minutes to be observed for possible allergic reactions. All medical charts of patients who have had previous anaphylactic reactions should be clearly marked with the

---

TABLE 7 SECONDARY TREATMENT OF ANAPHYLAXIS

If hypotensive after epinephrine therapy, administer IV normal saline or colloids to replace intravascular fluid loss

If hypotension persists, administer norepinephrine bitartrate 2–4 µg/min or dopamine 2–10 µg/kg/min to maintain blood pressure

If hypotension is due to β-blockage, administer glucagon 1–5 mg IV over 1 min and begin continuous infusion 1–5 mg/h

Administer specific antiarrhythmic agents if indicated

For persistent bronchospasm, administer aerosolized β$_2$ agonist every 2–4 h; if no improvement, aminophylline 6 mg/kg IV over 20 min, then continuous IV aminophylline drip at 0.9 mg/kg/h; monitor theophylline level

Keep patient in observation for at least 24 h in case of a protracted course

IV—intravenous.

TABLE 8 STEPS FOR PREVENTION OF ANAPHYLAXIS FOR THE PATIENT

Patient education about the incriminating agent and cross-reacting substances

Patients should discard all unused medications

Patients should avoid β-blocker agents and ACE inhibitors which might potentiate anaphylaxis

Patients should wear medical information jewelry stating anaphylactic sensitivities

Patients should be instructed in self-administration of epinephrine

Patients with food-induced anaphylaxis need to check all labels for the offending agent and to eat at restaurants where they can obtain information about ingredients used in foods on the menu

ACE—angiotensin-converting enzyme.

TABLE 9 STEPS IN PREVENTION OF ANAPHYLAXIS FOR THE PHYSICIAN

Take a detailed medical history noting past anaphylactic reactions

Mark all medical records clearly regarding past anaphylactic reactions

Require a clear indication of a drug's use

Administer chemically and antigenically non-cross-reacting medications

Administer medication orally if possible

Patients should be observed 30 min after an injection

Be prepared to treat anaphylaxis at all times

Have emergency equipment available

Use pretreatment and desensitization protocols when indicated

---

patient's sensitivities. Patients with a history of anaphylaxis should wear a medical identification bracelet (Medic-Alert; Turlock, CA) to inform others of their known allergies. They should be equipped and educated in the use of self-administered epinephrine such as Epi-Pen (Center Labs; Port Washington, NY) and ANA-KIT or ANA-Guard (Hollister Stier; Spokane, WA). If exposure to the anaphylactic agent occurs, patients should immediately use the epinephrine and promptly go to the nearest medical facility for evaluation.

REFERENCES AND RECOMMENDED READING

Recently published papers of particular interest have been highlighted as:
• Of interest
•• Of outstanding interest

1. Stark B, Sullivan T: Biphasic and protracted anaphylaxis. *J Allergy Clin Immunol* 1986, 78:76–83.

2. Schwartz L, Metcalfe D, Miller J, *et al.*: Tryptase levels as an indicator of mast-cell activation in systemic anaphylaxis and mastocytosis. *N Engl J Med* 1987, 316:1622–1626.

3. Weiss M, Adkinson N: Immediate hypersensitivity reactions to penicillin and related antibiotics. *Clin Allergy* 1988, 18:515–540.

4. Sullivan T, Wedner H, Shatz G, *et al.*: Skin testing to detect penicillin allergy. *J Allergy Clin Immunol* 1981, 68:171–180.

5. Yunginger J, Sweeney K, Sturner W, *et al.*: Fatal food-induced anaphylaxis. *JAMA* 1988, 260:1450–1452.

6.•• Sampson H, Mendelson L, Rosen J: Fatal and near-fatal food-induced anaphylaxis in children. *N Engl J Med* 1992, 316:1622–1626.

7. Hoffman D: Allergy to biting insects. *Clin Rev Allergy* 1987, 5:177–190.

8. Slater J: Rubber anaphylaxis. *N Engl J Med* 1989, 320:1126–1130.

9. Kelly K, Kurup V, Zacharisen M, *et al.*: Skin and serologic testing in the diagnosis of latex allergy. *J Allergy Clin Immunol* 1993, 91:1140–1145.

10. Sheffer A, Austen K: Exercise-induced anaphylaxis. *J Allergy Clin Immunol* 1984, 73:699–703.

11. Kidd J, Cohen S, Sosman A, Fink J: Food-dependent exercise-induced anaphylaxis. *J Allergy Clin Immunol* 1983, 71:407–411.

12.• Wong S, Dykewicz M, Patterson R: Idiopathic anaphylaxis. A clinical summary of 175 patients. *Arch Intern Med* 1990, 150:1323–1328.

13. Barach E, Nowak R, Lee T, *et al.*: Epinephrine for the treatment of anaphylaxis. *JAMA* 1984, 251:2118–2122.

14. Lieberman P: The use of antihistamines in the prevention and treatment of anaphylaxis and anaphylactoid reactions. *J Allergy Clin Immunol* 1990, 86:684–686.

15. Kaliner M, Sigler R, Summers R, Shelhamer J: Effects of infused histamine: analysis of the effects of H-1 and H-2 histamine receptor antagonists on cardiovascular and pulmonary responses. *J Allergy Clin Immunol* 1981, 68:365–371.

16. van der Linden P, Struyvenberg A, Kraaijenhagen R, *et al.*: Anaphylactic shock after insect-sting challenge in 138 persons with a previous insect-sting reaction. *Ann Intern Med* 1993, 118:161–168.

17. Toogood J: Risk of anaphylaxis in patients receiving beta-blocker drugs. *J Allergy Clin Immunol* 1988, 81:1–5.

18. Zaloga G, DeLaney W, Holmboe E, Chernow B: Glucagon reversal of hypotension in a case of anaphylactoid shock. *Ann Intern Med* 1986, 105:65–66.

19. Verresen L, Waer M, Vanrenterghem Y, Michielsen P: Angiotensin-converting-enzyme inhibitors and anaphylactoid reactions to high-flux membrane dialysis. *Lancet* 1990, 336:1360–1362.

20. Hunt K, Valentine M, Sobotka A, *et al.*: A controlled trial of immunotherapy in insect hypersensitivity. *N Engl J Med* 1978, 299:157–161.

SELECT BIBLIOGRAPHY

Atkinson TP, Kaliner MA: Anaphylaxis. *Med Clin North Am* 1992, 76(4):841–855.

Levy JH, Levi R: Diagnosis and treatment of anaphylactic/anaphylactoid reactions. *Monogr Allergy* 1992, 30:130–144.

Marquardt D, Wasserman S: Anaphylaxis. In *Allergy Principles and Practice*, edn 4. Edited by Middleton E, Reed C, Ellis E, *et al.* St. Louis: Mosby-Year Book; 1993:1525–1536.

Yungiger J. Anaphylaxis. *Ann Allergy* 1992, 69:87–96.

Insect and Arthropod Bites and Stings

Richard F. Lockey

10

Key Points

- Several kinds of reactions occur secondary to arthropod bites and stings including toxic reactions, large local reactions, and systemic allergic reactions.

- The most serious adverse reactions secondary to arthropod bites and stings are systemic IgE-mediated reactions that result in anaphylaxis.

- Systemic allergic reactions are primarily caused by Hymenoptera insects, which include honeybees, wasps, yellow jackets, hornets, and ants.

- Systemic allergic reactions secondary to Hymenoptera stings are treated with allergen immunotherapy. Such therapy, appropriately administered, reduces the risk of stinging anaphylaxis from 40% to 60% to less than 5%.

- Systemic non-life-threatening reactions induced by stings of bees, wasps, yellow jackets, and hornets confined to the skin (urticaria, angioedema, erythema, and generalized pruritus) do not require venom immunotherapy in children younger than 15 or 16 years of age.

Arthropod bites and stings inflicted by different species of insects, arachnids (spiders), and acarids (mites) cause several kinds of reaction in humans: 1) trauma inflicted by the puncture of the skin and feeding, and 2) reaction to the irritating toxic substances, antigenic substances, or both introduced into the host (Figs. 1, 2, and 3). The io caterpillar has stiff spines containing a poison that when touched pricks the skin and causes a severe local irritant reaction (Fig. 4) [1]. The most serious of these reactions, anaphylaxis, is allergic in origin (IgE mediated) and is caused by sensitization of the host to antigenic substances found in either the saliva or the venom.

Sensitization of the host can also lead to large local reactions thought to be caused by one or more allergic mechanisms. The first is IgE-mediated hypersensitivity, as in the cutaneous late-phase reaction; the second, cell-mediated hypersensitivity. Rarely, neurologic sequelae occur, and they also seem to be mediated by IgE or by an immune complex reaction.

BITES

Proteins isolated from the saliva of various arthropods may play a role in the pathogenesis of local and systemic reactions. For example, the high molecular weight protein designated F-1 seems to be the major skin-reactive substance of the mosquito *Aedes aegypti* [2•]. The substance appears to be homogenous on immunoelectrophoresis, contains 9% carbohydrate, has a minimum molecular weight of 33,000 kd, and contains a high percentage of glycine, alanine, and proline. When injected into the skin of sensitized individuals, it produces a linear dose-response of the skin reaction diameter versus the log of the amount of F-1 injected.

Papular urticaria to flea bites has been historically associated with two components of the oral secretions of the cat flea (*Ctenocephalides felis* [3,4••,5]). Component

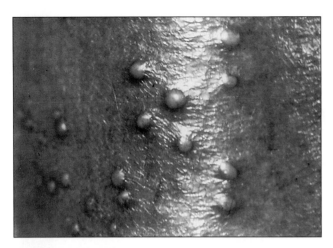

FIGURE 1 The sting of the imported fire ant results in an immediate wheal-and-flare response; within 24 hours, a characteristic sterile pustule appears at the sting site. If left undisturbed, the pustule usually resolves over 10 days. (*From* Lockey [14•]; with permission.)

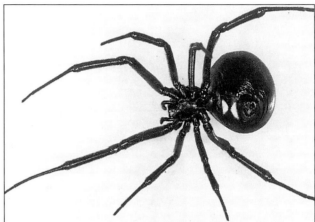

FIGURE 2 Black widow spider (*Latrodectus mactans*). Black widow spiders are usually found near buildings. Note the hourglass configuration on the abdomen, which is red. It is characteristic for the spider. These spiders like abandoned houses, water meter boxes, and areas under park benches or tables. The poison, primarily a neurotoxin, affects the nervous system. Antivenom for black widow spiders is available, although it is rarely necessary because most bites are self-limited. (*From* Lockey *et al.* [6]; with permission.)

A, a hapten, has a molecular weight of between 4 and 10 kd and becomes a complete antigen when it is coupled with skin collagen. Component B has a molecular weight of less than 1 kd. Most allergenic compounds, including histamine-like compounds and enzymes that have proteolytic, anticoagulant, cytolytic, and hyaluronidase-like activity, are found to have molecular weights of greater than 5 kd.

Local Reactions

People without a history of flea bites follow a sequence of skin reactions when they are repeatedly bitten over a 1-year period [2•,5]. In stage I, the induction period, there is no observable skin reaction or abnormality on skin biopsy. Stage II is characterized by a delayed skin reaction that occurs 18 to 24 hours after a bite and is accompanied by infiltration of lymphocytes and other mononuclear cells into the dermis and extending into the epidermis. These pruritic, erythematous, and indurated lesions may persist for 10 to 14 days. Stage III manifests as an immediate skin reaction (within 15 to 60 minutes) that clears in 4 hours and is followed by a delayed skin reaction. At the immediate phase of this stage, the primary infiltrating cells are eosinophils, whereas mononuclear cells characterize the delayed skin reaction. Stage IV is characterized by an immediate (within 20 minutes) skin reaction and eosinophilic response and a mild or absent delayed (within 24 hours) reaction with a mononuclear response. With continued challenge, both responses diminish. Stage V is the stage of nonreactivity, in which the biopsy site at 20 minutes and at 24 hours reveals little or no cellular responses.

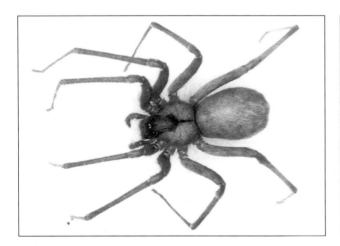

FIGURE 3 Brown recluse spider (*Loxosceles reclusa*). The venom of the brown recluse spider (also known as the fiddleback spider) is primarily cytotoxic, causing local tissue destruction and delayed wound healing. Treatment is symptomatic. (*From* Lockey *et al.* [6]; with permission.)

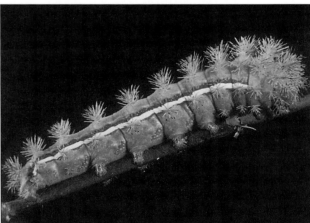

FIGURE 4 Io caterpillar (*Automeris io*). The io caterpillar is a beautiful caterpillar that is more than 2 in long. It is pale green with yellow spines, and along each side are a red stripe and a yellow stripe. The stiff spines contain a poison and can result in a severe stinging injury. Supportive care is indicated. (*From* Lockey *et al.* [6]; with permission.)

The role of the immune system in the pathogenesis of these reactions has not been resolved, although IgG antibodies and cell-mediated immunity against oral secretions of mosquitoes and fleas has been demonstrated.

Papular Urticaria

Papular urticaria in humans is characterized by pruritic erythematous papules, vesicles, or bullae grouped in clusters. They are associated with multiple flea, mosquito, and bed bug bites [2•,3,4••,5,6]. Papular urticaria develops only in subjects with delayed reactions to such bites, when previously unreactive bite sites flare. It commonly occurs in children 2 to 7 years of age and usually involves the extremities. Chigger bites can result in similar lesions (Fig. 5). Cetirizine, administered prophylactically, is effective in partially ameliorating papular urticaria [7].

Systemic Allergic Reactions

Anaphylactic reactions from bites are rare, and they have been most commonly associated with insects of the orders Hemiptera and Diptera (*see* Fig. 7). Kissing bugs, cone-nose bugs, or assassin bugs of the order Hemiptera, genus *Triatoma*, are commonly found from Texas to California in the United States (Fig. 6). A systemic allergic reaction has also been reported secondary to a brown spider bite [8]. Typically, these bugs bite at night, when the victim is asleep; the bite is painless and the victim is awakened by itching, respiratory distress, and other allergic symptoms. Several deaths have been reported from anaphylaxis in the United States, and there is evidence of IgE sensitization to the insect's saliva with such reactions. IgE antibody–induced anaphylaxis has also been reported to the western black-legged tick, *Ixodes pacificus*, in California. Similar kinds of reactions from the Australian paralysis tick, *Ixodes holocyclus*, have been reported in Australia [9].

The most commonly occurring insect bites are from the order Diptera, family Culicidae, or mosquitoes, and appear to cause rare systemic reactions. Insects of the same order, family Simuliidae, or black flies, are a plague in areas of the northern hemisphere; their bites have been associated with anaphylactic reactions. Horse flies and deer flies are large flies that administer painful bites that have been associated with verified systemic reactions. There is significant evidence that systemic reactions caused by some of the insects in the order Diptera are IgE mediated [3,4••].

INSECT STINGS

More than 16,000 species of Hymenoptera are found in the United States (Fig. 7) [10•,11••,12•,13••]. Many of the workers and adult females of this order have a modified ovipositor and venom sac for stinging. Humans stung by Hymenoptera insects suffer local cutaneous reactions at the sting site, ranging from transient erythema to edema with or without pain, extensive erythema, or edema and induration lasting for more than 48 hours (Fig. 8) [14•]. Systemic allergic reactions to Hymenoptera insect stings occur in 0.4% to 4% of the population. It has been estimated that up to 50 individuals die of Hymenoptera insect sting anaphylaxis yearly in the United States.

Members of three families of Hymenoptera are responsible for most insect sting reactions (Figs. 9, 10, and 11) [10•, 11••,12•,13••]. Apidae (honeybees and bumblebees), Vespidae (wasps, yellow jackets, and hornets), and Formicidae (native and imported fire ants and harvester ants) (Figs. 12 and 13). The apids and vespids are found in most regions of the United States. *Solenopsis invicta*, and the less prevalent and aggressive *Solenopsis richteri*, collectively referred to as the imported fire ant, have largely replaced the native fire ants (*Solenopsis geminata*, *Solenopsis aurea*, and *Solenopsis xyloni*) in the United States [15•,16,17]. Both species originated in South America, where they cause similar medical problems. The imported fire ant inhabits much of the

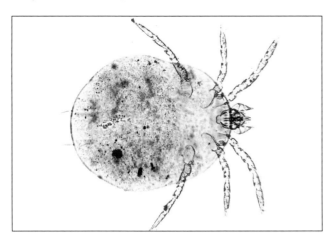

FIGURE 5 Chigger or red bug (*Trombicula* sp.). Chiggers or red bugs prefer to live in damp areas where the vegetation is thick. In these locations, they climb on plants and wait for a host to pass. Red bugs usually congregate on one's body where clothing is close to the body, such as under a belt or garter or shoe tops. They attach themselves to the skin with their mouth parts and inject salivary juices into the tissue. The mites feed on the damaged tissue, causing erythematous pruritic papules. Avoidance and supportive therapy are indicated. (*From* Lockey *et al.* [6]; with permission.)

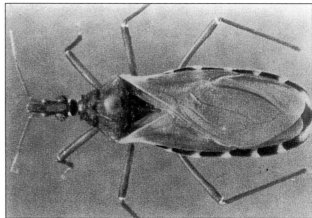

FIGURE 6 Kissing bugs, cone-nose bugs, or assassin bugs of the order Hemiptera, genus *Triatoma*, are commonly found from Texas to California in the United States. They typically bite at night, when the victim is asleep. IgE sensitization to the insect's saliva can occur, with subsequent anaphylaxis.

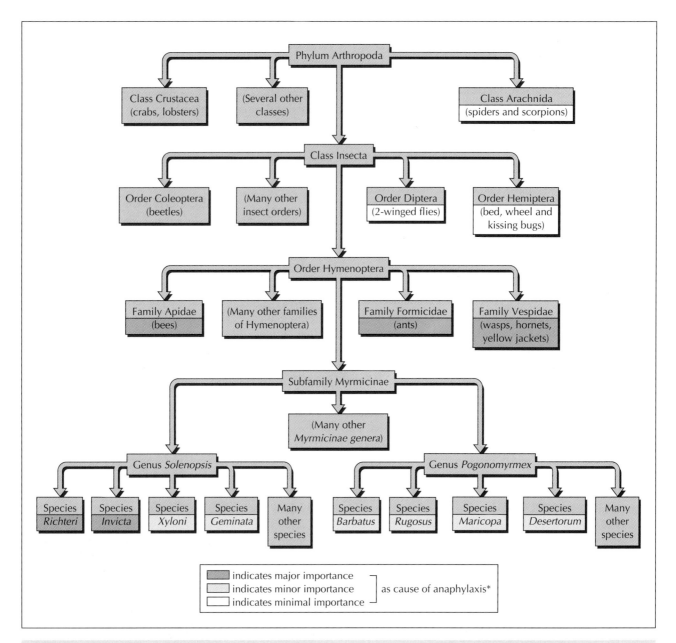

Figure 7 Taxonomy of the phylum Arthropoda. This diagram identifies insects that can cause systemic allergic reactions. Among them are the insects of the order Hymenoptera, which are most responsible for systemic allergic reactions. (*From* Levine and Lockey [4••]; with permission.)

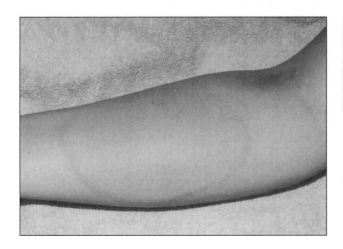

Figure 8 Large local reactions often result from the sting of the imported fire ant. In this patient, shown 6 hours after three stings from a single fire ant, much of the forearm is covered with an erythematous and edematous lesion that is pruritic and painful. The reaction peaked in size at 48 hours. (*From* Lockey [14•]; with permission. *Courtesy of* R. deShazo, Mobile, AL.)

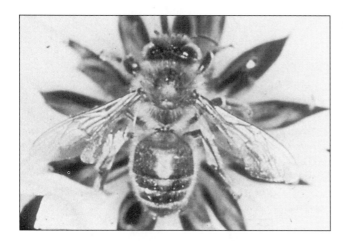

FIGURE 9 Honeybee (*Apis mellifera*). This Hymenoptera insect has a barb on its stinger and may leave its stinger in its victim's skin. The barbed stinger and the poison sac are torn from the bee after most stings. Care must be used in removing the stinger and the venom sac. If the venom sac is grasped, this action can squeeze venom remaining in the sac into the victim. The sting apparatus should be carefully scraped away with a fingernail or a knife blade. (*Courtesy of* Miles, Pharmaceutical Division–Allergy Products, Spokane, WA.)

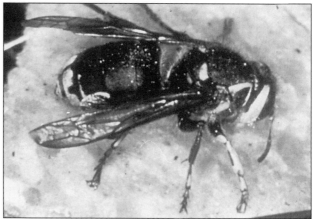

FIGURE 10 A hornet feeds on organic debris left on the ground. Hornets and yellow jackets are closely related insects. (*Courtesy of* Miles, Pharmaceutical Division–Allergy Products, Spokane, WA.)

southeastern United States, whereas harvester ants (genus *Pogonomyrmex*), which can also cause systemic reactions, are found primarily but not exclusively in the southwest and western parts of the country (Fig. 14). *Pogonomyrmex badius* is found east of the Mississippi.

Stingers of the various families of Hymenoptera are different in size but similar in design: they are ensheathed, barbed instruments with an attached venom sac located at the tip of the insect's abdomen. The larger barbs of the honeybee stinger firmly anchor into the human skin so that the stinger cannot be withdrawn by the insect. Thus, the stinger detaches when the animal flies away, resulting in its evisceration and death. Muscles associated with the remaining venom sac can continue to expel venom into the sting site for several minutes, delivering approximately 50 to 100 µL of venom. Most other Hymenoptera are able to withdraw their stinger from the skin, so they are able to sting again. The venoms are collected from Hymenoptera insects using several techniques (Fig. 15).

The imported fire ant grabs the victim's skin with its mandibles, and by pivoting about its neck, it makes numerous

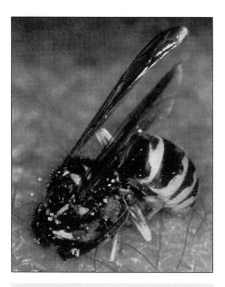

FIGURE 11 Hymenoptera insects are responsible for most insect sting reactions. Here, a member of the order Hymenoptera stings its victim. (*Courtesy of* Miles, Pharmaceutical Division–Allergy Products, Spokane, WA.)

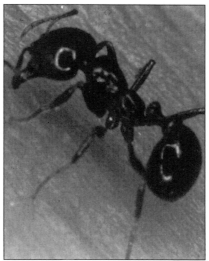

FIGURE 12 Imported fire ant (*Solenopsis invicta*). The fire ant worker is from 0.125 to 0.25 in long and varies in color from reddish-brown to dark brown. A sterile pustule forms at the site of each sting. Allergic reactions and secondary infections can be serious and can cause death. Neurologic problems are rare and transient.

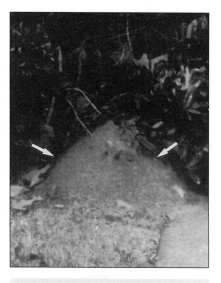

FIGURE 13 In firm soil, imported fire ant nests are large mounds as much as 10 to 15 in high, with a crustlike surface (*arrow*). In sandy soil, with little or no mound structure, nests may be present. Imported fire ants aggressively defend their nests and sting repeatedly when disturbed. (*Courtesy of* R. deShazo.)

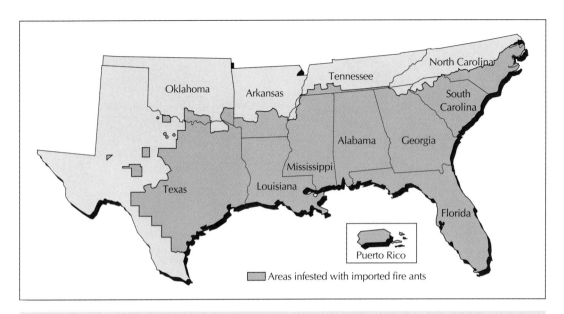

FIGURE 14 Parts of all of these southern states (and US Caribbean possessions) are infested with imported fire ants, which are spreading in the United States. They have also been found in Virginia, and isolated colonies have been found in New Mexico and Arizona. A cold-tolerant hybrid adds the possibility of greater spread. These ants also exist in their native habitat in South America. (*From* Lockey [14•]; with permission.)

stings in a semicircular distribution, injecting between 0.04 and 0.11 μL of venom with each sting. The harvester ant stings in a similar fashion.

Local Reactions
Nonallergic reactions
A nonallergic local reaction, which begins immediately after the sting, is a toxic response to venom constituents and induces mast cell degranulation that can provoke a wheal and flare and inflammation from other cell damage. Characteristically, erythema and edema associated with pain and pruritus occur. The reaction may persist for several hours and then resolve.

The venom alkaloids in imported fire ant venom are cytotoxic and cause a wheal-and-flare reaction followed by the development of a pustule within 24 hours. This pustule enlarges to 1 to 3 mm in diameter and, if undisturbed, becomes encrusted and resolves in 3 to 10 days; it may leave a superficial scar or pigmented macule [17,18]. No other insect leaves this characteristic lesion (Figs. 1 and 16). Harvester ants sting in a similar fashion, but the stings result in the wheal-and-flare reaction typical of reactions to other Hymenoptera stings, not the pustules that characterize the imported fire ant sting.

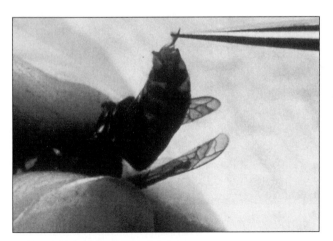

FIGURE 15 The venom sac is a thick-walled muscular reservoir that stores the venom produced in the acid glands. It is egg-shaped and approximately 1 to 2 mm in diameter. For vespid (yellow jacket, paper wasp, and hornet) venom production, thousands of nests must first be collected. Venom sac dissection is tedious and labor intensive. (*Courtesy of* Miles, Pharmaceutical Division–Allergy Products, Spokane, WA.)

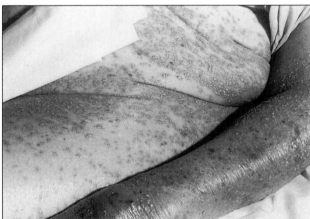

FIGURE 16 Fire ants invaded the home of this 84-year-old woman with senile dementia who was confined to bed because of a history of multiple hip fractures. She was stung at least 10,000 times, as illustrated by the typical pustular eruptions. She developed neither toxic nor immunologic sequelae from the stings. Lesions such as these can become secondarily infected. Patients can also become sensitized and develop subsequent anaphylaxis on re-sting. Transient neurologic sequelae from imported fire ant stings have also been reported. (*From* Diaz *et al.* [17]; with permission.)

Allergic reactions

Allergic local reactions to Hymenoptera stings are more extensive and last longer than nonallergic reactions. They develop in approximately 17% of subjects stung by bees, wasps, hornets, and yellow jackets and in 30% to 50% of subjects stung by the imported fire ant. These reactions, referred to as large local reactions, are also arbitrarily defined as local cutaneous reactions. They are pruritic and sometimes painful, with erythema and edema of more than 10 cm in diameter that persist for at least 48 to 72 hours (Fig. 8). They may last for up to 5 days and involve part or all of the extremity or face. Local reactions to Hymenoptera stings of any kind can become secondarily infected and have resulted in limb amputation, sepsis, and even death. Four percent to 5% of subjects with an imported fire ant sting may seek medical attention for a secondary infection. Prospective studies indicate that 5% to 10% of adults and 2% of children with a sting-induced large local reaction may be at risk for a systemic allergic reaction to a subsequent sting. Such patients are usually not thought to be at high risk for systemic reactions and therefore are not skin tested. If they are, many will have positive skin test reactions to Hymenoptera allergens, similar to those who have had a systemic reaction. Treatment of local reactions to Hymenoptera stings is outlined in Table 1.

Systemic Allergic Reactions

Most systemic allergic reactions begin within 30 minutes, and almost all reactions begin within the first 100 minutes after a sting, although reactions have been reported hours afterward [10•,19,20]. Urticaria and generalized pruritus are the most common clinical manifestations; however, generalized erythema, angioedema and upper airway edema, asthma, abdominal cramps, diarrhea, seizures, and hypoten-

sion secondary to vascular collapse can also occur and may result in death [4••,8•,21•]. When death occurs, it is almost always within 1 hour and more commonly in older persons, particularly in the presence of underlying diseases such as coronary artery disease or generalized atherosclerosis [4••].

Sustained reactions have persisted for 24 hours or longer despite appropriate therapy. Rarely, delayed reactions, which commonly involve the central nervous system, develop 24 to 96 hours after the sting and may not be associated with a preceding immediate reaction. Seizures, encephalitis, and various other neurologic manifestations have been described. Other unusual reactions include serum sickness, vasculitis, acute glomerulonephritis with renal failure, and nephrotic syndrome; the pathologic mechanisms that cause these reactions remain obscure.

DIAGNOSIS AND TREATMENT

Insect whole body extracts are used to evaluate patients with insect bite allergy because extracts of saliva are not currently available and probably will not be available in the near future. Interpreting the results of such tests requires care and comparison with control patients because biting insect saliva can cause irritant skin reactions. Patients with recurrent large local reactions, systemic reactions, or both have been placed on allergen immunotherapy; however, results are anecdotal because no controlled diagnostic or therapeutic studies have been done. Anaphylaxis should be treated in the same manner as any anaphylactic reaction. Antihistamines, topical steroids, topical antipruritics, and occasionally glucocorticosteroids are used to treat large local reactions.

Hymenoptera venoms (honeybee, wasp, yellow jacket, and hornet) and whole body extracts (ant) are used for the diagnosis of Hymenoptera hypersensitivity. Skin testing is the most sensitive method of diagnosing Hymenoptera sensitivity, although the *in vitro* radioallergosorbent test is also a reliable method of determining clinical sensitivity [10•,11••,12•,13••].

The treatment of systemic reactions caused by Hymenoptera insects is the same for any anaphylactic reaction, regardless of the cause, with epinephrine being the drug of choice (*see* Chapter 9).

Venom immunotherapy for stinging insect hypersensitivity will reduce the risk of stinging anaphylaxis from between 40% and 60% to less than 5%, and if an anaphylactic reaction occurs during maintenance venom therapy, it is usually mild [22]. Fatal reactions with stinging insects rarely occur in children and adolescents from 3 to 16 years of age. Most reactions in this age group are manifested by cutaneous symptoms, such as generalized erythema, pruritus, urticaria, or a combination, and repeated stings result in no reactions or in a repeated mild reaction, despite positive skin test results [23•,24]. Immunotherapy to appropriate venoms should be considered for all subjects older than 16 years of age who have a history of any systemic reaction and for those through 16 years of age who have moderate or severe systemic reactions and positive skin test or radioallergosorbent test findings. There is, however, evidence that adults with cutaneous reactions may be at minimal risk for a life-

Reaction	Treatment
TABLE 1 TREATMENT OF LOCAL REACTIONS TO HYMENOPTERA STINGS	
Nonallergic local	Remove stinger, if present
	Apply ice to slow rate of venom absorption and reduce edema and pruritus
	Cleanse with soap and water
	Lidocaine (topically or intradermally) for pain
	Oral or topical H_1-antagonist for edema and pruritus
Large local (allergic)	Ice, elevation of affected extremity, analgesics, and oral H_1-antagonist (possibly an H_2-antagonist)
	Prednisone (1 mg/kg/day) for 3–5 days, starting as soon as possible after sting

From Wright DN, Lockey RF [14]; with permission.

Table 2 Selection of Patients for Venom Immunotherapy

Sting reaction	ST/RAST	Venom immunotherapy
Systemic, non-life-threatening (child), immediate, generalized, confined to skin (urticaria, angioedema, erythema, pruritus)	+ or -	No
Systemic, life-threatening (child), immediate, generalized, may involve cutaneous symptoms, but also has respiratory (laryngeal edema or bronchospasm) or cardiovascular symptoms (hypotension/shock)	+	Yes
Systemic (adult)	+	Yes
Systemic*	-	No
Large local	+ or -	No
≤2 inches in diameter		
≤24 h in duration		
Normal local	+ or -	No
≥ in in diameter		
≥24 h in duration		

From Lockey RF [25]; with permission.
*The patient should be skin retested, with reconstituted extract, in 4 to 6 weeks. If still negative. RAST should be repeated to confirm the negative skin test. The opposite is true for a RAST-negative individual. in whom the skin test should confirm negative RAST results.
ST—skin test; RAST—radioallergosorbent test.

threatening reaction on a subsequent sting even without treatment (Table 2) [21•].

Increasing increments of venom are administered in a series of weekly injections until the patient can tolerate an injection of venom extract equivalent to the amount of venom delivered by one or more insect stings (Table 3). After 1 year

Table 3 Dosage Regimen for Venom Immunotherapy

Week	Dose, μg
1*	0.1
	1
	3
2	10
3	20
4	40
5	70
6	100
7	100
8	–
9	100
10, 11	–
12	100
13-15	–
16†	100

From Valentine MD [12]; with permission.
*Doses are administered at 20-minute intervals at the week-1 visit.
†Subsequent maintenance doses are administered every 4 weeks.
 The maintenance interval may be extended to 6 weeks if the serum antivenom IgG level is greater than 3.5 μg/mL.

of monthly injections, the interval can be increased to every 6 weeks or longer. In most patients, levels of venom-specific IgE eventually decrease and levels of venom-specific IgG (blocking antibody) increase [26]. Venom immunotherapy can be discontinued in 3 to 5 years if the results of repeated skin tests are negative. Some investigators recommend discontinuing venom immunotherapy after 3 to 5 years regardless of skin test results, particularly in patients who have mild to moderate systemic reactions [21•,27–29].

Initiating venom immunotherapy during pregnancy, especially during the developmentally sensitive first trimester, must be carefully considered in light of the relatively greater risk of allergic venom sting reactions as compared with reactions to inhaled allergens in subjects with respiratory allergic symptoms. Venom immunotherapy has been shown to be safe for use during pregnancy [30].

Although venoms have replaced whole body extracts for most Hymenoptera, whole body extracts are used for imported fire ant and harvester ant immunotherapy. There is good evidence that the whole body extracts contain sufficient amounts of venom antigens for effective immunotherapy, although there are no appropriate double-blind studies to show definitively that ant whole body extracts or venoms are efficacious [32,33].

Instructions on how to avoid being stung are necessary (Table 4). Patients with insect hypersensitivity should also carry an emergency insect sting kit containing aqueous epinephrine in a prefilled syringe. A bracelet or medallion that identifies the patient and the type of insect hypersensitivity may also be worn by the sensitive patient. Patients who have severe local reactions that do not respond to supportive therapy and those who have systemic reactions secondary to arthropod bites or insect bites or stings should be referred to an allergist-immunologist for evaluation and treatment.

TABLE 4 AVOIDANCE OF AND PROTECTIVE MEASURES AGAINST INSECT STINGS

Wasps usually nest under the eaves of homes or on overhangs, bushes, or trees.

Hornets nest in trees, and yellow jackets nest underground or in cavities of buildings.

The honeybee stinger is barbed. The honeybee venom sac remains in the skin of the stung victim. It should be removed carefully with a flick of the finger.

Insects seem to be less attracted to white or light khaki-colored clothing than to dark brown or black clothing.

Bright floral colors on clothing appear to attract insects and should be avoided.

Wearing long-sleeve shirts, socks, and shoes decreases the chances of being stung, whereas going barefoot increases the chances of being stung.

Scented sprays, soaps, suntan lotion, perfumes, and other cosmetics may increase the likelihood of attracting Hymenoptera insects.

Sweat bees are attracted to perspiration.

Food and beverages served outdoors attracts insects.

Lawn mowing, trimming hedges, sanding and painting homes, emptying garbage cans, and walking in wooded areas increases a person's chances of being stung.

Flower beds, fields covered with clover or other flowering plants, blooming fruit trees or trees that are bearing fruit, and areas in which fruits and vegetation are rotting should be avoided.

Windows should be closed and air conditioning used, whenever possible, while driving in a car.

Homes and cottages should be carefully screened and windows and doors checked for areas through which insects can enter the home.

Insects should be sprayed, whenever possible, around the home, particularly under the eaves.

Garbage cans should be kept clean, sprayed with insecticide where appropriate, and kept covered at all times.

When an insect is in the area, an individual should avoid sudden, rapid movements, which appear to antagonize Hymenoptera insects. The potential victim should slowly move away from an insect in an attempt to avoid an attack.

Subjects with a history of insect hypersensitivity who are not receiving treatment or who have not yet reached maintenance immunotherapy should carry an emergency sting kit containing aqueous epinephrine in an prefilled syringe. Instructions on how to use it should be provided by health care professionals.

REFERENCES AND RECOMMENDED READING

Recently published papers of particular interest have been highlighted as:
• Of interest
•• Of outstanding interest

1. Everson GW, Chapin JB, Normann SA: Caterpillar envenomations: a prospective study of 112 cases. *Vet Hum Toxicol* 1990, 32:114–119.

2.• Keunala T, Brummer-Korvenkontio H, Lappalainen P, *et al.*: Immunology and treatment of mosquito bites. *Clin Exp Allergy* 1990, 20:19–24.

3. Hoffman DR: Allergy to biting insects. *Clin Rev Allergy* 1987, 5:177–190.

4.•• Levine MI, Lockey RF, eds: *Monograph on Insect Allergy.* 3rd ed. American Academy of Allergy and Immunology. Pittsburgh, PA: Dave Lambert Associates; 1995.

5. Trudeau WL, Fernandez-Caldas E, Wright DN, Lockey RF: Fleas as a source of allergy. *Am J Asthma Allergy Pediatricians* 1990, 3:222–227.

6. Lockey RF, Stewart GE II, Maxwell LS: *Florida's Poisonous Plants, Snakes, Insects*, edn 3. Tampa, FL: Lewis S. Maxwell; 1992.

7. Reunala T, Brummer-Korvenkontio H, Karppinen A, *et al.*: Treatment of mosquito bites with cetirizine. *Clin Exper Allergy* 1993, 23:72–75.

8. Herman TE, McAlister WH: Epiglottic enlargement: two unusual cases. *Pediatr Radiol* 1991, 21:139–140.

9. Van Wye JE, Hsu YP, Lane RS, *et al.*: IgE antibodies in tick bite-induced anaphylaxis. *J Allergy Clin Immunol* 1991, 88:968–970.

10.• Mueller UR: *Insect Sting Allergy.* New York: Gustav Fischer; 1990.

11.•• Yuninger JW: Insect allergy. In *Allergy: Principles and Practice*, edn 4. Edited by Middleton E Jr, Reed CE, Adkinson R Jr, *et al.* St. Louis: Mosby; 1993:1511–1524.

12.• Valentine MD: Anaphylaxis and stinging insect hypersensitivity. *JAMA* 1992, 268:2830–2833.

13.•• Lockey RF: Immunotherapy for allergy to insect stings. *N Engl J Med* 1990, 323:1627–1628.

14.• Wright DN, Lockey RF: Local reactions to stinging insects (Hymenoptera). *Allergy Proc* 1990, 11:23–28.

15.• Lockey RF: The imported fire ant: immunopathologic significance. *Hosp Pract* 1990, 25:109–124.

16. deShazo RD, Butcher BT: Reactions to the stings of the imported fire ant. *N Engl J Med* 1990, 323:462–466.

17. Wright DN, Lockey RF: Adverse and allergic reactions to ant stings in the USA. *Int Pediatr* 1988, 3:250–255.

18. Diaz JD, Lockey RF, Stablein JJ, Mines HK: Multiple stings by imported fire ants (*Solenopsis Invicta*, Buren), without systemic effects. *South Med J* 1989, 82:775–777.

19. van der Linden PWG, Struyvenberg A, Kraaijenhagen RJ, *et al.*: Anaphylactic shock after insect-sting challenge in 138 persons with a previous insect-sting reaction. *Ann Intern Med* 1993, 118:161–168.

20. Müller U, Mosbech H, Blaauw P, *et al.*: Emergency treatment of allergic reactions to Hymenoptera stings. *Clin Exp Allergy* 1991, 21:281–288.

21.• Reisman RE: Natural history of insect sting allergy: relationship of severity of symptoms of initial sting anaphylaxis to re-sting reactions. *J Allergy Clin Immunol* 1992, 90:335–339.

22. Bousquet J, Müller UR, Dreborg S, *et al.*: Immunotherapy with Hymenoptera venoms. *Allergy* 1987, 42:401–413.

23.• Valentine MD, Schuberth KC, Sobotka AK, *et al.*: The value of immunotherapy with venom in children with allergy to insect stings. *N Engl J Med* 1990, 323:1601–1603.

24. Schuberth KC, Lichtenstein LM, Kagey-Sobotka A, *et al.*: An epidemiologic study of insect allergy in children: I. Characteristics of the disease. *J Pediatr* 1982, 100:546–551.

25. Wright DN, Lockey RF: Local reactions to stinging insects. *Allergy Proc* 1990, 11:27.

26. Golden DBK, Lawrence ID, Hamilton RH, *et al.*: Clinical correlation of the venom-specific IgG antibody level during maintenance venom immunotherapy. *J Allergy Clin Immunol* 1992, 90:386–393.

27. Reisman RE, Dvorin DJ, Randolph CC, Georgitis JW: Stinging insect allergy: natural history and modification with venom immunotherapy. *J Allergy Clin Immunol* 1985, 76:735–740.

28. Urbanek R, Forster J, Kuhn W, Ziupa J: Discontinuation of bee venom immunotherapy in children and adolescents. *J Pediatr* 1985, 107:367–371.

29. Reisman RE: Duration of venom immunotherapy: relationship to the severity of symptoms of initial insect sting anaphylaxis. *J Allergy Clin Immunol* 1993, 92:831–836.

30. Schwartz HJ, Golden BK, Lockey RF: Venom immunotherapy in the Hymenoptera-allergic pregnant patient. *J Allergy Clin Immunol* 1990, 85:709–712.

31. Nordvall SL, Johansson SGO, Ledford DK, Lockey RF: Allergens of imported fire ant. *J Allergy Clin Immunol* 1988, 82:567–576.

32. Freeman TM, Hylander R, Ortiz A, Martin ME: Imported fire ant immunotherapy: effectiveness of whole body extracts. *J Allergy Clin Immunol* 1992, 90:210–215.

Drug Reactions 11

John E. Erffmeyer

Key Points
- Adverse drug reactions are responsible for the majority of iatrogenic illnesses; allergic reactions are the most troublesome.
- Physician awareness is the most important factor in making a diagnosis.
- Diagnostic tests are of value, but are limited in number.
- Strategies and protocols exist for special situations when re-administration of a drug that had previously provoked an adverse reaction must be considered.
- Patient education and prevention of adverse reactions are the best treatment.

The multitude of allergic drug reactions may give the initial impression that any drug may cause any reaction. However, distinct patterns occur (Table 1). Any particular drug tends to cause a similar reaction in different individuals [1], but each individual's situation may be unique.

CLASSIFICATIONS

An adverse drug reaction is an unintended and undesired response that develops at appropriate doses of an appropriate drug administered for diagnostic, therapeutic, or prophylactic benefit [2••]. At least 80% of adverse drug reactions are predictable in that they are dose dependent and are related to known drug actions (Table 2) [2••]. The rest are unpredictable, and of those, approximately half are allergic reactions (Table 3). Because adverse drug reactions are responsible for the majority of iatrogenic illnesses, and because allergic reactions are the most troublesome, they are given the most attention in this chapter.

Allergic drug reactions are those that involve an immunologic mechanism. The following criteria may be of value in distinguishing allergic drug reactions from other adverse drug effects, even in the absence of direct immunologic evidence [2••]:

Allergic reactions occur in only a small percentage of individuals receiving the drug.
- The observed clinical manifestations do not resemble known pharmacologic actions of the drug.
- In the absence of prior drug exposure, allergic symptoms rarely appear during the first week of continuous therapy, and drugs that have been used with impunity for several months or longer are rarely responsible. This temporal relationship is often the most critical information in determining which of multiple drugs being administered needs to be considered most seriously as the cause of a suggested allergic drug reaction.
- The reaction may resemble other known allergic reactions (anaphylaxis, asthma, serum sickness–like reactions, urticaria). A variety of skin rashes (especially exanthems), fever, vasculitis, hepatitis, acute interstitial nephritis, pulmonary reactions (notably pulmonary infiltrates with eosinophilia), and the lupus syndrome have been attributed to drug hypersensitivity.

- The reaction may be reproduced by small doses of the suspected drug or other agents exhibiting similar or cross-reacting chemical structures.
- Blood or tissue eosinophilia may be suggestive of allergy.
- Occasionally, drug-specific antibodies or T lymphocytes have been identified that react with the suspected drug or relevant drug metabolite. This is seldom diagnostically useful in clinical practice, however, except for a limited number of therapeutic agents.
- The reaction usually subsides within several days following cessation of drug administration.

The induction of a drug-specific allergic response may be influenced by the age of the patient, underlying metabolic or genetic factors, the chemical properties of the drug (largely its protein reactivity), the dose and duration of therapy, and the route of drug administration [3]. Drug-induced allergic disease develops from a persistent drug-specific immune response and depends on the frequency of drug treatment, the amount of the dose, the duration of treatment, and probably on constitutional factors that are not clearly defined or understood (Table 4).

MANAGEMENT

The investigation and identification of a drug responsible for a suspected allergic drug reaction still depends largely on circumstantial evidence and the clinical skills of the physician [2••]. Physician awareness is the most important factor in making a diagnosis, being a suspicious detective and acknowledging likely suspects while not overlooking coexisting culprits such as nonprescription medications, foods, or other agents (for example, latex). With few exceptions, absolute proof that a drug is the causative agent is usually lacking, because conventional methods to diagnose allergic disorders are either unavailable or useless for determining a drug etiology [2••,4•].

Diagnostic Tests

In general, prick and intradermal skin testing for immunoglobulin E (IgE)-mediated allergic drug reactions has limited value, because many times it is not the drug molecule that sensitizes, but rather a drug metabolite or degradation product [2••]. This diagnostic technique may be employed for

TABLE 1 COMMON REACTIONS TO COMMON DRUGS

	Penicillins	Cephalosporins	Hormones	Vaccines	Captopril	Sulfonamides	Tetracyclines	NSAIDs	Thiazide diuretics
Maculopapular rash	X	X			X	X			X
Urticaria and angioedema	X	X			X	X		X	X
Serum sickness	X	X	X	X		X			
Anaphylaxis	X	X	X	X		X	X	X	
Interstitial nephritis	X	X			X	X	X	X	X
Anemia	X	X			X	X			
Granulocytopenia	X	X			X				

NSAIDs—nonsteroidal antiinflammatory drugs.

TABLE 2 PREDICTABLE ADVERSE DRUG REACTIONS

Type	Definition	Comments
Overdosage or toxicity	Observed effects are directly related to total amount of drug in body	May be expected in any patient provided a threshold level has been exceeded
Side effects	Pharmacologic actions developing at usual prescribed drug dosages while therapeutically undesirable, yet often unavoidable	May be expressed in an immediate or delayed manner
Secondary effects	Indirect, but not inevitable, consequences of pharmacologic actions of the drug	Alterations of normal microbial microenvironment (bacterial or yeast overgrowth); disease associated (Jarisch-Herxheimer phenomenon)
Drug interactions	Two or more drugs administered concurrently may act independently, or may interact to diminish or augment the expected response, or result in an unintended reaction	

Allergy and Immunology

TABLE 3 UNPREDICTABLE ADVERSE DRUG REACTIONS

Type	Definition	Examples
Intolerance	Reactions developing as a result of a lowered threshold to the normal pharmacologic action(s) of a drug in susceptible individuals	Tinnitus experienced at normal or small doses of aspirin
Idiosyncratic reactions	Qualitatively abnormal, unexpected drug reactions, which differ from the drug's known pharmacologic actions; susceptible individuals may possess a genetic enzymatic defect, not expressed under normal conditions, which is clinically manifested after administration of certain drugs	Glucose-6-phosphate dehydrogenase deficiency and the development of hemolytic anemia
Allergic reactions	Qualitatively aberrant reactions in which an immunologic mechanism, mediated via drug-specific antibodies and/or sensitized T lymphocytes, is involved in pathogenesis, or more often presumed to be involved	Urticaria due to IgE-mediated penicillin allergy; contact dermatitis due to cutaneously applied neomycin sulfate
Pseudoallergic reactions	Reactions that exhibit clinical manifestations similar to allergic reactions; however, the initiating event does not appear to involve a reaction between the drug, or its metabolite, and drug-specific antibodies and/or sensitized T lymphocytes	Urticaria subsequent to nonsteroidal antiinflammatory drugs
Non-drug-related reactions	Reactions that are unrelated to the drug itself, but attributable to events associated with and during its administration	Psychophysiologic reactions or reactions developing as manifestations of a possible underlying personality or psychiatric disorder (vasovagal reactions, hyperventilation, hysteria, Münchausen's, factitious); coincidental reactions (viral exanthem incorrectly attributed to the drug)

Treatment-related factors

Nature of the drug or drug metabolites

Cross-sensitization

  Once a patient is sensitized, cross-reactivity may occur to drugs or drug metabolites that are similar in chemical structure

Route of drug administration

  In order from most to least likely to sensitize: topical, intramuscular, intravenous, oral

Degree of exposure

  Dose, duration, and frequency of drug therapy

    In the case of penicillin (and other β-lactam antibiotic) sensitivity, frequent intermittent therapeutic courses, as opposed to prolonged treatment without drug-free intervals, are likely to result in drug sensitization; penicillin-induced hemolytic anemia generally requires high and sustained drug blood levels

Patient-related factors

Gender and age

  Women are more likely to react than men, in particular with regard to drug-induced cutaneous reactions; drug allergy tends to be less common at the extremes of age, with children less likely to react than adults

Constitutional and genetic factors

  An atopic constitution does not appear to predispose to allergic drug reactions, but it does appear to be associated with more serious allergic reactions once drug-specific IgE antibodies are present

Prior drug reactions

  Individuals who have previously developed allergic drug reactions may exhibit an increased tendency to develop reactions when new drugs are administered

Concurrent medical illness

high-molecular-weight drugs (proteins), including foreign antisera, hormones, toxoids, enzymes, and egg-containing vaccines, and for penicillin and other β-lactam antibiotics [5••,6]. The immunochemistry of penicillin has been studied in great detail. The immunogenic moieties' structures are known. When a drug's immunogenic determinants are unknown (as is currently the case with most other immunogenic drugs), skin tests may fail to detect a drug-specific immune response simply because the test antigen is not optimal [5••,6]. The method of skin testing is given in Table 5. Patch testing may be of value in cases of contact dermatitis due to topically applied medications. The radioallergosorbent test (RAST) is of limited value in IgE-mediated drug reactions, as it is generally less sensitive than the respective skin tests [6].

Drug-induced hemolytic anemia may be associated with a positive direct antiglobulin (Coombs') test. Measurement of serum complement levels and immune complex assays may be of benefit in serum sickness (foreign protein) or serum sickness-like (drug) reactions [6].

Penicillin and β-Lactam Antibiotics

Penicillin and other β-lactam antibiotics are reported to be the most common cause of anaphylaxis adverse drug reactions [7]. One to five anaphylactic reactions occur per 10,000 courses of treatment, with a fatality of approximately 1 every 50,000 to 100,000 courses of therapy. Fatal reactions develop within 60 minutes in 96% of cases, but may begin more than 1 hour after penicillin administration [8]. Most serious reactions are not preceded by an allergic reaction during previous penicillin therapy. Reactions may develop as a result of any form of drug exposure or administration. They may be more severe when penicillin has been injected. Individuals who have experienced anaphylactic reactions are at an increased risk for recurrence of anaphylaxis if penicillin is re-administered, even when IgE antibodies are undetectable by skin tests [3]. Atopic individuals who are allergic to mold and exhibit a positive skin test for the mold *Penicillium* are not at increased risk of experiencing an allergic reaction to the drug penicillin. Patients who use β-adrenergic antagonists may face increased risk of death if anaphylaxis occurs, because treatment of the anaphylactic reaction in these patients may be made more difficult. Inadvertent intravenous injection of procaine may result in the development of pseudoanaphylaxis, which may be distinguished by normotension and marked neuropsychiatric symptoms (which usually resolve within 30 minutes). Pseudoanaphylaxis is thought to occur as a result of the physiologic and chemical toxicity of procaine.

A recent study found a prevalence of 4% for drug-specific IgE, as documented by positive β-lactam immediate hypersensitivity skin tests, in patients with an unknown or negative history of penicillin allergy, indicating a substantial risk of

TABLE 5 SKIN TESTING FOR DRUG REACTIONS: IMMEDIATE HYPERSENSITIVITY SKIN TESTS ARE THE MOST RELIABLE AND RAPID METHOD OF DEMONSTRATING THE PRESENCE OF IgE ANTIBODY

Method

A drop of allergen testing solution is placed on the skin. Using a sharp needle (*eg*, 25 or 27 gauge), a prick (puncture) test is performed by passing the needle tip, bevel side up, through the drop of testing solution, contacting the skin at a 30° to 45° angle and gently breaking the superficial epidermis by pricking the skin with an upward motion. A negative saline control and positive histamine control may be performed using the same technique.

If negative after 15 to 20 min, an intradermal skin test should be performed by injecting 0.02 mL of solution intradermally, raising a small bleb. Intradermal tests are also evaluated 15 to 20 min after being performed.

A positive test is defined as 1 cm of erythema, with or without a wheal, with a negative saline control.

If the negative saline control elicits a cutaneous response (is positive), a skin test response would be considered positive if the reagent being tested produced a wheal 3 mm or greater in diameter, when compared with the saline control.

The prick test is safer but less sensitive. The intradermal test is more sensitive.

Precautions

Antihistamine administration during the 48 h before the performance of skin tests may diminish or suppress the skin test results and should be avoided. This is especially significant for astemizole, hydroxyzine, and terfenadine. Adrenergic drugs administered within 4 h of testing may also effect skin test results. Corticosteroid therapy (60 mg of prednisone, or the equivalent, daily) will not effect the skin test results.

The prick and intradermal skin test are safe and generally without risk. However, there are exquisitely allergic individuals who could develop a fatal anaphylactic reaction from prick or intradermal skin tests if the initial test concentrations are too high.

The physician should understand the theory and practice of these procedures. Consultation with a formally educated and experienced allergist may be necessary.

The skin tests should be performed in a setting where emergency treatment equipment is readily available and anaphylaxis can be treated promptly.

Astemizole may abolish or suppress skin reactivity to histamine for weeks (*eg*, 4 to 6 weeks, or longer). This may significantly interfere with skin test interpretation. If the positive histamine control skin test does not react (is negative), skin test results cannot be interpreted and are invalid.

If skin test reactions are equivocal, they should be repeated.

reactions [9]. Fortunately most allergic reactions to β-lactam antibiotics are cutaneous and not serious (Table 6).

When clinical circumstances create the need to determine whether a patient with a history of penicillin allergy would be at risk of developing a potentially serious IgE-mediated reaction if treated with penicillin, diagnostic penicillin skin testing may be performed. Skin testing with benzylpenicilloyl polylysine and penicillin G detects approximately 95% of patients at risk for an acute allergic reaction subsequent to penicillin administration. The incidence of positive skin tests among history-negative patients (false-positive) is low, 7% or less, and the incidence of significant immediate or accelerated reactions occurring in history-positive, skin test–negative patients (false-negative) is probably less than 1% [9]. Negative results are strong evidence that previous penicillin hypersensitivity has diminished or ceased to exist. However, negative results do not absolutely exclude the possibility of a significant reaction. A positive test to any of the reagents indicates that IgE antibodies are present to one of the antigenic determinants and places the individual at increased risk for the development of an anaphylactic or accelerated reaction.

The majority of patients with a history of penicillin allergy exhibit negative skin tests. Individuals with a recent history (within the last 12 months) of a documented reaction are likely to have positive skin tests [6]. Assuming no penicillin re-exposure, the rate of skin test reactivity in previously skin test–positive patients decreases by approximately 10% per year. The optimal treatment of an individual with definite β-lactam antibiotic allergy is avoidance of this class of antibiotics. If substitution is not possible, the cautious gradual administration of the drug (test dosing) or desensitization may be considered. These are risky procedures that should not be undertaken except in an intensive care setting.

Penicillin desensitization is not permanent. Patients who experience an allergic reaction during therapy or who exhibit positive skin tests should be told that penicillin should not be administered in the future without repeat skin tests being performed. Their medical records should be labeled as such. They should be encouraged to consider obtaining medical identification jewelry stating that they are allergic to penicillin.

Foreign Sera

Anaphylaxis and serum sickness may result from the injection of heterologous protein. Anaphylaxis develops less frequently than serum sickness and occurs most commonly in individuals with preexisting IgE specific for dander proteins of the corresponding animals. Serum sickness is dose dependent. It can be expected to develop in almost all patients who receive more than 70 mL of equine antivenin [10]. Primary serum sickness occurs 6 to 21 days (typically 7 to 14 days) after administration. Accelerated serum sickness may develop within 2 to 4 days in previously sensitized patients. Therapeutic indications for the use of foreign sera include snake bite, black widow spider bites, gas gangrene, botulism, and diphtheria. Negative skin tests virtually exclude anaphylactic sensitivity [2••,5••]. Should serum sickness develop, appropriate treatment with antipyretics, analgesics, antihistamines, and corticosteroids may be required. Plasmapheresis can be useful in the management of patients with severe serum sickness [11].

Insulin

Allergic reactions to insulin can be local and systemic [2••,12]. Generally, bovine insulin is more allergenic than porcine insulin, which is more allergenic than human recombinant DNA (rDNA) insulin [13]. Severe allergic reactions can develop to human rDNA insulin in susceptible individuals [14].

Most local insulin reactions are mild and transient, characterized by erythema, pruritus, burning, and induration of the injection site. They usually develop within 1 to 4 weeks after initiation of insulin therapy, unless the individual has previously received insulin therapy, in which case they may occur within the first few days of resuming treatment. They may occur within 20 minutes of the injection and subside rapidly, or may be delayed in appearance, developing 4 or more hours after the injection. The delayed reactions may evolve into

TABLE 6 ADVERSE REACTIONS TO PENICILLIN		
Type of reaction	**Time of onset**	**Clinical manifestations**
Immediate	Up to 1 h	Urticaria and angioedema
		Anaphylaxis
Accelerated	1 to 72 h	Urticaria and angioedema
		Laryngeal edema
Late	More than 72 h	Maculopapular rash
		Fever
		Vasculitis
		Serum sickness–like reactions
		Exfoliative dermatitis
		Stevens-Johnson syndrome
		Interstitial nephritis
		Immune cytopenias

painful local induration that may persist for days. Occasionally an individual may exhibit a biphasic response characterized by an immediate response that subsides within an hour, followed by a delayed local response 4 to 6 hours later.

Most patients with local allergic reactions improve within 3 to 4 weeks if they continue to use the insulin that is causing the reaction. However, if the reactions are quite troublesome it is not unreasonable to consider some of the following treatment options: substitute a different insulin preparation (the use of lente insulin eliminates the occasional local reaction due to protamine). If this is not successful, administering the total dose by two or three separate injections may be helpful. Administration of antihistamines (H_1 and H_2) for several weeks may provide symptomatic relief until the local reactions cease. Observe the patient's skin preparation and injection technique. Ensure that isopropyl alcohol used for skin cleansing is not irritating the skin and that the insulin is being injected subcutaneously, not intradermally. For especially symptomatic delayed local reactions, consideration may be given to administering a separate subcutaneous co-injection of dexamethasone (0.1 to 0.3 mg) in the insulin injection site [13]. Since local insulin allergy is almost always a self-limited process, periodic attempts to discontinue antihistamines and the subcutaneous steroid co-injections should be made. Do not stop insulin therapy because of troublesome local allergic reactions. Cessation of insulin treatment may increase the risk of a systemic reaction developing if insulin is subsequently re-instituted. Local insulin allergic reactions may persist and precede a systemic reaction. This occurs in a distinct minority of patients. Individuals with large local reactions may be given prescriptions for, and instructed in the use of, epinephrine for emergency treatment should a systemic allergic reaction develop [15].

Systemic allergic (IgE-mediated) reactions to insulin, manifested by urticaria and angioedema more frequently than bronchospasm, hypotension, or shock, are rare. Most commonly, an interruption in insulin therapy occurred, typically of several years' duration. Upon re-institution of insulin administration, allergic reactions occur, for example, the occurrence of progressively large local reactions at the injection site, ultimately followed by a systemic allergic reaction. Most frequently systemic reactions occur within 12 days of resumption of insulin treatment, usually developing within 30 minutes of the insulin injection. (It is not uncommon for women who received insulin therapy only when pregnant for gestational diabetes to be candidates for systemic reactions.) Patients allergic to insulin exhibit positive immediate hypersensitivity skin tests to insulin (Table 7). A positive skin test result does not establish a diagnosis of insulin allergy, because 40% to 50% of diabetics receiving insulin therapy develop a positive skin test for the insulin preparation used for their treatment. A negative insulin skin test does not rule out insulin allergy. Once the diagnosis of systemic insulin allergy has been established, an oral hypoglycemic agent may be substituted. If insulin therapy is essential, the patient may be desensitized to insulin [2••,12,16].

Latex (Natural Rubber)

The fact that products containing natural rubber could sensitize and cause contact dermatitis has been known for decades. Only since 1979 has it been widely appreciated that latex could sensitize and elicit IgE-mediated reactions, ranging from rhinitis, conjunctivitis, urticaria, and angioedema to fatal anaphylaxis [17–19]. Itching or swelling of hands after wearing rubber gloves, itching or swelling of lips after blowing up balloons, and itching or swelling of tongue or lips after dental examinations all suggest latex allergy. So does unexplained anaphylaxis or hypotension immediately before or during diagnostic or surgical procedures. Medical sources of exposure are gloves, rubber stoppers in multidose vials, injection ports in intravenous tubing, catheters, and adhesives. Nonmedical sources include balloons, condoms, gloves, tires, toys, sporting goods, and rubber bands. Strict avoidance is optimal, but difficult.

Individuals with known latex sensitivity should consider obtaining medical identification jewelry and be instructed in the use of epinephrine to be self-injected in case of a severe allergic reaction. Patients should take nonlatex gloves (not "hypoallergenic") to all visits with health care providers, in case nonlatex gloves are not readily available. Patients with known latex allergy who require surgery should ideally be operated on in a latex-free surgical suite and as the first case in the morning. Consideration can be given, on an individual basis, to pretreatment with antihistamines and steroids, not to prevent anaphylaxis but with the hope of being able to modify the severity of any allergic reaction that may develop.

Avian-Derived Immunizing Agents

Egg-related or egglike proteins have been eliminated from most contemporary vaccines. Influenza vaccine is made from viruses grown in avian eggs, and the viruses used in measles and mumps vaccines and the measles-mumps-rubella (MMR) vaccine are prepared in cell cultures of chick embryo fibroblasts. (Rubella vaccine is grown in human diploid cell cultures.) Allergy to chicken feathers is not a contraindication to vaccine administration. Whether or not an individual with a history of egg allergy should be immunized with an avian-derived vaccine may, on occasion,

TABLE 7 INSULIN SKIN TESTING
Should more than 24 hours elapse since the systemic reaction, performing skin tests with serial dilutions of insulin preparations is required
The patient should be tested with human (rDNA) insulin, pork, and beef insulins
Initially, prick skin tests may be performed using regular insulin, at a dilution of 0.0001 unit
If the prick tests are negative, intradermal tests may be performed, starting with a dilution of 0.00001 units (0.02 mL)

Observe guidelines regarding skin testing and cautious drug administration.

Skin test

Prick: Use full-strength MMR vaccine. If negative, administer full, recommended dose of MMR vaccine. If positive, administer MMR in gradual incremental fashion. If deemed appropriate, prick skin tests may be performed initially with a 1:100 dilution of MMR vaccine.

Cautious gradual administration (subcutaneous)

The initial dose should represent a small fraction of the total dose (*eg*, 0.05 mL). If no reaction after 15 to 20 min, 0.15 mL may be administered. If tolerated, two additional 0.15-mL injections may be administered at 15-min intervals. Alternatively, 0.05 mL may continue to be administered at 15- to 20-min intervals until the total dose of 0.5 mL has been given. After the completion of the procedure, it has been recommended that the patient should be observed for 2 h.

Physicians should be aware that MMR vaccination has provoked immediate, systemic reactions in nonallergic individuals.

From Patterson and coworkers [5••]; *with permission.*
MMR—measles, mumps, and rubella

Observe guidelines regarding skin testing and cautious gradual drug administration.

Skin tests

Prick: Use 1:10 dilution of vaccine in normal saline. If negative, an intradermal test is performed.

Intradermal: 0.02 mL of a 1:100 dilution. If negative, the vaccine may be administered in the routine fashion.

Cautious gradual administration

If either skin test is positive, the decision to administer the vaccine may be reassessed.

If immunization is deemed essential, gradual administration may be performed as suggested below.

Injections are administered at 15- to 20-min intervals.

Route	Dose, mL	Dilution
Intramuscular	0.05	1:100
Intramuscular	0.05	1:10
Intramuscular	0.05	Undiluted
Intramuscular	0.10	Undiluted
Intramuscular	0.15	Undiluted
Intramuscular	0.20	Undiluted

The patient should be observed for 60 min after the completion of the procedure.

create concern for patient and physician. In general, individuals who eat eggs or egg-containing foods without incident can be vaccinated, even if they exhibit a positive skin test to egg protein.

Individuals who have experienced anaphylactic reactions after eating eggs may be considered for vaccine administration after appropriate evaluation. The MMR vaccine may be safely administered to children with documented egg hypersensitivity [20,21] (Table 8). Similarly, influenza vaccination has been safely administered to patients with histories of allergic reactions to eggs [22] (Table 9). Should concern exist regarding the administration of tetanus toxoid to an individual with a history of an adverse reaction attributed to "tetanus," skin testing and gradual administration of the vaccine may be performed [2••,5••,23] (Table 10). One may consider first obtaining a serum tetanus antitoxin titer and then proceeding with the above, if indicated.

Local Anesthetics

Many patients claim to be "allergic" to local anesthetics [2••,5••,12,24,25] (Table 11). Symptoms attributed to local anesthetic "allergy" may actually be manifestations of a vasovagal reaction, anxiety, epinephrine-induced side effects, or toxicity developing subsequent to inadvertent intravenous injection of the local anesthetic. On occasion, symptoms may be suggestive of an immediate hypersensitivity reaction. Reactions developing due to the presence of preservatives (parabens, sulfites) appear to be extremely rare. Topical application of local anesthetics may sensitize. Contact dermatitis can develop. Delayed hypersensitivity has been associated with the delayed onset of local swelling after injection. The existence of IgE-mediated mechanisms being responsible for the pathogenesis of local anesthetic-induced adverse reactions has not been confirmed. If such reactions do occur, they are quite rare. Table 12 suggests a

Skin testing

Utilize aqueous tetanus toxoid. Do not use alum precipitated toxoid. A prick test is performed. If negative, 0.1 mL is administered subcutaneously. If no local reaction develops within 30 minutes, the remaining 0.4 mL of tetanus toxoid is injected subcutaneously.

If the prick test is positive, a 1:1000 dilution of tetanus toxoid is prepared and administered according to the schedule below. All injections from a given dilution should be administered prior to advancing to the next stronger dilution.

1:1000	1:100	1:10	Undiluted
0.05	0.05	0.05	0.05
0.10	0.10	0.10	0.10
0.20	0.20	0.20	0.20
0.30	0.30	0.30	0.30
0.50	0.50	0.50	

Injections of doses are repeated if large local reactions occur. Frequency of injections: weekly or biweekly.

TABLE 11 REPRESENTATIVE LOCAL ANESTHETICS

Group 1 (benzoic acid esters)*	Group 2 (others)†
Butacaine	Bupivacaine
Butethamine	Cyclonine
Chloroprocaine	Dibucaine
Cyclomethycaine	Dicyclone
Hexylcaine	Etidocaine
Piperocaine	Lidocaine
Procaine	Mepivacaine
Tetracaine	Pramoxine
	Prilocaine

*By means of patch testing, group 1 drugs have been shown to be antigenic; group 1 drugs cross-react with one another.

†Group 2 drugs do not appear to cross-react with one another or with drugs in group 1.

method to determine whether an individual may receive and tolerate a local anesthetic [12].

Radiographic Contrast Media

Anaphylactoid (non–IgE-mediated anaphylactic) reactions develop in 1% or less of patients receiving radiographic contrast media (RCM). Individuals with a history of an RCM-induced anaphylactoid reaction are at increased risk of experiencing a subsequent reaction if RCM is re-administered. Repeat reaction rates range from 16% to 30% [12].

In patients with history of a reaction who must have another RCM study, it is important to document the fact that the study has been deemed essential, to explain the potential risk to the patient (and family, if indicated), and to obtain consent for re-administration. Document that the patient understands that the pretreatment protocol for anaphylactoid reactions may not prevent all RCM-related adverse reactions (for example, noncardiogenic pulmonary edema). Use a lower

osmolar RCM agent. Discontinue β-adrenergic antagonists, if possible. A pretreatment protocol should be employed [2••,12]. Administer prednisone, 50 mg orally, 13, 7, and 1 hour before the procedure; diphenhydramine hydrochloride, 50 mg orally or intramuscularly, 1 hour before the procedure; if not contraindicated (for example, angina, arrhythmia) ephedrine, 25 mg orally, 1 hour prior to the procedure; and at the discretion of the physician, an H_2-receptor antagonist may be administered orally, 3 hours before the procedure (300 mg ranitidine, or 300 mg cimetidine).

The recurrence rate of anaphylactoid reactions, employing such a pretreatment protocol, has been reduced to approximately 6% to 9%, when hyperosmolar RCM agents have been re-administered. When a lower osmolar RCM agent is employed, along with pretreatment, recurrence rates can be reduced even further. When an older, oil-based nonbenzene ring agent is used for myelography, such as iophendylate, pretreatment is not necessary. When myelography is performed using an isotonic, triiodinated benzene ring agent, pretreatment should be administered.

Should a high-risk patient (previous reactor) require an emergency radiographic procedure employing RCM, an emergency pretreatment protocol has been proposed [2••,12]. This includes the intravenous administration of hydrocortisone, 200 mg immediately and every 4 hours, until the procedure is performed, plus diphenhydramine, 50 mg intramuscularly, 1 hour before the procedure. If ephedrine is not contraindicated, 25 mg may be administered orally 1 hour before the procedure. Emergency equipment and medications should be immediately available to treat reactions.

Sulfonamides

Adverse drug reactions to sulfonamides have been recognized for years. Sulfa-associated Stevens-Johnson syndrome can be fatal. A history of any adverse sulfa reaction is a definite indication for future avoidance. Test dosing and desensitization are dangerous and rarely indi-

TABLE 12 LOCAL ANESTHETICS: SKIN TESTING AND TEST DOSING

Observe guidelines for performing skin tests and test dosing.

Ascertain from the patient's physician or dentist which local anesthetic will be administered. Use the concentration that will be employed by the doctor. The preparation to be used for skin testing must not contain vasoconstrictors (*eg*, epinephrine). If the patient's doctor believes that the local anesthetic plus vasoconstrictor is essential for the performance of the anticipated procedure, the test dosing may be performed using the same local anesthetic used for skin testing, but with a vasoconstrictor.

Preservative-free (parabens, sulfites) local anesthetic preparations may be evaluated if there is a concern regarding sensitivity to preservatives.

Route	Dose	Dilution
Skin test		
Prick	1 drop	Undiluted
Intradermal	0.02 mL	1:100
Test dosing		
Subcutaneous	0.10 mL	1:100
Subcutaneous	0.10 mL	1:10
Subcutaneous	0.10 mL	Undiluted
Subcutaneous	0.50 mL	Undiluted
Subcutaneous	1.0 mL	Undiluted

The skin tests and test dosing should be performed at 15-min intervals.

If the skin tests are negative, begin test dosing protocol.

The patient should be closely observed for 1 h after the completion of test dosing.

If the patient's history is that of a delayed reaction, the local anesthetic should not be administered until 24 to 48 h after the completion of the test dosing.

TABLE 13 ASPIRIN AND NONSTEROIDAL ANTIINFLAMMATORY DRUG CROSS-REACTIVITY IN ASPIRIN-SENSITIVE INDIVIDUALS

Minimal cross-reactivity (10% or less)

Acetaminophen

Choline salicylate

Choline magnesium salicylate

Salsalate

Sodium salicylate

Extensive cross-reactivity (90% or more)

Diclofenac

Diflunisal

Fenoprofen

Ibuprofen

Indomethacin

Ketoprofen

Meclofenamate

Mefenamic acid

Naproxen

Oxyphenbutazone

Phenylbutazone

Piroxicam

Sulindac

Tolmetin

cated [2••,5••,6]. Re-administration of sulfonamides to patients with a history of a severe exfoliative cutaneous reaction is not recommended [2••].

Aspirin

Adverse reactions to aspirin are typically characterized by urticaria, angioedema, bronchospasm, or hypotension and shock. These reactions are not IgE-mediated. The precise pathogenic mechanism has not been defined. Other nonsteroidal antiinflammatory drugs (NSAIDs) that also inhibit cyclooxygenase activity may cross-react with aspirin and evoke symptoms in susceptible individuals [2••,26] (Table 13).

TREATMENT AND PREVENTION

Usually, the treatment of adverse drug reactions results in a favorable outcome; prevention is even more desirable. Keep medication use to a minimum. Avoid prescribing drugs with a reputation for producing allergic reactions, if possible. Always inquire as to a prior reaction to any drug about to be prescribed. When appropriate, the oral administration of medication may be preferable to parenteral.

Educate patients regarding avoidance and possible modes of inadvertent exposure. Recommend medical identification jewelry when appropriate. If patients cannot remember names of drugs not tolerated, encourage (or insist) that they keep on their person at all times a card listing all drugs not tolerated and the nature of adverse reactions. Label the patient's medical records.

References and Recommended Reading

Recently published papers of particular interest have been highlighted as:
- Of interest
- •• Of outstanding interest

1. Reed CE: Drug allergy. In *Cecil Textbook of Medicine*, edn 19. Edited by Wyngaarden JB, Smith LH Jr, Bennett JC. Philadelphia: WB Saunders; 1992:1479–1483.

2.•• Deswarte RD: Drug allergy. In *Allergic Diseases. Diagnosis and Management*, edn 4. Edited by Patterson R, Grammer LC, Greenberger PA, Zeiss CR. Philadelphia: JB Lippincott; 1993:395–552.

3. Adkinson NF Jr: Risk factors for drug allergy. *J Allergy Clin Immunol* 1984, 74:567–572.

4.• Adkinson NF Jr: Tests for immunological drug reactions. In *Manual of Clinical Laboratory Immunology*, edn 4. Edited by Rose NR, deMacario EC, Fahey JL, *et al.*: Washington DC: American Society for Microbiology; 1992:717–722.

5.•• Patterson R, Deswarte RD, Greenberger PA, Grammer LC: Drug allergy and protocols for management of drug allergies. *N Engl Reg Allergy Proc* 1986, 7:325–342.

6. Anderson JA: Allergic reactions to drugs and biological agents. *JAMA* 1992, 268:2845–2857.

7. Bochner BS, Lichtenstein LM: Anaphylaxis. *N Engl J Med* 1991, 324:1785–1790.

8. Anderson JA, Adkinson NF Jr: Allergic reactions to drugs and biologic agents. *JAMA* 1987, 258:2891–2899.

9. Sogn DD, Evans R III, Shepherd GM, *et al.*: Results of the national institute of allergy and infectious diseases collaborative clinical trial to test the predictive value of skin testing with major and minor penicillin derivatives in hospitalized adults. *Arch Intern Med* 1992, 152:1025–1032.

10. Erffmeyer JE: Serum sickness. *Ann Allergy* 1986, 56:105–109.

11. Sullivan TJ: Drug allergy. In *Allergy Principles and Practice*, edn 4. Edited by Middleton E Jr, Reed CE, Ellis EF, *et al.* St. Louis: Mosby-Year Book; 1993:1726–1746.

12. Lieberman P: Difficult allergic drug reactions. *Immunol Allergy Clin North Am* 1991, 11:213–231.

13. Shuldiner AR, Roth J: Insulin allergy and insulin resistance. In *Current Therapy in Allergy, Immunology, and Rheumatology*, edn. 4. Edited by Lichtenstein LM, Fauci AS. St. Louis: Mosby-Year Book; 1992: 152–157.

14. Ganz MA, Unterman T, Roberts M, *et al.*: Resistance and allergy to recombinant human insulin. *J Allergy Clin Immunol* 1990, 86:45–52.

15. Galloway JA, deShazo RD; Insulin chemistry and pharmacology; insulin allergy, resistance, and lipodystrophy. In *Diabetes Mellitus. Theory and Practice*, edn. 4. Edited by Rifkin H, Porte D Jr. New York: Elsevier Science Publishing; 1990:497–513.

16. Grammer LC, Chen PY, Patterson R: Evaluation and management of insulin allergy. *J Allergy Clin Immunol* 1983, 71:250–254.

17. Slater JE: Allergic reactions to natural rubber. *Ann Allergy* 1992, 68:203–209.

18. Slater JE: Latex allergy—what do we know? *J Allergy Clin Immunol* 1992, 90:279–281.

19. Slater JE: Latex allergy. *Ann Allergy* 1993, 70:1–2.

20. Beck SA, Williams LW, Shirrel MA, Burks AW: Egg hypersensitivity and measles-mumps-rubella vaccine administration. *Pediatrics* 1991, 88:913–917.

21. Fasano MB, Wood RA, Cooke SK, Sampson HA: Egg hypersensitivity and adverse reactions to measles, mumps, and rubella vaccine. *J Pediatr* 1992, 120:878–881.

22. Kletz MR, Holland CL, Mendelson JS, Bielory L: Administration of egg-derived vaccines in patients with history of egg sensitivity. *Ann Allergy* 1990, 64:527–529.

23. Carey AB, Meltzer EO: Diagnosis and "desensitization" in tetanus hypersensitivity. *Ann Allergy* 1992, 69:336–338.

24. Chandler MJ, Grammer LC, Patterson R: Provocative challenge with local anesthetics in patients with a prior history of reaction. *J Allergy Clin Immunol* 1987, 79:883–886.

25. Grammer LC, Chandler MJ, Patterson R: Additives or preservatives in injectable anesthetics. *J Allergy Clin Immunol* 1988, 82:309–310.

26. Manning ME, Stevenson DD, Mathison DA: Reactions to aspirin and other nonsteroidal anti-inflammatory drugs. *Immunol Allergy Clin North Am* 1992, 12:611–631.

Select Bibliography

Greenberger PA, Patterson R: Management of drug allergy in patients with acquired immunodeficiency syndrome. *J Allergy Clin Immunol* 1987, 79:484–488.

Moscicki RA, Sockin SM, Corsello BF, *et al.*: Anaphylaxis during induction of general anesthesia: subsequent evaluation and management. *J Allergy Clin Immunol* 1990, 86:325–332.

Purdy BH, Philips DM, Summers RW: Desensitization for sulfasalazine skin rash. *Ann Intern Med* 1984, 100:512–514.

Reisman RE, Lieberman P: Anaphylaxis and anaphylactoid reactions. *Allergy Clin North Am* 1992, 12(3).

VanArsdel PP Jr: Drug allergy. *Immunol Allergy Clin North Am* 1991, 11(3).

White MV, Haddad ZH, Brunner E, Sainz C: Desensitization to trimethoprim sulfamethoxazole in patients with acquired immunodeficiency syndrome and *Pneumocystis carinii* pneumonia. *Ann Allergy* 1989, 62:177–179.

Systemic Mastocytosis 12

Dean D. Metcalfe

> ### Key Points
> - Mastocytosis is a rare disease caused by tissue mast cell hyperplasia and systemic release of mast cell–derived mediators.
> - Most cases are diagnosed because there are associated characteristic cutaneous lesions, or after evaluation for unexplained flushing and anaphylaxis, or cytopenia.
> - Most patients do well, but some develop aggressive disease or hematopoietic disorders.
> - Management is largely for symptoms and is planned in concert with specialists.

Symptoms of systemic mastocytosis include fatigue, flushing, pruritus, abdominal pain, diarrhea, and intermittent episodes of hypotension. One or all of these symptoms may occur; yet, systemic mastocytosis is rare, perhaps affecting fewer than one in 100,000 people. Thus, systemic mastocytosis is a frequently considered, but rarely confirmed diagnosis.

The disease occurs in all age groups. There is no family history of mastocytosis in most confirmed cases. Reports in which two closely related family members have been diagnosed as having mastocytosis suggest there may be an inherited pattern in rare instances. Atopy is not associated with mastocytosis [1].

DISEASE CATEGORIES

Tissue mast cell hyperplasia is the pathologic hallmark of mastocytosis. Symptoms result primarily from the release of associated mast cell mediators [2]. Clinical characteristics, including disease severity, rapidity of disease progression, and presence of associated dermatologic abnormalities, are used to classify mastocytosis into four clinical groups in Table 1 [3,4••]. These groups aid in assigning prognosis and selecting therapy.

Indolent Mastocytosis

Indolent mastocytosis is the most frequent form of mastocytosis. More than 70% of patients with mastocytosis referred to the National Institutes of Health have this form of the disease; elsewhere, the number may approach 95%. Urticaria pigmentosa is the most common cutaneous manifestation of mastocytosis and is the usual presenting feature of indolent mastocytosis in both children and adults. Lesions of urticaria pigmentosa appear as small yellow-to-tan to red-brown macules or slightly raised papules (Figs. 1, 2, and 3). Urticaria pigmentosa in children most often resembles the adult pattern (Figs. 4 and 5), although lesion size occasionally is variable and larger (Fig. 6). Darier's sign consists of urtication and erythema around and over macules after lesions are rubbed or scratched. Diffuse cutaneous mastocytosis is a second, less common form of cutaneous mastocytosis. The entire cutaneous integument is involved, resulting in thickened skin that may

TABLE 1 CLINICAL CLASSIFICATION OF MASTOCYTOSIS

Indolent mastocytosis
Cutaneous disease only
Systemic disease defined by internal organ involvement

Mastocytosis with an associated hematologic disorder
Myeloproliferative
Myelodysplastic

Aggressive mastocytosis

Mast cell leukemia

From Metcalfe [4**]; with permission.

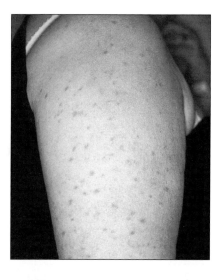

FIGURE 1
Urticaria pigmentosa in an adult. Discrete lesions are randomly distributed over the arm.

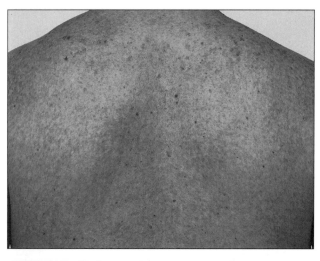

FIGURE 2 Urticaria pigmentosa in an adult. Discrete lesions are numerous and randomly distributed over the back.

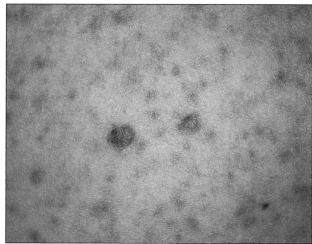

FIGURE 3 Close view of urticaria pigmentosa in an adult.

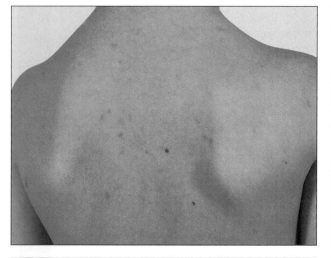

FIGURE 4 Urticaria pigmentosa in a young adult. Lesions are fewer and less intense than those seen in Figure 3. Lesions are randomly distributed.

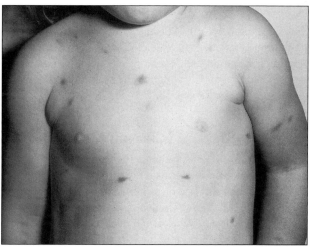

FIGURE 5 Urticaria pigmentosa in a child. Lesions are dark reddish-brown and widely scattered.

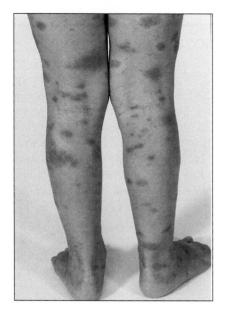

FIGURE 6 Urticaria pigmentosa in a child. Lesion size varies. With time, these lesions become less intense, although smaller lesions persist.

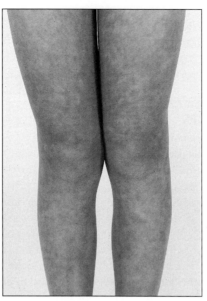

FIGURE 7 Diffuse cutaneous mastocytosis in a young adult. The skin has a mottled appearance and is diffusely thickened.

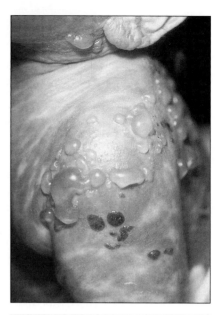

FIGURE 8 Bullous mastocytosis in a child.

appear yellow-brown (Fig. 7). Young children with urticaria pigmentosa or diffuse cutaneous mastocytosis may have bullous eruptions with hemorrhage (Fig. 8).

The diagnosis of systemic disease is made when mast cell hyperplasia is demonstrated in one or more internal organs [2]. Most commonly, this increase in mast cells and pathological characteristics are found in the bone marrow, followed by the gastrointestinal tract, liver, spleen, and lymph nodes. Systemic disease is common in adults but unusual in children.

Both children and adults with cutaneous or systemic disease may experience pruritus and spontaneous episodes of flushing or hypotension. Patients with systemic disease usually develop gastrointestinal symptoms, including abdominal pain, diarrhea, nausea, and vomiting [5]. These symptoms are associated with gastritis and peptic ulcer disease due to hyperhistaminemia; in more advanced cases, symptoms are associated with malabsorption due to mucosal infiltration with mast cells and other inflammatory cells. Pancreatic function remains normal. Bone pain is a complaint in advanced disease.

Mastocytosis with an Associated Hematologic Disorder

Fewer than 50% of patients diagnosed as having mastocytosis with an associated hematologic disorder present with urticaria pigmentosa [3,4••]. The remainder are given the diagnosis after a bone marrow examination in evaluation of an unexplained neutrophilia, eosinophilia, neutropenia, thrombocytopenia, or other peripheral blood abnormality that reveals characteristic mast cell infiltrates associated with a second hematologic disorder. These hematologic disorders include myelodysplastic syndromes and myeloproliferative disorders

such as de novo acute leukemia, chronic leukemia, and chronic neutropenia. These associated hematologic disorders are rarely seen in children, particularly if the onset of cutaneous disease is before 6 months of age.

Patients with both mastocytosis and an associated hematologic disorder may develop gastrointestinal disease, although apparently less frequently than that developed with indolent mastocytosis. Significant liver disease, splenomegaly, and ascites may occur, particularly with advanced disease. Hypersplenism may exacerbate thrombocytopenia and anemia. Pathologic fractures of the femurs and other weight-bearing bones have been reported.

Aggressive Mastocytosis

Patients with aggressive mastocytosis usually present with a several-month history of progressive flushing, gastrointestinal discomfort, and fatigue. Urticaria pigmentosa of recent onset is observed in less than 50% of cases. Hepatomegaly, splenomegaly, lymphadenopathy, and weight loss may be recorded on the initial examination or may develop in the first few months of disease progression. Mast cell infiltrates and fibrosis within the bone marrow may lead to marrow expansion. As the disease progresses, malabsorption develops, thus leading to weight loss. Compression fractures of the spine occur in advanced disease in association with generalized osteoporosis.

Mast Cell Leukemia

Mast cell leukemia is the most rapidly progressive form of mastocytosis and is the least common, occurring in less than 2% of cases [6]. The disease is accompanied by the presence of mast cells in the peripheral circulation to the extent that they comprise more than 10% of the nucleated cells. Bone marrow biopsy is required for diagnosis. Clinical findings center around a compromise of bone marrow function due to mast cell infiltrates in the marrow with anemia and thrombocytopenia.

PATHOLOGIC FEATURES

The clinical diagnosis of urticaria pigmentosa or diffuse cutaneous mastocytosis should be confirmed by biopsy of the skin. Mast cell hyperplasia (to fourfold) in the dermis may accompany other skin conditions such as eczema and chronic idiopathic hives. Mast cell hyperplasia in urticaria pigmentosa or in diffuse cutaneous mastocytosis is usually obvious, and the number of mast cells is, on average, 10 times greater than that in normal skin [7]. Thus, in the absence of characteristic macroscopic skin lesions, small increases in dermal mast cells are insufficient for diagnosis. By examining the bone marrow biopsy and aspirate, characteristic abnormal focal collections of mast cells can be identified and the hematopoietic marrow can be examined, providing information for diagnostic categorization [8,9•]. Biopsies of liver, spleen, and lymph nodes may also reveal mast cell hyperplasia [10].

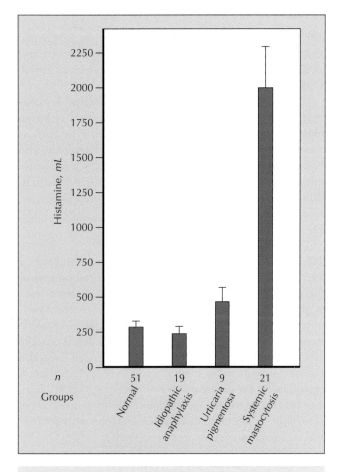

FIGURE 9 Plasma histamine levels in adults with mast cell disorders. Urticaria pigmentosa denotes patients with skin disease only. Systemic mastocytosis includes patients with indolent disease and patients with mastocytosis with an associated hematologic disorder. Plasma was obtained from patients with idiopathic disorders during asymptomatic periods. Data are presented as the mean ± standard error of the mean.

LABORATORY FINDINGS

Mastocytosis may be accompanied by elevations in plasma tryptase or histamine (Fig. 9), or urinary histamine or prostaglandin D_2 (PGD_2) metabolites [11,12]. Elevations in these mediators are not diagnostic. Elevations in tryptase, PGD_2 metabolites, and histamine also occur in association with severe systemic allergic reactions and in association with idiopathic anaphylaxis. However, elevations in one or more of these mediators should raise the suspicion of mastocytosis. Mastocytosis has also been diagnosed in the absence of demonstrable elevations in histamine or tryptase.

Although results of bone scans are usually normal early in disease progression, technetium bone scan results may become abnormal and offer some insight into disease severity and duration [13]. With time, bone scans progress from unifocal or multifocal to diffuse patterns (Fig. 10). These patterns are not specific for mastocytosis, but suggest systemic disease if present in a patient with urticaria pigmentosa or diffuse cutaneous mastocytosis. Radiographically detectable lesions, particularly of the proximal long bones, may also be present, followed by lesions of the pelvis, ribs, and skull.

A 24-hour urinary study of 5-hydroxyindoleacetic acid (5-HIAA) and urinary metanephrine helps eliminate the diagnosis of a carcinoid tumor or pheochromocytoma. Idiopathic anaphylaxis and flushing must also be considered. Patients with these disorders do not have histologic evidence of significant mast cell proliferation and have normal plasma histamine and tryptase levels between episodes of anaphylaxis.

TREATMENT

The treatment of indolent mastocytosis is principally for symptoms. H_1-receptor antagonists, such as hydroxyzine, reduce pruritus, flushing, and tachycardia. H_2-receptor antagonists, such as ranitidine, inhibit gastric hypersecretion and prevent gastritis and peptic ulcer disease, and may be recommended following an evaluation by a gastroenterologist. Hypotensive episodes are treated with epinephrine. Patients should be trained to medicate themselves with epinephrine and to promptly seek medical assistance if they experience a hypotensive episode. Prophylaxis with H_1- and H_2-antihistamines is valuable if hypotensive episodes are frequent. Hypotension has been observed after insect stings and administration of contrast media [14,15]. Aspirin and other nonsteroidal antiinflammatory drugs (NSAIDs) have therapeutic value in the treatment of recurrent hypotension and flushing in that they block the synthesis of PGD_2. However, aspirin and the other NSAIDs may exacerbate gastritis. Some patients also have a severe hypotensive response to aspirin ingestion. Because of these difficulties, aspirin should be added to the antihistamine regimen only when symptoms are severe and are otherwise uncontrolled. Aspirin should be administered initially under controlled circumstances and preferably under the care of an allergist-immunologist.

If skin involvement is extensive, patients may be referred to a dermatologist for methoxsalen with long-wave ultraviolet radiation. This treatment relieves pruritus and whealing after

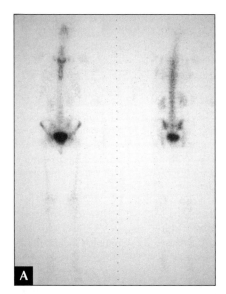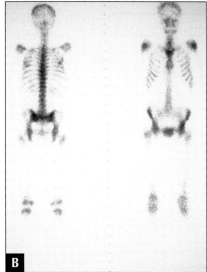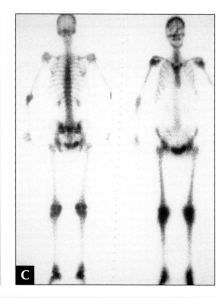

FIGURE 10 Skeletal scintigraphy showing a normal pattern **A**, multifocal abnormalities **B**, and a diffuse increase in scan intensity **C**. Images in **B** and **C** were obtained on two patients with indolent mastocytosis.

1 to 2 months of treatment. Pruritus recurs 3 to 6 months after therapy is discontinued. Patients may report a decrease in the number or intensity of cutaneous lesions after repeated exposure to natural sunlight. Topical steroids, as recommended by a dermatologist, may be applied under plastifilm occlusion for 8 h/d over 8 to 12 weeks in the treatment of urticaria pigmentosa or diffuse cutaneous mastocytosis. Lesions reappear within 1 year after therapy is discontinued.

The treatment of intestinal disease recommended in consultation with a gastroenterologist is determined by the degree of cramping, diarrhea, and malabsorption. Anticholinergics may give some relief. Oral cromolyn sodium is often useful in the management of abdominal symptoms [16]. Systemic glucocorticoids are effective in patients with severe malabsorption.

Patients with mastocytosis and an associated hematologic disorder are managed as dictated by the specific hematologic abnormality as diagnosed. Management is by a hematologist. Chemotherapy has not been shown to produce remission or to prolong survival in patients with mast cell leukemia, and it has no place in the treatment of indolent mastocytosis. One study suggests that splenectomy may improve the length of survival in patients with forms of mastocytosis associated with poor prognosis. Ascites is more often seen in mastocytosis with an associated hematologic disorder and in aggressive mastocytosis, and is difficult to control. Portal hypertension has been successfully managed with a portacaval shunt; exudative ascites has been successfully treated with systemic glucocorticoid therapy.

Aggressive mastocytosis is best managed by a hematologist-oncologist. Systemic steroids are used to control malabsorption and ascites. Anecdotal reports have described partial remissions in response to interferon γ and interferon α-2b.

NATURAL HISTORY

Patients with indolent mastocytosis who have only skin involvement have the best prognosis. Isolated urticaria pigmentosa in children resolves by adulthood in at least 50% of cases. Urticaria pigmentosa in adults with indolent mastocytosis usually progresses to systemic disease. Patients with mastocytosis with an associated hematologic disorder have a course that depends on the prognosis of the specific hematologic disorder. Survival of patients with aggressive mastocytosis is 2 to 4 years with intense symptom management. The mean survival expectation of patients with mast cell leukemia is usually less than 6 months.

ROLE OF THE GENERALIST

Mastocytosis is a rare disease and its management is not associated with the expertise of one specialty. After diagnosis of mastocytosis in a patient, symptomatic management often falls to a generalist. A hematologist should work in consultation with the generalist in selecting and implementing therapy for an associated hematologic disorder. The expertise of an allergist-immunologist helps in the management of episodes of hypotension and in managing the patient sensitive to insect sting. A dermatologist's advice may be sought in the management of skin disease, including the application of steroids and use of light therapy.

A generalist must not attribute new physical or psychological problems *a priori* to mastocytosis. Each new complaint must be evaluated thoroughly and treated appropriately. Most patients with mastocytosis have indolent disease and may be expected to have a reasonably normal and productive life.

References and Recommended Reading

Recently published papers of particular interest have been highlighted as:
- • Of interest
- •• Of outstanding interest

1. Müller U, Helbling A, Hunziker T, Wüthrich B, *et al.*: Mastocytosis and atopy: a study of 33 patients with urticaria pigmentosa. *Allergy* 1990, 45:597–603.

2: Metcalfe DD: The mastocytosis syndrome. In *Dermatology in General Medicine*, edn. 4. Edited by Fitzpatrick TB, Eisen AZ, Wolff K, *et al.* New York: McGraw-Hill; 1993, 2017–2023.

3. Travis WD, Li C-Y, Bergstrath EJ, *et al.*: Systemic mast cell disease: analysis of 58 cases and literature review. *Medicine* 1988, 67:345–368.

4.•• Metcalfe DD: Conclusions. *J Invest Dermatol* 1991, 96:64S–65S.

5. Cherner JA, Jensen RT, Dubois A, *et al.*: Gastrointestinal dysfunction in systemic mastocytosis: a prospective study. *Gastroenterology* 1988, 95:657–667.

6. Travis WD, Li C-Y, Hoagland HC, *et al.*: Mast cell leukemia: report of a case and review of the literature. *Mayo Clin Proc* 1986, 61:957–966.

7. Garriga MM, Friedman MM, Metcalfe DD: A survey of the number and distribution of mast cells in the skin of patients with mast cell disorders. *J Allergy Clin Immunol* 1988, 82:425–432.

8. Kettelhut BV, Parker RI, Travis WD, Metcalfe DD: Hematopathology of bone marrow in pediatric cutaneous mastocytosis: a study of seventeen patients. *Am J Clin Pathol* 1989, 91:558–562.

9.• Lawrence JB, Friedman BS, Travis WD, *et al.*: Hematologic manifestations of systemic mast cell disease: a prospective study of laboratory and morphologic features and their relation to prognosis. *Am J Med* 1991, 91:612–624.

10. Metcalfe DD: The liver, spleen, and lymph nodes in mastocytosis. *J Invest Dermatol* 1991, 96:455–465.

11. Friedman BS, Steinberg S, Meggs WJ, *et al.*: Analysis of plasma histamine levels in patients with mast cell disorders. *Am J Med* 1989, 87:649–654.

12. Schwartz LB, Metcalfe DD, Miller JS, *et al.*: Tryptase levels as an indicator of mast cell activation in systemic anaphylaxis and mastocytosis. *N Engl J Med* 1987, 316:1622–1626.

13. Rosenbaum RC, Frieri M, Metcalfe DD: Patterns of skeletal scintigraphy and their relationship to plasma and urinary histamine levels in mastocytosis. *J Nucl Med* 1984, 25:859–864.

14. Müller UR, Horat W, Wüthrich B, *et al.*: Anaphylaxis after Hymenoptera stings in three patients with urticaria pigmentosa. *J Allergy Clin Immunol* 1983, 72:685–689.

15. Scott HW Jr, Parris WCV, Sandidge PC, *et al.*: Hazards in operative management of patients with systemic mastocytosis. *Ann Surg* 1983, 197:507–514.

16. Horan RF, Sheffer AL, Austen KF: Cromolyn sodium in the management of systemic mastocytosis. *J Allergy Clin Immunol* 1990, 85:852–857.

Select Bibliography

Friedman BS, Germano P, Miletti J, Metcalfe DD: A clinico-pathologic study of ten patients with recurrent unexplained flushing. *J Allergy Clin Immunol* 1994, 93:53–60.

Friedman BS, Santiago ML, Berkebile C, Metcalfe DD: Comparison of azelastine and chlorpheniramine in the treatment of mastocytosis. *J Allergy Clin Immunol* 1993, 92:520–526.

Longley J, Morganroth GS, Tyrell L, et al.: Altered metabolism of mast cell growth factor (c-kit ligand) in cutaneous mastocytosis. *N Engl J Med* 1993, 328:1302–1306.

Weidner N, Horan RF, Austen KF: Mast cell phenotypes in indolent forms of mastocytosis: ultrastructural features, fluorescence detection of avidin binding, and immunofluorescent determination of chymase, tryptase, and carboxypeptidase. *Am J Pathol* 1992, 140:847–854.

Complement Deficiency Syndromes 13

James Holbert

Key Points
- Complement deficiencies are uncommon, but must be considered in specific disease settings.
- Deficiencies in the classical pathway of complement often manifest as immune complex diseases.
- Deficiencies in the alternative pathway often manifest as susceptibility to various pyogenic infections.
- The treatment of angioneurotic edema is divided into acute and chronic approaches.
- Paroxysmal nocturnal hemoglobinuria results from a complement deficiency.

Complement deficiency syndromes are uncommon [1] and result from inherited [2•,3•] or mutated genes that fail to code for adequate quantities of complement protein (null genes) or code for an abnormal or dysfunctional protein. Complement protein alleles demonstrate codominant behavior. Heterozygotes for null alleles generally have half the normal level of the particular protein; individuals with half-normal levels of protein are usually clinically normal. Deficiencies of each of the complement components occur with an autosomal recessive inheritance.

The complement cascade [4•,5] is depicted in Figure 1. Deficiencies of the complement system [6•] may be subdivided into two categories: 1) deficiencies of complement proteins; and 2) deficiencies of complement regulator proteins.

DEFICIENCIES OF COMPLEMENT PROTEINS

Functions of the complement system [7–9] are listed in Table 1. The function of the various complement components is related to the clinical syndrome that results from a specific protein's functional absence. Deficiencies of the complement proteins of the classical pathway of complement can generally be considered together (Table 2). Their absence is manifested clinically by immune complex diseases resembling lupus erythematosus [11] and rheumatoid arthritis. Patients with this group of complement deficiencies do not demonstrate increased susceptibility to infection. This absence of susceptibility to pyogenic infections results from the presence of an intact alternative pathway, through which potent humoral mediators are generated [12]. Autoimmune diseases that present as glomerulonephritis [13], rheumatoid arthritis, or systemic lupus–like syndromes are seen in more than half of patients with C2 or C4 deficiencies [14,15•]. The manifestation of autoimmune disease is possibly caused by the relationship of polymorphic genes encoding for C2 and C4 between the DR locus and the class I *MHC* genes [16], 5' to genes encoding the cytokines tumor necrosis factor and lymphotoxin. C2 deficiency has also been reported to be associated with increased susceptibility to *Hemophilus influenzae* septicemia in infancy, whereas other pyogenic infections are immunologically attenuated in a normal manner.

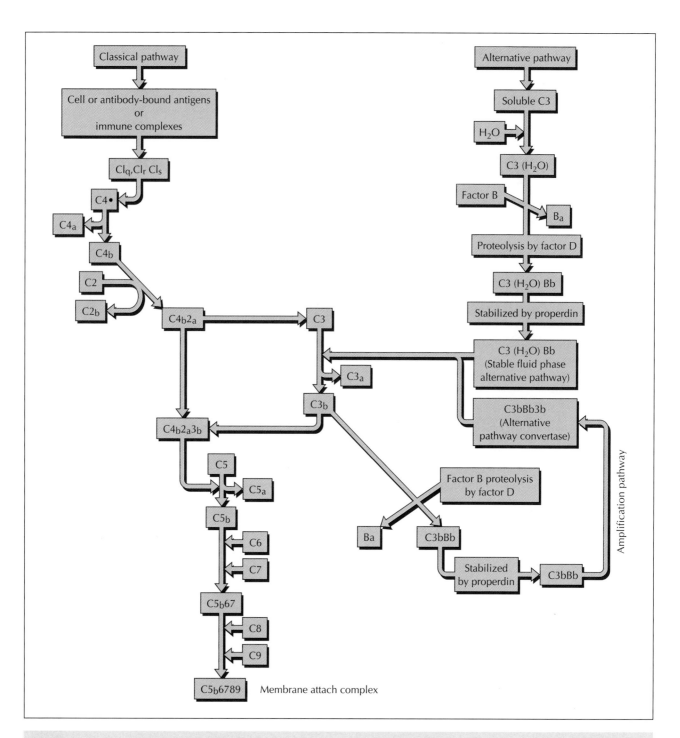

FIGURE 1 Complement cascade.

TABLE 1 PROTEIN COMPONENTS OF THE COMPLEMENT CASCADES

Component	Molecular size, *kd*	Serum concentration, μg/mL	Molecular size of subunit chains, *kd*	Activation products	Comments on function
Classical pathway					
C1 (C1qr$_2$s$_2$)	900				Initiates classical pathway
C1q	410	75	6 of A; 24 / 6 of B; 23 / 6 of C; 22		Binds to Fc portion of Ig
C1r	85	50	1	$\overline{C1r}$	$\overline{C1r}$ is a serine protease; cleaves $\overline{C1s}$
C1s	85	50	1	$\overline{C1s}$	$\overline{C1s}$ is a serine protease; cleaves C4 and C2
C4	210	200–500	1 of alpha; 90 / 1 of beta; 78 / 1 of gamma; 33	C4a C4b	C4a is an anaphylatoxin; C4b covalently binds to activating surfaces, where it is part of C3 convertase
C2	110	20	1	$\overline{C2a}$ C2b	$\overline{C2a}$ is a serine protease, part of C3 and C5 convertases
C3 (Also part of alternative pathway)	195	550–1200	1 of alpha; 110 / 1 of beta; 85	C3a C3b	C3a is an anaphylatoxin; C3b covalently binds to activating surfaces, where it is part of C3 and C5 convertases and also acts as opsonin
Alternative pathway					
Factor B	93	200	1	Ba $\overline{Bb}$	$\overline{Bb}$ is a serine protease, part of C3 and C5 convertases
Factor D	25	1–2	1	$\overline{D}$	Protease that circulates in active state; cleaves factor B
Properdin	220	25	4; 56		Stabilizes alternative pathway C3 convertase
Terminal lytic components					
C5	190	70	1 of alpha; 115 / 1 of beta; 75	C5a C5b	C5a is an anaphylatoxin
C6	128	60	1		C5b initiates MAC assembly
C7	121	60	1		Component of MAC
C8	155	60	1 of alpha; 64 / 1 of beta; 64 / 1 of gamma; 22		Component of MAC / Component of MAC
C9	79	60	1		Component of MAC; polymerizes to form membrane pores

MAC—membrane attack complex.
From Abbas *et al.* [10]; with permission.

TABLE 2 DEFICIENCY OF COMPLEMENT COMPLEX

Component deficiency	Associated disease	Inheritance	Treatment
C1q	Glomerulonephritis, SLE	AR	
C1r	SLE, glomerulonephritis, pyogenic infection	AR	
C1s	SLE, glomerulonephritis, pyogenic infection	AR	
C4	SLE, glomerulonephritis, pyogenic infection	AR	
C2	SLE, vasculitis glomerulonephritis, pyogenic infection, *Hemophilus influenzae* septicemia in infancy	AR	*Symptomatic* medical treatment
C3	Pyogenic infection, glomerulonephritis	AR	
Properdin	Pyogenic infection	XL	
Factor D	Pyogenic infection	?	
C5	Disseminated neisserial infections	AR	
C6	Disseminated neisserial infections	AR	
C7	Disseminated neisserial infections	AR	*Symptomatic* medical treatment (antibiotics)
C8	SLE, disseminated neisserial infections	AR	
C9	Normal, disseminated neisserial infections	AR	
C1INH	Hereditary angioneurotic edema (hereditary or acquired), SLE, B-cell immunoproliferative disease	AD	pooled plasma
Factor I	Pyogenic infections, vasculitis, glomerulonephritis		
Factor H	Pyogenic infections, vasculitis, glomerulonephritis, partial lipodystrophy		
DAF	PNH		none
HRF	PNH		
CD59 (MIRL)	PNH		none
CR1	SLE		
CR3	Pyogenic infections		

AD—autosomal dominant; AR—autosomal recessive; C1INH—C1 esterase inhibitor; DAF—decay accelerating factor; HRF—homologous restriction factor; MIRL—membrane inhibitor of active lysis; PNH—paroxysmal nocturnal hemoglobinuria; SLE—systemic lupus erythematosus; XL—X-linked.

Absence of the central complement component C3 results in failure to generate an appropriate response to pyogenic infections by disrupting the integrity of both the classical and alternative pathways. This disruption may occur through the absence of normal chemotactic factor (C5a) and leukocytosis promoting factor (C3e). The increased susceptibility to bacterial infections is manifested primarily as pneumonia, meningitis, otitis, and pharyngitis, which tend to recur. Early appropriate antibiotic therapy is indicated.

Deficiencies of the components of the alternative pathway of complement result in increased susceptibility to various pyogenic infections, probably as a result of a failure in the generation of C3-dependent opsonization [17]. Deficiencies of late complement components [18,19] that constitute the membrane attach complex (C5, 6, 7, 8 and 9) result in a significant increase in susceptibility to neisserial infections [20–22]. Patients with C9 deficiency are usually well clinically.

DEFICIENCIES OF COMPLEMENT REGULATORY PROTEINS

Hereditary angioneurotic edema results from deficiency of C1 esterase inhibitor (C1INH) [23] and is manifested by recurrent localized soft tissue swelling (Table 3). The absence of functional C1INH can result from a total or near-total absence of the inhibitor molecule or from production of a biologically ineffective molecule (Table 4).

Functional absence of C1INH permits continued or exaggerated activation of the C1s complex, which results in unregulated activation of C4 and C3. C1INH also regulates the activity of Hageman factor and kininogen. The interaction pathways of hereditary angioneurotic edema are depicted in Figure 2. Clinical manifestations of C1INH deficiency result from severe gastric edema, manifested as severe abdominal pain, vomiting and diarrhea, and from laryngeal obstruction and asphyxia.

Treatment for angioneurotic edema can be divided into acute and long-term therapeutic protocols. For preparation for an acute procedure (surgery), the following protocol is recommended:

1) 10 g of aminocaproic acid given intravenously slowly during the night before the procedure (1 to 2 g/h by intravenous constant infusion)
2) 5 g of aminocaproic acid given intravenously on the morning of the procedure
3) 2 U of fresh frozen plasma given intravenously after the aminocaproic acid and immediately before the procedure

TABLE 3 SURVEY OF CLINICAL FINDINGS IN INHERITED COMPLEMENT DEFICIENCY STATES*

Deficiency	Number of cases	Principal clinical findings
C1q	20	Inflammatory disease, mainly SLE or SLE-like conditions with or without
C1r(C1s)	10	glomerulonephritis (70%), bacterial infections (20%), apparent health (<20%)
C4	17	
C2	>100	Inflammatory disease, mainly SLE or SLE-like conditions (35%–75%), bacterial infections (35%–65%), apparent health (<20%)
C3	15	Bacterial infections, mostly recurrent (70%)
		SLE, vasculitis, glomerulonephritis (80%), apparent health (zero)
C5		Systemic neisserial infections, mostly meningococcal (>50%)
C6		
C7	>200	Recurrence rate high
C8		
C9	>200	Common in the Japanese population, probable association with meningococcal disease, but most cases healthy.
Factor D	3	Bacterial infections, including recurrent systemic neisserial infections
Properdin	53	
C1INH	>500	Heterozygous deficiency basis of hereditary angioedema. Secondary C4 and C2 deficiency; SLE-like disease in some patients
Factor I	8	Secondary C3 deficiency with susceptibility to bacterial infection and immune
Factor H	12	complex disease

*Figures include some unpublished cases known to the author.
C1INH—C1 esterase inhibitor; SLE—systemic lupus erythematosus.
From Sjoholm [2]; with permission.

TABLE 4 ABNORMALITIES AND DEFICIENCIES OF REGULATORY COMPLEMENT PROTEINS

Protein	Resulting complement activation abnormalities	Associated diseases pathology	Disease/syndrome name
Regulatory proteins			
C1 inhibitor	Deregulated classical pathway activation, consumption of C3	Acute, intermittent attacks of skin and mucosal edema	Hereditary angioneurotic edema
		Acute, intermittent attacks of skin and mucosal edema, systemic lupus erythematosus, B-cell lymphoproliferative diseases	Acquired angioneurotic edema
Factor I	Deregulated classical pathway activation, consumption of C3	Pyogenic infections, vasculitis, glomerulonephritis	
Factor H	Deregulated classical pathway activation, consumption of C3	Pyogenic infections, vasculitis, glomerulonephritis, partial lipodystrophy	
DAF	Deregulated C3 convertase activity	Complement-mediated intravascular hemolysis	Paroxysmal nocturnal hemoglobinuria
HRF	Increased susceptibility of erythrocytes to MAC-mediated lysis	Complement-mediated intravascular hemolysis	Paroxysmal nocturnal hemoglobinuria
CD59 (MIRL)	Increased susceptibility of erythrocytes to MAC-mediated lysis	Complement-mediated intravascular hemolysis	Paroxysmal nocturnal hemoglobinuria
Complement receptors			
CR1	Deregulated C3 convertase activity	Systemic lupus erythematosus	
CR3		Pyogenic infections	Leukocyte adhesion deficiency

DAF—decay accelerating factor; HRF—homologous restriction factor; MAC—membrane attack complex; MIRL—membrane inhibitor of reactive lysis.
From Abbas *et al.* [10]; with permission.

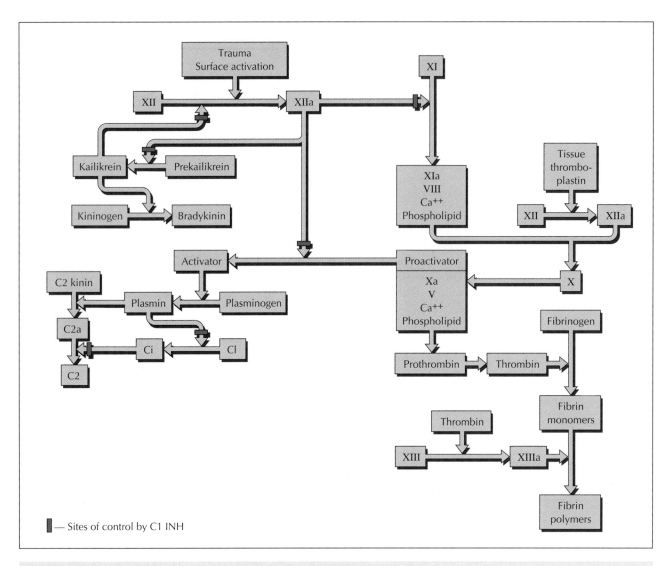

FIGURE 2 Interactions of clotting, fibrinolysis, kinin system, and complement pathways.

For long-term therapy, Danocrine (Winthrop, New York, NY) is given at 200 mg three times a day for 5 days, and then at 200 mg twice a day.

The recurrent episodes of acute circumscribed noninflammatory soft-tissue edema characteristic of angioneurotic edema are mediated by a vasoactive C2 fragment, designated C2 kinin, resulting from a heterozygous deficiency of C1INH gene product. Danocrine stimulates production of C1INH. Epsilon aminocaproic acid blocks plasmin-induced liberation of C2 kinin.

Paroxysmal nocturnal hemoglobinuria results from a deficiency of decay accelerating factor, which is responsible for dissociation and inactivation of C3 and C5 convertases of both complement activation pathways. Type II paroxysmal nocturnal hemoglobinuria results from a defect in production of decay accelerating factor. Type III paroxysmal nocturnal hemoglobinuria is associated with a deficiency of membrane attack complex–inhibitory factor. A summary of complement components is given in Table 1.

References and Recommended Reading

Recently published papers of particular interest are highlighted as:
- Of interest
- • Of outstanding interest

1. Morgan BP, Walport MJ: Complement deficiency and disease. *Immunol Today* 1991, 12:301–306.

2.• Sjoholm AG: Inherited complement deficiency states: implications for immunity and immunological disease. *APMIS* 1990, 98:861–874.

3.• Wurzner R, Orren A, Lachmann P: Inherited deficiencies of the terminal components of human complement. *Immunodefic Rev* 1992, 3:123–147.

4.• Kinoshita T: Biology of complement: The overture. *Immunol Today* 1991, 12:291–295.

5. Farries TC, Atkinson JP: Evolution of the complement system. *Immunol Today* 1991, 12:295–300.

6.• Kay PH, Papadimitriou JM: What's new in the role of complement in diseases. *Pathol Res Pract* 1990, 186:410–414.

7. Frank MM, Fries LF: The role of complement in inflammation and phagocytosis. *Immunol Today* 1991, 12:322–326.

8. Erdei A, Fust G, Gergely J: The role of C3 in the immune response. *Immunol Today* 1991, 12:332–337.

9. Gallinaro R, Cheadle WG, Applegate K, Polk HC: The role of the complement system in trauma and infection. *Surg Gynecol Obstet* 1992, 174:435–440.

10. Abbas AK, Lichtman AH, Pober JS.: *Cellular and Molecular Immunology.* Philadelphia: W.B. Saunders; 1991:262.

11. Syzuki Y, Ogura Y, Otsubo O, *et al.*: Selective deficiency of C1s associated with a systemic lupus erythematosus-like syndrome. *Arthritis Rheum* 1992, 35:576–579.

12. Muller-Eberhard HJ, Schreiber RD: Molecular biology and chemistry of the alternative pathway of complement. *Adv Immunol* 1980, 29:1–53.

13. Rother K, Hansch GM, Rauterberg EW: Complement in inflammation: induction of nephritides and progress to chronicity. *Int Arch Allergy Immunol* 1991, 94:23–37.

14. Lachman P: Complement deficiency and the pathogenesis of autoimmune immune complex disease. *Chem Immunol* 1990, 49:245–263.

15.• Lhotta K, Lonig P, Hintner H, *et al.*: Renal disease in a patient with hereditary complete deficiency of the fourth component of complement. *Nephron* 1990, 56:206–211.

16. Fronek Z, Timmerman LA, Alper CA, *et al.*: Major histocompatibility complex genes and susceptibility to systemic lupus erythematosus. *Arthritis Rheum* 1990, 33:1542–1553.

17. Fishelson Z: Complement C3: A molecular mosaic of binding sites. *Mol Immunol* 1991, 28:545–552.

18. Bhakdi S, Hugo F, Tranum-Jensen J: Functions and relevance of the terminal complement sequence. *Blut* 1990, 60:309–318.

19. Sanal O, Loos M, Ersoy F, *et al.*: Complement component deficiencies and infection: C5, C8 and C3 deficiencies in three families. *Eur J Pediatr* 1992, 151:676–679.

20. McBride SJ, McCluskey DR, Jackson PT: Selective C7 complement deficiency causing recurrent meningococcal infection. *J Infection* 1991, 22:273–276.

21. Morris JT, Kelly WJ: Recurrence of neisserial meningococcemia due to deficiency of terminal complement component. *South Med J* 1992, 85:1030–1031.

22. Zoppi M, Weiss M, Nydegger UE, *et al.*: Recurrent meningitis in a patient with congenital deficiency of the C9 component of complement. *Arch Intern Med* 1990, 150:2395–2399.

23. Zuraw BL, Altman LC: Acute consumption of C1 inhibitor in a patient with acquired C1-inhibitor deficiency syndrome. *J Allergy Clin Immunol* 1991, 88:908–918.

Vasculitis and Immune Complex Disease

14

Dennis K. Ledford

> **Key Points**
> - The spectrum of vasculitis includes numerous, heterogeneous syndromes and diseases with highly variable outcomes.
> - The diverse symptoms and signs of vasculitis introduce the diagnosis into the differential diagnosis of many common conditions, particularly infectious diseases, autoimmune diseases, and malignancy.
> - The cause of most forms of vasculitis is unknown.
> - The primary complication of vasculitis is ischemia; the more serious types of vasculitis affect medium to large arteries, resulting in greater tissue ischemia.
> - Laboratory tests only suggest or support the diagnosis of vasculitis; histologic evidence of the disease is the only proof of vasculitis.
> - The more virulent forms of vasculitis are treatable and have significant morbidity and mortality if untreated.

Vasculitis is a descriptive term for a diverse set of syndromes characterized by inflammation within blood vessel walls [1•]. The inflammation results in loss of vascular integrity with hemorrhage and edema, fibrin deposition with thrombosis, and ischemia from narrowing of the vascular lumen. Ischemia causes the major complications and determines the prognosis.

Although most vasculitic syndromes are relatively uncommon, the possibility arises frequently because the typical, vague constitutional symptoms of vasculitis are common to many diseases. Distinguishing vasculitis from infectious diseases and cancer is important because ill-advised treatment for presumed vasculitis can mask or aggravate these more treatable conditions (Table 1). Diagnostic criteria that distinguish between the major groups of vasculitic syndromes are outlined in Table 2, and therapeutic approaches are presented in Table 3.

HYPERSENSITIVITY VASCULITIS

Hypersensitivity vasculitis comprises 30% of all cases of vasculitis [2••]. Hypersensitivity vasculitis is a heterogeneous group of clinical syndromes characterized by immune complex deposition in capillaries, postcapillary venules, and occasionally arterioles (Table 4) [3].

The typical manifestations are dermatologic, and more than 95% of cases exhibit palpable purpura (Fig. 1). Other dermatologic manifestations include urticaria, erythema multiforme, and livedo reticularis. Comparison of histology of the dermatologic lesions from an affected subject generally shows a uniform stage of inflammation, implying that all lesions began simultaneously. The skin lesions are usually distributed symmetrically in dependent areas of the body. Visceral involvement is infrequent and is usually mild.

TABLE 1 DIFFERENTIAL DIAGNOSIS OF VASCULITIS

Infection
 Bacterial endocarditis
 Hepatitis B
 Human immunodeficiency virus
 Occult abscess
 Syphilis
Malignancy
 Lymphoma
 Hodgkin's disease
 Hypernephroma
 Metastatic carcinoma
 Multiple myeloma and macroglobulinemia

Autoimmune disease
 Rheumatoid arthritis
 Systemic lupus erythematosus
Marantic endocarditis
Multiple emboli/multiple cholesterol emboli
Drug allergy

TABLE 2 DIAGNOSTIC CRITERIA OF VASCULITIS

| Hypersensitivity vasculitis | Necrotizing vasculitis | | | |
	Polyarteritis nodosa	Allergic angiitis and granulomatosis	Wegener's granulomatosis	Temporal or giant cell vasculitis
≥3 of the following criteria (84% specificity and 71% sensitivity): 1. Age ≥16 years 2. Administration of a potential precipitating medicine 3. Palpable purpura 4. Maculopapular rash 5. Granulocytes around an arteriole or venule on biopsy ≥2 of the following criteria for Henoch-Schönlein purpura (88% specificity and 87% sensitivity): 1. Age <20 years 2. Palpable purpura 3. Abdominal pain 4. Granulocytes in the walls of small arterioles or venules on biopsy	>3 of the following criteria (52% specificity and 56% sensitivity): 1. ≥4-kg weight loss 2. Livedo reticularis 3. Testicular pain or tenderness 4. Diffuse myalgias (excluding proximal hip and shoulder area) 5. Mononeuropathy or polyneuropathy 6. Diastolic BP >90 mm Hg 7. BUN >40 mg/dL or creatinine >65 mg/dL 8. HB$_s$Ag, anti-HB$_s$Ag or anti-HB$_c$Ag 9. Arteriogram showing aneurysms or occlusion of visceral arteries 10. Arterial biopsy with neutrophils and monocytes infiltrating muscular artery	≥4 of the following criteria (99.7% sensitivity and 95% specificity): 1. Asthma 2. Peak blood eosinophil count >1.5 x 10^9/L or 10% of WBC 3. Mononeutopathy or polyneuropathy 4. Nonfixed pulmonary infiltrates 5. Patanasal sinus abnormalities 6. Tissue biopsy containing a blood vessel with extravascular eosinophils	≥2 of the following criteria (92% specificity and 88% sensitivity): 1. Oral or nasal inflammation manifested by oral ulcers or bloody nasal discharge 2. Chest radiograph with nodules, infiltrates, or cavities 3. Abnormal urine sediment with erythrocyte casts or microhematuria 4. Granulomatous inflammation within an arterial wall or in perivascular or extravascular area	≥3 of the following criteria (91% specificity and 94% sensitivity): 1. Age >50 years 2. New onset, localized headache 3. Erythrocyte sedimentation rate (Westergren's method) ≥50 mm/h 4. Arterial biopsy showing necrotizing arteries characterized by a predominance of mononuclear cell infiltrates or a granulomatous process with multinucleated giant cells 5. Temporal artery tenderness or decreased pulse

BP—blood pressure; BUN—blood urea nitrogen; HB$_c$Ag—hepatitis B core antigen; HB$_s$Ag—hepatitis B surface antigen WBC.

		TABLE 3 TREATMENT OF VASCULITIS			
	Necrotizing vasculitis				
Hypersensitivity vasculitis	**Polyarthritis nodosa**	**Allergic angiitis and granulomatosis**	**Wegener's granulomatosis**	**Temporal or giant cell vasculitis**	
Antihistamine therapy for pruritus	Glucocorticoid therapy (prednisone or equivalent, 1 mg/kg) in divided doses for 7–14 days			Glucocorticoid therapy (prednisone 1 mg/kg or equivalent) given as single daily dose	
Removal of offending drug	Single daily glucocorticoid therapy (prednisone or equivalent, 1 mg/kg) for 1 month if responding, longer if clinical response less convincing			Glucocorticoid therapy tapered slowly after clinical response and decrease in erythrocyte sedimentation rate	
Treatment of underlying disease	Taper to alternate day glucocorticoid therapy (prednisone or equivalent, 1 mg/kg) and reduce dose over 3–6 months if clinical response adequate			Treatment usually required for 8–18 months	
Glucocorticoid treatment reserved for renal disease	Cytotoxic therapy (cyclophosphamide 1–2 mg/kg/d) started with initial glucocorticoid therapy			Alternate day glucocorticoid therapy usually not effective	
	Adjust cytotoxic therapy to maintain white blood count ≥1– 1.5 x 10^9/L			Cytotoxic therapy reserved for relapses or for severe glucocorticoid side effects	
	Begin tapering cyclophospaamide after sustained remission, of approximately 12 months, reducing by 25 mg cyclophosphamide every 2 months				
	Use chlorambucil, azathioprine, or methotrexate if significant side effects occur				

TABLE 4 SELECTED HYPERSENSITIVITY VASCULITIS SYNDROMES
Autoimmune disease
Rheumatoid arthritis
Systematic lupus erythematosus
Sjögren's syndrome
Drugs
Cephalosporins
Penicillin
Sulfonamides
Infection
Endocarditis
Hepatitis B
Hepatitis C
Allergy
Urticarial vasculitis
Henoch-Schönlein purpura
Cryoglobulinemia
Hypocomplementemic urticarial vasculitis

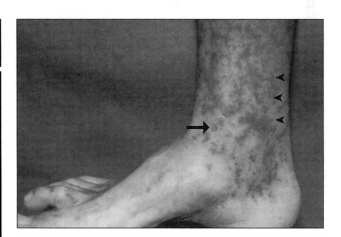

FIGURE 1 Hypersensitivity vasculitis exhibiting petechiae (arrow heads) and palpable purpura (arrow) in the typical location on the lower extremity.

Laboratory tests other than skin biopsy are often not helpful in making a diagnosis but may help exclude other diagnostic possibilities. The typical histology of cutaneous biopsies of hypersensitivity vasculitis is described as leukocytoclastic vasculitis.

The usual treatment for hypersensitivity vasculitis is reassurance; avoidance or removal of an offending antigen, such as a drug; or treatment of an underlying associated disease. Glucocorticosteroid therapy should be reserved for unusually severe forms of hypersensitivity vasculitis with significant renal involvement.

SYSTEMIC NECROTIZING VASCULITIS

The members of this broad class of vasculitis syndromes share an intense, destructive inflammation of small- to medium-sized muscular arteries, often resulting in major vascular obstruction and extensive tissue ischemia and infarction [4]. The propensity for infarction is responsible for the significant morbidity and mortality of this form of vasculitis, if untreated. Typical complications include stroke, renal ischemia with insufficiency, abdominal pain with bowel infarction, pulmonary necrosis with hemorrhage, and mononeuritis multiplex. Necrotizing vasculitis is divided into categories distinguished by the presence or absence of tissue granuloma and the distribution of vessel involvement (Table 5). All require aggressive treatment with glucocorticoids and cytotoxic agents to prevent complications [5].

Classic polyarteritis nodosa
Generalized involvement with sparing of the aorta, the primary branches of the aorta, and the elastic pulmonary arteries
  1- to 5-mm aneurysmal dilatation of affected vessels
Allergic angiitis and granulomatosis (Churg-Strauss Vasculitis)
Tissue and systemic eosinophilia
Soft tissue granulomas with eosinophilic infiltration
Occurs in atopic individuals with preceding history, often for many years, of asthma and upper airway disease
Frequent pulmonary involvement with less frequent renal involvement
Polyangiitis overlap syndrome
Necrotizing systemic vasculitis without classic features of either of the above or with some features of both

Polyarteritis Nodosa Group

Polyarteritis nodosa

Polyarteritis nodosa is the commonest of the three syndromes of the polyarteritis nodosa group of systemic necrotizing vasculitis (Table 5). It represents 7% of the vasculitic syndromes in the American College of Rheumatology prospective study of 1020 cases of vasculitis [2••]. The histology of affected vessels is characterized by transmural, pleomorphic (neutrophils, eosinophils, lymphocytes, monocytes, and macrophages) cellular infiltrate, fibrinoid necrosis, thrombosis, and aneurysm formation [6]. Palpable, aneurysmal nodules of the muscular arteries are uncommon, but small aneurysmal dilatations of affected arteries documented by arteriography are typical, although not diagnostic (Fig. 2).

The etiology of polyarteritis nodosa is unknown. A subset of cases, in some studies as large as 30% of the total, is associated with hepatitis B antigenemia [6]. In addition, antigens of streptococci, staphylococci, and mycobacteria have been recognized in the arterial lesions or the peripheral blood of affected subjects.

The presenting symptoms of patients with polyarteritis nodosa include malaise, fatigue, abdominal pain, fever, weight loss, peripheral nerve deficits (particularly foot drop from peroneal nerve involvement), and stroke. The frequency of organ system involvement during the course of the disease is listed in Table 6.

Allergic angiitis and granulomatosis

Allergic angiitis and granulomatosis, the second syndrome of the polyarteritis nodosa group, differs from polyarteritis nodosa by a history of preceding respiratory allergy and asthma, often for 5 to 15 years before the development of arteritis, a peripheral and tissue eosinophilia, and a frequent involvement of the pulmonary blood vessels [7]. Eosinophilia, elevated IgE level, and association with allergic disease suggest that an accelerated type I Gell-Coombs allergic mechanism plays an important role in the pathogenesis of allergic angiitis and granulomatosis. The primary role of the eosinophil is suggested by the observation that allergic angiitis and granulomatosis may occur in nonatopic, hypereosinophilic diseases, such as parasitic infestation, and may be cured by treating the underlying disease and resolving the hypereosinophilia [8].

Polyarteritis overlap syndrome

The occurrence of clinical features of polyarteritis nodosa and allergic angiitis and granulomatosis in a single individual is termed the polyangiitis overlap syndrome [9]. This observation suggests that polyarteritis nodosa and allergic angiitis and

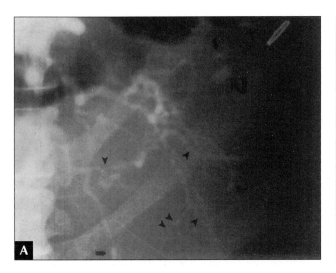

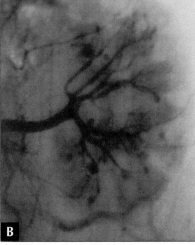

FIGURE 2 A, Arteriogram of polyarteritis that shows irregular narrowing of muscular arteries (arrow heads) with microaneurysms (arrow). **B,** Positive print of renal arteriogram, reversing light and dark in figure, that demonstrates multiple aneurysms typical of polyarteritis.

TABLE 6 ORGAN SYSTEM INVOLVEMENT IN SYSTEMIC NECROTIZING VASCULITIS

Organ system or signs	Involvement during disease course (%)
Kidney/renal	70
Musculoskeletal system	64
Arthritis/arthralgia	53
Myalgias	31
Cardiovascular	62
Hypertension	54
Congestive heart failure	12
Myocardial infarction	6
Pericarditis	4
Nervous system	60
Peripheral neuropathy	51
Stroke	11
Altered mental status	10
Seizure	4
Gastrointestinal tract	44
Abdominal pain	43
Nausea/vomiting	40
Cholecystitis	17
Bleeding	6
Perforation	5
Bowel infarction	1
Skin	43
Rash/purpura	30
Nodule	15
Livedo reticularis	4

granulomatosis have common pathophysiology mechanisms despite the histologic and clinical differences.

Diagnosis

The diagnosis of the polyarteritis type of systemic necrotizing vasculitis requires the histopathologic demonstration of necrotizing vasculitis of muscular arteries and compatible clinical manifestations. The selection of tissue for biopsy should be based on clinical evidence of involvement because findings from random biopsy have an unacceptably low yield. Useful biopsy sites include the sural nerve, skin, muscle, testicle, and rectum. More invasive, riskier biopsy sites, selected only if other laboratory findings indicate involvement, include the kidney, lung, and bowel. Angiography showing multiple 1- to 5-mm diameter aneurysms and irregular vessel narrowing may help in establishing the extent of disease and in suggesting the diagnosis (Fig. 2). Normal angiography does not exclude the diagnosis, because 20% of cases polyarteritis nodosa lack multiple aneurysms; conversely, the presence of multiple aneurysms does not guarantee the diagnosis because other conditions may show this finding (Table 7).

The 5-year survival rate for patients with untreated, polyarteritis-type systemic necrotizing vasculitis is 4% to 13% [7]. Monotherapy with systemic glucocorticoids increases the

5-year survival rate to approximately 80%. The addition of cytotoxic therapy enhances the therapeutic response of glucocorticoids and helps minimize side effects by permitting dose reduction (Table 3).

Wegener's Granulomatosis

Wegener's granulomatosis is a systemic necrotizing vasculitis characterized by the clinical triad of granulomatous vasculitis of the upper and lower respiratory tract, glomerulonephritis, and variable degrees of systemic small-vessel vasculitis [10]. However, limited forms of Wegener's granulomatosis occur with airway involvement only. Wegener's granulomatosis occurs with approximately the same frequency as polyarteritis nodosa and develops in all age groups, although characteristically appears in the fourth or fifth decade of life. Affected patients often present with complaints localized to the airway, most commonly sinusitis or nasal obstruction. Other common symptoms and signs include otitis media and ear pain, decreased auditory acuity, epistaxis and nasal septal cartilage necrosis (Fig. 3), laryngitis, tracheal stenosis, and cough with sputum production and hemoptysis.

The diagnosis of Wegener's granulomatosis depends on an adequate tissue biopsy specimen that shows necrotizing granulomas and vasculitis. An open lung biopsy is the most likely site for the characteristic pathologic findings. Other biopsy sites, such as the nasopharynx, sinus, gingiva, skin, or kidney, may also be helpful but frequently exhibit nonspecific, chronic inflammation or small vessel vasculitis. Other laboratory tests that may be of value are listed in Table 8.

Antineutrophil cytoplasmic antibodies are detected in 60% to 70% of people with Wegener's granulomatosis, and the level of this antibody fluctuates with the activity of disease [11]. The specificity of this antibody makes it a very useful diagnostic test. Although antineutrophil cytoplasmic antibodies have also been detected in patients with glomerulonephritis without Wegener's granulomatosis, the pattern of fluorescence is distinguished by perinuclear staining rather than by the granular, cytoplasmic fluorescence of Wegener's granulomatosis (Fig. 4). The role of antineutrophil cytoplasmic antibodies in the pathogenesis of vasculitis is unproven [12,13].

Untreated patients with Wegener's granulomatosis have a mean survival of 5 months and a 90% mortality in 2 years. With treatment, sustained disease remission occurs in 75% to 90% of patients, with apparent cure in some. The treatment regimen is the same as that used for necrotizing vasculitis of the polyarteritis nodosa type (Table 3). Improvement has been reported with trimethoprim-sulfamethoxazole therapy, but a

TABLE 7 NONVASCULITIC DISORDERS ASSOCIATED WITH MULTIPLE SMALL ANEURYSMS ON ARTERIOGRAPHY

Atrial myxoma
Fibromuscular dysplasia
Mycotic aneurysms with endocarditis
Pseudoxanthoma elasticum
Thrombotic thrombocytopenic purpura

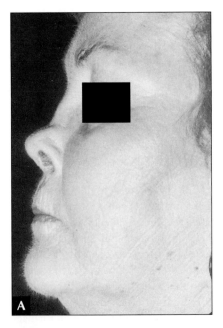

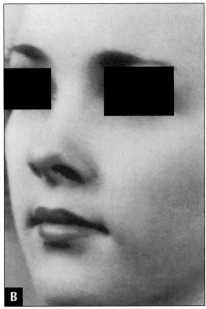

FIGURE 3 A, Profile of nasal septal collapse in patient with Wegener's granulomatosis. B, Patient before development of vasculitis.

TABLE 8 LABORATORY TEST RESULTS USEFUL IN DIAGNOSIS OF WEGENER'S GRANULOMATOSIS

Increase in acute-phase reactants
Rheumatoid factor (50% of cases)
Antineutrophil cytoplasmic antibody (60%–70% of cases)
Urinalysis
   Hematuria
   Proteinuria with or without casts
Chest radiographs (ill-defined infiltrates, single or multiple nodules, cavitary lesions)
Sinus radiographs or computed tomographic scan (95% have demonstrable sinusitis)

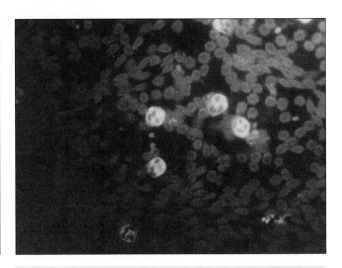

FIGURE 4 Fluorescent photomicrograph of antineutrophil cytoplasmic assay in Wegener's granulomatosis. (see Color Plate)

double-blind, controlled study for this treatment is lacking [14]. A study of the effectiveness of weekly methotrexate administration (15 to 25 mg) in patients with Wegener's granulomatosis suggests that this antimetabolite may be an option in patients who are intolerant to cytotoxic therapy [15]. Pulse cyclophosphamide, 10 to 20 mg/kg as a single infusion once every 3 to 4 weeks, was not effective, as reported in a controlled trial [16].

TEMPORAL ARTERITIS OR GIANT CELL VASCULITIS

Giant cell vasculitis, also referred to as temporal arteritis, is a generalized vasculitis affecting large- and medium-sized arteries with a well-defined elastic lamina [17]. Temporal arteritis is a misnomer because any arterial bed may be affected. Extracranial branches of the carotid arteries are most commonly affected, and ischemia from giant cell vasculitis is rarely seen below the neck.

Giant cell vasculitis rarely occurs before the age of 50 years, and its incidence increases by about 30 times from ages 50 to 80. Giant cell vasculitis is two to three times more prevalent in women than in men. The origin is unknown, but a cell-mediated autoimmune response against the vascular wall, particularly the elastic lamina, is a potential explanation.

The symptoms of giant cell vasculitis are listed in Table 9. Visual impairment, one of the most serious complications, occurs in more than one third of untreated subjects and is secondary to ischemia in the distribution of the retinal artery. Polymyalgia rheumatica is a syndrome that may be associated with giant cell vasculitis and is characterized by proximal myalgias, peri-articular stiffness and pain, weight loss, and fever. Forty percent to 50% of patients with polymyalgia rheumatica have giant cell vasculitis of the temporal artery, even without typical symptoms of headache, visual changes, or scalp tenderness. The symptoms of polymyalgia rheumatica usually respond to lower doses of antiinflammatory drugs than do the symptoms and ischemic manifestations of giant cell vasculitis.

The diagnosis of giant cell vasculitis is based on the results of a biopsy specimen, usually taken from the temporal artery, that demonstrate a granulomatous inflammation, with giant

TABLE 9 SYMPTOMS OF GIANT CELL OR TEMPORAL ARTERITIS
Headache (often described as boring, may be unilateral)
Visual impairment and diplopia
Jaw claudication
Dysphagia
Scalp tenderness
Anorexia
Fever
Fatigue
Polymyalgia rheumatica
Arthralgia
Myalgia
Aching stiffness in proximal musculature
Synovitis

cells focused on the elastic lamina of the vascular wall (Fig. 5). The biopsy yield is enhanced if the procedure is performed on palpable abnormalities of the vessel, but the pathologic diagnosis can be made from a biopsy specimen taken from clinically normal vessels in 30% to 40% of clinically suspected cases. The biopsy will yield definitive histologic findings even if treatment has been administered for 10 to 14 days before the biopsy [18••]. Other laboratory findings are nonspecific and include elevation of the erythrocyte sedimentation rate, mild normochromic, normocytic anemia, and minimal elevation of hepatic transaminases and alkaline phosphatase levels.

Within days of initiation of glucocorticoid therapy, the systemic symptoms and focal manifestations improve. This treatment also prevents the commonest cause of irreversible morbidity—visual loss. Treatment initially consists of 40 to 60 mg/d of oral prednisone, and the clinical findings and erythrocyte sedimentation rate are monitored. The dosage can usually be tapered to 5- to 10-mg per day over 6 to 12 months, but low-dose therapy may be necessary for several years. Cytotoxic therapy may be useful if glucocorticoid side effects are problematic.

MISCELLANEOUS SYNDROMES

Takayasu's Arteritis

Takayasu's arteritis resembles temporal arteritis histologically but affects young adults, usually 15 to 20 years of age, with a striking female preponderance (9:1) [19]. Takayasu's arteritis is rare in the United States, but the incidence is much higher in Asia [20••]. The disease typically has three phases: 1) systemic symptoms that last several weeks before resolving; 2) an ensuing arteritis, typically affecting the aortic arch and its major branches, which resolves over several months; and 3) a prolonged asymptomatic period, averaging 8 years, before symptoms and signs of vaso-occlusive disease develop. The pulmonary circulation is affected in up to 50% of cases. Arteriography is central to the diagnosis, and findings of irregular vessel narrowing, occlusion, and aneurysm formation are indicative of the disorder.

Although glucocorticoids are somewhat effective in suppressing arteritis, their efficacy in prolonging life and reducing morbidity and mortality is unknown. Initial oral prednisone therapy, 40 to 80 mg/d, is reduced to every-other-day therapy over several months and then tapered. Cytotoxic therapy and methotrexate treatment benefits selected patients with active disease who have not responded to glucocorticosteroids [21•]. Vascular surgery to relieve arterial obstruction should be considered after the inflammatory disease has abated.

Microscopic Polyarteritis

Microscopic polyarteritis is a small-vessel necrotizing vasculitis that usually affects the lung and results in serious pulmonary hemorrhage [22]. It also typically affects the kidney and abdominal viscera, and nasopharyngeal and oral involvement may occur. This vasculitis may be an atypical form of Wegener's granulomatosis. The typical renal involvement of microscopic polyarteritis is a rapidly progressive crescentic glomerulonephritis, often more fulminant than that occurring with Wegener's granulomatosis. Antineutrophil cytoplasmic antibodies are frequently detected in microscopic polyarteritis as well. Microscopic polyarteritis differs histologically from Wegener's granulomatosis in that granulomas are not seen. The prognosis is poor, perhaps worse than for Wegener's granulomatosis, and the treatment is the same as that for Wegener's granulomatosis.

Kawasaki's Disease

Kawasaki's disease is an acute vasculitis that primarily affects infants and young children, but may occur in young adults [23]. It occurs in endemic and epidemic form worldwide but is most prevalent in Japan. The epidemic form usually occurs in the fall or late winter, suggesting an undefined infectious etiology. The incidence seems to be increasing worldwide,

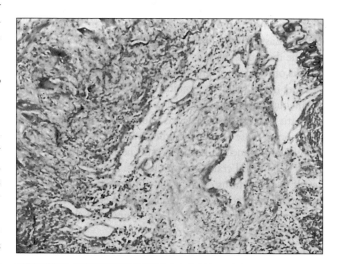

FIGURE 5 Low-power photomicrograph of biopsy of temporal artery that shows necrotizing inflammation with granuloma formation and giant cells. The most intense inflammation is focused on the internal elastic lamina, resulting in disruption of the elastic layer. Endothelial proliferation contributes to vessel narrowing and ischemia.

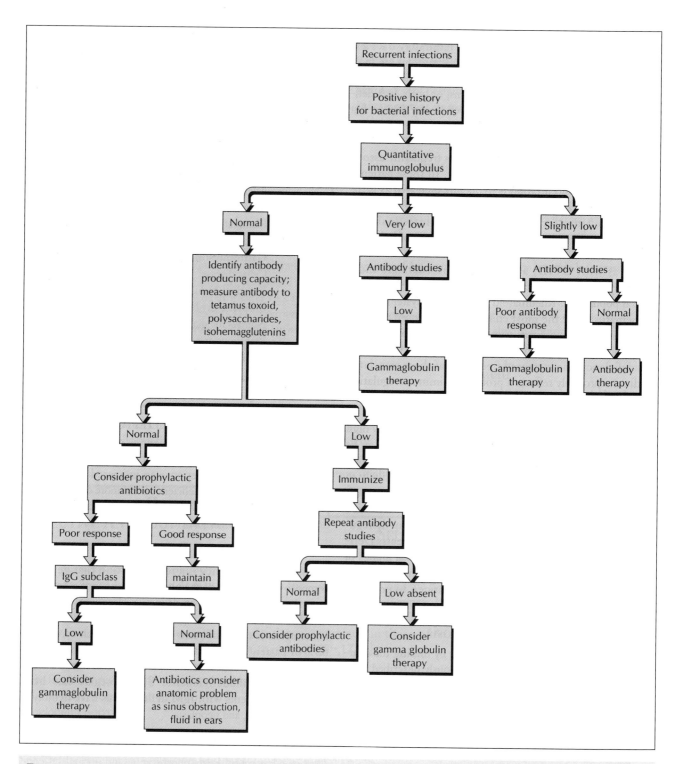

FIGURE 6 Algorithm for evaluating patients with recurrent infection.

References and Recommended Reading

Recently published papers of particular interest have been highlighted as:
- Of interest
- •• Of outstanding interest

1. Cunningham-Rundles C: Clinical and immunological analysis of 103 patients with common variable immunodeficiency. *J Clin Immunol* 1989, 9:22–33.

2. Spickett GP, Webster ADB, Farrant J: Cellular abnormalities in common variable immunodeficiency. *Immunodefic Rev* 1990, 2:199–219.

3. Yocum MW, Kelso JM: Common variable immunodeficiency: The disorder and treatment. *Mayo Clin Proc* 1991, 66:83–96.

4. Sneller MC, Strober W, Eisenstein E, *et al.*: New insights into common variable immunodeficiency. *Ann Int Med* 1993, 118:720–730.

5. Kersey JH, Shapiro RS, Filipovich AH: Relationship of immunodeficiency to lymphoid malignancy. *Pediatr Infect Dis J* 1988, 7(suppl):S10–S12.

6. Mori S, Kondo N, Motayoshi F, *et al.*: Diversity in DNA rearrangements and in RNA expressions of immunoglobulin gene in common variable immunodeficiency. *Eur J Immunogen* 1992, 19:273–285.

7. Baumert E, Wolff-Vorbeck G, Schlesier M, Peter HH: Immunophenotypical alterations in a subset of patients with common variable immunodeficiency. *Clin Exp Immunol* 1992, 90:25–30.

8.•• Schaffer FM, Monteiro RC, Volanakis JE, Cooper MD: IgA deficiency. *Immunodefic Rev* 1991, 3:15–44.

9. Olerup O, Smith CI, Bjorkander J, Hammarstrom L: Shared HLA class II associated genetic susceptibility and resistance, related to the HLA-DQB 1 gene, in IgA deficiency and common variable immunodeficiency. *Proc Natl Acad Sci* 1992, 89(22):10653–10657.

10. Tsukada S, Saffran DC, Rawlings DJ, *et al.*: Deficient expression of a B-cell cytoplasmic tyrosine kinase in human X-linked agammaglobulinemia. *Cell* 1993, 72:279–290.

11.• Berkman SA, Lee ML, Gale RP: Clinical uses of intravenous immunoglobulins. *Ann Intern Med* 1990, 112:278–292.

12. Buckley RH, Schiff RI: The use of intravenous immune globulin in immunodeficiency diseases. *N Engl J Med* 1991, 325:110–117.

13. Schiff RI, Sedlak D, Buckley RH: Rapid infusion of Sandoglobulin in patients with primary humoral immunodeficiency. *J Allergy Clin Immunol* 1991, 88:61–67.

14. Burks AW, Sampson HA, Buckley RH: Anaphylactic reactions after gamma globulin administration in patients with hypogammaglobulinemia: detection of IgE antibodies. *N Engl J Med* 1986, 3114:560–564.

15. Herrod HG: Management of the patient with IgG subclass deficiency and/or selective antibody deficiency. *Ann Allergy* 1993, 70:3–11.

16. Popa V, Kim K, Heiner DC: IgG deficiency in adults with recurrent respiratory infections. *Ann Allergy* 1994, 70:418–424.

17. Hong R, Ammann RJ: Disorders of the IgA system. In *Immunologic Disorders of Infants and Children*, 3rd edn. Edited by Stiehm ER. Philadelphia: WB Saunders; 1989:329–342.

18. Guill MF, Brown DA, Ochs HD, *et al.*: IgM deficiency, clinical spectrum and immunologic assessment. *Ann Allergy* 1989, 62:547–552.

19. Inove T, Okumura Y, Shirahama M, *et al.*: Selective partial IgM deficiency: functional assessment of T and B lymphocytes in vitro. *J Clin Immunol* 1986, 6:130–135.

Select Bibliography

Ammann AJ, Hong R: Selective IgA deficiency. Presentation of 30 cases and a review of the literature. *Medicine* 1971, 50:223–236.

Eisenstein EM, Chua K, Strober W: B cell differentiation defects in common variable immunodeficiency are ameliorated after stimulation with anti-CD40 antibody and IL-10. *J Immunol* 1994, 152:5957–5968.

Fischer MB, Hauber I, Vogel E, *et al.*: Effective interleukin-2 and interferon-γ gene expression in response to antigen in a subgroup of patients with common variable immunodeficiency. *J Allergy Clin Immunol* 1993, 92:340–352.

Gross S, Blaiss MS, Herrod HG: Role of IgG subclasses and specific antibody determinations in the evaluation of children with recurrent infection. *J Pediatr* 1992, 121:516–522.

Primary immunodeficiency diseases: report of a WHO scientific group. *Immunodeficiency Rev* 1992, 3:195–236.

HIV Infection: Diagnosis and Early Management

16

Gailen D. Marshall, Jr.

Key Points

- HIV infection can occur in men and women, homosexuals and heterosexuals, children and adults.

- Although often asymptomatic for years, HIV continues to proliferate (usually in the regional lymph nodes), making the HIV-positive patient infectious during the entire course of his or her disease.

- A high index of suspicion with early HIV testing must occur in patients in high-risk behavior groups and for individuals with unexplained chronic infections, any opportunistic infection, and even infections known to be prevalent in the HIV-positive population.

- Although most therapy in AIDS management is typically aimed at treating medical complications, retarding the progression of early HIV disease is a major therapeutic goal.

In the early 1980s, physicians began to see significant numbers of patients (primarily homosexual men) with life-threatening infections caused by opportunistic agents. Within a few years, the cause was identified as a retrovirus that was initially designated human T-cell lymphotropic virus type III and was subsequently renamed HIV (human immunodeficiency virus). The disease, dubbed AIDS (acquired immunodeficiency syndrome), was initially observed in select patient populations such as homosexual men and intravenous drug users [1]. From a world case incidence of 100,000 in 1982 to an estimated world incidence of 30 to 50 million by 2000, this disease has become the modern-day plague and has spread to involve all patient populations, including heterosexuals, women, and children [2]. Specific risk behaviors have been identified, and much effort is aimed at prevention, including the use of safer sexual practices, improved methods for blood product screening, and increased HIV testing, particularly for high-risk populations. However, no cure or even widely accepted treatment is currently available for this fatal disease.

Fortunately, although no definitive therapy yet exists, much can be done to aid the HIV-positive patient in his or her battle with the virus. Early detection is important in the overall management strategy of the disease. This chapter emphasizes the detection and early management of the disease. Specific therapy for later complications is considered elsewhere in this text.

PATHOPHYSIOLOGY

The human immune system is designed to protect the body from disturbances of homeostasis by foreign infections and effete or neoplastic self. This marvelous organ system functions as a well-rehearsed orchestra and accomplishes its goal, beginning in utero, by intricately distinguishing self from nonself, protecting the former and aggressively recognizing and destroying the latter through the production of soluble molecules such as antibodies, complement components, and cytokines, as well as activated cells such as macrophages and lymphocytes. B lymphocytes make and secrete antibodies, whereas certain T lymphocytes destroy intracellular parasites such as viruses, mycobacteria, and fungi and activate macrophages to contain and destroy infectious agents. The conductor of this immune orchestra is the cell type that most significantly controls the functions of other effector cells—the T helper cell.

T helper cells produce small-molecular-weight substances called cytokines, which are the messengers of the immune system. Without this activity, the immune system loses not only its message for action but also its regulatory signals. The result is a chaotic loss of defense against opportunistic infections and neoplastic transformations. The T helper cell is so susceptible because it carries the primary receptor for HIV infection—the CD4 molecule. HIV infects not only CD4$^+$ lymphocytes, but also mononuclear phagocytes of the

mononuclear phagocytic (reticuloendothelial) system, rapidly spreading throughout the body.

NATURAL HISTORY OF HIV INFECTION

Initial infection with HIV may be asymptomatic or can present as an acute viral syndrome characterized by fever, malaise, macular rash, sore throat, lymphadenopathy, headache, and arthralgia [3]. An aseptic meningitis can also occur. These symptoms typically resolve in a few weeks. Three weeks to 3 months after initial infection, patients seroconvert (*see* later discussion; Fig. 1). Patients then typically enter an asymptomatic phase, which lasts from months to years (median time in the United States is approximately 10 years). Patients may develop lymphadenopathy with or without constitutional symptoms such as weight loss, sweats, fatigue, and malaise within the asymptomatic period.

As the CD4 count decreases from normal preinfection levels (typically > 1000/mm^3) to less than 200/mm^3, patients begin to develop systemic complications, such as opportunistic infections, malignancies, neurologic complications (*eg*, progressive multifocal leukoencephalopathy), and cachexia. When the CD4 count decreases to less than 50/mm^3, death is likely within 24 months. The classification of the stages of HIV disease (Table 1) is important for both prognostic and therapeutic reasons (*see* later discussion). Of course, there are clinically well AIDS patients with CD4 counts of 10/mm^3 and others who die with CD4 counts near 500/mm^3. However, reports are very consistent regarding the natural history of HIV-induced disease in the majority of infected patients [4].

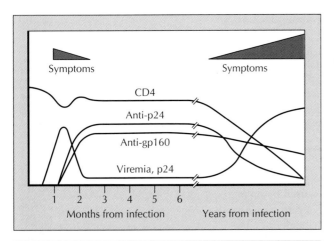

FIGURE 1 Serologic and cellular markers during HIV infection. (From Clark et al. [25]; with permission.)

RISK GROUP AND BEHAVIOR

With such a dismal clinical course as a result of HIV infection, considerable effort has been expended to identify patient

---

TABLE 1 CENTERS FOR DISEASE CONTROL AND PREVENTION CLASSIFICATION OF HIV-POSITIVE ADULT PATIENTS

CD4 count, *cells/mm³*	Clinical category		
	A*	B†	C‡
>500	A1	B1	C1§
200–499	A2	B2	C2§
<200	A3§	B3§	C3§

*Asymptomatic or acute HIV syndrome (viral).

†Symptomatic (bacterial infections, chronic vulvovaginal candidiasis, thrush, hairy leukoplakia, chronic shingles, nocardiosis, peripheral neuropathy, or constitutional symptoms (fever, weight loss, or diarrhea) for more than 1 month.

‡AIDS-defining illness (opportunistic infections or malignancies).

§All patients are reported as having AIDS with either AIDS-defining illness or an absolute CD4 count of less than 200/mm³.

TABLE 2 PATIENT POPULATIONS AT INCREASED RISK FOR AND DEFINED RISK BEHAVIORS FOR HIV TRANSMISSION

Patient population

Homosexual men who engage in anal intercourse

Intravenous drug abusers

Heterosexual or homosexual prostitutes

Anyone with multiple sexual partners

Persons who have received blood transfusions (particularly between 1978 and 1985)

Persons with a history of non-HIV sexually transmitted disease

Behaviors

Heterosexual or homosexual intercourse without condoms

Anal intercourse (heterosexual or homosexual intercourse)

Oral-genital intercourse (particularly with ejaculation)

Frequenting of prostitutes or other promiscuous individuals

---

populations at increased risk for becoming HIV positive, as well as behaviors that can put any individual at risk for acquiring the infection (Table 2). The goal of this approach is to modify behavior patterns that are present in high-risk populations and can appear in other people as well. It is not designed to discriminate against or persecute any individual or special population.

Homosexual men are at increased risk for infection. This risk is much higher if the subject has multiple sexual partners and practices unprotected sexual intercourse, including insertive and receptive anal, anal-oral, and genital-oral intercourse. Such risk is also present for promiscuous heterosexual intercourse [5]. The mistaken concept is that a negative HIV test result confers safety. Because an interval of up to 3 months may be present between infection and seroconversion, any individual with multiple sexual partners is at increased risk.

Other practices that introduce blood or blood products into the circulation are also capable of transmitting the virus. The most common is the sharing of needles by intravenous drug users (a common practice) [6]. It has been suggested that the casual transfer of minute amounts of blood (*eg*, from cuts or oral lesions) may be infectious, but such clinical cases have not been widely documented. Much concern remains about the individual rights of infected health care workers, athletes, food service workers, and so on versus the protection of the public [7]. Epidemiologic studies are ongoing to provide definitive answers to these dilemmas.

DIAGNOSIS

Clinical Suspicion

The major interventional step in the optimal management of HIV-positive patients is early detection. Because the presenting symptoms can often be confused with those of viral syndromes such as infectious mononucleosis, a high index of suspicion must exist for the clinician to pursue a diagnosis of HIV infection. Much social pressure still exists among clinicians against pursuing such a diagnosis in many patients. However, with the growing epidemic, clinicians must dispel such pressure and explain to patients that an HIV evaluation is in no way a judgmental statement on their lifestyle.

Patients who present with chronic infections of *any* nature must be considered for a diagnostic work-up [8]. This becomes increasingly true of those with opportunistic diseases and of those with infections known to be prevalent in the HIV-positive population (*eg*, tuberculosis) [9]. A history should then be obtained to look for factors such as risk behaviors, potentials for exposure (*eg*, in laboratory workers or health care givers), and other underlying illnesses that could account for presenting symptoms (Table 3). In the absence of a solid clinical reason to the contrary, particularly if risk behavior, exposure, or both can be established, HIV testing should be pursued.

TABLE 3 OBTAINING A PATIENT HISTORY
Ascertain the following:
Present symptoms and concerns
HIV risk factors
Common co-infections
Travel history
Past toxic reactions to drugs
Social situation
State of mind

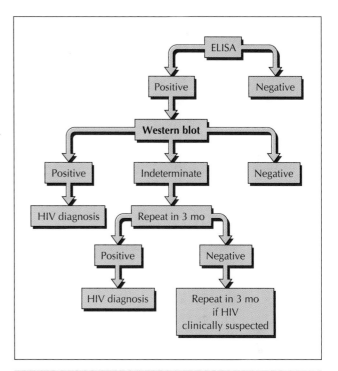

FIGURE 2 Algorithim for HIV testing. ELISA—enzyme-linked immunosorbent assay.

HIV Testing

It is important to consider that proper HIV testing may include multiple testing episodes (Fig. 2). Because of the 3-month window for seroconversion after infection, false-negative findings may lead away from the proper diagnosis. Thus, in patients in whom a high index of suspicion exists, an initial negative test should be followed by repeated testing within 3 months [10].

Circulating antibodies directed against various HIV proteins are detected in current screening tests for HIV infection. Enzyme-linked immunosorbent assays are the most common screen (Fig. 3). A negative test result has a high sensitivity (except as mentioned earlier) but less specificity. Thus, an enzyme-linked immunosorbent assay result positive for HIV must be confirmed, usually with Western blot technology (Fig. 4). Newer technologies designed to

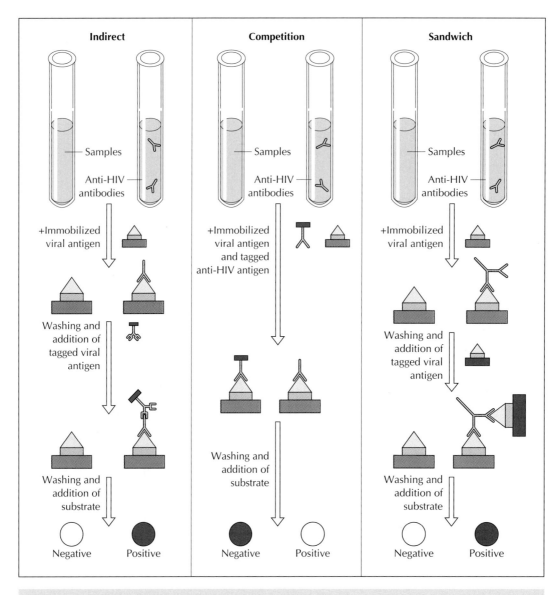

FIGURE 3 The different formats of enzyme-linked immunosorbent assay. (From Aldorini and Waller [26]; with permission.)

detect infection earlier rely on finding virus-specified proteins in patient's blood. These technologies include finding proteins such as p24, tat, and gp120; culturing of the virus; and more recently, using molecular techniques such as quantitative reverse transcriptase polymerase chain reactions to detect virus-specific nucleic acid material. Although they are still developmental, these tests will offer increased sensitivity of testing in the early phases of disease.

Other, less direct laboratory values that might spur a physician to pursue HIV testing in an otherwise-asymptomatic patient include a relative absolute lymphopenia ($<1500/mm^3$), a reduced peripheral CD4 count, and polyclonal gammopathy (often initially detected as an increased globulin fraction) [11]. If no specific explanation exists for such abnormalities, HIV testing should be considered. Other factors (including medical history and social behaviors) must also be considered.

Staging

Recently, controversy has emerged about the staging of HIV disease. However, for the clinician, relatively strong Centers for Disease Control and Prevention guidelines (Table 4) allow a practical staging for prognostic and therapeutic purposes [12]. It is rational that a patient with a life expectancy of months will be followed up differently than one who is expected to live a relatively normal life for some years with basic maintenance care.

The standard for the staging of HIV disease has revolved around the absolute peripheral blood CD4 count. Combining this count with the presence of various clinical parameters, from nonspecific constitutional symptoms such as weight loss, fevers, and adenopathy, to specific clinical entities such as opportunistic infections and malignancies, allows both the clinician and the patient to work toward effective management. As a rule, patients whose CD4 counts are greater than

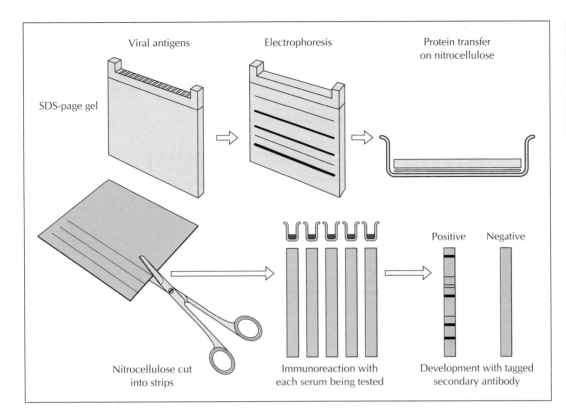

FIGURE 4
Western blotting
technique.
(From Aldorini
and Waller [26];
with permis-
sion.)

Viral antigens Electrophoresis Protein transfer on nitrocellulose

SDS-page gel

Nitrocellulose cut
into strips

Immunoreaction with
each serum being tested

Positive Negative

Development with tagged
secondary antibody

600/mm^3 and who are asymptomatic need to be followed up on a routine 6-month basis with repeated CD4 counts and clinical evaluations, including thorough examinations for constitutional symptoms (*eg*, weight loss and night sweats) occult opportunistic infection (*eg*, thrush) and malignancies (*eg*, skin lesions and adenopathy). As the CD4 count decreases to less than 500/mm^3, constitutional symptoms of progressive disease become more common. When this occurs, follow-up visits every 3 to 4 months become necessary, with attention being paid to the evaluation of constitutional symptoms. Once the HIV-positive patient's CD4 count drops below 200/mm^3, he or she is classified as having AIDS, regardless of the clinical presentation.

TABLE 4 BASELINE LABORATORY ASSESSMENT OF HIV-POSITIVE PATIENTS

Complete blood count with platelet count and differential
count
T-cell subsets (CD3, CD4, and CD8)
Liver function tests (AST, ALT, ALK-P, LDH, TB)
Renal function tests (electrolyte, blood urea nitrogen,
and creatinine levels)
Toxoplasma titer (IgG)
Hepatitis B screen (antigen and core antibody)
DTH with PPD and at least two controls (mumps,
trichophytosis, candidiasis)
Chest radiograph

AST—aspartate aminotransferase; ALT—alanine aminotransferase;
ALK-P—alkaline phosphatase; LDH—lactate dehydrogenase; TB—
total bilirubin levels; DTH—delayed type sensitivity; PPD—purified
protein derivative.

MANAGEMENT OF THE HIV-POSITIVE PATIENT

Basic Principles

Although HIV disease still appears to be uniformly fatal, the interval between seroconversion and death continues to increase. Thus, a positive outlook for both patient and physician can offer significant quality of life and hopefully prolong survival. There are three basic management principles for HIV-positive patients: 1) retard the progression of the disease, 2) manage the side effects of the disease and therapy, and 3) counsel the patient and family about how they can optimize patient comfort and survival. The clinician and the patient must establish and maintain a therapeutic partnership for optimal management to occur.

Use of Antiretroviral Agents

The use of antiretroviral agents to delay the progression of HIV disease is the mainstay of conventional therapy. Zidovudine is the first and still the most commonly used of these agents. It can prolong survival in HIV-positive patients with constitutional symptoms and may delay progression of the disease (including the development of neurologic complications) from seroconversion to AIDS [13]. Initial studies with zidovudine showed benefit with this agent versus placebo in patients who had CD4 counts of less than 200/mm^3 and opportunistic infections. Subsequent studies demonstrated benefit with limited toxicity in HIV-positive patients with or without symptoms who had CD4 counts of less than 500/mm^3. However, recent studies have suggested that early zidovudine therapy in asymptomatic patients with CD4 counts of greater than 500/mm^3 is not beneficial compared with placebo (*see* later discussion; Figs. 5 and 6). Thus, current efforts focus on when to begin zidovudine therapy.

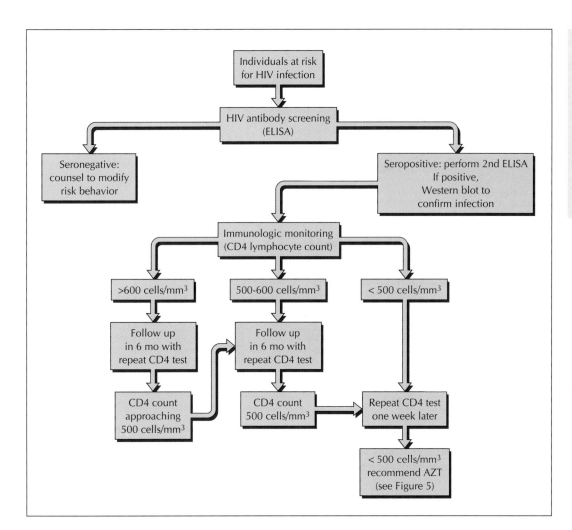

FIGURE 5
Guidelines for
the initiation
of zidovudine
therapy.
AZT—zidovu-
dine; ELISA—
enzyme-linked
immunosorbent
assay. (From
Volberding [27];
with permis-
sion.)

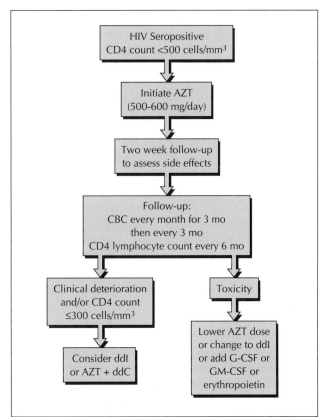

FIGURE 6 Zidovudine management protocol. AZT—zidovudine; CBC—complete blood count; ddI—dideoxyinosine;
ddC—dideoxycytidine; G-CSF—granulocyte colony-stimulating
factor; GM-CSF—granulocyte-macrophage colony-stimulating
factor. (From Volberding [27]; with permission.)

Aside from its considerable expense, zidovudine therapy can result in potentially dose-limiting toxicity, primarily bone marrow suppression. This effect appears to be dose related, having been observed commonly in patients receiving 1200 mg/d (200 mg every 4 hours). It manifests as anemia requiring transfusion and as neutropenia predisposing to acute life-threatening infections. Other documented side effects include hepatotoxicity, nausea and vomiting with anorexia, headache, myalgias, and insomnia. These effects are not seen as frequently with lower doses, but laboratory monitoring (complete blood count and liver function tests) must still be maintained.

Other antiretroviral agents have been developed. Their presence is justified by the toxicity of zidovudine and by the observation that significantly resistant strains of HIV emerge from patients after 6 to 12 months of zidovudine therapy and may well correlate with disease progression commonly seen after 2 to 3 years of therapy [14]. The drug resistance of HIV strains is well documented and almost uniformly occurs in patients with late-stage AIDS who are treated with high doses of zidovudine. These observations mandate a change in antiretroviral therapy, although resistant strains emerge against these new agents also.

The second major antiretroviral agent, dideoxyinosine, is a US Food and Drug Administration–approved alternative drug used in both adults and children with advanced HIV infection who are intolerant of zidovudine or show clinical immunologic deterioration while receiving zidovudine (eg, implying the emergence of drug-resist virus) [15]. Dideoxyinosine is taken on an empty stomach (metabolism begins in the gastric acid). It has minimal hematologic toxicity but can cause severe pancreatitis and peripheral neuropathy. The risk of pancreatitis from dideoxyinosine is dose dependent and is associated with previous pancreatitis episodes (from any cause) or exposure to intravenous pentamidine (see later). Other side effects include insomnia, diarrhea, and hyperuricemia (with gout and nephrolithiasis possible). Some children experience retinal hyperpigmentation. The use of dideoxyinosine as a first-line agent is currently being evaluated and might appropriately be considered in a patient with significant underlying marrow dysfunction (eg, anemia or thrombocytopenia).

Finally, other antiretroviral agents (eg, dideoxycytidine and foscarnet) are in various stages of development to be used in addition to or instead of zidovudine for advanced AIDS [16]. The goals are minimizing the side effects of zidovudine, treating resistant strains, and delaying the progression of disease on current therapy.

Recently, the National Institute of Allergy and Infectious Diseases issued preliminary recommendations for antiretroviral therapy (Table 5). These recommendations, developed by leading clinical researchers, divide HIV-positive patients into four major groups, depending on whether they have received previous antiretroviral therapy, are tolerant or intolerant of zidovudine, or have disease progression despite zidovudine therapy.

With all this in mind, controversy still exists about whether to start antiretroviral therapy in asymptomatic HIV-positive patients early or to wait until they demonstrate significant clinical symptoms indicative of progressive disease. Recent results from the Concorde trial cast doubt on the effectiveness of starting zidovudine (and thus perhaps all antiretrovirals) in early asymptomatic disease when the measured endpoint was survival, even though the CD4 count was relatively preserved in the treated patients [17]. In contrast, the Italian zidovudine Evaluation Group demonstrated a significant prolongation of the asymptomatic period in zidovudine-treated HIV-positive patients, even though their baseline CD4 counts were <200/mm^3 [18]. This controversy serves as an important reminder that therapy for early HIV disease is not fully established and that the National Institute of Allergy and Infectious Diseases recommendations will probably undergo revision (perhaps on an ongoing basis) as more information from these long-term clinical studies becomes available.

Prophylaxis for *Pneumocystis Carinii* Pneumonia

Pneumocystis carinii pneumonia is the most common opportunistic infection seen in HIV-positive patients. It has been one of the leading infectious causes of death in AIDS patients. This statistic has been altered by regular prophylaxis for *P. carinii* pneumonia [19]. HIV-positive patients with CD4 counts of less than 250/mm^3 should receive prophylaxis. The most cost-effective regimen consists of one trimethoprim-sulfamethoxazole tablet daily. Unfortunately, many patients cannot tolerate this, and immunologic sensitivity to trimethoprim-sulfamethoxazole is common in this patient population. Intravenous pentamidine is commonly used to treat *P. carinii* pneumonia in patients who are sensitive to trimethoprim-sulfamethoxazole. An inhaled form of pentamidine has been widely evaluated as a prophylactic agent. Although it is not as effective as trimethoprim-sulfamethoxazole, it is used in patients intolerant of oral regimens [20].

Use of Immunomodulators

Although most individuals are familiar with the concept that HIV causes immunodeficiency, fewer appreciate that a significant portion of the host immune response remains intact; particularly early in infection. Indeed, rheumatologic and allergic complications (both *hyper*immune responses) are more frequent in HIV-positive patients than in age- and sex-matched controls [21]. Thus, recognition of this fact allows the clinician to pursue two avenues of therapy—the use of vaccines against known infectious agents and the use of vaccines against HIV itself.

Basic recommendations depend largely on the relative risk of the target population and the form of the vaccine (ie, live versus killed versus recombinant protein). In general, the use of attenuated live vaccines is contraindicated because of the potential risk of reverting to the wild type [22]. Otherwise, the administration of the major antiviral vaccines, including hepatitis B, rubella (especially in women), mumps (especially in men) and measles vaccines is indicated in patients with a

Situation	Patient condition	Preliminary recommendations	Agent or agents
Initiation of therapy in patients who have never received antiretroviral therapy	Asymptomatic; CD4 count ≥ 500*	Observe, monitor clinical status and CD4 counts every 6 mo	No antiretroviral therapy
	Asymptomatic; CD4 count 200–500; stable over time	Initiate therapy *or* Observe†, monitor, initiate therapy if clinical or laboratory evidence of deterioration is present	Zidovudine in divided doses equal to 600 mg/d; may consider zidovudine and ddI or zidovudine and ddC combination‡
	Symptomatic; CD4 count 200–500	Start antiretroviral therapy	
	Symptomatic or asymptomatic; CD4 count ≤ 500	Start antiretroviral therapy†	
	AIDS or severe AIDS-related complex with any CD4 count	Start antiretroviral therapy	
Change of therapy in patients tolerating an initial therapy	CD4 count > 300; stable	Continue zidovudine	
	CD4 count < 300	Continue zidovudine *or* Change to ddI (especially if zidovudine therapy duration is > 4 mo)	
Therapy for patients intolerant of zidovudine	CD4 count ≥ 500; zidovudine intolerant	Discontinue antiretroviral therapy	No antiretroviral agent
	CD4 count 50–500; zidovudine intolerant	Switch antiretroviral agents	ddI
	CD4 count < 50; zidovudine intolerant	Switch antiretroviral agents or discontinue antiretroviral therapy	ddI or ddC or no antiretroviral agent
Therapy patients who experience disease progression despite zidovudine therapy	CD4 count 50–500; disease progression	Change antiretroviral regimen	ddI monotherapy or zidovudine and ddI or zidovudine and ddC
	CD4 count < 50; disease progression	Switch to alternative monotherapy or consider using combination therapy	ddI; ddC; zidovudine and ddI; or zidovudine and ddC

*All CD4 counts are in cells/mm³.
†Apparent inconsistencies are noted; finalized guidelines on antiretroviral treatment are expected to be published later in a peer-reviewed journal.
‡Clinical benefit of combination therapy has not yet been demonstrated.
ddC—dideoxycytidine; ddI—dideoxyinosine.

negative history of these diseases. In addition, influenza vaccination should strongly be considered, because it would be for any other susceptible individual. Tetanus-diphtheria vaccine should be given every 10 years. Pneumococcal vaccine is currently recommended for all HIV-positive patients, and revaccination is considered if the vaccine was given 6 or more years previously because the frequency of pneumococcal pneumonia and sepsis is increased 20- to 100-fold compared with the HIV-negative population. Vaccines for foreign travel are recommended as for normal individuals, with the exception of live viral vaccines.

Particularly with one-time vaccines, it is important to immunize as early in the course of disease as possible because protective immune responses have been correlated with the stage of the disease based on CD4 counts [23].

Recently, the development of therapeutic HIV vaccines has begun to undergo extensive clinical evaluation [24]. The goal is to induce the patient's impaired immune system to improve its recognition of and/or response to HIV antigens than it does in response to natural infection. Therapeutic strategies involve the use of attenuated HIV virus, inactivated virus, viral particles, and recombinant or synthetic proteins.

Many clinical trials are being conducted to look for efficacy of any of these vaccines in HIV patients.

Counseling the HIV-Positive Patient and Family

It is important for the clinician to recognize the needs of the HIV-positive patient for understanding, information, and reassurance. Although the disease is still fatal, many productive years can be expected in most HIV-positive patients. With clinical courses lasting for more than 10 years with relatively good health, proper education of the patient regarding realistic clinical expectations, recognition of early signs of reversible complications, and encouragement toward as normal a lifestyle as possible will all benefit the patient. Public health education to reinforce safe sexual practices for patients and their significant others and to dispel various myths about HIV transmission is also indicated. Finally, discussions with the patient about mortality issues, guilt, and despair can control situational depression and allow the clinician to differentiate depression from the dementia that can be seen with advancing disease.

The patient's family or support group should also be involved in educational and counseling efforts. Many clinical misconceptions exist among family members, particularly regarding the longevity and infectivity of the HIV-positive patient. This can produce an unintended banishment of the patient from loved ones because of their fear of being infected or lead to the erroneous assumption that the patient will soon be dead. Frank answers to questions and educating the family in the expected care that will be needed by the patient, as well as the recognition of complicating side effects to allow early intervention, are fundamental to the overall management of HIV disease.

ROLE OF THE GENERALIST

Much information on the pathophysiology of AIDS is being discovered, and new and potentially exciting therapies are currently being developed. However, AIDS is still a primary care disease requiring clinical acumen, compassion, and diligence to control the side effects of medications, recognize the clinical progression of the disease, and provide the support necessary to both patient and family. The primary care physician will ultimately be most successful in changing the attitude of medical professionals (and perhaps of society as well) with regard to the worthiness of therapy for patients with HIV-induced disease, particularly early in its course. Although practitioners may not agree with patients' individual choices that may have resulted in their acquiring the infection, they are obliged to provide the best care possible without prejudice.

Finally, the generalist should be active in counseling his or her HIV-negative patient population about the risks associated with acquiring HIV infection. This may take the form of written information, one-on-one counseling sessions, or even public forums. Clinicians must keep up with the latest developments regarding protective measures and new therapies so that they can serve as resources for their patients. The Hippocratic Oath demands nothing less.

REFERENCES AND RECOMMENDED READING

1. Libman H: Pathogenesis, natural history and classification of HIV infection. *Prim Care* 1992, 19:1–17.
2. Weiss PJ, Wallace MR, Olson PE, Rossetti R: Changes in the mix of AIDS-defining conditions. *N Engl J Med* 1992, 329:1962.
3. Levy JA: Human immunodeficiency virus and the pathogenesis of AIDS. *JAMA* 1989, 261:2997–3006.
4. Greenberg P: Immunopathogenesis of HIV infection. *Hosp Pract* 1992, 109–124.
5. Darrow WW, Echenberg DF, Jaffe HW, *et al.*: Risk factors of human immunodeficiency virus (HIV) infections in homosexual men. *Am J Public Health* 1987, 77:479–484.
6. Chaisson RE, Moss AR, Oniski R, *et al.*: HIV infection in heterosexual intravenous drug abusers in San Francisco. *Am J Public Health* 1987, 77:169–176.
7. Rothman DJ, Edgar H: AIDS, activism and ethics. In *AIDS: Problems and Prospects.* Edited by Corey L. New York: Norton; 1993:145–155.
8. McCarthy BD, Wong JB, Munoz A, Sonneberg FA: Who should be screened for HIV infection? A cost-effective analysis. *Arch Intern Med* 1993, 153:1107–1116.
9. Barnes PF, Block AB, Davidson PT, Snider DE: Tuberculosis in patients with human immunodeficiency virus infection. *N Engl J Med* 1991, 324:1644–1650.
10. Volberding PA, Cohen PT: Indications for use of HIV antibody testing. In *The AIDS Knowledge Base.* Edited by Cohen PT, Sande MA, Volberding PA. Waltham, MA: The Medical Publishing Group; 1990:2.1.1.
11. Haseltine WA: Silent HIV infections. *N Engl J Med* 1989, 320:1487–1489.
12. Bartlett JG: *The Johns Hopkins Guide to Medical Care of Patients With HIV Infection.* edn 3. Baltimore: Williams Wilkins; 1993.
13. Broder S: Antiretroviral therapy in AIDS. *Ann Intern Med* 1990, 113:604–618.
14. Richman DD: Antiretroviral drug resistance. *AIDS* 1991, 5:S189–S194.
15. Kahn J: New developments in the clinical use of didanosine. *J Acquir Immune Defic Syndr* 1993, 6:S47–S50.
16. Richman DD: Antiviral therapy of HIV infection. *Annu Rev Med* 1991, 42:69–90.
17. Concorde coordinating committee. Concorde: MRC/ANRS randomized double-blind controlled trial of immediate and deferred zidovudine in symptom-free HIV infection. *Lancet* 1994;343:871–881.
18. Vella S, Giuliano M, Dally LG, *et al.*: Long-term follow-up of zidovudine therapy in asymptomatic HIV infection: results of a multicenter cohort study. *J Acquir Immune Defic Syndr* 1994, 7:31–38.
19. Carr A, Penny R, Cooper DA: Prophylaxis of opportunistic infections in patients with HIV infection. *J Acquir Immune Defic Syndr* 1993, 6:S56–S60.
20. Torres RA, Barr M, Thorn M, *et al.*: Randomized trial of dapsone and aerosolized pentamidine for the prophylaxis of *Pneumocystis carinii* pneumonia and toxoplasmic encephalitis. *Am J Med* 1993, 95:573–583.
21. Zunich KM, Lane HC: Immunologic abnormalities in HIV infection. *Hematol Oncol Clin North Am* 1991, 5:215–228.
22. Rhoads JL, Birx DL, Wright DC, *et al.*: Safety and immunogenicity of multiple conventional immunizations administered during early HIV infection. *J Acquir Immune Defic Syndr* 1991, 4:724–731.
23. Recommendations of the Advisory Committee on Immunization Practices (ACIP): Use of vaccines and immune globulins for persons with altered immunocompetence. *MMWR Morb Mortal Wkly Rep* 1993, 42:1–18.

24. Redfield RR, Birx DL: HIV-specific vaccine therapy: concepts, status and future directions. *AIDS Res Hum Retroviruses* 1992, 8:1051–1058.

25. Clark SJ, Saag MS, Decker WG, *et al*.: High titers of cytopathic virus in plasma of patients with symptomatic primary HIV-1 infection. *N Engl J Med* 1991, 324:954–960.

26. Aldorini A, Waller BD, eds: *Technologies in HIV Research*. New York: Stockton Press; 1990.

27. Volberding PA: Strategies for antiretroviral therapy in adult HIV disease: the San Francisco perspective. In *Textbook of AIDS Medicine* Edited by Broder S, Morgan TC, Bolognesi D. Baltimore: Williams & Wilkins; 1994:773–787.

Immunotherapy and Immunomodulation 17

Leonard Bielory

Key Points

- Control of the immunologic reactions have become more specific over the past 20 years.

- Recent advances include development of anticytokine therapeutic modalities aimed at the production of cytokines (*eg*, cyclosporin) and their receptors (*eg*, interleukin-1 receptor), as well as infusion of specific cytokines (*eg*, interferons).

- The use of monoclonal antibodies for diagnosis and therapy is advancing with the identification of important peptides from human and bacterial sources.

- Use of immunomodulatory agents will increase in the realm of the primary care physician.

Immunomodulation is the control and regulation of the inflammatory immune response by a variety of techniques (Table 1) [1•,2•,3]. The primary function of the immune system is the development of an inflammatory response to a foreign or infectious antigen, which produces rubor (redness), dolor (pain), calor (heat), tumor (swelling), and *functio laesa* (loss of function). The archetype immunomodulatory agents nonspecifically affect various aspects of the immune response, whereas novel agents are more specific in their function (Fig. 1).

The mechanisms used in the modulation of the specific immune cells and their inflammatory responses are listed in Tables 2 and 3. Initially, the first generation of immunosuppressants—cyclophosphamide, azathioprine, and glucocorticosteroids— were thought to be equally inhibitory to every type of immune cell, but there may be a selective effect of each of these agents on cell-mediated immunity mediated by T lymphocytes and humoral immunity mediated by B lymphocytes. The use of general immunosuppression is associated with two major complications: increased susceptibility to infections and increased risk of malignancy.

IRRADIATION

The proliferative phase of the immune response is the most sensitive to radiation. High-dose irradiation (900 to 1200 rad) destroys the overall immune response, whereas low-dose irradiation preferentially decreases the primary (radiosensitive) immune response more than the secondary (radioresistant) immune response of the memory-type of cells.

Total lymphoid irradiation (TLI) delivers high doses of radiation to lymphoid tissue, whereas other tissues are shielded (Fig. 2). It is used in the treatment of lymphoid malignancies (*ie*, Hodgkin's disease) and has been attempted in other T-suppressor cell autoimmune disorders. The most common adverse effects of TLI are moderate constitutional symptoms including fatigue, anorexia, diarrhea, abdominal pain, nausea, weight loss, xerostomia, and herpes zoster. Ovarian sterility can occur unless the ovaries are operatively relocated to a position where they can be shielded. Hypothyroidism occurs in 20% of patients who do not receive shielding of their

TABLE 1 IMMUNOMODULATORY TECHNIQUES

Technique	Mechanism of action	Example	Disorder
Irradiation	Activates antiproliferative, lymphocytolytic, interference with DNA repair	Total lymphoid PUVA	Lymphomas
Pheresis	Removes circulating immunologically active components that can then be replaced by other biological fluids or returned in a transformed immune state	Lymphocytopheresis Plasmapheresis Lymphokine-activated killer cell Plateletpheresis	Leukemia Goodpasture's syndrome Melanoma Thrombocytosis
Surgery	Removes or transplants immunologically active tissue	Bone marrow Thymus Spleen	Leukemia Severe combined immunodeficiency
Alkylating agents	Reacts with the nucleophilic portion of DNA and RNA	Cyclophosphamide Busulfan Cisplatin Chlorambucil	Vasculitis Myeloproliferative disorders
Antimetabolites	Inhibits action of a variety of cytoplasmic and nuclear enzymes	Purine and pyrimidine analogues Folic acid antagonists Methylhydrazines Hydroxyurea Alkaloids Protein inhibitors	Myeloproliferative disorders
Steroids	Stabilizes lysosomes, impairs antigen recognition and processing, alters prostaglandin and leukotriene formation	Prednisone Methylprednisolone	All disorders associated with inflammation
NSAIDs	Alters prostaglandin and leukotriene formation	Aspirin Indomethacin	All disorders associated with inflammation
Immunotherapy	Activates immunotolerance	Penicillin allergy Bee venom Pollen immunotherapy	Drug allergy Asthma Allergic rhinoconjunctivitis Insect sting Hypersensitivity
Antibody	Activates cytolysis, reticuloendothelial system blockade	Heterologous anti-thymocyte globulin Monoclonal antibodies Human gamma globulin	Aplastic anemia Humoral immunodeficiency Prophylaxis of viral infections Organ rejection
Cytokines	Stimulates proliferation and differentiation	Interferon (α, β, γ) Colony-stimulating factors Thymopentin	Atopic dermatitis Viral hepatitis
Immunophilins	Blocks lymphocyte activation	Cyclosporine Rapamycin FK506	Uveitis Organ rejection

NSAIDs—nonsteroidal antiinflammatory drugs; PUVA—psoralen ultraviolet light (treatment).

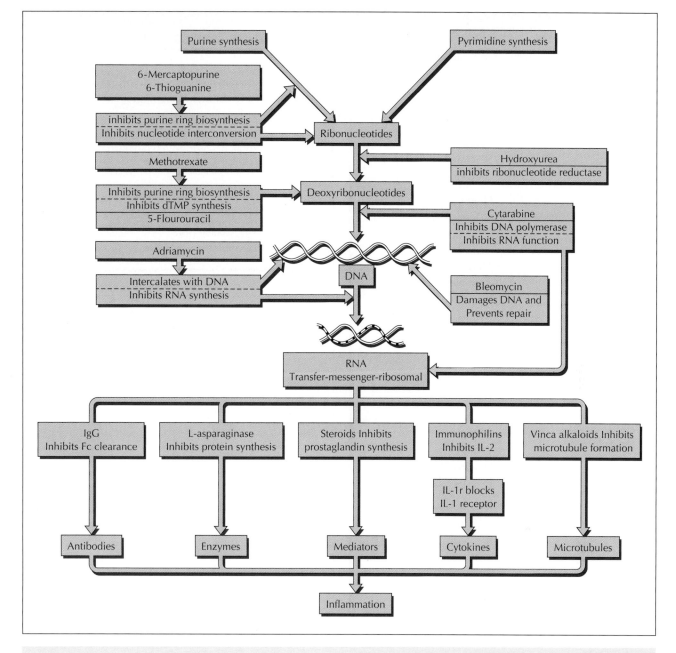

FIGURE 1 Immunomodulation interferes with the cell growth cycle of those cells involved in the inflammatory response.

A single agent can affect several points of the cell growth cycle. IL—interleukin; dTMP—deoxy-thymidine monophosphate.

thyroid. Bone marrow suppression, radiation carditis, pneumonitis or enteritis, and severe viral or bacterial infections can occur; secondary tumors rarely develop.

Ultraviolet light (UVL) irradiation produces depressed cellular immunity [4•]. The use of photoactivated chemical cross-linkers (*eg*, 8-methoxypsoralen) with long-wave UVL (UVA; 320–400 nm) is termed PUVA and has been used for treatment of specific T-cell-mediated disorders, such as erythrodermic cutaneous T-cell lymphoma and psoriasis. The delivery of the UVL is limited to the superficial dermis, that is, the treatment is only "skin deep" and has been effective in severe cases of atopic dermatitis.

PHERESIS

Pheresis is the discriminating removal of a specific blood component (*eg*, platelets, plasma, red blood cells, leukocytes, and lymphocytes). Within hours to days, plasmapheresis removes antibodies, immune complexes, hormones, drugs, and other plasma-soluble substances. The use of a special staphylococcal protein A pheresis column can selectively remove IgG and IgG-containing immune complexes. Plasmapheresis is used in the following immunologically mediated disorders: hyperviscosity syndromes associated with myelomas, mushroom poisoning, theophylline toxicity,

TABLE 2 INDICATIONS FOR IMMUNOSUPPRESSIVE THERAPY

Connective tissue disorders
Rheumatoid arthritis
Dermatomyositis
Temporal arteritis
Systemic lupus erythematosus
Polymyalgia
Polymyositis
Polymyalgia rheumatic

Gastrointestinal
Crohn's disease
Ulcerative colitis

Hepatic
Chronic active hepatitis
Primary biliary cirrhosis

Endocrinologic
Adrenal insufficiency
Hypercalcemia
Thyroid dysfunction
Graves' disease
Diabetes mellitus
  (juvenile onset)

Dermatologic
Eczema
Alopecia
Dermatomyositis
Erythema multiforme
Pemphigus
Pemphigoid
Psoriasis
Urticaria pigmentosa

Neurologic
Myasthenia gravis
Multiple sclerosis

Renal
Nephrotic syndrome
Glomerulonephritis

Hematologic
Aplastic anemia
Idiopathic thrombocy
  topenic purpura
Thrombotic thrombocy
  topenic purpura
Hemolytic anemias
Cold agglutinin diseas

Organ transplantation
Kidney
Liver
Heart/lung
Bone marrow

Allergic
Anaphylaxis
Stevens-Johnson syndrome
Urticara

Respiratory
Asthma
Pulmonary fibrosis

TABLE 3 CLASSIFICATION OF IMMUNOMODULATION

Specific
Active immunization (antigen ± adjuvant)
Passive transfer (cells, antiserum, transfer factor)
Physical removal of serum or blood components
Blocking of cell surface receptors
Hyposensitization, desensitization
Depressing mast cell reactivity
Nonspecific
Interleukin, interferon, bacille Calmette-Guerin
Blocking effector mechanisms and mediators
Interference with metabolism
Radiation, drugs, hormones, antisera

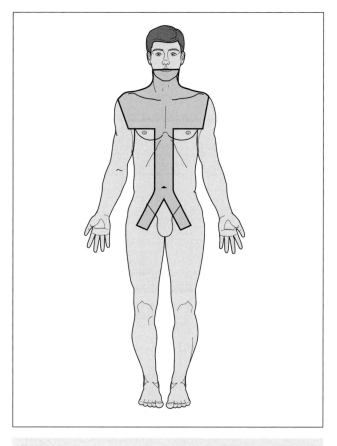

FIGURE 2 The primary location of lymphoid tissue (cervical, axillary, mediastinal, periaortic, and inguinal lymph nodes, thymus, and spleen in shaded area), which is the focus of total lymphoid irradiation.

Goodpasture's syndrome, autoimmune hemolytic anemia, myasthenia gravis, and systemic lupus erythematosus (life-threatening arteritis).

Plasma exchange is the process of separating and removing plasma, then replacing it with either fresh frozen plasma or plasma protein fractions. The exchanged plasma is used in the treatment of thrombotic thrombocytopenic purpura. In general, pheresis is associated with defibrination, thrombocytopenia, and hypogammaglobulinemia. Selective forms of cellular pheresis are used to treat a variety of disorders. For example, plateletpheresis is used for essential thrombocytosis, hemapheresis for sickle cell anemia, and lymphocytopheresis for leukemias. A special form of lymphocytopheresis, coupled with the incubation and reinfusion of interleukin-2 lymphokine-activated killer (LAK) cells, has resulted in a favorable clinical response in patients with renal cell carcinoma and melanoma (Fig. 3) [5]. Transfusions have also altered immune function by either improving renal allograft survival or decreasing bone marrow transplant engraftment survivals [6].

STEROIDAL ANTIINFLAMMATORY AGENTS

Glucocorticosteroids inhibit the arachidonic acid cascade (Table 4). The persistence of the steroid-induced response is dependent on the half-life of the steroid. The differential effect of glucocorticosteroids on circulating monocytes, which are depleted, and neutrophils, which are retained, has been exploited with the development of alternate-day steroid treatments for a variety of autoimmune and inflammatory disorders. In general, neutrophil function is minimally affected by phagocytosis. Steroid-induced lymphopenia reaches its maximum effect in 4 to 6 hours and lasts for 24 to 72 hours. Wound healing is retarded by glucocorticosteroids, but not by nonsteroidal antiinflammatory drugs (NSAIDs) or androgenic steroids.

Major complications associated with steroid use are primarily metabolic and include hyperglycemia, cataracts, hypercholesterolemia, osteoporosis, and adrenal suppression.

Pulse therapy, large daily doses of intravenous methylprednisolone (0.5 to 2.0 g) given for 1 to 3 days, limits the adverse reactions associated with chronic large oral steroid doses. Pulse therapy has been used in the reversal of renal transplant rejection and in some patients with autoimmune disorders (eg, systemic lupus erythematosus, optic neuritis). Common minor side effects include respiratory tract infections, facial flushing, a metallic taste in the mouth, palpitations, headaches, and sweating. Steroid-sparing agents include troleandomycin for asthma, methotrexate for psoria-

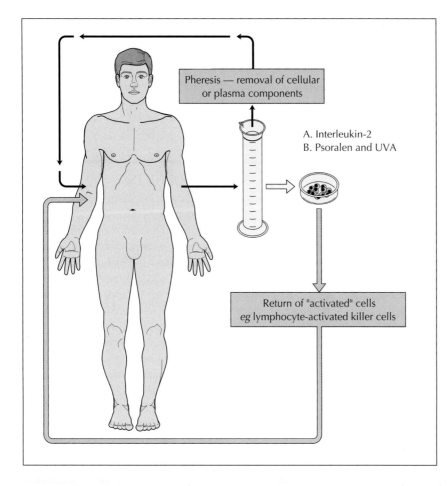

FIGURE 3 A special form of pheresis combined with removal of lymphocytes and incubation with growth factors such as interleukin-2 or photoactivated chemical cross-linkers (*eg*, 8-methoxypsoralen) and exposure to selective wavelengths have been used for the treatment of specific T-cell-mediated disorders and tumors (*eg*, renal cell carcinoma and melanoma). UVA—ultraviolet A light.

		TABLE 4 CORTICOSTEROID PREPARATIONS				
Corticosteroid	**Antiinflammatory potency***	**Equivalent pharmacologic dose (mg)**	**Mineralocorticoid activity**	**Increased appetite**	**Muscle myopathy**	**Biologic $T_{1/2}$ (h)**
Hydrocortisone	1.0	20.0	2+	2+	1+	8
Cortisone	0.8	25.0	2+	2+	1+	8
Prednisone	2.8	5.0	1+	3+	1+	12
Prednisolone	4.0	5.0	1+	3+	1+	12
Methylprednisolone	5.0	4.0	0	2+	1+	12
Triamcinolone	5.0	4.0	0	0	3+	24
Paramethasone	10.0	2.0	0	3+	2+	36
Dexamethasone	30.0	0.75	0	4+	2+	36
Betamethasone	30.0	0.6	0	4+	2+	36

*Relative to hydrocortisone, which is assigned a value of 1. The hypothalamic axis suppression directly correlates to the antiinflammatory potency of the drug. $T_{1/2}$—half-life.

sis, chrysotherapy (*ie*, gold salts therapy) for rheumatoid arthritis, and antimalarials for systemic lupus erythematosus.

NONSTEROIDAL ANTIINFLAMMATORY DRUGS

Nonsteroidal antiinflammatory drugs also modify the arachidonic acid that produces prostaglandins and thromboxanes. NSAIDs include salicylic acid (aspirin), pyrazolin (phenylbutazone), indoleacetic acid (indomethacin, sulindac), pyrrolic acid (ibuprofen, fenoprofen, naproxen), propionic acid (ketoprofen benoxaprofen), anthranilic acid (mefenamic acid), oxicam (piroxicam).

The enhancing inflammatory effects of prostaglandins include vascular permeability, granuloma formation, vasodilation, fever, and hyperalgesia [7]. Prostaglandins can also counteract the vasoconstriction caused by norepinephrine or angiotensin. Renal deterioration from NSAIDs occurs in patients with prostaglandin-dependent renal function, such as heart failure, cirrhosis, and renal insufficiency [8].

ALKYLATING AGENTS

Alkylating agents are radiomimetic because their effects resemble those of irradiation but are temporary, because lymphoid cells can repair their DNA.

Cyclophosphamide is the best known agent and is used at lower dosages (2 mg/kg/d) than when used for chemotherapy. Impaired renal function increases immunosuppression and drug toxicity, resulting in hemorrhagic cystitis, which necessitates drug dose reduction. Cyclophosphamide interacts with allopurinol, glucocorticosteroids, and barbiturates, thus requiring dose reduction when those agents are also at work.

Vinblastine and vincristine are *Vinca* alkaloids that are predominantly used in the treatment of hematologic malignancies as well as refractory cases of idiopathic thrombocytopenic purpura.

Hydroxyurea is well absorbed from the gastrointestinal track and is excreted unchanged in the urine within 12 hours. Its primary use is for treatment of myeloid proliferative disorders (*eg*, myelogenous leukemia and hypereosinophilia).

The thiopurines are one of the major antimetabolites used in clinical practice. Azathioprine, derived from 6-mercaptopurine, is the most frequently used drug in this class. Its primary target is proliferating lymphocytes. Clinical effects are seen within 3 to 4 weeks. The primary adverse effect is reversible bone marrow suppression, although infections may occur regardless of the degree of neutropenia (Table 5). Allopurinol increases the toxicity and warrants the reduction of the azathioprine dose by 75%. Another class of antimetabolites includes folic acid antagonists (*eg*, methotrexate), which interfere with a crucial enzyme, dihydrofolate reductase, involved in the synthesis of thymidine and purine nucleotides. Methotrexate, a folic acid antagonist, is reversibly bound to albumin and can be displaced by aspirin and sulfonamides.

IMMUNOPHILINS

Immunophilins are a family of cytoplasmic proteins that include the cyclical dodecapeptide cyclosporine, macrocyclic lactone FK506, and rapamycin. The immunophilins catalyze the folding of proline-containing proteins, which then interfere with DNA transcription required in T-lymphocyte activation, such as cell-mediated immunity, allograft rejection, and graft-versus-host reactions [9]. These agents appear to exert their influence on the humoral and cell-mediated hypersensitivity reactions by inhibiting the generation of interleukin-2 and other lymphokines and their receptors. Antibody production, neutrophil function, and wound healing are not affected. Reversible nephrotoxicity is associated with high-dose treatment. Low-dose use of cyclosporine (2 to 5 mg/kg/d) in the treatment of psoriasis, rheumatoid arthritis, or uveitis is not associated with as many adverse reactions.

TABLE 5 ADVERSE REACTIONS TO VARIOUS IMMUNOMODULATORY AGENTS				
Reaction	**Methotrexate**	**Azathioprine**	**Cyclophosphamide**	**Cyclosporine**
Infection	+	+	+	+/-
Myelotoxicity	+	+	+	+/-
Nephrotoxicity	+/-	-	-	++
Hepatotoxicity	++	+/-	+/-	+
Pneumonitis	+	+/-	+/-	+
Cystitis	-	-	++	-
Pancreatitis	-	+	-	-
Neoplasia	+/-	+	+	+/-
Infertility	+/-	+/-	++	-
Fetal toxicity	++	+/-	+/-	+/-

—none; +/—minimal; +—substantial; ++—major concern.

CYTOKINES

Activated immune cells release special hormones, called cytokines, which have been synthetically isolated and manufactured with molecular engineering techniques. Interferon, originally thought to be an antiviral agent, kills bacteria and protozoal pathogens. Adverse effects of interferon (ie, chills, myalgia, erythema, fever) are dose related. High-dose interferon treatment for cancer is associated with the development of an immune glomerulonephritis. Another cytokine, thymopoietin, is produced by thymic epithelial cells, induces phenotypic maturation of thymocytes, and promotes their differentiation. Cytokines can be synthetically manufactured. A clinical trial has shown some improvement in pruritus in patients with atopic dermatitis, erythema, and extent of body involvement in 66% of atopic dermatitis patients. Thymopentin, is the active pentapeptide of a thymic hormone that provided significant clinical improvement in severity and pruritus after 6 weeks of treatment in patients with atopic dermatitis. Both interferon and thymopentin must be given by injection; both are proteins and cannot be administered orally.

IMMUNOTHERAPY

Immunotherapy (or desensitization) is the administration of an offending antigen, specific antibody, or antigen–antibody complex to develop tolerance to an allergen or allograft, without the induction of generalized immunosuppression. This can be done within hours to days, starting with small doses as in penicillin desensitization. In IgE/mast cell mediated hypersensitivity (allergic) reactions, desensitization leading to tolerance is associated with reduced lymphocyte proliferation and basophil sensitivity to the specific antigen. IgG-blocking antibodies and T suppressor cells for IgE-committed B cells are increased with subsequent reduction of IgE production. The only indication for immunotherapy as a first line of therapy is for the treatment of patients with bee sting hypersensitivity reactions. Pollen immunotherapy should be considered as an adjunct to medical therapy and significantly lessens symptoms, medication usage, and cost for patients with allergic rhinitis, conjunctivitis, and asthma. Recent research has focused on the control of the T lymphocyte in its orchestration of the mast cell–mediated response with the experimental development T-cell–idiotype-specific immunotherapy.

ANTIBODY

Intravenous IgG is specifically indicated in the treatment of the following primary antibody deficiencies [10].

Erythroblastosis fetalis
Pediatric AIDS [11]
Prevention of infection in low birth-weight infants
Chronic lymphocytic leukemia
Idiopathic thrombocytopenic purpura
Kawasaki syndrome
Chronic inflammatory demyelinating neuropathies [12]
Guillain-Barré syndrome.

Antibodies can be used to effectively block an immune response (eg, Rh factor), inhibit an infection (eg, hepatitis), deplete unwanted cells (eg, antilymphocyte globulin), and block binding to receptors [eg, anti–interleukin-1 for sepsis or anti–interleukin-2 receptor-directed (anti-TAC) therapy].

Therapy with mouse-derived antiidiotypic antibodies has had limited success in the treatment of patients with lymphoma and renal transplants due to the immunological response directed at the heterologous origin of the antibodies. However, immunotoxins, which are hybrid proteins that combine the potent cytocidal actions of a toxin and are harnessed for the selective destruction of target cells by attachment to a specific monoclonal antibody or growth factor, are in clinical studies for a variety of disorders [13]. Transplanted organs undergoing rejection and hematologic malignancies such as cutaneous T-cell lymphoma, leukemia, and Hodgkin's and non-Hodgkin's lymphomas express the high-affinity interleukin-2 receptor (Table 6) [14]. The interleukin-2 receptor thus provides a target with restricted success for treatment with anti-TAC receptor antibodies or chimeric interleukin-2 toxins.

TABLE 6 CANDIDATES FOR INTERLEUKIN-2 RECEPTOR-DIRECTED (ANTI-TAC) THERAPY

Neoplasia	Autoimmune disease	Allograft protocols
T cell (adult T-cell leukemia, cutaneous T-cell lymphoma)	Rheumatoid arthritis	Prevent organ allograft rejection
B cell (hairy-cell leukemia)	Systemic lupus erythematosus	Treat graft-versus-host disease
Other mononuclear cells (Hodgkin's disease)	Aplastic anemia	
Granulocyte (chronic and acute myelogenous leukemia)	Type I diabetes	
	Crohn's disease	
	Sarcoidosis	
	Scleroderma	
	Noninfectious uveitis	
	Chronic active hepatitis	
	Tropical spastic paraparesis	

TABLE 7 IMMUNE SERUM GLOBULIN FOR TREATMENT OF INFECTIOUS DISORDERS

Hyperimmune globulin	Source	Comment
Black widow spider antivenin	Equine	
Diptheria antitoxin	Equine	
Immune globulin	Human	Hepatitis A Measles
Hepatitis B immune globulin	Human	Hepatitis B
Immune globulin IV	Human	
Rabies immune globulin	Human	
Antirabies serum	Equine	
Crotalid antivenin	Equine	Coral snake, rattlesnake, copperhead, and water moccasin
Tetanus immune globulin	Human	
Tetanus antitoxin	Equine and bovine	
Varicella immune globulin	Human	
Vaccinia immune globulin	Human	Available from the Centers for Disease Control

TABLE 8 VACCINES FOR ACTIVE IMMUNIZATION

Vaccine	Live	Attenuated	Killed	Toxoid	Component*	Avian derived
Adenovirus†	+	+				
Botulinum				+		
BCG	+	+				
Cholera			+			
Diphtheria				+		
Hemophilus					+	
Hepatitis B					+	
Influenza			+			+
Measles	+	+				+
Meningococcal					+	
Mumps	+	+				+
Pertussis			+			
Plague			+			
Pneumococcal					+	
Polio						
Sabin	+	+				
Salk			+			
Rabies	+	+				+‡
Rubella	+	+				
Tetanus				+		
Typhoid			+			+
Vaccinia	+	+				
Varicella	+	+				
Yellow fever	+	+				+

*Polysaccharide or protein.
†Given only to military personnel.
‡May be obtained from human tissue culture that is free of egg protein.
BCG—bacille Calmette-Guérin.

IMMUNIZATIONS

The goal of immunization is to either passively protect an individual by administering preformed immunoreactive serum or actively induce host immunity by an antigenic stimulus without causing significant adverse effects. Passive immunization introduces preformed serum antibodies titered against specific antigens to provide temporary immunity when active immunization is not possible (Table 7). These sera, raised in humans or animals, provide immediate but variable, short-lived protection (1 to 6 weeks), allow no booster effect, and are often associated with adverse reactions. Passive immunization is primarily used for postexposure prophylaxis. On the other hand, vaccines have been developed to provide active protection against bacterial and viral infections (Table 8) as well as against tumors [15].

REFERENCES AND RECOMMENDED READING

Recently published papers of particular interest have been highlighted as:

* Of interest

** Of outstanding interest

1.• Hadden JW, Smith DL: Immunopharmacology, immunomodulation, and immunotherapy. *JAMA* 1992, 268:2964–2969.

2.• Goust JM, Stevenson HC, Galbraith RM, Virella G: Immunosuppression and immunomodulation. *Immunology Series* 1990, 50:481–498.

3. Boch JF, ed: *Immunointervention in Autoimmune Disease.* New York: Academic Press; 1989.

4.• Pamphilon DH, Alnaqdy AA, Wallington TB: Immunomodulation by ultraviolet light. *Immunol Today* 1991, 12:119–123.

5. Rosenberg SA, Spiess P, Lafeniere R: A new approach to the adoptive immunotherapy of cancer, using tumor infiltrating lymphocytes. *Science* 1986, 233:1318–1321.

6. Blumberg N, Triulzi DJ, Heal JM: Transfusion-induced immunomodulation and its clinical consequences. *Transfusion Med Rev* 1990, 4:24–35.

7. Goodwin JS: Immunomodulation by eicosanoids and anti-inflammatory drugs. *Curr Opin Immunol* 1989, 2:264–268.

8. Murray MD, Brater DC: Adverse effects of nonsteroidal anti-inflammatory drugs on renal function. *Ann Intern Med* 1990, 112:559–560.

9. Erlanger BF: Do we know the site of action of cyclosporine? *Immunol Today* 1992, 13:487–489.

10. Consensus Conference on Intravenous Immunoglobulin. *NIH Conn Med* 1990 (Dec), 54(12):667–683.

11. Mofenson LM, Moye J: Intravenous immune globulin for the prevention of infections in children with symptomatic human immunodeficiency virus infection. *Pediatr Res* 1993, 33:80–89.

12. Soueidan SA, Dalakas MC: Treatment of autoimmune neuro-muscular diseases with high dose intravenous immune globulin. *Pediatr Res* 1993, 33(suppl):95–100.

13. Pietersz GA, McKenzie IFC: Antibody conjugates for the treatment of cancer. *Immunol Rev* 1992, 129:57–80.

14. Strom TB, Kelley VR, Woodworth TG, Murphy JR: Interleukin-2 receptor-directed immunosuppressive therapies: antibody or cytokine-based targeting molecules. *Immunol Rev* 1992, 129:131–164.

15. Stevenson FK: Tumor vaccines. *FASEB J* 1991, 5:2250–2257.

SELECT BIBLIOGRAPHY

Allison AC, Lafferty K, Eds.: Immunosuppressive and anti-inflammatory drugs. *Proc N Y Acad Sci* 1993, 696:1.

St. Georgiev V, Yamaguchi H, Eds.: Immunomodulating drugs. *Proc N Y Acad Sci* 1993, 685:1.

TABLE 1 MEDICAL ADVANCES LINKED TO THE INCREASE IN SEPSIS CASES

Prolonged survival time of chronically ill patients
More time spent in the hospital setting
Greater use of immunosuppressive techniques
Increased use of chemotherapy and radiation therapy
Greater use of catheters
Increased use of intubation for ventilatory support
Increased use of various types of surgical prostheses
Imprudent use of antibiotics

TABLE 2 DEFINITIONS OF SEPSIS

Infection

A microbial phenomenon characterized by an inflammatory response to the presence of microorganisms or the invasion of normally sterile host tissue by these organisms.

Bacteremia

The presence of viable bacteria in the blood. The presence of viruses, fungi, parasites, and other pathogens in the blood should be described in a similar manner (*ie*, viremia, fungemia, and parasitemia)

Septicemia

Previously, the presence of microorganisms or their toxins in the blood. However, this term has been used clinically and in the medical literature in various ways that have added to confusion and difficulties in data interpretation. *Septicemia* also does not adequately describe the entire spectrum of pathogenic organisms that may infect the blood. We therefore suggest that this term be eliminated from current usage.

Systemic inflammatory response syndrome

A new term that broadly encompasses the essential disease process. The term emphasizes the fact that not all cases of runaway systemic inflammation can be tied to a specific infection.

Sepsis

The systemic inflammatory response to infection. In association with infection, manifestations of sepsis are the same as those previously defined for systemic inflammatory response syndrome; they include, but are not limited to, more than one of the following: 1) a temperature of > 38°C or < 36°C, 2) an elevated heart rate of > 90 bpm, 3) tachypnea, manifested by a respiratory rate of > 20 breaths per minute, or hyperventilation, as indicated by a $PaCO_2$ of < 32 mm Hg, and 4) an altered leukocyte count of > 12,000 cells/mm^3 or < 4000 cells/mm^3, or the presence of > 10% immature neutrophils (bands). To help identify these manifestations as sepsis, it should be determined whether they are a part of the direct systemic response to the presence of an infectious process. Additionally, the physiologic changes measured should represent an acute alteration from baseline in the absence of other known causes of such abnormalities.

Severe sepsis

Sepsis associated with organ dysfunction, hypoperfusion abnormality, or sepsis-induced hypotension. Hypoperfusion abnormalities include lactic acidosis, oliguria, and an acute alteration in mental status.

Sepsis-induced hypotension

A systolic blood pressure of < 90 mm Hg or a reduction in blood pressure of 40 mm Hg from baseline, in the absence of other causes of hypotension (*eg*, cardiogenic shock).

Septic shock

Sepsis-induced hypotension, persisting despite adequate fluid resuscitation, along with the presence of hypoperfusion abnormalities or organ dysfunction. This is an exacerbation of sepsis and a subset of severe sepsis. Patients receiving inotropic or vasopressor agents may no longer be hypotensive by the time they manifest hypoperfusion abnormalities or organ dysfunction, but they would still be considered to have septic shock.

Multiple organ dysfunction syndrome

The presence of altered organ function in an acutely ill patient such that homeostasis can not be maintained without intervention.

Adapted from Bone and coworkers [15••]; with permission.
$PaCO_2$—partial arterial pressure of carbon dioxide.

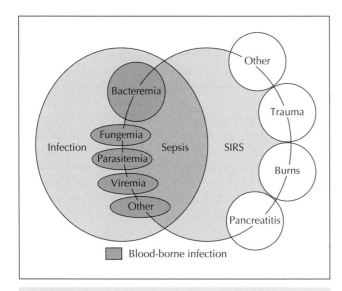

FIGURE 1 The relationship between sepsis and some associated conditions. SIRS—systemic inflammatory response syndrome. (*From* Bone and coworkers [15••]; with permission.)

most likely to improve patient survival. Although SIRS does not always involve infection and the activity of pathogenic organisms, it often does; thus, cultures should be performed immediately if the condition is suspected. However, even this technique cannot rule out occult infection, which often foments sepsis. The five most suggestive signs of sepsis are tachypnea, tachycardia, fever, hypotension, and mental status changes. The specific clinical criteria agreed on at the ACCP/SCCM conference can be found in Table 2 under the definition for *sepsis*.

Sepsis is, to some degree, a self-perpetuating disease: once the cascade of mediator releases involved in the inflammatory process has begun, both the mediators themselves and the injuries they cause may promote further release in what may become a vicious cycle. The sequelae to sepsis include septic shock, multiple organ dysfunction syndrome, and adult respiratory distress syndrome (ARDS).

The earliest, easy-to-recognize clinical signs of sepsis are shown in Table 3. Among certain groups of patients, fever—the normal response in inflammation—may be blocked or

altered. In any case, the absence of fever should not rule out a diagnosis of sepsis. Another early finding may be respiratory alkalosis, and chest radiographs may or may not show diffuse infiltrates. Coagulopathy may occur and is indicated by an increase in the prothrombin time and low levels of fibrinogen. As sepsis progresses, a metabolic acidosis may overtake the respiratory alkalosis, causing a low pH reading. Lactic acidosis, possibly in concert with renal dysfunction, results in an increased anion gap [2]. Chest radiographs show infiltrates indicative of acute lung injury.

Through mediator-induced tachycardia, cardiac output may increase early in sepsis; however, this is countered by profound peripheral vasodilation and possibly by a leaky capillary–induced hypovolemia. The result is hypotension that is usually treatable with volume replacement. However, as the disease progresses, myocardial contractility and cardiac output may decrease, which further exacerbates the hypotension. In very advanced sepsis, an α-adrenergic–mediated increase in peripheral resistance may occur. However, it may have little effect on the hypotension because of the progressive decrease in cardiac output. Additional signs of advanced sepsis include symptoms of organ dysfunctions, which may result at least in part from the previously mentioned cardiovascular events. These dysfunctions are important because as the number of involved organs increases, the patient's prognosis becomes increasingly grave (Table 4).

History, Physical Examination, and Laboratory Work

In making the diagnosis of sepsis, the patient's history can be very useful. The physician must determine whether the patient is immunocompromised, where the patient acquired the infection, and whether the patient has underlying diseases that may provide clues about an infective agent. It should be determined whether the patient is taking any medications or if any central nervous system effects such as confusion or

TABLE 3 EARLY CLINICAL SIGNS OF SEPSIS
Tachypnea
Tachycardia
Positive culture results
Observed site of infection
Hyperthermia
Hypothermia—particularly in patients who are
Elderly
Immunocompromised
Alcoholic
Suffering from hepatic or renal failure
Receiving immunosuppressive therapy

TABLE 4 ORGANS AFFECTED BY SEPSIS AND MULTIPLE ORGAN DYSFUNCTION SYNDROME	
Organ	**Symptoms**
Lung	Tachypnea [13]
	Respiratory alkalosis [13]
	Hypercapnia
	Hypoxia
	Adult respiratory distress syndrome [2]
Kidney	Oliguria
	Azotemia
	Proteinuria
Liver	Hyperbilirubinemia
	Increased serum transaminase levels
Central nervous system	Mental confusion
	Coma
Heart	Hypotensive increase in output initially
	Hypocalcemic or hypoxic-caused decrease in cardiac function

seizures have been experienced. Any other clues about the source of infection should be explored, including recent travel and occupational risks.

The physical examination is an important aspect of the patient work-up. Here, signs of infection may allow the physician to quickly administer antibiotics empirically in the hope that they will be specific for the microbe. All body openings should be examined thoroughly, along with the heart, lungs, abdomen, and skin. The patient's mental status should be determined.

Although laboratory work to identify the pathogen may take some time, other work can be done quickly and is useful in the patient's treatment (Table 5). Chest radiography and electrocardiography should be performed. Samples from any infected sites, along with the blood, urine, and sputum samples, should be carefully cultured. Because of the likelihood of contamination, at least two separate cultures should be performed [3].

Risk Factors

One of the risk factors for sepsis frequently seen in the hospital setting is recent surgery. Surgical patients recovering in the intensive care unit may be suspected of developing the condition. Table 6 lists a number of other risk factors for sepsis and its sequelae.

TREATMENT

Despite the knowledge that has accumulated since sepsis and its sequelae were first described, the goals of treatment have changed little to date. The essentials of treatment consist of antimicrobial therapy and supportive care; however, despite major advances in both of these fields, the mortality rate has changed little in the past two decades. To achieve the best outcome in sepsis, it is important to institute antibiotic therapy at the earliest possible moment during its course. If infection by pathogens can be arrested before systemic inflammatory mediators are released, sepsis and its sequelae should be allayed. One study indicated that the timely application of appropriate antibiotic therapy may decrease mortality and shock by 50% [4]. The localization and drainage or removal of an infected site can greatly improve a patient's outlook.

It is important for patients in the intensive care unit who are at risk for developing sepsis to be monitored; accurate monitoring can decrease the time delay before treatment. Despite their association with infection, it is appropriate to use invasive devices such as arterial catheters; they allow an accurate and rapid assessment of important parameters such as the blood gas level, hemodynamic changes, and acid-base changes. The pulmonary artery catheter can be used to assess changes in volume and should be used as a guide in fluid resuscitation.

Antibiotic Therapy

For numerous reasons, it is generally recommended that two forms of antibiotics be used concurrently in patients believed to have sepsis. One reason is that complete culture results may take 2 or 3 days—much too long to wait when sepsis is suspected—and the physician rarely knows which organism to target. Additionally, the use of two different agents may provide a synergistic effect, achieving better bactericidal action than either agent used alone. The possibility that a patient may be infected with more than one type of pathogen is also addressed with this method. When the source of infection is known, a variety of different drugs may be indicated, depending on the specific organism. Table 7 summarizes appropriate treatments for a number of specific infective conditions in sepsis. The probability of a favorable outcome increases appreciably when the organism is identified and specific antibiotics can be used [4].

Patients rendered neutropenic by disease or treatment (eg, chemotherapy) may benefit from the concurrent use of an antipseudomonal penicillin. Additionally, a third-generation cephalosporin may be used because these agents have strong antipseudomonal action. When a nonpseudomonal, aerobic pathogen is present, a combination of an aminoglycoside and

TABLE 5 LABORATORY WORK TO DETECT SEPSIS
Complete differential blood count
Coagulation assessment
Prothrombin time
Activated partial thromboplastin time
Fibrin assessment
Platelet count
Glucose level
Blood urea nitrogen level
Creatinine level
Lactic acid level
Blood gas levels
Bilirubin level
Serum transaminase level
Electrolyte levels

TABLE 6 CONDITIONS ASSOCIATED WITH SEPSIS	
Age	Surgery
Allergic response	Abdominal
Burns	Cardiac
Catastrophic illness	Trauma
Diabetes mellitus [14]	Aspiration
Drug overdose	Chest injury
Fat embolism	Hemorrhagic shock
Heatstroke	Massive transfusions
Hematologic malignancy	Multiorgan injury
Ischemia	
Infections	
Bacterial	
Disseminated fungal disease	
Disseminated viral disease	
Pancreatitis	

TABLE 7 ANTIBIOTIC THERAPY FOR INFECTIVE CONDITIONS IN SEPSIS

Infection	Organisms	Antibiotics
Community-acquired		
Urinary	Enterobacteriaceae	Ceftriaxone[†]
	Enterococccus spp	Ampicillin + gentamicin
Pulmonary	*Streptococcus pneumoniae*	Penicillin G
	Klebsiella spp, *Haemophilus influenzae*	Ceftriaxone[†]
	Staphylococcus aureus	Naficillin[‡]
Abdominal	Enterobacteriaceae, anaerobes, *Enterococcus* spp	Ampicillin + gentamicin[§] + clindamycin or metronidazole; ampicillin-sulbactam; ticarcillin-clavulanate; imipenem
Meningitis (adult)	*Streptococcus pneumoniae,* *Neisseria meningitidis*	Ceftriaxone[†]
Endocarditis (native valve)		
Non–intravenous drug abuser		
Subacute	*Streptococcus viridans, Streptococcus bovis, Enterococcus* spp	Penicillin G or ampicillin + gentamicin
Acute	*Staphylococcus aureus, Enterococcus* spp, *Streptococcus pneumoniae*	Nafcillin[‡] + gentamicin
Intravenous drug abuser	*Staphylococcus aureus,* Enterobacteriaceae	Nafcillin[‡] + gentamicin
Hospital-acquired		
Intravascular catheter sepsis	*Staphylococcus epidermidis, Staphylococcus aureus*	Vancomycin
Unspecified site	Enterobacteriaceae	Ceftriaxone[†] + gentamicin[§]; ticarcillin-clavulanate; ampicillin-sulbactam; imipenem
Neutropenic patient	Enterobacteriaceae, *Pseudomonas* spp	Piperacillin or ticarcillin + tobramycin[§]

Adapted from Rakel [17]; with permission.
[†]Or an equivalent.
[‡]Vancomycin should be used for penicillin-allergic patients or for methicillin-resistant staphylococci.
[§]Peak aminoglycoside levels should be at least 6–8 µg/mL.

cefazolin is appropriate, whereas ceftriaxone should be used instead of cefazolin if the infection is nosocomial in nature. In cases of pelvic and intraperitoneal infection, and in any other situation in which anaerobes are likely to be involved, the recommended therapy includes the use of an aminoglycoside coupled with a strong agent against anaerobes.

All sites of infection should be surgically débrided. This step is of critical importance because it greatly reduces the quantity of inflammation-inciting, bacterially produced mediators. Internal sites should be drained via catheters placed with the aid of imaging modalities such as computed tomography or ultrasonography. Other possible sources of infection, such as catheters, cannulas, or endotracheal tubes, should be replaced. Such devices can also be cultured to identify pathogens.

Supportive Treatment
Volume resuscitation

To combat the shock and hypotension characteristic of sepsis, volume replacement with intravenous fluids is recommended as a first endeavor. If the patient is not in the intensive care unit, fluids must be replaced empirically. In such a situation, extreme caution must be exercised. Capillary leakage into the lung may be exacerbated, seriously impairing pulmonary function. With accurate monitoring via the pulmonary capillary wedge pressure reading, leakage can be precisely controlled and large quantities of fluid may be used appropriately. If hypotension persists in the face of a pulmonary capillary wedge pressure that increases to 15 to 18 mm Hg, inotropic agents should be used.

Mechanical ventilation

If sepsis advances to the point at which organ dysfunctions become apparent, treatment should include measures to counter these effects. Because the lungs are often the first organ to be adversely affected by the inflammatory process, supportive therapy often includes the use of assisted ventilation. Such support should generally be instituted when the PaO_2 decreases below 50 to 60 mm Hg despite the use of supplemental oxygen. This sign also signals that the patient is developing ARDS, a sequela of sepsis and a condition that significantly decreases the chance of a favorable outcome.

Modern ventilators allow the clinician to control the flow of respiratory gases delicately. The technique of positive end-expiratory pressure should be used, and if possible, the pressure should be kept below 12 to 15 cm H_2O. Alternatively, the technique of constant positive airway pressure may be used. These techniques help to prevent—and may even reverse—the tendency toward alveolar collapse; the matching of ventilation and perfusion should be improved as well.

Figure 2 diagrams the effect of the positive end-expiratory pressure technique in the collapsed alveolus. The currently recommended treatment for ventilatory support in ARDS is summarized in Table 8. A less invasive improvement on the technique of intubation—use of the face mask to deliver constant positive airway pressure—can be used in many cases, although the possibilities of gastric insufflation and vomiting present dangers and should be watched for.

Because excess lung water leading to ventilation-perfusion mismatching is an important cause of hypoxemia in sepsis-associated ARDS, patients on the ventilator may still show gas exchange deficits. An exciting new treatment currently undergoing clinical trials is the use of inhaled nitric oxide. The recent discovery that this substance is produced in various cells and acts as a powerful vasodilator may lead to its use in ARDS patients [5]. When inhaled, it is distributed to ventilated alveoli, where it causes localized vasodilation. The net result is a significant improvement in ventilation-perfusion matching and better gas exchange [6••].

Supportive treatment may be possible for other organs that become dysfunctional. For example, in cases of renal dysfunction, which may develop at any time in sepsis, dialysis may be beneficial. Frequently, however, symptoms of dysfunction of more than one organ may not occur until the patient has advanced sepsis and may be near death.

Innovative Therapies

Several innovative therapies have been examined in clinical trials. As an anti-inflammatory measure, corticosteroids have been used in an attempt to arrest the inflammatory process because they appeared to be effective in animal models of sepsis [7]. However, clinical trials of these drugs have not provided consistently favorable results thus far [8,9], although they will be useful in patients whose adrenal function is known to be inadequate. Other attempts to block the better-known mediators of the inflammatory response have generally been unfavorable;

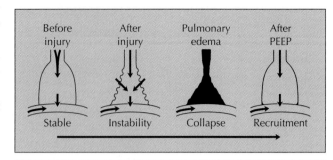

FIGURE 2 The effects of sepsis on the lung and correction with the positive end-expiratory pressure (PEEP) technique. (*From* Bone [16]; with permission.)

they include attempts to block the effects of histamine, endorphins, and coagulation [10–12].

In another direction, researchers have developed monoclonal antibodies to a variety of mediators involved in sepsis. For example, endotoxin, a cell surface molecule found on gram-negative bacteria, is believed to precipitate the inflammatory response in gram-negative sepsis [14•]. It has been the target of therapeutically administered monoclonal antibodies, although with inconsistent results [15••]. Efforts have also been underway to engineer receptor blockers that could alleviate the effects of various key endogenous septic mediators. These blockers include a soluble receptor for tumor necrosis factor-α, which binds to the mediator in circulation and blocks its activity, and a receptor antagonist for interleukin-1.

As understanding of the processes and mediators that cause sepsis improves, new therapeutic methods should become available. These methods will probably involve the blockage or inactivation of a variety of septic mediators or their cellular receptors. In many cases, specifically developed monoclonal antibodies may be used to achieve this goal. Figure 3 shows therapies that may someday be used in the clinical situation, along with a number of conventional treatments.

TABLE 8 A PRESSURE-TARGETED STRATEGY FOR VENTILATORY MANAGEMENT OF ADULT RESPIRATORY DISTRESS SYNDROME

Control alveolar pressure, not $PaCO_2$

Avoid large V_1 and use lowest PA possible to meet unequivocal therapeutic goals

Hold transalveolar pressure < 15 cm H_2O

Minimize oxygen demands

Use permissive hypercapnia as needed to prevent alveolar overdistention

Maintain end-expiratory PA (PEEP + AP) > 7 cm H_2O but < 15 cm H_2O

Make any necessary changes in mean Paw by changing T_1/T_{tot}, not by increasing PEEP

Consider specialized adjunctive measures to improve gas exchange and O_2 delivery*

Adapted from Marini [18]; with permission.

*In addition to standard measures such as skillful management of pulmonary vascular pressure, repositioning, use of cardiotonic agents, and minimizing O_2 demand, specialized adjunctive measures might include experimental methods such as intravenous or intratracheal catheter-assisted gas exchange or extracorporeal CO_2 removal if they are available.

AP—auto PEEP; PA—alveolar pressure; $PaCO_2$—partial pressure of carbon dioxide, arterial; Paw—airway pressure; PEEP—positive end-expiratory pressure; T_1/T_{tot}—inspiratory time fraction (duty cycle); V_1—tidal volume.

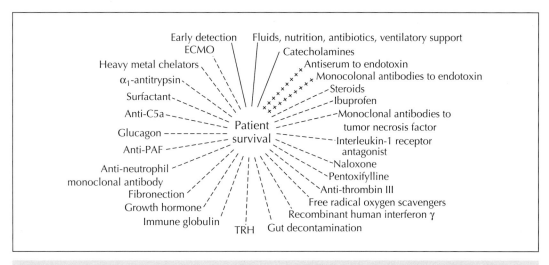

FIGURE 3 Various treatment modes for sepsis, including conventional treatments (*solid line*), those currently being developed and studied (*dotted line*), and those of questionable benefit following clinical trials (*plus signs*). ECMO—extracorporeal membrane oxygenation; PAF—platelet-activating factor; TRH—thyrotropin-releasing hormone.

REFERENCES AND RECOMMENDED READING

Recently published papers of particular interest have been highlighted as:

• Of interest

•• Of outstanding interest

1. Young LS: Gram-negative sepsis. In *Principles and Practice of Infectious Diseases*, edn 3. Edited by Mandell GL, Douglas RG Jr, Bennett JE. New York: Churchill Livingstone; 1990:611–636.

2. Lee RM, Balk RA, Bone RC: Ventilatory support in the management of septic patients. *Crit Care Med* 1989, 5:157–175.

3. Sheagren JN: Mechanism-oriented therapy for multiple system organ failure. *Crit Care Clin* 1989, 5:393–409.

4. Kreger BE, Craven DE, McCabe WR: Gram-negative bacteremia IV: re-evaluation of clinical features and treatment in 612 patients. *Am J Med* 1980, 68:344–355.

5. Palmer RMJ, Ashton DS, Mondcada S: Vascular endothelial cells synthesize nitric oxide from L-arginine. *Nature* 1988, 333:664–666.

6.•• Rossaint R, Falke KJ, Lopez F, *et al.*: Inhaled nitric oxide in the adult respiratory distress syndrome. *N Engl J Med* 1993, 328:399–405.

7. Sheagren JN: Corticosteroids for the treatment of septic shock. *Infect Dis Clin North Am* 1991, 5:875–882.

8. Bone RC, Fischer CJ, Clemmer TP, *et al.*: A controlled clinical trial of high-dose methylprednisolone in the treatment of severe sepsis and septic shock. *N Engl J Med* 1989, 317:653–658.

9. The Veterans Administration Systemic Sepsis Cooperative Study Group: Effect of high-dose glucocorticoid therapy on mortality in patients with clinical signs of systemic sepsis. *N Engl J Med* 1987, 317:659–665.

10. Jacobs R, Kaliner M, Shelhamer JH, *et al.*: Blood histamine concentrations are not elevated in humans with septic shock. *Crit Care Med* 1989, 17:30–35.

11. Demaria A, Hefferman JJ, Grindlinger GA, *et al.*: Naloxone versus placebo in treatment of septic shock. *Lancet* 1985, i:1363–1365.

12. Corrigan JJ, Kiernat JF: Effect of heparin in experimental gram-negative septicemia. *J Infect Dis* 1975, 131:138–143.

13. Harris RL, Musher DM, Bloom K, *et al.*: Manifestations of sepsis. *Arch Intern Med* 1987, 147:1895–1906.

14.• Bone RC: The pathogenesis of sepsis. *Ann Intern Med* 1991, 115:457–469.

15.•• Bone RC, Balk RA, Cerra FB, *et al.*: Definitions for sepsis and organ failure and guidelines for the use of innovative therapies in sepsis. *Chest* 1992, 101:1644–1655.

16. Bone RC: Treatment of severe hypoxemia due to the adult respiratory distress syndrome. *Arch Intern Med* 1980, 140:85–89.

17. Rakel RE, ed: *Conn's Current Therapy 1993*. Philadelphia: WB Saunders; 1993:65.

18. Marini JJ: Mechanical ventilation and newer ventilatory techniques. In *Textbook of Pulmonary and Critical Care Medicine*, vol 3. Edited by Bone RC, Dantzker DR, George RB, *et al.* St. Louis: CV Mosby; 1993:1–26.

SELECT BIBLIOGRAPHY

Bone RC: How gram-positive organisms cause sepsis. *J Crit Care* 1993, 8:51–59.

Bone RC: The systemic inflammatory response syndrome: does the new name mean new therapies? *Clinical Immunotherapeutics* 1994, 1:369–377.

Ruokonen E, Takala J, Kari A, *et al.*: Septic shock and multiple organ failure. *Crit Care Med* 1991, 19:1146–1151.

Sheagren JN: Mechanism-oriented therapy for multiple systems organ failure. *Crit Care Clin* 1989, 5:393–409.

Immunization of Adults 2

Marie R. Griffin
William Schaffner

> ### Key Points
> - An immunization history should be obtained routinely from all adult patients.
> - Make sure every patient has received a primary series of tetanus-diphtheria toxoid vaccine.
> - Hepatitis B vaccine is recommended for all adolescents and young adults.
> - Influenza and pneumococcal vaccines are recommended for all adults 65 years and older as well as younger persons with underlying pulmonary, cardiac, or metabolic disease.

Approximately 50,000 to 70,000 adults die each year in the United States from vaccine-preventable diseases, predominantly pneumococcal infection, influenza, and hepatitis B (Table 1). Although the efficacy of pneumococcal and influenza vaccines is only moderate, the impact of these vaccines could be great if they were used as recommended because of the high prevalence and substantial mortality associated with these diseases. Hepatitis B vaccine, in contrast, is highly efficacious. Routine use of this vaccine in children and young adults has the potential for drastically reducing the incidence and associated complications of this disease.

Unfortunately, physicians caring for adult patients generally have a poor record of immunization practices. There are numerous reasons for this, including skepticism about the efficacy and safety of vaccines, insufficient reimbursement, and uncertainty of the national standards of appropriate immunization practice. Increasingly, however, adult patients are interested in health promotion and disease prevention and expect their physicians to be skilled in these areas. Vaccines have been described as the most cost-effective preventive measure known, thus they are likely to play an increasing role in the routine care of adult patients in the future.

A history of immunizations should be obtained at the time of each new patient visit and reviewed periodically. This process should become as routine for physicians who treat adults as it is for pediatricians. Five vaccines used for routine immunizations of adults are listed in Table 2 and discussed in this chapter. Special considerations for immunizations must be given to HIV-infected persons, other immunocompromised individuals, health care workers, residents, the staff of other institutions (nursing homes, day care centers, postsecondary educational institutions), pregnant women, animal handlers, and international travelers. User-friendly guidelines for the immunization of adults including all the currently licensed vaccines are available [2•,3].

SPECIFIC VACCINES FOR ROUTINE IMMUNIZATION

Pneumococcal Vaccine

It has been estimated that about half of the estimated annual 40,000 deaths from invasive pneumococcal disease in the US adult population could be prevented by

TABLE 1 ESTIMATED ANNUAL DEATHS FROM VACCINE-PREVENTABLE DISEASE IN ADULTS IN THE UNITED STATES*

Diseases	Estimated annual deaths	Estimated deaths preventable by vaccine
Pneumococcal diseases	40,000	20,000
Influenza	10,000–30,000	5000–10,000
Hepatitis B	5000	4000
Measles, mumps, rubella	< 30	< 30
Tetanus/diphtheria	< 25	< 15

From Gardner and Schaffner [1]; with permission.
*The figures for estimated annual deaths in adults are from Williams *et al.* [13], the Centers for Disease Control and Prevention [3], and the American College of Physicians Task Force on Adult Immunization [2].

TABLE 2 ROUTINE IMMUNIZATION OF ADULTS

Vaccine	Recommendations
Pneumococcal	All adults at age 65 (or older)
	High-risk patients get first dose at any age
	Boosters every 6 years only for those with asplenia, nephrotic syndrome, or renal failure
Influenza	All adults yearly starting at age 65
	High-risk patients start at any age
	Offer vaccine to other healthy, younger adults
Hepatitis B	All young adults
	Special attention to high risk groups
Measles-mumps-rubella (MMR)	Adults born since 1956 who have no documentation of immunization or proof of immunity
	Special risk groups should get two doses
Tetanus-diphtheria (Td)	All adults every 10 years

TABLE 3 INDICATIONS FOR PNEUMOCOCCAL AND INFLUENZA VACCINES IN PERSONS UNDER AGE 65

Chronic cardiac disease
Chronic pulmonary disease
Anatomic or functional asplenia
Chronic liver disease
Alcoholism
Diabetes mellitus
Chronic renal failure
Hodgkin's disease
Chronic lymphatic leukemia
Multiple myeloma
Chemotherapy for malignancies
Organ transplantation
HIV infection

following current immunization recommendations. Both disease incidence and case fatality increase with age and with a variety of underlying medical conditions. The currently available 23-valent polysaccharide vaccine is inexpensive, safe, and moderately effective [4•]. Efficacy decreases from 93% in those under 55 years of age to 46% in those over 85 years, and is poor among immunocompromised patients [5]. Revaccination with a booster dose after 6 years is currently recommended only for those patients at highest risk for pneumococcal disease and for patients who are likely to have rapid declines in antibody levels: asplenic patients, patients with nephrotic syndrome or renal failure, and transplant recipients. Although the current vaccine is imperfect, it could have a considerable impact on prevention of serious pneumococcal disease if used as recommended.

The vaccine should be given as a single intramuscular or subcutaneous dose (0.5 mL) and may be given simultaneously with influenza vaccine, but at a different site. The vaccine is recommended for all adults over 65 years of age and for younger adults with high risk medical conditions (Table 3). Such "high risk" adults constitute over 30% of persons aged 50 to 64 (Fig. 1). Minor local side effects, such as pain or redness, may occur in 50% of persons, but more severe allergic or systemic reactions, such as fever or rash, occur in less than 1%. Local Arthus-type reactions have been reported infrequently following revaccination with the current vaccine.

Some authorities recently have advocated a substantially more aggressive use of pneumococcal vaccine. They suggest lowering the age of recommended pneumococcal immunization from age 65 to age 50, partly because of the high prevalence of high-risk conditions at this age, the histori-cally poor vaccine coverage in this group (only 8% of high-

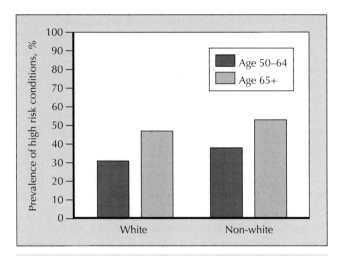

FIGURE 1 Self-reported prevalence of high-risk conditions among US adults 50 years of age and older by age group and race. (*Data from* American College of Physicians Task Force on Adult Immunization and Infectious Diseases Society of America [2•]; with permission.)

In addition, for those immunized at least 6 years earlier, a booster dose should be considered at age 65.

Influenza Vaccine

Influenza epidemics occur every few years in the United States and are associated with 10,000 to 40,000 deaths, 80% to 90% of which occur among those over 65 years, particularly those persons with underlying cardiac or pulmonary disease. Like pneumococcal vaccine, influenza vaccine efficacy decreases with advancing age, so that efficacy is only 30% to 40% in the elderly. The greatest benefit of the vaccine in older patients is in reducing the severity of disease and preventing hospital admission and death.

The vaccine should be given in a single intramuscular dose (0.5 mL) and may be given simultaneously with pneumococcal vaccine but at a different site. It is indicated yearly in all adults over 65 years, younger adults with high-risk conditions, and healthy younger adults at risk of transmitting infection to others, particularly health care workers or others with household or institutional contact with high-risk persons (Table 3). The vaccine should also be offered to other healthy adults who wish to reduce their risk of developing and transmitting influenza. Given these rather broad indications, it is evident that annual influenza immunization should be used much more widely than it is now.

The most frequent side effect of the vaccine is soreness at the injection site, which occurs in less than one third of patients. A mild "flu-like" illness beginning 6 to 12 hours after immunization and lasting 1 to 2 days occasionally occurs. More severe immediate hypersensitivity reactions are extremely rare. Since the association of Guillain-Barré syndrome with the 1976 "swine flu" vaccine, annual surveillance has revealed no convincing association with this neurologic disease. Vaccination is contraindicated in those with anaphylaxis to eggs.

risk persons 50 to 64 years of age report having received pneumococcal vaccine), and the increasing incidence of disease around age 50, especially in blacks (Fig. 2). The administration of the vaccine at age 50 would then occur at the same time as other screening and disease prevention activities for patients in their middle years; for example, sigmoidoscopy for men and women and mammography for women. Also, by immunizing at a younger age, enhanced antibody responses could be expected. Thus, some feel that by providing pneumococcal vaccine at age 50, this surge in disease occurrence could be prevented. Although these are not yet "official" recommendations, we believe it is likely that guidelines similar to these will be adopted in the future.

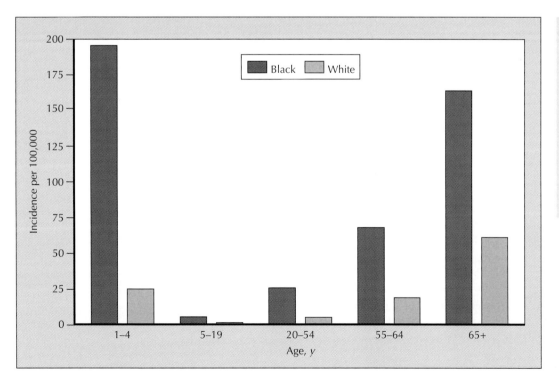

FIGURE 2 Incidence of pneumococcal bacteremia in blacks and whites 1 year of age and older, Monroe County, New York, 1985 through 1989. (*From* Bennett and coworkers [10]; with permission.)

Hepatitis B Vaccine

In the United States, there are approximately 300,000 new infections with hepatitis B virus (HBV) each year, of which 6% to 10% result in a chronic carrier state; about 25% of carriers develop chronic active hepatitis. Some of these persons eventually develop hepatocellular carcinoma. It is estimated that HBV causes about 5000 deaths per year in the United States from fulminant hepatitis, cirrhosis, and liver cancer. Recombinant hepatitis B vaccine, which is free of the theoretic concern of contamination with HIV or other viruses associated with the earlier plasma-derived vaccine, has been available for use in the United States since 1986. Hepatitis B vaccine is 85% to 95% effective in preventing infection in healthy young adults [6]. Antibody response to vaccine declines with advancing age and with the presence of renal failure, diabetes, chronic liver disease, HIV infection, smoking, and obesity. Of those patients who do not have an adequate response to the initial series, 25% respond after a single additional dose and 50% to 70% respond after a further full three-dose series.

Hepatitis B infection has long been recognized as a health risk associated with the practice of male homosexuality and the illicit use of injectable drugs. Increasingly, however, it has become apparent that these lifestyle characteristics cannot account for nearly half of all the recorded cases of hepatitis B. Although maternal-fetal transmission and occupational acquisition of infection by health care workers account for some cases, it now has been determined that up to 40% of infections are acquired heterosexually [7]. This realization has prompted a substantially increased interest in providing hepatitis B vaccine to virtually the entire young adult population.

Hepatitis B vaccine has now been incorporated into the routine infant immunization schedule, with the goal of interrupting transmission. However, because most infections occur in young adults, there is also a new emphasis on immunizing pre-adolescents, adolescents, college students, and other young adults. Indications for hepatitis B vaccine are given in Table 4. Serologic screening for evidence of immunity before vaccine administration is cost-effective only for members of very high risk groups (*eg*, homosexual men or persons from countries where hepatitis B infection is endemic).

Hepatitis B vaccination requires a three-dose series—the second and third doses are given 1 and 6 months following the first. For adults aged 20 and older, the dose of both available recombinant vaccines is 1.0 mL. For adolescents, the dose is 0.5 mL for Recombivax HB (Merck, Rahway, NJ) but 1.0 mL for Engerix-B (SmithKline, Philadelphia, PA). Immunosuppressed patients and those on renal dialysis require larger doses. Age, underlying medical conditions, sex, obesity, and smoking influence seroconversion rates (Table 5). Neither booster doses nor routine serologic testing to determine postimmunization antibody status is currently recommended for younger persons with normal immune function. Some experts recommend serologic testing of persons over 30 years and those at especially high risk of infection to assure immunity. Annual follow-up serologic testing is recommended for hemodialysis patients, with revaccination of those whose antibody level falls below 10 mU/mL.

The recombinant vaccines produce mild soreness at the injection site for 1 to 2 days in 15% to 20% of persons. Fewer persons experience mild constitutional symptoms. No severe reactions have been clearly attributed to these vaccines.

Measles-Mumps-Rubella Vaccine

Outbreaks of measles and mumps in high schools and colleges, the occurrence of small clusters of congenital rubella syndrome, and outbreaks of all these vaccine-preventable diseases among health care workers have focused attention on young adults as important in the trans-

---

TABLE 4 INDICATIONS FOR HEPATITIS B IMMUNIZATION

Population	Comments
All infants	Routine immunization
Adolescents, young adults	Routine immunization should be considered
	Those who are sexually active should be immunized
Occupational risk	All who have potential exposure to blood, including health care workers; morticians; police, fire, and corrections personnel
	Ideally, vaccine should be given early in training, before blood exposure
Lifestyle risk	Multiple sex partners (more than one in previous 6 months, heterosexual or homosexual)
	Homosexuality or bisexuality
	Any prior sexually acquired disease
	Injecting drug user
Special patient groups	Hemodialysis patients
	Hemophiliacs
Environmental risk	Household and sexual contacts of HBV carriers
	Clients and staff of institutions for developmentally disabled persons
	Prisoners and corrections personnel
	International travelers to HBV-endemic areas

HBV—hepatitis B virus.

TABLE 5 FACTORS INFLUENCING SEROCONVERSION AFTER THREE DOSES OF HEPATITIS B VACCINE	
Factor	**Seroconversion**
Age, y	
20–29	95%
30–39	90%
40–49	85%
50–59	71%
60+	47%
Underlying medical illness	
HIV infection	50%–75%
Diabetes	70%–80%
Renal failure	60%–70%
Chronic liver disease	60%–70%
Other factors	
Gender	Female > male
Obesity	Decreased
Smoking	Lower antibody titers in smokers

From American College of Physicians [2•]; with permission.

mission of these viruses. Many adults born after 1956 did not have natural infection with these viruses and were either not vaccinated or had primary vaccine failure (about 5% for each of the three viral antigens).

Measles-mumps-rubella (MMR) vaccine is recommended for adults born after 1956 unless there is evidence of immunity to both measles and mumps (*ie*, physician-diagnosed disease, documentation of immunization with live virus vaccine, or laboratory evidence of immunity). In addition, all women of childbearing potential should be vaccinated with MMR unless there is documentation of rubella vaccination after their first birthday or a positive serologic test for rubella antibody. Although the incidence of rubella has dropped dramatically in the United States, a recent increase in cases among young adults—accompanied by an increase in congenital rubella syndrome—emphasizes the importance of immunization of young adults (Fig. 3). Because of the theoretic risk to the developing fetus, MMR (a live, attenuated viral vaccine) should not be given to pregnant women or women who are considering becoming pregnant within 3 months of vaccination. Also, the vaccine should not be given to those who are immunocompromised as a result of malignancy or chemotherapy.

The routine childhood immunization series now includes two doses of MMR. Documentation of two doses of MMR for those born after 1956 is currently required by many post-secondary educational institutions. Immunity against these viruses is especially important for travelers to countries where these diseases are endemic, as well as for health care workers.

MMR vaccine, in a dose of 0.5 mL, is given subcutaneously; when two doses are required, they should be given at least 1 month apart. Adverse reactions occur only in susceptible vaccinees. Approximately 5% to 15% of recipi-

ents develop fever greater than 39.4°C (103°F), and 5% have a transient rash between 5 and 12 days after vaccination. Meningitis or encephalitis occurs rarely after immunization (resulting from the mumps component) and significantly less often than after natural infection. Up to 40% of adult vaccinees susceptible to rubella develop arthralgias; frank arthritis is much less frequent. Joint symptoms generally begin 3 to 25 days after immunization, persist 1 to 11 days, and rarely recur. Persistent joint symptoms have been reported in up to 5% of susceptible women vaccinated compared with 30% infected with the wild virus.

Tetanus-Diphtheria Toxoid Vaccine

Both tetanus and diphtheria are now rare in the United States and occur almost exclusively in adults who never completed a primary immunization series (Fig. 4). For adults, the current emphasis is on assuring primary immunization of older adults and pregnant women who never received their primary tetanus-diphtheria toxoid (Td) series and giving routine Td boosters every 10 years to all adults. Local reactions are common after Td injection (principally soreness at the inoculation site), but severe reactions are rare.

Because there are only rare reports of tetanus in persons who complete a primary series, the primary emphasis for the practicing internist should be to identify those persons who have never received tetanus vaccine. That task is easier stated than done, because most patients do not have a written record of their previous immunizations and their memories are vague. Prior military service provides secure assurance that a patient was immunized. If patients cannot give a confident history, it is prudent to give such persons a primary immunization series.

The current recommendation to give boosters every 10 years is presently under review by national advisory groups [8•]. An alternative schedule under consideration is to provide a primary series in childhood (virtually all children in the United States receive this now) with boosters only in adolescence or young adulthood (age 15 to 25) and again at age 50. This schedule would establish a mid-adult focus for a series of health maintenance activities.

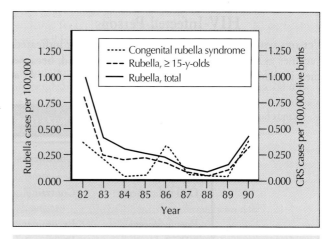

FIGURE 3 Incidence of rubella and congenital rubella syndrome (CRS) in the United States, 1982–1990. (*Data from* Centers for Disease Control [11]; with permission.)

TABLE 8 FUTURE VACCINES

Vaccine	Comments
Near licensure	
Varicella-zoster	Live, attenuated viral vaccine
	> 90% effective
	May reduce occurrence of herpes zoster (shingles)
	Target groups: susceptible health care workers, teachers
Hepatitis A	Killed viral vaccine
	> 98% effective
	Target groups: international travelers, day care staff, food handlers, military
Future	
Influenza	Live, cold-adapted vaccine can be given by nasal drops—no longer need injections
Pneumococcal	Protein-conjugated for enhanced efficacy
Diarrheal diseases	
Rotavirus	A common cause of gastroenteritis worldwide
	Vaccine must include several serotypes
Shigella	Causes institutional and community-wide epidemics
	Vaccine could prevent day-care center outbreaks
Enterotoxicogenic *Escherichia coli*	Another major cause of enteritis in the world
	Vaccine could prevent some cases of traveler's diarrhea

REFERENCES AND RECOMMENDED READING

Recently published papers of particular interest have been highlighted as:
• Of interest
•• Of outstanding interest

1.   Gardner P, Schaffner W: Immunization of adults. *N Engl J Med* 1993, 328:1252–1258.

2.• American College of Physicians Task Force on Adult Immunization and Infectious Diseases Society of America: *Guide for Adult Immunization*, edn 3. Philadelphia: American College of Physicians; 1994.

3.   Centers for Disease Control: Update on adult immunization. Recommendations of the immunization practices advisory committee (ACIP). *MMWR Morb Mortal Wkly Rep* 1991, 40:1–94.

4.• Musher DM, Watson DA, Dominguez EA: Pneumococcal vaccination: work to date and future prospects. *Am J Med Sci* 1990, 300:45–52.

5.   Shapiro ED, Berg AT, Austrian R, *et al.*: The protective efficacy of polyvalent pneumococcal polysaccharide vaccine. *N Engl J Med* 1991, 325:1453–1460.

6.   Hadler SC, Francis DP, Maynard JE, *et al.*: Long-term immunogenicity and efficacy of hepatitis B vaccine in homosexual men. *N Engl J Med* 1986, 315:209–214.

7.   Alter MJ, Hadler SC, Margolis HS, *et al.*: The changing epidemiology of hepatitis B in the United States. Need for alternative vaccination strategies. *JAMA* 1990, 262:1218–1222.

8.• LaForce FM: Routine tetanus immunization for adults: once is enough. *J Gen Intern Med* 1993, 8:459–460.

9.   Centers for Disease Control: *Health Information for International Travel*. Washington, DC: US Government Printing Office; 1993. [HHS publication No. (CDC) 93-8280.]

10. Bennett NM, Buffington J, LaForce FM: Pneumococcal bacteremia in Monroe County, New York. *Am J Public Health* 1992, 82:1513–1516.

11. Centers for Disease Control: Increase in rubella and congenital rubella syndrome—United States, 1988–1990. *MMWR Morb Mortal Wkly Rep* 1991, 41:93–99.

12. Prevots R, Sutter RW, Strebel PM, *et al.*: Tetanus surveillance—United States, 1989–1990. *MMWR Morb Mortal Wkly Rep* 1992, 41:1–9.

13. Williams WW, Hickson MA, Kane MA, *et al.*: Immunization policies and vaccine coverage among adults: the risk for missed opportunities. *Ann Intern Med* 1988, 108:616–625.

SELECT BIBLIOGRAPHY

Howson CP, Howe CJ, Fineberg HV: *Adverse Effects of Pertussis and Rubella Vaccines*. Washington, DC: National Academy Press; 1991.

Plotkin SA, Mortimer EA: *Vaccines*. Philadelphia: WB Saunders Company; 1988.

Root RK, Griffis JMc, Warren KS, *et al.*: *Immunizations*. New York: Churchill Livingstone; 1989.

Schaffner W, ed: Immunization in Adults I and II. *Infect Dis Clin North Am* 1990, 4:1–354.

Stratton KR, Howe CJ, Johnston RB Jr: *Adverse Effects Associated with Childhood Vaccines*. Washington, DC: National Academy Press; 1993.

Antibacterial Agents—General 3
Jay P. Sanford

> ### *Key Points*
> - Antibacteral therapy may be either empirical, based on clinical and laboratory findings, or definitive, based on cultures and sensitivities.
> - Selection of an empirical antibiotic should be based on following a logical sequence of probabilities.
> - Depending on the likely infection and the patient's condition, for many infections the best course may be to delay treatment until culture results are available.
> - Considerations of a specific antibiotic must include its spectrum of antibacterial activity, clinical pharmacology, potential adverse effects, and drug-drug interactions.
> - Failure of the patient to respond to an "appropriate" antibiotic poses a new series of considerations, which also should be based on logical sequence of studies and resultant findings.

The plethora of new antibacterial agents, with the concomitant recognition of previously nonpathogenic microorganisms as pathogens in the immunocompromised host and the emergence of antibacterial resistance to many agents of choice, has created new problems for the physician and patient, both in the empirical early selection and in the subsequent definitive selection of antibacterial agents.

Antibacterial therapy is either empirical (*ie*, based on clinical symptoms and signs, laboratory findings, and epidemiologic information) or definitive (*ie*, based on the results of bacteriologic cultures and antimicrobial susceptibilities). A decision to initiate empirical antibacterial treatment should follow a sequence of thoughts and actions. The usual symptom or sign that suggests infection is fever. The clinician performing the evaluation should determine whether the fever is likely to be of infectious cause, a result of drug fever, or a manifestation of neoplastic or collagen vascular disease [1•]. If it is probably of infectious origin, is the infection more likely to be bacterial or nonbacterial (*ie*, viral, fungal, or of other microbial etiology)? If it is likely to be bacterial in origin, what is the anatomic site? Given the site, what are the most likely causative organisms [2•]? Are there modifying circumstances that would predispose the patient to specific organisms (*eg*, fever in a patient 3 weeks after receiving a prosthetic aortic valve)? After the considerations have been narrowed to the most likely organisms, the physician must consider what antibacterial agents are most likely to be effective [3••]; to be nontoxic or least toxic; and if other considerations are equal, to be least expensive in terms of the agent and its administration. However, before proceeding with the empiric prescription of an antibiotic, the physician should consider whether review of previous records can identify culture results and susceptibilities that might be helpful; whether stained smears of body fluids, secretions, or aspirates can provide information that reduces the degree of empiricism [4]; and whether the patient is receiving other drugs that may interact with the antibiotic selected, or vice versa. For example, the patient who is receiving a nonsedating antihistamine such as terfenadine should not receive erythromycin [5•]. Appropriate cultures should be obtained before an antibacterial agent is started: cultures are likely to be of much less value if they are obtained 3 days later, when the patient may not be responding as anticipated. Other points to consider before empiric antibiotic treatment is started are whether the patient has a site of undrained pus that will need to be drained to facilitate response and whether imaging studies will be of value.

For many bacterial infections, it is better to delay the initiation of treatment until definitive therapy can be selected based on the results of blood, aspirate, or body fluid cultures. For example, empiric treatment should not be initiated in the nonimmunocompromised patient who has chronic osteomyelitis, asymptomatic bacteriuria, or suspected infective endocarditis without accompanying cardiac failure.

Once the clinician has gone through a rational thought process and reached the decision to initiate empiric antibacterial treatment, the next considerations are as follows:
- What drugs are available (classification)?
- Is the agent likely to be active against the suspected organism or organisms (spectrum of activity) [6••,7•,8••,9]?

- Will the agent arrive at the site of infection in active form (clinical pharmacology)?
- What are the potential adverse effects [10]?
- Will other drugs interfere with the agent's effectiveness or increase its toxicity, or vice versa (drug-drug interactions)[10]?

The following sections address these general considerations to facilitate individualization and optimal agent selection. Recommendations for specific infections are made in the chapters dealing with individual diseases.

CLASSIFICATION OF ANTIBACTERIAL AGENTS

Because antibacterial agents have been discovered, synthesized, and introduced like "Topsy," classification has been retrospective and inconsistent among groups of agents. For example, the penicillins are grouped by structure, whereas the cephalosporins are grouped by a composite of sequence of introduction, structure, and spectrum of antibacterial activity (Table 1).

TABLE 1 CLASSIFICATION OF ANTIBACTERIAL AGENTS

β-Lactam antibiotics	Aminoglycosides and spectinomycin	Lincosamides
Penicillins	Streptomycin	Lincomycin
Natural penicillins	Neomycin	Clindamycin
Aminopenicillins	Kanamycin	
Penicillinase-resistant	Gentamicin	**Quinolones**
penicillins	Amikacin	Nalidixic acid group
Carboxypenicillins	Tobramycin	Nalidixic acid
Ureidopenicillins	Netilmicin	Oxolinic acid
Cephalosporins	Spectinomycin	Cinoxacin
First generation		Carboxyfluoroquinolones
Second generation	**Tetracyclines**	Norfloxacin
Third generation	Tetracycline	Ciprofloxacin
Fourth generation	Minocycline	Ofloxacin
Other β-lactam antibiotics	Doxycycline	Pefloxacin
Carbapenems		Enoxacin
Imipenem	**Chloramphenicol**	Lomefloxacin
Monobactams		Rufloxacin
Aztreonam	**Macrolides**	
β-Lactamase inhibitors	14-Membered ring	**Polymyxins**
Clavulanate	Erythromycins	Polymyxin B
Sulbactam	Oleandomycin	Colistimethate (polymyxin E)
Tazobactam	Clarithromycin	
	Roxithromycin	**Rifamycins**
Glycopeptides	Dirithromycin	Rifampin
Vancomycin	15-Membered ring (azalide)	Rifabutin
Teicoplanin	Azithromycin	
	16-Membered ring	**Nitroimidazoles**
	Josamycin	Metronidazole
		Folic acid antagonists
		Sulfonamides
		Trimethoprim

β-Lactam Antibiotics

The β-lactam antibiotics include the penicillins, cephalosporins, carbapenems, and monobactams.

Penicillins

The penicillins are divided into classes primarily on the basis of their antibacterial activity. Penicillin G and penicillin V are the two natural penicillins; the other penicillins are partially synthesized.

Aminopenicillins have more activity than the natural penicillins against *Enterococcus faecalis* and many aerobic and anaerobic gram-negative bacilli, including *Haemophilus influenzae*, *Escherichia coli*, *Salmonella* and *Shigella* spp, and some strains of *Bacteroides fragilis*. *Pseudomonas* spp, *Klebsiella* spp, *Enterobacter* spp, and most strains of *B. fragilis* are resistant. The aminopenicillins are susceptible to inactivation by multiple β-lactamases. The frequency of resistant strains, even among community-acquired bacterial strains, is becoming an increasingly important problem that can no longer be ignored in the selection of antibacterial agents.

The penicillinase-resistant penicillins can be considered primarily as the antistaphylococcal penicillins. This class of penicillins inhibits staphylococci (both *Staphylococcus aureus* and *Staphylococcus epidermidis*), *Streptococcus pyogenes*, and *Streptococcus pneumoniae*. None of the penicillinase-resistant penicillins is active against *Enterococcus faecalis* or aerobic or anaerobic gram-negative bacilli. Unfortunately, strains of staphylococci that have emerged with altered penicillin-binding proteins (methicillin-resistant *S. aureus* and methicillin-resistant *S. epidermidis*) are resistant to all penicillins and cephalosporins.

The carboxypenicillins and ureidopenicillins can be grouped as the antipseudomonal penicillins. Both the carboxypenicillins and the ureidopenicillins are susceptible to β-lactamases, but they are more resistant to the β-lactamases from *Pseudomonas*, *Enterobacter*, and *Morganella* spp than are the natural penicillins and the aminopenicillins. The carboxypenicillins are less active than ampicillin against *S. pyogenes*, *S. pneumoniae*, and *E. faecalis*. The ureidopenicillins are derivatives of ampicillin, an aminopenicillin, and hence have better activity against streptococci and enterococci than do the carboxypenicillins.

Cephalosporins

The cephalosporins have been classified as first-, second-, third-, and most recently, fourth-generation agents. The members of each group and the salient features of their antibacterial activity are summarized in Table 2 [11••].

TABLE 2 FEATURES OF FIRST, SECOND, THIRD, AND FOURTH GENERATION CEPHALOSPORINS		
Generation	**Drugs**	**Antibacterial activity**
First	Cephalothin, cefazolin, cephapirin, cephradine, cephalexin, cefadroxil	Most active against gram-positive cocci (but enterococci resistant)
		Limited activity against aerobic gram-negative bacilli: *Escherichia coli*, *Klebsiella pneumoniae*, *Proteus mirabilis*
Second		
Cefuroxime subgroup	Cefuroxime, cefamandole, cefonicid, ceforanide, cefaclor, cefuroxime axetil, cefprozil, loracarbef (a carbacephem not a cephalosporin)	About equal to first-generation agents against gram-positive cocci
		More active against *E. coli*, *K. pneumoniae*, *P. mirabilis*
		Active against *Haemophilus influenzae*, *Neisseria* spp, some *Enterobacter* spp, *Serratia* spp, anaerobes
		Not active against *Pseudomonas* spp
Cephamycin subgroup	Cefoxitin, cefotetan, cefmetazole	Less active than first-generation agents against gram-positive cocci
		Active against *E. coli*, *K. pneumoniae*, *P. mirabilis*
		Not active against *Enterobacter*, *Serratia*, and *Pseudomonas* spp
		Most active against *Bacteroides* spp
Third		
Modest antipseudomonal activity (cefotaxime subgroup)	Cefotaxime, ceftizoxime, ceftriaxone, moxalactam, cefixime, cefpodoxime proxetil	Less active than first-generation agents against gram-positive cocci
		Most active against *E. coli*, *K. pneumoniae*, *Proteus* spp
		Inconsistent against *Enterobacter*, *Serratia*, *Acinetobacter*, and *Pseudomonas* spp
		Modest activity against anaerobes
Enhanced antipseudomonal activity	Ceftazidime, cefoperazone	Least active against gram-positive cocci
		Similar to agents in the cefotaxime subgroup against aerobic gram-negative bacilli
		Most active against *Pseudomonas aeruginosa*
Fourth	Cefepime, cefpirome	Activity against gram-positive cocci is about equal to that of first-generation agents
		Limited activity against enterococci
		More active than agents in the cefotaxime subgroup against *Enterobacter* and *Serratia* spp
		Equal to ceftazidime against *Pseudomonas aeruginosa*

Adapted from Sader and Jones [11••]; with permission.

β-Lactamase Inhibitors

The β-lactamase inhibitors are compounds that are structurally related to the β-lactam antibiotics [12•]. They have minimal inherent antibacterial activity but have been developed to have an affinity for binding the destructive β-lactamase enzymes in the bacterial periplasmic space that is higher than the affinity of the β-lactam antibiotics. The β-lactamase inhibitors in clinical use have pharmacokinetics that are similar to those of penicillins or cephalosporins, enabling them to be combined with and to protect a β-lactamase–susceptible penicillin (ampicillin, amoxicillin, piperacillin, or ticarcillin) or cephalosporin. Because multiple β-lactamase enzymes exist and more are being recognized, there are some that are not inhibited by current β-lactamase inhibitors. If the mechanism of antimicrobial resistance is not the production of β-lactamases but an alteration in membrane penetration or a decrease in binding to the penicillin-binding protein, combination with a β-lactamase inhibitor will not increase the activity of the antibiotic.

Choice of Agent

A broad overview of the antibacterial activity of the common classes of antibacterial agents provides an initial guideline to the question of whether the agent selected is likely to be effective against the probable causative organism or organisms (Table 3). However, it is essential to appreciate that regional, interhospital, and even intrahospital differences occur in the frequency of susceptible and resistant strains of specific organisms such as *H. influenzae*, *S. aureus*, and *Klebsiella pneumoniae* [7•]. The clinician must keep these differences in mind in selecting an empiric antibiotic. These differences also underlie the critical importance of obtaining culture results and determining sensitivities of individual specific isolates.

CLINICAL PHARMACOLOGY

Once an antibiotic has been selected that is likely to have antibacterial activity against the causative organism or organisms, it is essential to decide by which route it should be given and how often it should be given. It is also important to know whether the agent is likely to reach the site of infection and what the influence of host factors will be on the clinical pharmacology.

Choice of Route

The choice of the route of administration usually lies between oral and intravenous. The oral administration of antibacterial agents, except for that of antimycobacterial agents, has generally been reserved for infections that are mild and are treated on an outpatient basis. With the increasing emphasis on hospital cost containment, changes are occurring: intravenous drugs are increasingly being administered in the home or in the outpatient setting, and regimens are being developed in which drugs are initially given intravenously and then alternative agents are given orally to complete a course of treatment [13•]. When drugs are to be administered orally, it is important to know whether absorption is decreased by food or by other drugs such as antacids (Table 4) [10]. For drugs that are

not absorbed from the gastrointestinal tract or in seriously ill patients in the United States, the intravenous route is preferred because immediate high serum concentrations can be ensured.

However, serum concentrations adequate to treat many infections are achieved after intramuscular administration. Intramuscular regimens were more common in the United States in the past and remain commonly used in Europe. From the standpoint of cost, it is important not to get caught in the cycle of initially giving the antibiotic intravenously because the patient needs to be rehydrated and intravenous access is in place, and then, after the patient has been rehydrated, maintaining the intravenous line with its attendant risks just to give the antibiotic.

Reaching the Site of Infection

The amount of drug that reaches the extravascular tissues in which the infection is present depends on the protein binding in plasma, the concentration gradient from plasma to tissues, and the diffusibility of the agent. In most infections, if the local inhibitory concentration of the antibacterial agent exceeds the minimal inhibitory concentration for the infecting microorganism, cure results, but only in areas of the body in which adequate host defenses such as polymorphonuclear leukocytes, complement, and antibody are present. In areas in which these factors are inadequate or absent—such as in the spinal fluid, in vegetations on heart valves, or in abscess cavities—concentrations of at least four times the minimal inhibitory concentration or even the minimal bactericidal concentration are required for cure.

Large abscesses usually require drainage to be cured. The diffusion of an antibiotic across the semipermeable abscess wall is often limited. Local factors within the abscess cavity may further diminish antibacterial activity. In mixed infections, the β-lactamases from anaerobic organisms may destroy a β-lactamase antibiotic being used to treat infection with aerobic gram-negative bacilli. Abscess cavities have a pH of less than 7.0, are anaerobic, and are filled with the nucleoproteins from disintegrating leukocytes. Aminoglycosides are inactive in an anaerobic environment, are less active at a pH of less than 7.4, and are complexed to nucleoproteins. As a result, aminoglycosides have little if any activity against organisms in undrained abscesses. In this clinical setting, their usefulness is limited to preventing the spread of infection.

With the introduction of the newer macrolide antibiotics azithromycin and clarithromycin, the relationship between antibacterial effectiveness and serum concentrations has become obfuscated. These agents diffuse rapidly from the intravascular compartment into the extravascular tissue spaces, including intracellularly into neutrophilic leukocytes, monocytes, and pulmonary alveolar macrophages. The clinician is no longer even roughly able to correlate serum concentrations with clinical effectiveness.

Frequency of Administration

The frequency of administration of antibacterial agents is also undergoing reevaluation and revision [14••]. With the natural penicillins, which have serum half-lives of approximately 30

TABLE 3 ANTIBACTERIAL AGENTS: SPECTRA OF *IN VITRO* ACTIVITY

Drugs	Streptococci	Enterococci	Staphylococci	Haemophilus influenzae, Moraxella catarrhalis	Escherichia coli, Proteus mirabilis	Klebsiella, Enterobacter, and Serratia spp	Pseudomonas spp	Bacteroides spp
β-Lactams								
Penicillins								
Natural penicillins	+*	±	0	0	0	0	0	0
Aminopenicillins	+*†	+	0	±†	+†	0	0	±
Penicillinase-resistant	+	0	+	0	0	0	0	0
Carboxypenicillins	±	0	0	+	+	±	+	+
Ureidopenicillins	+†	+	0	+	+	+	+	+
Cephalosporins								
First generation	+‡	0	+	+	+	0	0	0
Second generation								
Cefuroxime	+	0	+	+	+	+	0	+§
Cefoxitin	+	0	+	+	+	±	0	+
Third generation								
Cefotaxime	+	0	+	+	+	+	±	+
Antipseudomonal	+	0	+	+	+	+	+	0
Fourth generation								
Cefepime	+‡	±	+	+	+	+	+	0
Imipenem	+	+	+	+	+	+	+	+
Aztreonam	0	0	0	+	+	+	+	0
With β-lactamase inhibitors								
AM/CL	+	+	+	+	+	±	0	+
TC/CL	+	0	+	+	+	+	+	+
AM/SB	+	+	+	+	+	+	+	0
P/T	+	+	+	+	+	+	+	+
Vancomycin	+	+	+	0	0	0	0	0
Aminoglycosides	0	0	+	+	+	+	+	0
Tetracyclines	+¶	0	0	+	±	0	0	±
Chloramphenicol	+	0	0	+	+	0	0	+
Macrolides								
Erythromycins	+¶	0	+	±	0	0	0	0
Azithromycin	+**	0	+	+	0	0	0	0
Clarithromycin	+**	0	+	+	0	0	0	0
Clindamycin	+	0	+	0	0	0	0	+
Fluoroquinolones	±	0	+	+	+	+	+	0
Polymyxins	0	0	0	+	+	±	+	0
Rifampin	+	±	+	+	0	0	0	0
Metronidazole	0	0	0	0	0	0	0	+
TMP/SMX	+	+	+	+†	+	±	0	0

*Streptococcus pneumoniae strains resistant to β-lactams are increasing in the United States (15%–30% in 1993). All are sensitive to vancomycin and rifampin.
†β-Lactamase–producing strains are increasing in the United States (*H. influenzae*, 25%–30%; *M. catarrhalis*, 90%).
‡First- and fourth-generation cephalosporins are most active against staphylococci.
§Cefuroxime subgroup of agents is not as active as the cephamycin subgroup against *B. fragilis*. (*see* Table 2).
¶*Streptococcus pyogenes* (group A and other groups) is often resistant to tetracyclines and macrolides, especially in Europe.
**Organisms that are resistant to erythromycin show cross-resistance to other macrolides.
AM/CL—amoxicillin clavulanate; TC/CL—ticarcillin clavulanate; AM/SB—ampicillin sulbactam; P/T—piperacillin tazobactam;
  TMP/SMX—trimethoprim-sulfamethoxazole; +—most isolates sensitive *in vitro*; ±—variable in sensitivities; 0—resistant, fewer than 10% sensitive.

TABLE 4 PHARMACOKINETIC PROPERTIES OF ANTIBACTERIAL AGENTS

Drug	Routes of administration	Oral		Serum half-life, *h*	Dose and route	Peak serum level, *μg/mL*
		With food	Absorption, %			
Penicillins						
Natural penicillins						
Penicillin G	IV, IM, PO	N	15	0.5	12 g qd IV	16
Penicillin V	PO	Y	35	1.0	500 mg PO	3–4
Benzathine penicillin G	IM			>168 (1 wk)	1.2 MU IM	0.07
Aminopenicillins						
Ampicillin	IV, IM, PO	N	40	1.0	500 mg PO	2.5–4.0
					2.0 g IV	109–150
Amoxicillin	PO	Y	60	1.0–1.3	250 mg PO	1.0–6.4
Bacampicillin	PO	Y	75	1.0	400 mg PO	6–8
Penicillinase-resistant penicillins						
Nafcillin	IV, IM			0.5	500 mg IV	11
Oxacillin	IV, IM, PO	N	30	0.5	500 mg IV	43
Cloxacillin	PO	N	35	0.5	500 mg PO	2–9
Dicloxacillin	PO	N	40	0.5	250 mg PO	9–18
Carboxypenicillins						
Ticarcillin	IV, IM			1.2	3.0 g IV	190
Ureidopenicillins						
Mezlocillin	IV, IM			1.1	3.0 g IV	263
Piperacillin	IV, IM			1.0	4.0 g IV	350
Imipenem	IV, IM			1.0	500 mg IV	40
Aztreonam	IV, IM			2.0	1.0 g IV	125
With β-lactamase inhibitors						
Amoxicillin clavulanate	PO	Y	60	1.3	250 mg PO	4
Ampicillin sulbactam	IV, IM			1.0	3.0 g IV	109–150
Piperacillin tazobactam	IV			1.0	3.375 g IV	240
Cephalosporins						
First generation						
Cephalothin	IV, IM			0.5	2.0 g IV "push"	80–100
Cefazolin	IV, IM			1.9	1.0 g IV	188
Cephapirin	IV, IM			0.6	1.0 g IV	70
Cephradine	IV, IM, PO	N	90	1.3	500 mg PO	16
Cephalexin	PO	Y	90	1.3	500 mg PO	18–38
Cefadroxil	PO	Y	90	1.5	500 mg PO	16
Second generation						
Cefaclor	PO	N	50	0.8	500 mg PO	13
Cefamandole	IV, IM			1.0	2.0 g IV	165
Cefoxitin	IV, IM			0.8	1.0 g IV	110
Cefuroxime	IV, IM			1.5	1.5 g IV	100
Cefuroxime axetil	PO	Y	52	1.2	250 mg PO	4.1
Cefonicid	IV, IM			4.0	1.0 g IV	220
Cefmetazole	IV			1.2	1.0 g IV	77
Cefotetan	IV, IM			4.2	1.0 g IV	124
Cefprozil	PO	Y	94	1.2	500 mg PO	10.5
Loracarbef	PO	N	~90	1.2	200 mg PO	8

(Continued)

TABLE 4 PHARMACOKINETIC PROPERTIES OF ANTIBACTERIAL AGENTS (CONTINUED)

Drug	Routes of administration	Oral		Serum half-life, h	Dose and route	Peak serum level, μg/mL
		With food	Absorption, %			
Third generation						
Cefoperazone	IV, IM			1.9	1.0 g IV	153
Cefotaxime	IV, IM			1.5	1.0 g IV	100
Ceftizoxime	IV, IM			1.7	1.0 g IV	132
Ceftriaxone	IV, IM			8.0	1.0 g IV	150
Ceftazidime	IV, IM			1.8	1.0 g IV	60
Cefixime	PO	Y	50	3.1	400 mg PO	3–5
Cefpodoxime proxetil	PO	Y	46	2.3	200 mg PO	2.9
Fourth generation						
Cefpirome	IV			2.0	1.0 g IV	87
Cefepime	IV			2.0	2.0 g IV	193
Vancomycin	IV, PO	N	< 1		125 mg PO	"None"
	IV			6.0	1.0 g IV	20–50
Aminoglycosides						
Amikacin	IV, IM			2.0	7.5 mg/kg IV	38
Gentamicin or tobramycin	IV, IM			2.0	1.25 mg/kg IV	5–7
Tetracyclines						
Doxycycline	PO, IV	Y	93	18.0	100 mg PO	1.8–2.9
Minocycline	PO	Y	95	16.0	200 mg PO	2.2
Chloramphenicol	PO, IV, IM	N	80	1.5–3.5	500 mg PO	8–14
Macrolides						
Azithromycin	PO	N	37	12.0/68.0*	500 mg PO	0.4
Clarithromycin	PO	Y	50	5.0–7.0	500 mg PO	2–3
Erythromycin				1.4		
Base	PO	N	40		500 mg PO	0.4–1.8
Stearate	PO	N	30–65			
Ethylsuccinate	PO	N	OK			
Estolate	PO	Y	OK		500 mg PO	1.4–5.0
Lactobionate or gluceptate	IV				500 mg IV	10
Clindamycin	PO, IV, IM	Y	90	2.4	150 mg PO	2.5
					600 mg IV	15
Fluoroquinolones						
Norfloxacin	PO	N	30–40	4.0	400 mg PO	1.4–1.8
Ciprofloxacin	PO, IV	Y	70	4.0	500 mg PO	1.8–2.8
					400 mg IV	4.6
Ofloxacin	PO, IV	N	98	7.0	400 mg PO	3.5–5.3
					400 mg IV	4.0–4.5
Enoxacin	PO	N	60	6.0	400 mg PO	2.0
Lomefloxacin	PO	Y	> 95	8.0	400 mg PO	1.4
Pefloxacin†	PO	Y	~100	9.0	400 mg PO	3.8–5.6
Polymyxin B	IV, IM			6.0–7.0	500,000 U IM	1–8
Rifampin	PO	N	Well	2.0–5.0	600 mg PO	4–32 (7)‡
Metronidazole	PO, IV	Y	90	6.0–14.0	250 mg PO	6.2
					500 mg IV	20–25
TMP/SMX	PO, IV		90–100	11.0/9.0§	1 single-strength tablet	TMP, 1–3 SMX, 20–50
					2 ampules IV (160 mg TMP/ 800 mg SMX)	TMP, 3–9 SMX, 45–100

Adapted from Sanford and coworkers [10]; with permission.

*Twelve h is the initial distribution; 68 h, the terminal half-life.

†Not available in the United States.

‡Seven is the mean level.

§Eleven hours is the half-life for trimethoprim; 9 h, the half-life for sulfamethoxazole.

IM—intramuscular; IV—intravenous; N—no; PO—oral; qd— every day;
   TMP/SMX—trimethoprim-sulfamethoxazole; Y—yes.

to 60 minutes, it was dogma to give a dose every third or fourth half-life, unless this drug was combined with an agent to delay absorption from an intramuscular site or unless an agent such as probenecid was given to block renal excretion. A series of laboratory and clinical observations have modified this dogma. The most far-reaching of these has been the recognition of the phenomenon of "postantibiotic effect," which is the delayed regrowth of surviving bacteria after limited exposure to an antimicrobial agent [15•]. Although the mechanisms of this effect have not been proved, the observations are of clinical relevance, at least with aerobic gram-negative bacilli and the aminoglycosides. Considerable evidence now indicates that a single daily dose of an aminoglycoside is as effective as, and may be less nephrotoxic than, multiple divided daily doses [16••]. The postantibiotic effect may apply to the quinolones, although clinical data are lacking. β-Lactam antibiotics produce the postantibiotic effect on gram-positive bacteria but rarely on gram-negative organisms (except for imipenem, which acts on both). The newer macrolides have prolonged tissue half-lives, with the terminal half-life of azithromycin being 68 hours. The clinical implications of such prolonged half-lives in terms of dosing frequency remain unclear, although the length of therapy has been reduced. Nowhere is the issue of frequency of dosing more variable than with the oral cephalosporin drugs [17•]. Cephalexin, which has a half-life of 0.9 to 1.1 hours, is recommended to be given four times daily, and cefprozil, cefuroxime axetil, and loracarbef, which have half-lives of 1.2 hours, are recommended twice daily. However, the efficacy of each in clinical trials, such as in the treatment of acute otitis media, is comparable.

Influence of Host Factors

The influence of host factors on the clinical pharmacology of antibacterial agents is also important in achieving efficacy while avoiding toxicity. Many antibacterial agents, including the β-lactams and the aminoglycosides, are removed by renal excretion. The dosage must be adjusted as renal function decreases. Glomerular filtration decreases approximately 1% per year after 30 years of age. In the elderly, dosage adjustment is required, even with normal serum creatinine concentrations.

Some antibacterial agents are metabolized and removed primarily by hepatic mechanisms. Although drugs removed by hepatic mechanisms less commonly require dosage adjustment even with advanced liver disease, such adjustments need to be considered for clindamycin, cefoperazone, chloramphenicol, erythromycin, metronidazole, and nafcillin.

Many of the mechanisms by which drugs are excreted have not matured in the neonate; hence, dosage adjustment is required. Because disease processes such as cystic fibrosis increase the clearances of many antibiotics, higher than usual doses are required to achieve adequate serum levels.

ADVERSE EFFECTS

Every antibacterial agent that is administered orally or parenterally has produced one or more adverse effects in some patients [10]. In reviewing the product labeling on any antibacterial agent, the clinician should recall that when untoward events, even if rare, occur in the single given patient, they represent all-or-nothing occurrences. Under some circumstances, adverse effects are predictable. Patients with glucose-6-phosphate dehydrogenase deficiency may develop hemolysis when exposed to the following antibacterial agents: sulfonamides, trimethoprim, nalidixic acid, and nitrofurantoin.

DRUG-DRUG INTERACTIONS

The list of reported drug-drug interactions, many of which are potentially life threatening, is long. Before writing a prescription, the physician should review with the patient all drugs, including over-the-counter drugs, that the patient is taking. It is also important to remember that the patient may be taking a drug or drugs prescribed by another physician. After having ascertained what the patient is taking, the clinician should look up (ie, should not assume that he or she knows) all the potential drug-drug interactions [10].

FAILURE OF ANTIBACTERIAL THERAPY

There are few bacteria that are not susceptible to one or more of the available antimicrobial agents, yet infections remain an important proximate cause of death. Apparent failures of antibacterial therapy may reflect the outcome of physiologic processes initiated by infection that have progressed beyond the point of physiologic recovery despite bacteriologic cure. For example, the mortality rate during the first 24 hours of pneumococcal bacteremia has not decreased with the administration of penicillin [18]. Failures are often the consequence of inadequate host defense mechanisms.

In the patient with reasonably intact host defense mechanisms who fails to respond to an "appropriate" antibiotic, a number of possibilities should be considered. The infection being treated may be viral or fungal in etiology rather than bacterial. The patient may have developed drug fever resulting from the antibiotic or another drug. The patient may have a focus of infection that has not been drained, such as maxillary sinusitis in the postoperative patient who has had a nasogastric tube in place for several days. There may be an obstruction to anatomic drainage, such as a ureter or a foreign body that has not been removed. Failure can also occur if appropriate attention has not been given to the selection of definitive rather than empiric therapy, to the clinical pharmacology of the agent, and to drug-drug interactions that may block absorption or cause accelerated metabolism or excretion.

References and Recommended Reading

Recently published papers of particular interest have been highlighted as:
- Of interest
- • Of outstanding interest

1. • Knockaert DC, Vanneste LJ, Vanneste SB, Bobbaers HJ: Fever of unknown origin in the 1980's. *Arch Intern Med* 1992, 152:51–55.

2. • Fang GD, Fine M, Orloff J, *et al.*: New and emerging etiologies for community-acquired pneumonia with implications for therapy. *Medicine* 1990, 69:307–316.

3. •• Jacoby GA: Prevalence and resistance mechanisms of common respiratory pathogens. *Clin Infect Dis* 1994, 18:951–957.

4. Flournoy DJ, Davidson LJ: Sputum quality: can you tell by looking? *Am J Infect Control* 1993, 21:64–69.

5. • Honig PK, Woosley RL, Zamani K, *et al.*: Changes in the pharmacokinetics and electrocardiographic pharmacodynamics of terfenadine with concomitant administration of erythromycin. *Clin Pharmacol Ther* 1992, 52:231–238.

6. •• Sanders CV, Aldridge KE: Current antimicrobial therapy for anaerobic infections. *Eur J Clin Microbiol Infect Dis* 1992, 11:999–1011.

7. • Meyer KS, Urban C, Eagan JA, *et al.*: Nosocomial outbreak of *Klebsiella* infection resistant to late generation cephalosporins. *Ann Intern Med* 1993, 119:353–358.

8. •• Breiman RF, Butler JC, Tenover FC, *et al.*: Emergence of drug-resistant pneumococcal infections in the United States. *JAMA* 1994, 271:1831–1835.

9. Frieden TR, Munsiff SS, Low DE, *et al.*: Emergence of vancomycin resistant enterococci in New York City. *Lancet* 1993, 342:76–77.

10. Sanford JP, Gilbert DN, Sande MA: The Sanford Guide to Antimicrobial Therapy 1995. Dallas: Antimicrobial Therapy, Inc.: 1995.

11. •• Sader HS, Jones RN: Historical overview of the cephalosporin spectrum: four generations of structural evolution. *Antimicrobic Newsletter* 1992, 8:75–82.

12. • Payne DJ, Cramp R, Winstanley DJ, Knowles DJC: Comparative activities of clavulanic acid, sulbactam and tazobactam against clinically important β-lactamases. *Antimicrob Agents Chemother* 1994, 38:767–772.

13. • Paladino JA, Sperry HE, Backes JM, *et al.*: Clinical and economic evaluation of oral ciprofloxacin after an abbreviated course of intravenous antibiotics. *Am J Med* 1991, 91:462–470.

14. •• Nightingale CH, Quintiliani R, Nicolau DP: Intelligent dosing of antimicrobials. *Current Clinical Topics in Infectious Disease* vol 14. Edited by Remington JS, Swartz MM. Cambridge, MA: Blackwell Scientific Publications; 1994:252–265.

15. • MacKenzie FM, Gould IM: The post-antibiotic effect. *J Antimicrob Chemother* 1993, 32:519–537.

16. •• Gilbert DN: Once-daily aminoglycoside therapy. *Antimicrob Agents Chemother* 1991, 35:399–405.

17. • Pichichero ME: Assessing the treatment alternatives for acute otitis media. *Pediatr Infect Dis J* 1994, 13:527–534.

18. Austrian R, Gold J: Pneumococcal bacteremia with special reference to bacteremic pneumococcal pneumonia. *Ann Intern Med* 1964, 60:759–776.

Select Bibliography

Murray BE: The life and times of the eneterococcus. *Clin Microbiol Rev* 1990, 3:46–65.

Neu HC: General therapeutic principles. In *Infectious Diseases*. Edited by Gorbach SL, Bartlett JF, Blacklow NR. Philadelphia: WB Saunders; 1992:153–160.

Neu HC: The 10 most commonly asked questions about cephalosporins. *Infect Dis Clin Pract* 1994, 3:209–211.

Petersdorf RG, Beeson PB: Fever of unexplained origin: report on 100 cases. *Medicine* 1961, 40:1–30.

Fever of Unknown Origin

John T. Sinnott IV
Douglas A. Holt
Evelyn Kim

Key Points

- The physician must first determine if the patient meets the criteria for a true fever of unknown origin.

- Most fevers of unknown origin can be attributed to treatable disease presenting in an uncommon manner.

- The diagnosis of a patient with fever of unknown origin must begin with a complete and meticulous history and physical examination.

- Repeat physical examinations can reveal changes in the patient's clinical status that may lead to a definitive diagnosis.

- Laboratory studies should not be performed blindly but be directed toward discovering possible causes of fever.

The feaver is to the Physitians, the eternal reproach. John Milton (1608–1674)

Although fever in the modern era may no longer carry the stigma of fatal disease, it still possesses the potential to vex even the most astute clinician. Fever is associated with a multitude of pathologic processes and has been a sentinel of illness throughout history. In most patients, an elevation in body temperature accompanies a recognized disease process, with the fever resolving either independently or after therapeutic intervention. A patient suffering from protracted fever with no diagnosis following the initial evaluation presents the challenging syndrome of fever of unknown origin (FUO).

In most patients, the cause of fever will be diagnosed after the initial history taking, physical examination, laboratory studies, and microbiologic evaluation. To be considered a candidate for FUO evaluation, a patient must meet the following criteria: the illness must be of more than 3 weeks' duration; the patient's temperature must exceed 101°F (38.3°C) on several occasions; and no diagnosis can have been made after 1 week of rigorous investigation [1,2]. Restricting the definition of FUO to these parameters, in accordance with the seminal study conducted by Petersdorf and Beeson [1] in 1961, excludes the more readily diagnosed febrile illnesses.

ETIOLOGY

Multiple studies have determined that the majority of diseases responsible for FUO can be divided into four discrete categories: 1) infection (30%), 2) neoplasm (25%), 3) collagen vascular disease (15%), and 4) granulomatous disease (10%). The remaining 10% of cases of FUO are attributable to miscellaneous causes. Recent studies have suggested that neoplastic processes are increasing and collagen vascular disorders declining in frequency [2]. The most common causes of FUO are intra-abdominal abscess, lymphoma, urinary tract infection, endocarditis, tuberculosis, granulomatous hepatitis, Still's disease, cytomegalovirus infection, systemic lupus erythematosus, Crohn's disease, and factitious fever. Other causes of FUO are listed in Table 1. In approximately 10% of individuals with FUO, a definitive cause is never identified. Fortunately, the prognosis for patients with undiagnosed conditions is generally favorable.

During the initial patient evaluation, the physician must first approach the junction of probability and epidemiology. The clinician should recall the relative frequencies of diseases associated with FUO and then integrate this information with the characteristics of the patient population at hand. Age, hospital setting, lifestyle, race, and gender can provide the initial guidance for the direction of the evaluation. After this synthesis, the diagnostician must review the established causes of FUO and target the most likely etiologies. A conceptual grasp of possible etiologies pursued by a systematic approach assists in formulating a limited differential diagnosis.

Infections

Infections comprise one third of the diseases responsible for FUO. Infections may manifest either in an insidious manner with a meek prodrome or as an unrelenting fever of acute onset. These infections may be the result of a common agent presenting atypically, an atypical pathogen, or an uncommon agent mimicking a common illness.

Abscesses

In order of descending frequency, abscesses arise from the liver and biliary tract, subphrenic region, the spleen, and the colon [3]. A history of abdominal trauma, surgery, cholecystitis, diverticulitis, or inflammatory bowel disease may predispose a patient to abscess formation. Symptoms of shoulder pain and physical findings of an elevated hemidiaphragm or a hepatic friction rub suggest a hepatic process. A transient elevation in liver enzyme levels suggests Charcot's fever of intermittent cholangitis [4,5,6•].

Genitourinary infections

Perinephric abscesses may exhibit no growth on urine culture. Urinary tract abnormalities, such as bladder reflux in children,

papillary necrosis, and caliectasis, may also be underlying noninfectious sources of fever [7•]. Prostatic, pelvic, and perirectal abscesses also occur. Patients with leukemia, diabetes mellitus, inflammatory bowel disease, and diverticulitis are at highest risk for perirectal abscess.

Endocarditis

Infective endocarditis usually does not present a diagnostic dilemma, but all patients with FUO must be evaluated with blood cultures. Because endocarditis may be subacute in onset and culture negative, a heart murmur or peripheral stigmata of endocarditis should be tenaciously pursued. A meticulous examination to identify a portal of entry is essential, and antibiotics should be avoided during the diagnostic period unless the patient is septic or at risk for acute valvular dysfunction.

Mycobacterial and fungal infections

Extrapulmonary tuberculosis can present with few localizing signs or symptoms, normal roentgenographic findings, a nonreactive tuberculin skin test result, and none of the classic symptoms of pulmonary tuberculosis. In patients with miliary tuberculosis, subsequent chest roentgenograms usually show the development of interstitial miliary lesions [8]. Elderly patients and those with HIV infection are at increased risk for both primary infection and reactivation disease with *Mycobacterium tuberculosis*. Peritoneal or genitourinary tract involvement is particularly subtle, and often anemia, thrombocytosis, or monocytosis may be the only clue. Biopsy with the histologic evaluation and mycobacterial culture of suspected tissue is the most effective diagnostic approach.

The deep fungal infections—histoplasmosis, blastomycosis, cryptococcosis, and coccidioidomycosis—can mimic tuberculosis. Again, extrapulmonary infection is often subtle, and tissue biopsy is usually needed for diagnosis.

Mycobacterium avium complex infection should be suspected in any febrile patient with significant immunosuppression, including HIV infection [9••]. Abdominal pain and diarrhea are clues suggesting disseminated *M. avium* complex infection.

TABLE 1 MISCELLANEOUS CAUSES OF FEVER OF UNKNOWN ORIGIN	
Etiology	**Clues to the diagnosis**
Common	
Drug fever	—
Thromboembolism	Dyspnea, chest pain (blood gas measurements may remain normal)
	Patient recovering from pelvic surgery or parturition at greatest risk
Alcoholic liver disease	Hepatomegaly, increased serum aspartate aminotransferase levels
Factitious fever	Absence of diurnal temperature variation, discrepancy between concomitant oral and rectal temperature measurements
Cryptic hematoma	Recent history of blunt trauma or anticoagulant therapy
Rare	
Occult dental infection	Poor dentition, history of recent dental procedure
Familial Mediterranean fever	Episodic fever with abdominal pain, serositis, skin rash, arthritis
Idiopathic pericarditis	
Subacute granulomatous thyroiditis	

Viral infections

Viral infections are usually self-limited, but Epstein-Barr virus, cytomegalovirus (CMV), and HIV infection may be associated with protracted fever. In the older adult, atypical presentations of infectious mononucleosis can obfuscate an otherwise straightforward diagnosis. Elderly patients may complain only of fever, malaise, and pharyngitis, without having the classic findings of atypical lymphocytosis, splenomegaly, or lymphadenopathy [10]. The delay in serologic response characteristic of the elderly may further obscure an otherwise readily diagnosed case of Epstein-Barr virus infection.

In healthy individuals, CMV infection may produce a mononucleosis-like illness with prolonged fever. Patients who have undergone solid organ or bone marrow transplantation, who have received blood products, or who are HIV positive are at risk for CMV-associated gastritis, hepatitis, pneumonitis, or FUO. Leukopenia or atypical lymphocytes may be the only finding suggestive of CMV disease.

The symptoms of primary HIV infection mimic those found in mononucleosis-like illnesses and may on occasion present as FUO. Because this disease can manifest with nonspecific symptoms and patients may lack obvious risk factors, HIV serology should be included in the initial evaluation. Diagnostic clues suggestive of HIV infection include rashes, lymphadenopathy, sore throat, oral ulcers, and an enanthema in conjunction with urticaria [11].

Vertebral osteomyelitis

A patient with the diagnostic triad of lower extremity weakness, back pain, and a history of urinary tract infection should be evaluated for vertebral osteomyelitis [3]. Osteomyelitis of hematogenous origin may cause symptoms of local pain or swelling.

Uncommon infections

Uncommon infections causing FUO are listed in Table 2.

Neoplasm

Malignancy is the underlying disease in approximately one fourth of patients with FUO (Table 3). Although any neoplastic process can elevate body temperature, lymphoma, leukemia, and localized abdominal carcinoma are the most often encountered. In patients with malignancy, infection must always be excluded as a cause of fever.

Collagen Vascular Disease

Approximately 15% of FUO cases are eventually diagnosed as connective tissue disorders. Prominent diagnostic clues include a markedly increased erythrocyte sedimentation rate, recurrent cutaneous lesions, synovitis, and serositis (Table 4). In patients with atypical presentations, prolonged fever may be the only symptom.

Granulomatous Disease

Approximately 5% to 10% of cases of FUO can be attributed to granulomatosis. This most commonly occurs in the liver, but any organ system may be involved. Although many infectious processes can trigger granuloma formation and fever, idiopathic granulomatous diseases are most commonly encountered with FUO.

TABLE 2 UNCOMMON INFECTIONS CAUSING FEVER OF UNKNOWN ORIGIN

Agent	Risk factors	Clinical features
Brucella species	Occupational exposure to farm animals, travel to endemic areas	Arthritis, hepatitis, subacute endocarditis
Coxiella burnetii (Q fever)	Contact with cats and farm animals, ingestion of contaminated dairy products	Atypical pneumonia, hepatitis, splenomegaly; endocarditis with hepatosplenomegaly
Leptospira species	Exposure to dog, farm animal, or rodent urine	Weil's syndrome (icterus, jaundice, renal failure, myocarditis)
Listeria monocytogenes	Disseminated disease occurs in pregnant women, neonates, and immuno-compromised patients	Subacute endocarditis, osteomyelitis, peritonitis, cholecystitis
Borrelia burgdorferi (Lyme disease)	Travel to endemic areas, camping, exposure to ticks	Fever occurs during dissemination (second stage) or late infection (third stage); widespread systemic manifestations
Plasmodium species (malaria)	Febrile relapse may occur years after an untreated primary infection	"FAST" diagnosis: fever, anemia, splenomegaly, travel
Chlamydia psittaci (psittacosis)	Contact with birds	Atypical pneumonia, persistent cough
Streptobacillus moniliformis or *Spirillum minus* (rat-bite fever)	History of exposure to rats is not mandatory for diagnosis	Vomiting, pharyngitis, endocarditis
Francisella tularensis (tularemia)	Contact with rabbits; tick bites	High fever; ulceroglandular, glandular, typhoidal, or oculoglandular syndrome
Salmonella typhi (typhoid fever)	History of achlorhydria, hemolysis, cirrhosis, splenectomy, or HIV infection	Cough, headache, rose spots, splenomegaly, leukopenia

TABLE 3 MALIGNANCIES CAUSING FEVER OF UNKNOWN ORIGIN

Malignancy	Comments
Hodgkin's lymphoma	Most frequent neoplasm producing recurrent fever as an initial symptom; fever may precede recognizable lymph node enlargement by months
Non-Hodgkin's lymphoma	Prolonged fever and thrombocytopenia may predate lymphadenopathy
Leukemia	Fever may present as part of preleukemic syndrome: anemia, leukopenia, and absence of blast cells
Abdominal tumor	Most commonly renal cell, hepatic, or colorectal carcinoma
Other malignancy	Atrial myxoma (not to be confused with infectious endocarditis)

Granulomatous hepatitis

Granulomatous hepatitis presents with a vague history and a paucity of physical findings, which delays the diagnosis of this disease. Laboratory studies may show an increased alkaline phosphatase level. The diagnosis is made by histologic examination (Table 5). Generally, patients with idiopathic disease have a favorable prognosis, with spontaneous or steroid-induced resolution [12].

Inflammatory bowel disease

Inflammatory bowel disease may present with few or no gastrointestinal symptoms, so the presence of fever may be the initial complaint of a patient with Crohn's disease [13]. Diagnosis requires invasive procedures.

Trophyrema whippeli infection (Whipple's disease) is a syndrome of diarrhea, serositis, dementia and, at times, fever. Jejunal or lymph node biopsy showing periodic acid–Schiff stain positive macrophages is used for the diagnosis.

Sarcoidosis

Sarcoidosis is suggested by uveitis, hilar adenopathy, arthralgia, erythema nodosum, and elevated angiotensin-converting enzyme activity. Noncaseating granulomas in tissue biopsy confirm the diagnosis.

Other Causes

Most of the disorders in this category are simply abnormal presentations of relatively common phenomena. A few conditions by virtue of their obscurity may require protracted evaluation before identification. Only drug fever is discussed here; other etiologies are mentioned in Table 1. Drug fever may present with only fever, without rash or eosinophilia. Additionally, drugs such as phenytoin, methyldopa, and isoniazid may be tolerated for months or even years before producing a febrile response. Other drugs that cause FUO include quinidine, penicillin, procainamide, and salicylates. A meticulous medication history is crucial to establishing a diagnosis of drug fever. On cessation of therapy, a patient should defervesce in 48 to 72 hours [14].

DIAGNOSIS

A patient with FUO provides a prime opportunity to sharpen diagnostic acumen and refine the bedside manner. A physician willing to accept this challenge must make a long-term commitment to the patient. Although carefully selected diagnostic tests may ultimately find a cause, only the history and physical examination can direct the evaluation. In most cases, the primary care physician can determine the cause of FUO.

History and Physical Examination

Initially, fever with no apparent explanation on several occasions should be confirmed. Next, the diagnostic categories and most common causes of FUO should be recalled. The history taking and physical examination may not immediately yield a diagnosis, but this portion of the evaluation is crucial and will guide future decisions. Thorough questioning with thoughtful analysis allows the most strategic approach to the directed evaluation. Finally, the diagnostician must conduct repeated history takings and physical examinations in search of omitted clues and new developments.

TABLE 4 COLLAGEN VASCULAR DISEASES CAUSING FEVER OF UNKNOWN ORIGIN

Disease	Comments
Giant cell arteritis (most common cause of fever of unexplained origin in elderly patients)	Associated with an elevated erythrocyte sedimentation rate, visual disturbance, jaw claudication; diagnosis is with temporal artery biopsy
Rheumatoid arthritis (Still's disease)	Notable absence of joint involvement; presence of evanescent maculopapular rash on trunk, lymphadenopathy, splenomegaly; diagnosis is often by exclusion
Systemic lupus erythematosus	Atypical disease may present with negative serologic findings
Other	Rheumatic fever, mixed connective tissue disease, polymyositis, polyarteritis nodosa

TABLE 5 GRANULOMATOUS HEPATITIS FEVER

Infectious	Noninfectious
Tuberculosis	Sarcoidosis
Brucellosis	Hodgkin's lymphoma
Tularemia	Giant cell arteritis
Listeriosis	Crohn's disease
Histoplasmosis	Drug reaction
Cytomegalovirus and Epstein-Barr virus infection	
Q fever	
Syphilis	

TABLE 6 HISTORICAL CLUES IN FEVER OF UNKNOWN ORIGIN

Exposure	Disease
Bird	Salmonellosis, psittacosis, tuberculosis
Cat	Cat-scratch fever, Q fever, toxoplasmosis
Dog	Leptospirosis
Cattle	Brucellosis, Q fever, leptospirosis
Rodents	Leptospirosis, relapsing fever
Tick	Ehrlichiosis, Lyme disease
Spelunking	Relapsing fever
Dairy product	Salmonellosis, listeriosis, yersinial infection, brucellosis, Q fever
Chicken or pork	Salmonellosis, yersinial infection
Shellfish	Salmonellosis

History

The onset of illness, its chronology, associated symptoms, and any previous medical evaluations should be elicited. The clinician should seek information on pertinent exposures, such as travel, occupation, tuberculosis risk, diet, animal contact, sexual contact, and drug use (Table 6). An inventory of all medications, including nonprescribed drugs, should be taken.

In reviewing the patient's past medical history, the clinician should ask about previous surgery, prosthetic device implantation, trauma, or metabolic disorders. Cholecystitis, diverticulitis, or appendicitis should alert the clinician to possible abscess formation, whereas arthritis and carpal tunnel syndrome should suggest a collagen vascular disorder [15]. A review of systems improves patient recall and elicits further information.

Physical examination

Table 7 and Figure 1 show the types of examinations that should be performed.

Laboratory and Diagnostic Studies

Only a thorough history taking and physical examination ensure efficient use of laboratory and diagnostic studies. If a diagnosis is suggested by the findings of the initial examination, laboratory tests can be very focused. If no diagnosis is suggested, initial laboratory screening studies should be ordered. Once a diagnostic direction has been established from the history, physical examination findings, and initial tests results, carefully selected laboratory studies and diagnostic procedures are initiated. This evaluation should begin with noninvasive studies.

Initial screening

The routine laboratory evaluation of FUO includes the following: a complete blood count with differential, determination of the erythrocyte sedimentation rate, measurement of liver function enzyme levels, the Venereal Disease Research Laboratory test, an HIV antibody screen, urinalysis with culture, culture of stool for ova and parasites, blood cultures, chest roentgenography, and the Mantoux skin test.

TABLE 7 PHYSICAL FINDINGS IN FEVER OF UNKNOWN ORIGIN

Finding	Disease
Erythema nodosum	Tuberculosis, yersinial infection, SLE, sarcoidosis, Crohn's disease, any granulomatous disease
Proptosis	Lymphoma, Wegener's granulomatosis, thyroid disease
Conjunctivitis	Tuberculosis, Still's disease, cat-scratch fever
Band keratopathy	Sarcoidosis
Uveitis	Sarcoidosis, toxoplasmosis, syphilis, tuberculosis, Still's disease
Murmur	Endocarditis
Hepatomegaly	Lymphoma, hepatic abscess, hepatitis, hepatoma
Splenomegaly	Lymphoma, malaria, SBE, SLE, CMV infection, EBV infection
Adenopathy	Hodgkin's disease, toxoplasmosis, CMV infection, EBV infection

CMV—cytomegalovirus; EBV—Epstein-Barr virus; SBE—subacute bacterial endocarditis; SLE—systemic lupus erythematosus.

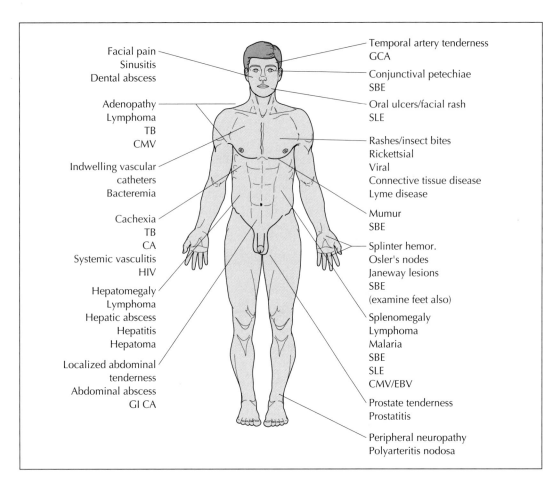

Facial pain
Sinusitis
Dental abscess

Adenopathy
Lymphoma
TB
CMV

Indwelling vascular
catheters
Bacteremia

Cachexia
TB
CA
Systemic vasculitis
HIV

Hepatomegaly
Lymphoma
Hepatic abscess
Hepatitis
Hepatoma

Localized abdominal
tenderness
Abdominal abscess
GI CA

Temporal artery tenderness
GCA

Conjunctival petechiae
SBE

Oral ulcers/facial rash
SLE

Rashes/insect bites
Rickettsial
Viral
Connective tissue disease
Lyme disease

Mumur
SBE

Splinter hemor.
Osler's nodes
Janeway lesions
SBE
(examine feet also)

Splenomegaly
Lymphoma
Malaria
SBE
SLE
CMV/EBV

Prostate tenderness
Prostatitis

Peripheral neuropathy
Polyarteritis nodosa

FIGURE 1 Clues from the physical examination: clinical clues and their differential diagnosis. CA—cancer; CMV—cytomegalovirus; EBV—Epstein-Barr virus; GCA—giant cell arteritis; GI—gastrointestinal; hemor.—hemorrhage; SBE—subacute bacterial endocarditis; SLE—systemic lupus erythematosus; TB—tuberculosis.

Specific diagnostic techniques

Serologic tests
IgM titers to CMV, Epstein-Barr virus, and toxoplasmosis may be helpful in the patient with a mononucleosis-like illness. Other serologic tests that are useful in certain clinical settings include *Brucella* agglutination, a streptozyme screen (rheumatic fever), a *Coxiella burnetii* antibody titer (Q fever endocarditis), and an antinuclear antibody screen (collagen vascular disease).

Noninvasive scanning procedures
Ultrasonography visualizes the liver, kidney, pancreas, and pelvis. Computed tomography is particularly useful for imaging the retroperitoneum, the abdominal cavity, and the pelvis, whereas magnetic resonance imaging is preferred for the central nervous system and the skeleton. Radionuclide scintigraphy with either indium-111–labeled leukocytes or gallium-67 can be used, but both studies may produce false-positive results in up to 30% of patients [16,17].

Gastrointestinal studies
Contrast studies with small bowel follow through, barium enema, and sigmoidoscopy may elucidate gastrointestinal abnormalities. These studies could also be included in the initial screening.

Tissue biopsy
Directed tissue biopsy offers the best opportunity to confirm a diagnosis. Most biopsies pose little risk and yield high bene-

fits, especially if the specimen is cultured for mycobacteria as well as histologically examined. Direct fluorescent antibody staining and polymerase chain reaction are becoming available for tissue testing. Typical sites and indications for biopsy are given in Table 8.

PATIENTS WITH SPECIAL CONSIDERATIONS
Both elderly patients and immunocompromised patients require a slightly different approach to the evaluation of prolonged fever. The parameters of the corresponding evaluation, as well as its pace and intensity, may need to be altered. Travelers may have exotic infections requiring more specific evaluations.

Patients with HIV Infection
Causes of FUO in the HIV-seropositive patient are tuberculosis, *Mycobacterium avium* complex infection, cytomegalovirus infection, *Pneumocystis carinii* pneumonia, primary HIV infection, histoplasmosis, cryptococcosis, salmonellosis, lymphoma, and tumor.

Elderly Patients
Prolonged fever is of great concern in the elderly. Not only do these individuals tend to have serious disease underlying the FUO, but they are more likely to have comorbid conditions that can be exacerbated by elevations in temperature. These mandate an expeditious evaluation. An elderly patient should be hospitalized for evaluation if signs of severe debilitation or rapid weight loss are present.

TABLE 8 TYPICAL SITES AND INDICATIONS FOR BIOPSY

Site or indication	Comment
Lymph node enlargement	Computed tomographic direction assists in the evaluation of the abdominal and retoperitoneal lymph nodes [17]
Liver function abnormalities	Biopsy may also be undertaken as a specific diagnostic procedure in problematic patients
Bone marrow	Bone marrow biopsy is performed if hematologic abnormalities are present; lymphoma, disseminated infection, and granulomatous disease may be identified
Temporal artery pain or visual symptoms	These symptoms should suggest biopsy
Skin lesions	Biopsy of skin lesions should be performed

In addition to being subject to the common causes of FUO and those listed in Table 1, elderly patients may also suffer from temporal arteritis, pulmonary emboli, infectious mononucleosis, polyarteritis nodosa, and polymyalgia rheumatica.

The history taking and physical examination should be conducted in the same manner as the standard FUO evaluation. Age-relevant medical factors, such as prostatic disease, diverticulitis, diabetic sequelae, and integumentary dysfunction, should be emphasized.

Travelers

A thorough travel history combined with knowledge of the diseases endemic to pertinent areas of travel is crucial to evaluating FUO in the traveler (Table 9). Further information on this topic is provided elsewhere in this volume.

MANAGEMENT

For patients whose evaluation yields a diagnosis, fever should abate on appropriate treatment. In the patient whose condition is stable, antimicrobial therapy should be withheld while the patient is repeatedly reexamined. Empiric antimicrobial therapy should be used only when the clinician has no feasible diagnostic alternatives and a high degree of clinical suspicion, or when the patient is seriously ill from a suspected bacterial process such as endocarditis.

Therapeutic trials of antibiotics or corticosteroids should be avoided because they are associated with side effects and may delay the diagnosis of the underlying illness. In the elderly or immunocompromised patient, antituberculous

therapy may be considered while awaiting biopsy or culture results. Patients with granulomatous hepatitis may initially be given a trial of antituberculous therapy followed by corticosteroids if culture results are negative and there is no response in 4 to 6 weeks. A cautious trial of prednisone therapy for clinically diagnosed temporal arteritis may be considered if biopsy is not available. Finally, a trial of naproxen has been advocated to differentiate between fever caused by tumor and fever caused by infection [18].

If the source of fever in a patient remains obscure, the clinician can prescribe salicylates, acetaminophen, or ibuprofen. Follow-up care with planned reevaluation for FUO is vital to ensure that a more serious disease is not progressing unchecked.

REFERENCES AND RECOMMENDED READING

Recently published papers of particular interest have been highlighted as:
• Of interest
•• Of outstanding interest

1. Petersdorf RG, Beeson PB: Fever of unexplained origin: report on 100 cases. *Medicine* 1961, 40:1–30.
2. Petersdorf RG: Fever of unknown origin: an old friend revisited. *Arch Intern Med* 1992, 152:21–22.
3. Larson EB, Featherstone HJ, Petersdorf RG: Fever of undetermined origin: diagnosis and follow up of 105 cases, 1970–1980. *Medicine* 1982, 61:269–292.
4. Knockaert DC, Vanneste LJ, Vanneste SB, Bobbaers HJ: Fever of unknown origin in the 1980s: an update of the diagnostic spectrum. *Arch Intern Med* 1992, 152:51–55.
5. Barbado FJ, Vasquez JJ, Pena JM, *et al.*: Pyrexia of unknown origin: changing spectrum of diseases in two consecutive series. *Postgrad Med* 1992, 68:884–887.
6.• Kazanjian PH: Fever of unknown origin: review of 86 patients treated in community hospitals. *Clin Infect Dis* 1992, 15:968–973.
7.• Dinarello CA, Wolff SM: Fever of unknown origin. In *Principles and Practice of Infectious Diseases*, edn 3. Edited by Mandell GL, Douglas RG Jr, Bennett JE. New York: Churchill Livingstone; 1990:468–479.
8. Van Scoy RE: Fever, and fever of unknown origin. In *Infectious Diseases: A Modern Treatise of Infectious Processes*, edn 4. Edited by Hoeprich PD, Jordan MC. Philadelphia: JB Lippincott; 1989: 94–100.

TABLE 9 CAUSES OF FEVER OF UNKNOWN ORIGIN IN TRAVELERS

Location	Disease
South America	Trypanosomiasis, amebic liver abscess
Africa	Malaria, visceral leishmaniasis
Southeast Asia	Malaria, tuberculosis, hepatitis
North America (sylvan areas)	Lyme borreliosis, ehrlichiosis, babesiosis, tularemia, leptospirosis

9.•• Durack DT, Street AC: Fever of unknown origin: reexamined and redefined. *Curr Clin Top Infect Dis* 1991, 11:35–51.

10. Axelrod P, Finestone AJ: Infectious mononucleosis in older adults. *Am Fam Physician* 1990, 42:1599–1606.

11. Kinloche-de Loes S, de Saussure P, Saurat JH, *et al.*: Symptomatic primary infection due to human immunodeficiency virus type 1: review of 31 cases. *Clin Infect Dis* 1993, 17:59–65.

12. Zoutman DE, Ralph ED, Frei JV: Granulomatous hepatitis and fever of unknown origin: an 11-year experience of 23 cases with three years' follow-up. *J Clin Gastroenterol* 1991, 13:69–75.

13. Wolff SM, Fauci AS, Dale DC: Unusual etiologies of fever and their evaluation. *Annu Rev Med* 1975, 26:277–281.

14. Mackowiak PA, LeMaistre CF: Drug fever: a critical appraisal of conventional concepts. An analysis of 51 episodes in two Dallas hospitals and 97 episodes reported in the English literature. *Ann Intern Med* 1987, 106:728–733.

15. Scully RE, Mark EJ, McNeely BU: Weekly clinicopathological exercises: case 35-1986. *N Engl J Med* 1986, 315:631–639.

16. Saitoh-Miyazaki C, Itoh K: Comparative findings between ^{111}indium-labeled leukocytes and ^{67}gallium scintigraphy for patients with acute and chronic inflammatory diseases. *Prog Clin Biol Res* 1990, 355:141–150.

17. Rowland MD, Del Bene VE: Use of body computed tomography to evaluate fever of unknown origin. *J Infect Dis* 1987, 156:408–409.

18. Chang JC: Neoplastic fever: a proposal of diagnosis. *Arch Intern Med* 1989, 148:1728–1780.

SELECT BIBLIOGRAPHY

Knockaert DC: Fever of unknown origin: a literature survey. *Acta Clin Belg* 1992, 47:42–57.

Mackowiks PA, ed: *Fever: Basic Mechanisms and Management*. New York: Raven Press; 1991.

Oizumi K, Onuma K, Watanade A, Motomaya M: Clinical study of drug fever induced by parenteral administration of antibiotics. *Tohoku J Exp Med* 1989, 159:45–56.

Respiratory Infections: Outpatient

5

Kurt B. Stevenson
Steven L. Berk

Key Points

- History and physical examination in the office setting may provide important clues to the etiology of community-acquired pneumonia.
- The need for hospitalization after the diagnosis of pneumonia is heavily dependent upon the patient's severity of underlying illness; patients with heart failure, diabetes, cancer, or HIV disease generally require hospitalization.
- *Streptococcus pneumoniae* and *Mycoplasma pneumoniae* are the most common causes of community-acquired pneumonia. Other agent include *Chlamydia* species, viruses, *Haemophilus influenzae*, *Legionella* species, and *Staphylococcus aureus*. In many cases no pathogen is identified.
- Patients treated in the outpatient setting for pneumonia must be carefully monitored to ensure compliance and clinical improvement.
- Elderly patients and those with chronic cardiac, pulmonary, and renal disease should receive both influenza and pneumococcal vaccines.

Infections of the respiratory tract constitute one of the most frequent infectious disease problems facing primary care physicians as well as specialists. It is estimated that pneumonia develops in 3 million persons in the United States each year resulting in 500,000 hospital admissions and 50,000 deaths [1]. Pneumonia can affect patients of all ages causing varied presentations caused by numerous etiologic agents. Although infections of the respiratory tract can also be acquired in the hospital setting, most patients develop their infection in the community and will initially be evaluated as outpatients. The examining physician will need to determine whether infection is limited to the bronchi or whether true pneumonia exists. Bronchitis can generally be managed in the outpatient setting whereas pneumonia may require hospitalization. The clinical state of the patient's pulmonary function and the potential for respiratory decompensation requiring hospitalization and supportive measures will need to be assessed. The establishment of an etiologic diagnosis is an important element of treating patients with respiratory tract infections and is critical to initiating appropriate therapy. Treatment in the outpatient setting mandates that the patient be closely followed to insure compliance and clinical improvement.

OFFICE EVALUATION

The patient suspected of having pneumonia should provide a comprehensive history and receive a complete physical examination. The nature and duration of the patient's symptoms should be elucidated. A study conducted by the British Thoracic Society Research Committee of 453 patients with pneumonia demonstrated cough in 88%, dyspnea in 77%, sputum production in 69%, chest pain in 64%, hemoptysis in 17%, and confusion in 17% [2]. These classic symptoms may be absent in the elderly who may present with only constitutional complaints, central nervous system symptoms, tachypnea, or low-grade fever [3]. Upper quadrant abdominal pain with guarding or ileus may be seen in either very young or elderly patients [4]. An acute process with rapidly progressive symptoms demands a different approach than chronic or indolent symptoms.

The history should focus on underlying medical conditions. In patients with preexisting chronic diseases the incidence of pneumonia is higher, the etiologic possibilities broader, and the case fatality rate is greater than in otherwise healthy patients. Patients with cerebrovascular or other neurologic diseases may experience aspiration because of altered mentation or swallowing dysfunction. Patients with pulmonary diseases experience ineffective cough, defective ciliary action, or alveolar macrophage dysfunction. Cardiac diseases often result in pulmonary congestion and wet alveoli. Chronic liver or renal diseases may result in relative abnormalities of host defense whereas malignancies, chemotherapy, and other immunosuppressive conditions present definite defects in immune function. A careful "exposure" history will examine epidemiologic issues that may have placed the patient at risk for acquisition of unusual or opportunistic pathogens (Table 1).

The physical examination must assess the stability of the patient and the extent of pulmonary involvement. Rales and wheezes found in the chest may be nonspecific and can be heard with other conditions such as bronchitis, asthma, or congestive heart failure. Specific signs such as bronchial breath sounds, egophony, tactile fremitus, or dullness to percussion may appear only late in the illness and may not be completely present at the initial examination. The physical examination should also detect the presence of other systemic diseases or extrapulmonary manifestations of the pulmonary infection.

The chest radiograph may provide some clues to the etiology of the respiratory tract infection. The presence of an infiltrate on the chest film will first distinguish pneumonia from bronchitis and, secondly, the pattern of the infiltrate will indicate the likely pathogens. Focal alveolar or lobar infiltrates suggest "typical" bacterial infection whereas diffuse interstitial or patchy infiltrates are more typical of viral, mycoplasmal, chlamydial, or other "atypical" pneumonic processes. Interestingly, a recent prospective study examining guidelines for ordering chest films in an emergency department demonstrated that no single symptom or sign was a reliable predictor of pneumonia [5]. Table 2 summarizes radiographic as well as other features of these two pneumonia "syndromes."

Sputum studies should be performed on all patients with suspected pneumonia. The nature of the sputum production can provide helpful clues to the etiology of the pneumonia. For examples, "rusty" sputum suggests *Streptococcus pneumoniae*, "foul smelling" sputum implies anaerobic bacteria, or "dry" cough may indicate an atypical agent of pneumonia such as *Mycoplasma pneumoniae* or *Legionella pneumophila*. Expectorated samples for Gram stain and culture will be reliable only if they contain large numbers of polymorphonuclear leukocytes, small numbers of epithelial cells, and mucus strands [6]. Additional sputum stains such as fluorescent antibody staining for *Legionella* or acid-fast staining for *Mycobacteria* should be obtained if clinically indicated. The value of sputum culture

TABLE 1 EPIDEMIOLOGIC ISSUES IMPORTANT IN THE EXAMINATION OF A PATIENT WITH OUTPATIENT PNEUMONIA

Recent travel
Exposure to animals and birds
Exposure to tuberculosis
Smoking history
Occupational hazards
High risk behavior for acquisition of HIV infection
Recent antibiotic administration
Recent hospitalization
History of similar illness in family members
    or household contacts

TABLE 2 CHARACTERISTICS OF BACTERIAL VERSUS "ATYPICAL" PNEUMONIA

	Type of Pneumonia	
Characteristic	Bacterial	"Atypical"
Age	Older	Younger
Presentation	Sudden onset	Insidious onset
Cough	Productive, purulent, or bloody sputum	Nonproductive, paroxysms
Myalgias, headache, photophobia	Not prominent	Prominent
Fever	High	Moderate
Rigors	Common	Rare
Pleuritic chest pain	Common	Rare
Physical findings	Dullness with bronchial or tubular breath sounds	Often minimal
Chest radiograph	Lobar consolidation	Patchy, interstitial
Effusion	May be large	Small, if present
Abscess	Rare	Rare
Leukocyte count	$> 15 \times 10^9 \backslash L$	$< 15 \times 10^9 \backslash L$

Adapted from Rodnick and Gude [4]; with permission.

remains controversial and may often be even misleading but should be obtained if the sputum sample is considered microscopically meaningful [7]. Culture on selective media such as charcoal yeast extract agar for *L. pneumophila* will need to be requested at the time of sputum collection.

Leukocyte count and blood cultures may provide useful information particularly if the patient is considered ill enough to warrant hospitalization. The leukocyte count and differential may help to distinguish between pneumonia of viral and bacterial cause. Total counts greater than 15,000 per μL often indicate a bacterial etiology [4]. Blood cultures are positive in 25% to 40% of patients with pneumococcal pneumonia but have a lower sensitivity for other types of bacterial pneumonia [2,4,8]. Other laboratory tests may be less meaningful during the initial evaluation. Tests for cold agglutinins, for example, are positive in up to 50% of patients with infection caused by *M. pneumoniae* [9]. This test is easy to perform, inexpensive, and provides rapid data but may have a low sensitivity and specificity especially early in the course [10]. Serology is also often very useful but requires acute and convalescent testing delaying the diagnosis and providing little information for initial management.

The most useful diagnostic tests for outpatients suspected of having pneumonia, therefore, are the chest radiograph, leukocyte count, and sputum Gram stain [4]. Other diagnostic tests such as blood cultures, special sputum stains and cultures, or serologies should be undertaken only if clearly clinically indicated, if the patient requires hospitalization, or if therapy fails.

INDICATIONS FOR HOSPITALIZATION

The major consideration in the treatment of a patient with pneumonia is the need for hospitalization, and this decision is based primarily on the severity of the patient's illness. Recent studies by several investigators have delineated risk factors associated with increased mortality from pneumonia (Table 3) [1,2,11,12]. Underlying conditions such as alcoholism,

congestive heart failure, diabetes mellitus, cancer, or other immunodeficiency (especially HIV infection) are also associated with a less favorable outcome. Under most circumstances, patients with any of these conditions should be initially treated in the hospital setting.

Additional indications for hospitalization include likely patient noncompliance, uncertain diagnosis, pulmonary cavitation or abscess, and extrapulmonary spread such as meningitis, septic arthritis, or endocarditis [3]. The availability of home intravenous therapy has made the need for parenteral antibiotics less of an issue when considering hospitalization. The patient who demonstrates a good clinical response to parenteral therapy, a stable chest film, no evidence of metastatic foci of infection, and absence of sepsis can be discharged on oral antibiotics or continue to receive parenteral therapy at home. Continued outpatient therapy after discharge mandates close patient follow-up to insure compliance and ongoing clinical improvement.

ETIOLOGIC AGENTS

Studies examining the infectious causes of community-acquired pneumonia in patients from the United States, France, the United Kingdom, and Sweden have recently been reviewed [4]. The spectrum of pathogens were similar for both inpatients and outpatients (Table 4). *S. pneumoniae* is the

TABLE 3 RISK FACTORS ASSOCIATED WITH INCREASED MORTALITY FROM PNEUMONIA
Advanced age
Male sex
Confusion
Fever (38.3° C)
Tachypnea (rate > 30/min)
Hypotension
Hypoxemia (O$_2$ saturation < 88%)
Leukopenia or pronounced leukocytosis
Bacteremia
Bilateral or multilobar infiltrates
Large pleural effusions
Staphylococcal or gram-negative infection
Steroids, cytotoxic drugs, or other immunosuppressive therapy

TABLE 4 ETIOLOGIC AGENTS OF COMMUNITY-ACQUIRED PNEUMONIAS
Bacterial or "typical" pneumonias
Streptococcus pneumoniae
Streptococcus pyogenes
Streptococcus agalactiae
Staphylococcus aureus
Haemophilus influenzae
Klebsiella pneumoniae
Proteus, Enterobacter, Pseudomonas, and other gram-negative bacilli (usually in hospitalized patients)
Legionella pneumophila
"Atypical" pneumonias
Mycoplasma pneumoniae
Chlamydia pneumoniae
Chlamydia psittaci
Legionella pneumophila
Other *Legionella* species
Francisella tularensis
Coxiella burnetti
Viruses
Mixed or aspiration pneumonias
Other
Mycobacterium tuberculosis
Histoplasma capsulatum
Blastomyces dermatitidis
Cryptococcus neoformans
Coccidioides immitis

most common pathogen in either setting accounting for 9% to 42% of cases. The second most commonly recognized organism was *M. pneumoniae* causing up to 36% of infections. Other agents included viruses, *Haemophilus influenzae*, *Chlamydia* species, *Legionella* species, *Staphylococcus aureus*, and gram-negative bacteria. Interestingly, no pathogen was identified in 45% to 51% of outpatients and 29% to 35% of inpatients. This disturbing inability to isolate a causative organism in a large proportion of patients has been confirmed by other investigators [13]. Additionally, as many as 10% of patients may have more than one pathogen [3].

Pneumonia caused by *S. pneumoniae* is the prototype of lobar pneumonia or "typical" bacterial pneumonia. The onset is usually abrupt with chills, fever, pleuritic chest pain, and the development over 6 to 24 hours of purulent sputum described as pinkish or "rusty" in color. The patient is usually acutely ill with obvious respiratory distress and findings on examination of consolidation. Chest radiographs show alveolar filling and lobar consolidation often with air bronchograms. Occasionally subsegmental infiltrates occur indicating bronchopneumonia. Pneumococcal pneumonia can be complicated by sepsis,

shock, respiratory failure, empyema, meningitis, septic arthritis, purulent pericarditis, and endocarditis. Other bacteria capable of causing a similar syndrome of acute lobar pneumonia include *Klebsiella pneumoniae*, other gram-negative bacilli, *S. aureus*, and *Streptococcus pyogenes* and *Streptococcus agalactiae*. These pathogens can be distinguished from each other during the initial stages of diagnosis based on the clinical setting, host factors, and Gram stains of sputum and pleural fluid (Fig. 1).

Haemophilus influenzae is a common cause of meningitis, otitis media, epiglottitis, and pneumonia in young children typically caused by encapsulated, type B strains. Bronchitis and pneumonia in adults caused by this agent is increasing and is primarily seen in patients with underlying chronic pulmonary disease or alcoholism. In contrast to children, many of the causative strains in adults are nontypeable and nonencapsulated. Community-acquired lobar pneumonia secondary to *K. pneumoniae* is virtually limited to adult patients with severe underlying problems such as alcoholism, diabetes mellitus, and chronic obstructive pulmonary disease. Pulmonary necrosis with development of cavitation, abscess formation, and empyema are common and sputum is

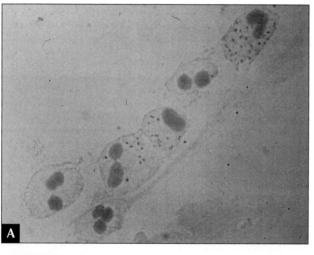
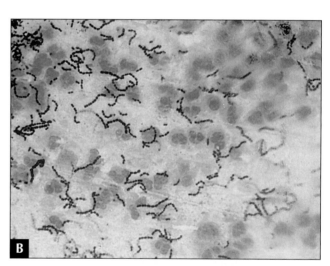
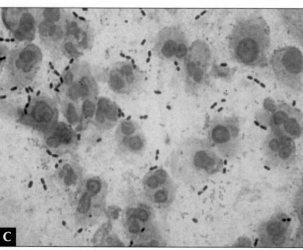
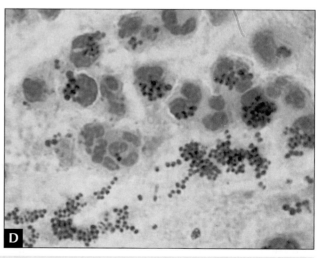

FIGURE 1 **A**, Gram-negative intracellular diplococci suggesting *Moraxella catarrhalis*. **B**, Gram-positive cocci in chains. This patient had pneumonia caused by group B beta-hemolytic streptococci. **C**, Mixed bacterial pneumonia. In addition to the gram- positive diplococci (*Streptococcus pneumoniae*), small gram-negative coccobacilli of *Haemophilus influenzae* are seen in the background. **D**, Gram-positive cocci in clumps in a patient with *Staphylococcus aureus* pneumonia.

described as "currant jelly" in nature. Other gram-negative bacilli capable of causing community-acquired pneumonia in debilitated hosts include *Enterobacter* species, *Serratia marcescens*, and *Pseudomonas aeruginosa*. These organisms, however, more typically cause hospital-acquired pneumonia. *Moraxella catarrhalis* is a gram-negative diplococcus capable of causing exacerbations of chronic bronchitis or pneumonia in patients with underlying pulmonary disease [14].

Aspiration pneumonia in the community usually is caused by *Bacteroides melaninogenicus* and other oral anaerobes and is seen in the setting of a patient who is obtunded or has a defective cough reflex. Primarily, inhalation pneumonia due to *S. aureus* in the community usually occurs after influenza or in the setting of obstruction caused by bronchogenic carcinoma. It has a high propensity to develop abscesses and pleural empyema. Hematogenous pneumonia secondary to *S. aureus* is associated with endocarditis or high-grade bacteremia. Pneumonia due to *S. pyogenes* is rare and is usually the complication of influenza, measles, varicella, or chronic pulmonary disease.

Mycoplasma pneumoniae is the classic cause of the "atypical" pneumonia syndrome [15,16]. The term "atypical pneumonia" was first used in 1938 to describe tracheobronchopneumonia and severe systemic symptoms, which are often more prominent than the respiratory complaints. Other pathogens capable of causing atypical pneumonia include *Chlamydia pneumoniae*, *Chlamydia psittaci*, *L. pneumophila*, *Coxiella burnetti*, and *Francisella tularensis*. A number of viruses, including influenze A and B, adenovirus, and respiratory syncytial virus, have also been associated with this syndrome.

Mycoplasma pneumoniae causes mild pneumonia, tracheobronchitis, and pharyngitis with gradual onset of illness associated with headache, malaise, low-grade fever, and an intractable, nonproductive cough in 90% to 100% of patients. Patients may also experience chest pain due to protracted coughing, pharyngitis with cervical adenopathy, sinusitis, and hemorrhagic bullous myringitis. Chest radiograph usually reveals unilateral segmental pneumonia of the lower lobes but can be complicated by multilobe and lobar involvement, pleural effusions, abscess, pneumatocele formation, hilar adenopathy, and diffuse pulmonary infiltrates. Sputum Gram stain will show polymorphonuclear leukocytes, mononuclear cells, and no organisms.

Extrapulmonary manifestations of *M. pneumoniae* infection are often noted and of varied severity [16]. Hemolytic anemia is a complication of IgM antibodies directed against the I antigen of the erythrocyte membrane (cold hemagglutination production). Reported complications of the central nervous system include aseptic meningitis, meningoencephalitis, transverse myelitis, neuropathies, cerebrovascular thrombosis, cerebellar ataxia, cranial nerve palsies, and sensorineural hearing loss. Stevens-Johnson syndrome and other dermatologic manifestations have been noted and cardiac complications, including myopericarditis, have been reported.

Definitive diagnosis of *M. pneumoniae* infection is made by either isolation of the organism by culture on artificial media or demonstration of an appropriate serologic response. A fourfold or greater rise in specific antibody on complement fixation testing is the most common diagnostic modality. Cold agglutinin titers may be helpful but may also be positive in cases of rubella, infectious mononucleosis, adenovirus infections, influenza, psittacosis, peripheral vascular disease, and illnesses associated with dysproteinemias [16].

A recently recognized human respiratory pathogen is *C. pneumoniae*, which causes up to 10% of all cases of pneumonia [15,17]. It causes a mild respiratory illness in teenagers and young adults that may be biphasic. Patients may have severe pharyngitis often with hoarseness followed by a subsegmental pneumonitis 1 to 3 weeks later. Bronchitis, sinusitis, and pharyngitis may all occur in the absence of pneumonia. In adults, symptoms of this pneumonia are difficult to distinguish from other lower respiratory tract infections. A more severe, even fatal, illness may occur in the elderly, especially those with underlying illnesses. Definitive diagnosis of *C. pneumoniae* infections requires either isolation of the organism on culture or an appropriate serologic response.

Psittacosis, caused by *C. psittaci*, is a worldwide zoonosis [15]. Parrots are the main reservoir but almost any bird species is capable of hosting the organism. It is a systemic illness associated with high fever followed by severe headache, myalgias, nonexudative pharyngitis, and epistaxis. Pulmonary complaints, especially a persistent cough, become the most predominant features often complicated by tachypnea, pleuritic chest pain, hemoptysis, pleural rub, and severe pneumonia with the potential for acute respiratory failure. Reported extrapulmonary complications consist of rash (Horder's spots), erythema nodosum, disseminated intravascular coagulation, splenomegaly, encephalitis with seizures, hemolytic anemia, endocarditis, pericarditis, hepatitis, pancreatitis, acute renal failure, and reactive arthritis. Definitive diagnosis is established with an appropriate serologic response.

Legionella pneumophila can cause a wide spectrum of clinical illness ranging from a mild, self-limited atypical pneumonia to potentially fatal pulmonary and opportunistic infection in immunocompromised hosts [18]. Extrapulmonary manifestations are common. Nausea, vomiting, diarrhea, abdominal pain, confusion, and renal dysfunction, according to some studies, may be helpful clues to the diagnosis. The definitive diagnosis is made by isolation of the organism on charcoal yeast extract agar. Direct fluorescent antibody testing and DNA probes of sputum samples have been shown to be helpful diagnostic tools. *Legionella* antigen can also be detected in the urine with high sensitivity and specificity. Serologic tests are also available but are less important in the setting of cultures and special stains.

Q fever is a zoonotic clinical illness caused by the rickettsial pathogen *C. burnetti* [15]. The most common reservoirs are sheep, goats, cattle, and ticks. This organism is a highly contagious primary respiratory pathogen capable of causing three distinct pulmonary presentations: atypical pneumonia, rapidly progressive pneumonia, and an asymptomatic infiltrate in a febrile patient. The organism can also cause endocarditis, hepatomegaly with jaundice and granulomatous hepatitis, hemolytic anemia, myopericarditis, optic neuritis, uveitis, iritis, neuropathy, meningitis, encephalitis, osteomyelitis, and glomerular nephropathy. Diagnosis is usually based on serologic data given that the isolation of *C. burnetti* is difficult and hazardous.

Many viruses are capable of producing upper and lower respiratory infections including adenoviruses, influenza viruses, respiratory syncytial virus, and parainfluenza viruses. Influenza is an important predisposing factor for the development of bacterial pneumonia, particularly *S. pneumoniae, H. influenzae,* and *S. aureus.* Other organisms ranging from *Mycobacterium tuberculosis* to fungi (*Histoplasma capsulatum, Blastomyces dermatitidis, Cryptococcus neoformans,* and *Coccidioides immitis*) will cause community-acquired pulmonary infections in the appropriate setting and host.

OUTPATIENT THERAPY

In addition to the initiation of appropriate antibiotics for all patients suspected of having a treatable pneumonia, there are certain general principles of management that should be implemented. Expectorants may loosen sputum and adequate hydration will help to clear secretions. Cough suppressants may be beneficial in patients with severe paroxysms of coughing that produce respiratory fatigue or pleuritic and chest wall pain. Fever can be controlled with aspirin or acetaminophen given regularly. Oxygen therapy may be indicated for hypoxemia but these patients are usually better monitored in the hospital setting.

Antibiotics for the outpatient treatment of pneumonia are outlined in Table 5. Most of the antibiotics listed are standard agents that have been historically proven to be effective. Newer agents, however, have been developed and will receive specific mention.

New macrolide agents, clarithromycin and azithromycin, are similar in structure to erythromycin [19]. Compared with erythromycin, clarithromycin has increased activity against streptococci, *S. aureus, L. pneumophila, M. catarrhalis,* and *Chlamydia trachomatis.* It also has *in vitro* activity against *Mycobacterium avium* complex and *Toxoplasma gondii.* Gastrointestinal side effects are less common when compared with erythromycin therapy. Azithromycin, when compared with erythromycin, has increased gram-negative activity against *H. influenzae* while maintaining gram-positive activity. Initial data demonstrate that these drugs are effective in the treatment of upper and lower respiratory tract infections and may be appropriate for the outpatient treatment of community-acquired pneumonia. The role of these agents will be better defined as results of clinical trials become available for evaluation.

Fluoroquinolones have also received recent attention as potential agents for the treatment of outpatient pneumonia [20–22]. These agents probably have a limited role in the treatment of community-acquired pneumonia because established antibiotic regimens have proven so effective. Additionally, most quinolones have poor activity against *S. pneumoniae,* the most common cause of community-acquired pneumonia.

TABLE 5 ANTIBIOTIC THERAPY FOR PNEUMONIA IN OUTPATIENTS*		
Organism	**Drug of choice**	**Alternative drugs**
Streptococcus pneumoniae (pneumococcus)	Penicillin	Cephalosporins
Streptococcus pyogenes		Erythromycin
Streptococcus agalactiae		Clindamycin
Haemophilus influenzae	Amoxicillin	TMP-SMX
	Amoxicillin-clavulanic acid	Tetracycline
	(If β-lactamase positive)	Cefaclor
		Cefuroxime axetil
		Ciprofloxacin
Moraxella catarrhalis	Amoxicillin-clavulanic acid	TMP-SMX
		Tetracycline
		Cefaclor
		Cefuroxime axetil
		Ciprofloxacin
		Erythromycin
Legionella pneumophila	Erythromycin	TMP-SMX
	± Rifampin	Clarithromycin
Mycoplasma pneumoniae	Erythromycin	Azithromycin
Chlamydia pneumoniae	Erythromycin	Tetracycline
Chlamydia psittaci	Tetracycline	Tetracycline
Coxiella burnetti (Q fever)	Tetracycline	
Mixed or aspiration pneumonias	Clindamycin	Amoxicillin-clavulanic acid

*Antibiotic choice should always be based on available antimicrobial susceptibility data.
TMP-SMX—trimethoprim-sulfamethoxazole.

The gram-stained sputum sample and chest radiographs provide the best guides for instituting therapy in the outpatient setting (Table 6). Empiric combination therapy may be necessary to cover all potential organisms. The newer macrolides, because of broader spectrum, may provide single agent coverage in this setting.

Amantadine is an effective therapeutic agent in appraising influenza A if begun within 1 to 2 days of symptoms. More rapid defervescence and improvement in peripheral airway disease have been demonstrated in controlled studies. The use of aerosolized ribavirin in children with respiratory syncytial virus disease has been shown to reduce viral shedding and improve symptoms. Effects on mortality in life-threatening disease of the elderly are not well documented.

PATIENT FOLLOW-UP

Patients treated in the outpatient setting for pneumonia must be carefully monitored to ensure compliance and clinical improvement. Telephone contact with the patient or a return clinic visit within 48 to 72 hours is mandatory. Failure to improve indicates a need for reassessment and probable hospitalization. Patients who show good clinical response should be scheduled, after an appropriate length of therapy, for a return appointment to document clinical cure.

Resolution of pneumonia on chest radiograph may take 6 to 16 weeks especially in patients with underlying obstructive pulmonary disease. Failure of chest radiograph to return to normal indicates the need for further studies looking for endobronchial lesions, tuberculosis, or another secondary process. Repeat blood work and sputum testing are usually not indicated unless the patient fails to respond to therapy. Many patients with pneumonia will be discharged from the hospital to continue therapy as outpatients. They should be monitored in a similar fashion.

PREVENTION

Elderly patients, residents of long-term care facilities, or those with chronic cardiac, pulmonary, renal, or hematologic illnesses are candidates for the influenza vaccine each year. It is protective in 70% to 80% of cases but less than 20% of those eligible patients are immunized each year [7]. A single dose of the 23-valent pneumococcal vaccine is likewise indicated for the same patients. Patients with asplenia, sickle cell anemia, multiple myeloma, cirrhosis, and cerebrospinal fluid leaks should also receive the vaccine. It appears to reduce the risk of pneumococcal pneumonia in 60% to 80% of healthy elderly persons but may be less effective in those with underlying conditions [23].

TABLE 6 USE OF SPUTUM GRAM STAIN IN SELECTION OF ANTIBIOTIC THERAPY IN OUTPATIENT PNEUMONIA

Gram stain result	Organism suspected	Empiric antibiotic selection[†]
Neutrophils and gram-positive lancet-shaped diplococci	Pneumococci	Penicillin (erythromycin)[‡]
Neutrophils and small gram-negative rods	Haemophilus influenzae	Amoxicillin, amoxicillin-clavulanic acid if β-lactamase suspected (TMP-SMX)[‡]
Few leukocytes, no predominant organism	Viral, mycoplasmal, chlamydial, or other "atypical" pneumonia	Erythromycin (tetracycline)[‡]
Neutrophils and gram-negative diplococci	Moraxella catarrhalis	TMP-SMX
Neutrophils and large gram-positive cocci in clusters	Staphylococcus aureus	Amoxicillin-clavulanic acid
Neutrophils and gram-negative rods	Gram-negative	Admit for intravenous therapy Naficillin (vancomycin)[‡]
Neutrophils and mixed flora	Unclear type, suspect possible anaerobic pneumonia in appropriate clinical setting	Admit for intravenous therapy TMP-SMX plus metronidazole or amoxicillin-clavulanic acid or clindamycin

Adapted from Rodnick and Gude [4]; with permission.
[†]Refer also to Table 3.
[‡]Parentheses represent alternative empiric antibiotic selection.
TMP-SMX—trimethoprim-sulfamethoxazole.

References and Recommended Reading

Recently published papers of particular interest have been highlighted as:
* Of interest
** Of outstanding interest

1. Fine MJ, Smith DN, Singer DE: Hospitalization decision in patients with community-acquired pneumonia: a prospective cohort study. Am J Med 1990, 89:713–721.

2. British Thoracic Society Research Committee: Community-acquired pneumonia in adults in British hospitals in 1982–1983: a survey of aetiology, mortality, prognostic factors and outcomes. Q J Med 1987, 62:195–220.

3. Brown RB: Community-acquired pneumonia: diagnosis and therapy of older adults. Geriatrics 1993, 48:43–50.

4. Rodnick JE, Gude JK: Diagnosis and antibiotic treatment of community-acquired pneumonia. West J Med 1991, 154:405–409.

5. Gennis P, Gallagher J, Falvo C, et al.: Clinical criteria for the detection of pneumonia in adults: guidelines for ordering chest roentgenograms in the emergency department. J Emerg Med 1989, 7:263–268.

6. Geckler RW, Grellion DH, McAllister CK, et al.: Microscopic and bacteriologic comparison of paired sputa and transtracheal aspirates. J Clin Microbiol 1977, 6:396–399.

7. LaForce FM: Community-acquired lower respiratory tract infections—prevention and cost control strategies. Am J Med 1985, 78(suppl 6B):52–57.

8. Levy M, Dromer F, Brion N, et al.: Community-acquired pneumonia—importance of initial noninvasive bacteriologic and radiographic Investigations. Chest 1988, 92:43–48.

9. Levine DP, Lerner AM: The clinical spectrum of *Mycoplasma pneumoniae* infections. Med Clin North Am 1978, 62:961–978.

10. Mansel JK, Rosenow EC III, Smith TF, et al.: Mycoplasma pneumoniae pneumonia. Chest 1989, 95:639–646.

11. Siegel D: Management of community-acquired pneumonia in outpatients. West J Med 1985, 142:45–48.

12. Marrie TJ, Durant H, Yates L: Community-acquired pneumonia requiring hospitalization: 5-year prospective study. Rev Infect Dis 1989, 11:586–599.

13. Bates JH, Campbell GD, Barron AL, et al.: Microbial etiology of acute pneumonia in hospitalized patients. Chest 1992, 101:1005–1012.

14.• Verghese A, Berk SL: Moraxella (Branhamella) catarrhalis. Infect Dis Clin North Am 1991, 5:523–538.

15.• Martin RE, Bates JH: Atypical pneumonia. Infect Dis Clin North Am 1991, 5:585–601.

16. Murray HW, Masur H, Senterfit LB, et al.: The protean manifestations of Mycoplasma pneumoniae infection in adults. Am J Med 1975, 229:240.

17. Grayston JT, Diwan VK, Cooney M, et al.: Community- and hospital-acquired pneumonia associated with Chlamydia TWAR infection demonstrated serologically. Arch Intern Med 1989, 149:169–173.

18. Nguyen MH, Stout JE, Yu VL: Legionellosis. Infect Dis Clin North Am 1991, 5:561–584.

19. Piscitelli SC, Danziger LH, Rodvold KA: Clarithromycin and azithromycin: new macrolide antibiotics. Clin Pharm 1992, 11:137–152.

20. Peugeot RL, Lipsky BA, Hooton TM, et al.: Treatment of lower respiratory infections in outpatients with ofloxacin compared with erythromycin. Drugs Exp Clin Res 1991, 17:253–257.

21. Chodosh S: Temafloxacin compared with ciprofloxacin in mild to moderate lower respiratory tract infections in ambulatory patients. A multicenter, double-blind, randomized study. Chest 1991, 100:1497–1502.

22. Bayer AS: Clinical utility of new quinolones in treatment of osteomyelitis and lower respiratory tract infections. Eur J Clin Microbiol Infect Dis 1989, 8:1102–1110.

23. Broome CV, Facklam RR, Fraser DW: Pneumococcal disease after pneumococcal vaccination: an alternative method to estimate the efficacy of pneumococcal vaccine. N Engl J Med 1980, 303:549–552.

Select Bibliography

Brown RB: Management of pneumonia in outpatients. In *Infections in Outpatient Practice, Recognition and Management.* Edited by Gleckman RA, Gantz NM, Brown RB. New York and London: Plenum Medical Book Company; 1988:89–100.

Mandell GL, Douglas RG, Bennett JE: *Principles and Practice of Infectious Diseases,* edn 3. New York, Edinburgh, London, Melbourne: Churchill Livingstone; 1990.

Simon HB: Approach to the patient with acute bronchitis or pneumonia in the ambulatory setting. In *Primary Care Medicine,* edn 2. Edited by Goroll AH, May LA, Mulley AG Jr. Philadelphia: JB Lippincott Company; 1987:206–213.

Tillotson JR: Pneumonia. In *Current Therapy in Infectious Diseases-3.* Edited by Kass EH, Platt R. Toronto and Philadelphia: BC Decker Inc.; 1990:105–118.

Wallace RJ, ed: Lower Respiratory Tract Infections. *Infect Dis Clin North Am* 1991, 5:437–738.

Winterbauer RH: Atypical pneumonia syndromes. *Clin Chest Med* 1991, 12:203–413.

Infections of the Sinuses, Pharynx, and Larynx

Wafeeq A. Mahmood
Anthony W. Chow

6

Key Points

- The clinical presentation and microbial etiology of acute and chronic sinusitis are vastly different, as are the goals of management. Nasal cultures are misleading and should not be used to guide antimicrobial therapy.

- The throat culture remains the gold standard for the diagnosis of group A streptococcal pharyngitis. However, a positive culture is not always correlated with clinical infection because the carrier rate of group A streptococci in healthy individuals approaches 20%.

- The presentation and clinical course of epiglottitis in adults is different from that in children, in whom the disease is more acute in onset and fulminant in nature.

- All patients suspected of acute epiglottitis should be admitted to the hospital for careful monitoring, preferably in an intensive care unit.

The paranasal sinuses (maxillary, frontal, anterior and posterior ethmoid, and sphenoid) are a group of air-containing spaces that are lined with pseudocolumnar ciliated epithelium and drain through the ostia into the nasal cavity (Fig. 1). Sinusitis affects an estimated 3.5 million Americans per year. Most infections occur within the sinuses that open into the middle meatus between the lower and middle turbinates (maxillary, anterior ethmoid, and frontal). Interestingly, the middle meatus bears the major part of the inspiratory nasal airflow causing many inspired particles to impact there. The ciliated epithelial lining of the sinuses is contiguous with the nasal cavity. The cilia beat towards the ostia, effectively propelling antral contents toward this opening and clearing the sinus. Conditions that impair this activity ultimately result in microbial invasion and suppuration. Factors leading to the production of sinus-related symptoms include mucosal inflammation with sinus ostial obstruction (barotrauma, mucosal hypertrophy, vasomotor and allergic rhinitis, or viral upper respiratory tract infections), defects in mucociliary clearance (Kartagener's syndrome, cystic fibrosis, IgA deficiency, ciliary dysmotility, or idiopathic), colonization by abnormal organisms (immunodeficiency states [including AIDS], collagen vascular disease, or instrumentation), and structural abnormalities and mechanical obstruction (choanal atresia, nasal polyps or tumors, deviated nasal septum, foreign body, or trauma) [1]. Obstruction or reduction in the patency of the ostia appears to be the most important factor. Dental extraction or periapical infections of the maxillary molar teeth are particularly important causes of maxillary and chronic sinusitis.

Etiology

The paranasal sinuses are considered to be sterile, although transient colonization by the resident upper respiratory flora does occur. Most cases of acute purulent sinusitis result from bacterial causes (Table 1) [2••]. *Streptococcus pneumoniae* and *Haemophilus influenzae* account for over 50% of all cases of acute maxillary sinusitis in adults. Obligate anaerobes and *Staphylococcus aureus*, a common nasal contaminant, are

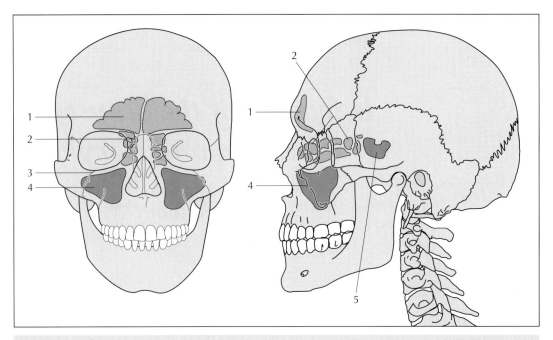

FIGURE 1 Paranasal sinuses. Frontal view (**left**) and sagittal view (**right**). 1) Frontal sinus, 2) ethmoid sinus, 3) maxillary ostium, 4) maxillary sinus, and 5) sphenoid sinus.

infrequent causes of acute sinusitis. Although an antecedent viral upper respiratory infection is an important predisposing cause of acute sinusitis, viruses are isolated infrequently in antral aspirates [3•].

Acute sphenoid sinusitis differs from maxillary sinusitis in that streptococci and *S. aureus* are the major pathogens, followed by pneumococci and *H. influenzae*. Nosocomial sinusitis secondary to prolonged nasotracheal intubation is commonly caused by polymicrobial gram-negative bacilli (*Pseudomonas aeruginosa, Klebsiella pneumoniae, Escherichia coli,* and *Proteus mirabilis*), *S. aureus,* as well as anaerobes [4••].

The microbiology of chronic sinusitis is usually polymicrobial, with *Bacteroides, Peptostreptococcus, Fusobacterium,* and *Veillonella* spp being the predominant anaerobic isolates, whereas viridans streptococci and nonencapsulated *H. influenzae* are the major facultative isolates. Fungal sinusitis is rare, but *Aspergillus, Mucor, Candida, Pseudallescheria boydii,* and other saprophytic fungi may cause invasive disease—usually in the debilitated host.

Clinical Presentation

Acute sinusitis is clinically defined as infection with symptoms and signs existing less than 1 month, chronic sinusitis

Pathogen	Mean percentage of cases (range)	
	Adults	**Children**
Bacteria		
Streptococcus pneumoniae	31 (20–35)	36
Haemophilus influenzae (unencapsulated)	21 (6–26)	23
Staphylococcus pneumoniae and *Haemophilus influenzae*	5 (1–9)	—
Anaerobes (*Bacteroides, Fusobacterium, Peptostreptococcus, Veillonella*)	6 (0–10)	—
Staphylococcus aureus	4 (0–8)	—
Streptococcus pyogenes	2 (1–3)	2
Moraxella catarrhalis	2	19
Gram-negative bacteria	9 (0–24)	2
Viruses		
Rhinovirus, adenovirus, influenza, parainfluenza	3–15	0–2

TABLE 1 MICROBIAL CAUSES OF ACUTE MAXILLARY SINUSITIS

From Chow and coworkers [2••]; with permission.

as symptoms and signs existing more than 3 months, and subacute sinusitis as symptoms and signs existing between 1 and 3 months. Symptoms of acute sinusitis include nasal obstruction, nasal discharge (initially clear, later turning cloudy), postnasal drainage (nausea, productive cough, halitosis), facial pain exacerbated by straining and leaning forward, headache (forehead in frontal sinusitis, suboccipital in sphenoid sinusitis, and retroorbital in ethmoid sinusitis), fever (less than 50% of cases), malaise, popping sounds in ears, and muffled hearing. Also, other signs of acute sinusitis to look for include tenderness over the involved sinus, edema of the soft tissue overlying the affected sinus, visible pus in the nares or nasopharynx, and the presence of edema and hyperemia of the nasal mucosa or purulent discharge from ostial openings observed during rhinoscopy. Symptoms associated with chronic sinusitis are usually less intense but are more protracted. Fever is uncommon, whereas fatigue, general malaise, and an ill-defined feeling of unwellness and irritability are more prominent. A chronic nonproductive cough may be present.

In maxillary sinusitis, the findings of caries and signs of associated infection may suggest a dental source for the sinusitis. In ethmoid sinusitis, edema of the eyelids and excessive tearing are present. Swelling of the periorbital tissues, proptosis, or limitation of extraocular movement may occur in more fulminant cases, suggesting the possibility of an orbital extension of infection [5•].

Sphenoid sinusitis is rare but can be disastrous if recognition is delayed. The sphenoid sinus lies in close proximity to the dura, optic nerves, pituitary gland, and cavernous sinus (Fig. 2) [6]. Sphenoid sinusitis is often misdiagnosed as ophthalmic migraine, aseptic meningitis, cavernous sinus thrombosis, trigeminal neuralgia, or retroorbital tumor. Headache is the most common initial symptom, and one third of patients have hypo- or hyperaesthesia of the ophthalmic or maxillary branches of the fifth cranial nerve [5•].

Nosocomial sinusitis may be relatively silent except for unexplained fever [4••]. Sinusitis in HIV-infected patients is common. Patients with a CD4 count less than 200/mm³ are prone to infection involving multiple sinuses that respond incompletely to antibiotic therapy, often resulting in chronic sinusitis [7]. Complications of acute and chronic sinusitis are summarized in Table 2.

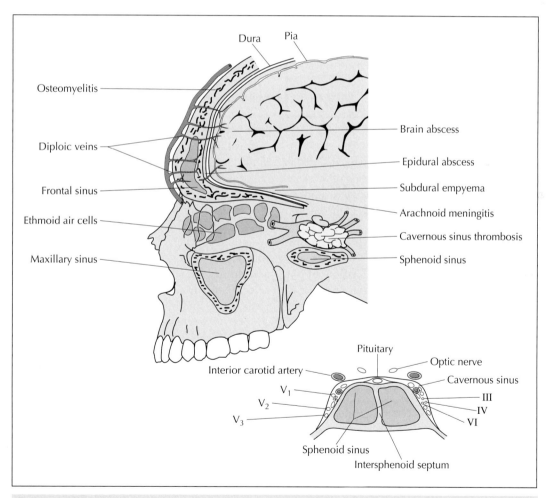

FIGURE 2 Major routes for intracranial extension of infection, directly or via the vascular supply. The coronal section demonstrates the structures adjoining the sphenoid sinus. (*From* Vortel and Chow [6]; with permission.)

TABLE 2 COMPLICATIONS OF ACUTE AND CHRONIC SINUSITIS

General
Facial and orbital cellulitis or abscess
Cranial osteomyelitis
Cavernous sinus thrombosis
Subdural or epidural empyema
Intracerebral abscess
Acute bacterial meningitis

Specific
Maxillary sinuses
    Osteomyelitis of anterior orbital plate
    Infection of parapharyngeal and infratemporal spaces
    Pneumonia and lung abscess
Frontal and ethmoid sinuses
    Osteomyelitis of the frontal bone
    Frontal subperiosteal abscess (Potts' puffy tumor)
    Orbital cellulitis
Sphenoid
    Ptosis
    Ophthalmoplegia
    Diplopia
    Proptosis
    Decreased visual acuity

TABLE 3 LABORATORY DIAGNOSIS OF SINUS INFECTION	
Procedure	**Application**
Transillumination	Maxillary and frontal sinusitis
Radiography	Mainstay procedure for the diagnosis of sinus infection
Computed tomography or magnetic resonance imaging	Complicated sinusitis, ethmoid and sphenoid sinusitis
Sinus aspiration and culture	Microbic etiology in the following situations: Complicated sinusitis Failure of empiric antimicrobial therapy Severe immunosuppression Nosocomial sinusitis in nasally intubated patients
Endoscopic sinoscopy	Chronic and complicated sinusitis

Laboratory Diagnosis

Various diagnostic procedures and their applications are listed in Table 3. The finding of normal light transmission of the sinus on transillumination is good evidence for the absence of infection. Conversely, the finding of complete opacity of the sinus on transillumination correlates strongly with active infection. Transillumination is less helpful in patients with chronic sinusitis because of persistent mucosal abnormalities.

Standard four-view radiographic examination of the paranasal sinuses may demonstrate air fluid levels, mucosal thickening, or opacification of the sinus that correlates well with active infection.

Computed tomography and magnetic resonance imaging are especially valuable in the evaluation of neoplasms and complicated infections that have extended beyond the sinuses, such as osteomyelitis, periorbital extension, and intracranial suppuration. They are also useful for examination of the ethmoid and sphenoid sinuses, which are not well visualized by standard radiography [8].

Culture of nasal pus or sinus exudate obtained by irrigation is unreliable because of contamination by the indigenous nasal flora. Sinus aspiration remains the gold standard for establishing the microbic etiology [2••]. However, it is debatable whether sinus aspiration needs to be performed in every patient with sinusitis because the microbial etiology of acute maxillary sinusitis is well characterized and relatively predictable in most immunocompetent patients. Indications for sinus aspiration and culture are summarized in Table 3. Quantitative cultures are useful in distinguishing colonization or contamination from true infection. Bacterial titers of 10^4 colony forming units per mL or greater generally correlate well with active sinus infection.

Endoscopic sinoscopy allows direct visualization of the sinus mucosa, appropriate microbiologic sampling, and histopathologic evaluation [9]. It also facilitates drainage by limited resections to relieve ostial obstruction.

Treatment

The goals of antimicrobial therapy for acute sinusitis are 1) eradication of the causative pathogens, 2) provision of symptomatic relief, 3) restoration and improvement of sinus function, and 4) prevention of intracranial complications and chronic sequelae. Initial antimicrobial therapy is usually selected empirically and directed against the most likely pathogens, including *H. influenzae*, *S. pneumoniae*, and *Moraxella catarrhalis*. An oral regimen with a β-lactam antibiotic such as ampicillin or amoxicillin for 10 to 14 days is generally considered standard therapy for acute sinusitis in both children and adults. A favorable clinical response rate of 70% to 80% can be expected [2••,10]. In penicillin-allergic patients, a second-generation cephalosporin, a new macrolide, or trimethoprim-sulfamethoxazole are alternatives that provide adequate coverage against *S. pneumoniae*, *H. influenzae*, and *M. catarrhalis*. Penicillin plus a β-lactam inhibitor or extended-spectrum cephalosporins have not yielded superior results in controlled trials of acute maxillary sinusitis, even though the prevalence of β-lactamase-producing strains among respiratory pathogens appears to be increasing (up to 20% of *H. influenzae* strains, 50% to 70% of *M. catarrhalis* strains, and 20% to 30% of respiratory anaerobes) [2••]. In addition to antibiotic therapy, nasal decongestants are useful in acute sinusitis to reduce antral swelling and increase the ostial diameter.

The role of anti-infective agents in chronic sinusitis is not as clear as that in acute sinusitis. Conservative antimicrobial therapy and sinus irrigations without surgical intervention are successful in only one third of cases. Surgery is performed to facilitate sinus drainage through the creation of an artificial ostium and submucosal resection of diseased tissue. With combined medical and surgical treatment, the cure rate for chronic maxillary sinusitis is greater than 60% after 3 years of follow-up. Anti-infective agents useful for chronic sinusitis should have broad-spectrum activity against respiratory anaerobes as well as viridans streptococci, *S. pneumoniae*, *H. influenzae*, and *M. catarrhalis*.

Nosocomial sinusitis in patients with prolonged transnasal intubation should be strongly suspected and presumed to be present if concurrent purulent rhinorrhea or otitis media is also present. In such patients, the nasal tube should be removed, and broad-spectrum antibiotics, as well as nasal decongestants, should be initiated while the search continues for other causes of fever. If fever persists and no other cause is found, a computed tomography scan of the paranasal sinuses should be obtained. If computed tomography reveals evidence of sinusitis, maxillary sinus aspiration

should be performed and additional antibiotic therapy initiated based on culture results (Fig. 3) [11]. Empiric antibiotic therapy for patients with nosocomial sinusitis should include agents that are active against gram-negative rods and staphylococci, as well as anaerobes.

Specific antimicrobial therapy for fungal sinusitis is required only if the disease is invasive or the patient is severely immunocompromised and the risk of progressive disease is high. Noninvasive disease usually responds to surgical débridement alone. Most patients with invasive disease should be treated with amphotericin B in cumulative doses exceeding 2 g. The role of azole antifungal agents (*eg*, fluconazole or itraconazole) for invasive fungal sinusitis remains unclear at present.

When to Refer

Patients with complicated sinusitis that has extended beyond the sinuses should be hospitalized for aggressive evaluation; ear, nose, and throat consultation; and parenteral antibiotic therapy. In patients with chronic sinusitis, surgical procedures to facilitate sinus drainage through the creation of an artificial ostium and submucosal resection of diseased tissue are the mainstays of treatment. Patients with fixed anatomic obstructions, such as deviated nasal septum or nasal polyps, may require surgical correction if sinusitis becomes recurrent.

PHARYNGITIS AND TONSILLITIS

Pharyngitis is one of the most common medical problems that brings patients to physicians' offices and is a significant cause of absence from work. Table 4 shows the most common infectious and noninfectious causes of pharyngitis [12•].

Etiology

Respiratory viruses are by far the most common infectious causes of pharyngitis (Table 4) [12•]. Among bacterial pathogens, group A β-hemolytic streptococci remains the most important (95% in pharyngitis and as high as 38% in acute tonsillitis). *Mycoplasma pneumoniae* and *Chlamydia pneumoniae* (TWAR) are recognized as important causative agents in pharyngitis in both children and adults [12•]. *H. influenzae* affects pediatric patients predominantly and only rarely causes pharyngitis in adults. Pharyngeal and tonsillar infection associated with a mixture of anaerobic bacteria and spirochetes can occur rarely as a complication of acute necrotizing gingivitis (*ie*, Vincent's angina or "trench mouth"). *Candida albicans*, which is part of the normal flora, can produce painful oropharyngeal thrush and esophagitis, usually in immunosuppressed patients receiving steroids or antibiotics.

Peritonsillar abscess (quinsy) is a complication of tonsillitis most often seen in adolescents and young adults. Although group A streptococci are the primary pathogens, anaerobic microorganisms such as *Bacteroides*, *Fusobacterium*, and *Peptostreptococcus* spp are commonly implicated.

In about one third of patients with pharyngitis or tonsillitis, a microbial etiology is not detected despite the use of

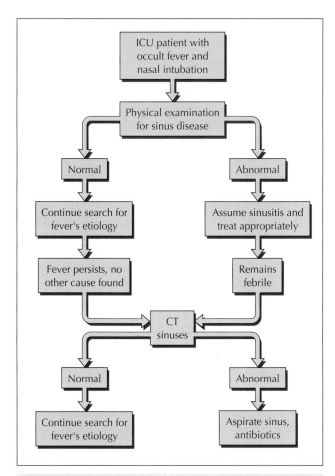

FIGURE 3 Algorithm for the treatment of intensive care unit (ICU) patients with occult fever and nasal intubation. (*From* Deresinski [11]; with permission.)

TABLE 4 ETIOLOGY OF PHARYNGITIS

Selective infectious causes

Bacterial

    Group A streptococcus (*Streptococcus pyogenes*)

    Non-group A streptococcus (Group C and G)

    Mycoplasma pneumoniae

    Chlamydia pneumoniae (TWAR strain)

    Corynebacterium hemolyticum

    Corynebacterium diphtheriae

    Haemophilus influenzae

    Neisseria gonorrhoeae

    Neisseria meningitidis

    Treponema pallidum

    Anaerobes (Vincent's angina)

Fungal

    Candida albicans (moniliasis)

Viral

    Rhinovirus

    Influenza and parainfluenza

    Adenovirus (pharyngoconjunctival fever)

    Coxsackie A (herpangina)

    Herpes simplex virus

    Epstein-Barr virus

    Cytomegalovirus

    HIV

Selective noninfectious causes

Pemphigus vulgaris

Aphthous stomatitis

Erythema multiforme

Neutropenia

Systemic lupus erythematosus

From Vukmir [12•]; with permission.

tococcal pharyngitis. It should always be suspected in a homosexual man or any patient who has symptoms of a urogenital infection. *H. influenzae* pharyngitis is very painful and usually associated with otitis media, laryngotracheitis, or epiglottitis—a life-threatening complication. *Corynebacterium hemolyticum* has been associated with a syndrome of pharyngitis associated with a scarlatiniform erythematous rash particularly in teenagers and young adults. Diphtheria caused by *Corynebacterium diphtheriae* is characterized by a "bull neck" with anterior cervical lymphadenopathy and a grey membrane that is firmly adherent to the tonsil and pharyngeal mucosa. Myocarditis, cranial nerve paralysis, and peripheral neuropathy may be present. Vincent's angina is characterized by odynophagia and fetid breath associated with gingivobuccal ulceration, membranous exudate, and submandibular lymphadenopathy.

Viral pharyngitis is usually associated with upper respiratory tract symptoms such as cough and rhinorrhea. On examination, the pharynx may show mild erythema and edema, but pharyngeal and tonsillar exudates and cervical lymphadenopathy are usually absent. Infectious mononucleosis resulting from Epstein-Barr virus (EBV) is characterized by exudative pharyngitis or tonsillitis associated with cervical lymphadenopathy and systemic complaints of fever, headache, malaise, and fatigue. Although mild cases of herpetic pharyngitis are indistinguishable from those caused by other respiratory viruses, severe cases are characterized by vesicles and shallow ulcers of the palate, which may be associated with gingivostomatitis. A distinguishing feature of adenovirus pharyngitis is an associated conjunctivitis, which occurs in one third to one half of cases. Herpangina resulting from coxsackievirus is characterized by 1- to 2-mm vesicles involving the posterior oropharynx, which subsequently rupture to become small white ulcers.

Oropharyngeal candidiasis is characterized by a white cheesy exudate with focal bleeding points that can be scraped off to demonstrate yeast forms by Gram stain or culture.

Peritonsillar abscess is suggested by the development of severe pain that is often referred to the ear in a patient with remitting pharyngitis. Fever and dysphagia resulting in drooling are common, and trismus occurs in some patients. On examination, the affected tonsil is displaced medially, the soft palate is erythematous and displaced forward, and the uvula is edematous and displaced to the opposite side.

Laboratory Diagnosis

Various diagnostic procedures and their applications are listed in Table 6. Throat culture remains the gold standard for the diagnosis of group A streptococcal pharyngitis. However, it has a false negative rate of 5% to 10%. In addition, a positive culture is not always correlated with clinical infection because the carrier rate of group A streptococci in healthy persons approaches 20%.

A number of rapid diagnostic kits for streptococcal pharyngitis based on the extraction and identification of streptococcal antigens from throat swabs are currently available. The sensitivity of these rapid tests varies from 62% to 95% whereas the specificity ranges from 88% to 100% [2••,14].

sophisticated culture techniques. Finally, pharyngitis can occur as a manifestation of systemic diseases resulting from noninfectious causes (Table 4) [12•].

Clinical Presentation

A thorough history and a careful physical examination is important in the patient that complains of sore throat because there are many possible causes and some can be distinguished clinically (Table 5) [13]. Group A streptococcal pharyngitis is suggested by fever, oropharyngeal exudate, and anterior cervical lymphadenopathy. It may also present as mild pharyngitis that is clinically indistinguishable from that caused by common respiratory viruses. The possibility of mycoplasma and chlamydial pharyngitis should be considered in a patient with persistent pharyngitis, negative throat culture, and coexisting symptoms of lower respiratory tract infection. Although gonococcal infection of the pharynx is usually asymptomatic, it can produce symptomatic pharyngitis that cannot be readily distinguished clinically from strep-

Organism	Fever	Tonsillar exudate	Tender cervical nodes	Enanthem	Exanthem	Other associations
Group A streptococcus	++*	++	++	Petechiae (+) Strawberry tongue (+)	Scarlet fever (+)	History of exposure
Mycoplasma pneumoniae	+	—	+	—	+	Prominent respiratory symptoms, myringitis
Chlamydia pneumoniae (TWAR)	++	+	+	—	—	Nonproductive cough
Corynebacterium hemolyticum	+	+	+	—	++	10 years of age
Corynebacterium diphtheriae	++	Membrane (++)	+	—	—	Incomplete immuniza-tion, outbreak
Haemophilus influenzae	++	—	+	—	—	Dysphagia, "cherry red" epiglottis
Mixed anaerobes	—	Membrane (+)	+	Ulcerative gingivitis (+)	—	Foul odor
Candida albicans	—	Thrush (+)	—	Thrush (+)	—	Antibiotic use, steroids, immunodeficiency
Viruses						
Rhinovirus, influenza, parainfluenza	+	—	—	—	—	Winter-spring
Adenovirus	+	+	+	—	—	Conjunctivitis
Coxsackievirus	+	—	—	Herpangina (+)	+	Summer
Epstein-Barr virus	++	++	++	Petechiae (+)	Ampicillin (+)	Splenomegaly, atypical lymphocytosis, heterophile antibody
Herpes simplex virus	+	—	—	Ulcerative gingivitis (+)	—	Immunosuppressed

* ++-common, +-occasional, —-uncommon
From Todd [13]; with permission.

The heterophile antibody (monospot) test should be performed in patients with suspected Epstein-Barr virus mononucleosis and is usually positive within 2 weeks of the onset of illness. In individuals with a negative heterophile test, Epstein-Barr virus–specific serologic studies (*eg,* Epstein-Barr virus capsid antigen-IgM antibody) should be obtained. Mycoplasmal, chlamydial, and viral pharyngitis are confirmed mostly by serologic studies of acute and convalescent antibody titers. Virus isolation, with the exception of herpes simplex virus, is infrequently performed in clinical practice.

Treatment

Penicillin has been the treatment of choice for group A streptococcal pharyngitis (Table 7) [15,16]. Treatment should be initiated within 1 week of onset and continued for 10 days to prevent the subsequent development of acute rheumatic fever. Evidence that antibiotic therapy can prevent glomerulonephritis is lacking, however. Erythromycin or cephalosporins are alternative agents in penicillin-allergic patients. Antibiotic regimens for the treatment of other bacterial causes of pharyngitis are

TABLE 6 LABORATORY DIAGNOSIS OF PHARYNGITIS AND TONSILLITIS

Procedure	Application
Throat culture	Streptococcal pharyngitis and tonsillitis
Streptococcal antigen detection	Rapid diagnostic kit for identification of strepto-coccal infection to enable prompt treatment
Heterophile antibody (monospot) test	Infectious mononucleosis
Serologic studies (acute and convalescent sera)	Viral, mycoplasma, and chlamydial pharyngitis
Virus isolation	Herpetic pharyngitis

summarized in Table 7 [16]. Tonsillectomy is indicated for patients with repeated episodes of tonsillitis [12•]. Anti-toxin (20,000 to 50,000 U for mild to moderate disease

TABLE 7 THERAPEUTIC REGIMENS FOR BACTERIAL CAUSES OF PHARYNGITIS

Organism	Regimen of choice	Alternative regimens
Group A streptococcus*	Benzathine penicillin G <27.3 kg: 600,000 U intramuscular once ≥27.3 kg: 1,200,000 U intramuscular once Penicillin V (phenoxymethyl) 250 mg orally three times daily for 10 d	Erythromycin estolate 20–40 mg/kg/d (maximum 1 g) orally two to four times daily for 10 d Erythromycin ethylsuccinate 40 mg/kg/d (maximum 1 g) orally four times daily for 10 d
Mycoplasma pneumoniae	Erythromycin 500 mg orally four times for 7–10 d	Tetracycline 500 mg orally four times daily for 7–10 d
Chlamydia pneumoniae	Doxycycline 100 mg orally two times for 7–10 d	Erythromycin 500 mg orally four times daily for 7–10 d
Corynebacterium hemolyticum	Penicillin V 500 mg orally four times for 7–10 d	Erythromycin 500 mg orally four times daily for 7–10 d
Corynebacterium diphtheriae	Erythromycin 500 mg orally four times for 7 d	Clindamycin 450 mg orally three times daily for 7 d
Haemophilus influenzae	Ampicillin-sulbactam 500 mg orally four times daily for 7–10 d	Cefuroxime axetil 250 mg orally two times daily for 7–10 d
Mixed anaerobes	Metronidazole 500 mg orally three times daily for 7–10 d	Clindamycin 450 mg orally three times daily for 7–10 d

*Amoxicillin, dicloxacillin, oral cephalosporins, and clindamycin are acceptable alternative agents but usually are not recommended; sulfonamides, trimethoprim, tetracycline, and chloramphenicol are not acceptable for rheumatic fever prevention in the treatment of group A streptococcal pharyngitis.

From Dajani *et al.* [16]; with permission.

involving the tonsils and pharynx; 50,000 to 100,000 U for laryngeal involvement with severe disease) is the mainstay of therapy for diphtheria to prevent myocarditis and peripheral neuritis [17•]. Booster doses of tetanus–diphtheria toxoid should be administered to adults at least every 10 years. Treatment of gonococcal pharyngitis is described elsewhere (*see* Chapter 10, Sexually Transmitted Diseases).

Viral pharyngitis is managed symptomatically with warm saline gargles and supportive measures such as rest, aspirin, and liquids. Herpetic pharyngitis in immunocompromised patients should be treated with acyclovir.

When to Refer

The treatment of peritonsillar abscess consists of intravenous antibiotics and surgical drainage. Excellent results (85% to 95% cure rate) are obtained with needle aspiration and oral antibiotics followed by tonsillectomy when the acute infection has resolved (usually 4 to 6 weeks later) [18••,19•]. Traditionally, intravenous penicillin G has been the antibiotic of choice; but with the increasing rate of β-lactamase producing strains of oropharyngeal *Bacteroides* that are resistant to penicillin, this treatment may no longer be adequate in all cases. Intravenous clindamycin is probably the antibiotic of choice for very ill patients or those who respond suboptimally to penicillin. Unvaccinated individuals with characteristic tonsillar–uvular exudate who appear toxic should be hospitalized and treated presumptively for diphtheria with antibiotics and diphtheria antitoxin.

EPIGLOTTITIS AND LARYNGITIS

Acute epiglottitis, also known as supraglottitis, is an acute infection of the supraglottic structures including the false vocal cords, aryepiglottic folds, and the epiglottis (Fig. 4). It can result in severe, sudden, or progressive airway obstruction and is potentially fatal. Although it is considered to be mainly a pediatric emergency, the incidence in adults appears to be increasing [20]. Acute laryngitis is a common

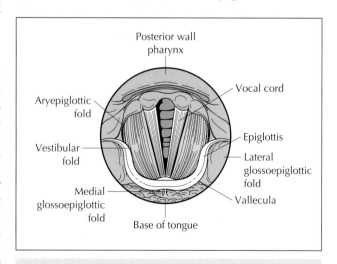

FIGURE 4 Horizontal view of the glottic and supraglottic structures. (*From* Sheikh and Mostow [20]; with permission.)

complication of viral upper respiratory tract infections and can be defined as hoarseness resulting from inflammation of the glottis. Although the disorder is self-limiting, it nevertheless is stressful for professional musicians and others who place great demands on their vocal cords.

Etiology

The common microbial causes of acute epiglottitis and laryngitis are shown in Table 8. *H. influenzae* type B is the major cause of epiglottitis in both children and adults; however, bacteremia in adults (15% to 30%) is less common than in children (95%).

Clinical Presentation

The presentation and clinical course of epiglottitis in adults is different from that in children, in whom the disease is more acute in onset and fulminant in nature. Severe sore throat and high fever progress rapidly, with systemic toxicity, increasing dyspnea, and respiratory obstruction occurring in a matter of hours. In contrast, the disease progression is more gradual and less dramatic in adults, usually extending over several days. The common presenting symptoms and signs of acute epiglottitis in adults are shown in Table 9. Conditions that may be confused with epiglottitis include angioneurotic edema of the larynx, foreign body aspiration, or impingement of the airway by an extrinsic mass. However, these conditions are readily distinguished from acute epiglottitis by the lack of toxic manifestations and negative radiographic findings. In children, it is important to distinguish between epiglottitis and croup, a viral infection causing obstruction of the subglottic rather than supraglottic structures. Croup usually affects younger children (aged 3 months to 3 years) with a slower progression of the clinical course, and patients present with hoarseness with a characteristic cough.

In acute laryngitis, patients usually have common cold symptoms before the onset of hoarseness and occasionally aphonia.

Laboratory Diagnosis

The diagnosis of acute epiglottitis is based primarily on the history and either abnormal findings on laryngoscopy or a confirmatory soft tissue radiograph of the lateral neck. Simple inspection of the pharynx is usually unrewarding. Furthermore, any instrumentation even with a tongue blade may provoke laryngeal spasm and total airway obstruction. There are several diagnostic procedures used for various applications. Lateral neck radiography is used for the diagnosis of acute epiglottitis. A patient should not be left alone in the radiography department during the procedure without someone capable of emergency intubation or tracheostomy in attendance. Laryngoscopy is the gold standard procedure for the diagnosis of acute epiglottitis. Blood culture is used for microbial diagnosis. Throat cultures are not useful because of contamination by the indigenous oropharyngeal flora. Confirmation of the causative organism requires a positive culture either from blood or aspirated contents from an epiglottic abscess.

Treatment

All patients suspected of acute epiglottitis should be admitted to hospital for careful monitoring, preferably in an intensive care unit. Empiric antibiotic therapy should be started once appropriate cultures are obtained. The initial choice should be an intravenous antibiotic effective against *H. influenzae* (including β-lactamase producing strains), *S. pneumoniae*, *S. aureus*, and other gram-negative bacilli. Suitable agents include β-lactamase resistant β-lactams such as penicillin plus β-lactamase inhibitor, an extended spectrum cephalosporin, or a carbapenem. Subsequent treatment should be guided by culture and sensitivity results. A total of 7 to 10 days of therapy is recommended. Patients usually improve within 24 to 48 hours after initiation of appropriate antibiotic therapy. The presence of continued fever suggests abscess development and mandates careful reexamination and consideration of surgical drainage.

The treatment of acute laryngitis is primarily supportive with humidification, hydration, and resting the voice until

TABLE 8 MICROBIAL CAUSES OF ACUTE EPIGLOTTITIS AND LARYNGITIS		
	Common	**Rare**
Acute epiglottitis	*Haemophilus influenzae* type B (60%–100% of cases)	*Streptococcus pneumoniae*
		Streptococcus pyogenes
		Staphylococcus aureus
		Klebsiella pneumoniae
		Haemophilus parainfluenzae
Acute laryngitis	Viruses	*Moraxella catarrhalis*
	Influenza	*Haemophilus influenzae*
	Rhinovirus	Tuberculosis
	Parainfluenza	Syphilis
	Respiratory syncytial virus	Candidiasis
	Coxsackievirus	Histoplasmosis

TABLE 9 SYMPTOMS AND SIGNS OF EPIGLOTTITIS IN ADULTS	
Symptoms and signs	**Patients, %**
Sore throat	90
Odynophagia	80
Dysphonia	50
Dyspnea	30
Drooling	15
Fever	80
Inspiratory stridor	30
Respiratory distress	45
Cervical lymphadenopathy	—
Pharyngitis	—

TABLE 10 ACUTE EPIGLOTTITIS: THE FREIDMAN CLASSIFICATION

Stage I	Stage II	Stage III	Stage IV
No respiratory complaints	Subjective respiratory complaint	Moderate respiratory distress	Severe respiratory distress
Respiratory rate less than 20	Respiratory rate greater than 20	Stridor, retractions, perioral cyanosis	Stridor, retractions, cyanoses, delirium, decreased consciousness
		Respiratory rate greater than 30	Respiratory arrest

From Freidman and coworkers [25]; with permission.

TABLE 11 ACUTE EPIGLOTTITIS: AIRWAY MANAGEMENT

No respiratory complaints (Freidman Stage I)

Monitoring in intensive care unit

Humidified oxygen

Intravenous antibiotics

Intubation tracheostomy kit immediately available

Mild to moderate respiratory distress (Freidman Stage II, III)

Transport to operating room

Otolaryngologist standing by, set-up for tracheostomy

Attempt inhalational or modified inhalational induction

If airway obstructs, options include

Attempt intubation

Establish surgical airway

Needle cricothyrotomy, oxygenate, then perform intubation, retrograde intubation, or tracheostomy

Severe respiratory distress, impending arrest (Freidman Stage IV)

Immediate intubation, cricothyrotomy, or tracheostomy in the emergency room

Criteria for extubation

Normal temperature, resolution of systemic toxicity

Normal chest radiograph

Patient able to breathe around occluded endotracheal or tracheostomy tube with cuff deflated

Visual examination of supraglottic structures indicates decreased edema and inflammation

From Crosby and Reid [23]; with permission.

---

hoarseness and aphonia have subsided. Patients in whom the hoarseness has persisted beyond 2 weeks should have a laryngoscopic examination to exclude the presence of tumors and other chronic diseases of the larynx. Antibiotic therapy is not indicated unless secondary bacterial infection is present. Results of one double-blind study showed that treatment with penicillin V had no significant effect compared with placebo in shortening the duration of dysphonia or other respiratory symptoms [21••]. Erythromycin in oral doses of 0.5 g twice daily for 5 days, however, may be more effective [22•]. However, this disorder is self-limiting in most cases, and antibiotic therapy as a routine measure appears unwarranted.

When to Refer

The approach to airway management in an adult with acute epiglottitis is somewhat controversial. Whereas tracheostomy has been recommended for all patients in the past, recent studies indicate that no more than 10% to 30% of patients will require airway intervention [23,24]. Freidman *et al.* [25] classified adult acute epiglottitis into four clinical stages, which greatly facilitates airway management in these patients (Tables 10 and 11). Intubation rather than tracheostomy is the preferred procedure for provision of an artificial airway, and yields better results both in reducing mortality and shortening the duration of hospitalization. Humidified oxygen is essential. Steroids are commonly used, but their efficacy has not been studied in controlled trials.

REFERENCES AND RECOMMENDED READING

Recently published papers of particular interest have been highlighted as:

• Of interest

•• Of outstanding interest

1. Bruce HM: Diagnosis of sinusitis in adults: history, physical examination, nasal cytology, echo, and rhinoscope. *J Allergy Clin Immunol* 1992, 90:436–441.

2.•• Chow AW, Hall CB, Klein JO, *et al.*: General guidelines for the evaluation of new anti-infective drugs for the treatment of respiratory tract infections. *Clin Infect Dis* 1992, 15(suppl 1):S62–S88.

3.• Gwaltney JM, Scheld WM, Sande MA, *et al.*: The microbial etiology and antimicrobial therapy of adults with acute community-acquired sinusitis: a fifteen year experience at the University of Virginia and review of other selected studies. *J Allergy Clin Immunol* 1992, 90:457–462.

4.•• Borman KR, Brown PM, Mezera KK, Phaveri H: Occult fever in surgical intensive care unit patients is seldom caused by sinusitis. *Am J Surg* 1992, 164:412–416.

5.• Chow AW: Life-threatening infections of the head and neck. *Clin Infect Dis* 1992, 14:991–1004.

6. Vortel JJ, Chow AW: Sinus infections. In *Infectious Diseases*. Edited by Gorbach SL, Bartlett JG, Blacklow NR. Philadelphia: WB Saunders; 1992:431–437.

7. Godofsky EW, Zinreich J, Armstrong M, *et al.*: Sinusitis in HIV-infected patients. A clinical and radiographic review. *Am J Med* 1992, 93:163–170.

8. Zinreich SJ: Imaging of chronic sinusitis in adults: x-ray, computed tomography, and magnetic resonance imaging. *J Allergy Clin Immunol* 1992, 90:445–451.

9. Schaefer SD, Manning S, Close LG: Endoscopic paranasal sinus surgery. *Laryngoscope* 1989, 99:1–5.

10. Bamberger DM: Antimicrobial treatment of sinusitis. *Semin Respir Infect* 1991, 6:77–84.

11. Deresinski S: Sinusitis in surgical ICU patients. *Infect Dis Alert* 1993, 12:65–67.

12.• Vukmir RB: Adult and pediatric pharyngitis: a review. *J Emerg Med* 1992, 10:607–616.

13. Todd JK: The sore throat: pharyngitis and epiglottitis. *Infect Dis Clin North Am* 1988, 2:149–162.

14. Willis SE: Throat culture or rapid strep test? *Postgrad Med* 1990, 88:111–114.

15. Peter G: Streptococcal pharyngitis: current therapy and criteria for evaluation of new agents. *Clin Infect Dis* 1992, 14(suppl 2):S218–S223.

16. Dajani AS, Bisno AL, Chung KJ, *et al.*: Prevention of rheumatic fever. A statement for health professionals by the Committee on Rheumatic Fever, Endocarditis, and Kawasaki Disease of the Council on Cardiovascular Disease in the Young, the American Heart Association. *Circulation* 1988, 78:1082–1086.

17.• Kind AC, Williams DN: Antibiotic treatment of pharyngitis. *Semin Respir Infect* 1991, 6:69–76.

18.•• Ophir D, Bawnik J, Poria Y, *et al.*: Peritonsillar abscess. A prospective evaluation of outpatient management by needle aspiration. *Arch Otolaryngol Head Neck Surg* 1988, 114:661–663.

19.• Stringer SP, Schaefer SD, Close LG: A randomized trial for outpatient management of peritonsillar abscess. *Arch Otolaryngol Head Neck Surg* 1988, 114:296–298.

20. Sheikh KH, Mostow SR: Epiglottitis—an increasing problem for adults. *West J Med* 1989, 151:520–524.

21.•• Schalèn L, Christensen P, Ingvav E, *et al.*: Inefficacy of penicillin V in acute laryngitis in adults. Evaluation from results of a double-blind study. *Ann Otol Rhinol Laryngol* 1985, 94:14–17.

22.• Schalèn L, Ingvav E, Kamme C, *et al.*: Erythromycin in acute laryngitis in adults. *Ann Otol Rhino Laryngol* 1993, 102:209–214.

23. Crosby E, Reid D: Acute epiglottitis in the adult—is intubation mandatory? *Can J Anaesth* 1991, 38:914–918.

24. Rivron RP, Murray JAM: Adult epiglottitis: is there a consensus on diagnosis and treatment? *Clin Otolaryngol* 1991, 16:338–344.

25. Freidman M, Toriumi DM, Grybauskas V, *et al.*: A plea for uniformity in the staging and management of acute epiglottitis. *Ear Nose Throat J* 1988, 67:837–880.

SELECT BIBILIOGRAPHY

Bluestone CD: The diagnosis and management of sinusitis in children. Proceedings of a closed conference. *Ped Infect Dis* 1985, 4(suppl 6):S49–S81.

Klein JO, Teele DW, Pelton SI: New concepts in otitis media: results of investigations of the Greater Boston Otitis Media Study Group. *Adv Ped* 1992, 39:127–156.

Marchant CD, Carlin SA, Johnson CE, Shurin PA: Measuring the comparative efficacy of antibacterial agents for acute otitis media—the "Pollyanna phenomenon". *J Pediatr* 1992, 120:72–77.

Melen I, Lindahl L, Andreasson L: Short- and long-term treatment results in chronic maxillary sinusitis. *Acta Otolaryngol* 1986, 102:282–290.

Williams RL, Chalmers TC, Strange KC, *et al.*: Use of antibiotics in preventing recurrent acute otitis media and in treating otitis media with effusion—a meta-analytic attempt to resolve the brouhaha. *JAMA* 1993, 270:1344–1351.

Nosocomial Pneumonia 7

Brian E. Scully

Key Points

- Aspiration of oropharyngeal and gastric flora is the major factor leading to the development of nosocomial pneumonia.

- "Intestinalization" of the oral flora often occurs in the hospital due to use of antimicrobials and loss of cell surface fibronectin.

- Diagnosis is often uncertain due to the presence of confounding and sometimes multiple pulmonary conditions.

- Especially important in choosing empiric therapy are a knowledge of the local flora and a review of recent antimicrobial use in the patient.

- Useful preventive measures include scrupulous attention to the principles of infection control, particularly with regard to ventilator use and the timely removal of nasogastric and endotracheal tubes; antimicrobial prophylaxis remains controversial.

Nosocomial pneumonia is the leading cause of infection-related mortality in hospitalized patients. It comprises 13% to 18% of all nosocomial infections, and more than 250,000 patients are affected annually in the United States. When all medical and surgical patients are included, the incidence is from 0.8% to 0.9%. Rates are 10- to 20-fold higher among intubated and intensive care unit patients and higher still in those who have had recent head trauma.

Mortality varies greatly, according to the severity of the underlying disease. Reported mortality rates vary from 20% to 50%. Patients who are bacteremic or are infected with virulent organisms, such as *Pseudomonas aeruginosa*, do especially poorly.

PATHOGENESIS

The main route of infection is through microscopic or gross aspiration of bacteria from the oropharynx (Fig. 1) [1,2••,3•]. Bacteremic infection of the lungs occurs but is rare. The risk of aspiration is increased in patients with altered consciousness or impaired gag reflex and in patients with delayed gastric emptying. The presence of an endotracheal tube may lead to pooling of secretions, which can leak around the cuff into the lower airways. Nasogastric tubes provide a conduit for regurgitation of gastric contents, particularly if the tube is used for feeding or is improperly placed. Loss of cell-surface fibronectin in the oropharynx allows gram-negative bacilli to colonize and displace the normal flora (Fig. 2).

Mechanical trauma to the tracheal and bronchial epithelium from suctioning or from the endotracheal tube itself allows organisms, especially *Pseudomonas aeruginosa*, to attach themselves and multiply in the lower airways. Finally, a biofilm of organisms forms within the endotracheal tube, from which particles can be dislodged and blown into the distal airways. Table 1 summarizes these mechanisms.

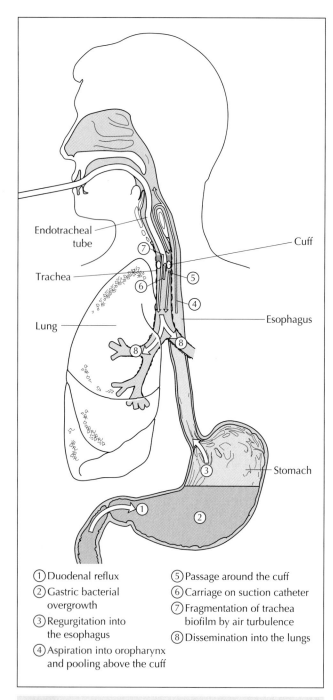

① Duodenal reflux
② Gastric bacterial overgrowth
③ Regurgitation into the esophagus
④ Aspiration into oropharynx and pooling above the cuff
⑤ Passage around the cuff
⑥ Carriage on suction catheter
⑦ Fragmentation of trachea biofilm by air turbulence
⑧ Dissemination into the lungs

FIGURE 1 Bacterial colonization of the ventilated lung.

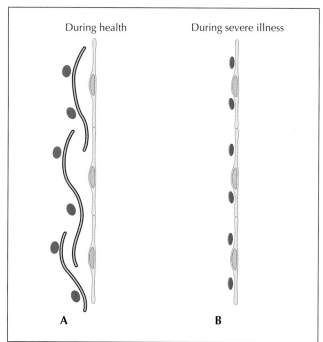

FIGURE 2 A, Normally, fibronectin coats the squamous epithelium of the oropharynx, and gram-positive cocci bind to it, thus colonizing the upper airways. **B**, During severe illnesses, there is loss of cell-surface fibronectin for a variety of reasons, and gram-negative bacilli through their pili can attach to the squamous cells, colonizing the airway.

TABLE 1 PATHOGENIC FACTORS IN NOSOCOMIAL PNEUMONIA
Basic mechanism: microscopic or gross aspiration
Loss of fibronectin in oropharynx, allowing attachment of gram-negative bacteria
Mechanical trauma to trachea
Presence of tube, encouraging aspiration
Reduced ability to cough
Lung damage secondary to edema, infarction, atelectasis, adult respiratory distress syndrome
Immune factors

BACTERIOLOGY

Bacteria are the most important pathogens [4,5]. Because of the changes in oropharyngeal colonization that occur during hospitalization, it is useful to classify nosocomial pneumonias as either early onset (within the first 72 hours) or late onset. Table 2 lists the most probable pathogens by probable time of onset. Gram-negative organisms, especially *Pseudomonas* and *Klebsiella* species, are the most frequently found pathogens and occur usually in patients who have been hospitalized.

Staphylococcus aureus can occur in either group. It is particularly common in patients who have had recent head

injury [6•]. Methicillin-resistant *S. aureus* (MRSA) infection occurs often in patients who received extensive courses of antibiotics and in outbreaks. Many pneumonias are caused by more than one organism. The exact incidence of anaerobes is unknown, but they are especially important when gross aspiration has occurred. They are not major pathogens in intubated patients.

Viruses are uncommon. Influenza and respiratory syncytial virus are sometimes encountered in the winter months in the setting of an epidemic. Cytomegalovirus and adenoviruses are restricted to immunocompromised patients, especially organ transplant recipients.

TABLE 2 BACTERIOLOGIC CLASSIFICATION OF NOSOCOMIAL PNEUMONIA

Time of onset	%
Early (<72 hours)	
Streptococcus pneumoniae	5–10
Haemophilus influenzae	< 5
Late (>72 hours)	
Pseudomonas aeruginosa	15
Klebsiella spp	10
Enterobacter spp	10
Acinetobacter spp	5
Escherichia coli	1–5
Serratia marcescens	1–5
Proteus spp	1–5
Xanthomonas maltophilia	1–5
Early and late	
Staphylococcus aureus (methicillin-resistant *S. aureus* especially in late onset)	20–25
Anaerobic bacteria	
Legionella spp	0–10
Aspergillus spp	< 1
Pneumocystis carinii	< 1
Viruses	< 1

Fungi are also uncommon except in immunocompromised patients. Isolation of *Candida* species from the sputum usually represents colonization in the setting of recent broad-spectrum antibiotic therapy. *Aspergillus* species are the most common pathogens; they affect granulocytopenic patients and transplant recipients especially. *Pneumocystis carinii* occasionally may complicate the hospitalization of patients with acquired immunodeficiency syndrome.

CLINICAL FEATURES AND DIAGNOSIS

The diagnosis of nosocomial pneumonia is often difficult to make [7]. Recent Centers for Disease Control and Prevention criteria for diagnosis depend on various combinations of clinical, laboratory, and radiographic findings (Table 3). Typically, a patient is febrile, has a cough, and has either diffuse or focal findings on examination and radiograph. Chest pain and signs of sepsis may or may not be present. Many of these signs may also be present in atelectasis, pulmonary embolism, congestive heart failure, or pericarditis, or the patient with an extrapulmonary source of infection may have pulmonary findings related to adult respiratory distress syndrome (ARDS) or fluid overload [8,9,10]. Severely debilitated patients may not mount a febrile response, and leukopenic patients may have minimal clinical and radiographic findings. Several recent studies show that clinical and radiologic criteria lead to overdiagnosis and treatment [7,10•]. Joshi [7], for example, found that 80% of new infiltrates occurring in an intensive care unit (ICU) setting could be cleared by vigorous chest postural drainage alone. Conversely, pneumonia may develop in patients who have ARDS and often goes undiagnosed [8,9].

Microbiologic diagnosis is also fraught with difficulty: patients are only rarely bacteremic, many cannot produce good sputum specimens, and they may be colonized but not infected with gram-negative and gram-positive bacteria in the lower airway. However, the absence of these bacteria in secretions is evidence against their presence in the lung because they are easily cultured. Gram staining is useful. The presence of more than 25 polymorphs and fewer than 10 epithelial cells per low-power field in combination with a uniform population of organisms on Gram staining supports a diagnosis of bacterial pneumonia and is helpful in guiding therapy. Changes in the sputum Gram stain may sometimes precede the development of infiltrates on the radiograph.

Recently, there has been much interest in bronchoscopic techniques using protected-brush (PB) techniques or bronchoalveolar lavage to obtain specimens for quantitative culture [11,12]. Cultures containing more than 10^3 organisms per milliliter in PB specimens and more than 10^5 organisms per milliliter in bronchoalveolar lavage specimens correlate well with the presence of pneumonia (specificity and sensitivity, 90%). In my experience, the main use for these techniques appears to be in severely ill patients who are intubated and who may have other reasons for pulmonary infiltrates (*eg*, ARDS, fever, or immunocompromise).

TABLE 3 CENTERS FOR DISEASE CONTROL AND PREVENTION CRITERIA FOR DIAGNOSIS OF NOSOCOMIAL PNEUMONIA IN ADULTS

Either of the following criteria **must** be met:
•Rales or dullness to percussion on physical examination of the chest and **any** of the following:
  A) New onset of purulent sputum or change in character of sputum
  B) Organism isolated from blood culture
  C) Isolation of pathogens from transtracheal aspirate, bronchial brushing, or biopsy
•Chest radiographic examination shows new or progressive infiltrate consolidation, cavity or pleural effusion, and **only** one of the following:
  A) A, B, or C, as above
  B) Isolation of virus or detection of viral antigen in respiratory secretions
  C) Diagnostic single antibody titer (IgM) or fourfold increase in paired serum samples (IgG) for pathogen

THERAPY

Therapy for nosocomial pneumonia is almost always empiric and should be directed toward the most likely pathogens in the given patient. To determine this, the following questions must be asked:

- How long has the patient been hospitalized?
- What are the resident flora and their antibiograms in the unit?
- What antimicrobial therapy has the patient received?
- What are the underlying diseases?
- Is the patient being ventilated?
- What is the Gram stain of the sputum?
- Is the patient likely to have aspirated?

Of these, it is critical to review any recent antimicrobial therapy that the patient may have received because it is likely that the infecting bacteria are resistant to it [13•].

Many effective regimens are available. Table 4 lists several therapies that I have found effective, in addition to comments regarding the advantages and disadvantages peculiar to each. Patients at high risk for aspiration should receive a regimen that is efficacious against anaerobic organisms. Patients who are critically ill and may be septic or immunosuppressed should receive an aminoglycoside, particularly in the third-generation cephalosporin or penicillin-containing regimens. This is for purposes of possible synergy and also to ensure coverage. Aminoglycosides should be administered in doses that are on the high side to optimize penetration into the lung [14]. In units with a high prevalence of MRSA, particularly if the Gram stain is suggestive or if recent β-lactam therapy has been given, vancomycin should be included initially. If

Legionella species seem likely because of the local epidemiology of the host, erythromycin should be added or a quinolone-containing regimen prescribed [15]. Finally, imipenem is active against some of the pathogens that tend to be selected out by other β-lactams (*ie, Enterobacter cloacae, Acinetobacter* species, *P. aeruginosa*, and *Enterococcus faecalis*) and should be considered for such patients [16].

In addition to choosing the correct antibiotic regimen, it is critically important to optimize pulmonary drainage, fluid balance, electrolytes, and nutritional status. Occasionally, patients require repeated therapeutic bronchoscopies to clear secretions. Consideration should be given to aspiration of significant pleural effusions to exclude empyema. In selected cases, infectious disease or pulmonary consultants are helpful, as follows:

- In renal or hepatic failure to guide dosing and choice of antimicrobials
- In complex cases to guide diagnostic tests and choice of antibiotics
- In immunocompromised patients
- In persistently febrile patients

PREVENTION

The prevention of nosocomial pneumonia requires strict adherence to general principles of infection control and the judicious, timely use of invasive devices and equipment [17•]. Recently the continuous suctioning of subglottic secretions has been shown to result in a 50% reduction in early onset pneumonia due to organisms such as *Haemophilus influenzae*, streptococci, and *Straphylococcus aureus* [18]. Table 5 details a

---

TABLE 4 THERAPIES FOR NOSOCOMIAL PNEUMONIA

Regimen	Advantage	Disadvantages
Cefoxitin, 2 g q 6 h IV ± gentamicin, 2.5 mg/kg q 12 h IV	Anaerobic coverage is good	Does not cover *Pseudomonas* or *Enterobacter* spp without the aminoglycoside; nephrotoxicity of aminoglycoside-containing regimen
Ceftazidime or cefotaxime, 1–2 g q 8 h IV ± gentamicin	Excellent activity against Enterobacteriaceae, *Pseudomonas* spp (ceftazidime), and some oral flora (cefotaxime)	Ceftazidime has poor staphylococcal and anaerobic activity; risk of superinfection
Clindamycin, 600–900 mg q 8 h IV + aztreonam, 1–2 g q 8 h	Excellent anaerobic and gram-negative activity, including many strains of *Pseudomonas aeruginosa*	Many *Enterobacter* and *Acinetobacter* spp are resistant; risk of superinfection
Piperacillin, 3–4 g q 6 h + gentamicin	Excellent anaerobic, streptococcal, and gram-negative activity	Poor staphylococcal coverage; nephrotoxicity
Ticarcillin/clavulanate, 3.1 g q 6 h + gentamicin	Good staphylococcal, anaerobic, and gram-positive coverage, especially if gentamicin is included	Many Enterobacteriaceae are resistant to ticarcillin/clavulanate; gentamicin is required in critical or complex cases
Imipenem, 50 mg q 6–8 h	Excellent broad spectrum activity, including anaerobes, staphylococci, and gram-negative organisms	Risk of superinfection; dosing critical if renal insufficiency is present
Ciprofloxacin or ofloxacin, 400 mg q 12 h IV ± clindamycin	Excellent broad activity, good tissue penetration of quinolones; ability to use orally	Clindamycin necessary for anaerobic coverage; staphylococcal efficacy of quinolones is poor

IV—intravenously; q—every.

TABLE 5 STRATEGIES FOR THE PREVENTION OF NOSOCOMIAL PNEUMONIA

Good postoperative care (*eg*, early mobilization, breathing exercises, cautious sedative use)

Early removal of nasogastric tubes

Maintenance of ventilated patients at 30° elevation to lessen risk of aspiration

Limited stress ulcer prophylaxis; preferential use of cytoprotective agents to lessen gastric colonization

Evaluation of the need for enteral versus parenteral feeding; continuous rather than bolus feeding

Careful handwashing and glove usage

Proper care of the ventilator (*eg*, suctioning to prevent backflow of tubing condensate, timely circuit changes)

Consideration of selective decontamination of the digestive tract

number of the most important measures. Hospitals with effective infection control programs have significantly lower rates of nosocomial pneumonia than hospitals that do not. In these institutions, awareness among nursing and medical staff of basic infection control principles, such as hand washing and use of gloves, is high.

Selective decontamination of the digestive system of patients in the ICU has received much attention in the past 5 to 10 years [19•]. Many regimens have been tried—often cefotaxime systemically and a combination of tobramycin, amphotericin B, and polymyxins in a paste to the mouth and in a solution through the nasogastric tube. Reduced rates of respiratory infections have been found in some studies, but there has been little effect on mortality or length of ICU stay. Surgical patients may benefit more than medical patients, but there is no clear consensus regarding the benefits of selective decontamination of the digestive system and much concern regarding the potential for the long-term selection of resistant flora.

Finally, the use of cytoprotective agents rather than compounds that reduce gastric acidity appears to be associated with a reduced risk of nosocomial pneumonia. [20•,21].

REFERENCES AND RECOMMENDED READING

Recently published papers of particular interest have been highlighted as:
• Of interest
•• Of outstanding interest

1. Johanson WG, Pierce AK, Sanford JP: Changing pharyngeal bacterial flora of hospitalized patients: emergence of gram-negative bacilli. *N Engl J Med* 1969, 281:1137–1140.

2.•• Torres A, Serra-Batlles J, Ros E, *et al.*: Pulmonary aspiration of gastric contents in patients receiving mechanical ventilation: the effect of body position. *Ann Intern Med* 1992, 116:540–543.

3.• Heyland D, Mandel LA: Gastric colonization by gram-negative bacilli and nosocomial pneumonia in the intensive care patients: evidence for causation. *Chest* 1992, 101:187–193.

4. Bates JH, Campbell G, Barron AL, *et al.*: Microbial etiology of acute pneumonia in hospitalized patients. *Chest* 1992, 101:1005–1012.

5. Bartlett JG, O'Keefe P, Tally FP, *et al.*: Bacteriology of hospital-acquired pneumonia. *Arch Intern Med* 1986, 146:868–871.

6.• Rello J, Ausina V, Castella J, *et al.*: Nosocomial respiratory tract infections in multiple trauma patients: influence of level of consciousness with implications for therapy. *Chest* 1992, 102:525–529.

7. Joshi M, Ciesla N, Caplan E: Diagnosis of pneumonia in critically ill patients. *Chest* 1988, 94:4S.

8. Andrews CP, Coalson JJ, Smith JD, Johanson WG Jr: Diagnosis of nosocomial bacterial pneumonia in acute, diffuse lung injury. *Chest* 1981, 80:254–258.

9. Bell RC, Coalson JJ, Smith JD, Johanson WG Jr: Multiple organ system failure and infection in adult respiratory distress syndrome. *Ann Intern Med* 1983, 99:293–298.

10.• Wunderink RG, Woldenberg LS, Zeiss J, *et al.*: The radiologic diagnosis of autopsy proven ventilator-associated pneumonia. *Chest* 1992, 101:458–463.

11. Fagon JY, Chastre J, Hance AJ, *et al.*: Detection of nosocomial lung infection in ventilated patients: use of a protected specimen brush and quantitative culture techniques in 147 patients. *Am Rev Respir Dis* 1988, 138:110–116.

12. Chastre J, Fagon JY, Soler P, *et al.*: Diagnosis of nosocomial bacterial pneumonia in intubated patients undergoing ventilation: comparison of the usefulness of bronchoalveolar lavage and the protected specimen brush. *Am J Med* 1988, 85:499–506.

13.• Scheld WM, Mandell GL: Nosocomial pneumonia: pathogenesis and recent advances in diagnosis and therapy. *Rev Infect Dis* 1991, 13(Suppl 9):S743–S751.

14. Moore RD, Smith CR, Leitman PS: Association of aminoglycoside plasma levels with therapeutic outcome in gram-negative pneumonia. *Am J Med* 1984, 77:657–662.

15. Scully BE: Therapy of respiratory tract infections with quinolone antimicrobial agents. In *Quinolone Antimicrobial Agents*. Edited by Wolfson J, Hooper, D. Washington, DC: American Society of Microbiology; 1983:339–363.

16. Acar JF: Therapy for lower respiratory tract infections with imipenem/cilastin: a review of worldwide experience. *Rev Infect Dis* 1985, 7(Suppl 3):S513–S517.

17.• Mahul PH, Auboyer C, Jospe R, *et al.*: Prevention of nosocomial pneumonia in intubated patients: respective role of mechanical subglottic secretions drainage and stress ulcer prophylaxis. *Intensive Care Med* 1992, 18:20–25.

18. Valles J, Artigas A, Rello J, *et al.*: Continuous aspiration of subglottic secretions in preventing ventilator associated pneumonia. *Ann Intern Med* 1995, 122:179–186.

19.• Craven DE: Use of selective decontamination of the digestive tract: is the light at the end of the tunnel red or green? *Ann Intern Med* 1992, 117:609–611.

20.• Cook DJ, Laine LA, Guyatt GH, Raffin TA: Nosocomial pneumonia and the role of gastric pH: a meta-analysis. *Chest* 1991, 100:7–13.

21. Tryba M: Prophylaxis of stress ulcer bleeding. A meta-analysis. *J Clin Gastroenterol* 1991, 13(Suppl 2): S44–S55.

SELECT BIBLIOGRAPHY

Lode H, Craven DE, Stoutenbeek ChP, eds: Nosocomial pneumonia: prevention and treatment. *Intensive Care Med* 1992, 18 (S1).

Tablan OC, Anderson IJ, Arden NH, *et al.*: Guidelines for prevention of nosocomial pneumonia—1994. *Infect Control Hosp Epidemiol* 1994, 15:587–590.

Cellulitis 8

Richard Allen Johnson

Key Points
- Soft tissue infections are relatively common in healthly individuals and in the increasing population of immunocompromised individuals.
- The traditional etiologic agents of cellulitis are *Staphylococcus aureus* and group A streptococcus; in the immunocompromised host, a much broader spectrum of agents must be suspected.
- Successful response to therapy depends on early diagnosis, initiation of adequate antibiotic therapy, correction of risk factors such as neutropenia, and surgical debridement when indicated.

Cellulitis, which is also referred to as *soft-tissue infection*, is characterized by an acute, diffuse, spreading, edematous inflammation of the dermis and subcutaneous tissues, often associated with systemic symptoms of malaise, fever, and chills. *Erysipelas* is a superficial cellulitis that spreads rapidly via extension within lymphatic channels. *Necrotizing soft tissue infections* (NSI) are characterized by necrosis of the dermis, hypodermis, fascia, or muscle and are, in turn, classified as necrotizing cellulitis, necrotizing fasciitis, or myonecrosis. *Staphylococcus aureus* and group A β-hemolytic *Streptococcus pyogenes* (GAS) are the infectious agents that cause cellulitis; however, a wide variety of bacteria and some fungi are capable of causing soft-tissue infections. If treatment is delayed, cellulitis can spread extensively both in contiguous tissues and by lymphatic and blood vessels; it can be complicated by metastatic infection in other organs; can result in necrosis of the overlying epidermis with bulla formation and ulceration of the hypodermis, fascia, and muscle; and can result in shock and death.

ETIOLOGY AND PATHOGENESIS

Cellulitis often follows a detectable break in the integrity of the skin associated with a great variety of underlying dermatoses, a traumatic or operative wound, a burn, venous access devices [1], or other cutaneous lesions (Table 1). Pathogens invade the dermis and subcutis, and the host immune system mounts an acute inflammatory response to their presence. In most cases, the number of invading organisms is small, such that their isolation is not possible in the majority of cases, suggesting that the majority of the clinical findings are mediated by a variety of cytokines [2].

Cellulitis occurs in otherwise healthy individuals but tends to be more severe in those with a wide variety of predisposing causes (Table 2).

Neutropenia is common in individuals undergoing cancer chemotherapy and is associated with *Pseudomonas aeruginosa* cellulitis, also called *ecthyma gangrenosum*, as well as aspergillosis of soft tissues. Cirrhosis and diabetes mellitus predispose an individual to *Vibrio vulnificus* cellulitis, following ingestion of contaminated seafood. Diabetes with ketoacidosis is associated with mucormycosis.

TABLE 3 SYNOPSIS OF NECROTIZING INFECTIONS

Organism	History	Physical examination	Laboratory	Course
Staphylococcus aureus	Skin trauma or underlying dermatosis	Portal of entry usually apparent Deeper infections with ill-defined borders Toxin syndromes: SSSS, TSS	Culture: skin, ±blood	May become superinfected with gram-negative organisms Endocarditis can follow bacteremia
GAS				
Erysipelas	Age: children, elderly Portal of entry: secondarily infected dermatoses, traumatic or surgical wound, tinea pedis	Face most common site High fever Rapidly enlarging cellulitis; ±bullae; well-demarcated borders	Respiratory tract colonization Bacteremia follows skin infection Culture GAS from skin ±blood	Most do well with intravenous antibiotics
Cellulitis	Portal of entry: surgical or traumatic wounds Previous episodes at same site, injecting drug use Calf cellulitis can follow coronary bypass surgery at saphenous vein donor site Local pain	Cellulitis extending from portal of entry Tenderness Regional lymphan-denopathy High fever	Culture GAS from skin ±blood	Prognosis varies with predisposing conditions
GBS				
Puerperal sepsis	Historically occurred following childbirth	High fever Anogenital cellulitis extending to pelvic organs	Culture: skin, ±blood	Significant morbidity and mortality
Streptococcus pneumoniae	Connective tissue disease, HIV disease, corticosteroid therapy, drug or alcohol abuse	Cellulitis without portal of entry	Culture: blood, ±skin	High morbidity and mortality associated with predisposing conditions
Erysipelothrix rhusiopathiae Erysipeloid	Portal of entry: break in skin while handling edible animal products Onset: 2–7 days after puncture	Fever: low grade Violaceous erythema at break in skin Most commonly on hand Cellulitis spreads slowly	Culture: wound	Resolves spontaneously
Haemophilus influenzae	Age: <2 y Rapidly progressive Incidence decrease due to Hib vaccine	Fever: moderate to high Site: periorbital, buccal Color: violaceous, red-blue	Culture: oropharynx, blood	Responds well to antibiotics
Pseudomonas aeruginosa Ecthyma gangrenosum	Neutropenia Pain: moderate to severe	Fever: high NSI with "gun-metal" gray color, well-demarcated borders Sites: anogenital, axillary	Culture: skin, ±blood Histology: septic vasculitis	High morbidity and mortality unless neutropenia corrected G-CSF improved prognosis

(Continued)

TABLE 3 SYNOPSIS OF NECROTIZING INFECTIONS (*CONTINUED*)

Organism	History	Physical examination	Laboratory	Course
Mycobacterium fortuitum complex	Recent surgery, injection, penetrating wound	Low-grade cellulitis	Culture: skin Biopsy: acid-fast bacilli	Responds well to antibiotics
Vibrio vulnificus	Diabetic, cirrhotic Ingestion of raw or under-cooked seafood	Fever: high NSI	Culture: blood, skin Biopsy: NSI	High morbidity and mortality
Aeromonas spp	Trauma in aquatic environment Most patients immuno-competent More common in males	Fever: high NSI	Culture: skin, blood Biopsy: NSI	Significant morbidity, even in healthy individuals
Cryptococcus neoformans	Chronically immunocom-promised	Low-grade cellulitis	Culture: skin Biopsy: large yeast forms	Usually responds well to amphotericin B Diagnosis often delayed
Mucormycosis	Diabetes/ketoacidosis Neutropenia	Rapidly progressive NSI	Culture: skin Biopsy: large mycelial forms	High morbidity and mortality

GAS—group A β-hemolytic *Streptococcus pyogenes*; GBS—group B β-hemolytic *Streptococcus pyogenes*; G-CSF—granulocyte-colony stimulating factor; Hib—*Haemophilus influenzae* type b; NSI—necrotizing soft-tissue infection; SSSS—staphylococcal scalded skin syndrome; TSS—toxic shock syndrome.

the onset of EG and may result in metastatic spread of *P. aeruginosa* infection to a distant site. Septic vasculitis occurs early in EG with resultant tissue infarction and hematogenous dissemination.

Clinically, EG is characterized by an initial cellulitis, followed by central infarction occurring within the first hours or days. If effective antibiotic therapy is not initiated promptly following onset of fever and cellulitis, the EG may extend rapidly, with associated sepsis and shock. Early use of granulocyte-colony stimulating factor has markedly reduced the morbidity and mortality of EG.

Haemophilus influenzae

Haemophilus influenzae type b (Hib) colonizes the upper airways of infants and young children and is the most common cause of cellulitis of the head and neck in this age group [8]. Typically a child presents with swelling and erythema of the face or arm following an ear or respiratory infection. Secondary bacteremia in this setting is not uncommon. In this age group, *H. influenzae* cellulitis must be differentiated from erythema infectiosum, the "slapped cheek" of infection with primary human parvovirus B19. Hib vaccine is given during childhood immunization and has dramatically reduced the incidence of Hib infections in young children. Household contacts of patients with Hib infection should receive chemoprophylaxis if a second child under the age of 4 is at home.

Erysipelothrix rhusiopathiae

Erysipelothrix rhusiopathiae causes erysipeloid, a mild suba-cute cellulitis that resembles erysipelas. The infection is an occupational disease, transmitted in those who handle foods such as saltwater fish, shellfish, meat, or poultry. Clinically, the lesion appears as a tender violaceous area around the portal of entry, which slowly extends peripherally as the center clears. The diagnosis is usually made by the typical clinical appearance on the hand of an individual who handles fish or meat. Diagnosis can be made by isolating the organism from a biopsy specimen taken from the edge of the lesion. Erysipeloid must be differentiated from "seal finger," which occurs in aquarium workers and veterinarians following trauma associated with working with seals. Erysipeloid resolves spontaneously or with antibiotic therapy; uncommonly, bacteremia and aortic valvulitis occur with significant mortality (38%).

Mycobacterium chelonei

Mycobacterium chelonei subspecies *abscessus*, surgical wound infections have been reported after contaminated gentian violet solution is used to mark the skin prior to surgery [9]. Similar infections have also followed the use of jet injectors. Patients presented with cellulitis 1 to 2 weeks after the procedure. *M. fortuitum* has been reported to cause infection following penetrating injury [10] and electromyography.

Vibrio vulnificus

Vibrio vulnificus and other *Vibrio* species are free-living gram-negative rods occurring naturally in the marine environment and capable of contaminating oysters and other shellfish. Individuals with cirrhosis, diabetes mellitus, and other chronic illnesses are predisposed to infection with *Vibrio* species and are advised to avoid eating raw seafood. Ingestion of seafood contaminated with *V. vulnificus* can result in gastroenteritis, primary septicemia, or NSI, which occur following bacteremia as well as inoculation of the organism into the skin. Most reported cases have occurred in Florida and the Gulf Coast (Alabama, Louisiana, and Texas), with a peak incidence in May through October. *V. vulnificus* and *V. alginolyticus* usually infect compromised hosts; *V. damsela*, however, can cause fulminant necrotizing infections in immunocompetent patients.

Clinically, *V. vulnificus* cellulitis that occurs following ingestion and septicemia often involves the legs bilaterally. Involved sites usually show findings of a necrotizing soft-tissue infection with formation of hemorrhagic bullae [11].

Aeromonas hydrophila

Aeromonas hydrophila and other *Aeromonas* species are also found naturally in aqueous environments and are capable of causing soft-tissue infections with necrosis. In some series, *A. hydrophila* cellulitis occurred subsequent to injuries such as punctures, abrasions, and lacerations sustained in an aquatic environment or the "outdoors." In other reports, this was not the case [12]. Infections occur much more often in males than in females, in healthy as well as immunocompromised individuals, and the lower limb is involved most commonly. Clinically, infections with *Aeromonas* spp arise around the portal of entry with initial findings of cellulitis, which can progress to NSI.

Gram-negative bacteria

Other gram-negative bacteria have also been reported to cause cellulitis, with or without necrosis, including *Klebsiella pneumoniae*, *Campylobacter fetus*, *Proteus mirabilis* [13], *Escherichia coli*, *Serratia marcescens* [14], and *Legionella* spp [15].

Variation of Clinical Findings by Disease
Mucormycosis

Mucormycosis, an invasive necrotizing phycomycosis of the soft tissues, is an increasing cause of morbidity and mortality in patients with impaired immunity [16•]. Of the Phycomycetes, the members of the family Mucoraceae are the most common human pathogens. Burn victims, trauma patients, and diabetics are particularly susceptible to these infections. Progressive infection despite extensive debridement and broad-spectrum antibacterial coverage may be indicative of mycotic rather than bacterial infection. Phycomycotic vascular invasion and destruction result in infarction and hematogenous mycotic dissemination. As in bacterial deep necrotizing infections, rapid invasion and high mortality are characteristic. Early diagnosis can be made by examination of frozen tissue or fungal wet preparation slides. Histologically, the Phycomycetes have broad branching nonseptate, gram-

negative hyphae. Once mucormycosis is identified, urgent surgical debridement and administration of high dose amphotericin B are indicated.

Necrotizing soft-tissue infections

Necrotizing soft-tissue infections differ from other variants of cellulitis because of significant tissue necrosis, lack of response to antimicrobial treatment alone, and the need for surgical debridement of devitalized tissues. The elaboration of proteases, which degrade extracellular matrix and fat, in combination with exotoxins and endotoxins account for the rapid extension of these infections [17•,18•]. NSIs can be divided into three categories based on their depth of involvement: necrotizing cellulitis [19], necrotizing fasciitis, and myonecrosis. Since the presence of necrosis of fascia can be determined only by surgical exploration and histopathologic examination of the infected site, necrotizing cellulitis cannot be differentiated from necrotizing fasciitis on clinical grounds alone. Necrotizing fasciitis is a progression of necrotizing cellulitis, *ie*, necrotizing cellulitis with additional involvement of adjoining fascia.

Necrotizing cellulitis

Necrotizing cellulitis can be caused by a single microorganism or by several acting in synergy. In immunocompetent hosts, organisms capable of acting alone in causing necrotizing cellulitis include GAS, *Vibrio* spp, *Aeromonas* spp, and *Clostridium* spp. In immunocompromised hosts, *P. aeruginosa* and opportunistic fungi such as *Mucor* or *Rhizopus* spp can produce necrotizing cellulitis. Progressive synergistic cellulitis (gangrene) requires the joint action of an anaerobic streptococcal species with either *S. aureus* or *Proteus* spp. It usually occurs in surgical or traumatic wounds and is slowly but relentlessly progressive. Since fascial planes are not involved, undermining of skin is limited to the edges of the lesion. Clostridial cellulitis is a crepitant anaerobic infection that is limited to the subcutaneous tissues, with less systemic toxicity than clostridial myonecrosis.

Necrotizing fasciitis

Necrotizing fasciitis can be caused by a single microorganism such as GAS, *Vibrio* spp, or Zygomycetes. The majority of cases, however, are caused by polymicrobial infections with synergistic facultative aerobic (*Streptococcus* or *Enterobacter* spp) and anaerobic gas-forming organisms (*Bacteroides* or *Peptostreptococcus* spp). In contrast to necrotizing cellulitis, in which skin changes demarcate the extent of disease, necrotizing fasciitis initially extends deeply along fascial planes with relative sparing of the overlying epidermis. Bacterial necrotizing fasciitis is characterized by local erythema, marked edema, and moderate tenderness, followed by secondary gangrenous skin changes as nutrient dermal vessels undergo thrombosis. Local tenderness is replaced by anesthesia as a consequence of cutaneous nerve necrosis. "Dishwater pus" is characteristic of synergistic polymicrobial necrotizing fasciitis. Severe systemic toxicity is usually out of proportion to the cutaneous findings. Unlike necrotizing cellulitis, necrotizing fasciitis often requires debridement well beyond the margin of normal-appearing skin.

Bacterial myonecrosis

Bacterial myonecrosis has been classified into two etiologic types: clostridial and nonclostridial. *C. perfringens*, *C. novyi*, and *C. septicum*, the etiologic agents of clostridial myonecrosis, thrive in the devitalized tissue of a traumatized wound. The clinical course of infection progresses rapidly, with high morbidity and mortality in spite of adequate treatment. The earliest clinical lesion of myonecrosis is characterized by tenderness and tense edema with little epidermal change. A distinctive foul-smelling, serosanguineous discharge exudes from eroded areas within the infected site. Crepitance is often present, but it may be masked by the tense edema. Older lesions may have areas of yellow-bronze or green-black necrosis, at times with bulla formation. Nonclostridial crepitant myonecrosis may be caused by anaerobic streptococci, other anaerobes acting in synergy, and *Aeromonas hydrophila*. Independent of the etiologic agent of bacterial myonecrosis and even with aggressive management, the prognosis is grave.

DIFFERENTIAL DIAGNOSIS

The differential diagnosis of cellulitis and erysipelas is outlined in Table 4. The differential diagnosis of NSI, which includes that of dermal gangrene, is shown in Table 5.

DIAGNOSIS

The diagnosis of cellulitis must be made initially on clinical findings and data from Gram stain of exudates or aspirates; diagnosis is later confirmed or modified by the cultural isolates.

Gram Stain

Gram stain of exudate, pus, bulla fluid, aspirate, or touch preparation may be obtained from an apparent portal of entry. Clusters of gram-positive cocci are seen with *S. aureus* cellulitis, and chains of gram-positive cocci are seen with GAS infection. Probably more reflective of the cause of the cellulitis is examination of any fluid, aspirate, or touch preparation from the cellulitic lesion. A wound exudate showing gram-positive rods yet few neutrophils is nearly pathognomonic of clostridial infection.

"Touch" Preparation

The back of a lesional biopsy specimen is touched to glass microscope slides. Potassium hydroxide solution is applied to the specimen, which is then examined for yeast or mycelial forms. Fungal forms can be seen in disseminated candidal infection, cryptococcal cellulitis, or phycomycoses. Specimens can be Gram stained and examined for bacteria, as can touch preparations. Touch preparations can also be examined by the cytology laboratory using a number of special stains.

Hematologic Studies

In the report by Hook and colleagues [4], only 46% of patients had elevated leukocyte counts (≥10,000/μL) and 59% had an elevated erythrocyte sedimentation rate (≥25 mm/h).

Culture

The "gold standard" of etiologic diagnosis of cellulitis is isolation of the infecting organism by culture of the infected site as well as of blood. Isolation of a pathogen from culture of a primary lesion (portal of entry) is helpful, in that the isolated organism is usually the cause of the invasive infection. In the study by Hook and colleagues [4], a potential pathogen was isolated in only 26% of cases of cellulitis in adults using culture of a punch biopsy specimen, aspirate, or blood.

Culture of a *primary lesion*, defined as any break in the integrity of the skin (*ie*, ulcers, fissures, abrasions) in continuity with the area of cellulitis, is often helpful in identification of the pathogen [4].

Culture of exudate, erosions, ulcerations, abscesses, or surgical wounds overlying the cellulitis has the highest yield in isolation of the infecting organism.

Needle aspiration has been used in cases of early cellulitis in which the epidermis is intact and abscess formation has not occurred [20]. Aspiration should be attempted with a syringe and needle, with the needle tip placed into the advancing border. If no fluid is obtained, 1 to 2 mL of nonbacteriostatic normal saline can be injected into the site and aspiration can be attempted again. The aspirate can be Gram stained and cultured. The reported yield of needle aspiration ranges from 5% to 100% [21]. Needle aspiration has a higher yield in patients with diabetes mellitus or underlying malignancies [22].

TABLE 4 DIFFERENTIAL DIAGNOSIS OF CELLULITIS AND ERYSIPELAS
Acute allergic contact dermatitis (*eg*, poison ivy)
Giant urticaria and angioedema
Deep venous thrombosis
Erythema nodosum and a variety of panniculitides
Carcinoma of the breast with diffuse lymphatic invasion
Early herpes zoster infection
Erythema migrans
Insect bite
Fixed drug eruption

TABLE 5 DIFFERENTIAL DIAGNOSIS OF NECROTIZING SOFT-TISSUE INFECTION
Vasculitis
Thromboembolic phenomenon
Peripheral vascular disease
Purpura fulminans
Calciphylaxis
Warfarin necrosis
Traumatic injury
Brown recluse spider bite

Culture of lesional biopsy specimens has been reported to have a higher yield than cultures of aspirate or blood, the rate being equal to or less than 20% with relatively few organisms present [23].

Dermatopathology

A lesional biopsy specimen is often helpful in ruling out cellulitis-simulating noninfectious inflammatory lesions such as erythema nodosum, vasculitis, and eosinophilic cellulitis. In ecthyma gangrenosum, a septic vasculitis is seen. Direct visualization using tissue Gram stain can demonstrate the infecting organism in some cases. However, in cases of infections caused by *S. aureus* or GAS, organisms are rarely seen. Direct immunofluorescent techniques have been reported to identify streptococcal pathogens in 19 of 27 cases of erysipelas and 10 of 15 cases of cellulitis. In cases of cryptococcal cellulitis, large yeast forms can be identified in the dermis and hypodermis. Hyphal forms are easily seen in mucormycosis and aspergillosis.

Incisional skin biopsy and surgical exploration with histopathologic examination of frozen sections has been shown to improve mortality in necrotizing fasciitis by expediting treatment. Necrosis and dense polymorphonuclear infiltration confined to the hypodermis and fascia, in association with obliterative vascular thrombosis, are classic findings in necro-

tizing fasciitis. The gloved finger or surgical probe easily undermines the surrounding skin in necrotizing fasciitis but not in necrotizing cellulitis.

Imaging

Magnetic resonance imaging has been reported to be helpful in the diagnosis of severe acute infectious cellulitis, distinguishing pyomyositis, necrotizing fasciitis, and infectious cellulitis with or without subcutaneous abscess formation [24]. Radiographic examination of involved sites is helpful in identifying air within soft tissue and extensive soft tissue involvement.

MANAGEMENT

Individuals with prior episodes of cellulitis are particularly predisposed to future episodes of cellulitis, especially at sites of chronic lymphedema. Support stockings, antiseptics to skin, and chronic secondary antibiotic prophylaxis (penicillin G, dicloxacillin, or erythromycin, 500 mg daily [25•]) should be considered for these patients. Individuals who have had saphenous veins harvested for coronary artery bypass angioplasty are at risk for cellulitis in the donor leg and should be advised about maintaining the integrity of pedal skin and washing with a benzoyl peroxide bar. Those

---

TABLE 6 DRUGS OF FIRST CHOICE AND ALTERNATIVE DRUGS FOR TREATMENT OF SOFT TISSUE INFECTIONS

Infecting organism	Drug of first choice	Alternative drugs
Staphylococcus aureus or *epidermidis*		
nonpenicillinase-producing	Penicillin G or V	A cephalosporin; vancomycin; imipenem; clindamycin; a fluoroquinolone
penicillinase-producing	A penicillinase-resistant penicillin	A cephalosporin; vancomycin; amoxicillin/clavulanic acid; ticarcillin/clavulanic acid; piperacillin/tazobactam; ampicillin/sulbactam; imipenem; clindamycin; a fluoroquinolone
methicillin-resistant	Vancomycin± gentamicin±rifampin	Trimethoprim-sulfamethoxazole; minocycline; a fluoroquinolone
Streptococcus pyogenes (group A) and groups C and G	Penicillin G or V	An erythromycin; a cephalosporin; vancomycin; clarithromycin; azithromycin; clindamycin
Streptococcus, group B	Penicillin G or ampicillin	A cephalosporin; vancomycin; an erythromycin
Streptococcus pneumoniae	Penicillin G or V	An erythromycin; a cephalosporin; vancomycin; rifampin; trimethoprim-sulfamethoxazole; azithromycin; clarithromycin; clindamycin; chloramphenicol
Haemophilus influenzae	Cefotaxime or ceftriaxone	Cefuroxime; chloramphenicol
Pseudomonas aeruginosa	Ticarcillin, mezlocillin, or piperacillin + tobramycin, gentamicin, or amikacin	Ceftazidime, imipenem, or aztreonam + tobramycin, gentamicin, or amikacin; a fluoroquinolone
Vibrio vulnificus	A tetracycline	Trimethoprim-sulfamethoxazole; a fluoroquinolone
Aeromonas spp	Trimethoprim-sulfamethoxazole	Gentamicin or tobramycin; imipenem; a fluoroquinolone
Clostridium perfringens	Penicillin G	Metronidazole; clindamycin; imipenem; a tetracycline; chloramphenicol
Mycobacterium fortuitum (complex)	Amikacin + doxycycline	Cefoxitin; rifampin; a sulfonamide
Cryptococcus neoformans	Amphotericin B ± flucytosine	Fluconazole; itraconazole; amphotericin B
Mucormycosis	Amphotericin B	No dependable alternative

---

with tinea pedis should be advised to apply topical antifungal agents.

Antibiotic regimens are chosen by the findings of the initial assessment and altered according to later cultural data (Table 6) [26,27]. Superinfection of a gram-positive cellulitis with gram-negative organisms can require alteration of antibiotic therapy. In that the most common agents causing cellulitis and erysipelas are *S. aureus* and GAS, antibiotic therapy initially should be directed at adequate treatment of these two pathogens (Table 6). The incidence of methicillin-resistant *S. aureus* infections, both nosocomial and community-acquired, is increasing; these infections are treated with intravenous vancomycin [28,29]. Immobilization and elevation of an infected limb reduces edema and speeds recovery.

The key to treatment of NSI is early diagnosis, followed by complete surgical debridement of necrotic tissue in combination with high-dose antibiotics. Broad antibiotic coverage is recommended until microbiologic cultures identify the infecting organisms. Adjunctive hyperbaric oxygen therapy may reduce morbidity and mortality in both clostridial and nonclostridial necrotizing infections.

COMPLICATIONS AND PROGNOSIS

Complications of cellulitis include abscess formation, superficial and deep gangrene, superficial thrombophlebitis, deep thrombophlebitis, acute glomerulonephritis (GAS), septicemia, endocarditis, and death. Malnutrition, hypertension, old age, and intravenous drug use are predictors of high mortality.

REFERENCES AND RECOMMENDED READING

Recently published papers of particular interest have been highlighted as:

• Of interest

•• Of outstanding interest

1. Groeger JS, Lucas AB, Thaler HT, *et al.*: Infectious morbidity associated with long-term use of venous access devices in patients with cancer. *Ann Intern Med* 1993, 119:1168–1174.

2. Sachs MK: Cutaneous cellulitis. *Arch Dermatol* 1991, 127:493–496.

3. Sigurdsson AF, Gudmundsson S: The etiology of bacterial cellulitis as determined by fine-needle aspiration. *Scand J Infect Dis* 1989, 21:537–542.

4. Hook EW III, Hooton TM, Horton CA, *et al.*: Microbiologic evaluation of cutaneous cellulitis in adults. *Arch Intern Med* 1986, 146:295–297.

5. Fleisher G, Ludwig S, Campos J: Cellulitis: bacterial etiology, clinical features, and laboratory findings. *J Pediatr* 1980, 97:591–593.

6. Schwartz B, Schuchat A, Oxtoby MJ, *et al.*: Invasive group B streptococcal disease in adults. A population-based study in metropolitan Atlanta. *JAMA* 1991, 266:1112–1114.

7. Lawlor MT, Crowe HM, Quintiliani R: Cellulitis due to *Streptococcus pneumoniae*: case report and review of the literature. *Clin Infect Dis* 1992, 14:247–250.

8. Israele V, Nelson JD: Periorbital and orbital cellulitis. *Pediatr Infect Dis J* 1987, 6:404–410.

9. Safranek TJ, Jarvis WR, Carson LA, *et al.*: *Mycobacterium chelonei* infections after plastic surgery employing contaminated gentian violet skin-marking solution. *N Engl J Med* 1987, 317:197–201.

10. Subbarao EK, Tarpay MM, Marks MI: Soft-tissue infections caused by *Mycobacterium fortuitum* complex following penetrating injury. *Am J Dis Child* 1987, 141:1018–1020.

11. Tyring SK, Lee PC: Hemorrhagic bullae associated with *Vibrio vulnificus* septicemia. Report of two cases. *Arch Dermatol* 1986, 122:818–820.

12. Isaacs RD, Paviour SD, Bunker DE, Lang SDR: Wound infection with aerogenic *Aeromonas* strains: a review of twenty-seven cases. *Eur J Clin Microbiol Pathol* 1988, 7:355–360.

13. Musher DM: Cutaneous and soft-tissue manifestations of sepsis due to gram-negative enteric bacilli. *Rev Infect Dis* 1980, 2:854–866.

14. Bornstein PF, Ditto AM, Noskin GA: *Serratia marcescens* cellulitis in a patient on hemodialysis. *Am J Nephrol* 1992, 12:374–376.

15. Waldor MK, Wilson B, Swartz M: Cellulitis caused by *Legionella pneumophila*. *Clin Infect Dis* 1993, 16:51–53.

16.• Virden CP, Lynch FP, Hansbrough JF: Invasive necrotizing phycomycoses. *Infect Med* 1993, 10:30–33.

17.• Stevens DL, Musher DM, Watson DA, *et al.*: Spontaneous nontraumatic gangrene due to *Clostridium septicum*. *Rev Infect Dis* 1990, 12:286–296.

18.• Reed MJ, Annand VK: Odontogenic cervical necrotizing fasciitis with intrathoracic extension. *Otolaryngol Head Neck Surg* 1992, 104:596–600.

19. Salvino C, Harford FJ, Dobrin PB: Necrotizing infections of the perineum. *South Med J* 1993, 86:908–911.

20. Uman SJ, Kunin CM: Needle aspiration in the diagnosis of soft tissue infections. *Arch Intern Med* 1975, 135:959–961.

21. Sachs MK: The optimum use of needle aspiration in the bacteriologic diagnosis of cellulitis in adults. *Arch Intern Med* 1990, 150:1907–1912.

22. Kielhofner MA, Brown B, Dall L: Influence of underlying disease process on the utility of cellulitis needle aspirates. *Arch Intern Med* 1988, 148:2451–2452.

23. Duvanel T, Auckenthaler R, Rohner P, *et al.*: Quantitative cultures of biopsy specimens from cutaneous cellulitis. *Arch Intern Med* 1989, 149:293–296.

24. Saiag P, Le Breton C, Pavlovic M, *et al.*: Magnetic resonance imaging in adults presenting with severe acute infectious cellulitis. *Arch Dermatol* 1994, 130:1150–1158.

25.• Kremer M, Zuckerman R, Avraham Z, Raz R: Long-term antimicrobial therapy in the prevention of recurrent soft-tissue infections. *J Infect* 1991, 22:37–40.

26. The choice of antibacterial drugs. *Med Lett Drugs Ther* 1994, 36:53–60.

27. Systemic antifungal drugs. *Med Lett Drugs Ther* 1994, 36:16–18.

28. Bradley SF, Terpenning MS, Ramsey MA, *et al.*: Methicillin-resistant *Staphylococcus*: colonization and infection in a long-term care facility. *Ann Intern Med* 1991, 115:417–422.

29. Goetz MB, Mulligan ME, Kwok R, *et al.*: Management and epidemiologic analyses of an outbreak due to methicillin-resistant *Staphylococcus aureus*. *Am J Med* 1992, 92:607–614.

Urinary Tract Infections: Uncomplicated, Complicated, and Nosocomial

9

Jack D. Sobel

Key Points

- A valuable new diagnostic and management approach to urinary tract infections (UTIs) is to view episodes as uncomplicated and complicated.

- Most episodes of UTI in young adult women can be managed without pre- and posttreatment urine cultures and do not require urologic investigation.

- Uncomplicated bacterial cystitis is effectively treated with 3 days of antimicrobial therapy; uncomplicated pyelonephritis should be treated for a total of 14 days.

- Most adults with asymptomatic bacteriuria do not require therapy except during pregnancy and prior to urinary tract instrumentation.

- Catheter-associated bacteriuria should be treated only in the presence of symptoms.

EPIDEMIOLOGY

At least 10% to 20% of the female population experience a symptomatic urinary tract infection (UTI) at some time during their lives [1]. Although the prevalence of bacteriuria in men is low (0.1% or less), it rises dramatically in older men, mainly related to prostatic enlargement. Men with bacteriuria frequently have anatomic abnormalities of the urinary tract. At least 10% of men and 26% of women over 65 years of age have bacteriuria. Hospitalized patients have the highest prevalence of bacteriuria, mainly because of the use of indwelling catheters and instrumentation. A single catheterization causes UTI in 1% of ambulatory persons; however, after catheterization of hospitalized patients, infection occurs in at least 10% [2•].

PATHOGENESIS

Bacteria invade and spread within the urinary tract usually by the ascending route and rarely by the hematogenous and lymphatic pathways [1]. Even in the presence of catheterization, most UTIs occur in structurally and functionally normal urinary tracts. Urinary tract infections tend to be preceded by periurethral and distal urethral colonization with uropathogens. Susceptibility to UTI depends upon genetic and behavioral risk factors [1]. Congenital and acquired structural and functional abnormalities such as calculi, neurogenic bladder, strictures, and diabetes mellitus all cause major susceptibility to infection. In the presence of predisposing abnormalities, bacterial pathogens readily invade and ascend the urinary tract, requiring the minimal expression of virulence factors to cause disease. Virulence factors allow for selection of clones of uropathogenic coliforms from the fecal flora. These factors enable the pathogens to persist in the face of efficient defense mechanisms and enhance their ability to cause disease [3•]. Virulence factors of bacterial uropathogens and host defense mechanisms are shown in Table 1.

Because most UTIs occur in otherwise healthy young women, most of our knowledge about the pathogenesis of UTIs is derived from this population [4]. The

TABLE 1 VIRULENCE FACTORS OF UROPATHOGENIC BACTERIA AND NORMAL HOST DEFENSE MECHANISMS IN THE URINARY TRACT

Virulence factors	Host defense mechanisms
Clonality (O, K, H serotypes)	Flushing effect of micturition
Adherence to vaginal and uroepithelial cells	Antibacterial constituents of urine
Hemolysin production	Antiadherence mechanisms
Aerobactin production	Urinary IgA, IgG
Resistance to phagocytosis	Tamm-Horsfall protein
Resistance to serumcidal activity	Bladder mucopolysaccharide layer
Bacterial generation time in urine	Antibacterial activity of mucosa
Bacterial ureteroplegic factor	IL-6
	Phagocytic cells

short female urethra allows bacteria colonizing the distal urethra to enter the bladder after urethral massage, such as occurs during intercourse [5,6]. Although the fecal flora offers the primary source and reservoir of uropathogens, the vagina and periurethral regions are colonized prior to onset of the UTI [7]. Factors facilitating colonization of the vagina include diaphragm and spermicide use, which in part accounts for the increased risk of UTI associated with sexual activity [8]. In contrast to *Escherichia coli*, resident vaginal lactobacilli are highly sensitive to nonoxynol 9 spermicide. Antibiotics, especially β-lactams, also promote introital colonization with *E. coli*. Estrogen hormone replacement therapy may protect against UTI in postmenopausal women by preserving a lactobacillus-dominant vaginal flora. Genetic factors may operate at a cellular membrane level to explain the unique susceptibility of some women to recurrent UTI in the absence of structural changes in the urinary tract. Genetic predisposition is because of the presence of certain blood group antigens on vaginal and uroepithelial cells that act as receptors for uropathogens [1].

Uncomplicated UTIs occur in normal urinary tracts, tend to develop in the community, are usually caused by sensitive *E. coli*, and respond well to antibiotic therapy. In contrast, complicated UTIs occur in urinary tracts that have structural or functional abnormalities or are nosocomial in origin, with a tendency to more diverse and resistant microorganisms. The latter infections respond less well to conventional therapy and require more prolonged treatment (Tables 2 and 3).

The majority of UTIs are caused by a single species of bacteria. *E. coli* is by the far the most common infecting organism in acute uncomplicated infection [1,4]. In complicated UTIs, there is an increased likelihood of *Proteus*, *Pseudomonas*, *Klebsiella*, and *Enterobacter* species and enterococci. The hospital environment frequently selects for resistant organisms and structural anomalies; catheters further select for polymicrobial infections. *Corynebacterium* group D_2 has recently been recognized as an important nosocomial pathogen. *Staphylococcus aureus* bacteriuria often indicates metastatic infection of the kidney following *S. aureus*

TABLE 2 COMPARISON OF UNCOMPLICATED AND COMPLICATED URINARY TRACT INFECTION

	Uncomplicated UTI	Complicated UTI
Age	Adults	Any age
Pathogens	*Escherichia coli*	*Escherichia coli*
	Staphylococcus saprophyticus	*Klebsiella* spp
		Proteus spp
		Pseudomonas aeruginosa
		Enterococci
Source	Community-acquired	Often nosocomial
Upper tract involvement	Infrequent	Frequent
Structural and functional abnormalities	Absent	Common
Instrumentation and catheters	Absent	Often
Susceptibility to antimicrobials	Yes	Variable
Response to short-course therapy	Good	Poor

UTI—urinary tract infection.

TABLE 3 COMPLICATED URINARY TRACT INFECTIONS

Pregnancy	Calculi
Nosocomial	Diabetes mellitus
Catheter and instrumentation	Structural anomalies
Postrenal transplantation	Vesicoureteral reflux
Chronic bacterial prostatitis	Neurogenic bladder

bacteremia. Occasional episodes of UTI are due to *Haemophilus influenzae*, *Ureaplasma urealyticum*, and *Mycobacterium hominis*.

SIGNS AND SYMPTOMS

The classic symptoms of cystitis include dysuria, urgency, and frequency of micturition (small volumes), often accompanied by suprapubic discomfort or lower back pain. The urine may be turbid and occasionally frankly bloody. Cystitis makes up 95% of outpatient visits for UTIs. Upper tract involvement is indicated by the onset of fever, rigors, flank pain, and vomiting. Clinical correlation between anatomic localization of infection and symptoms is poor, in that one third of patients with signs and symptoms of cystitis have only occult or silent kidney involvement. Similarly, numerous patients with pyelonephritis have no concomitant or antecedent symptoms of cystitis.

The majority of elderly patients with bacteriuria are asymptomatic, and pyuria may be absent. When present, symptoms are often nonspecific especially because frequency, urgency, nocturia, and incontinence may have multiple causes in the elderly. Bacteremia and septic shock more commonly complicate pyelonephritis in the elderly. Catheterized patients have few or no symptoms referable to the bladder when they develop bacteriuria but usually present with fever and sepsis.

Cystitis in women must be differentiated from other conditions in which dysuria is a prominent symptom, namely vulvovaginitis because of *Candida* and trichomoniasis and urethritis because of genital herpesvirus, *Neisseria gonorrhoeae*, and *Chlamydia trachomatis*; hence the necessity of performing a gynecologic evaluation in most women with dysuria. When, however, other symptoms are also prominent (*eg*, frequency and suprapubic pain or tenderness), the likelihood of bacterial cystitis is increased, especially in the presence of macroscopic or microscopic hematuria. The poorly understood entity of interstitial cystitis should be considered in women, particularly when the dominant symptom is frequency of micturition (mainly nocturnal) and in the absence of positive urinary cultures.

The clinical spectrum of ascending pyelonephritis ranges from mild disease compatible with home management to severe rigors, hypotension, and septic shock. Bacteremia and its consequences are more common in the elderly and diabetics and in the presence of urinary obstruction. Other infrequent complications include intrarenal suppuration and perinephric abscesses.

DIAGNOSIS OF URINARY TRACT INFECTION

Culture, usually of a voided midstream specimen, remains the most reliable modality of diagnosing UTI, although pretreatment cultures are not routinely required in uncomplicated UTIs. Culture is directed not only at identifying the causal microorganism but also at quantitation of bacteria isolated. This allows for differentiation between true infection and perineal contamination of urine [1,4]. Urethral catheterization is infrequently used to obtain uncontaminated urine and is generally inadvisable, because even in-and-out catheterization is expensive and not without complications. Although Kass originally demonstrated that 10^5 bacteria/mL of voided urine reliably distinguished between contaminated and infected urine, several more recent studies have shown that about one third of women with acute cystitis caused by *E. coli* and *Staphylococcus saprophyticus* have colony counts of between 10^2 to 10^4 colony-forming units (CFU)/mL (Table 4). Because similar findings have been observed in acute pyelonephritis, a more reasonable cutoff in acutely symptomatic women for defining significant or relevant bacteremia is greater than or about 10^2 CFU/mL of known uropathogen [4]. Nevertheless, because most microbiology laboratories use culture methodologies that accurately detect 10^3 but not 10^2 CFU/mL, a cutoff of 10^3 CFU/mL is now generally used [8]. Notably, the 10^5 CFU/mL criterion still applies to patients with asymptomatic bacteriuria.

Several screening technologies using photometry or bioluminescence have become available; these are valuable within a short period (2 hours) in identifying patients with a high concentration of bacteria in urine (10^5/mL) but are not sufficiently sensitive to detect low concentrations of bacteria, between 10^2 and 10^4 CFU/mL.

Pyuria detected microscopically is a valuable rapid screening method that physicians have traditionally used, although familiarity with the microscope has declined and there is more dependence on alternative screening tests. The hemocytometer method utilizing uncentrifuged urine is a highly sensitive indicator of UTI in acutely symptomatic women but is infrequently used. Instead, most laboratories use centrifuged urine sediment and count leukocytes per high power field—a method that is far less accurate. The leukocyte-esterase

TABLE 4 DIAGNOSTIC CRITERIA FOR URINARY TRACT INFECTION

	Significant bacteriuria, CFU/mL
Acute cystitis	$\geq 10^3$ (? $\geq 10^2$)
Acute uncomplicated pyelonephritis	$\geq 10^4$
UTI in males	$\geq 10^4$
Asymptomatic bacteriuria	$\geq 10^5$ x 2

CFU—colony-forming units; UTI—urinary tract infection.
Adapted from Rubin *et al.* [18]; with permission.

dipstick method, although less sensitive than hemocytometer counting, is nevertheless a reasonable rapid alternative to microscopy. Regardless of the method used, pyuria is less reliable in diagnosing complicated UTIs. Microscopic bacteriuria and hematuria lack sensitivity but are specific and when present in a patient with urinary symptoms are highly predictive of bacterial UTI. Failure to detect erythrocytes or bacteria by microscopy should not exclude a diagnosis of UTI, because bacteria are not easily detected in low-colony-count UTI (10^2 to 10^4 CFU/mL).

Pretreatment urine cultures should be obtained for all patients with complicated UTIs, all males, females with recurrent UTIs, patients in whom there is suspicion of upper tract infection, and, finally, when the diagnosis is in doubt (Table 3). Accordingly, adult females with cystitis can be treated empirically with antimicrobial agents without culture after the diagnosis is confirmed microscopically. This is because the spectrum and susceptibility of infecting bacteria are highly predictable in uncomplicated cystitis.

TREATMENT
Asymptomatic Bacteriuria

The majority of adults with asymptomatic bacteriuria do not require antimicrobial therapy, because untreated, uncomplicated UTIs uncommonly result in significant morbidity [9]. Exceptions are shown in Table 5. Moreover, in the absence of urologic abnormalities, there is little indication that asymptomatic bacteriuria leads to renal dysfunction or hypertension. In women, the prevalence of asymptomatic bacteriuria increases with rising age by 1% per decade, reaching 6% among women in their sixties but rising more rapidly thereafter to reach 20% among those in their ninth decade [10]. Although several studies in the 1960s and 1970s hinted that asymptomatic bacteriuria in the elderly was associated with a higher mortality rate [11], a more recent study failed to find any difference in life expectancy among bacteriuric and nonbacteriuric elderly individuals [12].

On the other hand, bacteriuria in pregnancy is associated with a high risk of developing acute pyelonephritis (25%) and may jeopardize the pregnancy. Hence women should be screened for bacteriuria during pregnancy, promptly treated, and carefully followed for recurrence of bacteriuria. Asympto-

TABLE 5 INDICATIONS FOR TREATMENT OF ASYMPTOMATIC BACTERIURIA
Preschool children
Pregnant women
Diabetics*
Neutropenia
Postrenal transplantation
Patients undergoing urologic procedures
Staghorn calculus*
*Controversial.

matic bacteriuria should not be treated in most catheterized patients, particularly those with chronic indwelling catheters and hospitalized patients.

Acute Cystitis

In the past, treatment for cystitis with an oral antibiotic was continued for 2 weeks [1]. Single-dose therapy (SDT) was introduced approximately 15 years ago based on proven efficacy, cost savings, and fewer complications. The effectiveness of SDT is the consequence of the superficial nature of the mucosal infection. Despite the convenience of SDT, this form of treatment is, however, inferior to a 3-day course using the same antibiotics (Table 6). Three-day therapy provides results almost identical to those of more prolonged therapy, at considerably less expense and with fewer side effects [13••]. The earlier efficacy studies of SDT probably suffered from sample size errors, and the greater efficacy with 3-day therapy most likely reflects enhanced capacity to eradicate occult renal parenchymal infection. The superior therapeutic results obtained with trimethoprim-sulfamethoxazole (TMP-SMX) and oral quinolone SDT in comparison with β-lactam antimicrobials reflects several pharmacokinetic advantages of the former, including more prolonged therapeutic concentrations in the urine and kidney as well as higher drug concentrations in the vagina, eradicating the potential for reinfection from this important reservoir. Three-day regimens effective for cystitis are shown in Table 7 but should be reserved for patients with uncomplicated cystitis only. (Excludes patients shown in Table 3.)

TABLE 6 DURATION OF THERAPY FOR ACUTE CYSTITIS

	Eradication of bacteriuria			Adverse effects of antibiotics	
Duration	TMP-SMX	β-Lactams	Duration	TMP-SMX	β-Lactams
Single dose	89%	68%	Single dose	7%	12%
3 d	95%	82%	3 d	7%	12%
≥5 d	96%	88%	≥5 d	25%	17%

TMP-SMX—trimethoprim-sulfamethoxazole.
Adapted from Norrby [13••]; with permission.

Antibiotic	Cystitis, %	Acute pyelonephritis, %	Complicated UTI, %
Ampicillin	65	72	30
First generation cephalosporins	87	81	51
Third generation cephalosporins		90	95
Gentamicin		100	81
Antipseudomonal penicillin		82	
Nitrofurantoin	86		
Sulfonamide		73	
Tetracycline	62		
Trimethoprim	93		
Trimethoprim-sulfamethoxazole	95	100	63
Ciprofloxacin	99	98	95

UTI—urinary tract infection.
From Johnson J, Stamm WE [19]; with permission.

Acute Pyelonephritis

Patients with mild, uncomplicated, acute pyelonephritis can be managed in the outpatient setting. Patients in this category are able to tolerate oral antimicrobial therapy; they are hemodynamically stable, compliant, and reliable enough to report lack of improvement early. Pregnant patients, diabetics, and others listed in Table 2 should be managed as inpatients. Based on the microbiology of acute uncomplicated pyelonephritis, outpatient antibiotic therapy includes TMP-SMX, amoxicillin-clavulanic acid, and quinolones. Admission to an overnight observation unit associated with an emergency room is a useful strategy.

The majority of patients require hospitalization, intravenous fluids, and parenteral antibiotics. Initial empiric therapy pending urine cultures has traditionally been ampicillin and aminoglycoside. Empiric therapy should, however, be directed by the results of a Gram stain examination of the infected urine. Ampicillin has a role only if gram-positive cocci are visualized, because this finding is usually indicative of enterococci. The majority of gram-negative uropathogens are now resistant to ampicillin, hence its role in UTIs has markedly diminished. In the presence of gram-negative bacilli, single-drug intravenous therapy with TMP-SMX, aminoglycosides, third-generation cephalosporins, aztreonam, extended-spectrum penicillins, or quinolones is adequate for uncomplicated pyelonephritis. Selection of therapy should be based on cost considerations and local antibiotic susceptibility patterns. Following the availability of sensitivity testing results, therapy can be modified. Parenteral therapy should be continued for at least 24 hours after fever resolves and the patient tolerates oral therapy. A combined course of 14 days is considered the minimal effective regimen if recurrences due to relapse are to be minimized [14].

Complicated cases of acute pyelonephritis are more likely to be caused by resistant microorganisms and are also associated with increased risk of bacteremia, septic shock, and local suppurative complications. Fortunately, gram-negative bacteremia secondary to UTI has a low mortality (5%) compared to bacteremia that is secondary to other causes. In this group, more aggressive antibacterial therapy is indicated, especially initially, when the empirically selected regimen must take into consideration increased risk of bacterial resistance. Hence a third-generation cephalosporin, a quinolone, or an aminoglycoside, alone or in combination is recommended until the susceptibility pattern is known and one agent can be stopped. Not all patients with acute pyelonephritis should have an ultrasound examination performed to exclude an obstruction. Patients with complicated disease, however, require, in addition to more aggressive therapy, earlier investigation and possibly also computed tomography and excretory urography, particularly when a calculus is suspected. Posttherapy urine cultures should be obtained in all patients with pyelonephritis.

RECURRENT URINARY TRACT INFECTION

Recurrent UTIs may be due to relapse or reinfection. Relapse infers failure of antimicrobials to completely eradicate bacteria from the urinary tract and tends to occur in structurally or functionally abnormal tracts. Relapsing infections (often pyelonephritis) tend to be caused by the same bacterial species, and bacteriuria reappears shortly after cessation of antibiotics. The source of relapsing infections is usually a structurally abnormal kidney, calculus, or chronic bacterial prostatitis in males. Three or more relapsing infections per year merit continuous maintenance suppressive antibiotic therapy with an agent selected on the basis of susceptibility pattern. A proven relapse after short-course therapy should be treated with 14 days of therapy. Prior to implementation of continuous maintenance therapy, a 6-week regimen is required. Relapsing infections also require thorough urologic evaluation.

In contrast, frequent reinfections tend to occur in adult women with structurally normal urinary tracts. In some women, reinfections are temporally related to sexual intercourse or diaphragm use and attacks tend to cluster in time. Three antibiotic strategies are effective in preventing reinfection: 1) continuous low-dose prophylaxis is highly effective, utilizing agents such as TMP, TMP-SMX, nitrofurantoin, and quinolones; 2) self-administered short-course treatment following self-diagnosis, applicable in a minority of women only; and 3) postcoital single-dose prophylaxis [15]. The choice of prophylaxis depends on the individual patient and factors associated with pathogenesis. Most regimens are initially prescribed for at least 6 months. However, UTIs tend to return at the preprophylaxis rate when the drug is withdrawn.

CATHETER-ASSOCIATED URINARY TRACT INFECTIONS

The urinary tract is the most common site of nosocomial infections (35% to 40%), most of which occur in patients who have undergone urologic manipulation [16]. Approximately 10% to 15% of patients in community hospitals have indwelling catheters. The majority of these infections are asymptomatic; symptoms of cystitis may supervene, but the most important consequence is ascending infection, pyelonephritis, bacteremia, and urosepsis, including septic shock. Catheter-associated UTI is the most common source of nosocomial gram-negative bacteremia and is associated with considerable mortality and prolonged hospital stays [2•,6].

Risk of infection increases with the use of the semiclosed drainage system, when the closed drainage system is disconnected, and with duration of catheterization. Accordingly, infection can be prevented by the use of a closed, sterile drainage system. Provided that this system is not violated, bacteriuria can usually be prevented for up to 10 days. The protective benefit of topical antibiotics applied to the urethral meatus is still controversial, as is the use of silver-impregnated urethral catheters. Systemic antibiotics have a short-term protective effect, but widespread and long-term use selects for infection by resistant strains and is not recommended for periods of catheterization longer than 7 days.

Asymptomatic bacteriuria should not be treated in patients with long-term or permanent urinary catheters. In contrast, asymptomatic bacteriuria in postoperative patients with short-duration catheters uncommonly resolves following removal of the catheter, and symptomatic UTI often follows. Hence, in this context, bacteriuria may be treated prior to removal of the catheter [17•]. Otherwise catheter-associated bacteriuria should be treated only in the presence of symptoms. Antibiotic therapy should be preceded by changing the catheter, because concretions may function as a site for bacterial persistence. Upper tract or constitutional manifestations require parenteral therapy, total duration of therapy being at least 7 days [2].

REFERENCES AND RECOMMENDED READING

Recently published papers of particular interest have been highlighted as:
• Of interest
•• Of outstanding interest

1.   Stamm WE, Hooton TM, Johnson JR, et al.: Urinary tract infections from pathogenesis to treatment. J Infect Dis 1989, 159:400–406.

2.• Stamm WE: Catheter-associated urinary tract infections: epidemiology, pathogenesis and prevention. Am J Med 1991, 91:65–71.

3.• Johnson JR: Virulence factors in Escherichia coli urinary tract infection. Clin Microbiol Rev 1991, 4:80–128.

4.   Johnson JR, Stamm WE: Urinary tract infections in women: diagnosis and treatment. Ann Intern Med 1989, 111:906–917.

5.   Strom BL, Collins M, West SL, et al.: Sexual activity, contraceptive use, and other risk factors for symptomatic and asymptomatic bacteriuria: a case-control study. Ann Intern Med 1987, 107:816–823.

6.   Buckly RM, McGukin M, MacGregor RR: Urine bacterial counts after sexual intercourse. N Engl J Med 1978, 298:321–326.

7.   Stamey TA, Sexton CC: The role of vaginal colonization with Enterobacteriaceae in recurrent urinary tract infection. J Urol 1975, 113:214–217.

8.   Fihn SD, Latham RH, Roberts P, et al.: Association between diaphragm use and urinary tract infection. JAMA 1985, 254:240–245.

9.   Zhanel GG, Harding GKM, Guay DRP: Asymptomatic bacteriuria: which patients should be treated? Arch Intern Med 1990, 150:1389–1395.

10. Boscia JA, Kobasa WD, Knight RA, et al.: Epidemiology of bacteriuria in an elderly ambulatory population. Am J Med 1986, 80:208–214.

11. Dontas AS, Kasviki-Charvati P, Paponayiotou PC, Marketon SG: Bacteriuria and survival in old age. N Engl J Med 1981, 304:939–943.

12. Nordenstam GR, Brandberg CA, Oden AS, et al.: Bacteriuria and mortality in an elderly population. N Engl J Med 1986, 314:1152–1156.

13.•• Norrby SR: Short-term treatment of uncomplicated lower urinary tract infections in women. Rev Infect Dis 1990, 12:458–467.

14. Johnson JR, Lyons MF II, Pearce W, et al.: Therapy for women hospitalized with acute pyelonephritis: a randomized trial of ampicillin versus trimethoprim-sulfamethoxazole for 14 days. J Infect Dis 1991, 163:325–330.

15. Nicolle LE, Harding GKM, Thomson M, et al.: Efficacy of 5 years of low-dose trimethoprim-sulfamethoxazole prophylaxis for urinary tract infection. J Infect Dis 1988, 57:1239–1247.

16. Schaeffer AJ: Catheter-associated bacteriuria. Urol Clin North Am 1986, 13:735–747.

17.• Harding GK, Nicolle LE, Ronald AR, et al.: How long should catheter-acquired urinary tract infection in women be treated? A randomized controlled study. Ann Intern Med 1991, 114:713–719.

18. Rubin RH, Shapiro ED, Andriole VT, et al.: Evaluation of new anti-infective drugs for the treatment of urinary tract infection. Clin Infect Dis 1992, 15(suppl):216–227.

19. Johnson JR, Stamm WE: Diagnosis and treatment of acute urinary tract infections. Infect Dis Clin North Am 1987, 1:773–792.

SELECT BIBLIOGRAPHY

Hooton TM, Stamm WE: Management of acute uncomplicated urinary tract infection in adults. Med Clin North Am 1991, 75:339–357.

Ronald AR, Nicolle LE, Harding GK: Standards of therapy for urinary tract infections in adults. Infection 1992, 20(suppl 3):S164–170.

Stamm WE, Counts GW, Running KR, et al.: Diagnosis of coliform infection in acutely dysuric women. N Engl J Med 1982, 307:463–468.

Stapleton A, Latham RH, Johnson C, Stamm WE: Post-coital antimicrobial prophylaxis for recurrent urinary tract infections: a randomized, double blind, placebo-controlled trial. JAMA 1990, 264:703–706.

Stapleton A, Nudelman E, Clausen H, et al.: Binding of uropathogenic Escherichia coli R45 to glycolipids extracted from vaginal epithelial cells is dependent on histo-blood group secretor status. J Clin Invest 1992, 90:965–972.

Sexually Transmitted Diseases 10
Byron E. Batteiger

Key Points

- The diagnosis of any one sexually transmitted disease (STD) indicates risky, unprotected sexual activity; a high risk of coexistent infection with another STD pathogen; and risk of acquiring HIV infection.

- Sexual behaviors that influence the risk of acquiring STDs include number of partners, rate of acquiring partners, casual partners, recent new partners, sexual preference, and type of sexual practice.

- Although many STDs present with typical symptoms and signs, asymptomatic infections are frequent, particularly in women.

- Women and newly born children bear a disproportionate burden of serious morbidities and complications associated with STDs.

- Vaccines currently are not available for preventing any STD other than hepatitis B. Control strategies consist of reducing new partner acquisition and modifying risky sexual behavior; reducing susceptibility by using condoms; and reducing infectivity and thereby disease spread by prompt diagnosis, treatment, and contact tracing.

Sexually transmitted diseases are a diverse group of disorders caused by protozoa, bacteria, viruses, and ectoparasites sharing the common thread of transmission by human sexual activity. Because sexual behavior is personal, studying its behavioral determinants is difficult, yet only by understanding them can effective ways be devised to change risky behaviors and to prevent and control these diseases. Sexual behaviors influencing the risk of acquiring sexually transmitted diseases include number of sexual partners, rate of acquiring partners, casual partners, sexual preference, and type of sexual practice. Health care behaviors that contribute to acquiring or complicating sexually transmitted diseases include failure to use condoms, noncompliance with therapy, delay in seeking medical care, and failure to refer infected partners.

The diseases listed in Table 1 include conditions not commonly thought of as being sexually transmitted, and they range from mild illnesses, readily treatable or with little associated morbidity, to HIV disease.

The diagnosis of any one sexually transmitted disease indicates risky, unprotected sexual activity; a high risk of coexistent infection with another sexually transmitted pathogen; risk of acquiring HIV infection; and an opportunity to influence the patient's behaviors to reduce risk. In developed countries the burden of these diseases falls on persons living in poverty, persons of color, and illicit drug users.

Some sexually transmitted diseases can be asymptomatic initially, yet produce major long-term morbidity and mortality. Chlamydial infections in women can produce silent salpingitis complicated by involuntary infertility and increased risk of ectopic pregnancy. Therefore, clinicians must obtain a sexual history, especially during the peak years of disease prevalence (roughly ages 14 to 35 years), and focus the physical examination accordingly (Tables 2 and 3). Sexually transmitted diseases must also be considered in older persons whose behaviors place them at risk. Screen-

TABLE 1 SEXUALLY TRANSMITTED DISEASES

Disease	Causative agent	Associated conditions
Gonorrhea	*Neisseria gonorrhoeae*	Cervicitis, salpingitis, urethritis, dermatitis-arthritis, conjunctivitis, proctitis
Chlamydia	*Chlamydia trachomatis*	Cervicitis, salpingitis, urethritis, conjunctivitis, neonatal pneumonia, proctitis
Syphilis	*Treponema pallidum*	Primary: genital ulcer
		Secondary: rash, lymphadenopathy
		Tertiary: neurosyphilis, others
Chancroid	*Haemophilus ducreyi*	Genital ulcer, regional lymphadenopathy
HIV disease	HIV types 1 and 2	Late stage: AIDS
Genital herpes	Herpes simplex virus type 2	Genital vesicles, ulcers
Genital warts	Human papillomavirus	Genital warts, cervical intraepithelial dysplasia
Cytomegalovirus disease	Cytomegalovirus	Asymptomatic infection
		Occasional mononucleosis syndrome
Molluscum contagiosum	Molluscum contagiosum virus (*Poxviridae*)	Skin papules
Enteric pathogens	*Salmonella, Shigella, Campylobacter* species	Proctocolitis, enteritis, diarrhea
Enteric protozoa	*Giardia lamblia, Entamoeba histolytica*	Diarrhea, abdominal pain
Trichomoniasis	*Trichomonas vaginalis*	Vaginitis
Ectoparasites	*Phthirus pubis, Sarcoptes scabiei*	Crab lice, scabies
Hepatitis	Hepatitis A, B, and C viruses	Hepatocellular disease

TABLE 2 ELEMENTS OF A SEXUAL HISTORY

Number of sexual partners: since past evaluation, past 30 d, past 60 d, past y, lifetime

Sexual preference: men only, women only, both men and women

Types of partners: regular partners, casual partners

Recent new sexual partner: within 30 to 60 d

Sexual practices: active or receptive vaginal, oral, or rectal intercourse

Type of contraception: barrier methods (condoms or diaphragm), consistency of use

History of sexually transmitted disease: chlamydiosis, gonorrhea, monogonoccocal urethritis, pelvic inflammatory disease, herpes, syphilis, warts

risk of sexual transmission of HIV. Worldwide control of sexually transmitted disease is a major key to control of HIV transmission.

Entire textbooks and monographs recently have been written about sexually transmitted diseases, and several sources cover topics in depth [1–4,5••,6•]. Drug regimens reflect the 1993 Sexually Transmitted Disease Treatment Guidelines from the Centers for Disease Control and Prevention [5••]. Table 5 summarizes treatments for sexually transmitted diseases, and Table 6 lists diagnostic tests.

CLINICAL SYNDROMES

Urethritis in Men

Urethral discharge and dysuria comprise this common clinical syndrome in men, although many infections are asymptomatic. The most common bacterial causes are *Neisseria gonorrhoeae* (gonococcal urethritis) and *Chlamydia trachomatis* (a frequent cause of nongonococcal urethritis).

The key diagnostic tool for distinguishing gonococcal and nongonococcal urethritis is a Gram stain of a smear made from an intraurethral swab specimen. In symptomatic gonococcal urethritis, neutrophils together with gram-negative intracellular diplococci are seen in 90% to 95% of men. A confirmatory culture is not needed because the Gram stain is highly specific. Because chlamydial coinfections are common in both men (15% to 20%) and women (35% to 40%) with gonorrhea, antibiotics active against chlamydia are given in addition to single-dose therapy for gonorrhea.

Because many sexual partners are infected, they should be identified, examined, and treated. Most women are minimally

ing for asymptomatic infections is appropriate for sexually active populations at especially high risk for *Chlamydia trachomatis* (Table 4).

Women and newly born children bear the burden of serious morbidities, including pelvic inflammatory disease resulting in chronic pelvic pain, infertility, and ectopic pregnancy; neonatal chlamydial conjunctivitis and pneumonia; congenital syphilis; and human papillomavirus–induced cervical intraepithelial neoplasia. Common symptoms and the diseases associated with them provide the framework for diagnosis and treatment. In persons with advanced HIV disease, certain sexually transmitted diseases are associated with increased severity, chronicity, and resistance to therapy. Certain STDs, especially those causing genital ulceration, are associated with increased

TABLE 3 ELEMENTS OF A PHYSICAL EXAMINATION

Women

Inspect pubic hair, external genitalia, and perirectal region for lesions, discharge
Inspect and palpate urethra, periurethral, and Bartholin's glands for swelling or discharge
Palpate inguinal region for lymphadenopathy
Speculum examination:
   Inspect vaginal mucosa, vaginal secretions, cervix
   Obtain endocervical swab specimens for chlamydia, gonorrhea tests
   Obtain posterior vaginal pool secretions for saline mount, potassium hydroxide preparation
   Perform Papanicolaou's test if not done during previous y
Bimanual examination:
   Examine for cervical motion tenderness
   Determine uterine size, position
   Palpate for adnexal swelling, mass, or tenderness
   Confirm findings with rectovaginal examination

Men

Inspect pubic hair, penis, scrotum, and perirectal region for lesions, discharge
Palpate scrotal contents: testes, adnexa, spermatic cord
Palpate inguinal regions for lymphadenopathy
Assess for urethral discharge and obtain two swab samples for Gram stain and gonorrhea culture and for chlamydia test

---

TABLE 4 SCREENING FOR ASYMPTOMATIC CHLAMYDIAL INFECTION IN WOMEN

Women visiting high prevalence facilities
Sexually transmitted disease clinics
Family planning clinics
Teen health clinics
Abortion clinics
Juvenile detention centers

Women with any of these risk factors in any setting
Sexually active adolescents
History of recent multiple or new sexual partners
Presence of another sexually transmitted disease
Use of nonbarrier methods of contraception

Routine testing suggested for:
Sexually active women under age 20 whenever a pelvic examination done
Sexually active women between ages of 20 and 25 annually

---

dipstick test can document pyuria when Gram stain is not available. *C. trachomatis* causes 23% to 55% of cases, *Ureaplasma urealyticum* 20% to 40%, and *Trichomonas vaginalis* 2% to 5%. Cultures for *N. gonorrhoeae* and a test for *C. trachomatis* should be obtained.

Women who are partners of men with nongonococcal urethritis are at high risk for chlamydial infection but are most often asymptomatic. They should have a speculum and bimanual examination, including tests for gonococcal and chlamydial infection, and receive treatment with a regimen likely to be effective for chlamydial infection.

It is important to distinguish between nongonococcal and gonococcal urethritis, because treatment differs. When examination of a gram-stained smear is not possible, single-dose therapy appropriate for gonorrhea along with 7 days of doxycycline or single-dose azithromycin therapy (1 g) for nongonococcal urethritis should be given. (Combined single-dose therapies—single-dose cefixime for gonorrhea and single-dose azithromycin for concurrent chlamydia—are not well studied, however.)

Posttreatment testing for cure of chlamydial and gonococcal urethritis is not necessary since available therapies are highly effective.

Complications of urethritis in men are relatively rare but include epididymitis manifest by pain, unilateral swelling, and tenderness of the testicular adnexa. The major complication of urethritis in men is transmission to women.

Pelvic Inflammatory Disease

The major morbidity of chlamydial and gonococcal infections is related to ascending tubal infection after an initial lower genital tract infection at the endocervix, the latter

symptomatic, and Gram stain of cervical secretions is much less sensitive or specific for gonococci and should not be done routinely. Cultures for gonococcal infection from the endocervix and the rectum, and a chlamydia test from the endocervix should be obtained before treatment.

In nongonococcal urethritis, the presence of five or more neutrophils per oil immersion field without gram-negative intracellular diplococci is diagnostic, with or without visible urethral discharge. Urinalysis or a positive leukocyte esterase

TABLE 5 TREATMENT OF SEXUALLY TRANSMITTED DISEASES

Disease	Recommended drugs	Dosage	Alternative
Uncomplicated chlamydial infection: urethritis, cervicitis, proctitis, conjunctivitis	Doxycycline or azithromycin	100 mg orally, twice daily for 7 d 1 g orally once	Erythromycin base, 500 mg orally four times daily for 7 d; or ofloxacin, 300 mg orally twice daily for 7 d
Chlamydial infection in pregnancy	Erythromycin	500 mg orally four times daily for 7 d	Erythromycin, 250 mg orally four times daily for 14 d; amoxicillin, 500 mg three times daily for 10 d
Nongonococcal urethritis	Doxycycline or azithromycin	100 mg orally, twice daily for 7 d 1 g orally once	Erythromycin base, 500 mg orally four times daily for 7 d; or ofloxacin, 300 mg orally twice daily for 7 d
Uncomplicated gonorrhea	Ceftriaxone or cefixime or ciprofloxacin or ofloxacin plus doxycycline	125 mg intramuscularly once 400 mg orally once 500 mg orally once 400 mg orally once 100 mg orally twice daily for 7 d	For β-lactam allergy: spectinomycin, 2 g intramuscularly once plus doxy-cycline, 100 mg orally twice daily for 7 d
Disseminated gonococcal infection (dermatitis-arthritis)	Ceftriaxone for 24–48 h after improved, then cefixime or ciprofloxacin	1 g intravenously every 24 h 400 mg orally twice daily 500 mg orally twice daily to complete 7 d	Cefotaxime or ceftizoxime, 1 g every 8 h; for β-lactam allergy: spectino-mycin, 2 g intramuscularly every 12 h
Epididymitis	Ceftriaxone and doxycycline	250 mg intramuscularly once 100 mg orally twice daily for 10 d	Ofloxacin, 300 mg orally twice daily for 10 d
Pelvic inflammatory disease, inpatient regimen	Cefotetan or cefoxitin and doxycycline until improved, then doxycycline	2 g intravenously every 12 h 2 g intravenously every 6 h 100 mg intravenously or orally every 12 h 100 mg orally for 12 h to complete 14 d	Clindamycin, 900 mg every 8 h, and gentamicin, 2 mg/kg load, then 1.5 mg/kg every 8 h until improved; then doxycycline, 100 mg orally twice daily, or clin-damycin, 450 mg orally four times daily to complete 14 d
Pelvic inflammatory disease, outpatient regimen	Ceftriaxone then doxycycline	250 mg intramuscularly once 100 mg orally twice daily for 14 d	Ofloxacin, 400 mg orally twice daily for 14 d, plus clindamycin, 450 mg orally four times daily, or metron-idazole, 500 mg orally twice daily for 14 d
First episode genital herpes	Acyclovir	200 mg orally five times daily for 7–10 d or until resolution	
Severe first episode genital herpes	Acyclovir	5 mg/kg intravenously every 8 h for 5–7 d	
First episode herpes proctitis	Acyclovir	400 mg orally five times daily for 10 d or until resolution	
Recurrent episode genital herpes	Acyclovir	200 mg orally five times daily or 400 mg orally three times daily or 800 mg orally two times daily for 5 d	
Prevention of frequent recurrences of genital herpes	Acyclovir	400 mg orally twice daily for 1 y, then discontinue to assess for recurrence rate	

(Continued)

TABLE 5 TREATMENT OF SEXUALLY TRANSMITTED DISEASES (CONTINUED)

Disease	Recommended drugs	Dosage	Alternative
Chancroid	Azithromycin or ceftriaxone or erythromycin base	1 g orally once 250 mg intramuscularly once 500 mg orally four times daily for 7 d	Ciprofloxacin, 500 mg orally twice daily for 3 d, or amoxicillin, 500 mg, with clavulanate, 125 mg orally three times daily for 7 d
Early syphilis (primary or secondary, or latent less than 1 y)	Penicillin G benzathine	2.4 million U intramuscularly once	Doxycycline, 100 mg orally twice daily for 14 d
Vaginal infection:			
Trichomoniasis	Metronidazole	2 g orally once	500 mg orally twice daily for 7 d
Bacterial vaginosis	Metronidazole	500 mg orally twice daily for 7 d	Metronidazole gel or clindamycin cream intravaginally nightly for 7 d
Candidiasis	Clotrimazole, miconazole, tioconazole, terconazole	Multiple-dose forms for 3-d or 7-d regimens	

TABLE 6 DIAGNOSTIC TESTS FOR SEXUALLY TRANSMITTED DISEASES

Test	Types	Use	Comments
Chlamydia culture	Cell culture	Diagnostic testing, screening; testing where specificity is crucial (cases of suspected abuse, rape); rectal site	Preferred test because of sensitivity and specificity, but expensive and not widely available; stringent sample handling required
Chlamydia nonculture tests*	Enzyme immunoassay, direct fluorescence test, DNA hybridization	Diagnostic testing, screening	Affordable and widely available but less sensitive than culture; should be used only at endocervical and urethral sites
Chlamydia polymerase chain reaction or ligase chain reaction assays	DNA amplification	Diagnostic testing, screening	May prove to match sensitivity of culture with less stringent handling requirements
Gonorrhea culture	Standard agar culture	Diagnostic testing, screening	Sensitive, specific, widely available, and inexpensive
Herpes culture	Cell culture	Diagnostic testing for lesions or asymptomatic shedding	Preferred test because of sensitivity and specificity
Herpes nonculture tests	Enzyme immunoassay, direct fluorescence, DNA detection	Diagnostic testing for lesions only	Less expensive and more available than cell culture but less sensitive
Nontreponemal serologic tests (reaginic tests)	VDRL, RPR, ART	Screening tests for syphilis, determination of disease activity by titer	May be falsely positive in many illnesses [8]; titers fall with treatment of early syphilis
Treponemal serologic tests	FTA-ABS MHA-TP	Confirms positive reaginic test	More specific than reaginic tests; may remain positive indefinitely
Tests for bacterial vaginosis	Amine odor on 10% potassium hydroxide mount; vaginal pH > 4.5; saline mount with clue cells; homogeneous adherent white discharge	Three of four establishes clinical diagnosis	High vaginal pH and fishy odor on potassium hydroxide preparation may be seen with trichomoniasis; cultures for *Gardnerella vaginalis* not useful

*See reference 6 for detailed consideration of chlamydia tests.
ART—automated reagin test; FTA-ABS—fluorescent treponemal antibody absorption; MHA-TP—microhemagglutination-*Treponema pallidum*; RPR—rapid plasmin reagin.

most often asymptomatic. The risk of infertility rises with each episode of salpingitis. Many cases of salpingitis caused by *C. trachomatis* are minimally symptomatic and go undetected until the woman comes to medical attention because of involuntary infertility or ectopic pregnancy. In addition to gonococcal and chlamydial pelvic inflammatory disease, some cases are caused by mixed infections with enteric gram-negative rods and anaerobes.

Preventing pelvic inflammatory disease with its resulting infertility and ectopic pregnancy is the major goal of controlling gonococcal and chlamydial infection. Primary prevention is accomplished by behavioral change or barrier contraception to prevent cervical infection, secondary prevention by screening for and treating cervical infection to prevent ascending infection. This is a very important strategy among sexually active women younger than 25, who are at high risk for acquiring chlamydial infection, and once infected, have a greater risk of pelvic inflammatory disease than do older women. Tertiary prevention consists of aggressive therapy for established symptomatic salpingitis; although treatment resolves symptoms, it is uncertain whether it reduces the risk of sequelae.

Pelvic inflammatory disease should be a prime diagnostic consideration among women, particularly adolescents, who have pelvic or lower abdominal pain. A careful sexual history ensures that the diagnosis is not overlooked. Unfortunately, many conditions can mimic the disease, including ectopic pregnancy, acute appendicitis, endometriosis, and functional pain. Laparoscopy is the gold standard of diagnosis but is often not readily available, is invasive and expensive, and does not diagnose early disease manifest by endometritis. Therefore, clinical diagnosis is the rule, based on the minimum criteria [5••] of lower abdominal tenderness, adnexal tenderness, cervical motion tenderness, and lack of other established causes of the symptoms.

Treatment requires combination antibiotics because of the range of bacteria involved. Pelvic inflammatory disease may be particularly difficult to treat in women with AIDS.

Vaginal Discharge

Vaginal discharge is occasionally seen with sexually transmitted cervicitis. Sexually active women with vaginal discharge should receive a pelvic examination, examination of vaginal fluids for vaginitis-associated organisms, and tests from the endocervix for chlamydia and gonorrhea. Herpes simplex virus can occasionally cause cervicitis and vaginal discharge; a culture or antigen test should be performed if ulcerative cervical or vaginal lesions are seen.

Among the causes of vaginitis, candidiasis is common but is not usually sexually transmitted. Most often, white curd-like vaginal exudate is found and shows typical pseudohyphae on potassium hydroxide preparation. Preferred treatments consist of 3- to 7-day courses of intravaginal creams or tablets. Nystatin preparations are not recommended because of inferior efficacy compared with the newer azole antifungal agents. Women with AIDS may have recalcitrant or frequently recurring disease.

Bacterial vaginosis, although not definitely sexually transmitted, is associated with sexual activity. It is characterized by an altered vaginal microbial flora, particularly anaerobic flora. Symptoms include vaginal discharge and odor, and

findings include homogeneous adherent whitish-yellow vaginal secretions with fishy odor and vaginal wall hyperemia. Treatment of sexual contacts is not necessary.

Trichomoniasis is a sexually transmitted protozoal infection, and it indicates an increased risk of other sexually transmitted diseases, including chlamydial infection, gonorrhea, and syphilis. The infection is characterized by odor, frothy yellowish-green profuse vaginal secretions, and sometimes punctate exocervicitis. Laboratory diagnosis relies on saline mount of secretions showing motile trichomonads (only 40% to 80% sensitive) or on culture, which is not widely available. Single-dose treatment for definite cases is preferred. Male partners should be examined for other sexually transmitted diseases and should receive a single dose of metronidazole.

Because of the insensitivity of laboratory tools, the clinician will not always be able to definitely classify clinically obvious vaginitis. In symptomatic women, treatment with an oral regimen suitable for bacterial vaginosis, also sufficient for trichomoniasis, should be considered.

Genital Ulcer Disease

Genital ulcer disease is associated with an increased risk of acquiring HIV infection. Although genital ulcer disease is less common in the United States than in developing countries, herpes simplex virus disease is endemic, and recent outbreaks of syphilis and chancroid have occurred.

Herpes simplex virus type 2

Herpes simplex virus type 2 (HSV-2) is the most common cause of genital ulcers in the United States. The first clinical episode is characterized by clusters of vesicles that rupture to form painful shallow ulcers that crust and gradually resolve in about 3 weeks. Severe cases can be accompanied by local lymphadenopathy, malaise, low-grade fever, and occasionally aseptic meningitis. The virus then establishes a life-long latent infection in dorsal root ganglia. Recurrent episodes are common and often heralded by a prodrome of pain or paresthesia; lesions are usually milder and resolve more quickly than those of first episodes. Lesions many occur on genital or perirectal skin or epithelium of vulva, vagina, cervix, urethra, or rectum. Autoinoculation to other skin areas or the eye can occur. Individuals are most infectious while lesions are present, but asymptomatic virus shedding between episodes serves as a frequent means of transmission. Many adults have serologic evidence of infection with no clinical history of outbreaks. Some periodically shed virus, serving as a reservoir for continued transmission.

Documenting the virus by culture or antigen test establishes a definite diagnosis. Acyclovir therapy is suppressive only and neither eradicates latent virus nor decreases the risk of subsequent recurrence. Treating recurrent episodes is less useful because lesions resolve more quickly. Acyclovir ointment is not useful for treating either primary or recurrent episodes. Persons with six or more recurrences per year benefit from chronic suppression, which is considered safe and effective for up to 5 years. After 1 year of suppressive therapy, acyclovir should be withheld temporarily to verify continuing need, because some patients inexplicably cease having recurrences.

Perinatal transmission of HSV occurs. Fully established HSV disease in neonates, although infrequent, is devastating. Pregnant women with genital herpes should be carefully examined at the time of labor. Women with visible lesions should undergo cesarean section. If lesions are not present, vaginal delivery is recommended. Genital culture of mother and child should be done. If either is positive, vigilance for early signs of infection in the neonate is warranted. Acyclovir therapy is reserved for definite clinical disease. Recombinant HSV-2 vaccines are currently in clinical trial, but efficacy is not yet established.

Syphilis

Syphilis is a treponemal infection with protean manifestations. Untreated primary or secondary syphilis can progress to neurosyphilis and other tertiary manifestations [1,2]. Only early disease is considered here.

Treponema pallidum typically produces genital ulcers (chancres) during primary infection. These are often single but may be multiple; they can affect the skin or oral, vulvar, vaginal, or rectal epithelia. Chancres often have indurated edges and are less commonly painful than herpetic ulcers or chancroid. Regional adenopathy is common. Secondary syphilis is a systemic disease resulting from dissemination of *T. pallidum* following untreated or inapparent primary disease. It is often accompanied by a rash.

Definitive diagnosis of early syphilis requires observing motile treponemes by darkfield microscopy of touch preparations of lesion exudate. Expertly prepared and interpreted tests are not available in many outpatient facilities, and patients should be referred to a clinic specializing in sexually transmitted diseases. Presumptive diagnosis makes use of nontreponemal serologic tests (VDRL, RPR) followed by confirmatory specific treponemal serologic testing (FTA-Abs, MHA-TP). However, 13% to 41% [7] of patients with chancres may have negative results in serologic tests initially, making follow-up testing necessary after about 2 weeks.

Penicillin is the preferred treatment for all stages of syphilis. Alternative regimens should be used with great caution, with adequate provision for follow-up nontreponemal serologic testing to document an adequate response. Many authorities advocate penicillin desensitization for treating a pregnant woman with syphilis because of the potential for congenital syphilis if treatment or follow-up is inadequate [5••].

Patients with syphilis should be tested for HIV infection; likewise, HIV-infected persons should be screened for syphilis. Severe disease, early progression to neurosyphilis, resistance to therapy, or relapse after presumed adequate therapy has been documented in HIV-infected persons. All contacts of patients with early syphilis should be evaluated and treated.

Chancroid

Chancroid is a genital ulcer disease caused by *Haemophilus ducreyi*, which is common in parts of Africa and Asia and has increased in frequency during the 1980s in the United States, particularly in urban areas. It is characterized by a papule at the inoculation site that evolves to a pustule and then to frank ulceration. The ulcers are typically painful and are associated with inguinal adenopathy. Definitive diagnosis requires isolating the causative bacterium, but culture is relatively insensitive and not widely available. Probable diagnosis is indicated by the painful ulcer, negative darkfield examination, negative results of nontreponemal serologic tests (VDRL, RPR), and atypical appearance for HSV ulcers or a negative HSV-2 culture or antigen test. Suppurative lymphadenopathy associated with ulcer is highly suggestive of chancroid.

Patients should be reexamined 3 days after treatment to be certain of improvement, especially when culture diagnosis is not possible. Fluctuant nodes may require aspiration in spite of appropriate antibiotics. HIV-infected persons with chancroid have a high rate of failure with standard short-course regimens.

Other sexually transmitted diseases causing genital ulceration or inguinal lymphadenopathy are lymphogranuloma venereum and donovanosis. Both are rare in the United States.

Sexually Transmitted Hepatitis

Hepatitis A and B frequently are sexually transmitted, and evidence suggests that some cases of hepatitis C are as well. In the United States, the most common means of hepatitis B transmission is by heterosexual contact. Although expensive, hepatitis B vaccine is effective and safe, and should be recommended for high-risk persons, who include sexually active homosexual and bisexual men, persons with another recently acquired sexually transmitted disease, and persons who have had more than one sex partner in the preceding 6 months [5••]. Treatment of a susceptible partner of a patient with known hepatitis B should consist of a single dose of hepatitis B immune globulin (HBIG, 0.06 mL/kg) along with the standard three-dose immunization series with hepatitis B vaccine.

ASSOCIATED CONDITIONS

Rash

Syphilis is always a diagnostic consideration in any sexually active patient with a generalized rash. The varied patterns of rash in secondary syphilis may resemble those of a large number of other skin diseases [8]. The rash of secondary syphilis is classically maculopapular with involvement of palms and soles. Drug eruptions and viral exanthems such as primary HIV infection and hepatitis B may also cause maculopapular rash. Other patterns of skin involvement in secondary syphilis include papulosquamous rash (with scaling) that may be confused with guttate psoriasis or pityriasis rosea; pustular or crusting lesions that can be confused with folliculitis, impetigo, or ectoparasite infestation; and hypopigmented lesions that resemble vitiligo or tinea versicolor.

A sexual history is essential for evaluating generalized rash, and blood tests for syphilis should be done. In virtually all immunologically normal people and in most HIV-positive patients, the nontreponemal test (VDRL, RPR) will be positive if secondary syphilis is causing the rash. Treatment for secondary syphilis is the same as for primary syphilis.

Localized, pruritic rashes may be associated with a variety of non-sexually transmitted infections, including tinea cruris and erythrasma [6•]. Scabies is characterized by intensely pruritic papular lesions in the genital region and between the fingers. Crab lice may also produce a pruritic genital rash associated with active crab lice or nits along hair shafts.

Arthritis

In general internal medicine practice, monoarticular or pauciarticular arthritis in young sexually active patients is often associated with a sexually transmitted disease. The classic presentation of tenosynovitis, associated in about two thirds of patients with a scattered pustular rash on the extremities, is highly suggestive of disseminated gonococcal infection. The primary genital, rectal, or oropharyngeal infection is often asymptomatic. Obtaining cultures for *N. gonorrhoeae* from blood, pharynx, urethra in men, and endocervix and rectum in women before treatment is key to diagnosis. Homosexual men who practice receptive anal intercourse should have rectal cultures as well. Definitive diagnosis requires a positive culture from blood, synovial fluid, or skin lesion aspirate (fewer than 50% of cases), but a probable diagnosis can be based on a positive culture from a mucosal site (more than 80% of cases) together with a compatible clinical history. Synovial fluid obtained by arthrocentesis is most often culture negative but excludes septic arthritis caused by other organisms. Brief hospitalization is appropriate to observe response to parenteral therapy, followed by an outpatient course of oral antibiotics.

Chlamydial infection is associated with reactive arthritis, in some cases with fully developed Reiter's syndrome, a syndrome that occurs in genetically predisposed persons with gastroenteritis or urethritis, the latter often chlamydial. The full syndrome is characterized by pauciarticular arthritis, skin and mucous membrane lesions, and conjunctivitis or uveitis. Initial therapy consists of treating the underlying urethritis with antibiotics appropriate for nongonococcal urethritis and anti-inflammatory drugs. Reiter's syndrome often resolves in 2 to 6 months but occasionally persists for more than 1 year.

Genital Growths

The most common genital growths are condyloma acuminata, or genital warts, caused by certain subtypes of sexually transmitted human papillomaviruses (HPV). Warts are found on genital or perineal skin; on the mucosa of the urethra, vagina, or rectum; and occasionally in the oropharyngeal region. In HIV-infected men and women, florid warts may occur. There is no effective antiviral treatment for HPV disease. Warts are usually removed by cryotherapy either with liquid nitrogen or a cryoprobe. Intravaginal or perianal warts are best managed surgically. Topical podophyllin and other topical therapies are only modestly effective.

Women with a history of sexually transmitted disease are at increased risk for cervical cancer. Certain subtypes of HPV that usually do not produce overt warts are associated with cervical intraepithelial neoplasia, which can progress rapidly in women with HIV infection. Appropriate yearly screening by Papanicolaou smear with referral of women with abnormal smears remains the mainstay for preventing cervical carcinoma arising from HPV-induced cervical intraepithelial neoplasia.

Molluscum contagiosum is another cutaneous viral infection manifest by papular lesions with a typically umbilicated center. These infections are passed by close personal contact and are not necessarily sexually transmitted. They can be treated with cryotherapy, although many will resolve spontaneously over a period of months. HIV-infected persons may have multiple or frequently recurrent lesions.

Proctitis, Proctocolitis, and Enteritis

Gonococcal, chlamydial, and HSV-2 infections and syphilis can cause symptomatic proctitis (involving the distal 10 cm of the rectum) in persons who practice receptive anal intercourse. The symptoms consist of anorectal pain, pruritus, tenesmus, and rectal discharge. Patients should undergo anoscopy to examine the mucosa and obtain appropriate cultures. Antigen detection tests for chlamydia should not be used because of their lack of specificity for diagnosing rectal infections. Empiric treatment while awaiting cultures and syphilis serology includes ceftriaxone, 125 mg intramuscularly, followed by doxycycline, 100 mg twice a day for 7 days.

Proctocolitis, which has symptoms of abdominal cramping and diarrhea, may be caused by *Campylobacter* species, *Shigella* species, and *Entamoeba histolytica*. It can occur in persons who have receptive anal intercourse or fecal-oral contact. Enteritis occurs from fecal-oral contact and is most frequently caused by *Giardia lamblia*. Treatment of these illnesses is found elsewhere in this volume.

DISEASE CONTROL

When diagnosing and treating a patient with a sexually transmitted disease, contact tracing is essential so that the chain of transmission can be interrupted and asymptomatic cases can be treated before sequelae develop. All states require reporting of HIV, syphilis, and gonorrhea, and many states require reporting of chlamydiosis, nongonococcal urethritis, and pelvic inflammatory disease. In most instances public health authorities can assist in notifying and treating contacts and provide specialized diagnostic services for all patients regardless of ability to pay.

Immunoprophylaxis is not available for sexually transmitted diseases other than hepatitis B. Control strategies are to reduce new partner acquisition and modify risky sexual practices, to reduce susceptibility by using barrier contraceptive devices, and to reduce infectivity and spread of disease by prompt diagnosis, treatment, and contact tracing.

REFERENCES AND RECOMMENDED READING

Recently published papers of particular interest have been highlighted as:
• Of interest
•• Of outstanding interest

1. Holmes KK, Mardh P-A, Sparling PF, *et al.*, eds: *Sexually Transmitted Diseases*, edn 2. New York: McGraw-Hill; 1990.

2. Mandell GL, Bennett JE, Dolin R, eds: *Principles and Practice of Infectious Diseases*, edn 4. New York: Churchill Livingstone; 1995.

3. Martin DH, ed: Sexually Transmitted Diseases. *Med Clin North Am* 1990, 74:1339–1697.

4. Cohen MS, Hook EW III, Hitchcock PJ, eds: Sexually transmitted diseases in the AIDS era: part 1. *Infect Dis Clin North Am* 1993, 7:739–873.

5.•• Centers for Disease Control and Prevention: 1993 Sexually transmitted diseases treatment guidelines. *MMWR Morbid Mortal Wkly Rep* 1993, 42(RR-14):1–102.

6.• Centers for Disease Control and Prevention: Recommendations for the prevention and management of *Chlamydia trachomatis* infections. *MMWR Morbid Mortal Wkly Rep* 1993, 42(RR-12):9–21.

7. Mroczkowski TF: Common nonvenereal genital lesions. *Med Clin North Am* 1990, 74:1507–1528.

8. Hutchinson CM, Hook EW III: 1990. Syphilis in adults. *Med Clin North Am* 1990, 74:1389–1416.

SELECT BIBLIOGRAPHY

Cohen MS, Hook EW III, Hitchcock PJ, eds: Sexually transmitted diseases in the AIDS era: part 2. *Infect Dis Clin North Am* 1994,

Infective Endocarditis 11

Michael H. Picard
Robert H. Rubin

Key Points

- Although the designations of *subacute* and *acute* are useful in defining clinical events and the need for surgery, these terms are no longer organism specific.

- Although the incidence of infective endocarditis has not changed significantly over the years, the age of affected patients has increased and the underlying cardiac disease has changed.

- Clinical manifestations and presentation of infective endocarditis are dependent on the virulence of the infecting organism and the duration of the disease prior to diagnosis.

- Prosthetic cardiac valves are far more susceptible to microbial seeding than native valves and have a much greater range of infecting microorganisms.

- The cornerstone of diagnosis in patients with suspected endocarditis remains the demonstration of sustained, high level bacteremia; the detection of valvular vegetations by echocardiography can assist in the confirmation of the disease, delineate the extent of disease, and identify complications of the infection.

- Pathologic consequences of infective endocarditis include those due directly to microbial invasion, those due to embolization of vegetation, those due to immunologic events, and those arising from hemodynamic consequences of the disease; the most common complication is symptomatic congestive heart failure.

- The goal of antibiotic treatment of infective endocarditis is the maintenance of a prolonged course of bactericidal antimicrobial therapy.

Infective endocarditis can involve any aspect of the endocardial surface of the heart—typically the heart valves, but also septal defects, mural endocardium, and intracardiac thrombi. Traditionally, the terms *subacute* and *acute* have been used to describe the clinical events. Subacute endocarditis describes the patient with a preexisting cardiac lesion who presents with a several-week history of fevers, night sweats, anorexia, weight loss, malaise, increased fatigability, and musculoskeletal complaints. In contrast, acute endocarditis has a far more fulminant course, with the patient presenting within a few days of the onset of hectic fevers and rigors, systemic toxicity, deteriorating cardiac function (even without a previous history of structural cardiac abnormalities), and a high rate of systemic complications.

EPIDEMIOLOGY

Although the incidence of infective endocarditis has not changed significantly over the past 50 years (2 to 5 cases/100,000 people/year), the age and underlying cardiac disease of patients developing endocarditis have changed substantially [1,2]. At present, approximately half of the cases occur in individuals between ages 31 and 60, with approximately 25% in the younger and older age groups—a marked change from the preantibiotic era when the median age was less than 30. The number of cases of endocarditis in the elderly is increasing, with many cases caused by nosocomial exposures associated with the use of vascular access devices within the hospital [3–5].

At present, rheumatic heart disease accounts for less than 25% of the cases of endocarditis, with congenital heart disease (primarily ventricular septal defects, patent ductus arteriosus, coarctation of the aorta, tetralogy of Fallot, bicuspid aortic valve, and pulmonic stenosis) accounting for an additional 15% of cases. So-called degenerative cardiac lesions are particularly common in the elderly and probably account for many cases of endocarditis that develop without previously recognized cardiac lesions.

Two forms of cardiac abnormality that have been recognized only during the past two decades are quite susceptible to the development of endocarditis. The first of these, idiopathic hypertrophic subaortic stenosis (IHSS, or hypertrophic obstructive cardiomyopathy), carries a 5% risk of endocarditis. The risk of endocarditis is greater in patients with greater hemodynamic abnormalities [6]. The second form is mitral valve prolapse (MVP). Approximately 40% to 50% of endocarditis cases occurring in patients with mitral regurgitation without other cardiac abnormality may represent instances of preexisting mitral valve prolapse. The subgroup of patients with mitral valve prolapse at risk for endocarditis are those with thickened valves and sufficient hemodynamic turbulence to produce a murmur [7].

Finally, endocarditis can develop in the setting of unusual forms of cardiac disease such as luetic heart disease, intracardiac fistulas, and the presence of pacemaker wires. Patients with cardiac prosthetic devices, particularly valves, are at highest risk for the development of endocarditis.

MICROBIAL ETIOLOGY

Streptococci and staphylococci account for 80% to 90% of native valve endocarditis and 60% to 70% of prosthetic valve infection. Whereas the streptococci predominate with native valve disease, staphylococcal infection is more prominent with prosthetic valve infection (Table 1). Speciation of the bacteria isolated from patients with endocarditis can be quite useful in identifying the portal of entry for the invading organism.

Appropriate care of the patient with endocarditis includes not only eradication of the cardiac infection, but also identification and correction of the problem that provided a portal of entry to the bloodstream [8–10].

Some patients will present with typical clinical manifestations of endocarditis but negative blood cultures—so-called culture-negative endocarditis. Such noninfectious processes as an atrial myxoma, systemic lupus erythematosus (and other collagen vascular diseases, including acute rheumatic fever), certain malignancies, and other conditions that excite a systemic inflammatory response can mimic endocarditis and should be excluded. Circumstances in which true infective endocarditis is present but blood cultures are negative include:

Patients who have received previous antibiotic therapy
Infection with fastidious, slow growing organisms such as *Haemophilus* spp, *Cardiobacterium hominis*, nutritionally deficient streptococci, and *Actinobacillus* species
Fungal infection
Infection with such unusual organisms as rickettsiae (particularly *Coxiella burnetii*, the causative agent of Q fever) and chlamydiae
Right-sided or mural endocarditis caused by a nonvirulent organism
Infection of long duration
Uremia resulting from immune complex glomerulonephritis

PATHOGENESIS AND PATHOLOGY

The critical first step in the pathogenesis of endocarditis is the deposition of platelet-fibrin thrombi on the valvular surface, the generation of so-called *nonbacterial thrombotic endocarditis* (Fig. 1). This most commonly occurs at sites of maximal hemodynamic turbulence and maximal mechanical stress. In addition, it may be induced by immune complex deposition, wasting illnesses (such as those caused by pancreatic, gastric, and lung carcinoma), various metabolic derangements, and trauma induced by intracardiac catheters (particularly Swan-Ganz catheters). Valvular surfaces altered in this fashion are far more susceptible to bacterial adherence than are valves that have not been so "prepared" [11,12].

TABLE 1 MICROBIAL ETIOLOGY OF INFECTIVE ENDOCARDITIS			
	Percentage of cases due to particular microorganisms		
Microorganism	Native valve	"Early" prosthetic valve	"Late" prosthetic valve
Nonenterococcal streptococci	40–70	5	20
Enterococci	10	<1	5–10
Staphylococcus aureus	20	10–20	10
Staphylococcus epidermidis	5	25	30
Gram-negative bacilli	5	1–5	5–10
Diphtheroid	1	5	5
Miscellaneous organisms	5	5–10	5
Polymicrobial	<1	1–5	1–5
Culture negative	5–10	5–10	5–10

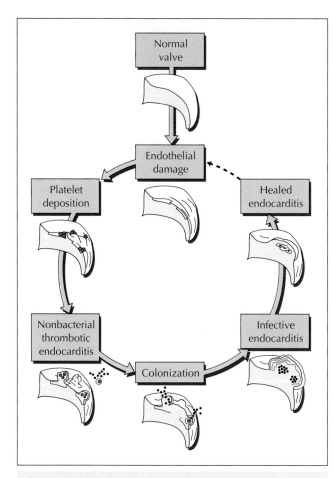

FIGURE 1 Diagram illustrates the main events in pathogenesis of subacute bacterial endocarditis.

As the second step, circulating organisms colonize these areas of thrombus. Transient, low-level bacteremia is a not uncommon event in association with chewing, toothbrushing, flossing, or the use of an oral irrigation device, particularly in individuals with periodontal disease. In addition, any manipulation of the mucosal surfaces of the gastrointestinal and genitourinary tracts, as well as infected cutaneous surfaces, can introduce the resident microbial flora into the circulation [11–17].

Once the bacteria have adhered to the valve surface, the bacteria stimulate further platelet aggregation, which amplifies the extent of the vegetation, providing a protected site for the bacterial colonies.

The pathologic consequences of infective endocarditis are caused by several processes, all of which can be present simultaneously. Thus, one needs to recognize the pathology and clinical events that result directly from microbial invasion, those that result from embolization of material from the vegetation, those that result from immunologic events that occur during the course of this illness, and, finally, those that result from the hemodynamic consequences of the process [12].

Acute bacterial endocarditis is associated with rapidly progressive suppurative disease that results in larger, more friable vegetations with a propensity for embolization, progressive local infection of the heart resulting in perforation of the valve, rupture of the chordae tendineae, valve ring abscesses, and intramyocardial extensions of infection that can result in fistula formation or catastrophic rupture. In addition, metastatic spread of infection is common, affecting the central nervous system, skeletal system, and soft tissues. Acute bacterial endocarditis is typically caused by *Staphylococcus aureus* but also is associated with *Streptococcus pneumoniae*, *S. milleri*, *Neisseria gonorrhoeae*, *Salmonella* spp, and, on occasion, enterococci, as well as other bacterial species. In contrast, subacute bacterial endocarditis is typically caused by viridans streptococci. The vegetations are smaller, resulting in a lower rate of embolization; local spread of infection within the heart is uncommon, and metastatic spread of infection is rare [12].

CLINICAL MANIFESTATIONS

Presentation

Acute infective endocarditis begins explosively, with fever, rigors, and systemic toxicity. Cardiac murmurs may be absent on presentation, appearing later in the clinical course. The early development of embolic events and congestive heart failure are not uncommon.

Patients with more subacute disease demonstrate the classical manifestations of endocarditis: constitutional symptoms of moderate fever, night sweats, arthralgias, malaise, anorexia, weight loss, and easy fatigability. Heart murmurs are almost always present, but changing murmurs are uncommon. The incidence of splenomegaly (approximately 30%), petechiae (30%), clubbing (15%), Osler nodes (15%), Janeway lesions (5%), and Roth spots (5%) is determined by the duration of the infection—increasing in incidence with disease of greater than 4 weeks' duration.

Neurologic complications, particularly emboli, occur in approximately one third of patients, with fully 10% of patients presenting with a chief complaint of a neurologic event rather than inflammatory or cardiopulmonary complaints (Table 2). Emboli to the spleen, kidneys, and other organs occur in about 30% of cases, with coronary artery embolization being a particular feature of aortic valve endocarditis. Many of these emboli, because of their small size, are silent. Emboli to major vessels such as the femoral, brachial, or renal arteries can occur, and, when they do, raise the possibility of fungal endocarditis. The risk of embolization decreases as a function of the duration of treatment [19•].

Renal disease during the course of endocarditis can result from embolic infarction, abscess formation caused by metastatic infection, diffuse glomerulonephritis resulting from immune complex deposition, or antibiotic-induced nephrotoxicity. Frank uremia is uncommon in the present era, and, when present, is usually caused by one of the latter two processes [3,12,20].

Approximately half of all patients with native valve endocarditis will develop some evidence of congestive heart failure, which usually responds to conventional therapy. Particularly at risk are patients with regurgitant murmurs, as more than 90% of these develop heart failure [12].

A special subgroup of patients with endocarditis comprises intravenous drug abusers. In these patients, right-sided endo-

TABLE 2 NEUROLOGIC COMPLICATIONS OF INFECTIVE ENDOCARDITIS SEEN IN 218 PATIENTS*	
Neurologic complication	**Occurrences, *n***
Cerebral infarction in territory of middle cerebral arteries	34
Meningeal signs and symptoms	33
Seizures	23
Multiple microemboli	23
Microscopic brain abscesses	8
Visual disturbances†	6
Cranial or peripheral neuropathy	5
Subarachnoid hemorrhage (without identifiable mycotic aneurysm)	5
Cerebral infarction in territory of vertebrobasilar arteries	4
Mycotic aneurysm	4
Psychiatric disturbance	4
Intracerebral hemorrhage	4
Cerebral infarcts in "watershed areas" due to hypotension	3
Subdural hemorrhage	2
Macroscopic brain abscess	1

From Pruitt and coworkers [18]; with permission.
*More than one complication was frequently observed in a single patient. Each complication is listed separately.
†Retinal artery emboli (4), retinal artery hemorrhage (1), and cortical blindness (1).

carditis is the rule, with the tricuspid valve being infected in approximately 50% of cases, the aortic valve in 25%, the mitral valve in 20%, and combined right- and left-sided disease in 5%. In those patients with tricuspid involvement, complaints and physical findings involving the chest predominate, including pleurisy and pleural friction rubs, dyspnea and signs of consolidation, and a variety of abnormalities on chest radiograph (elevated hemidiaphragm, pleural effusion, pulmonary infiltrate that may cavitate quite rapidly, and so forth). Patients usually have normal cardiac examinations on admission. Cutaneous *Staphylococcus aureus* accounts for approximately two thirds of cases, with such unusual organisms as *Pseudomonas aeruginosa*, other gram-negative bacilli, and *Candida* spp accounting for 15% of cases (presumably because of microbial contamination of the drugs being injected) [21].

Complications

More than half of the patients presenting with infective endocarditis will develop complications over the course of their illness (Table 3) [22•]. In addition to the effects resulting from bacteremia and systemic infection, there are specific influences on cardiac function. Most of these adverse effects are caused by the presence of valvular vegetations, and they have important clinical implications because these cardiac complications represent the major reasons for valve replacement.

Vegetations, particularly with virulent or inadequately treated organisms, can result in a variety of abnormalities ranging from valve destruction and regurgitation, to valve obstruction, to emboli. The most common of these abnormalities is significant aortic or mitral regurgitation resulting in sympto-

matic congestive heart failure. In fact, the most common cause of death in endocarditis patients is hemodynamic deterioration resulting from valvular regurgitation [3,20].

In both aortic and mitral endocarditis with associated regurgitation, two-dimensional echocardiography and Doppler ultrasound can confirm the presence of the vegetation and the extent of regurgitation.

PROSTHETIC VALVE ENDOCARDITIS

Prosthetic cardiac valves are far more susceptible to microbial seeding than are natural valves, with a much greater range of microorganisms causing endocarditis on the artificial valve (Table 1). The incidence of prosthetic valve endocarditis (PVE) is approximately 3% at 1 year after implantation and 5% at 4 years. There appears to be no significant difference in the incidence of endocarditis between mechanical and bioprosthetic values.

Patients with PVE are traditionally divided into two groups—those with infection presenting in the first 60 days following valve insertion ("early PVE"), and those presenting later ("late PVE"), when endothelialization of the valve has occurred. *Staphylococcus epidermidis*, gram-negative diphtheroid, and fungal infections predominate in the early group, reflecting perioperative contamination; viridans streptococcal infection occurs in the late group, consistent with a pathogenesis more akin to native valve endocarditis (*ie*, seeding during a transient bacteremia) [23,24].

The clinical findings in patients with PVE differ somewhat from those in patients with native valve endocarditis: the inci-

Echocardiographic finding	Number	Any cx (%)	FTR	CHF	Systemic embolism	Pulmonary embolism	CNS embolism	Surg	Mortality
Mitral vegetation	51	27 (52.9)	7	10	5	0	14	11	6
Aortic vegetation	34	21 (61.8)	0	10	6	0	5	12	4
Tricuspid vegetation	13	10 (76.9)	3	1	0	9	1	1	1
Prosthetic valve endocarditis	56	34 (60.7)	2	10	4	0	10	19	5
Nonspecific thickening	14	8 (57.1)	1	5	1	0	3	2	4
Aortic valve disease	4	3 (57.1)	1	1	0	0	1	1	1
Mitral valve disease	3	2 (66.7)	1	1	0	0	1	1	0
Mitral valve prolapse	3	1 (33.3)	0	1	0	0	0	0	0
No abnormality	26	7 (26.9)	0	0	4	0	4	0	2
Total number (%)	204	113 (55.4)	15 (7.4)	38 (8.6)	20 (9.8)	9 (4.4)	39 (19.1)	47 (23.0)	23 (11.3)

From Sanfilippo and coworkers [22•]; with permission.

Any cx—development of any complications; CHF—congestive heart failure; CNS—central nervous system; FTR—failure to respond to antibiotic treatment; Surg—surgical valve replacement.

dence of new or changing murmurs resulting from valve dehiscence or dysfunction (and moderate or severe heart failure) is far higher (more than 50%); the incidence of skin findings, splenomegaly, and immunopathologic processes is significantly lower (presumably because the patient comes to attention sooner); and patients with PVE (especially of the mitral valve) may develop functional stenosis caused by obstruction of the valve orifice or restriction in valve movement. In patients with PVE, those with viridans streptococcal infection closely resemble patients with native valve endocarditis, with similar infections in terms of signs, symptoms, and response to therapy [23,24].

The mortality rate of PVE is considerably higher than that of native valve endocarditis. Patients at high risk for a poor outcome include those with 1) infection with fungi, gram-negative bacilli, or staphylococci; 2) persistent fever while receiving appropriate antimicrobial therapy; 3) changing murmurs; 4) increasing heart failure; and 5) conduction system abnormalities.

Although native valve endocarditis primarily involves the leaflets, infections in prosthetic valves occur predominantly at the intersection of the sewing ring and the valve annulus.

DIAGNOSIS

The cornerstone of diagnostic efforts in the patient with suspected endocarditis is the demonstration of a sustained, high-level bacteremia; that is, more than 50% of four to six blood cultures drawn over a time period of greater than 2 hours should be positive for the same organism. Other laboratory tests are less helpful. In patients with acute disease, the leukocyte count is usually increased, whereas it is usually normal in the patient with subacute disease. A normochromic, normocytic anemia is usually present in patients with subacute disease, as is an increased erythrocyte sedimentation rate. In patients with disease of sufficient duration for immunologic phenomena to occur, positive rheumatoid factor and evidence of circulating immune complexes are common, as well as hyperglobulinemia, cryoglobulinemia, hypocomplementemia, proteinuria, and microscopic hematuria.

By far the most useful diagnostic technique, other than blood culturing, is echocardiography. Two-dimensional echocardiography and Doppler ultrasound are of particular use in 1) prospective identification of abnormal valves with a predisposition to infection, 2) early diagnosis of culture-negative endocarditis, 3) identification of complications of infection, 4) decisions regarding the surgical management of an infected valve (timing and type of operation), and 5) evaluation of endocarditis in the presence of prosthetic valves or complex congenital heart disease. Physical characteristics of vegetations assessed by echocardiography are used to assess prognosis both during and after treatment [22•,25].

Vegetations typically appear on the echocardiogram as one or more discrete echo-producing masses adherent to a leaflet surface yet distinct from the remainder of the leaflet (Fig. 2). The reported sensitivity of the two-dimensional echocardiogram to detect native valve vegetations ranges from 54% to 83% for the transthoracic approach and 95% to 100% for the transesophageal technique [26,27]. The ability of transthoracic echocardiography to detect vegetations increases in direct proportion to the size of the lesion [28]. For prosthetic valve infections, reflections from the prosthetic material reduce the sensitivity of transthoracic echocardiography for vegetation detection to 30%. The resolution is improved with transesophageal echocardiography to 77% [26].

Echocardiography can be used to *confirm* the presence of vegetations, but it has limited utility for routinely "ruling out" endocarditis in unselected patients with bacteremia, since the prevalence of endocarditis in such patients without risk factors is low [29]. *Diagnosis* of endocarditis by early echocardiogra-

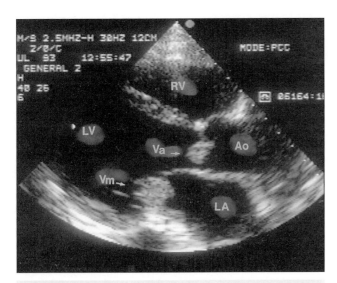

FIGURE 2 Native valve endocarditis by transthoracic echocardiography. Parasternal long axis view of heart revealing vegetations involving posterior leaflet of mitral valve (Vm) and one cusp of aortic valve (Va) in patient with lactobacillus endocarditis. Ao—ascending aorta; LA—left atrium; LV—left ventricle; RV—right ventricle.

phy can be of benefit, however, in those in whom culture-negative endocarditis is suspected. Transthoracic echocardiography cannot consistently differentiate infected from healed vegetations or detect the smallest lesions present in the earliest phases of the illness. In addition, other causes of valve thickening, such as the residua of old rheumatic disease or senile calcification can confound the detection of vegetations.

At present, the major value of echocardiography and Doppler ultrasound is in the identification of the complications associated with valvular infections such as valve regurgi-

tation, obstruction, aneurysm, and abscess (Fig. 3A). Assessment of regurgitation by color Doppler flow mapping can confirm the degree and etiology of regurgitation, and this information assists in the surgical planning (Fig. 3B). The ability of the transthoracic echocardiogram to detect paravalvular abscesses in either native or prosthetic valves is limited (sensitivity 30%); however, imaging from the transesophageal approach raises the detection rate to over 90% (Fig. 4) [30•].

As with all diagnostic tests, the major indication for use of transesophageal echocardiography is in cases in which the information obtained will have an impact on management. For native valve endocarditis this includes patients in whom there is a high suspicion for endocarditis yet the transthoracic echocardiogram is negative or of nondiagnostic quality, and those with persistent fever in whom extravalvular infection (abscess) is suspected. For prosthetic valves, the yield of vegetation detection is so improved that transesophageal echocardiography should be considered in all cases in which the diagnosis of prosthetic valve endocarditis is uncertain or when complications such as paravalvular regurgitation, valve obstruction, or abscess are suspected.

The *presence* of vegetations alone is a relatively nonspecific marker of risk for subsequent complications, since 80% of patients with a diagnosis of infective endocarditis will have vegetations detected by echocardiography [22•]. Physical characteristics of vegetations such as size, mobility, and extent of infection act as independent markers of a more complicated course during initial treatment [22•,26,31,32••,33]. As shown in Figure 5, as vegetations approach 10 mm in diameter, the rate of complications rises significantly. In successfully treated infections, the presence of irreversible structural damage to the valve leaflets, as evidenced by severe valvular regurgitation, is the strongest predictor of the need for late valve surgery [25].

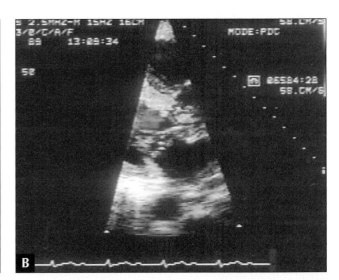

FIGURE 3 Transthoracic echocardiographic detection of paravalvular abscess and severe aortic regurgitation in *Staphylococcus aureus* aortic valve endocarditis. **A**, Parasternal long axis view of heart in early diastole demonstrating vegetation, prolapse, and destruction of an aortic valve cusp (*arrow*), and thickening of posterior aortic

wall caused by abscess (a). Extension of infection onto anterior leaflet of mitral valve is also present. **B**, Color flow Doppler map of same image revealing severe aortic regurgitation (aquamarine region) into the dilated left ventricle. (*see* Color Plate). Ao—ascending aorta; LA—left atrium; LV—left ventricle; RV—right ventricle.

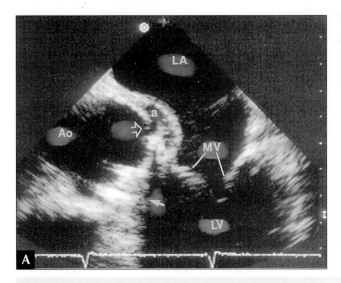

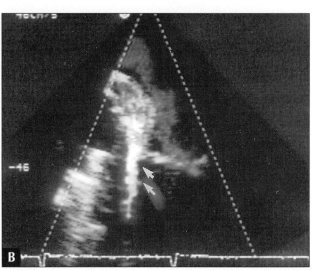

FIGURE 4 Transesophageal echocardiographic demonstration of paravalvular abscess and fistula in prosthetic valve endocarditis. **A,** Two-dimensional image of long axis of left ventricular base and aorta. Bright reverberations of a single disk valve are noted (*solid arrow*). There is a lucent distended region of the posterior aortic wall caused by abscess formation (a). The wall of the abscess is disrupted and the abscess communicates with the aorta (*hollow arrow*). **B,** Color flow Doppler map of the same region reveals an aortoventricular fistula with blood flow into the abscess from the ascending aorta and into the left ventricle (*arrows*) (*see* Color Plate). Ao—ascending aorta; LA—left atrium; LV—left ventricle; MV—mitral valve.

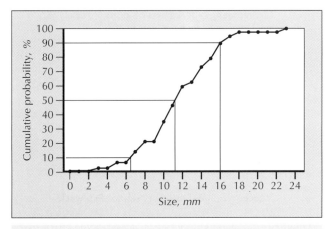

FIGURE 5 Plot of cumulative occurrence of complications in acute native valve endocarditis as a function of vegetation size measured on transthoracic echocardiogram within 5 days of diagnosis. As the maximum diameter of the vegetation exceeds 10 mm, the rate of complications rises. (*From* Sanfilippo and coworkers [22•]; with permission.)

MANAGEMENT

Principles of Antimicrobial Therapy

Because of the high titers of organisms found in the protected environment of vegetations in patients with endocarditis, there is an absolute requirement for a prolonged course of bactericidal antimicrobial therapy. If such a regimen is not possible, and only bacteriostatic therapy is available, then early surgical intervention in conjunction with such bacteriostatic therapy should be considered. To cure endocarditis, experience has shown that a peak serum bactericidal level of at least 1:8 is necessary (Table 4). Precise knowledge of the *in vitro*

antimicrobial susceptibility of the infecting organism is of great importance in choosing the antimicrobial regimen, particularly in deciding whether or not two or more drugs are needed to achieve synergistic killing of the infecting organisms or in treating relatively antibiotic-resistant infection [34].

The therapy for streptococcal infection should be considered in two categories: nonenterococcal infection and enterococcal infection. The mainstay of therapy for nonenterococcal streptococci remains penicillin. The precise regimen used depends on the level of susceptibility of the isolate to penicillin as outlined in Table 4 [35–38]. For patients allergic to penicillin, vancomycin, 15 mg/kg given every 12 hours, is substituted; first-generation cephalosporins offer another option.

Enterococci differ from the other streptococci in that penicillin, ampicillin, and vancomycin do not have a bactericidal effect and thus must be combined with an aminoglycoside. Because of resistance to streptomycin, gentamicin has become the aminoglycoside of choice at many centers. Unfortunately, the number of patients resistant to all aminoglycosides is increasing, and optimal therapies for this situation, including early surgery or constant infusion of high-dose ampicillin, are under investigation [39,40].

The therapy of choice for methicillin-sensitive *S. aureus* is nafcillin, although many centers use nafcillin plus gentamicin in patients with a particularly virulent clinical course [41,42]. With native valve infection caused by *S. epidermidis*, the same general approach as for *S. aureus* is taken.

For gram-negative infection, the therapy of choice is usually a β-lactam plus aminoglycoside combination for 4 to 6 weeks, with the precise choice of drugs being determined by the results of *in vitro* antimicrobial testing. For the fastidious gram-negative coccobacillary organisms (*Haemophilus* spp, *Actinobacillus actinomycetemcomitans*, and *Cardiobacterium hominis*), ampicillin plus gentamicin appears to be the therapy of choice.

TABLE 4 ANTIMICROBIAL THERAPY FOR INFECTIVE ENDOCARDITIS

Microorganism	MIC	Treatment
Penicillin-susceptible nonenterococcal streptococci*	<0.2 µg/mL	Pencillin G, 2–3 M U every 4 h for 4 weeks OR
		Penicillin G, 2–3 M U every 4 h IV for 4 weeks PLUS
		Streptomycin, 7.5 mg/kg every 12 h for 2 weeks OR
		Gentamicin, 1 mg/kg every 8 h for 2 weeks OR
		Penicillin plus streptomycin or gentamicin, both for 2 weeks
Relatively penicillin-resistant nonenterococcal streptococci*	0.2–0.5 µg/mL	Penicillin G, 4 M U every 4 h for 4 weeks PLUS
		Streptomycin, 7.5 mg/kg every 12 h for 2 weeks OR
		Gentamicin, 1 mg/kg every 8 h for 2 weeks
Relatively penicillin-resistant nonenterococcal streptococci*	>0.5 µg/mL	Penicillin G, 4 M U every 4 h for 4 weeks PLUS
		Streptomycin, 7.5 mg/kg every 12 h for 4 weeks OR
		Gentamicin, 1 mg/kg every 8 h for 4 weeks
Enterococci*		Penicillin G, 4 M U every 4 h OR
		Ampicillin, 2 g every 4 h for 4–6 weeks PLUS
		Gentamicin, 1 mg/kg every 8 h for 4–6 weeks
Staphylococcus aureus* (methicillin sensitive)		Nafcillin, 2 g IV every 4 h for 4–6 weeks
Staphylococcus aureus (methicillin resistant)		Vancomycin, 500 mg every 6 h for 4–6 weeks
Gram-negative bacilli		Two-drug bactericidal regimen for 4–6 weeks
Culture-negative endocarditis		Ampicillin, 2 g every 4 h for 4–6 weeks OR
		Vancomycin, 500 mg every 6 h for 4–6 weeks PLUS
		Gentamicin, 1 mg/kg every 8 h for 4–6 weeks

*In patients allergic to penicillin, vancomycin, 500 mg IV every 6 h, is substituted for the pencillin; gentamicin is added when the infecting organism is an enterococcus.
IV—intravenously; MIC—minimum inhibitory concentration.

Fungal infection should be treated surgically, in conjunction with amphotericin therapy.

For PVE, the recommendations are similar to those above, except that two drug regimens (cell wall active agent plus gentamicin) are usually used.

Empiric trials of antibiotics for presumed culture-negative endocarditis that is thought to be of bacterial origin are sometimes necessary. In patients with suspected native valve disease, a regimen of ampicillin or vancomycin plus gentamicin is usually used; for patients with suspected prosthetic valve disease, vancomycin, ampicillin, and gentamicin is recommended.

Surgical Management

Valve surgery for endocarditis is considered the treatment of choice for hemodynamic instability, intracardiac invasion, and poor response to medical therapy. Although valve replacement has dramatically improved outcome in endocarditis, in individual patients the risks of surgery must be weighed against potential benefits [23,43]. These risks include operative mortality, recurrent infection resulting in prosthesis infection, and long-term risks such as degeneration of bioprosthetic valves and the risks resulting from the anticoagulant therapy required in mechanical valves.

Valve replacement typically occurs at one of two stages of the disease: early (during active infection) resulting from acute complications or late (months to years after completion of antibiotic therapy) caused by the cumulative effects of chronic regurgitation. The operative risks are particularly increased in the setting of acute bacteremia and endocarditis when cardiac, renal, and other organ function may be compromised [44]. Although a period of antibiotics is desirable before surgery, the length of antibiotic treatment does not influence surgical outcome [44,45]. Rather, the degree of heart failure at the time of valve replacement is the most important determinant of success at surgery [45,46].

The major cardiac indications for valve replacement in infective endocarditis are listed in Table 5. Because heart failure is the major cause of death in infective endocarditis, the primary indication for valve replacement is significant heart failure, typically resulting from moderate or severe valve regurgitation.

Because of the difficulty in eradicating many of the infections associated with prosthetic valves, surgery is a common adjunct to antibiotic therapy for prosthetic valve endocarditis. This is particularly important for late prosthetic valve endocarditis, where a survival benefit has been shown with valve replacement [47]. However, valve replacement is not required in all cases of early prosthetic valve infection. Regardless of the timing of infection, surgery should be considered in the following situations: new regurgitation, moderate to severe heart failure, nonstreptococcal organism, extravalvular extension of infection (persistent fever, recurrent infection,

paravalvular abscess, or atrioventricular conduction abnormality), embolization, and fungal endocarditis [48].

PREVENTION

The prevention of infective endocarditis should be vigorously sought by the practitioner. There are three steps in achieving this goal: 1) assessing the cardiac risk of the patient for endocarditis (patients with prosthetic valves, a previous history of endocarditis, and a significant degree of intracardiac turbulence are at particularly high risk); 2) correcting underlying disease that could lead to transient bacteremia during the activities of daily life (eg, intensive dental care of patients with gingival disease or aggressive therapy for eczema or other skin conditions that could provide a portal of entry for bacteria); and 3) the use of prophylactic antibiotics at the time of an invasive procedure during which a bacteremia that could seed the heart is likely to occur (Table 6) [49,50]. Table 7 outlines the regimens that are recommended for this purpose. Our own preference is the use of parenteral regimens of prophylaxis for patients deemed to be at high risk, reserving oral regimens for patients who are believed to be at lesser risk.

TABLE 5 INDICATIONS FOR VALVE SURGERY IN INFECTIVE ENDOCARDITIS
Congestive heart failure resistant to medications
Moderate or severe valvular regurgitation
Valve obstruction
Persistent or recurrent infection
Invasive infection
Abscess
Fistula
Progressive heart block
Prosthetic infection
New regurgitation
Moderate to severe heart failure
Nonstreptococcal organism
Extravalvular extension of infection (persistent fever, recurrent infection, paravalvular abscess, and/or atrioventricular conduction abnormality)
Embolization
Fungal endocarditis
Systemic emboli

TABLE 6 DENTAL AND SURGICAL PROCEDURES FOR WHICH ENDOCARDITIS PROPHYLAXIS IS RECOMMENDED
Dental procedures known to induce gingival or mucosal bleeding
Tonsillectomy
Surgical manipulations that invade intestinal or respiratory mucosa
Bronchoscopy
Sclerotherapy for esophageal varices
Esophageal dilatation
Gallbladder surgery
Cystoscopy
Urethral dilatation
Urinary tract catheterization or surgery if infection is present
Prostatic surgery
Incision and drainage of infected tissue
Vaginal hysterectomy
Vaginal delivery in the presence of infection

Adapted from the American Heart Association recommendations, Dajani and coworkers [49]; with permission.
It should be emphasized that in patients at high risk for endocarditis, even low-risk procedures such as gastrointestinal endoscopy merit prophylaxis. Patients at high risk for endocarditis include those with prosthetic heart valves, those with a previous history of endocarditis, and those with systemic-pulmonary shunts or conduits.

TABLE 7 PROPHYLACTIC ANTIMICROBIAL REGIMENS FOR THE PREVENTION OF INFECTIVE ENDOCARDITIS

Site of procedure	Cardiac risk	Regimen*
Oral and upper respiratory tract	High*	30 min before procedure: Intravenous or intramuscular ampicillin, 2 g PLUS Gentamicin, 1.5 mg/kg PLUS (after the procedure) Amoxicillin, 1.5 g orally 6 h after initial dose OR Repeat parenteral therapy 8 h after initial dose
Oral and upper respiratory tract	Standard	Amoxicillin, 3 g orally 1 h before procedure; then 1.5 g 6 h after initial dose OR Erythromycin ethylsuccinate, 800 mg orally, or erythromycin stearate, 1 g orally 2 h before procedure; 1/2 the dose 6 h later OR Clindamycin, 300 mg orally 1 h before procedure; 150 mg orally 6 h later
Genitourinary/gastrointestinal		Same as high risk oral and upper respiratory tract program

Adapted from The American Heart Association Recommendations, Dajani and coworkers [49]; with permission.
*High-risk patients include those with prosthetic heart valves, a history of endocarditis, or systemic-pulmonary shunts or conduits.

REFERENCES AND RECOMMENDED READING

Recently published papers of particular interest have been highlighted as:
• Of interest
•• Of outstanding interest

1. Durack DT, Peterdorf RG: Changes in the epidemiology of endocarditis. In *Infective Endocarditis. An American Heart Association Symposium.* Edited by Kaplan DL, Taranta AV. Dallas: American Heart Association; 1977:3–14.

2. Griffin MR, Wilson WR, Edwards WD, *et al.*: Infective endocarditis. Olmsted County, Minnesota, 1950 through 1981. *JAMA* 1985, 254:1199–1202.

3. Weinstein L, Rubin RH: Infective endocarditis–1973. *Prog Cardiovasc Dis* 1973, 16:239–274.

4. Kaye D: Definitions and demographic characteristics. In *Infective Endocarditis.* Edited by Kaye D. Baltimore: University Park Press; 1976:1–10.

5. Watanakunakorn C: Changing epidemiology and newer aspects of infective endocarditis. *Adv Intern Med* 1977, 22:21–47.

6. Chagnac A, Rudniki C, Loebel H, *et al.*: Infectious endocarditis in idiopathic hypertrophic subaortic stenosis. Report of three cases and review of the literature. *Chest* 1982, 81:346–349.

7. Nishimura RA, McGoon MD, Shub C, *et al.*: Echocardiographically documented mitral valve prolapse: long term follow-up of 237 patients. *N Engl J Med* 1985, 313:1305–1309.

8. Venezio FR, Westenfelder GO, Cook FV, *et al.*: Infective endocarditis in a community hospital. *Arch Intern Med* 1982, 142:789–792.

9. Sussman JI, Baron EJ, Tenenbaum MJ, *et al.*: Viridans streptococcal endocarditis: clinical, microbiological, and echocardiographic correlations. *J Infect Dis* 1986, 154:597–603.

10. Mylotte JM, McDermott C, Spooner JA: Prospective study of 114 consecutive episodes of *Staphylococcus aureus* bacteremia. *Rev Infect Dis* 1987, 9:891–907.

11. Scheld WM: Pathogenesis and pathophysiology of infective endocarditis. In *Endocarditis.* Edited by Sande MA, Kaye D, Root RK. London: Churchill Livingstone; 1984:1–32. [Contemporary Issues in Infectious Disease.]

12. Weinstein L, Schlesinger JJ: Pathoanatomic, physiologic and clinical correlates in endocarditis. *N Engl J Med* 1974, 291:832–837;1122–1126.

13. Lopez JA, Ross RS, Fishbein MC, *et al.*: Nonbacterial thrombotic endocarditis: a review. *Am Heart J* 1987, 113:773–784.

14. Sullam PM, Drake TA, Sande MA: Pathogenesis of endocarditis. *Am J Med* 1985, 78(suppl 6B):110–115.

15. Everett ED, Hirschmann JV: Transient bacteremia and endocarditis prophylaxis: a review. *Medicine* 1977, 56:61–77.

16. Scheld WM, Valone JA, Sande MA: Bacterial adherence in the pathogenesis of endocarditis. Interaction of bacterial dextran, platelets, and fibrin. *J Clin Invest* 1978, 61:1394–1404.

17. Crawford I, Russell C: Comparative adhesion of seven species of streptococci isolated from the blood of patients with subacute bacterial endocarditis to fibrin-platelet clots in vitro. *J Appl Bacteriol* 1986, 60:127–133.

18. Pruitt AA, Rubin RH, Karchmer AW, Duncan GW: Neurologic complications of bacterial endocarditis. *Medicine* 1978, 57:329–343.

19.• Sterkelberg JM, Murphy JG, Ballard D, *et al.*: Emboli in infective endocarditis: the prognostic value of echocardiography. *Ann Intern Med* 1991, 114:635–640.

20. Lerner PI, Weinstein L: Infective endocarditis in the antibiotic era. *N Engl J Med* 1966, 274:388–393.

21. Reisberg BE: Infective endocarditis in the narcotic addict. *Prog Cardiovasc Dis* 1979, 22:193–204.

22.• Sanfilippo AJ, Picard MH, Newell JB, *et al.*: Echocardiographic assessment of patients with infectious endocarditis: prediction of risk for complications. *J Am Coll Cardiol* 1991, 18:1191–1199.

23. Calderwood SB, Swinski LA, Karchmer AW, *et al.*: Prosthetic valve endocarditis: analysis of factors influencing outcome of therapy. *J Thorac Cardiovasc Surg* 1986, 92:776–778.

24. Ivert TSA, Dismukes WE, Cobbs CG, *et al.*: Prosthetic valve endocarditis. *Circulation* 1984, 69:223–232.

25. Vuille C, Nidorf M, Weyman AE, *et al.*: Natural history of vegetations during successful medical treatment of endocarditis. *Am Heart J* 1994, 128 (6 Pt 1):1200–1209.

26. Mugge A, Daniel WG, Frank G, *et al.*: Echocardiography in infective endocarditis: reassessment of prognostic implications of vegetation determined by transthoracic and the transesophageal approach. *J Am Coll Cardiol* 1989, 14:631–638.

27. Aragam JR, Weyman AE: Echocardiographic findings in infective endocarditis. In *Principles and Practice of Echocardiography*, edn 2. Edited by Weyman AE. Philadelphia: Lea & Febiger; 1993:1178.

28. Erbel R, Rohmann S, Drexler M, *et al.*: Improved diagnostic value of echocardiography in patients with infective endocarditis by transesophageal approach. A prospective study. *Eur Heart J* 1988, 9:43–53.

29. Stratton JR, Werner JA, Pearlman AS, *et al.*: Bacteremia and the heart: serial echocardiographic findings in 80 patients with documented or suspected bacteremia. *Am J Med* 1982, 73:851–858.

30.• Daniel WG, Mugge A, Martin RP, *et al.*: Improvement in the diagnosis of abscess associated with endocarditis by transesophageal echocardiography. *N Engl J Med* 1991, 324:795–800.

31. Robbins MJ, Frater RWM, Woiero G, *et al.*: Influence of vegetation size on clinical outcome of right-sided infective endocarditis. *Am J Med* 1986, 80:165–171.

32.•• Jaffe WM, Morgan DE, Pearlman AS, Otto CM: Infective endocarditis, 1983-1988: echocardiographic findings and factors influencing morbidity and mortality. *J Am Coll Cardiol* 1990, 15:1227–1233.

33. Hecht SR, Berger M: Right-sided endocarditis in intravenous drug users: prognostic features in 102 episodes. *Ann Intern Med* 1992, 117:560–566.

34. Wolfson JS, Swartz MN: Drug therapy: serum bactericidal activity as a monitor of antibiotic therapy. *N Engl J Med* 1985, 312:968–975.

35. Karchmer AW, Moellering RC Jr, Maki DG, *et al.*: Single antibiotic therapy for streptococcal endocarditis. *JAMA* 1979, 241:1801–1806.

36. Bisno AL, Dismukes WE, Durack DJ, *et al.*: Treatment of infective endocarditis due to viridans streptococci. *Circulation* 1981, 63:730A–733A.

37. Wolfe JC, Johnson WD: Penicillin-sensitive endocarditis: in vitro and clinical observations on penicillin-streptomycin therapy. *Ann Intern Med* 1974, 81:178–181.

38. Wilson WR, Thompson RL, Wilkowske CJ, *et al.*: Short term therapy for streptococcal infective endocarditis. *JAMA* 1981, 245:360–363.

39. Bisno AL, Dismukes WE, Durack DT, *et al.*: Antimicrobial treatment of infective endocarditis due to viridans streptococci, enterococci, and staphylococci. *JAMA* 1989, 261:1471–1477.

40. Fernandez-Guerro ML, Barros C, Rodriguez Tudela JL, *et al.*: Aortic endocarditis caused by gentamicin-resistant *Enterococcus faecalis*. *Eur J Clin Microbiol Infect Dis* 1988, 7:525–527.

41. Abrams B, Sklaver A, Hoffman T, *et al.*: Single or combination therapy of staphylococcal endocarditis in intravenous drug abusers. *Ann Intern Med* 1979, 90:789–791.

42. Korzeniowski O, Sande MA: Combination antimicrobial therapy for *Staphylococcus aureus* endocarditis in patients addicted to parenteral drugs and in nonaddicts: a prospective study. *Ann Intern Med* 1982, 97:496–503.

43. Dinubile MJ: Surgery in active endocarditis. *Ann Intern Med* 1982, 96:650–659.

44. Stinson EB, Griepp RB, Vosti K, *et al.*: Operative treatment of active endocarditis. *J Thorac Cardiovasc Surg* 1976, 71:659–665.

45. Stinson EB: Surgical treatment of infective endocarditis. *Prog Cardiovasc Dis* 1979, 22:145–168.

46. Wilson WR, Danielson GK, Guiliani ER, *et al.*: Cardiac valve replacement in congestive heart failure due to infective endocarditis. *Mayo Clin Proc* 1979, 54:223–226.

47. Saffle J, Gardner P, Schoenbaum SC, Wild W: Prosthetic valve endocarditis: the case for prompt valve replacement. *J Thorac Cardiovasc Surg* 1977, 73:416–420.

48. Karchmer AW, Dismukes WE, Buckley MJ, Austen WG: Late prosthetic valve endocarditis: clinical features influencing therapy. *Am J Med* 1978, 64:199–206.

49. Dajani AS, Bisno AL, Chung KJ, *et al.*: Prevention of bacterial endocarditis: recommendations by the American Heart Association. *JAMA* 1990, 264:2919–2922.

50. Durack DT: Current issues in the prevention of infective endocarditis. *Am J Med* 1985, 78(suppl 6B):149–156.

SELECT BIBLIOGRAPHY

Baumgartner WA, Miller DC, Reitz BA, *et al.*: Surgical treatment of prosthetic valve endocarditis. *Ann Thorac Surg* 1983, 35:87–104.

Bayer AS, Theofilopoulos AN: Immunopathogenetic aspects of infective endocarditis. *Chest* 1990, 97:204–212.

Clemens JD, Horwitz RI, Jaffe CC, *et al.*: A controlled evaluation of the risk of bacterial endocarditis in persons with mitral valve prolapse. *N Engl J Med* 1982, 307:776–781.

DiNubile MJ, Calderwood SB, Steinhaus DM, *et al.*: Cardiac conduction abnormalities complicating native valve active infective endocarditis. *Am J Cardiol* 1986, 58:1213–1217.

Erbel R, Rohmann S, Drexler M, *et al.*: Improved diagnostic value of echocardiography in patients with infective endocarditis by transesophageal approach. A prospective study. *Eur Heart J* 1988, 9:43–53.

Hutter AM, Moellering RC: Assessment of the patient with suspected endocarditis. *JAMA* 1976, 235:1603–1605.

Lee DC, Johnson RA, Bingham JB, *et al.*: Heart failure in outpatients: a randomized trial of digoxin versus placebo. *N Engl J Med* 1982, 306:699–705.

Lutas EM, Roberts R, Devereux RB, Prieto LM: Relation between the presence of echocardiographic vegetations and the complication rate in infective endocarditis. *Am Heart J* 1986, 112:107–113.

Mann T, McLaurin L, Grossman W, Craige E: Assessing the hemodynamic severity of acute aortic regurgitation due to infective endocarditis. *N Engl J Med* 1975, 293:108–113.

Marks AR, Choong CY, Chir MBB, *et al.*: Identification of high risk and low risk subgroups of patients with mitral valve prolapse. *N Engl J Med* 1989, 320:1031–1036.

McKinsey DS, McMurray TI, Flynn JM: Immune complex glomerulonephritis associated with *Staphylococcus aureus* bacteremia: response to corticosteroid therapy. *Rev Infect Dis* 1990, 12:125–127.

Morganroth J, Perloff JK, Zeldis SM, *et al.*: Acute severe aortic regurgitation: pathophysiology, clinical recognition, and management. *Ann Intern Med* 1977, 87:223–232.

Pesanti EL, Smith IM: Infective endocarditis with negative blood cultures. An analysis of 52 cases. *Am J Med* 1979, 66:43–50.

Phair JP, Clarke J: Immunology of infective endocarditis. *Prog Cardiovasc Dis* 1979, 22:137–144.

Steckelberg JM, Melton LJ III, Ilstrup DM, *et al.*: Influence of referral bias on the apparent clinical spectrum of infective endocarditis. *Am J Med* 1990, 88:582–588.

Stratton JR, Werner JA, Pearlman AS, *et al.*: Bacteremia and the heart: serial echocardiographic finding in 80 patients with documented or suspected bacteremia. *Am J Med* 1982, 73:851–858.

Van Scoy RE: Culture-negative endocarditis. *Mayo Clin Proc* 1982, 57:149–154.

Walterspiel JN, Kaplan SL: Incidence and clinical characteristics of "culture-negative" infective endocarditis in a pediatric population. *Pediatr Infect Dis* 1986, 5:328–332.

Meningitis: Diagnosis and Treatment

Carole A. Sable
Brian Wispelwey

12

Key Points

- A high index of suspicion is required to make the diagnosis of bacterial meningitis, particularly in patients at the extremes of life; empiric antibiotic therapy should be administered until a firm diagnosis is made.

- The increasing antimicrobial resistance of the common meningeal pathogens has altered recommendations for the empiric therapy for bacterial meningitis and necessitates the determination of antibiotic susceptibilities in all cases.

- Administration of adjunctive dexamethasone in infants and children with bacterial meningitis resulted in decreases in moderate and severe sensorineural hearing loss in several studies and is now standard practice. Similar data in adults are not available; however, if vancomycin is the required therapy, dexamethasone may need to be withheld.

- Immunization of children against *Haemophilus* influenzae type B has produced a dramatic decrease in the incidence of *H. influenzae* meningitis in children.

- Aseptic meningitis is due to a variety of infectious and noninfectious causes, and specific therapy must be directed against the underlying cause.

Bacterial meningitis remains a significant clinical entity; the annual attack rate is approximately three per 100,000 population, and the overall mortality remains greater than 10% despite advances in antimicrobial therapy (Fig. 1). In survivors, the incidence of long-term neurologic sequelae in the form of sensorineural hearing loss, seizures, and mental retardation is unacceptably frequent. Treatment of viral meningitis is limited by the lack of active antiviral agents against the common viral meningeal pathogens. Rapid diagnosis and appropriate therapy are essential to optimize outcome in this potentially devastating disease.

CLINICAL PRESENTATION

Obtaining an adequate history is essential in evaluating the risk and likely causes of meningitis in any patient. Symptoms, including otitis media and sinusitis, should be noted. Additionally, history of trauma or surgery, preexisting medical conditions (including asplenia, immunocompromise including malignancy and neutropenia, alcoholism, and diabetes mellitus), HIV risk factors, travel, and exposures (insects, animals, tuberculosis, other illnesses in the household) should be considered. A high index of suspicion is warranted in specific groups including infants less than 1 year old, the elderly, and the immunocompromised.

Bacterial

Patients with bacterial meningitis usually present concomitantly with, or report a history of, an upper respiratory infection. Classically, patients have fever, headache, meningismus, and central nervous system (CNS) dysfunction (lethargy, stupor, and

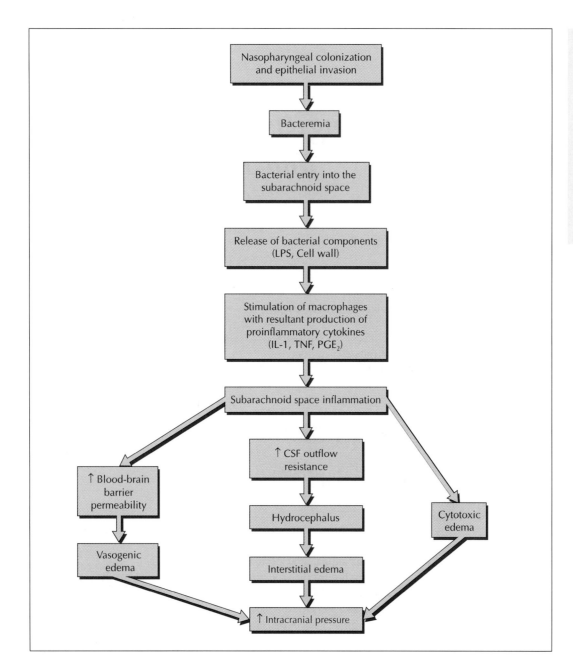

FIGURE 1
Proposed sequence of events in the development of bacterial meningitis. CSF—cerebrospinal fluids; IL-1—interleukin-1; LPS—lipopolysaccharide; PGE$_2$—prostaglandin E$_2$; TNF—tumor necrosis factor.

seizures). Other symptoms include nausea, vomiting, rigors, sweats, weakness, myalgias, and photophobia.

Symptoms in elderly patients may be more subtle, with a low-grade fever or no elevation in temperature. Confusion is often predominant in the elderly and many patients will have a coincident pneumonia.

Seizures prior to admission do not predict an adverse outcome and can be seen with either bacterial or viral meningitis. However, focal deficits at any time or generalized seizures after 3 days of therapy may signify an abnormality in the CNS and are associated with an abnormal neurologic examination on follow-up.

On physical examination, 80% of patients will have nuchal rigidity or a Kernig's or Brudzinski's sign. Up to 50% of patients are obtunded or comatose on presentation; if present, this is the most suggestive sign of bacterial meningitis. Twenty-five percent of patients will present with symptoms for less than 24 hours, but approximately 50% will have a more protracted course with symptoms for 1 to 7 days. A petechial or purpuric rash is an important diagnostic finding. It is most commonly associated with meningococcal disease (Fig. 2). Petechia or purpura is also seen with diseases caused by rickettsia, Streptococcus pneumoniae, Staphylococcus aureus, echoviruses, and some gram-negative bacilli.

Viral/Aseptic

Patients present with acute onset of symptoms with fever, malaise, pharyngitis, nausea, vomiting, and meningismus. Headache is commonly the predominant symptom. The patient may have an altered mental status, but focal neurologic signs are uncommon.

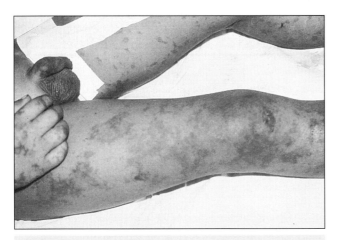

FIGURE 2 Meningococcal purpura (*see* Color Plate).

occlusion of the foramen magnum by herniating brain can result in a normal pressure. If the opening pressure falls to zero after a minimal amount of spinal fluid is removed, the diagnosis of spinal block must be considered.

Appearance

The normal appearance of CSF is clear. As few as 400 erythrocytes/μL or 200 leukocytes/μL can cause the CSF to appear cloudy, and 6000 erythrocytes/μL can make CSF appear bloody. Xanthochromia (yellow discoloration) occurs because of the breakdown of erythrocytes or protein and appears 2 to 4 hours after subarachnoid hemorrhage and 1 to 2 hours after a traumatic lumbar puncture if the specimen is not centrifuged.

Cell Count

Adults normally have fewer than 5 leukocytes/μL and these are small lymphocytes. One neutrophil may be considered normal only if all other CSF parameters are normal and the patient does not have symptoms of meningitis. More than one neutrophil is abnormal. The cells in the CSF are primarily lymphocytes, but in bacterial meningitis the vast majority (greater than 80%) are neutrophils. In aseptic meningitis neutrophils constitute approximately one third of the leukocytes. Note that subarachnoid hemorrhage can present with an increase in CSF leukocytes and, rarely, with a decreased glucose level accompanying the persistently elevated concentration of erythrocytes.

Glucose Concentration

Glucose enters the CNS by facilitated transport across the choroid plexus and capillaries. The normal ratio of CSF to

LABORATORY DIAGNOSIS

The cerebrospinal fluid (CSF) parameters that help differentiate bacterial from aseptic meningitis include the following (Tables 1 and 2).

Opening pressure

Pressure must be measured with the patient lying supine. It cannot be measured accurately with the patient sitting upright. Normal opening pressure in an adult is 50 to 195 mm CSF (4 to 15 mm Hg). It can be falsely elevated by the Valsalva maneuver and lowered by hyperventilation, leakage around the needle, or a delay in measuring the pressure. A normal opening pressure does not rule out herniation because

TABLE 1 CEREBROSPINAL FLUID PARAMETERS IN MENINGITIS		
	Bacterial	**Viral**
Cell count	1000 to 10,000 WBC/mm3	10 to 1000 WBC/mm3
Glucose	Predominantly PMNs	Usually lymphocytes, 1/3 PMNs
Protein	<40, ratio <0.4	Normal to slight decrease
Other	100 to 500 mg/dL	50 to 100 mg/dL
	Gram Stain, bacterial antigens	—

Gram stain: the most valuable single test

Positive in 60% to 80% of patients who have not received prior treatment

Sensitivity is decreased to 40% to 60% with prior treatment

Accuracy varies with etiologic agent, number of organisms, and the technique used

The sensitivity is 95% if at least 105 CFU/mL are present

Gram-negative bacilli and *Listeria* spp have a positive Gram Stain in only 50% of patients

Bacterial antigens: various methods

Counter immunoelectrophoresis—variable sensitivity, 32% to 95%

Latex agglutination—80% to 100%

Immunofluorescence—84%

Coagglutination—53% to 95%

Sensitivity is greatest for *Haemophilus influenzae* and lower for *Neisseria meningitidis* and *Streptococcus pneumoniae*

CFU—colony-forming units; PMN—polymorphonucleocytes; WBC—leukocyte.

TABLE 2 CEREBROSPINAL FLUID ABNORMALITIES AND ASSOCIATED DISEASES

Xanthochromia	**CSF eosinophilia**
Subarachnoid hemorrhage	Classically thought to represent parasitic infections but in the United States
Trauma	more common with fungi (*Coccidioides immitis*)
Uncommon causes	Mycobacteria
Protein >150 mg/dL	Rickettsia
Bilirubin >10 mg/dL	Viruses (LCM, mumps)
Melanoma metastatic to meninges	Bacteria (*Treponema pallidum*)
Hypoglycorrachia	Noninfectious diseases: malignancy, vasculitis, hypersensitivity, idiopathic,
Bacteria (especially if glucose <20 mg/dL)	and others
Mycobacteria	Parasites include *Trichinella, Ascaris, Toxoplasma, Cysticercus,*
Fungi	*Toxocara, Angiostrongylus cantonensis, Gnathostoma, Schistosoma,*
Less common causes	*Echinococcus,* and others
Viral meningoencephalitis	
Mycoplasma	
Noninfectious	
Sarcoid	
Carcinomatous meningitis	
Subarachnoid hemorrhage	

CSF—cerebrospinal fluid; LCM—lymphocytic choriomeningitis.

blood glucose is 0.6 (0.3 for patients with diabetes mellitus). In the ventricles the concentration of glucose is approximately 5 to 20 mg/dL higher than in the lumbar fluid. Equilibration of CSF glucose with blood takes 2 to 4 hours so blood should optimally be drawn prior to lumbar puncture. The decrease in glucose levels results primarily because of altered transport, but glucose consumption by leukocytes and bacteria also contributes. Hypoglycorrachia is commonly seen with meningitis caused by bacteria, fungi, and mycobacteria (*see* Table 2). A glucose level less than 20 mg/dL is very suggestive of bacterial meningitis. With resolution of meningitis, glucose levels correct more rapidly than either protein concentration or cell counts.

Protein

The normal mean protein concentration is approximately 25 to 40 mg/dL. The protein concentration in the cisterna magna is lower (15 to 30 mg/dL); this is an important fact to remember if CSF is obtained by a cisternal puncture. Protein concentrations can be abnormal for months after resolution of infection and cannot be followed as a measure of adequate therapy.

Gram Stain

The Gram Stain is the most valuable single test and is positive in 60% to 80% of patients not treated prior to lumbar puncture (Fig. 3). With prior treatment only 40% to 60% will test positive and the accuracy varies with the etiologic agent, the number of organisms, and the technique used. If there are at least 10^5 colony-forming units/mL, the sensitivity is 95%. *S. pneumoniae* is identified more commonly than *Neisseria meningitidis*, probably because of the difficulty in

identifying the small gram-negative diplococci. Other gram-negative bacilli and *Listerias* spp have a positive Gram Stain in only 50% of cases.

Bacterial Antigens

There are different methods of determining bacterial antigens. The earliest method was counter immunoelectrophoresis, which had variable sensitivity from 32% to 95%. The newer methods, including latex agglutination (LA), immunofluorescence (IF), and coagglutination, are more sensitive (LA, 80% to 100%; IF, 84%; and coagglutination, 53% to 95%). There is also variability with different etiologic agents; sensitivity is greatest for *Haemophilus influenzae* and lower for for *N. meningitidis* and *S. pneumoniae*.

A presumptive diagnosis of the type of meningitis can be made if all CSF parameters as well as the patient's symptoms are considered [3••].

In bacterial meningitis there is typically a neutrophilic pleocytosis, with hypoglycorrachia and an increased protein concentration. There are exceptions, and about one in seven patients will have predominantly lymphocytes, especially if the meningitis is caused by gram-negative bacilli or *Listeria* spp. A small minority of patients may have a normal glucose concentration, and a normal CSF profile can rarely be seen at the onset of disease, particularly in severely immunocompromised patients.

A diagnosis of partially treated bacterial meningitis is a special consideration. Antibiotics have little effect on the CSF cell count, protein, or glucose level during the first 2 to 3 days of therapy. Occasionally, the leukocyte differential will change to a lymphocyte predominance in this time. Antibiotics also decrease the yield of the Gram Stain and culture.

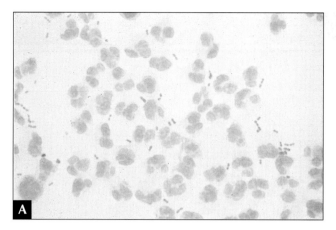

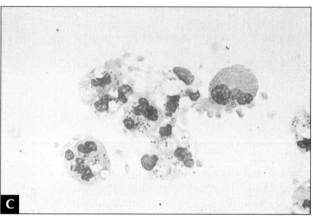

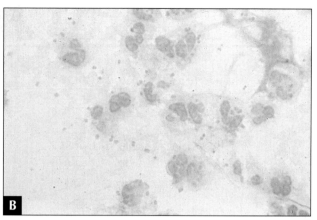

FIGURE 3 Gram stain of the three major meningeal pathogens. A, *Streptococcus pneumoniae*. B, *Neisseria meningitidis*. C, *Haemophilus influenzae*. (*See* Color Plates.)

Viral meningitis frequently presents with fewer cells, primarily lymphocytes; mildly elevated protein; and a normal glucose concentration. A neutrophil predominance may be seen in the first 24 to 36 hours and can exceed 50% of the leukocytes present.

Occasionally the glucose level is decreased, but is unlikely to be less than 20 mg/dL. Isolation of a virus from the CSF is rarely useful because of the low sensitivity and duration required for a positive viral culture.

TREATMENT

The selection of appropriate antimicrobial therapy for patients with bacterial meningitis must take into consideration the need for bactericidal activity, adequate penetration into the CNS, and reliable activity of the antimicrobial agent in purulent CSF. CSF antimicrobial concentrations of at least 10 to 20 times the minimal bactericidal concentration of the agent against the implicated pathogen are needed to ensure successful therapy because of the relative deficiency of host defenses in the CSF. Penetration of antimicrobial agents is determined primarily by the status of the blood-brain barrier, with increased permeability associated with enhanced penetration of the drug. Entry is also enhanced by a low molecular weight and simple chemical structure, a low degree of ionization at physiologic pH, high lipid solubility, and a low degree of protein binding [4•].

Combinations of different antimicrobials may result in antagonism (a bacteriostatic plus a bactericidal agent) or synergy (a β-lactam plus an aminoglycoside) and can therefore influence the outcome of therapy.

The ultimate selection of antimicrobial therapy is influenced by the patient's age and medical condition as well as an examination of the CSF. The ideal therapy would be specifically directed against a known pathogen. However, because of the serious consequences of delaying treatment, initial therapy is often empiric (Table 3). Treatment should be initiated immediately if bacterial meningitis is suspected and certainly if there is a delay in obtaining CSF or if the CSF Gram Stain is unrevealing [5••].

The greatest risk for bacterial meningitis is during the neonatal period, considered the first 30 days of life. More than 75% of cases in this age group are caused by *Escherichia coli* and group B streptococci. Other less frequent causes are enterococci, staphylococci, and nontypable *H. influenzae*.

The relative frequency of β-lactamase production by H. influenzae necessitates the use of a third-generation cephalosporin as empiric therapy in children. Cefotaxime is preferred over ceftriaxone because of the displacement of bilirubin from albumin seen with ceftriaxone.

Because of the increasing concern about *S. pneumoniae* isolates that are relatively or absolutely resistant to penicillin, authorities recommend the use of a third-generation cephalosporin (cefotaxime or ceftriaxone) empirically in adults with bacterial meningitis. In addition, if there are pneumococci with high-level resistance to penicillin in the region, vancomycin should be administered until antibiotic susceptibility is known.

Meningitis in postneurosurgical patients is most commonly caused by enteric gram-negative bacilli and staphylococci, including both *Staphylococcus aureus* and coagulase-negative staphylococci. Empiric therapy should include vancomycin plus a third-generation cephalosporin. Ceftazidime is frequently employed because of the concern of infection caused by *Pseudomonas aeruginosa*. Coagulase-negative staphylococci are the most common cause of infection with CSF shunts in place. Therapy is parenteral vancomycin, often in combination with rifampin, but frequently the hardware must be removed to effectively cure the infection.

TABLE 3 EMPIRIC THERAPY FOR SUSPECTED BACTERIAL MENINGITIS BY AGE GROUP

Age	Common pathogens	Therapy
Neonates (0 to 4 wk)	Escherichia coli group B streptococci Listeria monocytogenes	Ampicillin plus a third-generation cephalosporin or ampicillin plus gentamicin
Infants (4 to 12 wk)	Escherichia coli group B streptococci Listeria monocytogenes Haemophilus influenzae Streptococcus pneumoniae	Ampicillin plus a third-generation cephalosporin
Children (3 mo to 18 y)	Haemophilus influenzae Neisseria meningitidis Streptococcus pneumoniae	A third-generation cephalosporin
Adults (18 to 50 y)	Streptococcus pneumoniae Neisseria meningitidis	Third-generation cephalosporin plus vancomycin
Elderly (older than 50 y)	Streptococcus pneumoniae Listeria monocytogenes Gram-negative bacilli Haemophilus influenzae	Third-generation cephalosporin plus ampicillin plus vancomycin

SPECIFIC THERAPY

Once an etiologic agent is identified, therapy can be specifically directed toward that pathogen (Tables 4 and 5). There are special concerns about some of the etiologic agents implicated in bacterial meningitis.

All blood and CSF isolates of S. pneumoniae should be tested for susceptibility to penicillin. Although sensitive pneumococci [minimum inhibitory concentration (MIC) <0.06 µg/mL] can be treated effectively with high-dose penicillin or ampicillin, it is difficult to achieve adequate bactericidal concentrations of penicillin with current treatment regimens

TABLE 4 TREATMENT FOR SPECIFIC MENINGEAL PATHOGENS

Organism	Therapy
Haemophilus influenzae	
β-lactamase negative	Ampicillin
β-lactamase positive	Third-generation cephalosporin
Neisseria meningitidis	Penicillin G or ampicillin
Streptococcus pneumoniae	
MIC <0.06 µg/mL	Penicillin G or ampicillin
MIC 0.1 to 1.0 µg/mL	Third-generation cephalosporin
MIC >1.0 µg/mL	Vancomycin
Listeria monocytogenes	Penicillin G or ampicillin*
Enterobacteriaceae	Third-generation cephalosporin
Pseudomonas aeruginosa	Ceftazidime*
Staphylococcus aureus	Nafcillin or oxacillin
MRSA	Vancomycin
Coagulase-negative staphylococci	Vancomycin
Group B streptococci	Penicillin G or ampicillin*

*Consider the addition of an aminoglycoside in the treatment of these infections.
The third-generation cephalosporins most extensively studied are cefotaxime and ceftriaxone. Ceftazidime should be reserved for infections caused by Pseudomonas species.
MIC—minimum inhibitory concentration; MRSA—methicillin-resistant Staphylococcus aureus.

TABLE 5 ANTIBIOTICS AND DOSING INTERVALS FOR ADULTS WITH NORMAL RENAL FUNCTION

Antibiotic	Dose	Interval
Ampicillin	2 g	Every 4 h
Cefotaxime	2 g	Every 6 h
Ceftriaxone	2 g	Every 12 h*
Ceftazidime	2 g	Every 8 h†
Nafcillin	1.5–2 g	Every 4 h
Oxacillin	1.5–2 g	Every 4 h
Penicillin G	4 MU	Every 4 h‡
Vancomycin	1 g	Every 12 h§

*The dosage studied was 50 mg/kg every 12 hours.
†A higher dose may be needed.
‡Or 20–24 MU/day as continuous intravenous infusion.
§Adjust for appropriate peak and trough.

to effectively treat pneumococci with MICs to penicillin greater than 0.1 µg/mL [6].

Although isolates of N. *meningitidis* have been reported to be absolutely resistant to penicillin, clinical failures have not been reported with penicillin or ampicillin and there is no recommendation to alter therapy at this time. The earlier use of cefuroxime has been abandoned because of reports of delayed sterilization of the CSF in children with *H. influenzae* meningitis treated with cefuroxime [7]. Meningitis caused by gram-negative aerobic bacilli had been associated with a mortality of 40% to 80% prior to the introduction of the third-generation cephalosporins; current mortality rates are less than 23% [8].

Listeria monocytogenes meningitis should be treated with penicillin or ampicillin because *Listeria* is resistant to cephalosporins. Aminoglycosides have been shown to be synergistic with penicillins *in vitro* and in animal models and can be added to therapy in patients with *L. monocytogenes* meningitis [9].

Staphylococcus aureus is an uncommon cause of meningitis, and usually occurs after trauma or a neurosurgical procedure. The treatment of choice is an antistaphylococcal penicillin such as nafcillin sodium. Vancomycin should only be used for patients with a documented penicillin allergy or for infections caused by methicillin-resistant *S. aureus* [10].

DURATION OF THERAPY

The standard duration of therapy for bacterial meningitis in the United States has been 10 to 14 days. Cases of gram-negative and *Listeria* meningitis should be treated for 21 days because of a higher relapse rate associated with shorter courses of therapy in these infections [11]. Recent investigations have suggested the utility of shorter course therapy (7 days) in specific circumstances, including meningococcal meningitis and bacterial meningitis in children (with most infections caused by *H. influenzae*). There may be other cases in which shorter courses of therapy are adequate, but these must be individualized. If *L. monocytogenes* is associated with rhomboencephalitis and the production of discrete abscesses, at least 4 weeks of antibiotic therapy is often required.

VIRAL MENINGITIS

Viral agents implicated in meningitis include the enteroviruses, mumps, lymphocytic choriomeningitis, herpes simplex virus type 2 and varicella zoster virus (Tables 6 and 7). Treatment for viral meningitis is supportive [12•]. The only therapy that can be considered is acyclovir for meningitis caused by herpes simplex virus, and potentially for varicella zoster virus. The efficacy of acyclovir in this infection is not proven, and most cases are self-limited illnesses for which specific therapy is not indicated. Typically, patients are not treated with antiviral therapy.

ADJUNCTIVE THERAPY

Dexamethasone, which is directed at modifying the inflammatory response in the subarachnoid space, is the best studied adjunctive therapy for bacterial meningitis.

Most data in humans with bacterial meningitis involve studies of infants and children. Several randomized, placebo-controlled studies have demonstrated a decrease in the incidence of sensorineural hearing loss in children (with infections almost entirely due to *H. influenzae*) when adjunctive dexamethasone was administered with antibiotics [13–15]. An

---

TABLE 6 INFECTIOUS AND NONINFECTIOUS ETIOLOGIES OF ASEPTIC MENINGITIS

Infectious etiologies		Noninfectious etiologies	
Viruses	Mycobacteria	Malignancy	Medications
Enteroviruses	*Mycobacterium tuberculosis*	Lymphoma	Antibiotics (trimethoprim,
Arboviruses		Carcinomatous meningitis	sulfamethoxazole, INH)
Herpes simplex type 2	Spirochetes	Intracranial tumors or cysts	Nonsteroidal anti-inflamma-
HIV	*Borrelia burgdorferi*		tory agents (ibuprofen,
Lymphocytic choriomeningitis	*Treponema pallidum*	Systemic illnesses	naprosyn, sulindac,
Mumps		Vasculitis (CNS or systemic)	tolmetin)
(Rare: Herpes simplex type 1,	Other	Sarcoid	Immunosuppressants (OKT3,
VZV, CMV, influenza,	Paramceningeal infections	Behçet's	azathioprine, ara-C)
parainfluenza, measles)	Partially treated bacterial		Others include carba-
Postvaccination	meningitis	Other	mazepine, immunoglobulin
Postviral illness	*Mycoplasma pneumoniae*	Postprocedure (eg, neuro-	
	Listeria monocytogenes	surgery, spinal anesthesia)	Other
Fungi			Heavy metal poisoning
Cryptococcus neoformans			Migraine
Coccidioides immitis			Seizure
Histoplasma capsulatum			

ara-C—arabinosylcytosine; CMV—cytomegalovirus; CNS—central nervous system; INH—isonicotine hydrazine; VZV—varicella-zoster virus.

TABLE 7 COMMON ETIOLOGIES OF ASEPTIC MENINGITIS

Organism	Mode of transmission	Seasonality	Diagnosis	Comments
Enteroviruses (picornavirus)	Fecal-oral	Temperate climates, warmer months	No rapid diagnosis Culture CSF 40%–80% Throat and stool culture provide supportive data Serology	Includes Coxsackie A and B, Echovirus, enterovirus, and poliovirus Clues include epidemic disease in the community, exanthem, myopericarditis, and conjunctivitis Classic syndromes of pleurodynia, hand-foot-mouth disease, and herpangina
Mumps (paramyxovirus)	Respiratory droplets, direct contact, fomites	Late winter, early spring	No rapid diagnosis Culture, serology	Male-to-female ratio about 5:1 Age 2 y to 9 y most common Usually follows parotitis by days to weeks but may appear first
LCM (arenavirus)	Contact with rodents or their excreta	Late fall, early winter	No rapid diagnosis Culture CSF and blood and later, urine Serology	Young adults Late complications include orchitis, arthritis, myopericarditis, and alopecia
HSV 2 (herpesvirus)	Sexually transmitted	—	Cultures of CSF, buffy coat is positive in some	Primary genital herpes
HIV (group D retrovirus)	Blood, body fluids	—	HIV antibody may be negative at time of initial symptoms p24Ag, culture, PCR	HIV risks (injection drug use, homosexual behavior in men, blood transfusion, and sexual contact with those at risk) Symptoms of mononucleosis
Arthropod borne California group (bunyavirus) St. Louis (flavivirus)	Insect vector *Aedes triseriatus* *Culex* mosquitos	Warmer months (contact with insects)	Serology	Usually encephalitis but milder disease can present as meningitis
Mycobacterium tuberculosis	Respiratory droplets	—	Culture, AFB smear History +/- CXR often normal ppd (–) in a variable percent (up 50%)	Altered mental status SIADH Hypoglycorachia
Lyme disease (*Borrelia burgdorferi*)	Tick vector *Ixodes dammini*	Any time (meningitis can present in different stages)	CSF anti-Borrelia antibodies CSF culture Serology in serum aids diagnosis	Early or second stage disease Usually mild and resolves but occasionally chronic and relapsing Palsies of CN(VII), peripheral nerves

AFB—acid-fast bacillus; CN(VII)—cranial nerve; CSF— cerebrospinal fluid; CXR—chest radiograph film; LCM—lymphocytic choriomeningitis; PCR—patient contact record; SIADH—syndrome of inappropriate antidiuretic hormone.

additional study included both adults and children, but again demonstrated a benefit only in a subset of patients (those with pneumococcal meningitis) [16].

There is increasing evidence that dexamethasone may be beneficial in patients with bacterial meningitis. Side effects, including gastrointestinal hemorrhage, are uncommon. Earlier concerns about delayed sterilization of the CSF or side effects in patients with aseptic meningitis (diagnosed after treatment) have not been realized [17]. Current recommendations are to employ adjunctive dexamethasone in infants and children older that 2 months of age just prior to, or concomitantly with, the first dose of antimicrobial therapy at a dose of 0.15 mg/kg intravenously every 6 hours for 4 days. However, if vancomycin is required, as is increasingly the case, dexamethasone may need to be withheld. Penetration of vancomycin through the blood-brain barrier is marginal, even in the presence of inflammation.

Generalized recommendations cannot be made for adults based on the current data. Dexamethasone may be more useful in the subsets of patients with altered mental status,

increased intracranial pressure, or cerebral edema on computer tomography scan. Further studies in adults are under way.

CHEMOPROPHYLAXIS

Chemoprophylaxis is intended to prevent the transmission and development of disease in susceptible persons [19]. *N. meningitidis* is associated with a high incidence of secondary infections, with household contacts having 500 times the risk of the general population of developing meningococcal disease. The prophylaxis of choice in the United States is rifampin given as a dose of 10 mg/kg (maximum 600 mg) every 12 hours for 2 days. Failure to eradicate carriage of *N. meningitidis* has been reported in 10% to 20% of cases. Prophylaxis is not generally recommended for neighborhood or hospital contacts because the risk of disease is much lower. Ciprofloxacin has also been shown to be effective in adults but is not approved for use in children.

For all household contacts of *H. influenzae* disease, the current recommendation is rifampin prophylaxis if there are children younger than 4 years of age in the household and if exposure was less than 2 weeks earlier. If prophylaxis is used, all contacts and the index case must be treated regardless of immunization status as soon after the exposure as possible. The dose of rifampin is 20 mg/kg (maximum 600 mg) given once daily for 4 days. Prophylaxis in day care centers is more controversial.

Prophylaxis of contacts of *S. pneumoniae* disease is not recommended because the risk of secondary disease has not been defined.

IMMUNOPROPHYLAXIS

Hyperimmune bacterial polysaccharide globulin preparations (BPIG) were developed because of the poor immunogenicity of the early polysaccharide vaccines in children less than 2 years of age. Studies demonstrated higher titers of antibody during the first year of life, but titers that were not protective at 15 to 18 months. The new conjugate vaccines will, it is hoped, obviate the need for BPIG (Table 8).

TABLE 8 GENERAL GUIDELINES FOR IMMUNIZATIONS

Haemophilus influenzae

Begin at age 2 mo

Use the same vaccine for each dose because of differences in immunogenicity

Children who have invasive *H. influenzae* disease prior to 2 y should complete immunizations on schedule because development of immunity in this age group is uncertain

Children exposed to invasive *H. influenzae* disease should receive chemoprophylaxis regardless of immunization status (vaccines are not 100% effective)

Neisseria meningitidis

High-risk individuals (terminal complement deficiencies and asplenia)

Military recruits

Persons travelling to a region where disease is hyperendemic or epidemic

Consideration in certain outbreaks or epidemics

NOT routinely used in the United States (does not protect against serogroup B disease, does not provide lasting immunity in children, and the overall risk of disease is low)

Streptococcus pneumoniae

Persons 65 y or older

Chronic illness (includes cardiovascular and pulmonary disease, diabetes mellitus, alcoholism, cirrhosis, and CSF leaks)

Immunocompromised adults and children older than 2 y (asplenia, Hodgkin's disease, nephrotic syndrome, multiple myeloma, and chronic renal insufficiency)

HIV-infected adults and children older than 2 y

CSF—cerebrospinal fluid

REFERENCES AND RECOMMENDED REading

Recently published papers of particular interest have been highlighted as:
• Of interest
•• Of outstanding interest

1. Tunkel AR, Scheld WM: Pathogenesis and pathophysiology of bacterial meningitis. *Clin Microbiol Rev* 1993, 6:118.
2. Tunkel AR, Wispelwey B, Scheld WM: Pathogenesis and pathophysiology of meningitis. *Infect Dis Clin North Am* 1990, 4:555.
3.•• Greenlee JE: Approach to diagnosis of meningitis: cerebrospinal fluid evaluation. *Infect Dis Clin North Am* 1990, 4:583.
4.• Sable CA, Scheld WM: Theoretical and practical considerations of antibiotic therapy for bacterial meningitis. In *Bacterial Meningitis.* Edited by Schonfeld H, Helwig H. Basel, Switzerland: Karger; 1992:96.

5.•• Roos KL, Tunkel AR, Scheld WM: Acute bacterial meningitis in children and adults. In *Infections of the Central Nervous System*. Edited by Scheld WM, Whitley RJ, Durack DT. New York: Raven Press; 1991:335.

6. Appelbaum PC: World-wide development of antibiotic resistance in pneumococci. *Eur J Clin Microbiol Infect Dis* 1987, 6:367.

7. Arditi M, Derold BC, Yoger R: Cefuroxime treatment failure and *H. influenzae* meningitis: case report and review of the literature. *Pediatr* 1989, 84:132.

8. Cheruben CE, Corrado ML, Nair SR, *et al.*: Treatment of gram-negative bacillary meningitis: role of new cephalosporin antibiotics. *Rev Infect Dis* 1982, 4(suppl):s453.

9. Trautman M, Wagner J, Chahen M, *et al.*: Listeria meningitis: report of ten cases and review of current therapeutic recommendations. *J Infect* 1985, 10:107.

10. Schlesinger LS, Ross SC, Schaberg DA: *Staphylococcus aureus* meningitis: a broad based epidemiological study. *Medicine* 1987, 66:148.

11. Radetsky M: Duration of treatment in bacterial meningitis: a historical inquiry. *Pediatr Infect Dis J* 1990, 9:2.

12.• Connolly KJ, Hammer SM: The acute aseptic meningitis syndrome. *Infect Dis Clin North Am* 1990, 4:599.

13. Lebel MH, Freij BJ, Syrogiannopoulos GA, *et al.*: Dexamethasone therapy for bacterial meningitis: results of two double-blind, placebo controlled trials. *N Engl J Med* 1988, 319:964.

14. Lebel MH, Hoyt J, Waagner DC, *et al.*: Magnetic resonance imaging and dexamethasone therapy for bacterial meningitis. *Am J Dis Child* 1989, 143:301.

15. Odio CM, Faingezicht I, Paris M, *et al.*: The beneficial effects of early dexamethasone administration in infants and children with bacterial meningitis. *N Engl J Med* 1991, 342:1525.

16. Girgis NK, Farid Z, Mikhail IA, *et al.*: Dexamethasone treatment for bacterial meningitis in children and adults. *Pediatr Infect Dis J* 1989, 8:848.

17. Waagner DC, Kennedy WA, Hoyt MJ, *et al.*: Lack of adverse effects of dexamethasone therapy in aseptic meningitis. *Pediatr Infect Dis J* 1990, 9:922.

18.•• Recommendations of the Immunization Practice Advisory Committee: *Haemophilus influenzae* type B conjugate vaccine for prevention of *Haemophilus influenzae* type B disease in infants and children two months of age or older. *MMWR* Morb Mortal Wkly Rep 1991, 40No.RR-1:1.

19. Lieberman JM, Greenberg DP, Ward JI: Prevention of bacterial meningitis: vaccines and chemoprophylaxis. *Infect Dis Clin North Am* 1990, 4:703.

SELECT BIBLIOGRAPHY

Quagliarello V, Scheld WM: Bacterial meningitis: pathogenesis, pathophysiology, and progress. *N Engl J Med* 1992, 327:864.

Rotbart HA: Viral meningitis and the aseptic meningitis syndrome. In *Infections of the Central Nervous System*. Edited by Scheld WM, Whitley RJ, Durack DT. New York: Raven Press; 1991:19.

Sable CA, Scheld WM: Bacterial meningitis: a new look at an old foe. *Contemp Intern Med* 1992, 4:21.

Tunkel AR, Wispelwey B, Scheld WM: Bacterial meningitis: recent advances in pathophysiology and treatment. *Ann Intern Med* 1990, 112:610.

Tuomanen E: Advances in the diagnosis and management of bacterial meningitis. *Curr Opin Infect Dis* 1990, 3:596.

Infectious Diarrhea 13

Larry J. Goodman
Gordon M. Trenholme

> ### Key Points
> • Infectious diarrhea is acquired by ingesting the pathogen, usually as part of a contaminated meal.
> • A wide variety of agents, including viruses, bacteria, and parasites, cause diarrheal disease.
> • A careful history, physical examination, and microscopic examination of the stool are effective in narrowing the differential diagnosis.
> • Assessment of the state of hydration and careful rehydration are key early management points.
> • Widespread antimicrobial resistance complicates empiric treatment decisions.

Diarrhea, defined as three or more loose stools in a 24-hour period, is among the most common symptoms for which patients seek medical attention [1]. The reputation of many over-the-counter and home remedies has been enhanced by the short duration of illness (1 to 5 days) that is typical of most acute infectious diarrheas. Despite a usually benign course, diarrhea can rapidly lead to life-threatening dehydration, be associated with bacteremia, and have severe local complications such as toxic megacolon and intestinal rupture. Worldwide, diarrheal diseases account for over 5 million deaths in children under age 5 annually, and diarrhea is the most common infection complicating travel to many parts of the world [2].

The clinician must have a logical approach to the diagnosis and treatment of diarrhea to identify those patients with more serious illness or complications and to limit the cost of the evaluation. Problems in diagnosing and treating acute diarrhea are listed in Table 1.

PATHOGENESIS

A general understanding of the methods by which organisms associated with infectious diarrhea are acquired and cause disease is necessary to develop appropriate prevention and treatment strategies.

Acquisition

Most enteric infections are acquired by ingesting the pathogen orally. A contaminated food or beverage is the usual vehicle. Rarely, organisms are ingested via fecal-oral spread, with fomites or hands as intermediaries. Because the period from ingestion to symptoms may vary from several hours to over a week and because the contaminated food usually has no abnormal smell or taste, identifying the specific meal that caused an individual's illness is usually not possible. An exception occurs when a large number of people become ill after a common ingestion, particularly if they have previously shared no other common foods or beverages. Table 2 lists the most common vehicles for specific pathogens or toxins. Examples of less common methods of acquisition include person-to-person spread of pathogens in patient care institutions via fecal-oral spread—usually resulting from inadequate identification and isolation of the index case—or infection resulting from contamination of patient treatment materials.

Host Factors

The most important host factors that modify the risk of acquisition of an enteric pathogen are

- *Gastric acidity*—most organisms are killed by the low pH found in the stomach
- *Small-bowel motility*—constant movement limits the contact time of the organism to its potential attachment site
- *Indigenous microflora*—nonpathogens may take up attachment sites, compete for nutrients, and produce chemicals that are toxic for some pathogens

- *Coproantibody*—antibodies formed in the gut provide protection against some pathogens
- *Patient's age*—patients at the extremes of age are at the greatest risk for severe complications of diarrheal illness (*eg*, over half of all deaths resulting from diarrhea in the United States occur in patients over the age of 74)
- *The patient's general state of health*—persons who are malnourished or have an immune deficiency are at particular risk for a more severe infection and for infection with otherwise unusual organisms

The commonly observed finding that not all persons eating the same contaminated meal become ill is explained by differences in one or more of these factors [3].

Organism Factors

Table 3 lists some of the organisms that have been identified as enteric pathogens. Organism factors most associated with clinical symptoms result from the production of one or more exotoxins. An enterotoxin is an exotoxin that interacts with the intestinal epithelium at the level of cyclic AMP or GMP, leading to secretion of fluids into the lumen and a watery diarrhea. *Vibrio cholerae* and enterotoxicogenic *Escherichia coli* are examples of organisms that produce an enterotoxin. Cytotoxins are exotoxins that cause cell destruction. The cytotoxin of *Clostridium difficile*, the Shiga toxin of *Shigella dysenteriae*, and the Shiga-like toxins of enterohemorrhagic *E. coli* are associated with local cell destruction, bleeding, and, often, an inflammatory reaction.

AN APPROACH TO THE PATIENT WITH DIARRHEA

The first task in assessing a patient with acute diarrhea is to evaluate the severity of illness. Table 4 lists factors that are important in this evaluation, along with a suggested severity-

TABLE 2 COMMON FOOD VEHICLES FOR SPECIFIC PATHOGENS OR TOXINS

Vehicle	Pathogen or toxin
Undercooked chicken	*Salmonella* species, *Campylobacter* species
Eggs	*Salmonella* species (especially *Salmonella enteritidis*)
Unpasteurized milk	*Salmonella*, *Campylobacter*, and *Yersinia* species
Water	*Giardia lamblia*, Norwalk virus, *Campylobacter* and *Cryptosporidium* species, *Cyclospora*, *Aeromonas*, *Plesiomonas*
Fried rice	*Bacillus cereus*
Fish	
Shellfish	*Vibrio cholera*, *Vibrio parahemolyticus*, *Vibrio vulnificus*, other *Vibrio* species, neurotoxic shellfish poisoning, paralytic shellfish poisoning, Norwalk virus
Tuna, mackerel, mahi-mahi	Scombroid
Grouper, amberjack, snapper	Ciguatera
Sushi	*Anisakis* species (anisakiasis)
Beef, gravy	*Salmonella* species, *Campylobacter* species, *Clostridium perfringens*

TABLE 3 PATHOGENS ASSOCIATED WITH DIARRHEAL ILLNESS

Bacteria
  Campylobacter jejuni
  Salmonella spp
  Shigella sp
  Yersinia enterocolitica
  Vibrio cholera
  Vibrio parahemolyticus
Enterotoxicogenic *Escherichia coli*
Enterohemorrhagic *Escherichia coli*
Enteroinvasive *Escherichia coli*
Enteropathogenic *Escherichia coli*
  Plesiomonas shigelloides
  Aeromonas hydrophila
  Staphylococcus aureus
  Bacillus cereus
  Clostridium difficile
Viruses
  Rotavirus (mainly group A)
  Norwalk virus
  Adenovirus (serotypes 40 and 41)
  Calcivirus
  Astrovirus
Protozoa
  Giardia lamblia
  Entamoeba histolytica
  Cryptosporidium
  Isospora belli
  Enterocytozoon bieneusi (Microsporidium)
  Cyclospora

of-illness scale. Immediate management decisions are based on the results of this assessment.

Next, a more detailed history and a microscopic examination of a stool smear are obtained. Organisms are considered or rejected as possible pathogens based on the patient's syndrome and the history obtained. Laboratory studies are ordered to confirm or reject these preliminary conclusions. Table 5 lists common presenting syndromes and causative agents. Table 6 lists clinical "pearls" that may be useful in select cases. Photomicrographs demonstrating stool smears of leukocytes and erythrocytes, an *Entamoeba histolytica* trophozoite ingesting red cells, a *Giardia lamblia* trophozoite, *Cryptosporidium*, and *Cyclospora* are findings that may be diagnosed by careful microscopy (Figs. 1–5).

Differential Diagnosis

It is critical to understand that the clinical syndromes commonly associated with enteric pathogens may overlap and that patients may be infected with more than one pathogen. Also, many other illnesses may have diarrhea as part of the presenting symptom complex. Processes to consider in the differential diagnosis include sexually transmitted diseases (particularly *Neisseria gonorrhoeae*, herpes simplex, and syphilis), malaria, inflammatory bowel disease, bowel ischemia, pancreatitis, appendicitis, diverticulitis, laxative- or other drug-induced symptoms, and sprue.

Treatment

Fluids appropriate for rehydration include 5% dextrose/0.9% sodium chloride solution, lactated Ringer's solution, or oral rehydrating solutions (*eg*, Rehydralyte, Ross Laboratories, Columbus, OH). When indicated, antimicrobial therapy should be directed specifically against the causative agent. When empiric antibiotic therapy is indicated in an otherwise healthy outpatient with severe acute diarrhea, the agent

TABLE 4 FACTORS TO INCLUDE IN EVALUATING THE SEVERITY OF A DIARRHEAL ILLNESS*

	Degree of illness		
	Mild†	**Moderate†**	**Severe‡**
State of hydration	Normotensive; no orthostatic blood pressure/pulse changes or symptoms	Normotensive in lying position; mild orthostatic blood pressure or pulse changes with no or minimal orthostatic symptoms	Hypotensive; significant orthostatic blood pressure/pulse changes and orthostatic symptoms (*eg*, dizziness)
Frequency of diarrhea	1 to 4 loose stools/d	5 to 8 loose stools/d	> 8 loose stools/d
Abdominal symptoms and findings	Mild crampy pain, soft abdomen, no rebound, bowel sounds normal	Moderate pain; soft abdomen; occasional pain on palpation; normal or increased bowel sounds	Severe abdominal pain; increased pain with palpation; hypoactive or absent bowel sounds; rebound
Fever	Absent	< 101.5°F (< 38.6°C)	> 101.5°F (> 38.6°C)

*This table assists in focusing the history and physical examination in the assessment of the patient with diarrhea.
†Patients with mild to moderate illness can usually be managed successfully as outpatients. Empiric antibiotic therapy is given in select cases.
‡Patients with severe illness should be observed until symptoms and findings improve. They should be followed carefully for the development of bacteremia or the progression of abdominal findings. Abdominal radiographs, surgical evaluation, and empiric antibiotic use are often indicated.

TABLE 5 CLINICAL SYNDROMES FOR SPECIFIC ENTERIC PATHOGENS*

Syndrome	Incubation period	Fever	Stool exam for leukocytes/erythrocytes	Pathogens
Nausea and vomiting	5–15 min	No	Negative	Heavy metals, mass psychogenic illness†
Nausea, vomiting, diarrhea	1–18 h	No	Negative	Enterotoxicogenic *Escherichia coli*, *Clostridium perfringens*, *Bacillus cereus*, *Staphylococcus aureus*
Nausea, vomiting, diarrhea, myalgias, headache	12 h–3 d	Yes	Negative	Rotavirus, Norwalk virus, Norwalk-like viruses
Diarrhea and abdominal cramps	1–3 d	Yes	Positive‡	*Campylobacter jejuni*, *Shigella* species, *Entamoeba histolytica*, *Salmonella* species, *Yersinia* species, *Clostridium difficile*
Gastrointestinal bleeding	1–3 d	No	Gross blood	Enterohemorrhagic *Escherichia coli*§, cytomegalovirus¶
Malabsorptive diarrhea with bloating	1–2 wk	No	Negative	*Enterocytozoon bieneusi*, *Isospora belli*, *Giardia lamblia*, *Cryptosporidium*

*This table is a guide. Incubation periods and syndromes may overlap.
†Mass psychogenic illness is more common in adolescents. Rash may be part of the syndrome.
‡Gross blood and pus in stool is a clue for *Campylobacter jejuni*, *Shigella* species, or *Entamoeba histolytica*.
§Fever may be seen in approximately one third of cases.
¶Syndrome confined to compromised hosts, particularly bone marrow transplant recipients, and occurs 1 to 3 months posttransplantation.

TABLE 6 DIARRHEAL ILLNESSES—CLINICAL "PEARLS"

A stool Gram stain revealing many curved gram-negative rods is highly suggestive of *Campylobacter jejuni* or *Vibrio* spp as the pathogen

Nearly all cases of amebic colitis are associated with red cells in the stool

A patient with *Clostridium difficile* colitis who does not improve with oral vancomycin probably has a second process causing diarrhea. Although relapses are fairly common, primary treatment failures (particularly with vancomycin) are rare

Anoscopy or proctoscopy should be considered early in cases of severe colitis. Specimens for ova and parasites and culture may be obtained, as well as an immediate evaluation for the presence of pseudomembranes

Vibrio vulnificus causes a syndrome of diarrhea, bacteremia, hypotension, and hemorrhagic bullae. The organism is acquired from shellfish; the syndrome is usually seen in patients with severe liver disease

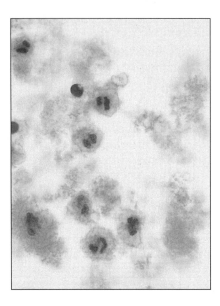

FIGURE 1 Stool smear demonstrating leukocytes and erythrocytes (trichrome stain) × 1000. (*Courtesy of* B. Harrison, Chicago, IL.)

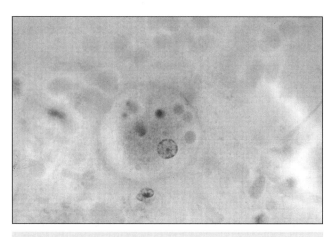

FIGURE 2 *Entamoeba histolytica* trophozoite ingesting erythrocytes (trichrome stain) × 1000. (*Courtesy of* B. Harrison, Chicago, IL.)

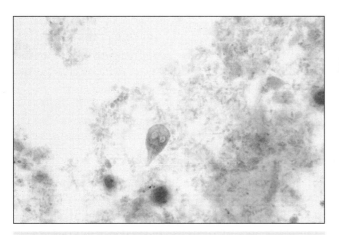

FIGURE 3 *Giardia lamblia* trophozoite (trichrome stain) × 1000. (*Courtesy of* B. Harrison, Chicago, IL.)

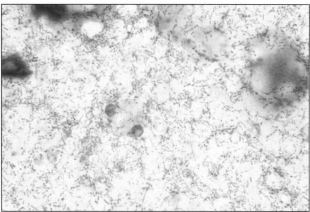

FIGURE 4 *Cryptosporidium* (modified Ziehl-Neelsen stain) × 1000. (*Courtesy of* B. Harrison, Chicago, IL.)

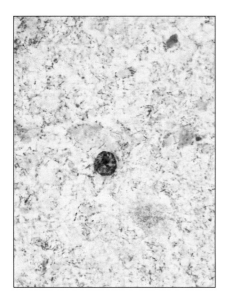

FIGURE 5
Cyclospora (modified Ziehl-Neelsen stain) × 1000. (*Courtesy of* B. Harrison, Chicago, IL.)

chosen should cover the most common treatable organisms (*Campylobacter jejuni, Salmonella, Shigella, E. coli*). *V. cholera* should also be covered if the travel or exposure history and the clinical syndrome are suggestive. Fluoroquinolones have activity against all of these pathogens and are currently a reasonable empiric treatment choice [4,5•]. However, increased quinolone resistance, particularly among *Campylobacter* isolates, requires careful attention to the clinical and microbiologic response. Five days of therapy is usually sufficient. If the patient received antimicrobial agents in the previous 3 weeks, *C. difficile* should also be covered, requiring the addition of metronidazole or vancomycin. In severely ill patients, empiric therapy should include coverage of bowel flora (primarily anaerobes) because of the risk of secondary bacteremia.

Antimotility agents have also been shown to shorten the duration of diarrhea in several settings. Loperamide reduced the incidence of diarrhea by approximately 80% in patients with traveler's diarrhea and appears to be associated with fewer side effects than diphenoxylate/atropine [6,7]. Antimotility agents are not generally recommended

for patients with fever, dysentery, or other evidence of an invasive syndrome.

Postinfectious Complications of Diarrhea

Reiter's syndrome includes a combination of an asymmetric arthritis, usually limited to larger joints and the axial skeleton, conjunctivitis/uveitis, keratoderma blennorrhagica (thickening of the skin of the palms and soles), and urethritis. Urethritis is the most common presenting symptom, with other parts of the syndrome following within 6 weeks of an enteric infection (*Salmonella, Shigella, Campylobacter, Yersinia* spp) or a sexually transmitted disease (gonorrhea, chlamydial, or mycoplasmal infection). Not all parts of the syndrome are necessary to make the diagnosis. Most patients are human leukocyte antigen (HLA)-B27–positive and are male. Nonsteroidal anti-inflammatory agents are the usual therapy.

Hemolytic-uremic syndrome may complicate diarrhea resulting from enteroviruses or *E. coli* producing Shiga-like toxins (enterohemorrhagic *E. coli*). Therapy is supportive.

Traveler's Diarrhea

Traveler's diarrhea is defined as diarrhea that occurs in a traveler from an industrialized country visiting a developing or semitropical area. The incidence of diarrhea may be as high as 50% in travelers in some areas. Approximately 80% of these cases result from bacterial pathogens. The most common organisms isolated from patients with traveler's diarrhea are enterotoxigenic *E. coli, Shigella* spp, *C. jejuni, Aeromonas* spp, *Plesiomonas shigelloides*, and *Vibrio* spp [5•].

The high incidence of disease, together with knowledge of the causative organisms and the most common methods of acquisition, make this illness an ideal target for prevention strategies. Fluoroquinolones—including norfloxacin (400 mg daily), ciprofloxacin (500 mg daily), ofloxacin (300 mg daily), and fleroxacin (400 mg daily)—have been effective in reducing the incidence of traveler's diarrhea and are currently the antimicrobial agents of choice for this purpose. Doxycycline (100 mg daily) and trimethoprim-sulfamethoxazole (160 mg as trimethoprim daily) are also effective but may be limited by more widespread resistance. Although antimicrobial agents are effective for this purpose, they are costly and may produce side effects more serious than a self-limited diarrhea. Concerns about allergic reactions, Stevens-Johnson syndrome, and antibiotic-associated diarrhea have limited the recommended use of antimicrobials for prophylaxis to patients with underlying illnesses that might be adversely affected by a diarrheal illness and those with an itinerary demanding peak performance each day.

Bismuth subsalicylate is less effective than antibiotic prophylaxis for traveler's diarrhea, but it has fewer side effects. The recommended dose is two tablets chewed four times daily. Neither bismuth subsalicylate nor antibiotic prophylaxis should be continued for longer than 3 weeks.

All travelers should be advised on simple and effective strategies to reduce exposure to enteric pathogens. These include drinking only bottled beverages and eating foods that are cooked and served hot. The advisory "boil it, cook it, peel it, or forget it" is a useful one for travelers to remember as they consider each meal.

Nosocomial Diarrhea

Diarrhea is common in hospitalized patients. Although many cases have a noninfectious etiology (*eg*, resulting from stool softeners or "preps" given for various procedures), all patients with diarrhea should be placed on enteric isolation until the cause is confirmed as a noninfectious one, a confirmed pathogen is eradicated, or the diarrhea abates. The most common infectious cause of diarrhea that begins during hospitalization is *C. difficile* [8,9]. Unless the patient has been exposed to someone with a known diarrheal pathogen or there is evidence of a nosocomial outbreak, the initial evaluation should be aimed primarily at this pathogen. Cultures for other bacterial pathogens and microscopic evaluations for ova and parasites have a very low yield in this setting. *C. difficile* can be treated with either metronidazole (250 mg four times daily) or vancomycin (125 mg four times daily) for 10 days. The drug chosen should be administered orally. Metronidazole is less expensive and, because of this, is recommended for the treatment of mild to moderate illness. For severe cases, vancomycin is recommended. As many as 25% of patients treated with either agent may relapse. Relapses should be re-treated. The addition of rifampin (600 mg twice daily) to vancomycin or 3 weeks of cholestyramine following antibiotic therapy have been suggested adjuvants in the therapy for relapsing disease. Treatment of asymptomatic carriage of *C. difficile* with either agent is not effective in permanently eradicating the organism from the stool [10].

Diarrhea in the Patient with HIV Infection

In the United States, nearly 50% of patients with AIDS have gastrointestinal symptoms, as compared with approximately 90% of AIDS patients having gastrointestinal symptoms in developing nations [11•]. In addition to common enteric pathogens, the differential diagnosis includes *Mycobacterium* spp (*Mycobacterium avium* complex, *Mycobacterium tuberculosis*), *Histoplasma capsulatum*, *Cryptosporidium* spp, *Isospora belli*, and *Enterocytozoon bieneusi* (microsporidium). Intestinal malignancies (lymphoma, Kaposi's sarcoma) and adrenal insufficiency may also produce gastrointestinal symptoms, including diarrhea. The evaluation can be focused by careful attention to the patient's degree of immunodeficiency (some infections are rare except in patients with severe immune compromise) and a full microscopic examination of the stool, including preparations for ova and parasite examination and acid-fast staining. Recurrent bacteremia with *Campylobacter* spp, *Salmonella* spp, enteroinvasive *E. coli*, and *Helicobacter cinaedi* has also been reported in patients with AIDS.

Unusual Food-Borne Illness Syndromes

Each of the organisms listed in Table 3 may be the causative agent of a food-borne outbreak. In addition, several toxin-associated processes may produce a confusing picture.

Ciguatera is a toxin found in fish, including bass, snapper, and grouper. Fish from the Caribbean and near the Indo-Pacific islands are particularly likely to be affected. The fish smell and taste normal. Within a few hours of ingestion, however, patients develop symptoms of paresthesias, weakness, headache, abdominal pain, and cardiovascular instability. Some patients later develop respiratory failure. Treatment is supportive. Patients should be observed until it is clear the symptoms are improving. Paralytic shellfish poisoning and puffer fish poisoning may cause similar symptoms.

Scromboid (histamine fish poisoning) is a chemical intoxication also associated with ingestion of fish (tuna, yellowfish, amberjack, mackerel). Within an hour of ingestion, patients develop symptoms of headache, dizziness, flushing, and cramps. Urticaria and bronchospasm occur in some patients. Antihistamine therapy is recommended.

CONCLUSIONS

The differential diagnosis of diarrhea is among the broadest of any common medical problem [12•,13•]. The cost of evaluating all patients for the large number of possible pathogens is prohibitive. Therefore, the clinician must focus the work-up to identify the most likely pathogens based on the patient's history, physical examination, and stool smear. For patients who are severely ill or who remain ill after an initially negative evaluation, consultation with an infectious disease or a gastroenterology specialist is appropriate.

REFERENCES AND RECOMMENDED READING

Recently published papers of particular interest have been highlighted as:
- Of interest
- Of outstanding interest

1. Hodgkin K: *Towards Earlier Diagnosis: A Family Doctor's Approach.* Baltimore: Williams & Wilkins; 1963.

2. WHO reports decry neglect of world health problems. *ASM News* 1990, 56:338–339.

3. Lew J, Glass R, Gangarosa R, *et al.*: Diarrheal deaths in the United States, 1979 through 1987. *JAMA* 1991, 265:3280–3284.

4. Goodman L, Trenholme G, Kaplan R, *et al.*: Empiric antimicrobial therapy of domestically acquired acute diarrhea in urban adults. *Arch Intern Med* 1990, 150:541–546.

5.• DuPont HL, Ericsson CD: Prevention and treatment of traveler's diarrhea. *N Engl J Med* 1993, 328:1821–1827.

6. van Loon FP, Bennish ML, Speelman P, Butler C: Double blind trial of loperamide for treating acute watery diarrhea in expatriates in Bangladesh. *Gut* 1989, 30:492–495.

7. Johnson PC, Ericsson CD, DuPont HL, *et al.*: Comparison of loperamide with bismuth subsalicylate for the treatment of acute traveler's diarrhea. *JAMA* 1986, 255:757–760.

8. Yannelli B, Gurevich I, Schoch PE, Cunha BA: Yield of stool cultures, ova and parasite tests, and *Clostridium difficile* determinations in nosocomial diarrheas. *Am J Infect Control* 1988, 16:246–249.

9. Siegel DL, Edelstein PH, Nachamkin I: Inappropriate testing for diarrheal diseases in the hospital. *JAMA* 1990, 263:979–982.

10. Johnson S, Hoomman DR, Bettin KM, *et al.*: Treatment of asymptomatic *Clostridium difficile* (fecal excretors) with vancomycin or metronidazole *Ann Intern Med* 1992, 117:297–302.

11.• Smith P, Quinn T, Strober W, *et al.*: Gastrointestinal infections in AIDS. *Ann Intern Med* 1992, 116:63–77.

12.• Guerrant R, Bobak D: Bacterial and protozoal gastroenteritis. *N Engl J Med* 1991, 325:327 328.

13.• Blacklow N, Greenberg H: Viral gastroenteritis. *N Engl J Med* 1991, 325:252–264.

SELECT BIBLIOGRAPHY

Blaser MJ, Berkowitz ID, La Force FM, *et al.*: *Campylobacter* enteritis: clinical and epidemiological features. *Ann Intern Med* 1979, 91:179–185.

Kelly CP, Pothoulakis C, LaMont JT: *Clostridium difficile* colitis. *N Engl J Med* 1994, 330: 257–262.

Klontz KC, Lieb S, Schreiber M, *et al.*: Syndromes of *Vibrio vulnificus* infections. Clinical and epidemiological features in Florida cases, 1981–1987. *Ann Intern Med* 1988, 109:318–323.

Intra-abdominal Infections 14

James S. Baldassarre
Matthew E. Levison

> ### *Key Points*
> - Intra-abdominal infection is due to the endogenous bacterial flora of the gastrointestinal tract; thus, most intra-abdominal infections are polymicrobial in nature.
> - Hospital-acquired intra-abdominal infection may include organisms resistant to multiple antibiotics.
> - Empiric, broad-spectrum antibiotic therapy is crucial, and delayed or inadequate antibiotic therapy may adversely affect survival.
> - Drainage of intra-abdominal infection is usually necessary: open surgical drainage allows for direct visualization of pathology, repair of diseased viscera, and débridement of necrotic tissue; percutaneous drainage entails less morbidity and is often appropriate.
> - Intra-abdominal abscess may result from previous intra-abdominal infection; visceral abscesses may be the result of contiguous spread within the abdomen or from hematogenous spread of bacteria.

PERITONITIS

Peritonitis refers to an infection of the peritoneal cavity [1]. The peritoneum is a serous membrane, and a small amount of fluid is normally contained within the peritoneal cavity; values for normal peritoneal fluid are given in Table 1.

Primary Peritonitis

Primary peritonitis is the infection of the peritoneal cavity not directly related to other intra-abdominal abnormalities [2]. It usually occurs in the presence of ascites from any of a variety of underlying conditions and can occur at any age.

Gram-negative enteric organisms are the most commonly identified pathogens in this illness, especially *Escherichia coli* and *Klebsiella pneumoniae*, followed by *Streptococcus pneumoniae* and other streptococci, including enterococci. *Staphylococcus aureus* accounts for 2% to 4% of isolates, and anaerobic and microaerophilic organisms are uncommon.

The clinical profile of primary peritonitis includes the abrupt onset of fever, abdominal pain, nausea, vomiting, and diarrhea. A physical examination often reveals diffuse abdominal tenderness, rebound tenderness, and diminished or absent bowel sounds in addition to ascites. The presentation may sometimes be insidious and the physical findings, limited; the diagnosis is confirmed by sampling the peritoneal fluid. Fluid obtained at paracentesis should be analyzed for cell count and differential and protein concentration, and a Gram stain and culture should be performed (Table 1). Cultures should be sent in an airless, capped syringe or injected directly into aerobic and anaerobic broth culture media; volumes of 10 mL or more will increase the yield of cultures. Results from Gram stains are often negative but are helpful in deciding initial therapy if positive. Measurement of lactate level and ascitic pH may also be

TABLE 1 CHARACTERISTICS OF NORMAL PERITONEALFLUID

Cell count	< 300/mm^3
Specific gravity	< 1.016
Total protein	< 3 g/dL
pH	> 7.35
Lactate	< 25 mg/dL

helpful. In the rare patient without ascites, peritoneal lavage with Ringer's lactate solution may be useful. In the patient with negative results of ascitic culture, an endoscopic or laparoscopic peritoneal biopsy may be necessary. Peritonitis secondary to other intra-abdominal causes should be excluded, particularly if the Gram stain or culture of peritoneal fluid reveals more than one organism. Patients with primary peritonitis tend to improve quickly when receiving appropriate antimicrobial therapy; failure to respond should prompt an examination for additional pathologic conditions.

The initial treatment is often empiric. Specific therapy should be based on the results of pathogen identification and susceptibility data. Initial therapy should be broad enough in spectrum to treat enteric gram-negative bacilli as well as streptococci. If peritonitis develops during hospitalization, therapy should also have activity against *Pseudomonas aeruginosa*. Appropriate antibiotic therapy is summarized in Table 2. Therapy is generally continued for 10 to 14 days, but short-course therapy for 5 days has been shown to be as efficacious

as the longer course. A clinical response should be evident by 48 hours. Surgery is usually not needed for primary peritonitis.

Rarely, primary peritonitis manifests with a subacute or chronic course. In this circumstance, other pathogens must be considered, including *Mycobacterium tuberculosis* or *Coccidioides immitis*. A biopsy of the peritoneum may be necessary to confirm the presence of these organisms.

Secondary Peritonitis
Diagnosis

Many intra-abdominal processes may cause secondary peritonitis (Table 3). Figure 1 is a diagram of the approach to the patient with suspected peritonitis.

Secondary peritonitis, like most types of intra-abdominal infections, is usually an endogenous polymicrobial infection. These organisms are derived from the polymicrobial flora at the site of the diseased or injured organs. Because the type of microflora that colonizes the mucosal surfaces normally varies at different sites along the gastrointestinal and genital tract, the microflora of secondary peritonitis correspondingly varies. The normal microflorae at various sites of the abdominal cavity are listed in Table 4.

The patient complains of moderate to severe abdominal pain that is increased by any movement. Pain may be localized to the area of underlying disease, such as right lower abdominal pain in appendicitis, or may be referred elsewhere, especially the back, chest, or shoulder. Anorexia, nausea, and vomiting are common. Chills, thirst, scant urine production, or the inability to pass stools or flatus may be noted.

The physical examination usually reveals an ill-appearing patient who lies quietly and has rapid shallow respirations.

TABLE 2 EMPIRIC ANTIMICROBIAL THERAPY FOR PRIMARY PERITONITIS

Outpatient acquired

Ampicillin, 2–3 g every 4 h plus aminoglycoside, 1.7 mg/kg every 8 h*

Ceftriaxone, 1–2 g every 24 h or other third-generation cephalosporin, 1–2 g every 8 h

Ampicillin/sulbactam, 3 g every 6 h

Piperacillin or other ureidopenicillin, 2–3 g every 4 h

Ticarcillin/clavulanic acid, 3.1 g every 6 h

Inpatient acquired

Ureidopenicillin, 2–3 g every 4 h plus aminoglycoside, 1.7 mg/kg every 8 h*

Ceftazidime, 1–2 g every 8 h plus aminoglycoside, 1.7 mg/kg every 8 h*

Ticarcillin/clavulanic acid, 3.1 g every 6 h plus aminoglycoside, 1.7 mg/kg every 8 h*

*Dose given is appropriate for gentamicin and tobramycin. Dosage modification is required for cases of renal insufficiency.

TABLE 3 COMMON CAUSES OF SECONDARY PERITONITIS

Perforated appendix

Suppurative cholecystitis

Diverticulitis

Perforated peptic ulcer

Intestinal perforation resulting from neoplasms, infarction, or obstruction

Pancreatitis

Operative contamination or anastomotic bowel leak

Trauma to the bowel, urinary tract, or female pelvis

Acute salpingitis or endomyometritis

Ruptured visceral abscess (hepatic or pancreatic)

Suppurative prostatitis

Peritoneal dialysis

Ventriculoperitoneal shunts

Fever or hypothermia may be seen, along with tachycardia. The pulse may be thready. Blood pressure is usually normal early in the illness, and a decrease in blood pressure signifies sepsis with shock. The bowel sounds are diminished or absent. Marked abdominal tenderness is present and is often maximal over the site of the abnormality. Rebound tenderness suggests inflammation of the parietal peritoneum, and muscular rigidity is present. In women, a pelvic examination is mandatory to

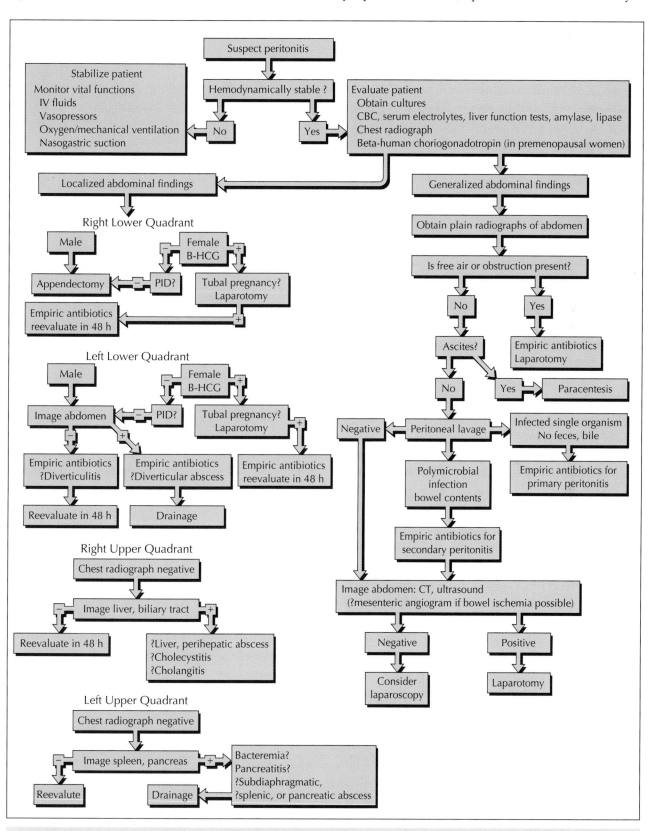

FIGURE 1 General approach to management of the patient with suspected peritonitis. B-HCG—beta-human choriogonadotropin; CBC—complete blood count; CT—computed tomography; IV—intravenous; PID—pelvic inflammatory disease.

TABLE 4 FEATURES OF NORMAL INTRA-ABDOMINAL FLORA

Site	Density, *mL*	Typical flora
Stomach	$\leq 10^3$	Oral streptococci
		Oral anaerobic gram-negative bacilli
		Lactobacilli
		Candida spp
Small bowel		Lactobacilli
Proximal	$< 10^4$	Facultative gram-negative bacilli (*eg*, *Escherichia coli*, *Klebsiella pneumoniae*, *Proteus* spp)
Distal	10^4–10^6	Anaerobic gram-negative bacilli (*eg*, *Bacteroides* spp, *Fusobacterium* spp)
Terminal ileum	10^6–10^7	Enterococci, anaerobic cocci
Large bowel	10^{11}–10^{12}	Anaerobic gram-negative bacilli
		Anaerobic gram-positive cocci
		Facultative gram-negative bacilli
		Clostridium spp
		Lactobacilli
		Enterococcus spp

exclude primary pelvic disease, as is a rectal examination in men (Fig. 2).

Typical physical findings may be absent in some patients, including those with lax abdominal musculature, such as those patients who have ascites or are postpartum. Patients taking glucocorticoids commonly fail to show typical signs or symptoms. A high index of suspicion is necessary in these cases.

Diagnostic evaluations must be brief but thorough. Laboratory studies should include the complete blood count, serum chemistry profile, liver profile, amylase measurement, and appropriate cultures, including blood and urine. Blood cultures are positive for a pathogen in 30% of cases. Radi-

ographs of the abdomen may reveal free intra-abdominal air or fluid, bowel distention, ileus, bowel wall edema, or other localizing signs. Radiographs of the chest should be obtained to exclude chest conditions that might simulate an intra-abdominal process. If free fluid is present, a needle aspiration biopsy of the peritoneal cavity is generally very safe and may be helpful. In patients without free peritoneal fluid, peritoneal lavage may be indicated. Typically, a liter of Ringer's lactate solution is infused into the peritoneum by using a peritoneal dialysis catheter placed through a small midline incision below the umbilicus. After dwelling for a few minutes, the fluid is drained by gravity back into the infusion

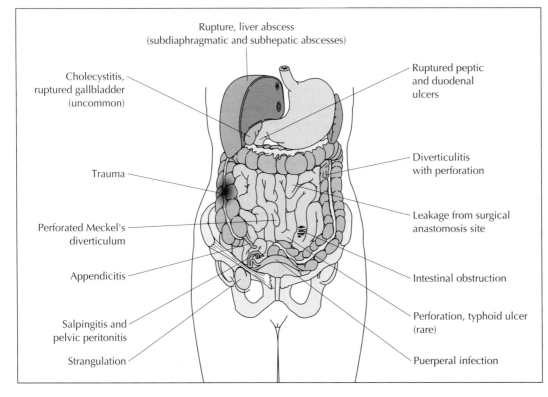

FIGURE 2
Various causes of peritonitis. (*From* Finegold [16]; with permission.)

bag. The fluid is then examined for the presence of neutrophils, bile, bacteria, or food particles.

The prognosis in secondary peritonitis is related to several factors, including the site and severity of the underlying condition, the age of the patient, the presence of contaminants in the peritoneum, the number and type of microbes involved, and the promptness of therapeutic intervention. Mortality rates range from 3.5% in those with early infection caused by penetrating trauma to higher than 60% in those with long-standing infection and multiorgan failure.

The initial steps in the management of the patient with peritonitis should be supportive. Patients with hemodynamic compromise require the infusion of intravenous fluids and, sometimes, vasopressors. Hypoxemia should be corrected with supplemental oxygen or mechanical ventilation, and electrolyte imbalances should be corrected. Nasogastric suction for the removal of gastrointestinal fluids and gas is necessary. Invasive monitoring with pulmonary artery, arterial, and urinary catheters is often appropriate.

Specific treatment involves both systemic antimicrobial therapy and surgery [3•,4]. Antibiotic therapy should be begun as soon as blood cultures have been collected, usually before cultures can be done on samples obtained from the intra-abdominal site. Intra-abdominal cultures should be done at the time of surgery or percutaneous drainage. Therapy is aimed at preventing bacteremia and minimizing the local spread of infection. Recent data suggest that survival in patients with intra-abdominal infections is diminished if initial therapy is inadequate, regardless of the adequacy of subsequent treatment [5•]; thus, empiric therapy must be broad spectrum. Although the ideal regimen remains controversial, it must always have activity against β-lactamase–producing anaerobes such as *Bacteroides fragilis* and facultative gram-negative enteric bacilli such as *E. coli*. The value of specific therapy directed against enterococci is uncertain, but it is often included. Therapy should always be given by the intravenous route until gastrointestinal function returns to normal.

Table 5 outlines several regimens of documented efficacy. The antibiotic regimen should be adjusted to include the most efficacious, least toxic, and least expensive combination of agents once cultures have been completed. Anaerobes are frequently not recovered in cultures despite their presence because of inadequate anaerobic culture techniques, and therapy against anaerobes must always be included. Therapy should be continued until the temperature, leukocyte count, and differential have normalized, and all drains have been removed.

When to Refer

Although some cases of secondary peritonitis may be managed without drainage, most will require drainage in some form: either open surgical drainage or percutaneous catheter drainage. Early intervention is crucial, and delay increases the mortality risk [6]. The specific aims of surgery include repair of the inciting event, drainage of pus and gastrointestinal contents from the peritoneum, and débridement of necrotic tissue. Leaving the peritoneal cavity packed and open, facilitated by the use of polypropylene mesh to avoid evisceration, and a planned return to the operating room for repeated débridement in patients with severe generalized peritonitis have been reported to be effective, but these results are yet to be confirmed by controlled prospective randomized trials. Surgery is not indicated for primary peritonitis, in moribund patients, or in patients with acute salpingitis.

Peritoneal Catheter-Related Peritonitis

Secondary peritonitis caused by contamination of an indwelling catheter, such as that used for chronic ambulatory peritoneal dialysis, deserves special consideration. This complication occurs at a rate of about one episode per patient per year and is usually a result of contamination of the catheter lumen by skin flora during manipulation of the tubing [7]. The most common isolates include *Staphylococcus epidermidis*, *S. aureus*, *Streptococcus* spp, and diphtheroids.

TABLE 5 EMPIRIC ANTIMICROBIAL THERAPY FOR SECONDARY PERITONITIS

Clindamycin, 600–900 mg every 8 h + aminoglycoside, 1.7 mg/kg every 8 h*

Ticarcillin, 3–4 g every 4–6 h ± aminoglycoside, 1.7 mg/kg every 8 h*

Piperacillin, 3–4 g every 4–6 h ± aminoglycoside, 1.7 mg/kg every 8 h*

Ampicillin/sulbactam, 3 g every 6 h ± aminoglycoside, 1.7 mg/kg every 8 h*

Aztreonam, 1–2 g every 8 h + clindamycin, 600–900 mg every 8 h ± aminoglycoside, 1.7 mg/kg every 8 h*

Cefoxitin or cefotetan, 2 g every 8 h ± aminoglycoside

Third-generation cephalosporin, 1–2 g every 8 h† ± aminoglycoside, 1.7 mg/kg every 8 h* *plus* metronidazole, 500 mg every 6–8 h, or clindamycin

Ticarcillin/clavulanic acid, 3.1 g every 6 h ± aminoglycoside, 1.7 mg/kg every 8 h*

Imipenem, 500–1000 mg every 6–8 h‡

Ciprofloxacin, 400 mg IV every 12 h + clindamycin

*Dose given is appropriate for gentamicin and tobramycin. Dosage modification is required for cases of renal insufficiency.
†Ceftriaxone is given as 1–2 g every 24 h.
‡Predisposes to seizures and may require dosage modification for cases of renal insufficiency.
IV—intravenous.

Other pathogens include *E. coli*, *Klebsiella* spp, *Enterobacter* spp, *Proteus* spp, and pseudomonads. Anaerobic bacteria and *Candida albicans* are occasionally seen.

Diagnosis

The diagnosis must be suspected in the appropriate setting when the patient reports abdominal pain with tenderness, nausea, vomiting, or diarrhea. Fever occurs in only 10% to 20% of cases. In samples of the dialysate, the fluid is cloudy with a leukocyte count of greater than 100/mm^3 and usually greater than 500/mm^3. Cultures of the fluid reveal the offending organism, but blood cultures are usually sterile.

Treatment

Treatment with the local instillation of antibiotic into the peritoneum with each bag of dialysate is usually adequate to eradicate the infection. Removal of the catheter is usually not necessary, except under the following circumstances:

    exit site or tunnel infection
    fungal, mycobacterial, or *P. aeruginosa* infection
    fecal contamination
    persistent or recurrent infection with the same organism
    peritoneal abscess
    catheter malfunction

The usual duration of therapy is 10 to 21 days and the prognosis for cure of infection is excellent.

INTRA-ABDOMINAL ABSCESS

Intraperitoneal Abscess

Intraperitoneal abscess can result from either primary or secondary peritonitis, with localization of the inflammatory process to one or several, usually dependent, areas. Abscesses also tend to be located at the site of the underlying condition (*eg*, periappendiceal or diverticular abscesses). Diseases resulting in intraperitoneal abscesses are similar to those that cause secondary peritonitis (Table 3). Secondary peritoneal abscesses are almost always polymicrobial in content, as previously noted.

Diagnosis

Clinical manifestations may be acute or chronic. In acute illness, the patient complains of fever with chills and abdominal pain and tenderness; however, some patients may have an indolent and protracted course with low-grade fever and progressive inanition. Abscesses in contact with the underside of the diaphragm may cause symptoms referred to the ipsilateral chest or shoulder.

Several noninvasive modalities are available to detect and localize the site of abscess. Plain radiographs are sometimes helpful. Gallium-67 and indium-111 tagged leukocytes localize in areas of inflammation and maybe useful in detecting abscesses within the abdomen. However, abscesses in liver or spleen may be difficult to detect solely by ^{67}Ga or ^{111}In-tagged leukocyte scans because normal accumulation in these organs may mask an adjacent inflammatory process. Ultrasonography is safe, rapid, and portable and can determine the size and shape of an abscess cavity. Ultrasound images are obscured by overlying bowel gas and therefore are sometimes of limited usefulness. Of all the currently available modalities, computed tomography (CT) appears to be the best [8]. It provides high-resolution anatomic images that are unaffected by bowel gas. By the use of intraluminal and intravascular contrast material, CT is able to differentiate bowel and vasculature from abscess cavity accurately (Fig. 3). It is also often able to guide percutaneous drainage procedures, sometimes obviating the need for surgery. Magnetic resonance imaging (MRI) may be somewhat better but is undoubtedly more costly, and experience is limited.

Treatment

The primary approach to the management of intraperitoneal abscesses is surgical or percutaneous catheter drainage, and the adequacy of drainage affects survival (*see* "When to Refer"). Percutaneous drainage is as effective as open drainage and carries less morbidity, necessitates a shorter length of hospitalization, and has a lower cost but is subject to many limitations [9•]. Percutaneous drainage does not allow direct visualization of the abdomen to confirm a diagnosis, and it does not allow for repair of the primary pathologic condition or the débridement of necrotic tissue. Many abscesses cannot be approached safely by the percutaneous route, and viscous purulent material may not drain freely through a small-bore catheter. Finally, multiple abscesses cannot be adequately drained. Thus, percutaneous drainage is appropriate only for those patients with a single or few well-delineated, accessible abscesses that can drain dependently through a percutaneously placed catheter, and who do not require tissue débridement or repair of abdominal viscera (Fig. 4). Surgical back-up must be available (Table 6). Initial antibiotic therapy is often empiric and should be modified by the culture results of appropriate specimens; appropriate therapy is as described for secondary peritonitis (Table 5).

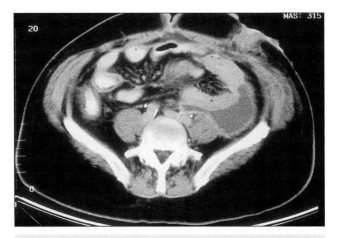

FIGURE 3 Intraperitoneal abscess in a patient with carcinoma of the colon.

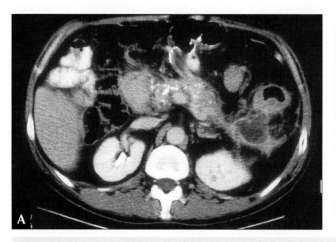 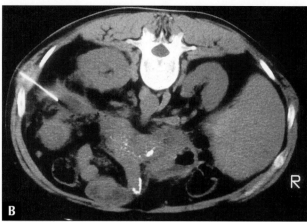

FIGURE 4 **A**, Abscess in the tail of the pancreas. **B**, With the patient prone, a needle is passed into the abscess cavity. A catheter is placed into the abscess cavity using a guidewire. When the patient lies supine, the abscess may drain dependently.

VISCERAL ABSCESS

Pancreatic Abscess

Pancreatic abscesses complicate 1% to 9% of cases of pancreatitis and occasionally arise from the secondary infection of a pancreatic pseudocyst. The pathogenesis is secondary infection of necrotic pancreatic tissue through the biliary tree or by hematogenous seeding [10].

Clinical detection of a pancreatic abscess can be difficult. Typically, the patient fails to respond to conservative treatment for pancreatitis; abdominal pain, nausea, and vomiting worsen, and fever commonly develops. Jaundice or an abdominal mass may be present. The diagnosis is readily made by imaging the abdomen, usually by CT or ultrasonography. Aspiration of the fluid-filled cavity may be necessary to differentiate true abscess from pseudocyst.

The primary therapy is prompt surgical or percutaneous drainage, combined with antimicrobial therapy aimed at gastrointestinal flora, especially enteric gram-negative bacilli and anaerobes. The mortality rate among patients with pancreatic abscess is relatively high but is often a result of underlying illness.

Hepatic Abscess

Pyogenic abscesses of the liver are relatively uncommon but do occur, often in patients with underlying biliary disease or sickle cell anemia [11]. Bacteria may reach the liver by any of several routes, including the biliary tree, the systemic or portal circulation, or by spread from an adjacent structure. Twenty-five percent of pyogenic liver abscesses are cryptogenic (*ie*, without discernible cause). Amebic liver abscess caused by *Entamoeba histolytica* infection also occurs in areas endemic for this pathogen but, for unknown reasons, is almost always in men.

The infecting organisms are again most often derived from the native intestinal flora by biliary, portal, or contiguous spread. Abscesses caused by *S. aureus* infection probably arise from bacteremia with or without concurrent infective endocarditis. Abscesses caused by infection by *Candida* spp, as part of the syndrome of hepatosplenic candidiasis, are seen in the setting of prolonged neutropenia during cancer chemotherapy.

Typical presenting symptoms of pyogenic liver abscess include chills and fever for days to weeks and dull right upper quadrant pain. The pain may be pleuritic or radiate to the right shoulder. Tender hepatomegaly is often present, but jaundice is absent unless there is concomitant cholangitis. The serum alkaline phosphatase level is usually elevated, and blood cultures are positive in 50% of all patients. The diagnosis can be confirmed by any of the imaging techniques already mentioned; ultrasonography is particularly useful in this circumstance. Aspiration for diagnosis may be done by CT or ultrasonographic guidance (Fig. 5).

The primary therapy for pyogenic liver abscess is antibiotic therapy. Many but not all such abscesses will require surgical

TABLE 6 REASONS FOR FAILURE OF PERCUTANEOUS DRAINAGE
Enteric fistula with ongoing contamination
Additional undrained abscesses
Thick pus
Phlegmon
Infected tumor
Bleeding

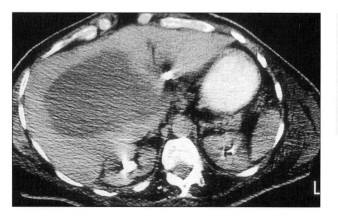

FIGURE 5 A single large abscess of the liver. *Escherichia coli* was found in a culture taken of the aspirated material.

drainage as well; some may be managed with percutaneous drainage if the lesion is amenable. Fever usually abates within 2 weeks, but antibiotic therapy should be prolonged, usually as long as 4 to 16 weeks. Periodic reimaging is useful for judging the progress of therapy. The overall prognosis for cure is very good, although the mortality rate remains high in those with significant underlying illness or advanced age.

Amebic liver abscess should be suspected in patients with a history of potential exposure, including travel to tropical areas or fecal–oral contact. Patients may note a history of diarrhea. There is right upper quadrant pain, but fever may be absent. CT or ultrasonography reveals the lesion. An aspirate of the abscess cavity is usually sterile in a routine culture, but amebic abscesses may be secondarily infected as well. The diagnosis is made by aspiration of the abscess or biopsy of the cavity wall; specific serologic tests for *Entamoeba histolytica* are usually positive as well. The therapy is metronidazole, 750 mg given orally three times daily for 5 to 10 days, followed by iodoquinol, 650 mg given orally three times daily for 10 days.

Splenic Abscess

Splenic abscesses are uncommon. Unlike what occurs in most other intra-abdominal infections, seeding of the spleen by microorganisms usually occurs by hematogenous spread from a distant source [12]. Patients often have infective endocarditis or inject illicit drugs parenterally. Reflecting this is the preponderance of gram-positive organisms isolated, with *S. aureus* and various streptococci being the most commonly isolated. Salmonella abscesses occur in patients with sickle cell anemia, and fungal abscesses (usually caused by *Candida* spp) are often part of a syndrome of hepatosplenic candidiasis in patients receiving cancer chemotherapy.

Patients usually note left upper quadrant abdominal pain and tenderness, and pain may be referred to the left shoulder. High fever is usually present. Imaging studies such as CT, ultrasonography, or MRI are all useful for confirming the diagnosis. The treatment is appropriate antibiotic therapy with splenectomy or surgical drainage. Initial therapy should be broad in spectrum, with adequate activity against *S. aureus* as well as enteric gram-negative bacilli and anaerobes; therapy should be adjusted when the offending organism has been identified.

SPECIFIC CAUSES OF INTRA-ABDOMINAL INFECTION

Appendicitis

Appendicitis presents as right lower quadrant pain associated with anorexia, nausea, and vomiting. Tenderness is present in the right lower quadrant with low-grade fever; however, normal variability in the location of the appendix may cause the physical findings to occur in other areas such as the back or suprapubic area. Rupture of a gangrenous appendix will lead to the findings of localized or generalized secondary peritonitis. The treatment of uncomplicated appendicitis is always surgical, with removal of the diseased organ; antibiotic therapy adds little. Imminent or actual rupture of the appendix is an indication for antibiotic therapy, as discussed for intraperitoneal abscesses.

An important differential diagnosis for acute appendicitis is mesenteric lymphadenitis, which may be the true pathologic condition in up to 20% of patients with suspected appendicitis. It is a self-limited, sometimes recurrent inflammation of mesenteric lymph nodes in the right iliac fossa. Physical findings are essentially the same as those for appendicitis, and exploration of the abdomen is necessary to exclude lymphadenitis; an appendectomy should be done at that time. Measles, infectious mononucleosis, and *Yersinia* infection may also mimic appendicitis. Actinomycosis of the appendix may present with subacute, chronic, or recurrent symptoms of appendicitis, with extensive fistula formation or fibrosis in the periappendiceal area. Table 7 lists the differential diagnosis for acute appendicitis.

Diverticulitis

Diverticula are outpouchings of the colonic mucosa through the muscular wall. They are usually located in the sigmoid and descending colon, and their occurrence increases with age. Obstruction of the opening of the diverticulum may lead to inflammation within the pouch, a process similar to that in appendicitis. The major clinical manifestations of acute diverticulitis are similar to those of appendicitis; however, it occurs in older patients, and symptoms are localized to the left lower abdomen. The major complication is rupture with formation of pericolonic abscesses or peritonitis. For uncomplicated diverticulitis, or diverticulitis with localized abscess formation, therapy consists of the administration of intravenous fluids, nasogastric suction, and appropriate intravenous antibiotics. Surgery may be necessary to remove the diseased portion of the bowel and drain the inflammatory process.

Regional Enteritis

Regional enteritis is a full-thickness inflammation of the bowel. This illness may mimic acute appendicitis or diverticulitis, and one of the complications is perforation of the bowel with secondary peritonitis, abscess, or fistula formation. The diagnosis may be made by seeing the characteristic findings of regional enteritis on contrast radiography. The management of this illness requires periodic antibiotic therapy, with judicious surgical intervention.

TABLE 7 DIFFERENTIAL DIAGNOSIS OF ACUTE APPENDICITIS
Diverticulitis
Mesenteric lymphadenitis
Acute salpingitis
Ectopic pregnancy
Ruptured ovarian cyst
Regional enteritis
Measles
Infectious mononucleosis
Yersinia enteritis
Cholelithiasis
Urolithiasis

Typhilitis

Typhilitis is a necrotizing enterocolitis seen in patients with neutropenia. It often affects the cecum and presents as appendicitis. The illness may progress quickly to acute peritonitis, and the mortality rate approaches 50%. Again, a combined approach with broad-spectrum antibiotics and surgery is probably most appropriate.

Acute Cholecystitis

Acute cholecystitis is usually caused by obstruction of the cystic duct by a stone or by inspissated secretions. Increased intraluminal pressure develops, leading to ischemia and necrosis; infection usually ensues.

The initial obstruction causes mild epigastric pain with nausea. Persistent obstruction leads to increasingly severe pain in the right upper quadrant, and pain may radiate to the right shoulder. Peritoneal signs may develop, moderate fever is common, and miminal jaundice may be present. The laboratory evaluation reveals a moderately elevated neutrophil count; mild increases in the total bilirubin and serum aspartate aminotransferase levels are common. The illness may resolve spontaneously over the course of days, but 25% to 30% will develop complications requiring surgery, including perforation with local abscess or peritonitis; if common duct obstruction also occurs, pancreatitis, cholangitis, or hepatic abscess may ensue.

Enteric gram-negative bacilli are the usual bacteriologic causes of cholecystitis, along with enterococci. Anaerobes may be present as part of a polymicrobial infection, especially in patients with prior biliary surgery or manipulation.

The diagnosis can usually be confirmed by ultrasonography or nuclear imaging. Ultrasonography will reveal a thickened gallbladder wall and the presence of stones. Hepatobiliary scanning with technetium-99 labeled compounds is also a rapid and accurate means by which to confirm this diagnosis; failure to visualize isotope in the gallbladder indicates cystic duct obstruction. CT is usually not necessary. The differential diagnosis of acute cholecystitis includes myocardial infarction, perforated peptic ulcer, pneumonia, hepatitis, and disease of the right kidney.

The treatment of complicated acute cholecystitis should always include broad-spectrum antibiotics appropriate for an intra-abdominal infection and should be continued through the time of surgery. The need for antibiotic therapy in uncomplicated cholecystitis is less certain. Perioperative antibiotic therapy at the time of cholecystectomy is useful to prevent postoperative infection. Monotherapy with a cephalosporin active against *E. coli* and *Klebsiella* spp is adequate for this purpose.

Cholangitis

Cholangitis refers to inflammation, usually with infection, of the common bile duct and intrahepatic bile ducts. This inflammation may occur in conjunction with acute cholecystitis and results from obstruction of the common bile duct. The onset of illness is usually acute, with high fever, chills, and diffuse pain and tenderness in the right upper quadrant. Jaundice is common and shock may also occur. Bacteremia occurs in 50% of cases, often with *E. coli* or anaerobes, including *Clostridium perfringens*. Complications include sepsis with shock, perforation with intraperitoneal infection, or hepatic abscess formation. The diagnosis can be confirmed by ultrasonographic evaluation of the biliary system, demonstrating common duct stones or dilatation. In patients with a previous history of cholangitis, fibrosis of the duct will prevent dilatation and thus limit the usefulness of the ultrasonographic findings.

Acute cholangitis is a life-threatening situation, necessitating immediate antibiotic therapy. Empiric therapy should again be targeted to enteric gram-negative bacilli and anaerobes to control bacteremia and sepsis. Surgery for decompression of the biliary tree is mandatory, and intraoperative cholangiography should be performed.

INFECTIONS OF THE FEMALE PELVIS

Infections of the female pelvis include endomyometritis and acute salpingitis, which may spread to result in peritonitis. The syndrome of infection of the fallopian tubes, endometrium, and pelvic peritoneum that is known as *pelvic inflammatory disease* (PID) is most often seen in sexually active young women. Endomyometritis is also a complication of childbirth.

Salpingitis

Salpingitis has many presentations, and confirmation of the diagnosis can be difficult. Acute salpingitis typically presents as marked lower abdominal pain, vaginal discharge, nausea, and vomiting; fever is present as the illness progresses. The patient is bent forward and moves gingerly. A physical examination reveals lower abdominal tenderness, and exquisite tenderness on cervical motion is present in a pelvic examination. An adenexal mass may also be palpable. A laboratory evaluation may reveal an elevated leukocyte count. A Gram stain of secretions from the cervical os will reveal neutrophils; the presence of intracellular gram-negative diplococci is suggestive of gonococcal infection, but this finding is neither sensitive nor specific.

This syndrome is seen most commonly in young women; the differential diagnosis must always consider acute appendicitis, ectopic pregnancy, adenexal torsion, and ruptured ovarian cyst. Because some patients will present with a subacute course, mild disease, or lack of fever, the diagnosis may be difficult to confirm clinically. Culdocentesis for a Gram stain and culture or laparoscopy may be necessary in some cases. Empiric therapy is often appropriate, and a close follow-up should be instituted.

The most common cause of acute salpingitis is *Neisseria gonorrhoeae*, especially in first episodes of salpingitis. Gonococcal salpingitis tends to occur around the time of menses and is associated with fever and cervical discharge. Subsequent episodes of salpingitis are more likely to be caused by a polymicrobial flora that includes streptococci and various anaerobic bacteria. Acute salpingitis caused by a native flora does not correlate with the menstrual cycle, is less likely to cause fever early in the course, and responds more slowly to therapy. In addition, *Chlamydia* and *Mycoplasma* spp have been implicated as infectious agents in salpingitis.

For women with mild disease, outpatient therapy can be attempted. Several regimens have been proposed, but most often the therapy is ceftriaxone, 250 mg administered intramuscularly once to treat the gonococcal infection, followed by oral doxycycline, 100 mg given twice daily to treat presumed concurrent chlamydial infection [13]. Patients must be followed up within the first 48 to 72 hours for assessment of improvement. Hospitalization must be recommended in several situations, including uncertain diagnosis, pregnancy, failure of outpatient therapy, inability to tolerate or comply with oral therapy, presence of an intrauterine device, or suspicion of a pelvic abscess. Any patient who appears acutely ill should also be hospitalized. Patients who are hospitalized should be treated with a parenteral antibiotic regimen. The combination of clindamycin with an aminoglycoside has been used extensively for this indication. Alternatively, the combination of cefoxitin or ceftriaxone with doxycycline is appropriate.

Patients who have a palpable mass or who fail to respond promptly to therapy should be evaluated for the presence of a tubo-ovarian abscess; this complication is usually seen only after the initial episode of salpingitis, where scarring has blocked the normal drainage of the fallopian tubes. The diagnosis can often be suggested by ultrasonography but can be confirmed only by laparoscopy or surgery. Tubo-ovarian abscesses may resolve with antibiotic therapy; occasionally, surgical extirpation of the diseased adnexa is necessary.

Endomyometritis

Unlike acute salpingitis, which occurs in outpatients, endomyometritis is usually seen in women after childbirth [14]. Risk factors for the development of this complication include cesarean delivery, prolonged labor, or prolonged rupture of the membranes (> 6 hours). The most important sign of infection is fever, and fever in the postpartum period should never be ignored. Additional signs include lower abdominal and uterine tenderness and foul-smelling vaginal discharge. Leukocytosis is common.

Several organisms may cause endomyometritis, and polymicrobial infection is common. Patients who develop illness within 48 hours of delivery are likely to be infected with group B or group A β-hemolytic streptococci. These patients often are extremely ill and have high fever; shock or a toxic-shock syndrome may ensue. Recovery of the β-hemolytic streptococci from the cervical secretions confirms the diagnosis. Therapy should be initiated as soon as this diagnosis is suspected.

Patients who develop illness more than 48 hours after delivery are more likely to have infection as a result of a polymicrobial colonic flora. Cultures of the cervical discharge for colonic organisms are not helpful, because these organisms are frequently present in the uterine mucosa post partum in the absence of disease. Blood cultures should be done in all patients with the clinical diagnosis of endomyometritis.

Therapy is most often empiric and should be active against the pathogens previously identified. Therapy should be continued until there has been clinical improvement and the patient has been afebrile for 48 to 72 hours.

A serious but uncommon complication of endomyometritis is suppurative pelvic thrombophlebitis, which should be suspected when the patient fails to respond to appropriate therapy within 48 to 72 hours of initiation or if pulmonary emboli develop [15]. Heparin should be added to the regimen. Rarely, plication of the inferior vena cava or ovarian vein is necessary.

ACKNOWLEDGMENT

The authors would like to thank Drs. A. Fisher, A. Dalke, and R. Konigsberg, Medical College of Pennsylvania, Department of Radiology, for their assistance in locating suitable radiographs.

REFERENCES AND RECOMMENDED READING

Recently published papers of particular interest have been highlighted as:
• Of interest
•• Of outstanding interest

1. Levison ME, Bush LM: Peritonitis and other intra-abdominal infections. In *Principles and Practice of Infectious Diseases*, edn. 3. Edited by Mandell GL, Douglas RD, Bennett JE. New York: Churchill Livingstone; 1990:636–669.

2. Wilcox CM, Dismukes WE: Spontaneous bacterial peritonitis: a review of pathogenesis, diagnosis and treatment. *Medicine* 1987, 66:447–456.

3.• Bohnen JMA, Solomkin JS, Dellinger EP, *et al.*: Guidelines for clinical care: anti-infective agents for intra-abdominal infections. *Arch Surg* 1992, 127:83–89.

4. Sawyer MD, Dunn DL: Antimicrobial therapy of intra-abdominal sepsis. *Infect Dis Clin North Am* 1992, 6:545–570.

5.• Mosdell DM, Morris DM, Voltura A, *et al.*: Antibiotic treatment for surgical peritonitis. *Ann Surg* 1991, 214:543–549.

6. Bohnen JMA: Operative management of intra-abdominal infections. *Infect Dis Clin North Am* 1992, 6:511–523.

7. Saklayen MG: CAPD peritonitis: incidence, diagnosis and management. *Med Clin North Am* 1990, 74:997–1010.

8. Mueller PR, Simeone JF: Intra-abdominal abscess: diagnosis by sonography and computed tomography. *Rad Clin North Am* 1983, 21:425–443.

9.• Levinson MA: Percutaneous versus open drainage of intra-abdominal abscesses. *Infect Dis Clin North Am* 1992, 6:525–544.

10. Stanten R, Frey CF: Comprehensive management of acute necrotizing pancreatitis and pancreatic abscess. *Arch Surg* 1990, 125:1269–1274.

11. Do H, Lambiase RE, Deyoe L, *et al.*: Percutaneous drainage of hepatic abscesses: comparison of results in abscesses with and without intrahepatic biliary communication. *AJR Am J Roentgenol* 1991, 157:1209–1212.

12. Nelken N, Isnatius J, Skinner M, *et al.*: Changing clinical spectrum of splenic abscess: a multicenter study and review of the literature. *Am J Surg* 1987, 154:27–34.

13. Centers for Disease Control: 1989 Sexually Transmitted Diseases Treatment Guidelines. *MMWR Morb Mortal Wkly Rep* 1989, 38(suppl S-8):1–43.

14. Cox SM, Gilstrap LC III: Postpartum endometritis. *Obstet Gynecol Clin North Am* 1989, 16:363–371.

15. Ledger WJ: Hospital-acquired obstetric infections. In *Infections in the Female*, edn. 2. Edited by Ledger WJ. Philadelphia: Lea & Febiger; 1986:249–278.

16. Finegold S: *Anaerobic Bacteria in Human Disease.* San Diego: Academic Press; 1977:272.

SELECT BIBLIOGRAPHY

Gorbach SL: Intraabdominal infections. *Clin Infect Dis* 1993, 17:961–967.

Hemming A, David NL, Robins RE: Surgical versus percutaneous drainage of intra-abdominal abscesses. *Am J Surg* 1991, 161:593–579.

Wilson SE, Finegold SM, Williams RA (eds): *Intra-abdominal Infection.* New York: McGraw-Hill; 1982.

Adult Osteomyelitis 15

Layne O. Gentry
Brandon Clint

Key Points

- The most common pathogens causing osteomyelitis in adults are *Staphylococcus aureus*, *Staphylococcus epidermidis*, and *Enterococcus faecalis*; however, antibiotic-resistant, gram-negative organisms are becoming more frequent, especially in posttraumatic infections.
- Although microbiologic culture of an open surgical biopsy specimen is the gold standard for diagnosis of osteomyelitis, culture of multiple specimens obtained by computed tomography (CT)-guided biopsy may also be reliable and less expensive.
- Intravenous antibiotics, usually administered for 4 to 6 weeks, are used to treat osteomyelitis; however, if the organisms are gram-negative and are susceptible, oral fluoroquinolones may be used for 6 to 8 weeks.

Osteomyelitis, a malady described in Egyptian and Aztec cultures more than a millennium ago, has continued as a medical problem, and promises to be even more of a challenge to clinicians as they become more sophisticated in managing bone, joint, and traumatic musculoskeletal disorders. Infection following traumatic fractures, insertion of joint and spinal prostheses, and bone infections of lower extremity ulcers associated with complications of diabetes mellitus are now the leading causes of osteomyelitis in adults. Before 1970 in adults (and currently in children) hematogenous dissemination of bacteria to bone from a distant site was the most common pathogenesis of this infection [1–4].

Bacteria remain the most common etiologic agents of osteomyelitis, followed by fungi. Unfortunately, nosocomially acquired gram-negative strains, often resistant to multiple antibiotics, are now causing infections after severe bone trauma and orthopedic prosthesis surgery. Infections caused by gram-positive bacteria are a continuing threat, although the incidence has decreased since 1970 [5]. Fungal infections of bone, rarely reported previously, have become more common and are difficult to manage because effective therapy has only recently improved.

Diagnosing osteomyelitis during the initial stage of the disease is often difficult; however, the availability of computed tomography (CT) and magnetic resonance imaging (MRI) technology has enhanced our ability to detect early bone infection. Radionuclide imaging, which has been available for much longer, continues to be adjunctive diagnostic aid [6]. Effective, safe, broad-spectrum antibiotic agents, the cornerstone of osteomyelitis treatment, have improved. The use of safe, long-term intravenous catheters and the introduction of home health services for antibiotic therapy have expedited the discharge of patients from the hospital and have dramatically cut costs. Fluoroquinolones have been established as effective and safe oral antibiotic agents on the basis of comparative clinical trials; however, the possibility of the emergence of resistant bacterial strains during prolonged therapy has raised concern [7].

PATHOGENESIS AND ETIOLOGY OF OSTEOMYELITIS

Risk factors and other important contributing factors in addition to trauma and surgery known to be associated with osteomyelitis are shown in Table 1. The initial bone infection, regardless of the route of entry (hematogenous dissemination or direct traumatic inoculation), causes inflammation, vascular compromise, local hypoxia, and eventually death of bone tissue. The bone infection may lead to areas of avascular tissue, or bone sequestrum. Because antibiotic penetration into this avascular area is impossible, surgical resection is imperative. If the infection dissects toward the periosteum, it may extend into the soft tissues and form a localized abscess or a sinus tract, or both, to drain fluids and necrotic tissue to the surface. These principles are shown schematically in Figure 1 [8•].

Etiology

Pathogens gain access to bone by extension from contiguous sites, by direct inoculation, or from hematogenous dissemination from a distant site. Shown in Table 2 are common examples of each of these three mechanisms of infection. Pathogens responsible for osteomyelitis are listed in Table 3. Note that *Staphylococcus aureus*, *Staphylococcus epidermidis*, and *Enterococcus faecalis* infections are the most common. Mixed aerobic and anaerobic infections are frequently seen in diabetics and with decubitus ulcerations. *S. aureus* is the major cause of hematogenous dissemination to bone.

Classification

Without an accurate, simple method to define osteomyelitis as to the exact site of infection, the duration of infection, the presence or absence of important host factors, or the outcome of clinical management, it has been impossible to accurately compile useful data obtained from individual clinical centers.

The differentiation between acute and chronic disease in the healthy host, and in the host with underlying diseases associated with greater risks for infection, is the basis for one of the two currently used methods of classifying osteomyelitis. Shown in Figure 2 is the anatomic site of bone infection [1,2,9]. If the bone infection site is localized (Stage III), but no adverse host factors are present, the classification would be IIIA. In contrast, if one or more of the important host factors are present, classification would be IIIB. Similarly, a diffuse anatomic lesion with adverse host factors would be IVB, and so on. The importance of this classification is that all cases, regardless of severity or site of infection, can be staged the same in every center where

---

TABLE 1 RISK FACTORS FOR OSTEOMYELITIS
Major risk factors Diabetes mellitus Peripheral vascular insufficiency Musculoskeletal trauma Orthopedic prosthetic devices **Other contributory factors** Malnutrition Sickle cell disease Hemodialysis Alcoholism Immunosuppression Advanced age Malignancy

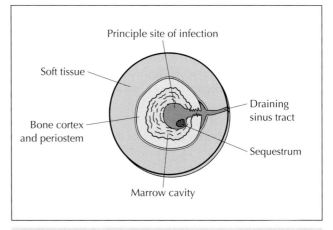

FIGURE 1 Schematic diagram of a cross section of bone and surrounding tissue showing the site of infection and the formation of a draining sinus tract.

TABLE 2 PATHOGENIC MECHANISM OF OSTEOMYELITIS AND ASSOCIATED FACTORS		
Extension from contiguous site	**Direct inoculation**	**Hematogenous spread**
Diabetic foot infections	Open fractures	Bacteremia from various sites (*ie*, genitourinary, pulmonary, endocarditis)
Decubitus ulcers	Orthopedic surgery	
Septic arthritis	Human bites	
Surgical wound infection	Penetrating trauma	
Abscess/septic bursitis		

TABLE 3 PATHOGENS IN ORDER OF FREQUENCY OF OCCURRENCE	
Direct inoculation and extension from contiguous site	**Hematogenous dissemination**
Posttraumatic	*Staphylococcus aureus*
Staphylococcus aureus	*Staphylococcus epidermidis*
Staphylococcus epidermidis	Gram-negative rods
Gram-negative rods	Mixed infections
Mixed infections	
Anaerobes*	
Mycobacterium spp	
Postsurgical	
Staphylococcus epidermidis	
Staphylococcus aureus	
Enterococcus faecalis	
Nosocomial gram-negative rods	
Mixed infections	
Candida spp	
Prosthetic joint	
Staphylococcus epidermidis	
Staphylococcus aureus	
Enterococcus faecalis	
Diabetic foot	
Mixed gram-positive/gram-negative infections, including anaerobes	

*Improved culture techniques have increased identification of anaerobes.

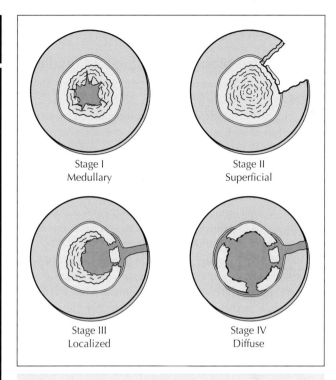

FIGURE 2 Schematic diagram of the anatomic site of bone infection showing the different stages of infection. (*From* Cierny [9]; with permission.)

osteomyelitis is treated—thus there is conformity of cases, with more precise treatment results.

A more functional classification has been suggested by Braun and Lorber [10] and is shown in Table 4. Chronic osteomyelitis is defined by meeting any one of the six listed criteria. There are several difficulties with this classification. A diagnosis of chronic osteomyelitis is easily made for several reasons. Radiographic changes in osteomyelitis are often nonspecific, especially in the early stages of infection, and frequently go undetected in patients with minimal symptoms. Six weeks of symptoms is therefore common, making a diag-

nosis of acute osteomyelitis unlikely. In addition, treatment results are not uniform, are dependent on early versus late diagnosis, and are often influenced by the presence of other important diagnoses, such as vascular insufficiency.

We have used a very simple classification of osteomyelitis that has served us well. Regardless of its source, acute osteomyelitis is defined as the first clinical episode complete with the signs, symptoms, and radiographic and histologic biopsy confirmation of bone infection. Chronic osteomyelitis is the diagnosis for all bone infections, based on the same signs, symptoms, and radiographic and biopsy-proven evidence, that have failed one or more treatment attempts.

DIAGNOSIS OF OSTEOMYELITIS

Diagnosis involves a combination of clinical suspicion, appropriate laboratory studies, and radiographic and radionuclide

TABLE 4 CRITERIA FOR CHRONIC OSTEOMYELITIS
Chronic osteomyelitis is defined as a bone infection that meets any of these criteria:
1. Clinical or radiographic evidence of infection with duration of ≥ 6 wk
2. Radiographic evidence of sequestrum formation or sclerosis plus bone destruction
3. Relapse or persistence following antibiotic therapy expected to be effective against pathogen(s)
4. Infection associated with foreign bodies, including surgical prostheses
5. Infection in the face of vascular insufficiency
6. Infection resulting from organisms that characteristically produce indolent, chronic disease (*Mycobacterium tuberculosis*, *Candida* spp)
Data from Braun and Lorber [10].

scanning techniques together with the histologic biopsy confirmation. A general algorithm is suggested in Figure 3.

Clinical Suspicion and Laboratory Studies

A dirty, open, comminuted fracture of a cortical bone such as the tibia is a likely place for osteomyelitis. Such cases are likely to be seen by the infectious diseases consultant, unless seen by the internist as part of a comprehensive evaluation for underlying medical problems. The internist is more likely to encounter patients with a postoperative surgical infection, an infection from a contiguous focus such as septic arthritis, a perinephric infection resulting from renal disease, or bacteremia developing into osteomyelitis at a distant site. Complications of diabetic foot infections and decubitus ulcers remain in the domain of the internist as well.

Patients may complain of localized pain at the site of bone infection unresponsive to typical nonsteroidals, heat, or rest. That is particularly true for patients with vertebral osteomyelitis, as they frequently have back pain. Infections of the larger cortical bones, such as the tibia and femur, or those in patients with peripheral neuropathy, may be painless, so clinical suspicion is paramount. Local tissue swelling and even cellulitis may be present as clues but are not required. For chronic osteomyelitis, it is not uncommon to have a draining sinus tract. Culture of this material is frequently misleading, as secondary contamination of wet wounds—especially of the lower extremity—is common, and organisms obtained from the bone biopsy often are less frequent in number and are different in genus and species.

In certain clinical situations, sinus tract or wound cultures are valuable as adjunct information in treating wound or soft tissue infection associated with osteomyelitis. A classic example might be a swollen diabetic foot with cellulitis and a purulent draining sinus tract. Temperature and leukocyte count may or may not be elevated and are unreliable indicators. The erythrocyte sedimentation rate, however, is elevated in a majority of cases and may be useful as an indicator of disease activity. If the patient appears actively ill or toxic, blood cultures should be taken as well, especially if hematogenous dissemination (ie, in intravenous drug abusers or patients with underlying endocarditis) is suspected. Blood isolates frequently correlate with the pathogen obtained at bone biopsy in such cases.

Radiographic Techniques

Diagnostic changes of osteomyelitis are not detectable on routine radiographs for at least 2 weeks. Within 4 weeks, however, nearly 100% of infected bones should demonstrate one or more of the following classic radiographic changes: periosteal elevation, bone destruction, sclerosis, sequestrum formation, and soft tissue swelling. Routine radiographs will fail to detect non-radiopaque foreign materials, and when trauma is involved, these materials may result in chronic recurrent symptoms if not detected. Although CT scanning is

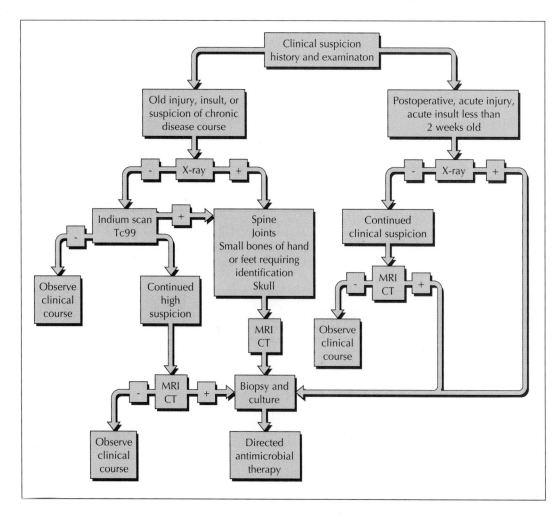

FIGURE 3 General algorithm for the diagnosis of osteomyelitis. CT—computed tomography; MRI—magnetic resonance imaging; Tc99—technetium-99.

more expensive, this technology demonstrates early bone and associated soft tissue changes resulting from infection and may be more useful in detecting foreign materials.

Magnetic resonance imaging is the most expensive technology and is not justified for routine imaging for osteomyelitis. MRI is, however, the most useful technique for determining the extent of infection. MRI is also very sensitive for early infection and adds increased specificity when the possibility of bone tumor or infarction may be in the differential diagnosis. MRI is the imaging technique of choice for detecting and assessing the site and extent of vertebral osteomyelitis.

Radionuclide Imaging

Imaging studies have been used for detecting osteomyelitis for many years. It must be emphasized, however, that none of these studies can reliably distinguish between infection, infarction, or tumor. A combination of clinical acumen and bone biopsy are necessary to confirm the diagnosis, despite an active focus demonstrated on a radionuclide scan. Illustrated in Table 5 is our interpretation of the comparison of the various radiographic and radionuclide imaging techniques for diagnosing osteomyelitis.

Technetium-99 is the most commonly available test and has excellent sensitivity; however, it has poor specificity when used alone. Gallium-67 scans may be useful for diagnosing osteomyelitis, but because they detect collections of actively phagocytic leukocytes, a significant soft tissue component in the osteomyelitis site is a critical criteria for diagnostic use. Indium-111 labeled leukocyte scans have recently been proposed as an important adjunct for detecting orthopedic prosthesis–associated infections, although a consensus has not been reached for this proposed use. Indium-111 scans are more sensitive to smaller foci of inflammation and are easier to interpret but are more expensive to perform.

Bone Biopsy

An open surgical biopsy obtained under direct vision (or alternatively, multiple needle biopsies done under radiographic guidance) and cultured aerobically and anaerobically is the gold standard diagnostic technique for osteomyelitis. Although direct vision during surgery is the most reliable technique, in our center, use of multiple fluoroscopic or CT-guided needle biopsies done by an experienced orthopedist or radiologist using a bone biopsy needle has been the least expensive, most reliable approach. Alternatively, if the patient requires surgical débridement—and many patients with cortical bone infections have sequestra that need to be removed—combining débridement, biopsy, and culture into one procedure is still more cost effective. (A note of caution: performed by an inexperienced person, needle biopsy of small bones of the hands and feet to confirm the presence of osteomyelitis may result in traumatic fracture as a complication.)

TREATMENT OF OSTEOMYELITIS

As noted in Figure 3, treatment is based on localizing the infection, appropriate biopsy and culture, antibiotics, surgical débridement, and stabilization, if necessary, followed by long-term outpatient therapy.

Surgical Support

Sequestered or dead bone with associated inflammatory debris is common in osteomyelitis and is a focus for persistent infection. In our 15-year experience, inadequate surgical débridement of devascularized tissue has been the most common cause for treatment failure. Surgical support is also important in providing the necessary mechanical support for the healing of the bone impaired by infection. If parenteral antibiotic therapy is necessary, placement of a long-term indwelling venous access line may be necessary for home intravenous therapy. Foreign bodies, whether bullets or orthopedic prosthetic devices, need to be removed, as osteomyelitis rarely, if ever, is successfully treated until such foci for persistent infection are removed. For hopeless cases of unrelenting osteomyelitis, or when underlying diseases such as diabetes mellitus and vascular insufficiency preclude a favorable outcome using standard therapy, major débridement or amputation may be necessary.

TABLE 5 COMPARISON OF RADIOGRAPHIC AND RADIONUCLIDE TECHNIQUES IN OSTEOMYELITIS			
Test	Sensitivity	Specificity for infection, infarction, or tumor	Cost
Radiographic			
Routine radiographs	Good after 3 wk (poor before)	Poor	Inexpensive
Computed tomography scan	Good in first 12 wk	Better	Expensive
Magnetic resonance imaging	Excellent in certain cases	Best	Very expensive
Radionuclide scans			
Technetium-99	Good in first 2 wk	Poor false negative in infection, false positive in infarction and tumor	Moderate
Gallium-67	Moderate only after 2 wk	Poor; good only in advanced cases	Moderate
Indium-111	Moderate even in first 2 wk	Acceptable; false positive in infarction; promise in diagnosis of infection of prosthesis	Expensive

TABLE 6 ANTIMICROBIAL THERAPY

Pathogen	Preferred therapy	Dosage	Comments
Gram-positive			
Staphylococcus aureus (methicillin-susceptible)	β-Lactamase-resistant penicillin		
	Nafcillin	2 g IV every 6 h	
	Oxacillin	2 g IV every 6 h	
	or		
	First-generation cephalosporin		Penicillin hypersensitive
	Cefazolin	2 g IV every 8 h	
	or		
	Oral fluoroquinolone		Less proven for *Staphylococcus aureus*
	Ciprofloxacin	750 mg orally every 12 h	
	Ofloxacin	400 mg orally every 12 h	Food and Drug Administration approval pending
Staphylococcus aureus (methicillin-resistant) or coagulase-negative *Staphylococcus*	Vancomycin	1 g IV every 12 h	Possible combination with rifampin
Streptococcus spp	Ampicillin	2 g IV every 6 h	Vancomycin for resistant *Enterococcus* or penicillin hypersensitivity
Gram-negative			
Pseudomonas aeruginosa	Third-generation cephalosporin		
	Ceftazidime	2 g IV every 12 h	
	Ceftriaxone	2 g IV every 24 h	
	or		
	Oral fluoroquinolone		Many advantages
	or		
	Semisynthetic penicillin		If resistant
	Piperacillin	3 g IV every 6 h	
	Mezlocillin	3 g IV every 6 h	
	or		
	Aminoglycoside		For highly resistant strains only, owing to possible nephrotoxicity
	Amikacin	15 mg/kg/d	
	Tobramycin	5 mg/kg/d	
Enterobacteriaceae and other gram-negative organisms	Oral fluoroquinolone		Clear first choice
	or		
	Third-generation cephalosporin		
	or		
	β-Lactamase inhibitor		
	Ticarcillin-clavulanic acid	3.1 g IV every 6 h	Proven in mixed infection
Anaerobes	Imipenem-cilastatin	1.0 g IV every 6 h	
	Clindamycin	0.9 g IV every 8 h	Anti-*Staphylococcus* activity also
	Metronidazole	0.5 g IV every 8 h	

From Gentry [11]; with permission.
IV—intravenous.

Antibiotic Therapy

If the diagnosis of osteomyelitis is supported by appropriate biopsy and culture, directed antibiotic therapy becomes the mainstay of management. In most instances, patients are not acutely ill or toxic, so that it is practical to wait for culture and antibiotic sensitivity results before initiating therapy. If, however, the patient is to have open biopsy and débridement at the same time, or is acutely ill, toxic, or possibly bacteremic, empiric therapy for the suspected organism is necessary. Antibiotics commonly used are given in Table 6. The new glycopeptide antibiotic, teicoplanin, is being studied in phase III trials for the treatment of infections with resistant gram-positive organisms. In a recent open-label trial, Weinberg reported clinical and bacteriologic cure rates of 88% in 34 patients with osteomyelitis who were treated with teicoplanin [12]. In cases in which resistant or unusual organisms are encountered or there is indecision about appropriate antibiotic therapy, an infectious disease consultation is necessary.

The gold standard for therapy is intravenous antibiotics for 4 or 6 weeks, given through a long-term indwelling venous access catheter. With current economic constraints, and if the organisms isolated are susceptible, it may be feasible to use one of the new oral fluoroquinolones for outpatient therapy for 6 to 8 weeks. Indeed, oral ciprofloxacin has Food and Drug Administration approval as monotherapy for osteomyelitis resulting from susceptible organisms. In a recent study of 17 adult patients with chronic osteomyelitis, treatment with oral ciprofloxacin (750 mg twice daily) resulted in clinical resolution in 13 patients (76%). In addition, the drug regimen was well tolerated [13]. Another new fluoroquinolone, fleroxacin, has been evaluated for the treatment of osteomyelitis in two recent noncomparative, multicenter studies. Combined results show that of a total of 39 patients with osteomyelitis, treatment with oral fleroxacin (400 mg per day) resulted in bacteriologic cure in 31 (79%) patients and in clinical cure in 24 (62%) patients [14,15].

The use of oral antibiotics could decrease complications associated with placing and maintaining indwelling catheters and toxicities associated with certain of the parenteral antibiotics, such as aminoglycosides. The economic savings is significant over a 6-week course of antibiotic therapy for osteomyelitis when parenteral administration is compared with oral, which is a strong incentive in favor of this newer form of therapy. If parenteral therapy is necessary, supervised administration of outpatient home health nursing services offers a significant savings over hospital confinement.

Outpatient Management

As proper coordination between medical, surgical, and radiologic services is needed in the hospital, the same coordination is needed for home health care services. While still in the hospital, patients are educated in the care, use, and administration of antibiotics via the catheter. Once discharged, they should be visited by a nurse at least once a week for inspection of the catheter sites, review of techniques, and inventory of supplies.

Laboratory examinations, which vary depending on the patient's age and renal function and the toxicity of the antibiotics used, are performed at 2- to 4-week intervals. A downward trend in the erythrocyte sedimentation rate may suggest improvement, but continued elevation may be nonspecific. Leukocyte count and differential with elevated eosinophils may provide early clues to allergic reactions to antibiotics that may occur with prolonged therapy. Radiography or scans need only be performed at a 4- to 6-month follow-up or as needed. Unless there is danger of a pathologic fracture resulting from destruction of bone by infection or surgical débridement, patients can be encouraged to maintain a normal schedule of activities, as full range of motion is the key to rehabilitation. Exceptions to this may be vertebral osteomyelitis, in which case a slightly longer course of bed rest may be needed [1,4].

PROGNOSIS

The key to a good prognosis is early detection and prompt institution of antimicrobial therapy. Acute osteomyelitis, detected early, is frequently treated effectively with antibiotics following débridement. Chronic disease, however, may develop a recurrent course over many years that may require continued antibiotic therapy and repeated surgeries, and may eventually lead to amputation.

REFERENCES AND RECOMMENDED READING

Recently published papers of particular interest have been highlighted as:
• Of interest
•• Of outstanding interest

1. Waldvogel FA Medoff G, Swartz MN: Osteomyelitis: a review of clinical features, therapeutic considerations and unusual aspects. *N Engl J Med* 1970, 282:198–206.
2. Gentry LO: Use of newer β-lactams in osteomyelitis. *Am J Med* 1985, 78:134–139.
3. Waldvogel FA, Papageorgiou PS: Medical progress: osteomyelitis: the past decade. *N Engl J Med* 1980, 303:360–370.
4. McHenry MC, Alfidi RJ, Wilde AH, Hawk WA: Hematogenous osteomyelitis: a changing disease. *Cleve Clin Q* 1975, 42:125–153.
5. Gentry LO: Approach to the patient with chronic osteomyelitis. In *Current Clinical Topics in Infectious Diseases*. Edited by Remington JS, Swartz MN. New York: McGraw-Hill; 1987:62–83.
6. Schawecher DS, Braunstein EM, Wheat JC: Diagnostic imaging of osteomyelitis. *Infect Dis Clin North Am* 1990, 4:441–463.
7. Gentry LO: Antibiotic therapy for osteomyelitis. *Infect Dis Clin North Am* 1990, 4:485–499.
8.• Sapico FL, Montgomerie JB: Vertebral osteomyelitis. *Infect Dis Clin North Am* 1990, 4:539–550.
9. Cierny G: The classification and treatment of adult osteomyelitis. In *Surgery of the Musculoskeletal System*. Edited by Evarts CM. New York: Churchill Livingstone; 1990:4337.
10. Braun TI, Lorber B: Chronic osteomyelitis. Orthopedic infection. In *Clinical Topics in Infectious Disease*. Edited by Schlossberg D. Springer-Verlag; New York: 1988.
11. Gentry LO: Osteomyelitis. In *Conn's Current Therapy*. Edited by Rakel RE. Philadelphia: WB Saunders; 1992:935.

12. Weinberg WG: Safety and efficacy of teicoplanin for bone and joint infections: results of a community-based trial. *South Med J* 1993, 86:891–897.

13. Yamaguti A, Trevisanello C, Lobo IM, *et al.*: Oral ciprofloxacin for treatment of chronic osteomyelitis. *Int J Clin Pharmacol Res* 1993, 13:75–79.

14. Green SL: Efficacy of oral fleroxacin in bone and joint infections. *Am J Med* 1993, 94:174S–176S.

15. Putz PA: A pilot study of oral fleroxacin given once daily in patients with bone and joint infections. *Am J Med* 1993, 94:177S–181S.

SELECT BIBLIOGRAPHY

Lipsky BA, Pecoraro RE, Wheat LJ: The diabetic foot: soft tissue and bone infection. *Infect Dis Clin North Am* 1990, 4:409–432.

Mader JT, Landon GC, Calhoun J: Antimicrobial treatment of osteomyelitis. *Clin Orthop* 1993, 295:87–95.

Infectious Arthritis 16
Mary T. Flood

Key Points
- Infectious arthritis afflicts all age groups and has a predilection for immunocompromised patients.
- The age of the patient and underlying medical condition provide important clues to the causative infectious agent.
- Successful management depends on prompt diagnosis, appropriate antimicrobial therapy, and drainage of the joint space.
- The choice of antibiotics for treatment is often empiric at the onset of therapy and may be changed as data become available.
- Definitive diagnosis in fungal and tuberculous arthritis is made by synovial biopsy and culture.

Infectious arthritis is an acute or chronic inflammation of a joint caused by direct invasion of the synovial space by microorganisms. Acute infections are generally caused by pyogenic bacteria and are termed *acute bacterial arthritis* or *septic arthritis.* Chronic infections are most often caused by mycobacteria or fungi. Sterile or reactive arthritis is an inflammatory reaction that is generally secondary to infection in another part of the body. A sterile arthritis may be associated with infection preceding the clinical syndrome, as in hepatitis B, or following infection, as with *Salmonella* or *Shigella* spp in gastrointestinal infections.

Infectious arthritis remains a major health problem in large urban medical centers, where the incidence can range between 0.034% to 13% of hospital admissions [1]. It afflicts all age groups and has a predilection for immunocompromised patients. The condition has a low mortality rate, but if not diagnosed early and treated promptly, it can cause severe, long-term morbidity.

ETIOLOGIC AGENTS

The age of the patient and underlying medical condition provide important clues to the probable infectious agent (Table 1). *Neisseria gonorrhoeae* infection is the most common cause of acute joint infection in healthy young adults aged 15 to 40 years, who account for most hospital admissions for acute bacterial arthritis in urban medical centers. In nongonococcal bacterial arthritis, *Staphylococcus aureus* is the causative agent in about 70% to 80% of cases; it is the predominant organism in children between the age of 2 years and the onset of sexual maturity and in persons over age 40 years. There have been several recent reports on the increased incidence of gram-negative organisms, especially *Escherichia coli* and *Pseudomonas aeruginosa* as causative agents of septic arthritis in the more debilitated elderly population [2].

Although *S. aureus* is the most common pathogen seen in septic arthritis in intravenous drug users, certain sections of the country have reported a higher incidence of gram-negative septic arthritis in these patients. Most cases of bacterial arthritis in

TABLE 1 FREQUENCY OF ETIOLOGIC AGENTS AS CAUSE OF BACTERIAL (SUPPURATIVE) ARTHRITIS

Organism	Children (%)* < 2 y	Children (%)* 2–10 y	Adults (%)
Staphylococcus aureus	7	25	70
Haemophilus influenzae, type B	40	5	< 1
Streptococcus spp[†]	15	15	15
Gram-negative bacilli	10	6	10
Anaerobes	0	1	< 1
Neisseria gonorrhoeae	4	11	[‡]

*In the neonate with prolonged hospitalization and instrumentation, consider coagulase-negative staphylococci, fungi, and gram-negative bacilli.
[†]Includes *Streptococcus pneumoniae*, groups A and B streptococci, viridans group streptococci, and microaerophilic and anaerobic streptococci.
[‡]50% of those aged 18 to 40 years.

HIV-positive patients who are intravenous drug users are caused by *S. aureus*. However, HIV infection predisposes patients to joint infections with opportunistic as well as common pathogens [3].

Staphylococcus aureus is also the primary pathogen recovered from about 80% of infected rheumatoid joints [4]. In patients with sickle cell disease, *Salmonella* spp and a variety of gram-positive and gram-negative organisms have been isolated from infected joints.

In the neonate, group B streptococci and gram-negative organisms are the most common pathogens in acute bacterial arthritis [5]. Gram-negative enteric organisms, coagulase-negative *Staphylococcus* spp, methicillin-resistant *S. aureus*, and fungi must be considered, however, in chronically hospitalized premature neonates. In children between 6 months and 2 years of age, infection with *Haemophilus influenzae* has accounted for about 40% of joint infections, although this number may decrease as children are vaccinated against *H. influenzae* [6].

PATHOGENESIS

The inflammatory process in infectious arthritis is caused by direct invasion of the joint cavity by pathogenic organisms. The initial site of involvement in septic arthritis is the synovium, a highly vascular connective tissue membrane that surrounds the joint space. The synovial membrane lacks a basement membrane, which facilitates the passage of pathogenic organisms from the blood to the synovial cavity in hematogenous dissemination [7••]. *N. gonorrhoeae* and *S. aureus* appear to have a predilection for the joint cavity and are likely to infect a joint during a bacteremic episode.

Pathogenic organisms may also enter the joint space by direct inoculation after a deep penetrating wound that violates the synovial cavity. In closed trauma, infection occurs through increased hyperemia, which provides increased exposure to microorganisms; damage to the local anatomy, which allows easier access of the microorganisms to the joint space; and hematoma formation, which provides a good culture medium [1]. Damage to the joint results from increased intraarticular pressure and the release of proteolytic enzymes from the polymorphonuclear leukocytes, which degrade the cartilage [1].

Endocrine factors appear to play a significant role in the pathogenesis of gonococcal infectious arthritis. There is a greater incidence of gonococcal arthritis in women, and women are particularly susceptible to gonococcal bacteremia during pregnancy, in the postpartum period, and during the first week of the menstrual cycle. Rubella arthritis occurs primarily in postpubertal women, and mumps arthritis is seen exclusively in postpubertal men, which suggests an endocrine-related factor in the pathogenesis of these forms of infectious arthritis [8••].

Recovery from various systemic infections has been associated with a reactive arthritis related to the immune response. Arthritis in patients with hepatitis B infection is a result of antigen-antibody complex formation; the postinfectious arthritis following *Shigella*, *Salmonella*, *Campylobacter*, and *Yersinia* gastrointestinal infections occurs most often in persons with HLA-B27 histocompatibility antigen.

PREDISPOSING FACTORS

Certain medical conditions are associated with an increased incidence of acute bacterial arthritis, especially in adults (Table 2). Chronic inflammation and joint damage, as is seen in rheumatoid arthritis, gout, pseudogout, and osteoarthritis, are predisposing factors for joint infection. These predisposing factors may be further enhanced by a postulated defect in granulocyte phagocytic function in these patients [9]. Osteoarthritis, joint trauma, and joint surgery are also risk factors for septic arthritis, because damaged joints are a nidus for bacterial infections.

TABLE 2 PREDISPOSING FACTORS IN INFECTIOUS ARTHRITIS

Adults
Long-term steroid therapy
Joint trauma
    Penetrating injury
    Intra-articular injections
    Pre-existing arthritis (including crystal arthritis)
Arthroscopic procedures (rare)

Children
Systemic illnesses
Trauma
Contiguous osteomyelitis

Data from Esterhai and Gelb [1] and Prober [5].

Other medical illnesses associated with an increased incidence of infectious arthritis include diabetes, systemic lupus erythematosus, neoplasms, renal failure, sickle cell disease, chronic liver disease, and HIV infection. Patients with these chronic underlying illnesses have suppressed or defective immune defenses and are susceptible to increased bacterial infections in general.

CLINICAL MANIFESTATIONS

Site of Infection

Although septic arthritis may involve any joint, the weight-bearing joints are most commonly affected (Table 3). In children and adults, bacterial arthritis is generally monarticular and involves the knee in about 50% of cases; the hip is the second most commonly infected joint [8••].

Polyarticular nongonococcal infectious arthritis, although rare, generally occurs in the setting of an underlying connective tissue disease; in patients with rheumatoid arthritis, 55% to 60% of cases of septic arthritis are polyarticular [10]. In

TABLE 3 FREQUENCY OF JOINT INVOLVEMENT IN BACTERIAL INFECTIOUS ARTHRITIS

	Children, %	Adults, %
Knee	40	50
Hip	20	25
Ankle	15	7
Elbow	15	10
Wrist	5	7
Shoulder	5	5
Interphalangeal and metacarpal	1	1
Sternoclavicular	1	8
Sacroiliac	0	2

disseminated gonococcal infections, more than 50% of patients present with polyarticular infectious arthritis with involvement of the knees, wrists, ankles, and small joints of the hands and feet. Polyarticular septic arthritis is also a frequent occurrence in intravenous drug users in whom there is increased involvement of axial, sternoclavicular, and shoulder joints [11].

Clinical Findings

The clinical findings in gonococcal and nongonococcal infectious arthritis in adults are outlined in Table 4. Most patients with nongonococcal infectious arthritis have fever and localized symptoms of warmth, pain, swelling, and tenderness over the involved joint. Frequently, there is a palpable joint effusion, and most patients experience decreased active and passive motion of the involved joint, a sign that often distinguishes septic arthritis from bursitis or cellulitis. Infections involving the axial joints, especially the sacroiliac joint, are often more difficult to diagnose; in these cases patients often have diffuse or localized pain in the neck, back, thigh, buttock, pelvis, or abdomen; the pain is often exacerbated by specialized maneuvers [1]. These patients may also have muscle spasms and tenderness to palpation over the infected area. In neurologically impaired or comatose patients, infectious arthritis may present as a fever of unknown origin.

Gonococcal bacterial arthritis occurs in about 30% to 40% of patients with disseminated gonococcal infection [4]. It generally presents as a very painful migratory polyarticular arthritis that is often function limiting and accompanied by fever, skin rash, urethral or vaginal discharge, and tenosynovitis.

In neonates, the clinical features of infectious arthritis are those of septicemia or fever of unknown origin. A careful physical examination may reveal localized swelling, pain on palpation or passive movement of the joint, and decreased movement of the extremity. Older children with septic arthritis can also present with signs of septicemia but will have pain at the involved joint, a joint effusion, and reluctance to move or bear weight on the infected joint.

DIAGNOSIS

The diagnosis of septic arthritis is made by the history, clinical findings, and isolation of the pathogenic organism from aspirated joint fluid. A suspicion of septic arthritis should mandate the use of arthrocentesis and careful examination of the synovial fluid if there is no contraindication (Table 5). The leukocyte count, the percentage of polymorphonuclear leukocytes, and the ratio of glucose in the synovial fluid to that in the peripheral blood correlate with the various diagnoses of infectious arthritis. A synovial fluid profile with a leukocyte count of greater than 50,000 mm^3, with greater than 90% polymorphonuclear leukocytes and a synovial fluid–to–fasting blood glucose ratio of less than 0.5 is highly suggestive of septic arthritis. However, various inflammatory arthritides, such as rheumatoid arthritis and Reiter's syndrome, and gout and pseudogout can also have a synovial fluid profile with more than 50,000 leukocytes/mm^3 with polymorphonuclear predominance.

TABLE 4 GONOCOCCAL AND NONGONOCOCCAL BACTERIAL ARTHRITIS: COMPARISON OF CLINICAL FINDINGS

Gonococcal	Nongonococcal
Generally affects healthy young adults	Generally affects elderly or immunocompromised persons
Polyarticular arthritis (> 50% of cases)	Monarticular arthritis (> 80% of cases)
Tenosynovitis common	Tenosynovitis rare
Rash common	Rash unusual
Blood cultures positive in < 10%	Blood cultures positive in > 50%
Joint cultures positive in < 25%	Joint cultures positive in > 90%

From Goldenberg and Reid [4]; with permission.

The definitive diagnosis of septic arthritis is made through microscopic identification of the infecting organism either by Gram stain of the synovial fluid or through culture. After arthrocentesis has been completed, the joint fluid should be brought to the microbiology laboratory promptly. If a delay is anticipated, the fluid should be inoculated into aerobic and anaerobic culture bottles. About 40% of patients with nongonococcal bacterial arthritis will have a positive Gram stain in a microscopic analysis of the synovial fluid, and approximately 95% will be diagnosed definitely from synovial fluid cultures. Synovial fluid in gonococcal bacterial arthritis is often sterile, and the cultures are positive in less than 25% of cases. Most patients with nongonococcal bacterial arthritis will have an elevated sedimentation rate, an elevated peripheral blood leukocyte count, and positive blood cultures. In gonococcal arthritis, the peripheral leukocyte count is within the normal range and blood cultures are positive in less than 10% of cases.

Although radiographs obtained within the first 10 days of joint infection generally have low diagnostic value, they provide a baseline evaluation of the infected joint and should be obtained, if possible, before arthrocentesis is performed. Early radiographs of an infected joint can demonstrate a joint effusion, joint space widening, and periarticular soft tissue swelling; they can also rule out the possibility of contiguous osteomyelitis (Fig. 1). The presence of intraarticular gas, although rare, would suggest a gas-forming organism such as *Clostridium* as the infecting agent. In prosthetic joint infections, radiographs can often demonstrate loosening of the prosthesis.

A three-phase radionuclide bone scan is the best earliest radiographic diagnostic test for septic arthritis. It will show diffuse increased activity around an infected joint in the blood-pool phase of the scan and increased uptake on both sides of the joint. However, these findings are nonspecific and can be found in other forms of noninfectious arthropathies.

Computed tomography (CT) can demonstrate the presence of a joint effusion within days of onset and detect joint destruction and abscess formation with high sensitivity. Magnetic resonance imaging (MRI) is also very sensitive in demonstrating the presence of a joint effusion, cartilage damage, and soft tissue involvement (Fig. 2). However, neither MRI nor CT can differentiate between infectious and noninfectious joint effusion.

ARTHROCENTESIS

Arthrocentesis, or joint aspiration, is the most important diagnostic procedure in the management of an infected joint, especially when an effusion is present. When aspirating the fluid, the physician should place the patient in a comfortable position in which both the anatomy of the joint can be studied and access to the joint can be achieved easily. After the anatomy of the joint is identified, the site of entry should be marked, and the area surrounding the planned site of entry should be thoroughly cleansed with povidone-iodine. Topical ethychloride spray or injectable lidocaine, 1%, can be used to anesthetize the site of needle entry. An 18- or 20-gauge needle attached to at least a 10-mL syringe

TABLE 5 ANALYSIS OF SYNOVIAL FLUID FOR DIFFERING FORMS OF INFECTIOUS ARTHRITIS

Condition	Leukocytes, *n/mm³*	Predominant cell type	Glucose ratio: synovial fluid to blood	Diagnostic smear, *% cases*
Normal	200–600	Mononuclear	0.8–1.0	0
Bacterial arthritis	10,000–100,000	> 90% PMN	< 0.5	> 90
Fungal arthritis	3000–30,000	70% PMN	≤ 0.5	< 20
Tuberculous arthritis	10,000–20,000	50%–70% PMN	0.5–1.0	< 20
Reactive	3000–10,000	Mononuclear	0.8–1.0	0

PMN—polymorphonuclear cells.

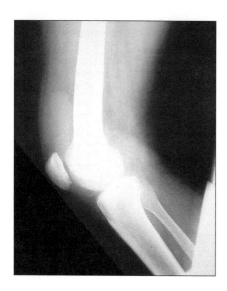

FIGURE 1 Lateral radiograph of the left knee. The large elliptical soft tissue mass represents synovial fluid or pus in the suprapatellar bursa. Soft tissue swelling and edema of the infrapatellar fat pad are also present.

Arthrocentesis of the shoulder joint is accomplished with the patient in a seated position, preferably with a back support and with the hands resting on the lap (Fig. 3B). With the needle directed superiorly and laterally, the joint should be entered anteriorly between the medial surface of the humeral head and the inferior tip of the coracoid process.

The synovial fluid of the elbow can be aspirated with the arm resting on a solid surface with the elbow flexed approximately 45 degrees (Fig. 3C). The needle should be inserted in the lateral aspect of the joint between the lateral epicondyle and the radial head.

Aspiration of the wrist is done on the dorsal surface of the joint with the hand slightly flexed (Fig. 3D). The joint can be aspirated from the medial, radial, or ulnar surface. To aspirate from the radial surface, one should insert the needle into the space on the ulnar side of the extensor tendon of the thumb; the ulnar and medial approaches are directed to the joint space between the border of the distal ulna and the carpal joint.

The ankle joint can be aspirated through either a medial or lateral approach (Fig. 3E). In the lateral approach, the needle is inserted into the joint space distal to the fibula; medially, the needle is inserted medial to the extensor hallucis longus tendon, which is identified by flexion of the great toe.

should be used for aspiration in accordance with the techniques discussed in the text that follows [12,13].

During aspiration of fluid from the knee, the leg should be placed on a solid surface with the knee maximally extended (Fig. 3A). The effusion should be palpated and the joint space entered medially or laterally, below the undersurface of the patella.

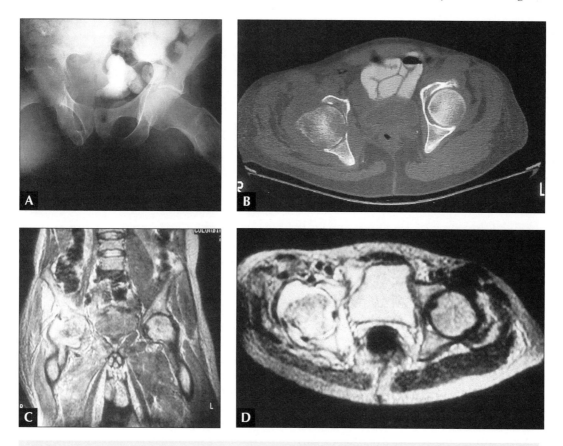

FIGURE 2 **A**, Radiograph of hips in frog lateral position. Right-sided joint space loss, irregularity of apposing cartilages, and marked osteopenia as compared with the left are indicative of a pyogenic infection. **B**, Computed tomographic scan of the same patient confirms the relative osteopenia and marked narrowing of the right hip joint, supporting the diagnosis of infection. **C** and **D**, Magnetic resonance imaging in the same patient. Coronal proton density (TR/TE:2020/50) (**C**) and axial T_2-weighted images (TR/TE:2020/100) with 5.2-slice thicknesses (**D**) reveal high signal within the right femoral head, acetabulum, and surrounding soft tissues representing marrow edema, synovitis, and synovial fluid or pus.

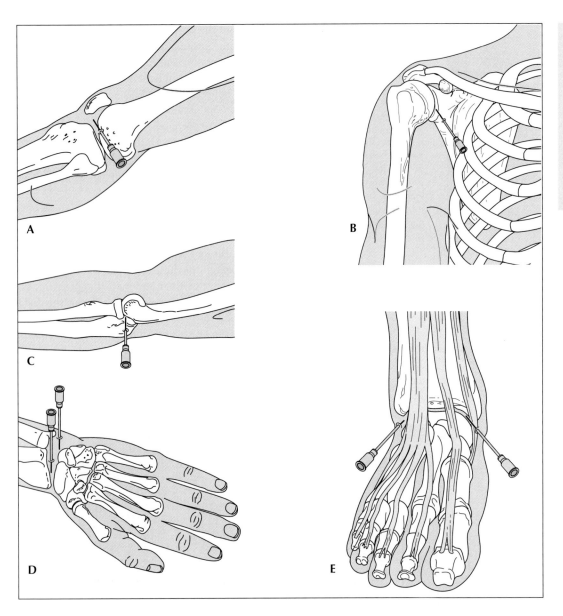

FIGURE 3
Diagrammatic representations of the technique of arthrocentesis in the knee (**A**), shoulder (**B**), elbow (**C**), wrist (**D**), and ankle (**E**). (*Adapted from* Stern [13]; with permission.)

Arthrocentesis of the hip joint should be performed by an orthopedist, because this procedure often requires arthroscopy to visualize the joint accurately. Aspiration of the small joints of the hands and feet also may require the intervention of an orthopedist because of the multiple joint spaces and the small amount of fluid that is present in these joints.

TREATMENT

Infectious arthritis should be considered a medical emergency that requires prompt diagnosis and treatment. Data presented by Goldenberg and Reid [4] in 1985 showed that successful recovery of patients with septic arthritis was notably better for those patients who were diagnosed and treated within 5 days of the onset of symptoms. The three elements of successful management are prompt diagnosis, appropriate antimicrobial therapy, and drainage of the joint space.

The choice of antibiotics is often empiric at the onset of therapy. It can be guided, however, by the most likely pathogen given the patient's age and medical condition and results of the Gram stain of the synovial fluid. Antibiotics can be subsequently tailored to the results of synovial fluid cultures. Drainage of the infected joint is important both to remove the inflammatory cells and debris and to decompress the joint. Knees, ankles, wrists, and elbows usually can be drained adequately by needle aspiration; deep joints such as hips and shoulders, axial joints, and the sternoclavicular joint generally necessitate open surgical drainage. Repeat aspiration may be required for 7 to 10 days until the leukocyte count decreases and the synovial fluid remains sterile. Arthroscopy provides better visualization during joint lavage and is particularly useful in more difficult-to-drain joints and in joints that are not responding clinically to repeated needle aspirations.

The route and duration of antibiotic therapy are controversial issues in the treatment of infectious arthritis (Table 6). Parenteral antibiotics should be given for a 1- to 2-week course until the infection has been eradicated. Parenteral antibiotics can be changed to oral antibiotics if there is a good clinical response, but serum and synovial fluid concentrations of oral antibiotics must be bactericidal for effective therapy. In

TABLE 6 TREATMENT REGIMENS FOR INFECTIOUS ARTHRITIS

Age	Gram stain	Drug of choice	Dosage	Interval
Infant (< 2 y)	+ cocci, pairs and chains	Penicillin-G*	100,000 U/kg/d, IV	Div. every 4–6 h
	+ cocci, clusters	Nafcillin†	150 mg/kg/d, IV	Div. every 6 h
	– bacilli	Cefotaxime *or*	200 mg/kg/d, IV	Div. every 6 h
		ceftriaxone	100 mg/kg/d, IV	Div. every 12 h
Children (2–13 y)	+ cocci, pairs and clusters	Penicillin-G*	250,000 U/kg/d, IV	Div. every 4–6 h
	+ cocci, clusters	Nafcillin †	150 mg/kg/d, IV	Div. every 6 h
	– coccobacilli	Cefuroxime	150 mg/kg/d, IV	Div. every 8 h
	– bacilli	Cefotaxime *or*	200 mg/kg/d, IV	Div. every 6 h
		ceftriaxone	100 mg/kg/d, IV	Div. every 12 h
Adolescents and adults	+ cocci, pairs and clusters	Penicillin-G*	1.2 MU/d, IV or IM	Div. every 4–6 h
	+ cocci, clusters	Nafcillin†	1–2 g, IV	Every 4 h
	– bacilli	Cefotaxime	1 g, IV	Every 8 h
	– cocci	Ceftriaxone	2 g, IV	Every 24 h
Healthy young adults	No organism seen	Ceftriaxone	2 g, IV	Every 24 h
Elderly	No organism seen	Ticarcillin + clavulanic acid *or*	3.1 g, IV	Every 6 h
		ampicillin/sulbactam *or*	1.5–3 g, IV	Every 6 h
		imipenem	0.5–1 g, IV	Every 6 h

*If penicillin resistant, use cefotaxime or ceftriaxone.
†Penicillinase-resistant synthetic penicillins; if methicillin resistant, use vancomycin.
Div.—divided dose; IM—intramuscular; IV—intravenous.

nongonococcal infectious arthritis, most antibiotics are administered intravenously for 2 weeks and are followed by 1 to 2 weeks of oral antibiotic administration. When the etiologic agent is difficult to eradicate, such as with *S. aureus* or a gram-negative bacilli, or if there is underlying structural joint disease, parenteral therapy should be given either for a full 4 weeks or for 2 weeks, followed by a 4- to 6-week course of oral antibiotics (*ie*, an oral quinolone). In gonococcal arthritis, parenteral antibiotics can be changed to oral therapy in 2 to 3 days if there is good clinical response; duration of therapy is generally 7 to 10 days.

FUNGAL ARTHRITIS

Fungal arthritis is rare and generally follows a chronic indolent course (Table 7) [14]. The organisms that cause fungal arthritis are divided into two groups, namely the mycotic agents that produce primary invasive systemic infections such as *Histoplasma*, *Coccidioides*, or *Blastomyces* and those fungi that produce opportunistic infection such as *Candida*, *Cryptococcus*, and *Sporothrix*. Fungal joint infection is a monarticular or oligoarticular arthritis, with the knee joint being the most commonly affected joint. The involved joints are swollen and have limited motion. Aspirated synovial fluid generally has an elevated protein content, a leukocyte count of 3000 to 30,000/mm^3 with polymorphonuclear cell predominance, and a normal serum-to-synovial-fluid–glucose ratio. The causative fungus can occasionally be isolated from the joint fluid, but definitive diagnosis is made by synovial biopsy and culture. The treatment of fungal arthritides usually requires open drainage,

débridement, and amphotericin B induction therapy [14]. Combination therapy with amphotericin B and flucytosine has also been effective. The newer oral antifungals, fluconazole and itraconazole, may be very effective in the long-term treatment of fungal arthritis, especially after induction therapy with amphotericin B [15,16].

VIRAL ARTHRITIS

Several viruses have been associated with the symptoms of infectious arthritis. The more commonly associated viruses include mumps, rubella, and erythema infectiosum; the less commonly associated include influenza, adenovirus, echovirus, rubeola, Epstein-Barr, varicella, and smallpox.

A painful, transient arthritis has been associated with naturally occurring rubella infections as well as rubella vaccination, especially in postpubertal women (Table 7). The joint symptoms usually occur within 7 days of the onset of the rash and last about 1 week. The arthritis is symmetric, additive, and occasionally migratory and most often involves the small joints of the hands, feet, wrists, and elbow. The arthralgias are generally self-limited, but symptoms may persist for several months, and carpal tunnel syndrome is a common complication. In rubella-associated arthritis, the synovial fluid has a leukocyte count of 10,000 to 20,000/mm^3 with a mononuclear cell predominance. The arthritis that occurs after rubella vaccinations resembles that seen with naturally occurring disease but is both age and sex related; it occurs in less than 3% of vaccinated children of both sexes and in more than 50% of vaccinated postpubertal women [9].

TABLE 7 CHARACTERISTICS OF INFECTIOUS ARTHRITIS CAUSED BY OTHER PATHOGENIC ORGANISMS

Infection	Fungus*	Rubella	Viral mumps	Parvovirus B19	Tubercular	Syphilitic
Occurrence	Rare	Mainly postpubertal women	Middle-aged men	10% children 60% adults with EI	Rare, but increasing	Congenital and tertiary; secondary rare
Affected joints	Knees, wrists, elbows	Small joints of hands and feet, knees, wrists, and ankles	Symmetric polyarthritis of large and small joints	Metocarpophalangeal, proximal interphalangeal, knees, wrists, ankles	Spine, hips, knees, ankles	Knees and elbows
Physical findings	Swollen joints, limited motion, chronic pain, migratory arthritis	Joint pains near onset of rash	Joint pains within 1 wk of parotitis	Rash characteristic of EI symmetrical polyarthritis	Monarticular arthritis, weight loss, low-grade fever	Joint effusion, gummatous osteoarthritis, neuropathic joints
Synovial fluid	3000–30,000 leukocytes/mm³;70% PMNs	10,000–20,000 leukocytes/mm³; mononuclear cells predominant	Effusions rare	3000 leukocytes/mm³; mononuclear cells predominant	10,000–20,000 leukocytes/mm³; 50%–70% PMNs	1000 leukocytes/mm³; mononuclear cells predominant
Treatment	Amphotericin B, IV 0.5 mg/kg/d	None	Steroids if symptoms persist	Anti-inflammatory drugs if necessary	Anti-tuberculosis medication for 18–24 mo; joint rest in acute stage†	Penicillin appropriate for stage of syphilis

*Causative fungi: *Histoplasma, Coccidioides, Blastomyces, Candida, Cryptococcus,* and *Sporothrix.*
†In populations with prevalence of multi–drug–resistant tuberculosis, use 4-drug therapy until culture results are available.
EI—erythema infectiosum; IV—intravenous; PMNs—polymorphonuclear cells.

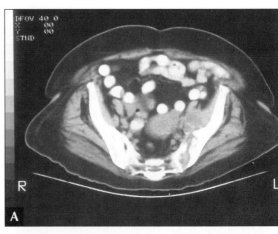

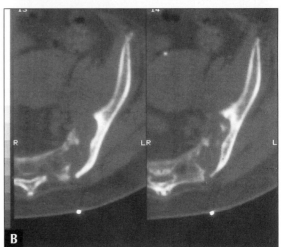

FIGURE 4 A, Computed tomographic scan of sacroiliac joints. The left joint is widened with irregular apposing surfaces. An anterior soft tissue mass due to a cold abscess and bony fragments are also noted in this case of tuberculous arthritis. B, Higher magnification of the infected joint.

Mumps is known to produce a symmetric polyarthritis of both the large and small joints within 1 week of the development of parotitis (Table 7). Mumps-associated arthritis is generally seen in middle-aged men and lasts about 1 month. There is no treatment for this arthritis, although corticosteroid therapy has been used in the more symptomatic cases.

Erythema infectiosum, or "fifth disease," a manifestation of parvovirus B19 infection, also has been associated with arthritis and arthralgias (Table 7) [17]. In one reported outbreak, as many as 60% of the affected adults reported pain and joint swelling; articular involvement is rarely reported in pediatric cases. The arthropathy is probably immune mediated, because its onset has been correlated with the appearance of circulating antibodies [18]. Affected patients generally experience the sudden onset of a symmetric peripheral polyarthropathy that affects the metacarpophalangeal joints, proximal interphalangeal joints, knees, wrists, and ankles. This arthropathy is self-limited and generally lasts about 2 weeks. There is no treatment; anti-inflammatory drugs may provide symptomatic relief.

TUBERCULOUS ARTHRITIS

Historically, tuberculous arthritis had been a rare form of infectious arthritis (Table 7). However, with the advent of AIDS, an increased incidence of articular involvement can be expected in these immunocompromised patients, with extrapulmonary manifestations of *Mycobacterium* tuberculosis and atypical tuberculosis infections.

Articular involvement is either the result of hematogenous dissemination of infection from a primary pulmonary focus or is secondary to reactivation of a previously seeded but dormant skeletal focus [18]. Factors that predispose an individual to the development of tuberculous arthritis are trauma and a compromised immune system. Patients generally present with an insidious monarticular arthritis. Joint pain and swelling may develop over months, with an average time from the onset of symptoms to diagnosis of 18 months.

The joints frequently involved in tuberculous arthritis are the spine, hips, knees, and ankles (Fig. 4). Tuberculous arthritis is unusual in children, in whom the hip and knee are the most commonly involved joints. In adults, vertebral joint involvement is more common and occurs secondarily to tuberculous vertebral osteomyelitis. The diagnosis of tuberculous arthritis is difficult to make because constitutional symptoms are uncommon, except for chronic weight loss and low-grade fever; initial radiographs are usually normal.

An open synovial biopsy establishes the diagnosis of tuberculous arthritis. An analysis of synovial fluid shows a nonspecific mild inflammatory reaction with a leukocyte count of about 20,000/mm³, with 50% polymorphonuclear leukocytes, and is nondiagnostic. Microscopic examination can detect acid-fast organisms in about only 20% of culture-positive joint effusions. Treatment consists of the administration of combination therapy for at least 18 to 24 months. Four-drug therapy with isoniazid, rifampin, pyrazinamide, and ethambutol is recommended until susceptibility patterns are available, at which time therapy can be reduced to two drugs to which the organism is susceptible.

SPIROCHETAL ARTHRITIS

Infectious arthritis has been associated with both syphilis and Lyme disease. Syphilitic arthritis can occur in congenital and tertiary syphilis; it is rarely seen in secondary syphilis (Table 7). Children and adolescents who present with congenital syphilis may have only a painless synovitis with an effusion (Clutton's joint), especially in the knees and elbows. These joints generally do not appear infected. Syphilitic arthritis may have a prolonged course if not diagnosed and treated; however, it generally follows a benign, self-limited course without residua.

Neuropathic joint disease (Charcot's arthropathy), most commonly involving the knees, and gummatous osteoarthritis of the large joints may occur in tertiary syphilis. In Charcot's arthropathy, the affected joint generally is painless and hypermobile with an effusion. Synovial fluid from a Charcot joint has a leukocyte count of 1000/mm³, with a mononuclear cell predominance. The treatment of syphilitic joint disease is penicillin given in a dosage appropriate for the particular stage of syphilis. The arthropathy associated with Lyme disease is discussed in Chapter 17.

PROSTHETIC JOINTS

Septic arthritis complicating prosthetic joint surgery has become an important surgical problem as the number of prosthetic joint replacements has increased. Patients with prosthetic joints have a 1% to 4% infection rate over 10 years; infection rates as high as 30% have been reported in cases of surgical revision of prosthetic joints [19].

Patients with prosthetic joint infections are often elderly with underlying chronic medical or joint conditions. A diagnosis of infection generally follows a prolonged period of indolent symptoms, especially pain, which often extends 2 to 8 months before diagnosis. These patients generally have a normal peripheral leukocyte count but elevated sedimentation rate, which often provides a significant clue to the diagnosis.

Intraoperative wound contamination is considered the portal of entry in early postoperative infections; late infections (more than 2 years postsurgery) are most likely hematogenously acquired [20]. *Staphylococcus* is the most common pathogen: *Staphylococcus epidermidis* accounts for 40% of prosthetic joint infections and *S. aureus*, for 20%. Multiple organisms as well as anaerobic organisms and fungi are occasionally found, especially in late infection. Since prosthetic joint infections are often caused by hematogenous seeding of the joint during a bacteremic episode, all patients with prosthetic joints should receive antibiotic prophylaxis when undergoing procedures known to cause bacteremia (Table 8).

Infection of a prosthetic joint generally necessitates that the prosthesis be removed to clear the infection. When the prosthesis is not removed, the patient is committed to lifelong antibiotic therapy. The decision to remove and replace a prosthetic joint is, however, a clinical judgment.

Type of procedure	Drug of choice	Dose/administration	Alternative therapy
Dental, oral, upper respiratory tract	Amoxicillin	3.0 g orally 1 h before procedure; 1.5 g orally 6 h later	Penicillin allergic: erythromycin stearate, 1.0 g before; 500 mg 6 h later *or* clindamycin, 300 mg before; 150 mg 6 h later
Genitourinary	Ampicillin/gentamicin then amoxicillin	If unable to take orally: ampicillin, 2.0 g IV or IM 30 min before procedure; 1.0 g IV 6 h later	Penicillin allergic: clindamycin, 300 mg IV 30 min before; 150 mg IV 6 h later
		Ampicillin, 2.0 g IV + gentamicin, 1.5 mg/kg IV 30 min before procedure; amoxicillin, 1.5 g orally 6 h later or IV regimen 8 h after first dose	Penicillin allergic: vancomycin, 1.0 g IV + gentamicin, 1.5 mg/kg 1 h before; may be repeated 8 h after first dose
Gastrointestinal (no specific recommendation)			Low risk: may use amoxicillin as above

Adapted from Dajani and coworkers [21]; with permission.
IM—intramuscular; IV—intravenous.

REFERENCES AND RECOMMENDED READING

Recently published papers of particular interest have been highlighted as:
• Of interest
•• Of outstanding interest

1. Esterhai JL, Gelb I: Adult septic arthritis. *Orthop Clin North Am* 1991, 22:503–514.

2. Vincent GM, Amirault JD: Septic arthritis in the elderly. *Clin Orthop* 1990, 251:241–245.

3. Hughes RA, Rowe IF, Shanson D, Keat CS: Septic bone, joint and muscle lesions associated with human immunodeficiency virus infection. *Br J Rheumatol* 1992, 31:381–388.

4. Goldenberg DL, Reid JI: Bacterial arthritis. *N Engl J Med* 1985, 312:764–771.

5. Prober CD: Current antibiotic therapy of community-acquired bacterial infections in hospitalized children: bone and joint infections. *Pediatr Infect Dis J* 1992, 11:156–159.

6. Green NE, Edwards K: Bone and joint infections in children. *Orthop Clin North Am* 1987, 18:555–576.

7.•• Goldenberg DL: Bacterial arthritis. In *Textbook of Rheumatology*, edn 4. Edited by Kelly WN, Harris ED Jr, Ruddy S, Sledge CB. Philadelphia: WB Saunders; 1993:1449–1466.

8.•• Smith JW: Bone and joint infections. In *Principles and Practices of Infectious Diseases*, edn 3. Edited by Mandell GL, Douglas RG Jr, Bennett JE. New York: Churchill Livingstone; 1990:911–918.

9. Turner RA, Schermacher HR, Myer AR: Phagocytic function of polymorphonuclear leukocytes in rheumatic diseases. *J Clin Invest* 1973, 52:1632–1635.

10. Barcos MA, Peris P, Miro JM, *et al.*: Septic arthritis in heroin addicts. *Semin Arthritis Rheum* 1991, 21:81–87.

11. Smith JW: Infectious arthritis. *Infect Dis Clin North Am* 1990, 4:523–538.

12. Parks DL: Joint aspiration and injection. In *Manual of Medical Therapeutics*, edn 26. Edited by Dunagan WC, Ridner ML. Boston: Little, Brown; 1989:459–462.

13. Stern R: Arthrocentesis and intraarticular injection. In *Manual of Rheumatology and Outpatient Orthopedic Disorders*, edn 3. Edited by Paget S, Pellicci P, Beary JF III. Boston: Little, Brown; 1993:33–37.

14. Cuellar ML, Silveira LH, Espinoza LR: Fungal arthritis. *Ann Rheum Dis* 1992, 51:690–697.

15. O'Meeghan T, Varcoe R, Thomas M, Ellis-Pegler R: Fluconazole concentration in joint fluid during successful treatment of *Candida albicans* septic arthritis. *J Antimicrob Chemother* 1990, 26:601–602.

16. Heller HM, Fuhrer J: Disseminated sporotrichosis in patients with AIDS: case report and review of the literature. *AIDS* 1991, 5:1243–1246.

17. Torok TJ: Parvovirus B19 and human disease. *Adv Intern Med* 1992, 37:431–455.

18. Berney S, Goldstein M, Bishko F: Clinical and diagnostic features of tuberculous arthritis. *Am J Med* 1972, 53:36–42.

19. Inman RD, Gallegos KV, Brause BD, *et al.*: Clinical and microbial features of prosthetic joint infection. *Am J Med* 1984, 77:47–53.

20. Gillespie WJ: Infection in total joint replacement. *Infect Dis Clin North Am* 1990, 4:465–484.

21. Dajani AS, Bisno AL, Chung KJ, *et al.*: Prevention of bacterial endocarditis: recommendations by the American Heart Association. *JAMA* 1990, 264:2919–2922.

SELECT BIBLIOGRAPHY

McCarty DJ, Koopman WJ, eds: *Arthritis and Allied Conditions*, vol 1 and 2, edn 12. Philadelphia: Lea and Febiger, 1993.

Lyme Disease 17

Benjamin J. Luft
Raymond J. Dattwyler

Key Points

- Erythema migrans is diagnostic of Lyme disease.
- Lyme arthritis most commonly affects the knee.
- Small joint involvement should suggest an alternative diagnosis.
- *Borrelia burgdorferi* invades the central nervous system early in the course of infection.
- For any patient suspected of having a central nervous system disorder a lumbar puncture should be done and the cerebrospinal fluid should be examined.
- All positive enzyme-linked immunosorbent assays (ELISAs) should be confirmed by Western blot.
- Amoxicillin is highly effective in patients with erythema migrans.

A new species of *Borrelia* was isolated from *Ixodes* ticks in 1982. Soon thereafter, this spirochete, *Borrelia burgdorferi*, was demonstrated to be the etiologic agent of Lyme disease. With this discovery, it became clear that a wide array of clinical syndromes, previously described in both Europe and the United States, resulted from infection with this pathogen and that Lyme disease was neither a new disease nor unique to North America. In 1992, the Centers for Disease Control and Prevention (CDC) reported 9677 cases from 45 states in the United States; the vast majority of cases were from four geographic regions: coastal areas in the Northeast, the Midatlantic region, the upper Midwest, and the Pacific coastal regions (Fig. 1) [1].

CLINICAL MANIFESTATIONS

Borrelia burgdorferi infection is a progressive infectious disease. Its major target organ systems are the skin, the musculoskeletal system, the nervous system, and to a lesser extent the heart (Table 1). Lyme disease is not chronic fatigue syndrome or fibromyalgia but rather an entity with objectively measurable abnormalities. Infection originates in the skin at the site of a bite from an infected tick. Early in the course of infection, spirochetes disseminate hematogenously, seeding multiple organs and producing both local manifestations and systemic signs and symptoms, including fever, malaise, arthralgias, and myalgias. As the infected host mounts an immune response, the infection can become latent or can progress to a chronic phase in which few, if any, systemic signs or symptoms are present but local inflammatory processes predominate. Therefore, clinicians should consider whether the disease is local or disseminated, acute or chronic.

Dermatologic

Three distinct dermatologic entities are associated with *B. burgdorferi* infection. The most common, erythema migrans, is identified with acute infection and is classically

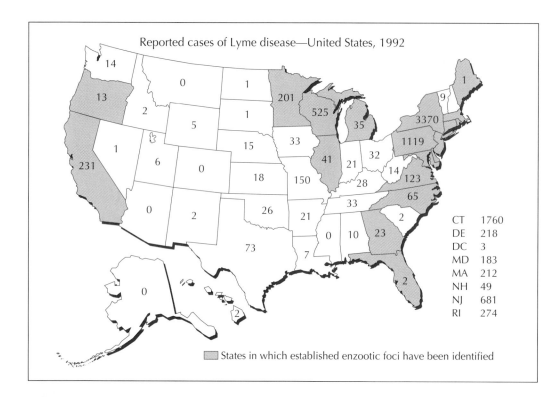

Reported cases of Lyme disease—United States, 1992

CT	1760
DE	218
DC	3
MD	183
MA	212
NH	49
NJ	681
RI	274

States in which established enzootic foci have been identified

FIGURE 1 Reported cases of Lyme disease in the United States in 1992 according to the Centers for Disease Control and Prevention case definition (Table 2). Reporting is mandatory in 49 states (all except Oregon) and in the District of Columbia. (*From* Centers for Disease Control and Prevention [18].)

TABLE 1 CLINICAL MANIFESTATIONS OF LYME DISEASE

Local infection

Erythema migrans
  Develops days to weeks after tick bite
  >5 cm in diameter
  Sites are usually the thigh, groin, and axilla
Erythema migrans with mild flu-like illness

Acute disseminated infection

Erythema migrans
  Multiple sites
  Severe systemic symptoms, other evidence of systemic
    spread (*eg*, abnormal liver function test results), or both
Neurologic
  Acute meningitis
  Acute encephalitis
  Cranial neuritis
  Radiculoneuritis (Bannwarth's syndrome)
  Peripheral neuropathy
Arthritis
Cardiac
  Atrioventricular block
  Myopericarditis

Chronic disseminated infection

Neurologic
  Peripheral neuropathy
  Chronic meningoencephalitis
  Chronic encephalitis
Arthritis
Acrodermatitis chronica atrophicans

---

described as an expanding, annular erythematous skin lesion with a central clearing area (Fig. 2) [2]. Erythema migrans can present in a variety of ways. The most common is a homogeneously erythematous annular lesion. Erythema migrans represents infection within the skin, with the primary lesion appearing at the site of the tick bite. Secondary lesions are observed in 10% to 15% of individuals. Untreated, erythema migrans will spontaneously clear within a few weeks to a month. A wide range of signs and symptoms can accompany this rash, varying from mild systemic signs and symptoms such as fever, transitory malaise, fatigue, and headache to more severe signs and symptoms such as debilitating, profound fatigue; lethargy; mild encephalopathy; meningeal irritation; and migratory musculoskeletal pain.

Two other dermatologic manifestations of *B. burgdorferi* infection, borrelia lymphocytoma and acrodermatitis chronica atrophicans (ACA), are much less common. Borrelia lymphocytoma, a solitary, bluish-red nodule consisting of dense lymphocytic infiltrates in the skin or subcutaneous tissue, typically develops in the areola in adults and in the lower portion of the ear lobe in children. It is associated with the acute disseminated phase of infection and is usually observed within the first 6 months of infection. Histologically, there are monotonous sheets of lymphocytes in the dermis or subcutaneous tissue, which can be confused with cutaneous lymphoma. However, it must be emphasized that although borrelia lymphocytoma is similar in appearance to a cutaneous lymphoma, *B. burgdorferi* does not cause true lymphoma.

Acrodermatitis chronica atrophicans, a chronic inflammatory skin condition leading to cutaneous atrophy, is rare in North America; most reports of it are from northern and eastern Europe. Initially, ACA is similar in appearance to the acute edematous phase of scleroderma. It may be mistaken for stasis dermatitis on occasion. Usually involving the distal

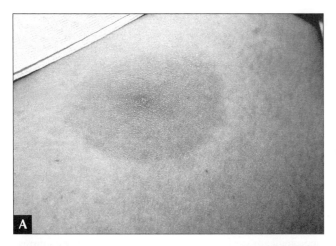

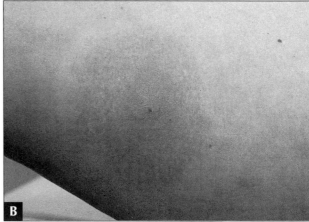

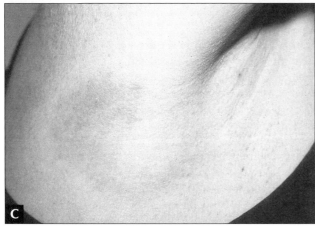

FIGURE 2 A–C, Erythema migrans lesions in patients with Lyme disease (see Color Plates).

extremities and less commonly the trunk, ACA is frequently violaceous to bluish-red in color, with a doughy consistency. Regions of inflammation may be multicentric, with various degrees of erythema and swelling. Areas of abnormal skin may be interspersed with areas of relatively normal looking skin. Most individuals with ACA are elderly and female.

Rheumatologic

Musculoskeletal complaints, including both arthralgias and arthritis, are common in *B. burgdorferi* infection. During the acute phase of infection, arthralgias predominate. Although frank arthritis can be observed in acute disease, it is usually associated with chronic infection. Approximately 50% of untreated individuals will develop a mono- or oligoarticular arthritis [3]. The course of Lyme arthritis is fairly stereotypic in both adults and children. Initially, patients experience episodic migratory pain in joints, tendons, bursae, muscle, or bone, usually without joint swelling or other evidence of frank arthritis. The pain can vary in intensity, affecting only one or two sites at a time and lasting from a few hours to, less commonly, a few days at any one site. As the disease progresses, intermittent episodes of frank arthritis develop. Characteristically, the arthritis is a mono- or oligoarticular large joint arthritis, with the knee being the most commonly affected joint. Polyarthritis is rare and should lead the physician to consider an alternative diagnosis, particularly if it is symmetric or if there is small joint involvement.

Although Lyme arthritis involves the knee in most cases, other large joints can be involved, including (in descending order) the shoulder, ankle, elbow, and hip. Except in individuals with ACA, small joint involvement is rare and is seen in the setting of large joint involvement. On examination, swelling and increased warmth of the affected joint are common, but there is generally little redness and the amount of swelling is disproportionately greater than the degree of pain. Large effusions, especially of the knee, are common, and Baker's cysts are observed. The arthritis is typically episodic in nature, with events lasting 1 or 2 weeks before spontaneously resolving. Systemic signs and symptoms other than fatigue and arthralgias are unusual in Lyme arthritis. Episodes of arthritis can recur for several years, with gradually increasing periods between occurrences. Eventually, even without treatment, most individuals have spontaneous resolution of their arthritis. Only approximately 10% of individuals develop chronic arthritis. However, the arthritis in these patients can be severe, with erosion of cartilage and bone. A few of these patients have required joint replacement.

Neurologic

Although controversy exists about the full range of the nervous system manifestations of *B. burgdorferi* infection, sound evidence of a causal relationship has been established for only a few neurologic disorders (Table 1) [4]. *B. burgdorferi* may invade the central nervous system (CNS) early in the course of infection, even in patients with minimal symptoms of meningitis [5••]. Clinically, it is often difficult to distinguish the headache and stiff neck in patients with true meningitis from those reported by patients with erythema migrans alone. Frequently, the only way to distinguish between the two is to examine the cerebrospinal fluid. The hallmark of patients with active CNS infection is the presence of cerebrospinal fluid abnormalities, including a mild pleocytosis largely consisting of mononuclear cells, a modest elevation in protein level, and a normal cerebrospinal fluid glucose level.

In chronic infection, local inflammatory CNS processes, including acute myelitis, localized encephalitis, and cerebellar ataxia, have been reported. However, in most patients with evidence of chronic disseminated B. burgdorferi infection, there are no objective neurologic abnormalities. Exceptions are listed in Table 1. As always, in any patient with suspected CNS infection the cerebrospinal fluid should be examined.

Meningopolyneuritis (Garin-Bujadoux, Bannwarth's syndrome) is the most dramatic involvement of the peripheral nervous system. However, the spectrum of disorders is wide, ranging in severity from meningopolyneuritis in acute infection to a milder and more common axonal neuropathy in chronic infection. Intense reticular pain, paresthesias, and hyperesthesias are characteristic of meningopolyneuritis, which is often associated with meningitis and a lymphocytic pleocytosis. No relationship has been observed between the neuritis and the site of the tick bite or erythema migrans rash, and the neuritis may be distributed asymmetrically, resembling polyneuritis multiplex. Paresis, spastic paraparesis, and neurogenic bladder may develop and may remain even after appropriate antibiotic therapy.

Forty percent of patients with late disease are reported to have abnormalities of two or more peripheral nerves. The spectrum of peripheral nerve involvement follows a continuum. The underlying pathologic mechanisms are the same but the degree of involvement is variable. The unifying characteristic in each is an axonopathy, probably secondary to vasculopathy.

Cranial nerve involvement is reported in up to 10% of patients with acute disseminated infection. Facial nerve palsy, either unilateral or bilateral, is the most common cranial neuropathy associated with this infection. Other cranial neuropathies occur but are less common. Evidence of polyneuritis or meningitis is frequently present in individuals with cranial neuritis; most patients require a lumbar puncture to define the extent of neurologic involvement. Papilledema with elevated cerebrospinal fluid pressure, producing a pseudotumor cerebri–like syndrome, has been reported. Although B. burgdorferi infection is associated with an array of neurologic manifestations, the clinician must take great care not to assume a cause-and-effect relationship between Lyme disease and neurologic entities. Nonspecific symptoms such as fatigue, depression, and memory disturbance should not be attributed to Lyme disease in the absence of other, objectively measurable abnormalities.

Cardiac

Cardiac involvement, which is less common than either musculoskeletal or neurologic abnormalities, has been reported to occur in up to 8% of adults with acute infection (Table 1). In our experience, however, it is noted in less then 1% of patients presenting with erythema migrans. It is usually self-limited.

DIAGNOSIS

Clinically, erythema migrans is the classic skin lesion of B. burgdorferi infection. The Centers for Disease Control and Prevention case definition includes the presence of erythema migrans or at least one objective sign of musculoskeletal, neurologic, or cardiovascular disease and laboratory confirmation of infection (Table 2). Unfortunately, erythema migrans is recognized in just two thirds of patients and only early in the course of infection. In the absence of erythema migrans, definitively diagnosing Lyme disease can be troublesome. B. burgdorferi is difficult to culture except from erythema migrans. In the chronic phase of the disease, the organism is rarely observed in clinical samples. Therefore, unlike most bacterial infections, which can be defined microbiologically by direct observation or culture of the pathogen, Lyme disease is defined indirectly. This situation frequently leads to misdiagnosis and confusion on both the part of the patient and that of the clinician. In the absence of an erythema migrans lesion, the diagnosis is based on the demonstration of an immune response to B. burgdorferi in an appropriate clinical setting. Making the diagnosis of Lyme disease requires that objective clinical abnormalities be documented.

When To Refer

The clinician must have a basic understanding of the immune response to B. burgdorferi in infected individuals to use serologic assays appropriately. As would be expected, at the onset of infection, levels of specific antibodies to B. burgdorferi are usually within the normal range. Antibody responses follow the usual pattern: IgM antibody appears first, then IgG and IgA [6,7]. Within 2 to 3 weeks after the onset of infection, a rise in the level of IgM antibody to one or more spirochetal antigens can be detected in most individuals. Approximately 70% of patients treated for erythema migrans will develop an antibody response to B. burgdorferi within 3 weeks. During the second and third months of infection, specific IgG and IgA responses gradually increase, and once established, they may remain detectable for years. Because spirochetes compose a portion of the normal human flora, most individuals have circulating antibodies that are cross-reactive with one or more B. burgdorferi antigens, which may complicate the assessment of the humoral response. Furthermore, prompt antimicrobial therapy, as in the case of syphilis, can abort the development of a mature humoral response [8,9].

In the clinical laboratory, antibodies to B. burgdorferi are usually detected by either indirect immunofluorescence assay or enzyme-linked immunosorbent assay (ELISA). Whole B. burgdorferi preparations are generally used for these assays.

TABLE 2 LYME DISEASE NATIONAL SURVEILLANCE CASE DEFINITION

Lyme disease is a systemic, tick-borne disease with protean manifestations, including dermatologic, rheumatologic, neurologic, and cardiac abnormalities. The best clinical marker for the disease is the initial skin lesion, erythema migrans, which occurs in 60% to 80% of patients.

Case definition for the national surveillance of Lyme disease
A person with erythema migrans
A person with at least one late manifestation and laboratory confirmation of infection

General definition
Erythema migrans: for purposes of surveillance, erythema migrans is a skin lesion that typically begins as a red macule or papule and expands over a period of days or weeks to form a large round lesion, often with partial central clearing. To be considered erythema migrans, a solitary lesion must measure at least 5 cm. Secondary lesions may also occur. Annular erythematous lesions developing within several hours after a tick bite represent hypersensitivity reactions and do not qualify as erythema migrans. In most patients, the expanding erythema migrans lesion is accompanied by other acute symptoms, particularly fatigue, fever, headache, mildly stiff neck, arthralgias, and myalgias. These symptoms are typically intermittent. The diagnosis of erythema migrans must be made by a physician. Laboratory confirmation is recommended for patients with no known exposure.

Late manifestations, which include any of the following when an alternative explanation is not found:

Musculoskeletal system: recurrent, brief attacks (lasting weeks or months) of objective joint swelling in one or a few joints, sometimes followed by chronic arthritis in one or a few joints. Manifestations that are not considered to be criteria for diagnosis include chronic progressive arthritis that is not preceded by brief attacks and chronic symmetric polyarthritis. Additionally, arthralgias, myalgias, or fibromyalgia syndromes alone are not accepted as criteria for musculoskeletal involvement.

Nervous system: lymphocytic meningitis; cranial neuritis, particularly facial palsy (may be bilateral); radiculoneuropathy; or rarely, encephalomyelitis alone or in combination. Encephalomyelitis must be confirmed with evidence of antibody production against *Borrelia burgdorferi* in the cerebrospinal fluid, shown by a higher titer of antibody in the cerebrospinal fluid than in the serum. Headache, fatigue, paresthesias, or mildly stiff neck alone are not accepted as criteria for neurologic involvement.

Cardiovascular system: acute-onset, high-grade (second- or third-degree) atrioventricular conduction defects that resolve in days to weeks and are sometimes associated with myocarditis. Palpitations, bradycardia, bundle-branch block, or myocarditis alone are not accepted as criteria for cardiovascular involvement.

Adapted from Rahn and Malawista [17]; with permission.

None of these assays are standardized. Consequently, there is wide variability among laboratories as to how assays are performed and reported [10•]. The sensitivity, specificity, and normal values are not comparable, and each laboratory must establish its own criteria. If tests are too sensitive, specificity becomes a problem because of the background of cross-reactive antibodies found in most individuals. This high level of cross-reactive antibodies is the reason that most laboratories performing the indirect immunofluorescence assay have established negative cutoffs of 1:64 or more. Laboratories using the ELISA have established their norms and negative cutoffs statistically, using absorbencies of 3 standard deviations (SDs) or more above the mean for healthy control subjects as the cutoff values.

Because current serologic assays use whole *B. burgdorferi* or flagellar antigen preparations, they have a relatively high false-positive rate of 2% or more. This high false-positive rate makes the assay unacceptable for disease screening in areas in which the incidence is low. In most areas, the incidence of Lyme disease is less than one in 1000, which results in a poor predictive value of a positive test result: there will be less than one true-positive result for every 20 false-positive results. Only in clinical situations in which the likelihood of disease is high do current serologic assays have any value. Western blot analysis should be used to confirm all positive ELISAs in which whole *B. burgdorferi* or flagellar antigen preparations were used. The CDC recently established guidelines for the performance and interpretation of Western blot in this disease.

The ELISA offers a marked advantage in testing the cerebrospinal fluid because of its greater sensitivity. The finding that an individual has significant amounts of anti–*B. burgdorferi* antibodies can be interpreted only in the context of the clinical setting, and the cerebrospinal fluid should be examined in all individuals suspected of having CNS disease. Alternatively, patients with CNS infection may have no evidence of anti–*B. burgdorferi* intrathecal antibody production, especially during the early phase of the infection. Individuals without diagnostic levels of antibody in either their serum or their cerebrospinal fluid are highly unlikely to have active *B. burgdorferi* infection, and other reasons for their signs and symptoms should be sought.

TREATMENT

Optimal treatment recommendations for *B. burgdorferi* infection have not been established because of a number of problems (Table 3). On the basis of current knowledge, we can state that β-lactams and tetracyclines are effective against *B. burgdorferi* (Table 4). Although the response to treatment with various tetracyclines and penicillins is good in patients with local infection, studies of early infection must be interpreted with caution [11]. No study to date has clearly defined whether amoxicillin or doxycycline is the gold standard for treatment of early *B. burgdorferi* infection [12–14]. However, our data show that amoxicillin is highly efficacious in preventing the short-term sequelae of Lyme disease (Luft and coworkers, Unpublished data).

Penicillin and ceftriaxone are the most widely used antibiotics for the treatment of serious *B. burgdorferi* infection (Table 4). Acute meningitis and meningoencephalitis resulting from *B. burgdorferi* are usually very responsive to high-dose penicillin therapy. However, there are several instances in which acute CNS infection has progressed despite penicillin therapy. For Bannwarth's syndrome, therapy usually halts the

TABLE 3 PROBLEMS AFFECTING TREATMENT RECOMMENDATIONS FOR LYME DISEASE

In vitro antimicrobial studies

In vitro sensitivity studies have not been conducted in a standardized manner, and their relationship to *in vivo* efficacy has not been established

Some strains of *B. burgdorferi* have a relatively high level of resistance to penicillin

B. burgdorferi is killed *in vitro* only after prolonged incubation with antibiotics

Clinical trials

Few randomized, prospective studies on the treatment of this infection have been published

Response to treatment must be assessed on clinical grounds and not on microbiologic criteria

It remains unclear whether persistent signs and symptoms result from continued infection, permanent tissue damage, or some undefined immune mechanism

TABLE 4 TREATMENT RECOMMENDATIONS FOR LYME DISEASE

Early Lyme disease

Primary agents (oral)

    Doxycycline, 100 mg twice daily for 21 d *or*

    Amoxicillin, 500 mg three times daily for 21 d

Alternative agents (not shown to be as effective as primary agents)

    Cefuroxime axetil, 500 mg twice daily for 21 d

    Clarithromycin, 500 mg twice daily for 21 d

    Azithromycin, 500 mg once daily for 14–21 d

Neurologic manifestations of Lyme disease

Facial nerve palsies

    If finding is isolated, oral doxycycline or amoxicillin as recommended for early disease may be adequate

    If finding is associated with other neurologic manifestations, intravenous therapy (ceftriaxone or penicillin G) is recommended

Lyme meningitis, encephalitis, radiculoneuropathy, and peripheral neuropathy

    Ceftriaxone, 2 g/d intravenously in a single dose for 21–28 d *or*

    Penicillin G, 20 MU/d intravenously in divided doses for 21–28 d

Lyme arthritis

Ceftriaxone, 2 g/d intravenously for 14–28 d

*Doxycycline, 100 mg orally, twice daily for 30 d *or*

*Amoxicillin plus probenecid, 500 mg of each orally, four times daily for 30 d

Lyme carditis

1st and 2nd degree heart block

    Doxycycline, 100 mg orally, twice daily for 21 d *or*

    Amoxicillin, 500 mg orally, three times daily for 21 d

3rd degree heart block

    Ceftriaxone, 2 g/d intravenously for 14–28 d *or*

    Penicillin G, 20 MU/d in four divided doses intravenously for 14–28 d

*Neurologic disease may develop after successful oral treatment of arthritis.

progression of the disease, but as many as 50% of patients continue to have severe neurologic signs, such as spastic paraparesis, after treatment. Similarly, approximately 50% or more of patients with arthritis secondary to *B. burgdorferi* fail to respond to intravenous penicillin therapy. Treatment of ACA with penicillin is successful in approximately 50% of patients, with a similar percentage experiencing continued extracutaneous manifestations. Thus, failure rates as high as 50% or more are commonly reported with penicillin treatment of chronic rheumatologic, dermatologic, or neurologic disease resulting from *B. burgdorferi*. It is not clear whether these treatment failures result from persistent, smoldering infection; immune autoreactivity triggered by the infection; the pathologic changes that occurred before treatment; or some combination of the three. In our experience, ceftriaxone is superior to penicillin in the treatment of late Lyme disease [15,16]. We currently recommend treating patients who have disseminated infection and significant organ involvement resulting from *B. burgdorferi* with ceftriaxone, 2 g once a day for 14 to 28 days.

References and Recommended Reading

Recently published papers of particular interest have been highlighted as:
• Of interest
• Of outstanding interest

1. Lyme disease: United States 1991–1992. *MMWR Morb Mortal Wkly Rep* 1993, 42:345–350.

2. Luft BJ, Dattwyler RJ: Lyme borreliosis: problems in diagnosis and treatment. In *Current Clinical Topics in Infectious Diseases*, vol 10. Edited by Remington JS, Swartz MW. New York: McGraw Hill Publishing Co.; 1989:56–81.

3. Steere AC, Schoen RT: The clinical evolution of Lyme arthritis. *Ann Intern Med* 1987, 107:725–731.

4. Finkel MJ, Halperin JJ: Nervous system Lyme borreliosis: revisited. *Arch Neurol* 1992, 49:102–107.

5.•• Luft BJ, Steinman CR, Schubach WH, *et al.*: Invasion of the central nervous system by *Borrelia burgdorferi* in acute disseminated infection. *JAMA* 1992, 267:1364–1367.

6. Dattwyler RJ, Volkman DJ, Halperin JJ, *et al.*: Specific immune response in Lyme borreliosis. Characterization of T and B cell responses to *Borrelia burgdorferi*. *Ann NY Acad Sci* 1988, 539:93–104.

7. Dattwyler RJ, Volkman DJ, Luft BJ: Immunologic responses in Lyme disease. *Rev Infect Dis* 1989, 6:S1494–S1498.

8. Dattwyler RJ, Volkman DJ, Luft BJ, *et al.*: Seronegative Lyme disease: dissociation of specific T- and B- lymphocyte responses to *Borrelia burgdorferi*. *N Engl J Med* 1988, 319:1441–1446.

9. Dressler F, Yoshnari NH, Steere AC: The T cell proliferative assay in the diagnosis of Lyme disease. *Ann Intern Med* 1991, 115:533–539.

10.• Bakken LL, Case KL, Callister SM, *et al.*: Performance of 45 laboratories participating in a proficiency testing program for Lyme disease serology. *JAMA* 1992, 268:891–895.

11. Steere AC, Hutchinson GJ, Rahn DW, *et al.*: Treatment of the early manifestations of Lyme disease. *Ann Intern Med* 1983, 99:22–26.

12. Massarotti EM, Luger SW, Rahn DW, *et al.*: Treatment of Lyme disease. *Am J Med* 1992, 92:396–403.

13. Dattwyler RJ, Volkman DJ, Conaty SM, *et al.*: Amoxicillin plus probenecid versus doxycycline in patients with erythema migrans. *Lancet* 1990, 336:1404–1406.

14. Nadelman RB, Luger SW, Frank E, *et al.*: Comparison of cefuroxime axetil and doxycycline in the treatment of early Lyme disease. *Ann Intern Med* 1992, 117:273–280.

15. Dattwyler RJ, Halperin JJ, Pass H, Luft BJ: Ceftriaxone as effective therapy in refractory Lyme disease. *J Infect Dis* 1988, 155:1322–1325.

16. Dattwyler RJ, Halperin JJ, Volkman DJ, Luft BJ: Treatment of late Lyme borreliosis: randomized comparison of ceftriaxone and penicillin. *Lancet* 1988, ii:1191–1194.

17. Rahn DW, Malawista SE: Lyme disease: recommendations for diagnosis and treatment. *Ann Intern Med* 1991, 114:472–481.

18. Centers for Disease Control and Prevention: Lyme disease— United States, 1991–1992 *MMWR Morb Mortal Wkly Rep* 1993, 42:345–348.

Select Bibliography

Coyle PK, Dattwyler RJ: Spirochetal infection of the central nervous system. *Infect Dis Clin North Am* 1990, 4:731–746.

Luft BJ, Bosler EM, Dattwyler RJ: Diagnosis of Lyme borreliosis. In *Lyme Disease: Molecular and Immunologic Approaches*. Cold Spring Harbor, NY: Cold Spring Harbor Laboratory Press; 1992:317–324.

Luft BJ, Jiang W, Munoz P, *et al.*: Biochemical and immunological characterization of the surface proteins of *Borrelia burgdorferi*. *Infect Immun* 1989, 57:3637–3645.

Tuberculosis 18

George M. Lordi
Lee B. Reichman

Key Points

- A high index of suspicion is needed for diagnosis of tuberculosis, which has nonspecific symptoms in general and atypical presentation in HIV-infected persons.
- Tuberculin skin test reaction size for positivity depends upon the population tested.
- Prophylactic therapy with isoniazid when indicated prevents the progression of tuberculosis infection to clinically active disease.
- An initial four-drug regimen (isoniazid, rifampin, pyrazinamide, ethambutol) is recommended in persons at risk for drug resistance pending drug susceptibility results.
- Patient compliance with an effective drug regimen is essential for cure.

The number of cases of tuberculosis reported annually in the United States declined from 1953 to 1985, but since 1986 yearly increases have occurred. The main factor in this resurgence of tuberculosis is the occurrence of tuberculosis in persons with HIV infection [1]. The impairment of cell-mediated immunity by the depletion of CD_4 lymphocytes renders this group especially vulnerable.

More than two thirds of cases of tuberculosis in the United States now occur in nonwhite ethnic and racial groups. High-risk minorities include Hispanics, Native Americans, and blacks. Immigrants from Asia, Africa, and Latin America where tuberculosis is prevalent are also at increased risk, as are the poor and residents of correctional facilities, homeless shelters, and nursing homes [2•].

CLASSIFICATION

The classification of tuberculosis is based on the concept of infection and active disease (Table 1) [3••].

CLINICAL MANIFESTATIONS

The symptoms of active tuberculosis are often nonspecific and obscure and are usually chronic. The lungs are the most common site of active disease. The apical and posterior segments of the upper lobe and the superior segments of the lower lobe are most frequently involved.

Extrapulmonary disease—such as tuberculous meningitis, pericarditis, renal tuberculosis, and tuberculous lymphadenopathy—is the major site of presentation in about 15% of cases. Table 2 lists the clinical manifestations of active tuberculosis.

In HIV-infected persons, the clinical presentation is often atypical, particularly in the latter stages of infection after AIDS is diagnosed [4]. In this group, extrapulmonary tuberculosis occurs in 60% to 70% of cases, especially lymphatic and disseminated (miliary) tuberculosis. In patients with pulmonary tuberculosis, apical cavitation is uncommon. Any portion of the lung can be involved, frequently with associated mediastinal or hilar adenopathy [5].

TABLE 1 CLASSIFICATION OF TUBERCULOSIS

Class	Description	Test results
1	Exposure with no evidence of infection	Negative tuberculin skin test
2	Tuberculosis infection without disease	Positive tuberculin skin test; negative bacteriologic and radiographic studies
3	Clinically active tuberculosis	Positive radiographic or clinical evidence; positive cultures

TABLE 2 CLINICAL MANIFESTATIONS OF ACTIVE TUBERCULOSIS

General
Fever
Weight loss
Anorexia
Malaise
Easy fatigability
Night sweats

Pulmonary disease
Chronic productive cough
Hemoptysis (may occur)
Chest pain and dyspnea (unusual)
Crackles over involved areas on physical examination
Dullness and decreased breath sounds on physical
    examination with pulmonary effusion

Extrapulmonary disease
Signs and symptoms vary with the site involved

DIAGNOSIS

Tuberculin Skin Test

A positive tuberculin skin test indicates tuberculous infection is present. The test is performed by injecting 0.1 cm^3 (5 tuberculin units) of purified protein derivative intracutaneously on the volar surface of the forearm. The test is read 48 to 72 hours later, with the diameter of induration determining positivity (Table 3).

A negative tuberculin skin test does not always exclude tuberculous infection or tuberculosis. Associated conditions such as viral exanthems, Hodgkin's disease, sarcoidosis, and overwhelming tuberculosis can decrease the tuberculin reaction. HIV-infected persons can have a false-negative reaction, and only about 33% of patients with AIDS and tuberculosis will have a positive tuberculin reaction [6]. Indications for tuberculin skin testing are summarized in Table 4.

Smears and Cultures

Pulmonary tuberculosis might be suspected by findings on the chest radiograph, but sputum smear and culture are essential for confirmation. Sputum culture is also essential for drug susceptibility studies. Three successive morning sputum specimens should be obtained. Susceptibility studies should be done routinely on all initial isolates. If the sputum smear is positive for acid-fast bacilli, treatment can be started while cultures are pending. Culture results usually take 3 to 6 weeks. Sputum smear and culture results usually correlate, but the culture can be positive even though the sputum smear is negative. It is hoped that gene probes specific for *Mycobacterium tuberculosis* will be routinely available in the future with identification possible within hours.

At times, saline aerosol nebulization may be necessary to induce sputum. Less commonly, fiberoptic bronchoscopy and bronchoalveolar lavage may be necessary to obtain specimens when smears are negative or sputum is unobtainable.

Extrapulmonary Tuberculosis

The diagnosis of extrapulmonary tuberculosis depends on the site. Though a lymphocytic predominance in pleural, peritoneal, or pericardial fluid may suggest tuberculosis, histologic examination and smear and culture of biopsy material are usually needed. With renal tuberculosis, the diagnosis will

TABLE 3 TUBERCULIN SKIN TEST RESULTS

Reaction size	Classification
5 mm	Positive in patients with HIV infection, close contacts of active cases, and persons with chest radiographs consistent with old tuberculosis
10 mm	Positive in intravenous drug users, high-risk minorities (blacks, Native Americans, Hispanics) in foreign born individuals from high-prevalence countries (Africa, Asia, Latin America), in residents of long-term facilities, and in persons with medical conditions that increase the risk of tuberculosis
15 mm	Positive in all other persons

From American Thoracic Society [3••]; with permission.

TABLE 4 INDICATIONS FOR TUBERCULIN TESTING

HIV infection

Chest radiographs consistent with past tuberculosis

Signs and symptoms suggestive of clinically active tuberculosis

Medical conditions that increase the risk of tuberculosis

Contact with persons with clinically active tuberculosis

Belonging to a group at high risk of recent infection with *Mycobacterium tuberculosis* (such as immigrants from Africa, Asia, Latin America, and Oceania; medically underserved populations; personnel and residents in some hospitals, nursing homes, mental institutions, and correctional facilities)

From American Thoracic Society [2•]; with permission.

usually be made by the culture of three consecutive morning urine specimens.

Treatment of tuberculous meningitis can be started based on spinal fluid findings pending culture results. For disseminated (miliary) tuberculosis, bone marrow, lung, or liver biopsies may be necessary.

TREATMENT

Preventive Therapy

The use of isoniazid therapy for persons with tuberculous infection (Class 2) is the mainstay of tuberculosis control in the United States. The aim is to prevent the development of clinically active tuberculosis (Class 3). The effect of isoniazid treatment persists for at least 20 years and presumably for life [7].

Adults are given a single daily dose of 300 mg; for children the dose is 10 mg per kilogram of body weight to a maximum of 300 mg per day. The duration of therapy is from 6 to 12 months. Twelve-month regimens are necessary for persons with HIV infection. Isoniazid cannot be given to everyone with tuberculous infection because of hepatotoxicity. The incidence of isoniazid-associated hepatitis increases with age, especially after age 35. Under that age, all persons with positive reactions should be considered for isoniazid therapy unless there is a contraindication such as liver disease.

Isoniazid is given to persons over age 35 if they are in a group at high risk for the development of active tuberculosis. At greatest risk are close contacts of a patient with an active case. During pregnancy, preventive therapy is postponed until after delivery.

Persons with a positive tuberculin test and with silicosis or with a chest radiograph showing fibrotic infiltration consistent with old, healed tuberculosis now receive 4 months of multidrug chemotherapy instead of preventive therapy.

Table 5 lists high-priority candidates for isoniazid preventive therapy. Once started on isoniazid preventive therapy, patients are monitored monthly for adverse effects, including signs and symptoms of liver damage, and for compliance with medication. Appropriate laboratory studies are done if toxicity is suspected. Ten percent to 20% of persons taking isoniazid will have serum transaminase elevations. The levels usually return to normal despite continuation of the drug. The drug should be discontinued if hepatitis is suspected or if transaminase levels are greater than three to five times normal. Baseline and periodic measurements of transaminase levels should be done for patients over 35 years of age.

Isoniazid can also cause peripheral neuropathy resulting from increased urinary pyridoxine excretion. Pyridoxine supplementation should be given to alcoholic patients, patients with seizure disorders, and pregnant patients.

TABLE 5 HIGH-PRIORITY CANDIDATES FOR TUBERCULOSIS PREVENTIVE THERAPY

Preventive therapy recommended with positive tuberculin tests, regardless of age, for:

Persons with HIV infection

Close contacts of persons with clinically active tuberculosis

Recent tuberculin skin test converters

≥10 mm increase within a 2-year period for those<35 years old

≥15 mm increase within a 2-year period for those >35 years old

Persons with medical conditions that increase the risk of tuberculosis (diabetes mellitus, corticosteroid therapy, immunosuppressive therapy, intravenous drug use, end-stage renal disease, some hematologic and reticuloendothelial diseases, and conditions associated with rapid weight loss)

From American Thoracic Society [2•]; with permission.

Clinically Active Disease

The treatment of pulmonary and extrapulmonary tuberculosis is essentially the same. The patient has to be compliant with an effective drug regimen. Characteristics of first-line drugs are summarized in Table 6.

Second-line antituberculous drugs are used in cases of treatment failure and drug resistance. All these drugs have limitations and are difficult to use. Their use requires subspecialty consultation. Characteristics of second-line agents are summarized in Table 7.

A combination of drugs is required to prevent the development of drug-resistant organisms. For adults, a 6-month drug regimen of isoniazid (300 mg per day) and rifampin (600 mg per day) with pyrazinamide (15–30 mg/kg per day) given during the first 2 months of the regimen is recommended. This regimen is highly effective, with very low relapse rates [9]. All three drugs are given in a single daily dose. Isoniazid and rifampin are given as a fixed dose combination.

For noncompliant patients, streptomycin as a parenteral agent is useful and can be given in place of pyrazinamide. Total dose should be limited to not more than 120 g [10]. Isoniazid and rifampin alone for 9 months is an alternative, but less useful, regimen.

Ethambutol is added to the basic regimen whenever primary drug resistance to isoniazid is suspected, such as in immigrants from Mexico and Southeast Asia. If drug susceptibility studies confirm resistance, treatment, including ethambutol, is continued for at least 12 months. If no resistance is found, ethambutol is discontinued.

Treatment of children is essentially the same as that of adults except for dosage adjustment [11]. Because visual acuity is difficult to monitor in children, ethambutol is not used.

In tuberculosis associated with pregnancy, the 9-month regimen of isoniazid and rifampin is preferred. Aminoglycosides such as streptomycin are not used because of the risk of fetal ototoxicity. Pyrazinamide is not used because its safety in pregnancy has not been determined. Breast feeding is not contraindicated during antituberculous treatment [12].

HIV Infection

HIV-infected and AIDS patients with tuberculosis resulting from susceptible organisms respond to the standard isoniazid, rifampin, and pyrazinamide regimen. Treatment with isoniazid and rifampin is continued for a minimum of 9 months and for at least 6 months after culture conversion. Ethambutol is added to the regimen if disseminated tuberculosis or central nervous system involvement is present or suspected [6]. It is best to administer ethambutol to all patients with HIV infection until the results of drug susceptibility studies are reported.

Monitoring Therapy

Sputum smears and cultures are the best guide to therapeutic response. More than 90% of patients on the 6-month regimen will have negative sputum cultures within 3 months. Responding patients will show weight gain, absence of fever, and diminished cough. Within 2 weeks, patients with susceptible organisms can be considered noninfectious [13]. Monthly monitoring for clinical progress and drug toxicity is standard after hospital discharge. In cases of pulmonary tuberculosis, a chest radiograph can be done at 3 months and at the conclusion of therapy to demonstrate clearing of infiltrate.

TABLE 6   DRUGS FOR THE INITIAL TREATMENT OF TUBERCULOSIS

Drug	Daily dose (adults)	Maximum daily dose	Selected adverse effects
Isoniazid	5 mg/kg	300 mg	Peripheral neuropathy
			Hepatic enzyme elevation
			Hepatitis
			Hypersensitivity
Rifampin	10 mg/kg	600 mg	Hepatitis
			Fever
			Nausea and vomiting
			Thrombocytopenia
			Orange discoloration of urine and secretions
Pyrazinamide	15–25 mg/kg	2 g	Hyperuricemia
			Hepatotoxicity
			Gastrointestinal distress
Ethambutol	15–25 mg/kg	2.5 g	Optic neuritis[†] (decreased visual acuity, red-green color discrimination)
			Skin rash
Streptomycin	15 mg/kg*	1 g*	Ototoxicity
			Nephrotoxicity

*If age >60, daily dose of streptomycin is 10 mg/kg, with maximum dose of 750 mg.
†Incidence is very low if a daily dose of 15 mg/kg is used [9].
From Centers for Disease Control, American Thoracic Society [8••].

TABLE 7 SECOND-LINE ANTITUBERCULOSIS DRUGS

Drug	Daily dose (adults)	Maximum daily dose	Selected adverse effects
Capreomycin	15–30 mg/kg	1 g	Renal toxicity Auditory and vesticular toxicity
Kanamycin	15–30 mg/kg	1 g	Renal toxicity Auditory toxicity
Ethionamide	5–20 mg/kg	1 g	Hepatotoxicity Gastrointestinal distress Hypersensitivity
Cycloserine	15–20 mg/kg	1 g	Personality change Psychosis Convulsions Rash
Para-aminosalicylate	150 mg/kg	12 g	Gastrointestinal distress Hepatotoxicity Hypersensitivity Sodium load

From Centers for Disease Control, American Thoracic Society [8••].

Failure of sputum conversion to negative within 3 to 4 months constitutes treatment failure and raises the possibility of drug-resistant organisms. The main cause of treatment failure, however, is noncompliance—the patient has not taken the medication properly.

Treatment regimens for drug-resistant tuberculosis—especially to drugs other than isoniazid—are complex, and subspecialty consultation is necessary in all cases of drug resistance. Treatment for drug-resistant tuberculosis is guided by drug susceptibility studies. At least two and preferably three drugs to which the organisms are sensitive are started. Second-line agents are usually necessary. Treatment regimens of 12 to 18 months are required. Directly observed supervised therapy can be used to enhance compliance.

MULTIDRUG RESISTANT TUBERCULOSIS

Outbreaks of tuberculosis resistant to multiple drugs are being reported. About 90% of such cases have occurred in HIV-infected patients. Noncompliance with medication results in the emergence of resistant bacilli, which are then transmitted to susceptible contacts, particularly in institutional settings such as prisons, hospitals, and homeless shelters.

The outbreaks have been characterized by rapid progression from infection to active disease and by high mortality (±80%). Most patients are resistant to the two best antituberculous drugs—isoniazid and rifampin; some have been resistant to all the first-line drugs [14].

Preventing transmission is essential. Centers for Disease Control and Prevention guidelines to prevent the transmission of tuberculosis in health care settings should be followed. Patients with suspected drug-resistant tuberculosis should be isolated until smears are negative for acid-fast bacillus [15•].

REFERENCES AND RECOMMENDED READING

Recently published papers of particular interest have been highlighted as:
• Of interest
•• Of outstanding interest

1. Barnes PF, Block AB, Davidson PT, Snider DE Jr: Tuberculosis in patients with human immunodeficiency virus infection. *N Engl J Med* 1991, 321:1644–1650.

2.• American Thoracic Society: Control of tuberculosis in the United States. *Am Rev Respir Dis* 1992, 146:1623–1633.

3.•• American Thoracic Society: Diagnostic standards and classification of tuberculosis. *Am Rev Respir Dis* 1990, 142:725–735.

4. Murray JR, Mills J: Pulmonary infectious complications of human immunodeficiency virus infection. Part I. *Am Rev Respir Dis* 1990, 141:1356–1372.

5. American Thoracic Society: Mycobacterioses and the acquired immunodeficiency syndrome. *Am Rev Respir Dis* 1987, 136:492–496.

6. Reider HL, Cauthen GM, Bloch AB, *et al.*: Tuberculosis and acquired immunodeficiency syndrome, Florida. *Arch Intern Med* 1989, 149:1268–1273.

7. Committee on Isoniazid Preventive Treatment, Daily WC, Chairman: Preventive treatment of tuberculosis. *Chest* 1985, 875:1285–1325.

8.•• Centers for Disease Control, American Thoracic Society: *Core Curriculum on Tuberculosis*, edn 2. Washington, DC: Government Printing Office; 1991.

9. American Thoracic Society: Treatment of tuberculosis and tuberculosis infection in adults and children. *Am Rev Respir Dis* 1986, 134:355–363.

10. Perez-Stable EJ, Hopewell PC: Current tuberculosis treatment regimens. *Clin Chest Med* 1989, 10:323–339.

11. Smith MHD: Tuberculosis in children and adolescents. *Clin Chest Med* 1989, 10:381–395.

12. Snider DE: Pregnancy and tuberculosis. *Chest* 1984, 865:105–135.

13. Rouillon A, Perdrizet S, Parrot R: Transmission of tubercle bacilli: The effects of chemotherapy. *Tubercle* 1976, 51:276–299.

14. Snider DE, Roper WL: The new tuberculosis. *N Engl J Med* 1992, 326:703–705.

15.• Centers for Disease Control: Nosocomial transmission of multidrug resistant tuberculosis among HIV-infected persons—Florida and New York, 1988–1991. *MMWR Morb Mortal Wkly Rep* 1991, 40:585–591.

SELECT BIBLIOGRAPHY

American Thoracic Society: Treatment of tuberculosis and tuberculosis infection in adults and children. *Am J Respir Crit Care Med* 1994, 149:1359–1374.

Barnes PF, Barrows SA: Tuberculosis in the 1990's. *Ann Intern Med* 1993, 119:400–410.

Iseman MD: Treatment of multidrug-resistant tuberculosis. *N Engl J Med* 1993, 329:784–791.

Schlossberg D, ed: *Tuberculosis*, edn 3. New York: Springer-Verlag; 1993.

Community-Acquired Fungal Diseases 19

George A. Sarosi

> **Key Points**
> - Community-acquired fungal diseases are the result of inhalation of the infecting aerosol; it is important that a careful history and laboratory examination be performed to provide accurate diagnosis.
> - The decision of whether to treat an individual with a community-acquired fungal infection requires an understanding of the natural history of the disease and the clinical illness in the individual.
> - Amphotericin B remains the most potent agent for the treatment for community-acquired fungal diseases, but because of its increased toxicity, the available oral agents are gaining increasing acceptance.
> - Ketoconazole, while still an effective agent, is hampered by its toxicity; the newer agents, fluconazole and itraconazole, have significant effectiveness and markedly reduced toxicity.

The endemic mycoses—histoplasmosis, blastomycosis, and coccidioidomycosis—are relatively common and seldom life-threatening illnesses in North America. The causative fungi share a number of characteristics: they are soil-dwelling organisms, they require organic nitrogen for growth, and their reproduction in nature is influenced by conditions of heat and moisture. All three organisms grow as molds in soil, and their spores are the infecting agents. They cause human or mammalian disease when the sites of growth are disturbed and an aerosol is produced that contains the infecting particles.

Following inhalation, these infecting particles lodge in the alveoli, where the spores convert to their respective pathogenic phase. For histoplasmosis and blastomycosis, this means conversion to the yeast phase, whereas for coccidioidomycosis, the conversion is to the giant spherule (the tissue phase of the infection).

The severity of symptoms after inhalation of the spores depends on the size of the infecting aerosol, as well as on the underlying immune state of the host. Most immunologically intact hosts who acquire their infection in open spaces (when the number of infecting organisms is likely to be small) will have either a very mild illness or no illness at all. Patients who inhale a large infecting aerosol (when the inhalation occurs in a closed, unventilated space) will develop extensive and potentially lethal airspace disease.

The vast majority of primary infections are restricted to the lung. Progressive dissemination outside the lung in normal hosts is infrequent, even in blastomycosis and coccidioidomycosis. When progressive dissemination occurs in histoplasmosis, the host is usually immunocompromised [1].

DIAGNOSIS

Generally speaking, the diagnosis of individual fungal infections depends on the diagnostic acumen of the examining physician. Because the vast majority of primary infections result in little or no symptomatology, most are not diagnosed during the acute illness. Most of what is known about the acute disease in these three fungal infections comes from careful study of large, usually community-wide, outbreaks. The entire clinical spectrum for all three is well described.

Although the acute, self-limited illness is seldom diagnosed, more chronic or disseminated forms of the infection usually result in greater symptomatology and thus lead to increased investigation. Most of these infections can be diagnosed by careful evaluation of available serologic information, study of respiratory secretions, or deep tissue biopsies.

Histoplasmosis

Although skin testing for histoplasmosis is well developed and a highly effective skin test antigen is available commercially, the histoplasmin skin test is not thought to be useful for the diagnosis of individual cases, and because of its propensity to influence the interpretation of the serologic test results, I recommend strongly against its use as a diagnostic test for sporadic cases of histoplasmosis. The skin test is best thought of as an excellent epidemiologic tool and should be so used (Table 1) [2].

If the diagnosis remains elusive or rapid progression of the disease precludes waiting for serologic confirmation, deep tissue biopsy is indicated. In addition to careful culturing of the specimen, the biopsy material should be examined using special stains. Most laboratories use one of the many variations of the silver stain. In my experience, the periodic acid–Schiff stain should also be used to increase the diagnostic yield.

Sporadically occurring acute histoplasmosis is exceedingly common. More than 99% of infected patients will have a self-limited disease [3]. Fewer than half of those infected will have any symptoms, and 10% to 15% will develop a symptomatic illness. When acute histoplasmosis is considered in the differential diagnosis, the best diagnostic test is serologic evaluation. The standard complement-fixing serologic test, although it takes approximately 3 to 6 weeks to reach its height, generally confirms the diagnostic impression. A titer rising to four times the initial titer or a single titer to the yeast phase of 1:32 or greater in the setting of a compatible illness is highly suggestive of acute histoplasmosis [2]. The more readily available immunodiffusion test unfortunately has an extremely high false-negative rate, and after 6 weeks, only approximately half of the patients with otherwise proven acute histoplasmosis will have positive test results. Although a positive test finding may be quite helpful, a negative finding cannot be taken as an indication of the absence of the disease. Recently, a new test that has become available in a single research laboratory appears to have much greater sensitivity and specificity [4]. This radioimmunoassay measuring the histoplasma polysaccharide antigen is unfortunately not available commercially.

The more chronic, indolent form of pulmonary histoplasmosis, an illness that mimics reinfection tuberculosis in that it involves the upper lobes of the lung, can usually be diagnosed quite readily by careful culturing of expectorated sputum [5]. The organisms are remarkably hardy, and if local facilities do not permit adequate culturing of the organism, the sputum may be mailed to regional reference laboratories without fear of losing the organism. Although isolation of the fungus is relatively simple, definite identification usually takes from 3 to 4 weeks. When the diagnosis is clinically suspected, therefore, the laboratory should be informed because it may be able to confirm or strongly suggest the presence of histoplasmosis earlier than the time required for definite laboratory diagnosis.

In patients whose T-cell–mediated immunity is compromised either by an underlying illness or by chemotherapy, the normal defenses against progressive dissemination of the fungus are lost. In these patients, the disease is a rapidly progressive, highly symptomatic illness in which the infection involves the cells of the reticuloendothelial system. The easiest and fastest way to diagnose suspected progressive disseminated histoplasmosis is with bone marrow biopsy and culture. The immediate staining of a bone marrow biopsy specimen with either Wright's stain or the periodic acid–Schiff stain

TABLE 1 PREFERRED MODALITIES FOR THE DIAGNOSIS OF COMMUNITY-ACQUIRED FUNGAL DISEASES IN NORTH AMERICA			
Type of infection	Histoplasmosis	Blastomycosis	Coccidioidomycosis
Acute			
No respiratory compromise	Serology	KOH	Serology
	±Culture	Culture*	PAP and silver stain[†]
			Culture*
Ventilatory failure	Lung biopsy	Lung biopsy	Lung biopsy
Chronic pulmonary	±Culture*	KOH	Serology
	Serology	Culture*	PAP and silver stain[†]
			Culture*
Progressive disseminated	Bone marrow and blood culture	KOH	Serology
		Culture*	PAP or silver stain[†]
			Culture*

*Culture of respiratory secretions or other biologic materials.
[†]Respiratory secretions or tissue.
KOH—10% potassium hydroxide digestion of respiratory secretions or other biologic material; PAP—Papanicolaou preparation; ±—with or without.

documents the yeast phase of *Histoplasma capsulatum* within phagocytes of the bone marrow [6]. Because of the high-grade fungemia, blood cultures using the lysis-centrifugation system, as well as bone marrow cultures, are likely to yield the organism [7•].

Blastomycosis

Blastomycosis is very similar to histoplasmosis except that it is far less common [8]. The ecologic niche for blastomyces is much more restricted; it appears to require a much more specific mixture of moisture and organic nitrogen and is likely to depend on other, as yet poorly defined soil conditions as well [9].

In patients suspected of having blastomycosis, an expectorated sputum sample (or other biologic material, such as pus aspirated from an abscess or bronchial washings) should be digested with 10% potassium hydroxide and examined under reduced light at 100 times magnification. The potassium hydroxide successfully digests all extraneous material and leaves the large yeasts visible. In addition, respiratory secretions obtained at the time of bronchoscopy can also be prepared with the Papanicolaou smear, which will also identify the large yeasts, thereby establishing the diagnosis [8]. Culture of these respiratory specimens is also an excellent way to recover the organism. The organism grows readily in standard laboratory mycologic media, but 3 to 4 weeks are required before the definitive diagnosis can be ascertained. As with histoplasmosis, the laboratory should be alerted to the possibility of blastomycosis. Frequently, a tentative diagnosis can be suggested in as few as 5 days.

The immunologic diagnosis of blastomycosis is not nearly as well developed as that of histoplasmosis. There is no commercially available blastomycin skin test. Serologic testing is not nearly as well developed in blastomycosis as in histoplasmosis. The standard complement fixation serologic test has an unacceptably high false-negative rate, and patients with histoplasmosis are also likely to have cross-reactive antibodies. The more recently available tests, such as the enzyme immunoassay, have increased diagnostic sensitivity at the cost of some decrease in specificity. Several new antigens are under investigation, but they are not available commercially. Even though a positive serologic test result should not be accepted as proof of the infection, all such positive results should be followed up by more invasive tests to establish the suspected diagnosis [2].

Because of the organism's propensity to involve the skin or bones, biopsy of all visible and suspected lesions frequently yields the organism. Careful histopathologic evaluation, especially with the periodic acid–Schiff stain, frequently reveals the large, budding yeasts of blastomycosis. The silver stain is also useful.

Coccidioidomycosis

During the acute infection, the organism is frequently recovered from the sputum of symptomatic patients. The density of the organisms is fairly high in involved lung parenchyma, and whenever this infection is suspected, sputum should be obtained, whether by expectoration, by induction with nebu-

lized saline, or by the use of invasive techniques, to allow immediate evaluation [10]. In my hands, the best single test is the Papanicolaou smear, but other investigators have obtained similar results with the methenamine silver technique. The potassium hydroxide technique is far less sensitive than the other available techniques. Histopathologic examination of all suspected biopsy material may yield the fungus. The large giant spherule is frequently seen on standard hematoxylin-eosin staining, but additional special stains should also be used.

Unlike in the other endemic mycoses, in which serodiagnosis is seldom timely and is recommended only in the context of an epidemiologic investigation, in coccidioidomycosis, serodiagnosis is highly developed and is helpful in diagnosis and management [11]. Moreover, serial testing not only provides excellent diagnostic results but also allows careful following of the course of the clinical infection and provides important prognostic information. A rising titer is worrisome and should lead to renewed efforts to define the extent of the disease. Although no single titer is truly diagnostic of extrapulmonary dissemination, most patients with high or rising titers are in danger of disease progression, with its attendant worsening prognosis.

Although most available literature deals with various older serologic tests, most material is now processed by immunodiffusion. Immunodiffusion testing allows recognition of both IgM and IgG antibodies. When IgM antibody is recognized, with or without IgG antibody, then the infection is acute, whereas if only IgG antibodies are recognized, the infection is usually either a longer-standing one or a reactivation from previous foci. Because the immunodiffusion test is not readily quantified, I recommend follow-up of all positive test results with the complement-fixing test in the reference laboratory of the University of California at Davis. Titers of 1:16 or higher should be followed up rigorously because in these patients, the risk of extrapulmonary dissemination is high [11].

When meningeal involvement is suspected, the cerebrospinal fluid should be submitted for immunologic testing. A titer of 1:2 (some authorities accept 1:1 dilution also) is diagnostic of coccidioidomycosis. The only exception is when vertebral osteomyelitis is present: occasionally, a weakly positive cerebrospinal fluid titer is noted without clinical meningitis.

Cultural recovery of the organism is not difficult, but it is quite hazardous. Only laboratories well equipped in biohazard management should be asked to grow specimens thought to contain *Coccidioides* spp because the risk for laboratory personnel is very high when inexperienced laboratories work on this material. Because of this increased risk, many laboratories have moved to the exoantigen testing, which allows growth of the organism without the cultures ever having to be opened.

There are two well-established skin tests for the diagnosis of coccidioidomycosis: one is coccidioidin, which is made from culture filtrates of the mycelial growth, and the other uses spherulin, which is made from the culture filtrates of the spherules. Although both skin tests are well standardized, the same caveat that applies to the other endemic mycoses should apply to coccidioidomycosis: a positive coccidioidin skin test result in the setting of a compatible chest syndrome does not conclusively establish the coccidioidal etiology of the disease; it could easily have been the residual of a previous infection. Only when the previous skin test status is known (*ie*, negative) can a positive skin test result be interpreted with certainty to represent a recent infection.

TREATMENT

In general, the vast majority of patients with acute community-acquired fungal disease do not require treatment. Clearly, the vast majority of patients (in excess of 99%) with acute histoplasmosis recover spontaneously without any drug therapy [3]. Although self-limited blastomycosis has been well recognized and accepted widely, it is still unclear what percentage of infected individuals with acute blastomycosis have self-limited disease [12]. Acute coccidioidomycosis tends to produce somewhat more acute and serious illness, and there is no sure way of identifying patients whose disease is likely to become worse when left untreated (Table 2) [10].

Histoplasmosis

Patients with acute pulmonary histoplasmosis whose illness is so extensive as to interfere with gas exchange should receive intravenous amphotericin B until clearing and clinical recovery occur. Complete clearing of the pulmonary infiltrate is not necessary, but immediate intervention may be life saving in patients who developed histoplasmosis following inhalation of a large aerosol. After successful stabilization of the illness with amphotericin B, many authorities recommend the additional use of an orally active agent, and clearly the best agent has

been itraconazole [13•]. Although ketoconazole is also effective, it is attractive mainly because of its lower price, and its limitations must be recognized [14].

Progressive disseminated histoplasmosis, especially in immunocompromised patients, should be treated with amphotericin B until improvement or stabilization occurs, and patients should then receive prolonged treatment with itraconazole. In patients coinfected with HIV, lifelong suppressive therapy with itraconazole is needed to prevent relapses [15•].

Blastomycosis

Although acute, self-limited pulmonary blastomycosis does occur, it is impossible to determine with certainty which patients will develop progressive disease and which are likely to have spontaneous resolution. For this reason, all patients whose air exchange mechanism is not seriously impaired might benefit from a period of watchful waiting [16]. If the patient's condition deteriorates, immediate antifungal therapy should be considered. In patients whose disease does not progress under observation, drug therapy is probably not warranted. Over the last few years, itraconazole has emerged as the drug of first choice for non–life-threatening, nonmeningeal blastomycosis. A relatively small dose (400 mg/d) is highly effective in immunologically intact and non–critically ill patients [13•]. Ketoconazole is also highly effective, but its greater gastrointestinal toxicity makes its use more problematic [14,17]. Amphotericin B remains the drug of choice for life-threatening or meningeal blastomycosis [8]. Coinfection with HIV is uncommon and always requires amphotericin B therapy, followed by lifelong suppressive treatment with itraconazole [18•].

TABLE 2 TREATMENT OF COMMUNITY-ACQUIRED FUNGAL DISEASES OF NORTH AMERICA			
Type of infection	Histoplasmosis	Blastomycosis	Coccidioidomycosis
Acute			
No respiratory compromise	Observation	Observation; if progressive, keto-conazole, 400–800 mg/d for 6 mo, *or* itraconazole, 400 mg/d for 6 mo	Observation; if high risk, flucona-zole, 400 mg/d, duration unknown
Ventilatory failure	Amphotericin B, 500–1000 mg *or* until stable	Amphotericin B, 500–1000 mg until stable, followed by ketoconazole or itraconazole for 6 mo	Amphotericin B, 1500–2000 mg until stable, followed by flucona-zole for 6 mo
Chronic pulmonary	Ketoconazole *or* itraconazole for 6 mo *or* Amphotericin B, 35 mg/kg total dose	Ketoconazole or itraconazole for 6 mo *or* amphotericin B, 2000 mg total dose	Fluconazole for 12 mo *or* ampho-tericin B, 2000–3000 mg
Progressive disseminated			
Normal host	Amphotericin B, 500–1000 mg, followed by itraconazole for 6 mo	Ketoconazole or itraconazole for 6 mo *or* amphotericin B, 2000 mg total dose	Amphotericin B, 2000–3000 mg total dose *or* fluconazole for 12 mo
T-cell immuno-suppressed	Amphotericin B, 500–1000 mg, followed by itraconazole for life	Amphotericin B, 2000 mg total dose, followed by itraconazole for life	Amphotericin B, 2000–3000 mg total dose followed by fluconazole for life
Meningeal	Amphotericin B, dose and duration unknown (rare)	Amphotericin B, 2000 mg or more, until clear	Fluconazole for 12 mo or more *or* amphotericin B, 2000–3000 mg total dose plus amphotericin B intrathecally

Coccidioidomycosis

As yet no clear evidence indicates that the treatment of symptomatic patients with acute coccidioidomycosis is useful [19••]. Nevertheless, in endemic areas, most practitioners do treat patients with acute disease, especially those who are at high risk for progression, such as blacks, Filipinos, diabetics, and immunocompromised patients. Currently, the treatment of choice appears to be fluconazole, 200 to 400 mg/d administered for weeks to months. A more specific recommendation cannot be made because the use of this drug in this syndrome is totally unproven and is based on more suggestive information in the use of fluconazole in the chronic illness. For patients whose acute coccidioidomycosis leads to air exchange problems, most authorities recommend the immediate use of amphotericin B, with a switch made to fluconazole after the patient's clinical condition has stabilized. Persistent pulmonary or extrapulmonary coccidioidomycosis requires treatment. When the meninges are involved, immediate treatment is mandatory. It is unclear whether any of the currently available modalities is likely to produce a lasting cure. In severely ill patients, amphotericin B intravenously, along with the intercurrent administration of amphotericin B intracisternally, is recommended. For patients with more stable conditions, the use of 400 to 800 mg of fluconazole daily has resulted in survival for long periods, with good quality of life [20••]. It is, however, highly unlikely that in the foreseeable future we will be able to talk about the "cure" of coccidioidomycosis with drug therapy.

REFERENCES AND RECOMMENDED READING

Recently published papers of particular interest have been highlighted as:
• Of interest
•• Of outstanding interest

1. Davis SF, Sarosi GA: Pulmonary mycoses. In *Pulmonary and Critical Care Medicine*, edn 1. Edited by Bone RC, Dantzker DR, George RB, *et al*. Chicago: Mosby–Year Book; 1993:1–24.

2. Davis SF, Sarosi GA: Role of serodiagnostic tests and skin tests in the diagnosis of fungal disease. *Clin Chest Med* 1987, 8:135–146.

3. Goodwin RA Jr, Lloyd JE, DesPrez RM: Histoplasmosis in normal hosts. *Medicine (Baltimore)* 1981, 60:231–266.

4. Wheat LJ, Kohler RB, Tewari RP: Diagnosis of disseminated histoplasmosis by detection of *Histoplasma capsulatum* antigen in serum and urine specimens. *N Engl J Med* 1986, 314:83–88.

5. Goodwin RA Jr, Ownes FT, Snell JD, *et al*.: Chronic pulmonary histoplasmosis. *Medicine (Baltimore)* 1979, 55:413–452.

6. Davies SF, Khan M, Sarosi GA: Disseminated histoplasmosis in immunological suppressed patients: occurrence in non-endemic areas. *Am J Med* 1978, 64:94–100.

7.• Wheat LJ, Connoly-Stringfield PA, Baker RL, *et al*.: Disseminated histoplasmosis in the acquired immunodeficiency syndrome: clinical findings, diagnosis and treatment, and review of the literature. *Medicine (Baltimore)* 1990, 69:361–374.

8. Sarosi GA, Davies SF: Blastomycosis: state of the art. *Am Rev Respir Dis* 1978, 117:929–956.

9. Klein BS, Vergeront JM, Weeks RJ, *et al*.: Isolation of *Blastomyces dermatitidis* in soil associated with a large outbreak of blastomycosis in Wisconsin. *N Engl J Med* 1986, 314:529–534.

10. Drutz DJ, Cantanzaro AZ: Coccidioidomycosis: state of the art. Part I. *Am Rev Respir Dis* 1978, 117:559–585.

11. Smith CE, Saito MT, Beard RR, *et al*.: Serologic tests in the diagnosis and prognosis of coccidioidomycosis. *Am J Hygiene* 1950, 52:1–21.

12. Sarosi GA, Hammerman JK, Tosh FE, *et al*.: Clinical features of acute pulmonary blastomycosis. *N Engl J Med* 1974, 290:540–543.

13.• Dismukes WE, Bradsher RW Jr, Cloud GC, *et al*.: Itraconazole therapy for blastomycosis and histoplasmosis. *Am J Med* 1992, 93:489–497.

14. Mycosis Study Group: Treatment of blastomycosis and histoplasmosis with ketoconazole. *Ann Intern Med* 1985, 103:861–873.

15.• Wheat LJ, Hafner R, Wulfsohn M, *et al*.: Prevention of relapse of histoplasmosis with itraconazole in patients with the acquired immunodeficiency syndrome. *Ann Intern Med* 1993, 118:610–616.

16. Sarosi GA, Davies SF, Phillips JR: Self-limited blastomycosis: a report of 39 cases. *Semin Respir Infect* 1986, 1:40–44.

17. Bradsher RW, Rice DC, Abernathy RS: Ketoconazole therapy for endemic blastomycosis. *Ann Intern Med* 1985, 103:872–875.

18.• Pappas PG, Pottage JC, Powderly WG, *et al*.: Blastomycosis in patients with the acquired immunodeficiency syndrome. *Ann Intern Med* 1992, 116:847–853.

19.•• Galgiani JN: Coccidioidomycosis. *West J Med* 1993, 119:28–35.

20.•• Galgiani JN, Catanzaro A, Cloud GA, *et al*.: Fluconazole therapy for coccidioidal meningitis. *Ann Intern Med* 1993, 119:28–35.

Infections in Cancer Patients 20

Kenneth V.I. Rolston
Gerald P. Bodey

Key Points

- Temperature of 101°F (38.3°C) that is not associated with the administration of pyrogenic substances indicates the presence of infection until proven otherwise.
- Characteristic manifestations are often absent or blunted; untreated infections can disseminate rapidly.
- More than half the infections are caused by gram-positive organisms, but gram-negative organisms remain a substantial threat.
- Organisms of "low virulence" or "nonpathogenic" organisms can cause serious infection and must not be ignored.
- The distribution of predominant pathogens and their susceptibility to antimicrobial agents varies in different institutions.
- Broad-spectrum antimicrobial therapy must be instituted promptly, as delays result in suboptimal responses.

Infections continue to be among the most common complications in patients with neoplastic disorders. The frequency of infection is related to the type of underlying malignancy and is often related to the degree and duration of neutropenia. Most infections occur in patients who are no longer responding to the therapy for their neoplasm, and multiple episodes of infection in the same patient are not uncommon. In addition, the spectrum of infection has been constantly changing because of alterations in chemotherapeutic regimens, the widening application of bone marrow transplantation, the increasing use of vascular access devices, and the development of newer antimicrobial agents for prophylaxis and therapy. Although it is now possible to treat most bacterial infections successfully, patients surviving these infections become susceptible to fungal, viral, and protozoal infections. The recent emergence of multidrug-resistant bacterial pathogens is beginning to cause concern. Future efforts need to be directed toward these challenging issues and toward strategies for the prevention of infection and the restoration of immune function.

THE SPECTRUM OF INFECTION

The tendency to lump all immunocompromised cancer patients into one category should be avoided because this implies that their infectious problems and the approaches to their treatment are similar. Table 1 lists the predominant defects in host defense mechanisms associated with various neoplastic disorders and the infectious agents most often found in patients who have these defects. The following examples illustrate the importance of recognizing the defects in host defense mechanisms and their impact on the predominant infections.

Patients with acute myelogenous leukemia and hairy cell leukemia are usually neutropenic; consequently, they often develop infections caused by gram-positive cocci, gram-negative bacilli, *Candida* spp, and *Aspergillus* spp (Fig. 1). Patients

TABLE 1 DEFECTS IN HOST DEFENSE MECHANISMS AND INFECTIOUS AGENTS ASSOCIATED WITH VARIOUS NEOPLASTIC DISORDERS AND THERAPIES		
Disease or therapy	**Predominant defect**	**Common infectious agents**
Acute leukemia, aplastic anemia	Neutropenia (< 500 neutrophils/mm³)	Gram-positive cocci, gram-negative bacilli, *Candida* spp, *Aspergillus* spp, *Fusarium* spp, Zygomycetes
Hairy cell leukemia	Neutropenia, monocytopenia, impaired lymphocyte function	Gram-positive cocci, gram-negative bacilli, mycobacteria (including nontuberculous)
Chronic lymphocytic leukemia, multiple myeloma	Hypogammaglobulinemia	Encapsulated organisms (*Streptococcus pneumoniae, Haemophilus influenzae, Neisseria meningitidis*)
Hodgkin's disease, AIDS	Impaired T-lymphocyte response	*Pneumocystis* spp, *Cryptococcus* spp, mycobacteria, *Toxoplasma* spp, *Cryptosporidium* spp, *Salmonella* spp, *Listeria* spp, *Candida* spp, herpesviruses
Bone marrow transplantation	Neutropenia, increased activity of suppressor T lymphocytes	Gram-positive cocci, gram-negative bacilli, herpesviruses, *Candida* spp, *Aspergillus* spp, *Fusarium* spp, Zygomycetes
Lung cancer, gynecologic malignancy	Local obstruction, tissue necrosis	Gram-negative bacilli, gram-positive cocci, anaerobes (mixed, polymicrobial infections)
Breast cancer	Tissue necrosis	Gram-positive cocci, gram-negative bacilli
Use of central venous catheters	Breach of integument	Gram-positive cocci and bacilli, gram-negative bacilli, *Candida* spp
Use of urinary catheters	Mucosal breach	Gram-negative bacilli, gram-positive cocci, *Candida* spp
Splenectomy	Impaired antibody production	*Streptococcus pneumoniae, Haemophilus influenzae, Capnocytophaga* spp, *Babesia* spp, *Neisseria* spp

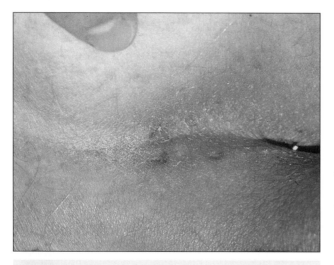

FIGURE 1 Cutaneous hemorrhagic lesions (ecthyma gangrenosum) in a neutropenic patient with *Pseudomonas aeruginosa* bacteremia (*see* Color Plate).

with hairy cell leukemia, however, also have impaired lymphocyte function and monocytopenia, resulting in an increased incidence of mycobacterial and viral infections. Anaerobic infections are uncommon in most patients with cancer, but they often play a significant role in patients with gynecologic and intestinal malignancies, who may have radiation damage to the bowel or infected tumor masses (Fig. 2). Bone marrow transplant recipients are susceptible to the usual infections associated with neutropenia during the immediate (20 to 30 days) posttransplant period. However,

several months after successful engraftment, they have increased suppressor T-lymphocyte activity, resulting in an increase in viral and in some bacterial and protozoal infections (*eg*, cytomegalovirus, other herpes viruses, *Pneumocystis carinii* infection). Thus, knowledge of the different types of infection associated with various defects in host defense mechanisms will lead to more appropriate approaches to their management. Table 2 lists the common infectious agents isolated from cancer patients.

NEUTROPENIA AND INFECTION

The importance of neutropenia as a major risk factor for the development of infection in cancer patients was recognized almost three decades ago, and it remains the most frequent predisposing factor [1]. Even in patients with other deficiencies in host defenses (*eg*, Hodgkin's disease), at least 30% to 35% of infections occur as a result of neutropenia. The risk of infection is related to the degree and the duration of neutropenia. The risk begins to increase when the neutrophil count dips below 1000/mm³ and is greatest at counts of less than 100/mm³. Most patients with solid tumors experience fewer than 7 days of severe neutropenia during each course of chemotherapy; they are at much less risk than are patients with acute leukemia and bone marrow transplant recipients, in whom severe neutropenia lasting 15 to 21 days is not uncommon. The treatment of patients who have impairment of other host defense mechanisms usually follows the standard infectious disease practice of making a specific diagnosis and administering specific therapy. The emphasis in

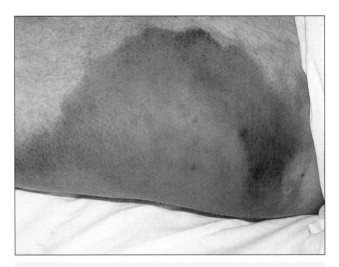

FIGURE 2 Rapidly progressive cutaneous infection caused by *Clostridium* spp in a patient with acute leukemia (*see* Color Plate).

MANAGEMENT OF FEVER IN NEUTROPENIC PATIENTS

When a cancer patient with a neutrophil count of less than 500/mm³ develops fever, he or she should be considered to have an infection unless the temperature elevation was associated with the administration of known pyrogenic substances [3]. A careful interview for historical information and a physical examination must be performed. Particular attention should be paid to sites that are frequently infected or serve as foci for the dissemination of infection, including the oropharynx, lower esophagus, lungs, skin, genitalia and perianal regions, fingernails, paranasal sinuses, and vascular catheter entry sites (Fig. 3). Before the initiation of empiric antibiotic therapy, at least two sets of blood culture specimens and culture specimens from other appropriate sites (eg, the throat, urine, or stools) should be obtained. In patients with central venous catheters, culture specimens should be obtained from the catheter and from a peripheral site. Blood cultures should be repeated daily while patients remain febrile. All febrile neutropenic patients should undergo chest radiography to identify pulmonary lesions (Fig. 4). In patients with severe neutropenia, radiographic findings may appear normal. Radiography or computed tomography of the paranasal sinuses

neutropenic patients is on the prompt administration of empiric, broad-spectrum antimicrobial therapy because any delay in therapy can result in the rapid dissemination of infection and in death [2].

| TABLE 2 COMMON INFECTIOUS AGENTS RECOVERED FROM PATIENTS WITH NEOPLASTIC DISORDERS |

Host defect	Infectious agent or agents	Host defect	Infectious agent or agents
Neutropenia	Bacteria	Cellular immune dysfunction	Bacteria
	Staphylococcus aureus		*Salmonella* spp
	Coagulase-negative staphylococci		*Mycobacterium tuberculosis*
	α-Hemolytic streptococci		*Mycobacterium avium* complex
	Enterococcus spp		*Listeria monocytogenes*
	β-Hemolytic streptococci		*Nocardia* spp
	Corynebacterium jeikeium		*Legionella* spp
	Bacillus spp		Fungi
	Escherichia coli		*Cryptococcus neoformans*
	Klebsiella spp		*Candida* spp
	Pseudomonas aeruginosa		*Histoplasma capsulatum*
	Enterobacter spp		*Coccidioides immitis*
	Xanthomonas maltophilia		Protozoa
	Acinetobacter calcoaceticus		*Pneumocystis carinii*
	Citrobacter spp		*Toxoplasma gondii*
	Serratia spp		*Cryptosporidium* spp
	Clostridium spp		*Isospora belli*
	Bacteroides spp		Viruses
	Fungi		Cytomegalovirus
	Candida spp		Herpes simplex virus
	Aspergillus spp		Varicella-zoster virus
	Zygomycetes		Helminth
	Torulopsis glabrata		*Strongyloides stercoralis*
	Fusarium spp	Humoral immune dysfunction	Bacteria (encapsulated)
	Trichosporon beigelii		*Streptococcus pneumoniae*
			Haemophilus influenzae
			Neisseria spp

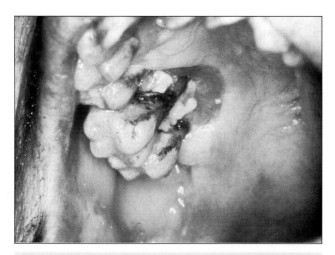

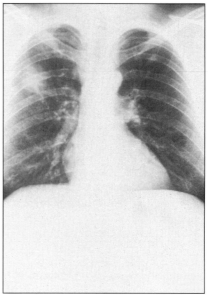

FIGURE 4 Characteristic rounded pulmonary infiltrate resulting from aspergillosis in a patient with acute myelogenous leukemia and persistent neutropenia.

FIGURE 3 Erosive gingival lesion resulting from *Pseudomonas aeruginosa* in a patient with prolonged neutropenia (*see* Color Plate).

should be performed in patients in whom these sites are potential sources of infection. Other laboratory investigations include complete blood counts and determination of baseline values for renal and hepatic functions. Invasive procedures such as lung, liver, or skin biopsies might be extremely useful in identifying sites of infection and isolating specific pathogens. The presence of thrombocytopenia, however, often precludes the performance of invasive procedures [4••,5•].

For many years, gram-negative bacilli accounted for more than 75% of all infections occurring in neutropenic patients. Now, approximately 60% of bacterial infections are caused by gram-positive organisms. Additionally, polymicrobial infections now account for up to 20% of documented bacterial infections and are associated with greater morbidity and mortality than are single-organism infections [6]. Organisms that are usually associated with low virulence and those that are considered nonpathogenic can cause serious, life-threatening infections in neutropenic patients. Consequently, antibiotic selection must provide broad-spectrum coverage that includes most gram-positive and gram-negative organisms.

Anaerobic coverage is generally not necessary in most neutropenic patients, except in patients with intestinal or genitourinary malignancies or in those with abdominal symptoms. Antibiotic regimens must be based on knowledge of the organisms that are most prevalent in a particular institution and on the antibiotic susceptibilies of these organisms, which can differ from institution to institution. Table 3 lists general principles that apply to the management of infections in neutropenic patients [7•,8•,9••].

ANTIBIOTIC THERAPY

Initial Therapy

Antibiotic regimens frequently used in neutropenic patients are listed in Table 4. No single regimen is optimal, and all provide broad antimicrobial coverage. The initial regimen may need to be altered during the course of a febrile episode depending on the susceptibility of microorganisms that might have been isolated; the development of bacterial, fungal, viral,

TABLE 3 GENERAL PRINCIPLES FOR MANAGING FEBRILE EPISODES IN NEUTROPENIC PATIENTS
A temperature of 101°F (38.3°C) persisting for 2 hours or more indicates the presence of infection unless it is associated with the administration of pyrogenic substances (*eg,* blood products)
Often the characteristic manifestations of infection are absent because of a blunted inflammatory response; failure to detect signs of infection does not indicate the absence of infection
A careful physical examination may reveal the site of infection and should be performed at least once a day
Untreated infection will disseminate rapidly and end fatally
Delayed administration of antimicrobial therapy results in suboptimal responses; therefore, antimicrobial regimens must be administered promptly
Nonpathogenic organisms cannot be ignored because they can cause serious illness
The distribution of predominant organisms and their antibiotic susceptibility might vary in different institutions; empiric antimicrobial regimens must be broad spectrum in their coverage and must take into consideration these local factors
Patients must be reevaluated frequently for the development of new superinfections, and appropriate therapeutic adjustments must be made promptly

TABLE 4 ANTIBIOTIC REGIMENS FREQUENTLY USED IN NEUTROPENIC PATIENTS

Combination regimens

Aminoglycoside + antipseudomonal penicillin

Aminoglycoside + extended-spectrum cephalosporin

Aminoglycoside + penicillin + cephalosporin

Aminoglycoside + carbapenem

Aminoglycoside + monobactam

Aminoglycoside + quinolone*

Vancomycin + antipseudomonal penicillin

Vancomycin + extended-spectrum cephalosporin

Vancomycin + monobactam or carbapenem

Vancomycin + quinolone*

Antipseudomonal penicillin + extended-spectrum cephalosporin[†]

Single-agent regimens (monotherapy)

Carbapenems

*Quinolones should not be used in empiric regimens in patients receiving these agents for prophylaxis.
[†]Extended-spectrum cephalosporins as single agents may not be adequate against resistant gram-positive bacteria.

or protozoal superinfections; or the lack of efficacy after administration of the regimen for 72 to 96 hours [10].

Combinations of aminoglycosides (*eg*, amikacin and tobramycin) and antipseudomonal penicillins (mezlocillin and piperacillin) are considered standard and are associated with overall response rates in the range of 70% to 85%. Aminoglycosides are also frequently combined with extended-spectrum cephalosporins (ceftazidime and cefoperazone) and newer β-lactams (aztreonam and imipenem). An important and often overlooked fact is that aminoglycosides by themselves are ineffective in patients with neutropenia, even against organisms that are susceptible to them *in vitro*. This fact is particularly of concern with the recent emergence of gram-negative bacilli that are resistant to β-lactams, and when aminoglycoside-containing regimens are used, it is important to ensure that the aminoglycoside is not the only drug to which the pathogen isolated is susceptible. In an attempt to circumvent aminoglycoside-associated toxicity, double–β-lactam combinations (penicillin plus a cephalosporin) have been evaluated. They have been found to be at least as effective as aminoglycoside-containing combinations but not as toxic [11]. Potential disadvantages of such combinations include their high cost and the selection of resistant organisms. With the increased incidence of gram-positive infections, many of which are caused by organisms resistant to β-lactam agents and aminoglycosides, the inclusion of vancomycin in the initial regimen might be considered. Alternatively, vancomycin may be added to the original regimen on isolation of a resistant gram-positive pathogen or if the original regimen has not produced a satisfactory response in 48 to 72 hours [12]. Certain broad-spectrum agents (imipenem and ceftazidime) have been used empirically as single agents in neutropenic patients and have produced response rates similar to those obtained with combination regimens [13•]. Patients receiving single-agent therapy need careful clinical monitoring, and antibiotic changes need to be made promptly if the clinical situation or microbiologic data indicate the need [14,15].

Recent advances have enabled us to evaluate not only the nature of initial empiric antimicrobial therapy but also the setting in which it is delivered. It is now possible to identify "low-risk" neutropenic patients when they present with fever and treat them in an ambulatory setting, without admission to hospital, with intravenous (IV), sequentially administered (IV followed by oral), or oral antibiotic regimens. Careful patient selection and close daily follow-up are essential for the success of this novel approach. Significant cost reduction, fewer resistant superinfections, and an improved quality of life for patients and their families are some of the advantages associated with outpatient antibiotic therapy.

Duration of Therapy

Some authorities recommend continuing antibiotic therapy in patients with documented infections until recovery from neutropenia [8•,9••]. This approach is expensive and may result in an increased number of superinfections by resistant bacteria or fungi, requiring numerous modifications of therapy. An alternative approach is to continue antibiotic therapy until all sites of infection have resolved; the causative pathogen, if isolated, has been eradicated; the patient has been treated for a minimum of 7 days; and the patient has remained afebrile and free of significant manifestations of infection for at least 4 days [7•]. Antibiotic therapy may be discontinued safely at this point despite the persistence of neutropenia and may be replaced with a prophylactic regimen. This approach is associated with a low relapse rate and fewer superinfections.

FEVER OF UNEXPLAINED ORIGIN

Patients with fever who display no clinical signs of infection and from whom no pathogen is isolated (fever of unexplained origin) form a most perplexing group. Many respond to antibacterial regimens, suggesting that they do have bacterial infections. Patients who remain febrile despite antibacterial therapy pose a difficult challenge. These patients might have bacterial infections that are resistant to therapy or nonbacterial infections (fungal, viral, or parasitic). Drug-related or tumor fever may also be present. An immediate and sustained response to the administration of nonsteroidal anti-inflammatory agents may indicate the presence of tumor fever. Aggressive, often invasive diagnostic maneuvers are sometimes necessary for the treatment of patients with fever of unexplained origin. In patients unable to tolerate invasive diagnostic procedures because of thrombocytopenia or other factors, the continuation of antibacterial therapy and the addition of empiric antifungal, antiviral, or antiparasitic therapy might be necessary. Figure 5 is an algorithm for treating febrile neutropenic patients.

OTHER THERAPEUTIC MODALITIES FOR IMPROVING HOST DEFENSES

Approximately 25% of infections in neutropenic patients fail to respond to appropriate antimicrobial therapy. In most cases, profound neutropenia persists. Patients with profound neutropenia and documented infections who fail to respond to optimal antibiotic therapy may benefit from granulocyte trans-

fusions. Recent technologic advances have provided several other means of strengthening host defenses. Among the many agents that improve defects in host defenses and stimulate hematopoiesis are polyclonal sera (J5 antiserum), monoclonal antibodies (HA-IA and E5), cytokines and hematopoietic growth factors (granulocyte-macrophage colony-stimulating factor, granulocyte colony-stimulating factor, and macrophage colony-stimulating factor), interleukins, and interferons [16•]. The toxicity associated with the agents may preclude their clinical usage. The role of polyclonal sera and monoclonal antibodies remains to be fully established, particularly in patients with neutropenia. The role of growth factors as adjuncts to antibiotic therapy for febrile neutropenic patients is under evaluation, and initial results are promising. These growth factors do not prevent neutropenia but do shorten its duration and reduce the number of infections associated with it. Other cytokines may potentiate the activity of neutrophils against specific pathogens [17•,18•].

PREVENTION OF INFECTION

The high frequency of infection in cancer patients during periods of myelosuppression has led to the development of programs for preventing infection. The two main strategies for preventing infection are 1) suppression of the endogenous microflora (from which most infections arise) and 2) prevention of the acquisition of new organisms from environmental sources. The former is usually achieved with the use of prophylactic antimicrobial regimens during periods of severe neutropenia. In patients at risk for fungal, viral, or protozoal

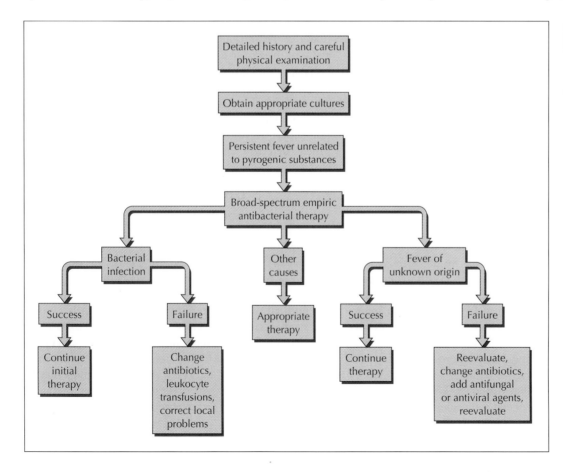

FIGURE 5
Treatment of febrile neutropenic patients.

infections, prophylaxis against these organisms is also provided. The acquisition of new organisms is prevented by various means, including strict hand washing, the use of well-cooked foods, and the use of various isolation techniques and protected environments [19,20].

Intravenous administration of immunoglobulins reduces the frequency of pulmonary infections in patients with impaired antibody production and may be useful in such patients [21•]. The use of growth factors, particularly in patients with prolonged neutropenia, may abbreviate the duration of severe neutropenia and reduce the incidence of neutropenia-associated infections. The judicious use of vaccines (*eg*, pneumococcal vaccine before splenectomy) may also reduce the incidence of specific infections in selected patients. Listed in Table 5 are the various means used for the prevention of infection.

It is likely that despite recent advances, infections will continue to plague patients with cancer because resistant bacteria and other organisms emerge as new threats to these susceptible patients. The greatest hope for control of infectious complications is the discovery of effective methods of providing adequate granulocyte replacement or of eliminating the risk that neutropenia will develop after chemotherapy by using nonmyelosuppressive antineoplastic regimens. Reducing the duration of myelosuppression and enhancing phagocytic activity appear to be attainable goals in the not-too-distant future. Eliminating the risk of myelosuppression appears to be a more distant goal.

TABLE 5 METHODS OF PREVENTING INFECTION

Suppression of endogenous flora
Oral nonabsorbable antibiotics
Oral absorbable antibiotics
Systemic antibiotics
Aerosolized antibiotics

Prevention of the acquisition of new organisms
Protected environments and other isolation techniques
Careful hand washing
Well-cooked foods with low bacterial content

Other modalities
Intravenous immunoglobulins
Vaccines
Growth factors (granulocyte-macrophage colony-stimulating factor, granulocyte colony-stimulating factor)

REFERENCES AND RECOMMENDED READING

Recently published papers of particular interest have been highlighted as:
• Of interest
•• Of outstanding interest

1. Bodey GP, Buckley M, Sathe Y, *et al.*: Quantitative relationships between circulating leucocytes and infections in patients with acute leukemia. *Ann Intern Med* 1966, 64:328–340.

2. Bodey GP, Jadeja L, Elting LS: Pseudomonas bacteremia: retrospective analysis of 410 episodes. *Arch Intern Med* 1985, 145:1621–1629.

3. Bodey GP: Infections in cancer patients: a continuing association. *Am J Med* 1986, 81(suppl 1A):11–26.

4.•• Hughes WT, Armstrong D, Bodey GP, *et al.*: Guidelines for the use of antimicrobial agents in neutropenic patients with unexplained fever: a statement by the Infectious Diseases Society of America. *J Infect Dis* 1990, 161:381–396.

5.• The design, analysis, and reporting of clinical trials on the empirical antibiotic management of the neutropenic patient: report of a consensus panel. *J Infect Dis* 1990, 161:397–401.

6. Elting LS, Bodey GP, Fainstein V: Polymicrobial septicemia in the cancer patient. *Medicine* 1986, 65:218–225.

7.• Rolston KVI, Bodey GP: Infections in patients with cancer. In *Cancer Medicine*, edn 3. Edited by Holland JF, Frei E, Bast RC, *et al*. Philadephia: Lea & Febiger; 1993:2416–2441.

8.• Pizzo PA: Empirical therapy and prevention of infection in the immunocompromised host. In *Principles and Practice of Infectious Diseases*, edn 3. Edited by Mandell GL, Douglas RG Jr, Bennett JR. New York:Churchill Livingstone; 1990:2303–2312.

9.•• Pizzo PA: Management of fever in patients with cancer and treatment induced neutropenia. *N Engl J Med* 1993, 328:1323–1332.

10. Bodey GP: Antibiotics in patients with neutropenia. *Arch Intern Med* 1984, 144:1845–1851.

11. Bodey GP, Fainstein V, Elting LS, *et al.*: β-Lactam regimens for the febrile neutropenic patient. *Cancer* 1990, 65:9–16.

12. Rubin M, Hathorn JW, Marshall D, *et al.*: Gram-positive infections and the use of vancomycin in 550 episodes of fever and neutropenia. *Ann Intern Med* 1988, 108:30–35.

13.• Rolston KVI, Berkey P, Bodey GP, *et al.*: A comparison of imipenem to ceftazidime with or without amikacin as empiric therapy in febrile neutropenic patients. *Arch Intern Med* 1992, 152:283–291.

14. Rolston KVI, Haron E, Cunningham C, *et al.*: Intravenous ciprofloxacin for infections in cancer patients. *Am J Med* 1989, 87(suppl 5A):261–265.

15. Rolston KVI, Bodey GP, Elting LS: Aztreonam in the prevention and treatment of infection in neutropenic cancer patients. *Am J Med* 1990, 88(suppl 3C):24–28.

16.• Ziegler EJ, Fisher CJ Jr, Sprung CL, *et al.*: Treatment of gram-negative bacteremia and septic shock with HA-IA human monoclonal antibody against endotoxin: a randomized, double-blind, placebo controlled trial. *N Engl J Med* 1991, 324:429–436.

17.• Roilides E, Walsh TJ, Pizzo PA, *et al.*: Granulocyte colony-stimulating factor enhances the phagocytic and bactericidal activity of normal and defective human neutrophils. *J Infect Dis* 1991, 163:579–583.

18.• Roilides E, Pizzo PA: Modulation of host defenses by cytokines: evolving adjuncts in prevention and treatment of serious infections in immunocompromised hosts. *Clin Infect Dis* 1992, 15:508–524.

19. Pizzo PA: Antimicrobial prophylaxis in the immunosuppressed cancer patient. *Curr Clin Top Infect Dis* 1983, 4:153–185.

20. Bodey GP: Antimicrobial prophylaxis for infection in neutropenic patients. *Curr Clin Top Infect Dis* 1988, 9:1–43.

21.• Dwyer J: Manipulating the immune system with immune globulin. *N Engl J Med* 1992, 326:107–116.

SELECT BIBLIOGRAPHY

Bodey GP: Empirical antibiotic therapy for fever in neutropenic patients. *Clin Infect Dis* 1993, 17(Suppl 2): S378–S384.

Bow EJ, Ronald AR: Antibacterial prophylaxis in neutropenic patients—where do we go from here? [Editorial]. *Clin Infect Dis* 1993, 17:333–337.

Roilides E, Pizzo PA: Perspectives on the use of cytokines in the management of infectious complications of cancer. *Clin Infect Dis* 1993, 17(Suppl):S385–S389.

Rubenstein EB, Rolston KVI, Benjamin RS, *et al.*: Outpatient treatment of febrile episodes in low-risk neutropenic patients with cancer. *Cancer* 1993, 71:3640–3646.

Sable CA, Donowitz GR: Infections in bone marrow transplant recipients. *Clin Infect Dis* 1994, 18:273–281.

Infection in the Organ Transplant Recipient

21

Nesli Basgoz
Robert H. Rubin

Key Points

- The risk of infection in the organ transplant patient, particularly opportunistic infection, is determined largely by the interactions between the patient's *net state of immunosuppression* and the *epidemiologic exposures* that he or she encounters.

- The net state of immunosuppression is a complex function determined by the presence of immunomodulating viral infection, metabolic factors, and technical issues, in addition to immunosuppressive therapy.

- There is an expected timetable for when different infections occur posttransplantation.

- The therapeutic prescription for the transplant patient consists of an immunosuppressive program to prevent and treat rejection and an antimicrobial program to make it safe.

- Prevention of infection is the goal in these patients; early recognition and aggressive therapy are required when prevention fails.

Each year 30,000 to 40,000 individuals throughout the world, half of them in North America, undergo organ transplantation to treat end-stage kidney, heart, liver, and lung disease. The success of these procedures, undeniably one of the great success stories of modern biomedical science, has, however, created an ever-increasing population of patients in whom three factors have combined to produce an array of clinical syndromes hitherto unknown in biology and medicine [1•,2]:

1. The presence in the allograft recipient of primarily vascularized organs that differ from the host at either or both major and minor histocompatibility loci.
2. The lifelong requirement for potent, broadly active immunosuppressive agents to prevent rejection of the transplanted organ.
3. The reactivation, systemic dissemination, and amplification of a group of viruses whose effects are modulated by the nature of the immunosuppressive therapy.

The net result is that allograft rejection and life-threatening infection, the two major barriers to successful organ transplantation, are closely linked.

RISK OF INFECTION

The risk of infection in the organ transplant recipient, as in other immunosuppressed hosts, is determined in large part by the interaction of epidemiologic exposures and the net state of immunosuppression.

Epidemiologic Exposures

Epidemiologic exposures for transplant patients should be considered in two categories: those occurring in the community and those occurring within the hospital (Table 1). Among important community-acquired infections, *Mycobacterium tuberculosis* and the systemic mycoses have a respiratory portal of entry. Immunity devel-

Community	Hospital
The geographically restricted, systemic mycoses (*Blastomyces dermatitidis*, *Coccidioides immitis*, *Histoplasma capsulatum*)	*Aspergillus* species
Mycobacterium tuberculosis	*Legionella* species
Strongyloides stercoralis	*Pseudomonas aeruginosa* and other gram-negative bacteria
Respiratory viruses (influenza, adenoviruses, respiratory syncytial virus)	*Pneumocystis carinii*
Food-borne bacteria (*Salmonella* species; *Listeria monocytogenes*)	

ops after the primary infection, but that immunity wanes with time and is markedly attenuated by the immunosuppressive drugs used in transplant patients. The end result is three epidemiologic patterns of infection with these agents:

- Reactivation of old infection, with secondary dissemination, after the onset of immunosuppression
- Progressive primary infection with systemic dissemination, after the initiation of the immunosuppressive therapy
- Reinfection in individuals previously immune whose immunity has been ablated with immunosuppressive therapy

In evaluating transplant patients with suspected infection, both a recent and remote detailed epidemiologic history are of critical importance [1•,3].

Strongyloides stercoralis, an intestinal nematode, can remain as an asymptomatic infestation of the gastrointestinal tract for decades after the infection was acquired (because of its unique autoinfection cycle). Following the initiation of immunosuppressive therapy, two potentially devastating clinical syndromes can develop: an accentuation of the normal effects of the organism, resulting in a hemorrhagic pneumonia or hemorrhagic enterocolitis, or both; or a disseminated strongyloidiasis syndrome throughout the body. The clinical presentation may be one of gram-negative bacteremia or meningitis. Recognition and treatment with thiabendazole before transplantation are essential.

There are increasing reports in organ transplant recipients of serious illness resulting from respiratory viruses that may circulate in the community. For example, during a community-wide epidemic of influenza A2 infection, a high rate of hospital admission was seen among stable organ transplant patients, with a relatively high rate of viral pneumonia and bacterial superinfection. Whether vaccination or rimantadine or amantadine prophylaxis has any protective value in this clinical situation is currently unknown [1•].

Finally, *Salmonella* gastroenteritis appears to be a more serious illness in this patient population, occurring with a higher rate of bacteremia and metastatic infection than in the general population. Transplant patients should be carefully counseled to avoid inadequately cooked foods and travel to developing countries where such infections are endemic [1•].

Even more important than epidemiologic exposures that occur in the community are those that occur within the hospital (Table 1). Two patterns of nosocomial exposure are recognized: *domiciliary* exposures, in which contaminated air is present in the room or on the ward where the patient is housed; and *nondomiciliary* exposures, which occur when the patient is taken from the ward to other sites in the hospital, for example, the radiology suite, operating room, catheterization laboratory, or endoscopy suite. Whereas domiciliary hazards are identified relatively easily because of clustering of cases in time and space, nondomiciliary hazards are both more common and more difficult to detect because of the absence of such clustering [4,5].

Immune Status

The net state of immunosuppression is a complex function determined by the interplay of several factors: the dose, duration, and temporal sequence of immunosuppressive therapies; the presence or absence of neutropenia, damage to the primary mucocutaneous barrier to infection, or foreign bodies such as catheters, drainage tubes, stents, or vascular access devices; the presence of such metabolic abnormalities as protein-calorie malnutrition, uremia (Table 2), and hyperglycemia; and the presence of infection with such immunomodulating viruses as cytomegalovirus, Epstein-Barr virus (EBV), and the hepatitis viruses. The importance of immunomodulating viruses is illustrated by the following observation: over the past 15 years more than 90% of the opportunistic infections that have occurred in organ transplant patients have been in patients with active infection with one or more of these viruses. Indeed, the exceptions to this observation have resulted from exposures to excessive environmental hazards, usually within the hospital environment [1•,3].

TIMETABLE OF INFECTION FOLLOWING ORGAN TRANSPLANTATION

The immunosuppressive programs used in all forms of organ transplantation resemble each other closely: cyclosporine or FK506 as the cornerstone of the antirejection prophylaxis program, accompanied by low-moderate dose prednisone therapy and azathioprine, with high-dose methylprednisolone pulses and antilymphocyte antibody therapy (either polyclonal or monoclonal) being used to treat acute rejection. As immunosuppressive programs have become standardized, the time course of infections has likewise become very standardized (Fig. 1). That is, although such infectious disease syndromes as pneumonia or fever can occur at any time posttransplant, the differential diagnosis is very different at different times in the posttransplant course. It is useful to divide the posttransplant course into three periods (Table 3).

TABLE 2 HOST DEFENSE DEFECTS CAUSED BY UREMIA OR ITS THERAPY

Defects caused directly by the uremic state

Depressed cell-mediated immunity (as exemplified by delayed rejection of skin and renal allografts and cutaneous anergy)

Delayed appearance of leukocytes at sites of inflammation

Attenuated antibody response to vaccines

Decreased bone marrow pool of granulocytes

Defects related to therapy

Abridgement of primary mucocutaneous barrier of infection by vascular and peritoneal access devices necessary for dialysis

Correctable nutritional deficiencies such as protein malnutrition and zinc and pyridoxine deficiency

Mobilization of iron stores by deferoxamine, thus increasing the risk of mucormycosis (and possibly other infections)

Complement activation and leukocyte dysfunction related to hemodialysis (membrane-blood interactions)

Chronic ambulatory peritoneal dialysis patients have a defect in opsonin activity in peritoneal effluent that correlates
   with risk of *Staphylococcus epidermidis* peritonitis

The First Month Posttransplant

Recognition of preexisting infection (*ie*, infection that was present in the recipient before the transplant and that continues, perhaps exacerbated by the transplant operation or the initiation of immunosuppressive therapy) is particularly important in patients undergoing liver and heart transplantation, as the gravity of their illness before transplant often requires intubation, vascular access lines, and other procedures that can lead to infection. Transplantation in the face of active infection is tantamount to disaster and should not be attempted.

Contamination of the allograft with *Staphylococcus aureus*, gram-negative bacilli, and *Candida* species can be equally catastrophic, as bloodstream infection at the time of harvest of either the donor or recipient will result in seeding of the vascular suture lines, mycotic aneurysm development, and vascular disruption at this site.

Routine postoperative infections, as seen in general surgical cases, comprise more than 95% of the infections occurring in this time period, although the consequences are far greater than in the normal host. The prime determinant of these

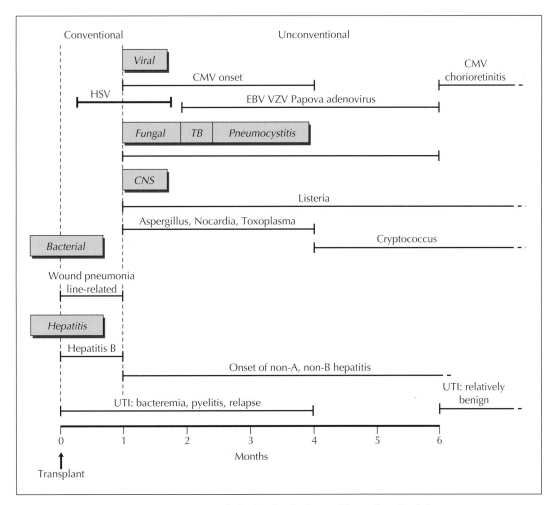

FIGURE 1
Timetable for the occurrence of infection in organ transplant recipients. CMV—cytomegalovirus; CNS—central nervous system; EBV—Epstein-Barr virus; HSV—herpes simplex virus; Papova—papovavirus; TB—tuberculosis; UTI—urinary tract infection; VZV—varicellazoster virus. (*Modified from* Rubin *et al.* [3]; with permission.)

TABLE 3 CHARACTERISTIC INFECTIONS FOLLOWING ORGAN TRANSPLANTATION

First month following transplantation
Preexisting infection
Contaminated allograft
Routine postoperative infections

1–6 months posttransplantation
Immunomodulatory viruses
   Cytomegalovirus
   Epstein-Barr virus
   Hepatitis viruses
   Human immunodeficiency virus
Opportunistic infections
   Pneumocystis carinii
   Listeria monocytogenes
   Aspergillus fumigatus
   Others

More than 6 months posttransplantation
General community infections
   Influenza
   Pneumococcal pneumonia
   Urinary tract infection
Opportunistic infections
   Pneumocystis carinii
   Listeria monocytogenes
   Cryptococcus neoformans
Chronic viral infection
   Cytomegalovirus
   Epstein-Barr virus
   Hepatitis viruses
   Papillomaviruses

More than Six Months Posttransplant

Approximately 75% of individuals will have had a good result from the transplant procedure and are on maintenance immunosuppression with satisfactory allograft function. Their infectious disease problems are those of the general community—influenza, pneumococcal pneumonia, and urinary tract infection.

Approximately 10% have had a relatively poor outcome from the transplant procedure, with ongoing acute and chronic rejection and too much acute and chronic immunosuppressive therapy (and, as a result, a high incidence of chronic immunomodulating virus infection). These patients are at the highest risk of any group for opportunistic infection with such agents as *Pneumocystis carinii*, *Listeria monocytogenes*, and *Cryptococcus neoformans*.

Patients who have chronic infection with cytomegalovirus, EBV, the hepatitis viruses, or the papillomaviruses may experience progressive organ destruction (*ie*, the liver by the hepatitis viruses or the retina by cytomegalovirus), develop full-blown AIDS, or present with viral-associated malignancies (*ie*, hepatoma from the hepatitis viruses, squamous cell carcinoma from the papillomaviruses, and lymphoma from EBV).

INFECTIONS OF PARTICULAR IMPORTANCE

Cytomegalovirus

Cytomegalovirus is the most important single cause of infectious disease morbidity and mortality in the organ transplant patient; it occurs almost exclusively in the period 1 to 4 months posttransplant. Three epidemiologic patterns of infection are described [1•,2,3,6]:

1. *Primary infection*, in which a cytomegalovirus-naive individual (who is serologically negative) receives cells harboring latent virus from a seropositive donor. Approximately 60% of individuals at risk for primary infection become clinically ill [7,8].
2. *Reactivation infection*, in which a cytomegalovirus-seropositive individual reactivates an endogenous virus.
3. *Superinfection*, in which a cytomegalovirus-seropositive individual receives an allograft from a seropositive individual, and the virus that reactivates is of donor rather than recipient origin.

The immunosuppressive program used has a major impact on cytomegalovirus infection. Among cytomegalovirus-seropositive individuals immunosuppressed with cyclosporine, prednisone, and azathioprine, the incidence of clinical disease is approximately 15%, whereas it rises to as high as 60% if antilymphocyte antibody therapy is utilized to treat rejection.

The clinical effects produced by cytomegalovirus are many and are similar in all forms of organ transplantation, with one notable exception: the organ transplanted is more severely affected than the native organ (Table 4). Thus, cytomegalovirus hepatitis is primarily a problem in liver transplant

infections is the technical skill with which the surgery is carried out and the endotracheal tube and invasive catheters are managed. This is the most important form of infection occurring in liver transplant recipients.

It is important to recognize that the first month posttransplant is the period when the highest daily doses of immunosuppressive drugs are being administered, but the net state of immunosuppression is not great. Thus, opportunistic infection is essentially unheard of.

One Month to Six Months Posttransplant

This is the period when the incidence of infection not related to technical aspects of the operation rises (Table 3). The combination of sustained immunosuppressive therapy and infection with immunomodulatory viruses (with cytomegalovirus being the most important) creates a net state of immunosuppression great enough for opportunistic infection to occur even without intense epidemiologic exposure.

Direct effects

Clinical infectious disease syndromes occurring predominantly 1–4 months
  posttransplant
  Fever
  Pneumonia
  Hepatitis
  Invasion of the gastrointestinal tract, producing inflammation, ulceration,
    or perforation
  Leukopenia, thrombocytopenia
  Myocarditis
Clinical infectious disease syndromes occurring more than 6 months
  posttransplant
  Chorioretinitis

Indirect effects

Contributes to the net state of immunosuppression resulting in an increased risk
  of opportunistic secondary infection
Plays a role in the pathogenesis of acute and chronic allograft injury

recipients; myocarditis is recognized only in heart transplant recipients; and pneumonia has its highest attack rate in lung and heart-lung recipients [1•,8].

To control active cytomegalovirus infection, intravenous ganciclovir is given at a dose of 5 mg/kg twice daily (with dose correction when renal dysfunction is present) in symptomatic disease, with concomitant cytomegalovirus hyperimmune globulin frequently administered in the face of severe disease (pneumonia, gastrointestinal bleeding or perforation, or significant neutropenia). Ganciclovir-resistant cytomegalovirus has not yet been an issue in the organ transplant patient. Because of its potential nephrotoxicity, there is little experience with foscarnet in this patient population [9•].

Prevention of cytomegalovirus infection has been a major goal, and partial protection has been achieved with prolonged courses of high-dose oral acyclovir and hyperimmune globulin [10,11]. Recently, three new approaches to the prevention of cytomegalovirus disease have been used: the combination of immunoglobulin with the antiviral; sequential therapy in which the more active compound, ganciclovir, is administered for 7 to 28 days, followed by high-dose oral acyclovir; and preemptive therapy in which ganciclovir is administered during periods of intensive anti-rejection therapy.

Epstein-Barr Virus

Although EBV produces fever and mononucleosis in the transplant patient, its major impact is in the production of the EBV-associated posttransplant lymphoproliferative disorder (PTLD). The usual site of EBV replication is the oropharynx, where the transformation and immortalization of B lymphocytes occurs. In transplant patients, immunosuppressive therapy, especially cyclosporine and antilymphocyte antibodies, suppresses the normal surveillance system in a dose-related

fashion, allowing EBV-immortalized B lymphocytes to escape.

The range of clinical disease classified as PTLD is broad, from a polyclonal lymphoproliferative disorder that is more akin to a mononucleosis syndrome, to a frankly malignant monoclonal lymphoma. Clinical manifestations include fever, invasion of the allograft, invasion of the abdominal viscera (presenting as hepatocellular dysfunction, gastrointestinal bleeding, or intestinal perforation), central nervous system disease (presenting with focal neurologic findings), tonsillar disease, as well as invasion of other lymphoid tissue. Unlike other forms of lymphoproliferative disease, purely extranodal disease may be observed [1•,12].

Management of this entity is currently controversial. Approximately 20% of individuals will have regression of their disease following significant reduction or cessation of immunosuppressive therapy. High-dose acyclovir or ganciclovir is commonly administered but may not have therapeutic benefit once established lymphoproliferative disease is present. Conventional lymphoma chemotherapy or radiotherapy has been difficult [13].

Hepatitis

The incidence of chronic liver disease in transplant patients is approximately 10% to 15%, with the two major causes being hepatitis B virus (HBV) and so-called non-A, non-B hepatitis (primarily hepatitis C virus [HCV]). With both of these forms of hepatitis, two epidemiologic patterns are observed. First, many individuals acquire asymptomatic chronic infection while on dialysis, and immunosuppression posttransplant then modulates viral proliferation and the effects on the liver. Alternatively, primary infection is acquired at the time of transplantation. In the case of HBV, this can result in overwhelming hepatic failure. More commonly, with both HBV and HCV, asymptomatic development of hepatocellular dysfunction first appears 1 to 4 months posttransplant and then continues for the life of the patient.

Immunosuppressive therapy has a direct stimulatory effect on the level of HBV replication. In the first 1 to 2 years posttransplant, HBV infection appears to contribute to the net state of immunosuppression, although overt manifestations of liver disease are unusual. Thereafter, progressive liver disease and hepatocellular carcinoma are seen [1•,14].

The most common cause of chronic liver disease in transplant patients is hepatitis C virus. The epidemiology of HCV appears to be similar to that of HBV: it is a chronic bloodborne infection, but it appears to be more slowly progressive than HBV. It also contributes to the net state of immunosuppression and may lead to the development of hepatocellular carcinoma [1•,14]. Treatment of hepatitis B or C with interferon alfa is far less effective than in the normal host and carries a risk of inducing rejection. Posttransplant, the hepatitis B vaccine is ineffective. Appropriate evaluation of the donor is the best method for preventing this form of infection [1•].

Bacterial Infections

The bacterial infections that occur in the organ transplant patient can be divided into three general categories: those resulting from common bacteria that affect the general population, mycobacterial infection, and opportunistic infection. In the first category, surgical issues and the posttransplant care are particularly important and dominate the infectious disease problems of the first month posttransplant (Table 3).

In the second category, mycobacterial infection in the transplant patient is caused by *M. tuberculosis* and atypical mycobacterial species. In tuberculosis, the use of isoniazid prophylaxis can be difficult because of the relatively high incidence of chronic liver disease. Thus, isoniazid should be administered for a minimum period of 1 year posttransplant, beginning approximately 3 weeks after the operation, to patients with a past history of active disease, patients with significant abnormalities on chest radiograph, and patients with positive tuberculin tests and an additional risk factor (malnutrition, some other immunosuppressing condition, and nonwhite racial background). Patients with positive tuberculin tests and no other risk factors are usually just followed closely [1•,15].

Listeria monocytogenes is a not infrequent cause of opportunistic infection in the transplant patient. This infection usually follows the ingestion of contaminated foodstuffs, particularly dairy products, and can cause a number of clinical syndromes: gastroenteritis, bacteremia, meningitis, meningoencephalitis, and cerebritis. This organism is the most common form of bacterial infection of the central nervous system in transplant patients. The widespread use of trimethoprim-sulfamethoxazole prophylaxis has markedly decreased the occurrence of this entity. Such prophylaxis is particularly important in patients 1 to 6 months posttransplant and in those individuals with a poor outcome from the transplant who are at high risk for opportunistic infection. When infection does occur, a meningeal dose of penicillin or ampicillin is the cornerstone of therapy [1•,16].

Nocardia asteroides produces invasive, opportunistic infection that closely resembles that produced by *M. tuberculosis*

and many of the fungi: a pulmonary portal of entry, with pneumonia as its most common presentation; a high incidence of hematogenous dissemination, with metastatic infection involving the skin, brain, skeletal system, and other sites occurring commonly. Nocardial infections have been particularly common in cardiac transplant recipients. Again, trimethoprim-sulfamethoxazole prophylaxis has greatly decreased their incidence [15]. If infection does occur, trimethoprim-sulfamethoxazole for 4 to 6 months is the basis of therapy; in individuals not tolerating this drug, alternative therapy with imipenem, minicycline, or other agents can be carried out.

Fungal Infections

In transplant patients the geographically restricted, systemic mycoses (blastomycosis, coccidioidomycosis, and histoplasmosis), which can infect any one, can occur, but these have a higher incidence of disseminated infection. The opportunistic fungal infections that rarely cause clinical disease in the normal host (*Pneumocystis carinii* pneumonia, invasive aspergillosis, invasive candidiasis, and cryptococcosis), however, are the major concerns.

Pneumocystis carinii occurs in approximately 10% of transplant recipients if no prophylaxis is administered. Its occurrence is closely linked with that of cytomegalovirus infection. *Pneumocystis* pneumonia is most common 1 to 6 months posttransplant and in patients with a poor outcome from the transplant procedure. In the transplant patient, *P. carinii* causes a progressive pneumonia over several days, usually interstitial in pattern, affecting predominantly both lower lung fields. Unlike what occurs in the AIDS patient, extrapulmonary pneumocystosis is extremely rare in the transplant recipient. Low-dose trimethoprim-sulfamethoxazole, aerosolized pentamidine, and such other regimens as pyramethamine and a sulfonamide are quite effective in preventing this infection [1•,17].

Invasive aspergillosis is a life-threatening condition that occurs when aerosolized organisms are delivered to the lower respiratory tract or sinuses of immunosuppressed individuals. Alternatively, invasion can occur at cutaneous sites that have been traumatized, as by macerating, occlusive dressings. The result of such inoculation is a necrotizing infection with characteristic blood vessel invasion. The latter event is responsible for the clinical and pathologic hallmarks of this infection: tissue infarction, hemorrhage, and metastatic spread. Although invasive *Aspergillus* infection localized to the primary site of infection can be cured with amphotericin therapy, once metastatic spread, particularly to the brain, has occurred, salvage of the patient is very doubtful. Prevention of disease because of attention to environmental hazards is particularly important with this entity. The new azole antifungal agent itraconazole has anti-*Aspergillus* activity, but at present should be regarded as being less effective than amphotericin in the treatment of this life-threatening infection [1•].

Invasive candidal infection in the transplant patient usually occurs as a consequence of wound infection, particularly in the liver transplant recipient, or as a consequence of a contaminated intravenous line. In addition, in the renal transplant patient, especially in diabetics and other individuals with poor bladder function, fungal balls may develop if candiduria is present, producing obstruction at the ureterovesical junction and ascending pyelonephritis. All three of these entities require therapy, either with amphotericin or fluconazole. It is particularly important to emphasize that the risk of visceral invasion in transplant patients with even transient candidemia is more than 50%, thus necessitating systemic antifungal therapy for even a single positive blood culture [1•].

Cryptococcal infection usually occurs more than 6 months posttransplant, particularly in patients who have had a poor outcome from the procedure. The clinical syndromes that occur in the transplant patient include an isolated, usually asymptomatic pulmonary nodule, pneumonia, cellulitis, meningitis, cerebritis, and the combination of meningitis and focal brain disease. In addition, metastatic spread to other sites such as the skeletal system and the urinary tract may occur. Cultures and the measurement of cryptococcal antigen in serum and cerebrospinal fluid have greatly facilitated diagnosis. Systemic antifungal therapy, with either amphotericin or fluconazole, is recommended [1•].

ANTIMICROBIAL STRATEGIES IN THE ORGAN TRANSPLANT RECIPIENT

The antimicrobial approach to the transplant patient is greatly influenced by the potential adverse effects of the antimicrobial drug interacting with cyclosporine. The key step in cyclosporine metabolism is mediated by hepatic cytochrome P-450–linked enzyme systems. Drugs that upregulate this function (ie, rifampin and, to a lesser extent, isoniazid) will decrease cyclosporine blood levels and increase the chance for allograft rejection. Drugs that downregulate this function (ie, erythromycin and the newer macrolides, clarithromycin and azithromycin, and the azole antifungal drugs, particularly ketoconazole and itraconazole) will increase cyclosporine blood levels, thus resulting in nephrotoxicity and overimmunosuppression. In addition, such drugs as vancomycin, the aminoglycosides, trimethoprim-sulfamethoxazole, and amphotericin can interact with cyclosporine to produce, idiosyncratically, severe nephrotoxicity. The end result is the use of third and fourth generation β-lactam drugs and fluconazole whenever possible in these patients [9•].

Antimicrobial agents, used in the transplant patient, can be prescribed in three ways: in the *therapeutic* mode, to treat established disease; in the *prophylactic* mode, given to all individuals to prevent a common infection; and in the *preemptive* mode, given to a subgroup of patients before the appearance of clinical disease. Because of the impact of infection on transplant recipients, and because of the potential for interactions with cyclosporine if full-dose therapeutic courses of antimicrobial agents are required, there is a particular emphasis on prophylactic and preemptive strategies of antimicrobial use in transplant patients [9•,18].

REFERENCES AND RECOMMENDED READING

Recently published papers of particular interest have been highlighted as:

• Of interest

•• Of outstanding interest

1.• Rubin RH: Infection in the organ transplant recipient. In *Clinical Approach to Infection in the Compromised Host* edn 3. Edited by Rubin RH, Young LS. New York: Plenum; 1994:629–705.

2. Rubin RH: Nephrology forum: infectious disease complications of renal transplantation. *Kidney Int* 1993, 44:221–236.

3. Rubin RH, Wolfson JS, Cosimi AB, Tolkoff-Rubin NE: Infection in the renal transplant recipient. *Am J Med* 1981, 70:405–411.

4. Hopkins C, Weber DJ, Rubin RH: Invasive aspergillus infection: possible non-ward common source within the hospital environment. *J Hosp Infect* 1989, 12:19–25.

5. Rubin RH: The compromised host as sentinel chicken. *N Engl J Med* 1987, 317:1151–1153.

6. Rubin RH: Impact of cytomegalovirus infection on organ transplant recipients. *Rev Infect Dis* 1990, 12(suppl 7):S754–S766.

7. Betts RF, Freeman RB, Douglas RG Jr, *et al.*: Transmission of cytomegalovirus infection with renal allograft. *Kidney Int* 1975, 8:385–392.

8. Ho N, Suwansirikul S, Dowling JN, *et al.*: The transplanted kidney as a source of cytomegalovirus infection. *N Engl J Med* 1975, 293:1109–1112.

9.• Rubin RH, Tolkoff-Rubin NE: Antimicrobial strategies in the care of organ transplant recipients. *Antimicrob Agents Chemother* 1993, 37:619–624.

10. Balfour HH Jr, Chace BA, Stapleton JT, *et al.*: A randomized, placebo-controlled trial of oral acyclovir for the prevention of cytomegalovirus disease in recipients of renal allografts. *N Engl J Med* 1989, 320:1381–1387.

11. Snydman DR, Werner BG, Heinze-Lacey B, *et al.*: Use of cytomegalovirus immune globulin to prevent cytomegalovirus disease in renal transplant recipients. *N Engl J Med* 1987, 317:1049–1054.

12. Stephanian E, Gruber SA, Dunn DL, Matas AJ: Posttransplant lymphoproliferative disorders. *Transplant Rev* 1991, 5:120–129.

13. Starzl TE, Nalesnik MA, Porter KA, *et al.*: Reversibility of lymphomas and lymphoproliferative lesions developing under cyclosporin-steroid therapy. *Lancet* 1984, 1:583–587.

14. Katkov WN, Rubin RH: Liver disease in the organ transplant recipient: etiology, clinical impact, and clinical management. *Transplant Rev* 1991, 5:200–208.

15. Sugar A: Mycobacterial and nocardial infection in the compromised host. In *Clinical Approach to Infection in the Compromised Host*, edn 3. Edited by Rubin RH, Young LS. New York: Plenum; 1994:239–273.

16. Hooper DC, Pruitt AA, Rubin RH: Central nervous system infection in the chronically immunosuppressed. *Medicine* 1982, 61:166–188.

17. Hibberd PL, Tolkoff-Rubin NE, Doran M, *et al.*: Trimethoprim-sulfamethoxazole compared with ciprofloxacin for the prevention of urinary tract infection in renal transplant recipients. *Online J Curr Clin Trials*, August 11, 1992 (Doc. No. 15).

18. Rubin RH: Preemptive therapy in immunocompromised hosts. *N Engl J Med* 1991, 324:1057–1059.

SELECT BIBLIOGRAPHY

Bird AG, McLochlin SM, Britton S: Cyclosporin A promotes spontaneous outgrowth in vitro of Epstein-Barr virus-induced B-cell lines. *Nature* 1981, 289:300–301.

Chou S: Acquisition of donor strains of cytomegalovirus by renal transplant recipients. *N Engl J Med* 1986, 314:1418–1423.

Grundy JE, Lui SF, Super M, *et al.*: Symptomatic cytomegalovirus infection in seropositive patients: reinfection with donor virus rather than reactivation of recipient virus. *Lancet* 1988, 2:132–135.

Hibberd PL, Tolkoff-Rubin NE, Cosimi AB, *et al.*: Symptomatic cytomegalovirus disease in the cytomegalovirus antibody seropositive renal transplant recipient treated with OKT3. *Transplantation* 1992, 53:68–72.

Marker SC, Ascher NL, Kalis JM, *et al.*: Epstein-Barr virus antibody responses and clinical illness in renal transplant recipients. *Surgery* 1979, 85:433–440.

Nemerow GR, Wolfert R, McNaughton ME, Cooper NR: Identification and characterization of the Epstein-Barr virus receptor on human B lymphocytes and its relationship to the C3d complement receptor (CR2). *J Virol* 1985, 55:347–351.

Preiksaitis JK, Diaz-Mitoma F, Mirzayans F, *et al.*: Quantitative oropharyngeal Epstein-Barr virus shedding in renal and cardiac transplant recipients: relationship to immunosuppressive therapy, serological responses, and the risk of post-transplant lymphoproliferative disorder. *J Infect Dis* 1992, 166:986–994.

Sixbey W, Nedrud JG, Raab-Traub N, *et al.*: Epstein-Barr virus replication in oropharyngeal epithelial cells. *N Engl J Med* 1984, 310:1225–1230.

Swinnen LJ, Costanzo-Nurdin MR, Fisher SG, *et al.*: Increased incidence of lymphoproliferative disorder after immunosuppression with the monoclonal antibody OKT3 in cardiac transplant recipients. *N Engl J Med* 1990, 323:1723–1728.

Yao QY, Rickinson AB, Gaston JS, Epstein MA: In vitro analysis of the Epstein-Barr virus: host balance in long-term renal allograft recipients. *Int J Cancer* 1985, 35:43–49.

Opportunistic Infections in HIV Disease

22

Jay Dobkin

> **Key Points**
> - Opportunistic infections (OIs) are the major sources of morbidity and mortality in AIDS patients.
> - Most OIs result from reactivation of latent infections due to deterioration of immune competence.
> - Effective treatment is available for many OIs, but relapse is common, necessitating long-term suppression.
> - Several of the major OIs are predictable based on the patient's count of CD4-positive T cells. Prophylactic regimens are well established for *Pneumocystis carinii* pneumonia, and others are being developed.

During the past decade, AIDS has increasingly become a condition relevant to general medical practice in the United States. The steady increase in new HIV infections, the progression of large numbers of those who are already infected to later states of AIDS, and the spread of the disease beyond its original geographic and subpopulation concentrations all mandate wider involvement by physicians in the United States.

Infections constitute the major complications in HIV-induced disease. Treatment and prevention of opportunistic infections have been areas of enormous progress during the first decade of the AIDS era, probably accounting for the bulk of improvements in morbidity and survival in AIDS. Primary medical care providers play the crucial role in timely diagnosis of HIV infection and institution of appropriate prophylaxis against opportunistic infections.

NATURAL HISTORY

Most infectious complications in AIDS occur in the late stages of the disease process, usually 10 or more years after HIV infection has occurred (Fig. 1). Progressive depletion of CD4-positive lymphocytes (or T4 cells) is the key pathogenetic process identified in AIDS. The strong association of many opportunistic infections with specific degrees of CD4 cell depletion forms the basis for staging HIV-infected patients. The quantitative degree of cell-mediated immunosuppression is predictive of the incidence and cause of secondary infectious complications. Several of these opportunistic processes are closely associated with specific levels of cell-mediated immunodeficiency, reflected by the level of circulating CD4-positive lymphocytes. Staging patients with CD4 cell counts provides a basis for starting preventive regimens and can also help clinicians better focus diagnostic evaluations.

INITIAL ASSESSMENT OF IMMUNE SYSTEM DAMAGE

After a patient tests positive for HIV, staging of immune system damage is done by quantitating T cells. Assessment should also be made for current infections requir-

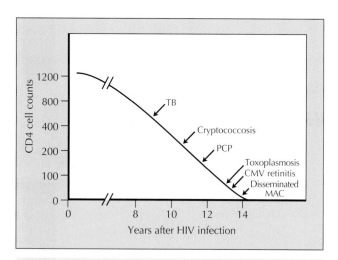

FIGURE 1 Pattern of opportunistic infections associated with declining CD4 cell counts. CMV—cytomegalovirus; MAC—*Mycobacterium-avium* complex; PCP—*Pneumocystis carinii* pneumonia; TB—tuberculosis.

ing treatment or for latent ones capable of reactivation. A baseline assessment for HIV-positive patients includes a complete history; physical examination including PAP smear and pelvic examination; complete blood count with differential; T cell subset analysis (*ie*, percentage of CD4 cells); purified protein derivative (PPD) test with controls; serologic tests for syphilis, hepatitis B, hepatitis C, and *Toxoplasma gondii*; and chest radiograph.

The enumeration of T cells is a crucial step in patient management, requiring some familiarity with laboratory procedures. The most widely used value, the absolute concentration of CD4-positive lymphocytes per cubic millimeter, is calculated:

$$Total\ leukocytes \times \%\ lymphocytes \times \%\ CD4^+\ cells$$

For example, if leukocytes = 5000, lymphocytes = 20%, and CD4+ = 20%, then absolute CD4 count = 200. The percentage of lymphocytes and total leukocytes are most variable. Time of day and intercurrent illness may affect the count [1,2•].

The initial CD4 count provides the critical basis for establishing the patient's stage of immune system damage and risk of AIDS-related complications (Fig. 1).

PRIMARY CARE: GENERAL CONSIDERATIONS

The substantial heterogeneity among AIDS patients has important medical consequences. For example, the effects of geographic background make disseminated histoplasmosis an important issue for midwesterners and Caribbean immigrants. Likewise, the risk of toxoplasmosis, as gauged by serologic status, varies widely based on country of origin. Perhaps most critical are gender and socioeconomic differences, which alter not only the pattern of medical complications but also the need for and access to medical and social services. Women with AIDS, a rapidly expanding group in the United States, have substantially different problems and needs. They are more likely to be economically and medically

indigent and to have dependents than are men with AIDS. Women appear to have shorter survival, which probably results from poorer accessibility and use of care, not from inherent biologic differences.

Special issues in HIV-positive women include recurrent or severe candidal vaginitis, cervical neoplasia, and safety of medications in pregnancy. Special social issues in HIV-positive women include poverty, poor access to care and services, care of dependents, and custody and guardianship issues.

Asymptomatic Patients

For some patients who seek testing and are found to be HIV positive while they are still asymptomatic, primary care is largely focused on health maintenance and timely prophylaxis as well as on counseling and education. Health maintenance strategies for asymptomatic HIV-positive patients include isoniazid prophylaxis for PPD-reactive patients, annual influenza vaccination, single vaccinations with pneumococcal and hemophilus vaccines, and hepatitis B vaccine series for susceptible, high-risk patients.

Repeat CD4 counts are obtained at regular intervals to gauge the course of the disease and appropriately time the introduction of opportunistic infection prophylaxis and antiretroviral therapy. Generally, patients with absolute CD4 cell counts of more than 600/mm³ should be tested every 6 months; patients with counts between 400/mm³ and 600/mm³ should be tested every 4 months. When a patient's count drops below 400/mm³, clinical and T-cell monitoring may be needed every 2 to 3 months.

Symptomatic Patients

Many patients are first identified as HIV positive when they are already symptomatic. They may present with one or more relatively benign prodromal processes that tend to predate the major opportunistic infections that define AIDS, such as herpes zoster, salmonellosis, bacterial pneumonia (especially bacteremic pneumococcal disease), oral hairy leukoplakia, and oral candidiasis. Some of these entities such as oral hairy leukoplakia (probably resulting from Epstein-Barr virus interacting with HIV) are not treated and are mainly important as indicators of the presence of HIV infection. Similarly, bacterial pneumonia may raise the diagnostic suspicion of HIV infection in an otherwise healthy young adult, but it usually responds to standard therapy.

MAJOR OPPORTUNISTIC INFECTIONS

The infectious complications associated with AIDS are well defined. They comprise a relatively small number of diseases predominantly caused by protozoan, fungal, viral, and mycobacterial pathogens, which are usually defended by the cell-mediated arm of the immune system (Table 1). Two striking features of AIDS-associated opportunistic infections are the frequent occurrence of several infections at once and a high tendency to relapse after initial successful treatment. Because of this tendency to relapse and because many opportunistic infections develop from reactivation of latent infection, prophylaxis and chronic suppression are key manage-

<table>
<tr><td colspan="2">

TABLE 1 MAJOR INFECTIOUS AGENTS IN AIDS COMPLICATIONS

</td></tr>
</table>

Fungi

Cryptococcus neoformans
Candida albicans
Histoplasma capsulatum

Protozoa

Pneumocystis carinii
Toxoplasma gondii
Cryptosporidia
Microsporidia

Viruses

Herpes simplex
Cytomegalovirus
Varicella zoster

Mycobacteria

Mycobacterium avium complex
Mycobacterium tuberculosis

Bacteria

Treponema pallidum
Streptococcus pneumoniae
Haemophilus influenzae

ment tools in the AIDS patient. Although many AIDS-related infections may be considered exotic and treatments are evolving quickly, general physicians backed up by appropriate specialists provide a great deal of primary care for HIV-infected patients.

Pneumocystis carinii Pneumonia

Pneumocystis carinii pneumonia (PCP) is the most frequent opportunistic infection with which AIDS patients present, affecting more than 80% of patients at some time. Major progress has recently been made in both prevention and treatment.

Prevention

Although the reservoir in nature and the epidemiology of PCP are incompletely understood, the degree of immune compromise associated with this infection is well defined in AIDS. Prospective natural history studies show that T-cell monitoring allows the institution of prophylaxis against PCP with a high degree of accuracy because most cases affect individuals whose absolute T4 lymphocyte count is substantially less than 200/mm^3. Two major modalities of prophylaxis (oral trimethoprim-sulfamethoxazole and aerosol pentamidine) have been well established, and several others have been used (Table 2) [3••,4].

A recent study comparing trimethoprim-sulfamethoxazole and aerosol pentamidine for prevention of recurrent PCP found trimethoprim-sulfamethoxazole clearly superior with a 1-year relapse rate of 4.5% compared to 18.5% for pentami-

TABLE 2 PROPHYLACTIC REGIMENS FOR *PNEUMOCYSTIS CARINII* PNEUMONIA

Agent	Dose and route of administration	Advantages	Disadvantages
First choice			
Trimethoprim-sulfamethoxazole	1 double-strength tablet 3 or 7 days per week	Highly effective	Associated with a high degree of adverse effects in AIDS patients: skin rash, leukopenia, and chemical hepatitis
Alternatives			
Pentamidine	Aerosol, 300 mg monthly (via Respirgard II nebulizer)*	Substantial efficacy	Substantial cost
		Deposition of drug in alveoli avoids the side effects associated with parenteral use	Possible association with pneumothorax
	Intravenous, 4 mg/kg once a month	May be used intermittently in patients with intolerance to trimethoprim-sulfamethoxazole, aerosol pentamidine, or dapsone	Occasional cases of extrapulmonary pneumocystis infection
			Severe side effects: renal and pancreatic damage, electrolyte abnormalities, rash, and cytopenias
		Efficacy similar to that of aerosol pentamidine	
Dapsone	50 mg daily or 100 mg on alternate days (oral)	Systemic effect	A potential oxidizer of G6PD-deficient erythrocytes: screening is needed for patients of African, Mediterranean, or Asian descent
		Lower cost	
		Ease of administration	

*Marquest Medical Products, Inc, Englewood, CO.

dine [5]. Although some side effects, such as rash, were more common with trimethoprim-sulfamethoxazole, overall tolerance was similar for the two drugs.

Diagnosis

Acute PCP in AIDS patients is often an indolent or subacute process as compared to PCP in non-AIDS patients, for whom it was originally described as fulminant. Often, AIDS patients with PCP have several weeks of fever, malaise and increasing cough, and shortness of breath before presentation. Hallmarks of PCP are nonproductive cough, fever, diffuse interstitial infiltrates on chest radiograph, and arterial hypoxemia. Diagnosis requires demonstration of cysts or trophozoites in sputum, bronchial secretions, or tissue sections. Saline-induced sputum is often adequate for diagnosis. Bronchoalveolar lavage is a sensitive technique.

Treatment

Treatment has been based on the use of either trimethoprim-sulfamethoxazole intravenously or by mouth or on the use of parenteral pentamidine therapy. Efficacy of the two regimens appears similar in AIDS, with about 80% of patients surviving a first episode of PCP [3••]. As noted, side effects of parenteral pentamidine are substantial and often severe. Many experts, therefore, prefer beginning therapy with trimethoprim-sulfamethoxazole and changing to pentamidine if side effects occur. Alternatives to trimethoprim-sulfamethoxazole or pentamidine include the combination of trimethoprim and dapsone or a recently approved drug, atovaquone, an antimalarial formerly designated as 566C80. Atovaquone was approved for treating mild to moderate PCP based on trials showing overall equivalent therapeutic efficacy to trimethoprim-sulfamethoxazole. As an oral non-sulfa drug that may also be effective in PCP prophylaxis and in prevention and treatment of toxoplasmosis, atovaquone appears to be a major therapeutic advance.

Several controversies arise in the patient who does not respond to initial therapy. Because the course of PCP in AIDS appears to be protracted, the designation of a patient as a treatment failure may be premature. Many patients require at least 1 week before hypoxemia improves and often require more than 1 week for fever and other signs to respond. Intubation and mechanical ventilation for patients with PCP has been debated, with some authorities suggesting that survival of such patients is too infrequent to warrant such an approach. Recently, most specialists in the field have agreed that assisted ventilation does have a role, at least in first episodes of PCP. Several controlled studies suggest that corticosteroids begun early in the course of severe PCP can substantially decrease the mortality rate [6•]. Patients with severe disease ($Po_2 < 70$ or A-a gradient > 35) should receive prednisone (40 mg twice daily for 5 days, then 40 mg per day for 5 days, then 20 mg per day for the remaining 11 days on PCP therapy).

Cryptococcal Meningitis
Diagnosis
Cryptococcal meningitis is one of the more frequent opportunistic infections seen in AIDS patients, but it occurs only about one tenth as often as PCP. Presentation in patients is often subtle with fever and headache the only features. Detection and measurement of cryptococcal antigen in serum and cerebrospinal fluid is the most rapid diagnostic test for cryptococcal meningitis, with greater than 90% sensitivity and specificity. Culture of the organism from body fluids or tissue is the gold standard of diagnosis. Cerebrospinal fluid cell counts may be normal or mildly abnormal. Computed tomography scans are usually normal or nonspecifically abnormal. Mass lesions are rare; other possible causes to consider in the differential diagnosis are lymphoma and toxoplasmosis.

Widespread dissemination of cryptococcal infection outside the central nervous system is relatively common. Lungs, pleura, and skin are frequent sites.

Treatment

Therapy for cryptococcal disease involves a standard regimen of intravenous amphotericin B with an acute total dose of about 1 g usually producing a good response. A high relapse rate is expected, so long-term suppression is strongly advised. Fluconazole (200 mg daily) is more effective than intermittent amphotericin for this purpose.

A shorter course of amphotericin (0.7 to 0.8 mg/kg/d for 2 weeks) with 5-fluorocytosine (100 mg/kg/d in 4 doses) followed by 8 to 10 weeks of high-dose daily oral fluconazole (400 mg) has been advocated as an alternative for acute management. Long-term suppression with fluconazole is then used as in the standard regimen. Although it is licensed for acute therapy, fluconazole should probably not be used this way because slower cerebrospinal fluid sterilization and a higher death rate are associated with this approach in comparative studies [7•].

Toxoplasmosis
Another AIDS-related complication involving the central nervous system is toxoplasmosis.

Prevention
Primary prophylaxis of toxoplasmosis has not been established. Trimethoprim-sulfamethoxazole PCP prophylaxis appears to offer some protection also against toxoplasmosis. A European study has shown effective primary prevention of both PCP and toxoplasmosis with a combination of dapsone and pyrimethamine given weekly. Azithromycin and atovaquone are being evaluated as prophylactic agents also.

Diagnosis
Toxoplasmosis usually presents as a progressive mass lesion with focal, brain abscess–like abnormalities on computed tomography or magnetic resonance imaging. The diagnosis is supported by the presence of IgG antibodies to *Toxoplasma gondii* in serum and can be confirmed by brain biopsy, although usually patients are diagnosed by response to a therapeutic trial of antitoxoplasmosis drugs.

Treatment
Response to therapy is often quite dramatic with resolution of intracerebral lesions and major improvement in neurologic

functioning. Long-term suppressive therapy appears to be required to prevent relapse [8,9]. First line treatment of toxoplasmosis uses sulfadiazine (1 to 2 g orally 4 times a day for 6 weeks) plus pyrimethamine (100 to 200 mg oral loading dose, then 50 to 100 mg daily for 6 weeks). Lower doses are maintained as suppressive therapy (sulfadiazine, 2 to 4 g/d, plus pyrimethamine, 25 to 50 mg/d). Folinic acid (10 mg/d during acute therapy; 5 mg/d during long-term suppression) is given to prevent the hematologic toxicity of pyrimethamine. As alternatives, the combination of clindamycin and pyrimethamine has similar efficacy to the sulfa-containing regimen, and azithromycin is being evaluated in combination with pyrimethamine.

Mycobacterium avium-intracellulare Infection

Disseminated *Mycobacterium avium* complex (MAC) infection, which was rare before the HIV epidemic, is a relatively common complication in AIDS. MAC is a grouping of two closely related mycobacteria, *M. avium* and *M. intracellulare*, which are recognized as uncommon causes of pneumonia in people with chronic lung disease. The organism, which is widely found in environmental water sources, produces an often massive invasion of the viscera including liver, spleen, and intestine, frequently with few symptoms. The major risk factor for developing disseminated MAC infection is immune status: affected patients have a mean CD4-positive lymphocyte count of less than 60/mm³, and MAC infection is rare in patients with counts greater than 100/mm³ [10,11••].

Diagnosis

The most common clinical presentation is persistent fever and weight loss. Hepatosplenomegaly with extensive elevation of hepatic alkaline phosphatase is a common MAC syndrome. Anemia or pancytopenia are often seen, possibly reflecting bone marrow infiltration. Rarely reported manifestations are localized pneumonia, arthritis, skin lesions, and endophthalmitis.

Culture of the peripheral blood on mycobacterial media has proven to be a reliable diagnostic technique. Acid-fast stains of stool are also often positive. Many patients appear to die with rather than of disseminated MAC infection.

Treatment

Efforts to treat this resistant organism have been disappointing, but recent studies report some success in suppressing mycobacteremia and improving symptoms. Combination regimens used in these studies included amikacin, ethambutol, ciprofloxacin, and rifampin or rifabutin. Clarithromycin, a new macrolide antimicrobial, has excellent *in vitro* activity against MAC and appears effective especially at high doses (2 g/d) in clearing the bloodstream and improving symptoms. Combination treatment with at least one additional agent (usually ethambutol or clofazimine) appears necessary because resistance may develop rapidly.

Prevention

Prevention of disseminated MAC infection has also been accomplished with the rifampin analog rifabutin (300 mg daily dose).

Cytomegalovirus Infections

Self-limited acute or subclinical cytomegalovirus (CMV) infection occurs frequently in normal hosts. In AIDS patients as well as others who are immunocompromised, reactivation of latent infection with widespread dissemination and organ damage may develop. Most AIDS-related cases occur in patients with fewer than 100 CD4 cells. Several varieties of severe CMV disease have been described in AIDS. CMV retinitis may occur along with other features of disseminated CMV disease or as the sole manifestation. Table 3 lists features of CMV retinitis and gastrointestinal disease and diagnostic methods. Widespread dissemination of CMV to other organs—including the pancreas, adrenals, and brain—has been reported, but CMV pneumonia appears to be a significantly less common manifestation in AIDS patients than in immunocompromised organ transplant recipients.

Treatment

Ganciclovir, the first agent approved for treating cytomegalovirus infection, has been joined by foscarnet as CMV therapy [12•]. Substantial experience supports the efficacy of drug treatment of CMV retinitis. Daily intravenous treatment

TABLE 3 DIAGNOSIS OF COMMON CYTOMEGALOVIRUS INFECTIONS		
Type of infection	**Features**	**Diagnosis made by**
Retinitis	Visual complaints	Characteristic morphology of the retina on fundoscopic examination
	"Floaters" or loss of peripheral vision (lesion far from optic nerve)	
	Scotoma (lesion close to optic nerve)	
	Hemorrhagic-exudative retinitis	
Gastrointestinal tract infection	Enterocolitis with bloody diarrhea and occasional intestinal perforation	Finding of characteristic inclusions on tissue biopsies
	Esophagitis or gastritis unresponsive to antifungal or antacid therapy	Culturation of the virus from peripheral leukocytes

	Ganciclovir	Foscarnet
Route of administration	IV	IV
Dosage		
Acute retinitis	5 mg/kg twice daily for 14 days	180 mg/kg/d either 2 or 3 times daily
Maintenance	5–7.5 mg/kg/d, 5–7 times per week	90–120 mg/kg/d
Toxicity profile	May induce leukopenia (may be life-threatening)	Nephrotoxic
		May cause calcium disturbances
How tolerated with AZT	Often not tolerated	Well tolerated
Other factors	New option: add G-CSF or GM-CSF for neutropenic patients	More expensive

AZT—azidothymidine; G-CSF—granulocyte colony-stimulating factor; GM-CSF—granulocyte-macrophage colony-stimulating factor; IV—intravenously.

is required with either drug. Table 4 compares these two agents. An oral form of ganciclovir is under development.

Candidiasis

Mucosal candidiasis is a nearly universal feature at some time during the course of HIV infection, with mild, if any, symptoms in most cases. Occasionally, severe oral and esophageal discomfort results [13].

Treatment

Because invasive disease with visceral involvement rarely occurs, treatment can be based on the extent of symptoms. Topical agents like nystatin and miconazole may be effective in mild cases, but oral systemic agents like ketoconazole or fluconazole are usually required when significant symptoms are present; occasionally, patients may respond only to a course of intravenous amphotericin B. Recently, relapses have been reported because of acquired fluconazole resistance in patients maintained on this drug.

Histoplasmosis

Disseminated histoplasmosis is a geographically limited AIDS complication affecting residents of the Ohio River Valley and some other areas of the United States. It is also encountered among immigrants from the Caribbean and Central America.

Treatment

Treatment with large doses of amphotericin B (2 g), followed by long-term suppression with this agent intermittently or an imidazole, such as fluconazole or itraconazole, has been generally successful [14]. Itraconazole has superior activity to older azoles against histoplasma and is recommended for long-term suppression. Its role in replacing amphotericin for acute therapy remains to be established.

Syphilis

There is a high rate of coinfection with other sexually transmitted agents in AIDS patients. An additional problem appears to be an alteration in the severity, natural history, or response to therapy, seen most strikingly in the case of syphilis. A number of cases have been described in which very rapid progression from primary or secondary syphilis to neurosyphilis occurred, sometimes despite standard therapy. Even more commonly, patients with HIV infection fail to demonstrate the expected serologic response to therapy.

Treatment

General guidelines call for standard intramuscular penicillin treatment for early syphilis, although many specialists advise a more aggressive approach, including lumbar puncture, even for neurologically asymptomatic patients. Daily intravenous or intramuscular penicillin is given for documented late syphilis, as in HIV-negative patients. A difficult issue is treatment for HIV-infected, syphilis-seropositive patients with nonspecific cerebrospinal fluid abnormalities that might be caused by either agent.

The Centers for Disease Control and Prevention guidelines strongly suggest careful follow-up of syphilis serology after treatment. Failure of non-treponemal tests (Venereal Disease Research Laboratory—VDRL; rapid plasma reagin—RPR) to turn negative or, especially, rising titers call for re-treatment. In some cases, long-term suppression with daily oral amoxicillin or intermittent parenteral penicillin may be useful.

Tuberculosis

Like other immunosuppressive conditions, HIV infection promotes tuberculosis reactivation and is strongly associated with rising rates of active tuberculosis in the United States and around the world. Primary infection and reinfection with tuberculosis also seem to be enhanced by HIV infection, and accelerated progression from infection to active disease has been documented. Two clinical features may differ in HIV-positive tuberculosis patients: noncavitary or otherwise atypical (even normal) chest radiographs may be found, and extrapulmonary disease occurs more commonly. Both of these features seem linked to the degree of immune compromise as reflected by CD4 cell depletion. Tuberculosis occurs predominantly in AIDS patients from subpopulations with higher background tuberculosis rates but can be spread nosocomially to other AIDS patients and is promoted by congregate care and housing or cough-inducing procedures such as sputum induction and aerosol pentamidine administration. Outbreaks of multidrug-resistant tuberculosis in several hospital AIDS units have had extremely high mortality rates. Promptly diagnosed, drug-sensitive tuberculosis responds well to standard therapy.

Prevention

Preventive therapy with isoniazid appears effective and is recommended for any HIV-positive patient with a purified protein derivative (PPD) reaction of 5 mm or more. Among many unsettled issues are how to approach tuberculosis prophylaxis in anergic patients or those exposed to drug-resistant strains [15].

Herpes Simplex Virus Infection

Chronic, nonhealing perianal or genital herpes simplex infection is an AIDS-defining event associated with advanced immune deficiency. Increasingly frequent recurrences of milder oral or genital herpes are common in earlier stages of HIV disease.

Treatment

Acute treatment with acyclovir is usually rapidly effective, but chronic suppression is often needed to control severe disease. Resistance to acyclovir has become increasingly common and should be suspected in those patients who fail to respond to aggressive intravenous acyclovir therapy. Treatment of these patients may necessitate the use of parenteral foscarnet.

Varicella-Zoster Virus Infection

Dermatomal herpes zoster is a common presenting feature of HIV infection, usually in patients with mild to moderate CD4 cell depletion. It rarely disseminates and may not need specific therapy.

Treatment

Some specialists advise acyclovir treatment in patients who are seen before lesion crusting has occurred. An odd variant seen in some AIDS patients is smoldering cutaneous zoster in which sparse, scattered lesions appear intermittently in a nondermatomal distribution. Although extensive cutaneous or visceral extension does not often occur in these patients, they may benefit from long-term oral acyclovir suppression.

Cryptosporidiosis and Microsporidiosis

Cryptosporidia and microsporidia are two intestinal protozoan pathogens first identified in the AIDS era that account for many cases of chronic and often severe diarrhea in advanced AIDS patients. Diagnosis can be made by special stool stains in the case of cryptosporidiosis, but microsporidiosis may require small bowel endoscopy and biopsy. Despite investigation of dozens of potential agents, treatment of cryptosporidiosis is nonspecific and symptomatic. Albendazole appears effective against some species of microsporidia.

REFERENCES AND RECOMMENDED READING

Recently published papers of particular interest have been highlighted as:
- Of interest
- •• Of outstanding interest

1. Kessler HA, Landay A, Pottage JC, *et al.*: Absolute number versus percentage of T-helper lymphocytes in human immunodeficiency virus infection. *J Infect Dis* 1990, 161:356–357.

2.• Lagakos SW, Hoth DF: Surrogate markers in AIDS: where are we? Where are we going? *Ann Intern Med* 1992, 116:599–601.

3.•• Masur H: Prevention and treatment of pneumocystis pneumonia. *N Engl J Med* 1992, 327:1853–1860.

4. Kovacs JA, Masur H: Prophylaxis for *Pneumocystis carinii* pneumonia in patients infected with human immunodeficiency virus. *Clin Infect Dis* 1992, 14:1005–1009.

5. Hardy WD, Feinberg J, Finkelstein DM, *et al.*: A controlled trial of trimethoprim-sulfamethoxazole or aerosolized pentamidine for secondary prophylaxis of *Pneumocystis carinii* pneumonia in patients with the acquired immunodeficiency syndrome. *N Engl J Med* 1992, 327:1842–1848.

6.• Bozzette SA, Sattler FR, Chiu J, *et al.*: A controlled trial of early adjunctive treatment corticosteroids for *Pneumocystis carinii* pneumonia in the acquired immunodeficiency syndrome. *N Engl J Med* 1990, 323:1451–1457.

7.• Saag MS, Powderly WG, Cloud GA, *et al.*: Comparison of amphotericin B with fluconazole in the treatment of acute AIDS-associated cryptococcal meningitis. *N Engl J Med* 1992, 326:83–89.

8. Luft BJ, Remington JS: Toxoplasmic encephalitis in AIDS. *Clin Infect Dis* 1992, 15:211–222.

9. Dannemann B, McCutchan JA, Israelski D, *et al.*: Treatment of toxoplasmic encephalitis in patients with AIDS. *Ann Intern Med* 1992, 116:33–43.

10. Nightingale SD, Byrd LT, Southern PM, *et al.*: Incidence of *Mycobacterium avium-intracellulare* complex bacteremia in human immunodeficiency virus-positive patients. *J Infect Dis* 1992, 165:1082–1085.

11.•• Horsburgh CR Jr: *Mycobacterium avium* complex infection in the acquired immunodeficiency syndrome. *N Engl J Med* 1991, 324:1332–1338.

12.• Studies of Ocular Complications of AIDS Research Group, in collaboration with the AIDS Clinical Trials Group: Mortality in patients with the acquired immunodeficiency syndrome treated with either foscarnet or ganciclovir for cytomegalovirus retinitis. *N Engl J Med* 1992, 326:213—220.

13. Wilcox CM: Esophageal disease in the acquired immunodeficiency syndrome: etiology, diagnosis, and management. *Am J Med* 1992, 92:412–421.

14. Wheat LJ, Connolly-Stringfield PA, Baker RL, *et al.*: Disseminated histoplasmosis in the acquired immune deficiency syndrome: clinical findings, diagnosis and treatment, and review of the literature. *Medicine* 1990, 69:361–374.

15. Cohn DL, Dobkin J: Treatment and prevention of tuberculosis in HIV infection. *AIDS* 1993, 7(suppl 1):S195–S202.

SELECT BIBLIOGRAPHY

Smith DK, Neal JJ, Holmberg SD: Unexplained opportunistic infections and CD4+ T-lymphocytopenia without HIV infection. An investigation of cases in the United States. The Centers for Disease Control Idiopathic CD4+ T lymphocytopenia Task Force. *N Engl J Med* 1993, 328:429–431.

Weiss RA: How does HIV cause AIDS? *Science* 1993, 260:1273–1279.

International Travel Advice for Adults

23

Harish Moorjani
Pierce Gardner

Key Points
- Preventive measures can reduce travel-related illness to a minimum.
- Individually tailored health advice to travelers is essential.
- Infections acquired during travel may not be manifested until the traveler has returned.
- Medical evaluation of an illness in the returning traveler requires an exhaustive and rational approach.

Preventive measures in the form of pretravel immunization and counseling regarding health maintenance strategies and an appropriate medical kit can reduce travel-related illness to a minimum. Travelers are a diverse group, including adventure backpackers, business executives, immigrants returning abroad to visit relatives, and tourists. Health advice to travelers should be tailored to the individual and should take into consideration a variety of factors including:

The areas to be visited and their indigenous health problems

The requirements of certain countries regarding yellow fever immunization

The lifestyle and type of accommodations anticipated during the trip

The duration of travel

The patient's status regarding routine immunizations

Special requirements for the extended traveler with close contact with indigenous population (*eg*, missionary groups, Peace Corps volunteers, and so forth)

Modifying factors, such as seasonal risks, altitude, and urban versus rural exposure

The patient's medical history, especially chronic problems that might disrupt foreign travel

Anticipated access to medical care during the trip

Malaria, hepatitis A, travel-associated diarrhea, and typhoid fever are the most significant infectious health hazards for American travelers. However, personal injury (*eg*, motor vehicle accidents) and chronic health problems (*eg*, cardiovascular disease) outweigh infectious diseases as causes of significant illness during travel [1]. A list of helpful resources for international travelers is provided in Table 1.

GENERAL MEASURES

Medical Kit

Recommendations for the traveler's medical kit will vary depending on the itinerary, length of stay, expected living conditions, the degree of medical sophistication of the traveler, and access to local medical facilities (Table 2).

Protection from Insect Bites

Mosquitoes and flies are vectors for a variety of parasites and for certain bacteria and viruses. A permethrin-containing insecticide spray can be applied to the external

TABLE 1 HELPFUL RESOURCES FOR TRAVELERS

Centers for Disease Control and Prevention: *Health Information for International Travel*, 1993 (revised annually). Atlanta, GA.
Obtained by writing:
   Centers for Disease Control
   Division of Quarantine
   Atlanta, GA 30333
World Health Organization: *International Travel and Health-Vaccination Requirements and Health Advice*, 1993
   (updated annually). Geneva, Switzerland.
Obtained by writing:
   WHO Publication Center
   49 Sheridan Avenue
   Albany, NY 12210
Centers for Disease Control and Prevention Voice Information System: Automated telephone system reached by dialing (404)
   332-4555. This system provides health information by region and advice on prevention of travel-related diseases.
Regional Information Centers maintained by the US Public Health Service.
International Association for Medical Assistance to Travelers (IAMAT): IAMAT, 417 Center Street, Lewiston NY 14092.
US Department of State, Overseas Citizens' Emergency Center, Washington DC 20520. (202) 647-5225 or (202) 647-1512.
Gardner P, ed: Health Issues of International Travelers. *Infectious Disease Clinics of North America*, vol 6, no 2.
   Philadelphia, WB Saunders, 1992.
Jong EC, Keystone JS, McMullen R, eds: *The Travel Medicine Advisor*, Atlanta, American Health Consultants, 1991.
Sakmar TP, Gardner P, and Peterson GN: *Health Guide for International Travellers*, Passport Books, NTC Publishing Group,
   Lincolnwood, IL, 1994.

surface of the clothing to create an effective shield against mites, chiggers, and mosquitoes. One application onto clothing will usually last through several washings.

During outdoor activities, an insect repellent containing diethyltoluamide (DEET) should be applied sparingly to exposed skin. At higher concentrations, absorption of DEET through the skin into the bloodstream may cause toxicity including skin rash, encephalopathy, seizures, insomnia, irritability, and confusion. This toxicity is of special concern in infants, children, pregnant women, and patients with skin conditions. Once the repellent is not needed, it should be washed off with soap and water. Protective clothing (long sleeves and pants) and mosquito netting are important barrier methods in areas with major insect risks.

Advice on Water and Food

The adage "Boil it, peel it, or forget it" captures the principles of avoiding enteric spread of pathogens. Practically, the traveler should be advised to eat hot cooked food and avoid salads and fruits that cannot be peeled after washing, foods that require handling after cooking, desserts that sit at room temperature for prolonged periods, food served by street vendors, and dairy products made from unpasteurized milk.

Drinks considered safe include hot drinks, carbonated beverages, pasteurized milk and milk products, beer, wine, and reliably boiled water. Emphasis should be placed on avoiding ice in beverages in places where tap water is unsafe.

There are many water purification devices and filters available commercially; the traveler should carry one suitable to the style of travel. Devices containing only a filter can remove most bacteria and parasites but not viruses. If water is likely to

be heavily contaminated, further chemical processing of filtered water with a commercially available preparation of tetraglycine hydroperiodine is recommended to kill viruses. Travelers who have iodine allergy or thyroid disease should avoid the iodine purification method.

In areas where schistosomiasis is endemic, swimming or wading in fresh water may be hazardous unless the water has been chlorinated.

Sexually Transmitted Diseases

The addition of potentially fatal infections (*eg*, AIDS, hepatitis B) to the traditional list of sexually transmitted diseases has heightened the need for precautionary sexual measures. Abstinence is the only completely sure way to avoid sexually transmitted diseases. The danger of sexually transmitted diseases can be decreased by employing barrier contraceptives. Spermicides may have additional protective effect against sexually transmitted diseases. Hepatitis B vaccination is advised for all travelers whose sexual activity involves even a small risk of hepatitis B exposure.

IMMUNIZATIONS

Please refer to the chapter on immunizations (Chapter 2) for details on vaccinations currently available for use in adults.

With rare exceptions, immunizations can be given simultaneously. Immune globulin preparations do not interfere with yellow fever or oral polio vaccines but should not be given with measles-mumps-rubella vaccine. Except in special high-risk situations, live virus vaccines should not be given to pregnant women or immunocompromised patients. Killed

TABLE 2 ITEMS IN A MEDICAL KIT

Adhesive bandages, sterile gauze pads (2 × 2 inches), adhesive tape, scissors, knife (a Swiss army–type with blade, scissors, and tweezers is especially useful)

Elastic bandage wrap

Bactericidal soap solution (*ie*, chlorhexidine gluconate)

Alcohol wipes

Thermometer

Pocket flashlight

Sunscreen (containing para-aminobenzoic acid)

Insect repellent spray and lotion (containing ≥ 20% diethyltoluamide)

Water purification tablets (preferably iodine)

Over-the-counter items

Acetaminophen

Ibuprofen

Hydrocortisone cream (0.5%)

Bismuth subsalicylate tablets

Toothache drops (benzocaine 5%, eugenol 9%)

Glucose-electrolyte mixture (Infalyte)* (recommended if traveling with infants or small children)

Topical solution for athlete's foot (*ie*, tolnaftate, haloprogin, clotrimazole)

Mild oral laxative

Nasal decongestant (*ie*, pseudoephedrine hydrochloride, 30- or 60-mg tablets)

Prescription items

Epinephrine (Epipen auto-injector† is most convenient; 0.3 mg intramuscular dose of 1:1000 epinephrine). One should suffice.

Scopolamine transdermal patches, 1 patch/3 d

Prochlorperazine, 10-mg tablets (20 tablets)

Antimalarial prophylaxis tablets; chloroquine, 500-mg tablets, or mefloquine, 250-mg tablets, 1 tablet per person per wk

Fansidar, 3 tablets/person

Loperamide hydrochloride, 2-mg capsules (16 capsules), or diphenoxylate hydrochloride-atropine, 2.5-mg tablets (16 tablets)

Trimethoprim-sulfamethoxazole double strength (160 mg/800 mg) tablets (14 tablets)

Doxycycline, 100-mg tablets (14 tablets)

Penicillin V, 250-mg tablets (40 tablets)

Fluoroquinolone capsules (norfloxacin, 400 mg; ciprofloxacin, 500 mg; ofloxacin, 400 mg) (14 tablets)

Mupirocin ointment (15 g, 1 tube)

From Sanford [2] and Mello and coworkers [15]; with permission.
*Mead Johnson Pediatrics, Evansville, IN.
†Center Laboratories, Port Washington, NY.

---

vaccines can be given simultaneously. Immunizations for travelers can be categorized into four groups:

1. Vaccines required for entry into specific countries (*eg*, yellow fever)
2. Vaccines indicated for people living in developed countries (*eg*, tetanus-diphtheria)
3. Immunizations for travelers planning extended trips to countries where purity of food and water is questionable (*eg*, typhoid vaccine)
4. Vaccines for special travelers such as Peace Corps volunteers and missionaries planning prolonged stays in remote areas (*eg*, rabies, hepatitis B)

Immunizations Required by Certain Countries

Under the International Health Regulations adopted by the World Health Organization, an international certificate of vaccination against yellow fever may be required for entry by certain countries. Certification for cholera vaccination is no longer required. Because the cholera vaccine is only partially protective (approximately 50%) and confers only short-term immunity (6 months or less), it is not routinely recommended for travelers. Even in areas endemic for cholera, the disease occurs mostly among those living in the poorest socioeconomic conditions. Therefore, the average traveler exercising good personal hygiene and care regarding food and water is at very little risk.

, Yellow fever is endemic in equatorial Africa and parts of South America, with occasional extension into Panama and the southern Caribbean islands. The yellow fever vaccine available in the United States is highly effective against both jungle and urban forms and provides long-lasting immunity (at least 10 years). The vaccine has a very good safety record and causes mild symptoms such as myalgia, headache, or low-grade fever in 2% to 5% of vaccine recipients. Serious complications, such as encephalitis, are exceedingly rare and occur almost exclusively in the very young (aged less than 6 months). The vaccine virus is highly thermolabile and must be stored and transported at subfreezing temperatures. Once the lyophilized vaccine is reconstituted, it must be used within 60 minutes. Only certain health facilities that agree to stringent conditions regarding transportation, handling, storage, and administration of the vaccine have been designated Yellow Fever Vaccination Centers and are authorized to validate the international certificate of vaccination. Although chloroquine inhibits replication of the yellow fever virus *in vitro*, it does not adversely affect antibody responses to yellow fever vaccination in humans.

Immunizations for People Living in Underdeveloped Countries

Travel concerns provide an opportunity to review and update immunizations currently recommended for all residents of the United States.

Poliomyelitis vaccine

For travelers to countries in which poliomyelitis is endemic, a one-time booster dose of either live attenuated oral polio vaccine or the enhanced-potency inactivated polio vaccine is indicated for adults who received a primary series during childhood. No cases of poliomyelitis caused by the wild-type virus have been reported in the western hemisphere since August 1991, and worldwide eradication is a likelihood in the next decade. The reduction of the wild-type disease highlights the uncommon problem of paralytic illness occurring after the administration of live attenuated oral polio vaccine. For adults who were not fully immunized as children, inactivated poliovirus vaccine is the preferred vaccine for a primary series, as it eliminates the risk of vaccine-associated paralytic illness.

Immunization for Travelers to Areas with Poor Sanitation and Uncertain Water Purity

The risk of infection by water-borne and fecal pathogens is dose-related and dependent on the degree to which food and water precautions are observed, as well as the duration of exposure.

The risk of typhoid fever exists primarily among travelers who spend extended periods living "close to the soil." The largest number of importations of *Salmonella typhi* are from Mexico and most often occur among travelers visiting small villages.

Among the three available typhoid vaccines, the Vi polysaccharide (Typhim V, Pasteur Mérieux) (a subunit vaccine) has equivalent protective efficacy (50% to 70%) but avoids the

endotoxin reactions of the previously available phenol-killed vaccine and is easier to administer than the four-dose oral attenuated live vaccine.

Passive immunization with immune globulin is protective against hepatitis A and is strongly recommended for individuals anticipating prolonged travel to areas of uncertain water and sanitary conditions. Doses should be repeated at 4- to 6-month intervals for up to 2 years. After 2 years, continued reimmunization is less beneficial, presumably because of the development of active and passive immunity from exposure to hepatitis A in highly endemic areas. An effective hepatitis A vaccine is nearing licensure and should reduce the role of immune globulin in the prevention of hepatitis A.

Immunizations Indicated in Special Situations

Hepatitis B is highly prevalent in many developing countries. The risk to the traveler is largely a function of lifestyle choices. Therefore, hepatitis B vaccine is recommended if sexual contact with high-risk persons is a possibility or if direct contact with blood or secretions is likely (*eg*, healthcare workers). Individuals planning prolonged residence in highly endemic areas should receive hepatitis B vaccine in anticipation of the need to utilize local dental or medical facilities.

For missionaries, Peace Corps members, and others anticipating prolonged residence in areas highly endemic for rabies (Africa, the Middle East, and Asia), preexposure immunization with rabies vaccine should be considered. Preexposure immunization does not preclude the need for postexposure wound care and additional rabies immunization. Concurrent chloroquine malaria prophylaxis may significantly impair antibody response to intradermally administered rabies vaccine.

Japanese encephalitis epidemics occur in the late summer and early autumn in the temperate regions and northern tropical zones in Asia and the Far East. Japanese encephalitis vaccine is recommended for travelers who are planning prolonged travel (longer than 1 month) to endemic areas, especially when the travelers' activities will include trips into rural farming areas or sleeping in unscreened quarters during the season when the mosquito populations are greatest.

Although meningococcal infection in American travelers is rare, meningococcal vaccine should be strongly considered for travelers to countries recognized as having epidemic meningococcal disease. The meningococcal polysaccharide vaccine currently available in the United States is a quadrivalent A/C/Y/W-135 vaccine.

MALARIA

Approximately 1000 cases of imported malaria are reported annually in the United States (not including travelers who get malaria while abroad). Most of these cases are preventable with pretravel advice and chemoprophylaxis [3].

The spread of drug-resistant strains of *Plasmodium falciparum* since the 1960s has reduced the efficacy of chloroquine prophylaxis. No currently available regimen of chemoprophylaxis against malaria is completely effective, and drug resistance continues to evolve.

For travelers, the risk of contracting malaria is greatest in sub-Saharan Africa, Papua New Guinea, and the Solomon Islands; intermediate on the Indian subcontinent and in Haiti; and low in the Far East and Latin America. Even in areas of low risk, there may be foci of intense transmission.

The essential strategy for the prevention of malaria is to prevent mosquito bites by using barrier methods and to obtain chemoprophylaxis (Tables 3 and 4).

Chemoprophylaxis

With the notable exception of chloroquine-resistant strains of *Plasmodium vivax* in areas of Indonesia and Papua New Guinea, all species of *Plasmodium* except *P. falciparum* have remained sensitive to chloroquine. Standard prophylactic doses of chloroquine are appropriate for travelers to the few areas where chloroquine-resistant strains of *P. falciparum* are not a problem (Central America north of Panama, Haiti, the Dominican Republic, the Middle East), or where *P. falciparum* malaria does not occur (Egypt, Iraq, Mauritius, and Turkey). A geographic distribution of malaria is shown in Figure 1. Chloroquine prophylaxis should be initiated 1 to 2 weeks before the traveler enters a malarious area. Prophylaxis should continue for 4 weeks after departure from such an area to cover the possibility of infection occurring on the day of departure and a long preerythrocytic phase of parasite development.

Mefloquine is highly effective against *P. vivax*, chloroquine-sensitive strains, and many multidrug-resistant strains of *P. falciparum*. Its whole-blood half-life of 6 to 23 days permits once-weekly dosing [4]. Side effects include nausea,

diarrhea, abdominal pain, palpitations, and occasional neuropsychiatric symptoms. Mefloquine is not recommended for patients taking β-blocker drugs or quinidine, for pilots or others whose activities require fine motor skills, or for pregnant women and children less than age 15 years. Patients with known neuropsychiatric disorders also should not take mefloquine. Transmission of mefloquine-resistant strains of *P. falciparum* has been reported in Eastern Thailand and Cambodia.

Doxycycline is active against the blood stages of *Plasmodium* species. It has a plasma half-life of 16 hours, necessitating daily administration. Doxycycline cannot be used in pregnant women or children less than age 8 years. Potential side effects include nausea, phototoxicity, and *Candida* vaginitis. Its use in malarial prophylaxis is limited to travelers to areas where mefloquine resistance is a problem or in whom mefloquine is contraindicated.

Chloroquine is generally well tolerated and has favorable pharmacokinetics, permitting once-weekly dosing. It is safe in pregnancy.

Proguanil is well tolerated and safe even in pregnant women, children, and others who cannot take mefloquine or doxycycline. Daily administration of proguanil combined with weekly chloroquine is less effective than mefloquine against most strains of *P. falciparum*. Proguanil is not licensed in the United States.

Early Treatment for Malaria

If professional medical care is not readily available, travelers who develop symptoms of malaria should initiate self-treatment [5].

Pyrimethamine-sulfadoxine—three tablets as a single dose—is effective against most strains of chloroquine-resistant *P. falciparum*. Pyrimethamine-sulfadoxine is not used for routine chemoprophylaxis because of rare but serious adverse events, including Stevens-Johnson syndrome, toxic epidermal necrolysis, agranulocytosis, and hypersensitivity hepatitis and pneumonitis.

Halofantrine has been used for self-treatment in areas where resistance to pyrimethamine-sulfadoxine occurs and is useful in travelers with hypersensitivity to sulfonamides. It will soon be available in the United States. It acts as a blood schizonticide and is effective for the treatment of chloroquine-resistant *P. falciparum* malaria.

TABLE 3 PERSONAL PROTECTION AGAINST MALARIA

Wear long-sleeved shirts and long trousers during evenings

Apply insect repellent to exposed skin during hours of risk and wash off afterwards

Spray aerosol insecticides in living and sleeping areas at dusk

Sleep in screened or air-conditioned areas

Use good-quality bed netting with small mesh impregnated with permethrin

Use mosquito coils or electric insecticides

TABLE 4 ADULT CHEMOPROPHYLAXIS AGAINST MALARIA

Drug	Adult dose
Mefloquine	250 mg (salt) once per wk beginning 1 wk before departure and for 4 wk after leaving the malarious area
Doxycycline	100 mg daily while in malarious area and for 4 wk after leaving the area
Chloroquine phosphate	500 mg (salt) once a wk beginning 2 wk before departure and for 4 wk after leaving the malarious area
Proguanil	200 mg once daily in combination with weekly chloroquine
Pyrimethamine-sulfadoxine	One tablet (25 mg pyrimethamine and 500 mg sulfadoxine) once a wk
Primaquine for terminal prophylaxis	26.3 mg (salt) once daily for 14 d

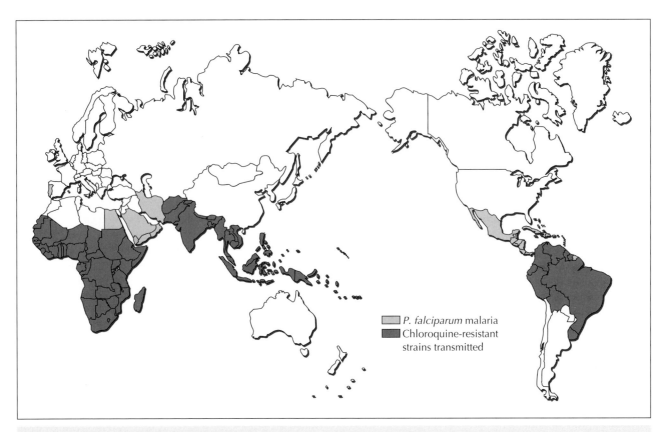

FIGURE 1 Geographic distribution of malaria. Regions where malaria is transmitted are shown as shaded areas. Regions where *Plasmodium falciparum* remains uniformly sensitive to chloro- quine are in light gray, and regions where chloroquine-resistant strains are transmitted are shown in dark gray. (*From* The Centers for Disease Control and Prevention [14].)

Legend: ▢ *P. falciparum* malaria ▢ Chloroquine-resistant strains transmitted

TRAVELER'S DIARRHEA

Etiologic Agents

The overwhelming majority of cases of traveler's diarrhea are caused by enteric pathogens, which are acquired by ingesting contaminated food or water. The most commonly identified pathogen is the diarrhea-inducing *Escherichia coli* (Table 5).

The most frequent cause of traveler's diarrhea is enterotox-icogenic *E. coli*, which produces toxins that stimulate intestinal secretions. Enteroinvasive *E. coli* invades epithelial cells, resulting in a shigella-like dysentery with mucosal inflamma- tion and ulceration. Shigellae account for approximately 10% of diarrheal illnesses among travelers to Latin America but are less frequent in Africa. *Salmonella* spp cause disease in almost 1% of persons with traveler's diarrhea in Latin America and 4% of those in Asia. *Campylobacter* spp cause disease by mucosal invasion and toxin production. They account for up to 15% of cases from Thailand and Bangladesh but are of little importance in Latin America. *Aeromonas hydrophila* is a water- borne agent commonly encountered in Asia.

The contribution of protozoa to traveler's diarrhea is vari- able. Protozoal diarrhea is uncommon in short-term travelers; these infections play a greater role in diarrhea associated with long-term adventurous travelers who stray from the usual tourist routes. *Entamoeba histolytica* and *Giardia lamblia* are the two most common protozoal etiologic agents of traveler's diarrhea. *Cryptosporidium parvum* is a common cause of diar- rhea in children in Latin America.

Gastroenteritis viruses of the Norwalk group, caliciviruses, adenoviruses, astroviruses, and rotaviruses are uncommon causes of traveler's diarrhea.

Risk of Developing Traveler's Diarrhea

Low-risk countries include Canada, the United States, north- ern Europe, Australia, and New Zealand. Intermediate-risk countries include most of southern Europe, the Far East, the former Soviet Union, and some Caribbean Islands. High-risk countries are found throughout most of Latin America, Africa, the Middle East, and Asia. Previous travel to a high- risk area is not associated with protection against traveler's diarrhea (Table 6) [7].

Traveler's diarrhea is usually a mild and manageable problem. The indications for antibiotic prophylaxis are not well established, and the drugs have potential side effects, including *Clostridium difficile* enterocolitis. There is concern that widespread antibiotic use will promote the emergence of drug-resistant pathogens and may also engender a false sense of security in travelers, resulting in carelessness and increased exposure to other enteric pathogens. Routine use of antibiotic prophylaxis has not been endorsed by the National Institute of Health Consensus Development Conference on Traveler's Diarrhea. Prophylaxis should be considered for some travelers, especially those with medical

TABLE 5 ETIOLOGY OF TRAVELER'S DIARRHEA		
Frequency	**Pathogen**	**Proportion of cases, %**
Common	ETEC	40–75
	EIEC	0–5
	Shigella spp	5–15
	Salmonella spp	0–15
	Giardia lamblia	0–3
	Entamoeba histolytica	0–3
	Campylobacter jejuni	Variable, often second only to ETEC
	Aeromonas spp	Uncertain, but generally low
	Vibrio parahemolyticus	0–2
Uncommon	*Cryptosporidium* spp	May be common in some areas
	Rotavirus	
	Norwalk virus	
Undiagnosed		10–25

From Farthing and coworkers [6]; with permission.
EIEC—enteroinvasive *Escherichia coli*; ETEC—enterotoxicogenic *Escherichia coli*.

TABLE 6 FACTORS PREDISPOSING AN INDIVIDUAL TO TRAVELER'S DIARRHEA AND COMPLICATING ITS COURSE
Epidemiologic factors
Adventurous style of travel
Lack of adherence to principles of preventing traveler's diarrhea
Lack of previous exposure to enteric pathogen
Host factors
Young age (< 6 y)
Gastric hypoacidity
Diabetes
Medications: diuretics, digitalis, lithium
Preexisting gastrointestinal disease
Immunodeficiency disorders

conditions putting them at higher risk and those who cannot tolerate even a 24-hour period of inactivity. The following groups of travelers might be considered for antibiotic prophylaxis:

Travelers with a record of repeated bouts of traveler's diarrhea

Those travelers with a diminished gastric barrier

Athletes and military personnel

Those with underlying medical disorders for whom the potential volume depletion of traveler's diarrhea might be poorly tolerated

Antibiotic prophylaxis is not recommended beyond 3 weeks. The drug should be started 1 day before departure and continued for 2 days after exposure.

Chemoprophylaxis

A variety of agents are effective for prophylaxis of traveler's diarrhea.

Bismuth subsalicylate seems to have both an antimicrobial action linked to the bismuth moiety and an antisecretory activity associated with the salicylate moiety. In high doses, it has moderate protective efficacy (about 65%). However, bismuth subsalicylate interferes with the absorption of doxycycline; therefore travelers should avoid taking the two drugs together.

Doxycycline, 100 mg/d, conferred 83% to 86% protection in travelers to Kenya and Morocco. Many recent surveys, however, have documented a rise in tetracycline resistance in different parts of the world (Mexico, Brazil, Egypt, Kenya, Thailand, and Honduras).

Trimethoprim-sulfamethoxazole (160 to 800 mg twice daily) conferred 71% protection over a period of 3 weeks in travelers to Mexico. Resistance to trimethoprim-sulfamethoxazole is also on the rise (Bangladesh, Thailand, Brazil), reaching approximately 40% in many developing countries.

Quinolones are the current drugs of choice for chemoprophylaxis of traveler's diarrhea. Ciprofloxacin, 500 mg/d, has provided a high degree of protection (79%) in various studies around the world. These drugs should not be given to young children or pregnant women.

Tables 7 and 8 portray self-therapy measures that may help patients who develop traveler's diarrhea.

EVALUATION OF THE RETURNING TRAVELER

Infections acquired during travel may not be manifested until the traveler has returned. For each presenting symptom, awareness of the distribution and incubation periods of the possible etiologic pathogens will help the evaluating physician to efficiently diagnose and treat the patient. Among the many afflictions of returning travelers, persistent diarrhea and febrile episodes most commonly lead to a request for medical evaluation.

Diarrhea in the Returning Traveler

The initial diagnosis and management of diarrhea will rely on an understanding of patient role factors and the prevalence of diarrheal pathogens in the environment of travel, along with detailed signs and symptoms of the current disease. Specific aspects of the history that may be helpful are listed in Table 9.

The median duration of diarrhea in travelers is 3 to 4 days. In 10%, diarrhea lasts more than 1 week, and in only 2% of travelers does it persist more than 1 month. Of all cases of diarrhea, 10% to 20% will involve more than one pathogen; several discrete episodes of diarrhea in the same patient may be caused by multiple organisms with different incubation periods acquired during the same contaminated meal.

Acute diarrhea

Acute diarrhea has a duration of 5 to 10 days. A strategy for the initial evaluation of acute diarrhea is shown in Figure 2. Two recent surveys have suggested that, among those who

TABLE 7 PHARMACOLOGIC SELF-THERAPY FOR TRAVELER'S DIARRHEA IN ADULTS BASED ON CLINICAL FEATURES

Clinical syndrome	Probable cause	Agent recommended
Watery diarrhea (no blood in stool or fever)	Bacteria	Antibacterial drug plus (for adults) 4 mg of loperamide initially, then 2 mg after each unformed stool, not to exceed 8 mg/d (over-the-counter dose) or 16 mg/d (prescription dose)
Dysentery (passage of bloody stools) or fever (temperature, >37.8°C [>100°F])	Invasive bacteria	Antibacterial drug*
Vomiting, minimal diarrhea	Viruses; preformed toxin (food poisoning)	Bismuth subsalicylate (for adults): 30 mL or 2 tablets (262 mg/tablet or 15 mL) every 30 min for 5 doses; may be repeated on day 2
Diarrhea in pregnant women	Bacteria	Fluids and electrolytes, can consider attapulgite: 3 g initially, repeated after unformed stools or every 2 h (whichever comes first), for total dosage of 9 g/d
Diarrhea despite trimethoprim-sulfamethoxazole prophylaxis	Unknown, possibly drug-resistant bacteria	Fluoroquinolone, with loperamide (see dose above) if no fever or blood in stool
Diarrhea despite fluoroquinolone prophylaxis	Unknown	Bismuth subsalicylate (see dose above) for mild-to-moderate disease; consult physician for moderate-to-severe disease or if disease persists

From Wood [8]; with permission.

*The recommended antibacterial drugs are as follows: trimethoprim (160 mg) and sulfamethoxazole (800 mg) for inland Mexico during the summer; and norfloxacin (400 mg), ciprofloxacin (500 mg), ofloxacin (300 mg), or fleroxacin (400 mg) for other areas in other seasons. The drugs should be taken in these doses twice daily for 3 days for more severe illness, particularly that associated with fever or the passage of bloody stools. For milder illness, single-dose therapy is effective. All patients should take oral fluids (Pedialyte, Ross Products Division, Columbus, OH; or flavored mineral water) plus saltine crackers.

TABLE 8 A REHYDRATION FORMULA FOR DIARRHEA SUFFERERS

Prepare two separate glasses of the following:

Glass number 1

    Orange, apple, or other fruit juice (rich in potassium), 8 ounces

    Honey or corn syrup (contains glucose necessary for absorption of essential salts), 1/2 teaspoon

    Table salt (contains sodium and chloride), 1 pinch

Glass Number 2

    Water (carbonated or boiled), 8 ounces

    Baking soda (contains sodium bicarbonate), 1/4 teaspoon

Drink alternately from each glass until thirst is quenched. Supplement as desired with carbonated beverages, water, or tea made with boiled or carbonated water. Avoid solid foods and milk until recovery occurs. It is important that infants continue breast feeding and receive water as desired while receiving these salt solutions.

From Centers for Disease Control and Prevention [9]; with permission.

need medical attention for diarrhea after returning from travel, *Campylobacter* and *Salmonella* infections are more common than enterotoxicogenic *E. coli* infections.

Diarrhea occurring with a short incubation period (< 12 hours) is most often caused by preformed toxins (eg, *Staphylococcus aureus* and *Bacillus cereus*). In the case of uncomplicated watery diarrhea with a short incubation period, observation and oral rehydration therapy are usually sufficient.

Characteristically, patients with watery diarrhea and cramps have enterotoxigenic *E. coli*, which will resolve without therapy in 3 to 5 days. Bismuth subsalicylate or antibiotics and

loperamide have been shown to shorten the duration of symptoms [11].

In patients with signs or symptoms of inflammatory diarrhea (fever, fecal blood, tenesmus, and the possible presence of fecal leukocytes), stools should be examined for fecal leukocytes. In patients with suspected parasitic causes of diarrhea, a modified acid-fast stain to look for *Cryptosporidium* and Cyanobacteria-like organisms and a trichrome strain for *E. histolytica* or *G. lamblia* should be obtained. Leukocytes may be absent from the stools of patients with *E. histolytica* because of lysis of leukocytes by the parasite.

TABLE 9 SPECIFIC ASPECTS OF THE HISTORY AND PHYSICAL EXAMINATION THAT SUGGEST A PARTICULAR ETIOLOGY OF TRAVELER'S DIARRHEA*

Exposures

Consumption of shellfish—*Vibrio* spp, Norwalk-like viruses, hepatitis A, *Plesiomonas shigelloides*

Prior antibiotic use—*Clostridium difficile*

Homosexual experience—proctitis with *Chlamydia trachomatis, Neisseria gonorrhoeae, Treponema pallidum, Entamoeba histolytica*

Outbreaks—*Staphylococcus aureus, Bacillus cereus, Vibrio cholerae*

HIV infection/immunocompromised host—cytomegalovirus, herpes simplex virus, coxsackievirus, rotavirus, *Salmonella* spp *Mycobacterium tuberculosis* or *M. avium-intracellulare, Cryptosporidium* spp, *Isospora belli, Strongyloides stercoralis, Entamoeba histolytica, Giardia lamblia, Microsporidium* spp

Developing countries—enterotoxicogenic *Escherichia coli, Shigella* spp, *Salmonella* spp, *Campylobacter jejuni*, rotavirus (children), *Entamoeba histolytica, Giardia lamblia, Cryptosporidium* spp

Developed countries—*Staphylococcus aureus, Bacillus cereus, Salmonella* spp, *Giardia lamblia, Campylobacter jejuni*

Specific areas: St. Petersburg (the former Leningrad)—*Giardia lamblia*; Mexico—*Shigella* spp; Thailand—*Aeromonas hydrophila*; mountain resorts, camping, or drinking unboiled well water—*Giardia lamblia*

Symptoms

Sudden onset with vomiting (incubation period < 6 h)— *Staphylococcus aureus, Bacillus cereus*

Watery diarrhea with or without low-grade temperature of acute onset—enterotoxicogenic *Escherichia coli*

Fever, abdominal cramps, tenesmus, bloody diarrhea—*Shigella* spp, *Entamoeba histolytica*

Chronic watery diarrhea—*Giardia lamblia, Cryptosporidium* spp

Chronic, intermittent diarrhea with abdominal bloating, flatulence, foul-smelling stool, and weight loss—*Giardia lamblia, Cryptosporidium* spp

Chronic inflammatory diarrhea, often with blood—*Entamoeba histolytica, Campylobacter jejuni, Yersinia enterocolitica*

Abdominal pain mimicking appendicitis—*Yersinia enterocolitica*

Watery diarrhea with neurologic complaints—*Clostridium botulinum*, ingestion of neurotoxin-producing fish or shellfish

From Kelsall and Guerrant [10]; with permission.

*The associations listed here are meant to provide some helpful clues for uncovering the most likely cause of diarrhea in travelers. Clearly, other organisms can cause diarrhea even when there is a history of either the exposures or the symptoms listed.

There is regionalization of risk for certain organisms. For example, infection rates are particularly high with *Shigella* spp in Mexico, *Vibrio parahaemolyticus* in Japan, and *A. hydrophila* in Thailand.

Persistent diarrhea

Chronic diarrhea has a duration of more than 10 to 14 days and may result from active, persistent infections (most often by a parasite), a disruption of normal architecture and functioning of the small bowel (possibly as a consequence of infection—tropical sprue, lactase deficiency), or overgrowth of organisms in normally sterile bowel. The most common infectious causes of chronic diarrhea and an approach to evaluation are presented in Figure 3.

Trips to mountain areas with exposure to untreated drinking water while camping and use of shallow wells as a source of water are thought to be risk factors for giardiasis. Many municipal water supplies in eastern Europe and Asia pose such risks. The diagnosis of giardiasis rests on the direct visualization of trophozoites or cysts. The time from ingestion of cysts to the detection of cysts in the stool is often longer than the incubation period, so newly symptomatic patients may have negative stool examinations.

Cryptosporidiosis is usually diagnosed by modified acid-fast examination of a stool specimen. The same stain will detect *Isospora belli* as well as Cyanobacteria-like organisms. Indirect immunofluorescence antibody staining is a more sensitive method for demonstrating *Cryptosporidium*.

The diagnosis of amebic intestinal infection is based on visualization of the trophozoites or cysts of *E. histolytica* in stool. Examination of fresh stool may show refractile trophozoites that have slow but directional motility. Smears of fecal samples preserved in formalin or polyvinyl alcohol can be stained with trichrome stain for the presence of trophozoites or cysts. Biopsy of involved mucosa with periodic acid–Schiff stain may be required for diagnosis of invasive amebic colitis. The indirect hemagglutination assay for antiamebic antibodies in the serum is positive in 85% of patients with invasive intestinal infection and in 95% of patients with extraintestinal amebiasis. The background rate of seropositivity in endemic areas can be up to 20%; therefore this test has limitations in persons originally from endemic areas or in those with a prior history of amebic colitis.

Disruption of the normal architecture of the small bowel can lead to diarrhea secondary to malabsorption. Disaccharidase deficiency after infection can lead to lactose intolerance.

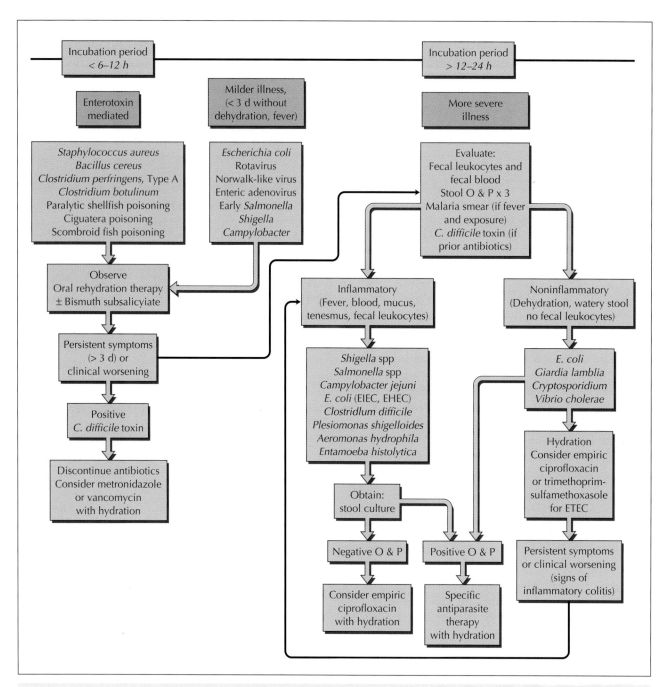

FIGURE 2 Evaluation of acute diarrhea in the returning traveler. This algorithm is a guide for initial evaluation of the patient with diarrhea of less than 5 to 10 days' duration. Asterisk (*) indicates agent should not be given if influenza or varicella infection is suspected, because of Reye's syndrome. EHEC—enterohemorrhagic *E. coli*; EIEC—enteroinvasive *E. coli*; ETEC—enterotoxicogenic *E. coli*; O & P—ova and parasites. (*From* Kelsall and Guerrant [10]; with permission.)

Small-bowel aspiration with mucosal biopsy should be considered in patients with persistent malabsorption and diarrhea despite three negative stool examinations for ova and parasites.

Fever in the Returning Traveler

In the returning traveler with fever but no localizing signs or symptoms, the following historic details may yield important diagnostic clues [12]:

Details regarding the area visited and the travel calendar

The types of accommodations used

The traveler's lifestyle and activities

The traveler's immunizations, medications, and adherence to indicated preventive measures

Knowledge of illness among fellow travelers or recognized exposures to communicable pathogens

The temporal relationship between possible exposures and onset of symptoms

The traveler's health history

Duration and time course of fevers

The incubation period for various pathogens is of diagnostic importance (Table 10 and Fig. 4). For instance, the minimum

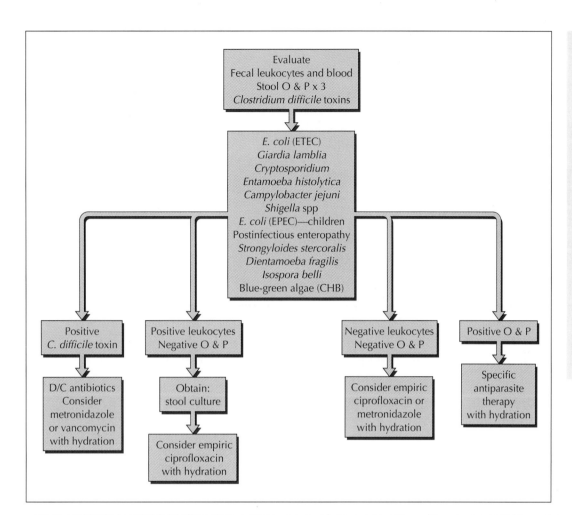

FIGURE 3
Evaluation of chronic diarrhea in the returning traveler. This algorithm is a guide for the initial evaluation of patients with diarrhea of greater than 14 days' duration. CHB—chronic hepatitis B; D/C—discontinue; EPEC—enteropathogenic *E. coli*; ETEC—enterotoxicogenic *E. coli*; O & P—ova and parasites. (*From* Kelsall and Guerrant [10]; with permission.)

TABLE 10 INCUBATION PERIODS FOR TROPICAL INFECTIOUS DISEASES	
Incubation period	**Infection**
Less than 21 d	Arboviral infections, including dengue and yellow fevers*
	Typhus fevers
	Typhoid and paratyphoid fevers
	Plasmodium falciparum infections†
	Plasmodium vivax, *Plasmodium ovale*, and *Plasmodium malariae* infections ‡
	Hemorrhagic fever agents, including Lassa fever and Ebola and Marburg viruses
	African trypanosomiasis
	Brucellosis
	Leptospirosis
	HIV
	Hepatitis A
More than 21 d	Viral hepatitis, including hepatitis A, B, C, and E
	HIV
	Tuberculosis
	Plasmodium falciparum infections
	Plasmodium vivax, *Plasmodium ovale*, and *Plasmodium malariae* infections‡
	Visceral leishmaniasis
	Amebic abscess of the liver
	Filariasis
	Typhoid and paratyphoid
	Brucellosis

*Three-day minimum incubation
†Eight-day minimum incubation
‡*Plasmodium ovale–vivax* may cause relapses for as long as 4 years after routine prophylaxis as a result of persistent liver stage
From Saxe and Gardner [13]; with permission.

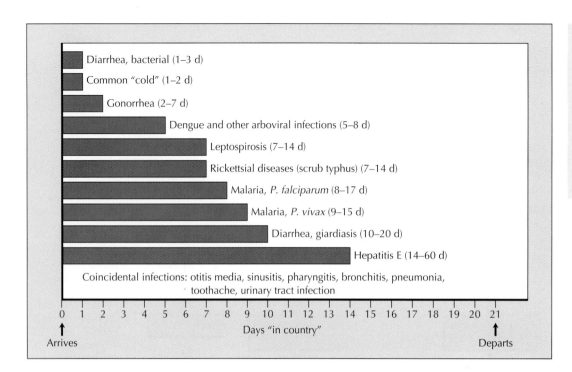

FIGURE 4
A time line for potential infectious diseases in travelers based on incubation periods and infection (exposure) on the first day. (*From* Sanford [2]; with permission.)

incubation period for malaria is 8 days; therefore, malaria is not a consideration in the traveler who develops fever within the first week following mosquito exposure. Similarly, an interval of more than 3 weeks between the last possible mosquito exposure and the onset of illness effectively rules out the diagnosis of viral hemorrhagic fever.

Fever patterns

It is helpful to determine whether there is a characteristic fever pattern, especially if malaria is being considered. Other fever patterns that may aid in the diagnosis of a particular infection are listed in Table 11. Fever patterns are never truly diagnostic and serve only as a hint of potential courses of fevers.

TABLE 11 FEVER PATTERNS AND POSSIBLE CAUSES

Fever pattern	Possible causes
Regular, periodic intermittent fever	
Fevers that occur at intervals of 48–72 h	Suggestive of *Plasmodium vivax* or *Plasmodium malariae* infections
Relapsing fever	
Febrile attacks lasting a few days, separated from each other by apyretic intervals of about the same length	Typical of the borrelioses; also seen in malaria, African trypanosomiasis, brucellosis, subacute bacterial endocarditis
Remittent fever	
Persistant fever in which the temperature is always elevated above normal	Typical of typhoid and other septicemic states; may be seen in *Plasmodium malariae* infections
Intermittent fever	
Persistent fever in which the temperature fluctuates between febrile and afebrile levels	Typical of pyrogenic infections, lymphomas, and miliary tuberculosis
Saddle-back or double-hump fever	
Fever that lasts a few days, followed by an afebrile period lasting a day or two, followed by a return of fever	Typical of a variety of viral infections, especially dengue fever
Double quotidian fever	
Two fever spikes per day (not related to antipyretics)	Typical of kala-azar, gonococcal endocarditis, early malaria

From Saxe and Gardner [13]; with permission.

Post-Trip Assessment

It is important to set priorities and to use laboratory tests judiciously in the evaluation of the febrile patient. If the physician takes the "shotgun" approach and orders all the possible relevant tests, the laboratory charges can be excessive.

The focus of the initial laboratory evaluation should be on diseases for which prompt diagnosis and correct treatment can be lifesaving. The chief considerations in this category are *P. falciparum* malaria and typhoid fever. Therefore, thick and thin blood smears for malaria and blood cultures, urine cultures, and stool cultures are important initial diagnostic steps in the evaluation of most febrile travelers. A rare, but important, consideration in travelers recently returned from West Africa is Lassa fever. This arenavirus can be diagnosed by blood culture, antigen detection, or immunofluorescent antibody measurement. Effective antiviral chemotherapy (ribavirin) is available for Lassa fever, and patients should be placed on strict isolation to prevent spread to hospital and laboratory workers.

Once the life-threatening diseases have been excluded, the physician can focus on the evaluation of the febrile patient in the same way that he or she would focus on a nontraveler.

Foreign travel may be a pertinent fact in a patient's past history for many years and should be part of the patient's permanent record. Amebic liver abscesses, echinococcal cysts, cysticercosis, and reactivation tuberculosis are examples of travel-related illness that may not be manifested for years or decades. These conditions are often difficult to diagnose and the travel history is often the critical diagnostic clue.

REFERENCES AND RECOMMENDED READING

Recently published papers of particular interest have been highlighted as:
- Of interest
- • Of outstanding interest

1. Steffen R, Lobel HO, Haworth J, *et al*.: *Travel Medicine*. Berlin:Springer-Verlag; 1989, 55–64.
2. Sanford JP: Self-help for the traveler who becomes ill. *Infect Dis Clin North Am* 1992, 6:405–412.
3. Winters RA, Murray HW: Malaria—the mime revisited: fifteen more years of experience at a New York City teaching hospital. *Am J Med* 1992, 93:243–246.
4. Lobel HO, Miani M, Eng T: Long-term malaria prophylaxis with weekly mefloquine. *Lancet* 1993, 341:848–851.
5. Krogstad DJ, Herwaldt BL: Chemoprophylaxis and treatment of malaria. *N Engl J Med* 1988, 319:1538–1540.
6. Farthing MJG, Keusch GT, eds: *Enteric Infection: Mechanisms, Manifestations, and Management*. New York: Raven Press; 1988:8.
7. Black RE: Epidemiology of travelers' diarrhea and relative importance of various pathogens. *Rev Infect Dis* 1990, 12(suppl 1):S73–S79.
8. Wood AJJ: Prevention and treatment of traveler's diarrhea. *N Engl J Med* 1993, 328:1821–1827.
9. Centers for Disease Control and Prevention: *Health Information for International Travel, 1988*. Atlanta: US Department of Health and Human Services; 1988. [Public Health Service, HHS publication no. (CDC) 88-8280.]
10. Kelsall BL, Guerrant RL: Evaluation of diarrhea in the returning traveler. *Infect Dis Clin North Am* 1992, 6:413–426.
11. Taylor DN, Sanchez JL, Candler W, *et al*.: Treatment of traveler's diarrhea: ciprofloxacin plus loperamide compared with ciprofloxacin alone. *Ann Intern Med* 1991, 114:731–734.
12. Manson-Bahr PEC, Bell DR: Diseases commonly presenting with fever. In *Manson's Tropical Diseases*, edn 19. London: Balliere Tindall; 1987:3.
13. Saxe SE, Gardner P: The returning traveler with fever. *Infect Dis Clin North Am* 1992, 6:427–439.
14. Centers for Disease Control and Prevention: *Health Information for International Travel 1994*. Atlanta: US Department of Health and Human Services; 1994. [Public Health Service, HHS publication no. (CDC) 94-8280.]
15. Mello KA, Gorbach SL, Koos EH, Platt R, eds: *Current Therapy in Infectious Disease*, vol 3. Philadelphia: BC Decker; 1990: 17–27.

SELECT BIBLIOGRAPHY

Dupont HL, Ericsson CD: Prevention and treatment of traveler's diarrhea. *N Engl J Med* 1993, 328:1821–1827.

Gardner P, ed: Health Issues of International Travelers. *Infectious Disease Clinics of North America*, vol 6. Philadelphia: WB Saunders; 1992.

Gardner PG, Schaffner WS: Immunization of adults. *N Engl J Med* 1993, 328:1252–1258.

Manson-Bahr PEC, Bell DR: *Manson's Tropical Diseases*, edn 19. London: Balliere Tindall; 1987.

Wyler DJ: Malaria chemoprophylaxis for the traveler. *N Engl J Med* 1993, 329:31–37.

Volume Index

Note: section numbers appear in boldface; page numbers followed by *f* indicate figures, and numbers followed by *t* indicate tables.

Alprazolam, for fibromyalgia, VI:11.7

Alprostadil, for digital ulcers in Raynaud's phenomenon, VI:5.3

Alternaria spp., and hypersensitivity pneumonitis, VII:4.2*t*

Aluminum toxicity, dialysis-associated, VI:13.6

Amantadine, for influenza, VIII:5.7

American College of Chest Physicians, definitions of sepsis and SIRS, VIII:1.1; 1.2*t*

Amikacin
    and doxycycline, for soft-tissue infections, VIII:8.8*t*
    for *Mycobacterium avium* complex infection, VIII:22.5
    for neutropenia, VIII:20.5
    for osteomyelitis, VIII:15.6*t*
    pharmacokinetics, VIII:3.7*t*

Aminoglutethimide, and theophylline dosage, VII:1.5*t*

Aminoglycosides, VIII:3.2*t*
    for acute pyelonephritis, VIII:9.5
    and anaerobic antibiotic, for septic pelvic or intraperitoneal infections, VIII:1.5
    and cefazolin, for sepsis, VIII:1.4–1.5
    and ceftriaxone, for nosocomial septic infection, VIII:1.5
    drug interactions, VIII:21.7
    efficacy, in abscesses, VIII:3.4
    for neutropenia, VIII:20.5; 20.5*t*
    for nosocomial pneumonia, VIII:7.4
    for osteomyelitis, VIII:15.6*t*
    pharmacokinetics, VIII:3.7*t*
    spectrum of *in vitro* activity, VIII:3.5*t*

Aminopenicillins, VIII:3.3
    pharmacokinetics, VIII:3.6*t*
    spectrum of *in vitro* activity, VIII:3.5*t*

Amiodarone
    adverse effects, V:17.5
    and hypersensitivity pneumonitis, VII:4.2*t*

Amitriptyline, for fibromyalgia, VI:11.6

Amoxicillin
    for bacterial sinusitis, VII:6.5–6.6
    for chlamydial infections in pregnancy, VIII:10.4*t*
    for common variable immunodeficiency, VII:15.6
    for endocarditis prophylaxis, VIII:11.10*t*
    for Lyme disease, VIII:17.6*t*
    pharmacokinetics, VIII:3.6*t*
    for pneumonia, VIII:5.6*t*
    and probenecid, for Lyme disease, VIII:17.6*t*
    for prosthetic joint infection prophylaxis, VIII:16.10*t*
    for sinusitis, VIII:6.4
    for syphilis in HIV-infected (AIDS) patient, VIII:22.6
    use with β-lactamase inhibitors, VIII:3.4

Amoxicillin/clavulanate (amoxicillin/clavulanic acid)
    for acute pyelonephritis, VIII:9.5
    for chancroid, VIII:10.5*t*
    for infected diabetic leg and foot ulcers, V:21.4
    pharmacokinetics, VIII:3.6*t*
    for pneumonia, VIII:5.6*t*
    for skin infections, V:2.3*t*
    for soft-tissue infections, VIII:8.8*t*
    spectrum of *in vitro* activity, VIII:3.5*t*

Amphotericin
    for *Aspergillus* infection in organ transplant recipients, VIII:21.6
    for candidiasis in organ transplant recipients, VIII:21.7

Amphotericin B
    for allergic bronchopulmonary aspergillosis, VII:3.5
    for blastomycosis, VIII:19.4; 19.4*t*

for coccidioidomycosis, VIII:19.4*t*; 19.5

for cryptococcal disease, VIII:22.4

and flucytosine, for soft-tissue infections, VIII:8.8*t*

for fungal arthritis, VIII:16.7

for fungal sinusitis, VIII:6.5

for histoplasmosis, VIII:19.4; 19.4*t*
    in HIV-infected (AIDS) patient, VIII:22.6

for soft-tissue infections, VIII:8.8*t*

Ampicillin
    for acute pyelonephritis, VIII:9.5
    and aminoglycoside
        for endocarditis, VIII:11.7
        for primary peritonitis, VIII:14.2*t*
    for bacterial sinusitis, VII:6.5–6.6
    dosage and administration, VIII:12.6*t*
    for endocarditis, VIII:11.8*t*
        prophylactic, VIII:11.10*t*
    and gentamicin
        for meningitis, VIII:12.6*t*
        for prosthetic joint infection prophylaxis, VIII:16.10*t*
        for sepsis, VIII:1.5*t*
    and gentamicin and clindamycin, for sepsis, VIII:1.5*t*
    and gentamicin and metronidazole, for sepsis, VIII:1.5*t*
    for osteomyelitis, VIII:15.6*t*
    pharmacokinetics, VIII:3.6*t*
    for sinusitis, VIII:6.4
    for soft-tissue infections, VIII:8.8*t*
    and sulbactam
        and aminoglycoside, for secondary peritonitis, VIII:14.5*t*
        for infectious arthritis, VIII:116.7*t*
        pharmacokinetics, VIII:3.6*t*
        for pharyngitis, VIII:6.8*t*
        for primary peritonitis, VIII:14.2*t*
        for sepsis, VIII:1.5*t*
        for soft-tissue infections, VIII:8.8*t*
        spectrum of *in vitro* activity, VIII:3.5*t*
    and third-generation cephalosporin, for meningitis, VIII:12.6*t*
    use with β-lactamase inhibitors, VIII:3.4

Amyloid
    lichen or papular, V:21.9–21.10
    macular, V:21.10
    nodular, V:21.10
    secondary localized cutaneous, V:21.10

Amyloidosis, V:21.9–21.10
    associated malignancies, V:19.7*t*
    classification, V:21.9
    clinical characteristics, V:19.7*t*
    in plasma cell dyscrasias, VI:17.3
    primary systemic, V:21.9

Anabolic steroids, for osteoporosis, VI:20.3

Anaerobes
    antibiotics for, VIII:3.3*t*
    neoplastic disorders and therapies associated with, VIII:20.2*t*
    in pharyngitis, VIII:6.6*t*
        treatment, VIII:6.8*t*
    in sore throat, differential diagnosis, VIII:6.7*t*
    sputum with, VIII:5.2

Analgesics
    for hemochromatosis, VI:13.5
    for osteoarthritis, VI:15.2

Anaphylactoid reactions, VII:9.1–9.6
    mechanisms, VII:9.1

Anaphylaxis, VII:9.1–9.6
    causative agents in, VII:9.2–9.4
    clinical manifestations, VII:9.3*f*
    differential diagnosis, VII:9.3*t*
    drugs causing, VII:9.3*t*

exercise-induced, VII:9.4
    food-dependent, VII:9.4

foods causing, VII:9.3*t*

idiopathic, VII:9.4
    plasma histamine levels with, VII:12.4*f*

mediators, VII:9.2*f*

miscellaneous causes, VII:9.4*t*

pathophysiology, VII:9.1

prevention, VII:9.5
    patient's approach, VII:9.5*t*
    physician's approach, VII:9.6*t*

signs and symptoms, VII:9.2

treatment, VII:9.4–9.5
    equipment for, VII:9.4*t*
    initial, VII:9.4*t*
    secondary, VII:9.5; 9.5*t*

Androgen-producing tumors, treatment, V:21.8

Aneurysms, multiple
    nonvasculitic disorders associated with, VII:14.5*t*
    in polyarteritis nodosa, VII:14.4*f*

Angiitis, allergic, VII:14.4
    diagnostic criteria for, VII:14.2*t*
    differential diagnosis, VII:14.4
    treatment, VII:14.3*t*

Angioedema, V:15.2*f*; VII:8.1–8.9; 8.2*f*
    acquired, VII:8.5
    characteristics, VII:8.1
    chronic idiopathic, treatment, VII:8.8*t*
    classification, VII:8.2–8.5; 8.3*t*
    clinical evaluation, VII:8.5–8.6
    cold-dependent
        diagnosis, VII:8.4*t*
        treatment, VII:8.4*t*
    delayed pressure
        diagnosis, VII:8.4*t*
        treatment, VII:8.4*t*
    drug-induced, V:17.2–17.3
    heat-induced
        diagnosis, VII:8.4*t*
        treatment, VII:8.4*t*
    hereditary, management, VII:8.5
    idiopathic, VII:8.5*f*
    signs and symptoms, VII:8.2–8.5
    sites of predilection, VII:8.1; 8.2*f*
    with systemic allergic insulin reactions, VII:11.6
    with systemic insect sting reactions, VII:10.7
    treatment, VII:8.6–8.9
    without urticaria, clinical examination in, algorithm for, VII:8.7*f*

Angiofibroma, V:7.6; 7.6*t*

Angiography, in differential diagnosis of vasculitis syndromes, VI:3.9

Angiokeratoma corporis diffusum legion, in Fabry's disease, VI:17.7*f*

Angiolipoma, V:7.5; 7.6*t*

Angioneurotic edema
    hereditary, VII:13.4
        interaction pathways, VII:13.6*f*
    treatment, VII:13.4–13.6

Angiotensin converting enzyme inhibitors
    for cardiac involvement in scleroderma, VI:5.8
    for renal involvement in scleroderma, VI:5.8–5.9

Angular cheilitis, V:4.6

Animal-derived sera, adverse effects, V:17.3

Ankle-brachial index, V:12.3

Ankle swelling, in Reiter's syndrome, VI:9.1; 9.2*f*

Ankle systolic blood pressure, measurement, V:12.3–12.4; 12.4*f*

Ankylosing hyperostosis, VI:8.6–8.7
    differential diagnosis, from ankylosing spondylitis, VI:8.6*t*
    ligament ossification in, VI:8.6; 8.6*f*

Aurothioglucose, for chronic arthritis in SLE, VI:4.3*t*

Aurothiomalate, for chronic arthritis in SLE, VI:4.3*t*

Auspitz sign, VI:10.1

Australian paralysis tick, VII:10.3

Autoantibodies

in differential diagnosis of idiopathic inflammatory myopathies, VI:6.6

in subsets of lupus erythematosus, V:14.5*t*

Autoantibody subjects, clinical utility, VI:3.6–3.7

Autoantibody tests, ordering, approach to, VI:3.7; 3.7*f*

Autoimmune disorders, and IgA deficiency, VII:15.7

Avascular necrosis

from corticosteroid hormone excess, VI:13.4

treatment, VI:13.4

Avian-derived immunizing agents, allergic reactions to, VII:11.6–11.7

Avian serum proteins, and hypersensitivity pneumonitis, VII:4.2*t*

Axial skeletal infections, VI:14.5

Azatadine

characteristics, VII:5.6*t*

dosage and administration, VII:8.8*t*

Azathioprine

adverse reactions to, VII:17.6*t*

for antirejection prophylaxis, VIII:21.2

for Behçet's disease, V:16.4*t*

for bullous pemphigoid, V:20.4

for chronic actinic dermatitis, V:13.6

for chronic arthritis in SLE, VI:4.3*t*

for cutaneous lupus erythematosus, V:14.5*t*, VI:4.6

for idiopathic inflammatory myopathies, VI:6.7

as immunomodulator, VII:17.6

for maintenance therapy in renal disease with SLE, VI:4.5

for musculoskeletal manifestations of scleroderma, VI:5.7

for myositis, V:14.8

for pemphigus vulgaris, V:20.6

for psoriatic arthritis, VI:8.9; 10.4*t*

for pyoderma gangrenosum, V:16.6

for Reiter's syndrome, VI:8.9

for rheumatoid arthritis, VI:2.8

side effects, VI:4.3*t*

for vasculitis, VII:14.3*t*

Azithromycin

for chancroid, VIII:10.5*t*

for chlamydial infections, VIII:10.4*t*

diffusion, VIII:3.4

drug interactions, VIII:21.7

for Lyme disease, VIII:17.6*t*

for nongonococcal urethritis, VIII:10.3; 10.4*t*

pharmacokinetics, VIII:3.7*t*

for pneumonia, VIII:5.6; 5.6*t*

for skin infections, V:2.3*t*

for soft-tissue infections, VIII:8.8*t*

spectrum of *in vitro* activity, VIII:3.5*t*

for toxoplasmosis, VIII:22.5

prophylactic, VIII:22.4

Aztreonam

for acute pyelonephritis, VIII:9.5

and amikacin, for soft-tissue infections, VIII:8.8*t*

and clindamycin and aminoglycoside, for secondary peritonitis, VIII:14.5*t*

and gentamicin, for soft-tissue infections, VIII:8.8*t*

for neutropenia, VIII:20.5

pharmacokinetics, VIII:3.6*t*

spectrum of *in vitro* activity, VIII:3.5*t*

and tobramycin, for soft-tissue infections, VIII:8.8*t*

B

Babesia spp., neoplastic disorders and therapies associated with, VIII:20.2*t*

Bacampicillin, pharmacokinetics, VIII:3.6*t*

Bacille Calmette-Guérin vaccine, VII:17.8*t*

Bacilli, gram-negative

aerobic, antibiotics for, VIII:3.3*t*

in endocarditis, VIII:11.2*t*

neoplastic disorders and therapies associated with, VIII:20.2*t*

Bacillus spp., in neutropenic patient, VIII:20.3*t*

Bacillus cereus

clinical syndrome from, VIII:13.4*t*

in diarrhea, VIII:13.3*t*

Bacitracin

ointment, for skin infections, V:2.3*t*

topical, for infected diabetic leg and foot ulcers, V:21.4

Back pain, VI:8.1–8.14

clinical evaluation, VI:8.11

diagnosis, VI:8.4–8.7

diagnostic testing in, VI:8.12–8.13

differential diagnosis, VI:8.5*t*; 8.5–8.7

referral for, emergency indications for, VI:8.14

related to disk degeneration, VI:8.9–8.10

treatment, VI:8.7–8.9; 8.13*f*; 8.13–8.14

Bacteremia

definition, VIII:1.2*t*

pneumococcal, incidence, VIII:2.3; 2.3*f*

Bacteria, gram-negative, in cellulitis, VIII:8.6

Bacterial infections

in organ transplant recipients, VIII:21.6

of skin, V:2.1–2.8

Bacteriuria. *See also* Urinary tract infections

asymptomatic, treatment, VIII:9.4

indications for, VIII:9.4*t*

in pregnancy, VIII:9.4

Bacteroides spp.

antibiotics for, VIII:3.3*t*; 3.5*t*

in chronic sinusitis, VIII:6.2

in neutropenic patient, VIII:20.3*t*

in peritonsillar abscess, VIII:6.5

in sinusitis, VII:6.5, VIII:6.2*t*

Bacteroides fragilis

antibiotic resistance, VIII:3.3

antibiotics for, VIII:3.3

Bacteroides melaninogenicus, in pneumonia, VIII:5.5

Bamboo spine, VI:8.4; 8.4*f*

Barbiturates, adverse effects, VII:17.4

Basal cell carcinoma, V:1.5*f*; 5.4–5.5

appearance, V:5.4–5.5

etiology, V:5.4

local invasion and metastases, V:5.5

nodular, V:5.2*f*

pigmented, V:6.5*f*

recurrence, V:5.5; 5.5*t*

superficial, V:5.2*f*

treatment, V:5.5

Bazex's syndrome

associated malignancies, V:19.7*t*

clinical characteristics, V:19.7*t*

B cells, differentiation, VII:15.2*f*

Beclomethasone

intranasal, for nasal polyps, VII:6.3

for rhinitis, VII:5.8*t*

Beclomethasone dipropionate, adverse effects, VII:1.6

Behçet's disease, V:16.3–16.4; 16.4*f*, VI:7.5–7.6, VII:14.8

clinical features, V:16.4

diagnosis, VII:14.8

differential diagnosis, VII:14.8

histopathology, V:16.4

management, VII:14.8

patient evaluation in, V:16.4

prognosis, V:16.4

treatment, V:16.4; 16.4*t*

Benoxaprofen, adverse effects, V:17.5

Benzalkonium, adverse effects, VII:1.5

Benzathine penicillin G

for early syphilis, VIII:10.5*t*

pharmacokinetics, VIII:3.6*t*

for pharyngitis, VIII:6.8*t*

Benzoates, contraindications to, in urticaria, V:15.3

Benzoyl peroxide

for acne conglobata, VI:10.5*t*

for acne vulgaris, VI:10.5*t*

Benzyl penicillin, for meningococcemia, V:18.6

Betamethasone, characteristics, VII:17.5*t*

Biphosphonates, for Paget's disease of bone, VI:20.7

Bismuth subsalicylate

contraindications to, VIII:23.7

for traveler's diarrhea, VIII:13.6; 23.8*t*

prophylactic, VIII:23.7

Bites

arthropod, VII:10.1–10.10

reactions to

local, VII:10.2–10.3

pathogenesis, VII:10.1

systemic allergic, VII:10.3

brown recluse spider, systemic allergic reaction to, VII:10.3

flea, V:11.2; 11.2*f*

papular urticaria with, VII:10.1–10.2

insect, protection from, VIII:23.1–23.2

mosquito, reactions to, VII:10.3

Bitolterol, for asthma, VII:1.4

Black flies, VII:10.3

Black-legged tick, VII:10.3

Black widow spider, VII:10.2*f*

Blastomyces, in fungal arthritis, VIII:16.7

Blastomyces dermatitides, in pneumonia, VIII:5.3*t*

Blastomycosis

diagnosis, VIII:19.3

preferred modalities for, VIII:19.2*t*

treatment, VIII:19.4; 19.4*t*

Blepharitis, VII:7.3*t*

Blepharoconjunctivitis, differential diagnosis, VII:7.4*t*

Blepharospasm, VII:7.3*t*

Blood, culture

in diagnosis of acute epiglottitis, VIII:6.9

in diagnosis of cellulitis, VIII:8.7

in pneumonia, VIII:5.3

Blood pressure, ankle systolic, measurement, V:12.3–12.4; 12.4*f*

Blood uric acid determination, in evaluation of monarthritis, VI:12.3–12.4

Bockhart's impetigo, V:2.4*t*; 2.4–2.5

Bone biopsy

in diagnosis of osteoporosis, VI:20.2–20.3

in osteomyelitis, VIII:15.5

Bone densitometry, in diagnosis of osteoporosis, VI:20.2

Bone diseases, metabolic, VI:20.1–20.8

Bone marrow transplantation, infectious agents in, VIII:20.2*t*

Bone scans, in diagnosis of systemic mastocytosis, VII:12.4; 12.5*f*

Cutaneous polyarteritis nodosa, VI:7.6; 10.12
Cutaneous vasculitis, symptoms associated with, VII:8.3
Cutis calcinosis, V:21.10f; 21.10–21.11
  dystrophic, V:21.10
    types, V:21.10
    treatment, V:21.11
Cyanosis, in asthma, VII:1.2
Cyclizine, characteristics, VII:5.6t
Cyclobenzaprine, for fibromyalgia, VI:11.6
Cyclophosphamide
  adverse effects, V:20.4, VII:17.6t
  for bullous pemphigoid, V:20.4
  for cicatricial pemphigoid, V:20.4
  for idiopathic inflammatory myopathies, VI:6.8
  as immunomodulator, VII:17.6
  for large vessel vasculitis, V:16.3
  for lung involvement in scleroderma, VI:5.8
  for maintenance therapy in renal disease with SLE, VI:4.5
  for myositis, V:14.8
  for pemphigus vulgaris, V:20.6
  for pyoderma gangrenosum, V:16.6
  for scleroderma, VI:5.8t
  for vasculitis, VII:14.3t
  for Wegener's granulomatosis, VI:7.4
Cycloserine, for tuberculosis, VIII:18.5t
Cyclospora, in diarrhea, VIII:13.3t; 13.5f
Cyclosporin A
  for chronic actinic dermatitis, V:13.6
  for pustular psoriasis, V:18.4
Cyclosporine
  adverse reactions to, VII:17.6t
  for antirejection prophylaxis, VIII:21.2
  for asthma, VII:1.7
  for Behçet's disease, V:16.4t
  for bullous pemphigoid, V:20.4
  dosage and administration, VII:17.6
  drug interactions, VIII:21.7
  and gout, VI:12.2
  for idiopathic inflammatory myopathies, VI:6.8
  low-dose, for resistant Behçet's disease, VII:14.8
  for myositis, V:14.8
  for psoriasis, VI:10.3t
  for psoriatic arthritis, VI:8.9; 10.4t
  for relapsing polychondritis, VI:18.4; 18.4f
  for scleroderma, VI:5.8t
Cyproheptadine
  characteristics, VII:5.6t
  dosage and administration, VII:8.8t
Cyproheptadine hydrochloride, for urticaria, V:15.3
Cyst(s)
  definition, V:1.3t
  epidermal inclusion, V:7.5; 7.5f; 7.5t
  trichilemmal, V:7.5; 7.5f
  types, V:7.5; 7.5t
Cystic fibrosis, differential diagnosis, VII:3.2–3.3
Cystitis
  acute, treatment, VIII:9.4–9.5
    duration, VIII:9.4t
  signs and symptoms, VIII:9.3
  in women, differential diagnosis, VIII:9.3
Cytarabine, adverse effects, V:19.11
Cytokines
  for cancer patient host defenses, VIII:20.6
  and immune system, VII:17.2t; 17.7
Cytomegalovirus
  clinical syndrome from, VIII:13.4t
  in fever of unknown origin, VIII:4.3
    in HIV-infected (AIDS) patient, VIII:4.6
  infection, in HIV-infected (AIDS) patient, VIII:22.5–22.6
    diagnosis, VIII:22.5t
    treatment, VIII:22.5–22.6

methicillin-resistant, VIII:7.2
  in neutropenic patient, VIII:20.3t
  in organ transplant recipients, VIII:21.4–21.5
    effects, VIII:21.4–21.5; 21.5t
    patterns, VIII:21.4
    prevention, VIII:21.5
    treatment, VIII:21.5
  in pharyngitis, VIII:6.6t
  sexually transmitted disease, VIII:10.1t
Cytomegalovirus hyperimmune globulin, for cytomegalovirus in organ transplant recipients, VIII:21.5
  prophylactic, VIII:21.5
Cytotoxics
  for meningoencephalitis and posterior uveitis, VII:14.8
  for vasculitis, VII:14.3t

D

Dactylitis, VI:9.1; 9.2f
Danazol
  for chronic autoimmune hemolytic anemia with SLE, VI:4.6
  for thrombocytopenia with SLE, VI:4.6
Danocrine, for angioneurotic edema, VII:13.6
Dapsone
  for Behçet's disease, V:16.4t
  for bullous pemphigoid, V:20.4
  for cicatricial pemphigoid, V:20.4
  for cutaneous lupus erythematosus, V:14.5t, VI:4.6
  for dermatitis herpetiformis, V:20.7
  for necrotizing venulitis, V:16.3
  oral, for recurrent aphthous ulcerations, VII:14.8
  for Pneumocystis carinii pneumonia, VIII:22.4
    prophylactic, VIII:22.3t
  for pustular psoriasis, V:18.4
  for pyoderma gangrenosum, V:16.6
  for Sweet's syndrome, V:16.3
  for toxoplasmosis prophylaxis, VIII:22.4
Darier's disease, V:3.5
Darier's sign, VII:12.1
Debridement
  for fungal arthritis, VIII:16.7
  for pyoderma gangrenosum, V:16.5
  for septic infections, VIII:1.5
Decongestants, VII:5.7t
  combinations with antihistamines and anti-cholinergics, VII:5.7
  for ocular allergic disorders, VII:7.5
  oral, side effects, VII:5.7
  for rhinitis, VII:5.7
  topical, side effects, VII:5.7
Deep tissue biopsy, in diagnosis of histoplasmosis, VIII:19.2
Deer flies, VII:10.3
Deferoxamine, for aluminum intoxication, VI:13.6
Degenerative disk disease, VI:8.9–8.10
  of ochronosis, VI:13.5
Degenerative joint disease, treatment, VI:12.7
Dehydroepiandrosterone sulfate, levels, in hyper-androgenemia, V:21.7
Dennie's line, VII:7.3
Deossification, V-shaped area, in osteoporosis, VI:20.8f
Dercum's disease, V:7.5
Dermatitis, V:9.1
  atopic, V:9.4t; 9.4–9.5
  chronic actinic, V:13.5–13.6; 13.7f
    clinical presentation, V:13.5
    management, V:13.6
    pathophysiology, V:13.6

photo tests for, V:13.6
  spectrum, V:13.6t
  clinical features, V:9.1
  contact, V:9.1–9.3
  eczematous, V:9.1
  exfoliative, V:9.8
    associated malignancies, V:19.7t
    clinical characteristics, V:19.7t
  hand and foot, V:9.5f; 9.5–9.6
  linear IgA, V:20.7
  stages, V:9.1
Dermatitis herpetiformis, V:20.6–20.7
  associated malignancies, V:19.7t
  clinical features, V:19.7t; 20.6–20.7
  diagnosis, V:20.7
  treatment, V:20.7
Dermatofibroma, V:1.6f; 7.3; 7.3f
  pigmented, V:6.5t
Dermatofibrosarcoma protuberans, V:7.3
Dermatographism, VII:8.3f
  diagnosis, VII:8.4t
  treatment, VII:8.4t
  in urticaria, V:15.2–15.3; 15.3f
Dermatologic diagnosis, V:1.1–1.11
Dermatologic tests, V:1.9–1.10
Dermatomyositis, V:14.6f; 14.6–14.9, VI:6.1–6.8.
    See also Idiopathic inflammatory myopathy(ies); Myositis
  in adults, clinical features, VI:6.2–6.3
  associated malignancies, V:19.7t
  classification, V:14.6
  clinical features, V:14.6–14.7; 19.7t, VI:6.1–6.4
  diagnostic criteria for, V:14.6
  electromyographic features, V:14.7
  juvenile, VI:6.4
  nail fold changes in, V:14.6; 14.7f
  prognosis, V:14.9
  rash in, VI:6.3; 6.3f
  systemic involvement in, V:14.7
Dermatomyositis-sine-myositis, diagnosis, V:14.6–14.7
Dermatopathy, diabetic, V:21.1–21.2
Dermatophytoses, V:4.1–4.6
  clinical features, V:4.1–4.4
  diagnosis, V:4.4
  treatment, V:4.5t; 4.5–4.6
Dermatosis, V:9.1
  life-threatening, V:18.1–18.7
  neutrophilic, V:16.1–16.6
  photoaggravated, V:13.6–13.7; 13.7t
Dermatosis papulosa nigra, V:7.2; 7.2f
Dexamethasone
  characteristics, VII:17.5t
  for meningitis, VIII:12.7–12.9
  for rhinitis, VII:5.8t
  topical
    for rhinitis, VII:5.8
    side effects, VII:5.8
Dexamethasone suppression test, in diagnosis of Cushing's syndrome, V:21.8
Dexchlorpheniramine, characteristics, VII:5.6t
Diabetes mellitus
  infections in, V:21.2–21.3
  leg and foot ulcers in, V:21.3f; 21.3–21.4
    infected
      evaluation, V:21.4
      treatment, V:21.4
      organisms causing, V:21.4
  musculoskeletal manifestations, VI:13.1
    management, VI:13.2t
  neuropathic leg ulcer in, V:12.4; 12.4f
  pruritus in, VII:11.2–11.3
  skin dermatoses in, V:21.1–21.4; 21.2t
    inflammatory, V:21.1–21.2; 21.2f

Itraconazole (*continued*)
    for histoplasmosis, VIII:19.4; 19.4*t*
        in HIV-infected (AIDS) patient, VIII:22.6
    for soft-tissue infections, VIII:8.8*t*
    spectrum of activity, V:4.5*t*

J

Japanese encephalitis vaccine, VIII:23.4
    for travelers, VIII:2.7*t*
Joint(s)
    drainage, for infectious arthritis, VIII:16.6
    lavage, for osteoarthritis, VI:15.4
    mycobacterial infections, treatment, VI:12.7
    protracted inflammation, VI:14.5–14.6
        joint damage from, VI:14.6; 14.6*f*
    trauma, consequences, VI:12.2; 12.2*f*
    tumors, VI:18.4
Joint fluid examination, in diagnosis of infectious
        arthritis, VI:14.2–14.3
Juxta-articular erosions, in hyperparathyroidism,
        VI:13.3*f*

K

Kanamycin, for tuberculosis, VIII:18.5*t*
Kaposi's sarcoma, V:1.6*f*
Kaposi's varicelliform eruption, V:3.5; 3.5*f*
Kasabach-Merritt syndrome, purpura fulminans
        from, V:18.5–18.6
Kawasaki's disease, VI:10.12–10.13; 10.13*f*;
        VII:14.7–14.8
    clinical course, VII:14.8
Kawasaki syndrome, V:18.5
    diagnostic criteria for, V:18.5; 18.5*t*
    treatment, V:18.5
Keloids, V:7.3–7.4; 7.4*f*
    treatment, V:7.4; 7.4*t*
Keratoacanthoma, V:5.3
Keratoconjunctivitis sicca, differential diagnosis,
        VII:7.4*t*; 7.5
Keratoderma blennorrhagica, on soles of feet, in
        Reiter's syndrome, VI:9.1; 9.3*f*
Kernig's sign, in meningitis, VIII:12.2
Ketanserin, for Raynaud's phenomenon, VI:5.3*t*
Ketoconazole
    for allergic bronchopulmonary aspergillosis,
        VII:3.5
    for blastomycosis, VIII:19.4; 19.4*t*
    for candidiasis, V:4.6–4.7
        in HIV-infected (AIDS) patient, VIII:22.6
    contraindications to, VII:5.6
    dosage and administration, V:4.5–4.6
    drug interactions, V:15.3, VIII:21.7
    for histoplasmosis, VIII:19.4; 19.4*t*
    spectrum of activity, V:4.5*t*
Ketoprofen, cross-reactivity, VII:11.9*t*
Ketorolac tromethamine, for allergic conjunctivitis,
        VII:7.5
Ketotifen, for asthma, VII:1.7
Kidney transplantation, for renal involvement in
        scleroderma, VI:5.8–5.9
Kinin system, VI:13.6*f*
Kissing bugs, VII:10.3; 10.3*f*
Klebsiella spp.
    antibiotic resistance, VIII:3.3
    antibiotics for, VIII:3.5*t*
    in catheter-related peritonitis, VIII:14.6
    in neutropenic patient, VIII:20.3*t*
    in nosocomial pneumonia, VIII:7.2
    in sepsis, VIII:1.5*t*
    in urinary tract infections, VIII:9.2; 9.2*t*

Klebsiella-Enterobacter spp., in leg and foot ulcers in
        diabetes, V:21.4
Klebsiella pneumoniae
    antibiotic resistance, variations in, VIII:3.4
    antibiotics for, VIII:3.3*t*
    in cellulitis, VIII:8.6
    in epiglottitis, VIII:6.9*t*
    in peritonitis, VIII:14.1
    in pneumonia, VIII:5.3*t*; 5.4–5.5
    in sinusitis, VIII:6.2
Knee
    effusions, benign, associated with adrenocorti-
        costeroid withdrawal, VI:18.4
    internal derangements, clinical features,
        VI:16.3*t*
    menisci
        functions, VI:16.4*t*
        torn, VI:16.3
Knee pain, VI:16.2–16.4
    treatment, VI:16.4*t*
Koebner phenomenon, V:1.10*f*

L

Laboratory tests
    predictive value, VI:3.4*f*
    sensitivity, VI:3.4*f*
    specificity, VI:3.4*f*
β-Lactam antibiotics, VIII:3.2*t*; 3.3–3.4
    adverse reactions to, VII:11.4–11.5
β-Lactamase inhibitors, VIII:3.4
    for osteomyelitis, VIII:15.6*t*
Laparoscopy
    disadvantages, VIII:10.6
    in pelvic inflammatory disease, VIII:10.6
    in salpingitis, VIII:14.9
Laryngitis, VIII:6.8–6.10
    acute, VIII:6.8–6.9
    clinical presentation, VIII:6.9
    etiology, VIII:6.8; 6.8*t*
    laboratory diagnosis, VIII:6.9
    treatment, VIII:6.9–6.10
Laryngoscopy, in diagnosis of acute epiglottitis,
        VIII:6.9
Lassa fever, VIII:23.13
Lateral cutaneous nerve, compression, symptoms,
        VI:16.6
Latex
    allergy to, VII:11.6
        surgery with, VII:11.6
    anaphylactoid reactions to, VII:9.4
Leg, sensory innervation, VI:16.6*f*
Legionella spp.
    in cellulitis, VIII:8.6
    in neutropenic patient, VIII:20.3*t*
    in pneumonia, VIII:5.3*t*
Legionella pneumophila
    infection
        diagnosis, VIII:5.5
        symptoms, VIII:5.5
    in pneumonia, VIII:5.3*t*; 5.5
    sputum with, VIII:5.2
Leg ulcers, V:12.1–12.9
    with antiphospholipid antibody syndrome,
        V:12.5*t*; 12.6
    arterial, V:12.2*t*; 12.3*f*; 12.3–12.4; 12.4*f*; 12.5*f*
        treatment, V:12.8
    atypical
        causes, V:12.4–12.7
        treatment, V:12.8; 12.8*t*
    causes, V:12.1; 12.2*t*; 12.2–12.4
    with cholesterol emboli, V:12.5*t*; 12.6; 12.6*f*
    cleansing, V:12.7

in cryoproteinemia, V:12.5*f*; 12.5*t*; 12.5–12.6
    diagnosis, V:12.1–12.2; 12.2*t*
    differential diagnosis, V:12.1; 12.2*t*
    factitial, V:12.6; 12.7*f*
    granulation tissue formation, V:12.7–12.8
    in neoplasia, V:12.7
    neuropathic, V:12.2*t*; 12.4; 12.5*f*
        treatment, V:12.8
    occlusive dressings for, V:12.7*f*; 12.7–12.8
    with pyoderma gangrenosum, V:12.5*t*; 12.6;
        12.6*f*
    treatment, V:12.7–12.8
    venous, V:12.2*t*; 12.2–12.3; 12.3*f*
        treatment, V:12.8; 12.8*f*
    vitamin A derivatives for, V:12.8
Lentigines, V:1.5*f*; 6.3*f*
Lentigo, V:6.3*f*; 6.4*f*
Leptospira spp., in fever of unknown origin, VIII:4.3*t*
Leser-Trélat sign, V:7.1
    associated malignancies, V:19.8*t*
    clinical characteristics, V:19.8*t*
Lesion biopsy
    in blastomycosis, VIII:19.3
    in cellulitis, VIII:8.8
Leukemia
    acute
        cutaneous infection in, VIII:20.3*f*
        infectious agents in, VIII:20.2*t*
    acute myelogenous, infections in, VIII:20.1
    arthritis associated with, VI:17.1–17.2
    chronic lymphocytic, infectious agents in,
        VIII:20.2*t*
    hairy cell
        infections in, VIII:20.1
        infectious agents in, VIII:20.2*t*
    mast cell, VII:12.3–12.4
Leukemia cutis, V:19.2; 19.3*f*
Leukemic synovitis, VI:17.1
    characteristics, VI:17.2*t*
Leukocyte count
    in cellulitis, VIII:8.7
    in pneumonia, VIII:5.3
    in urinary tract infections, VIII:9.3
Leukocyte-esterase dipstick method, in diagnosis
        of urinary tract infections, VIII:9.3–9.4
Leukocytoclastic vasculitis, V:16.1–16.2
Levocabastine, for ocular allergic disorders,
        VII:7.5; 7.6*t*
Lichenification, V:1.7*f*
    definition, V:1.3*t*
Lichen planus, V:1.9; 1.10*f*
Lichen sclerosus et atrophicus, V:14.9
Lidocaine
    for Behçet's disease, V:16.4*t*
    for local reaction to insect sting, VII:10.7*t*
    use in arthrocentesis, VIII:16.4
Lincosamides, VIII:3.2*t*
Lipodermatosclerosis, V:12.2–12.3; 12.3*f*
    treatment, V:12.9
Lipomas, V:7.5–7.6
Liposclerosis, V:9.9
Listeria spp., neoplastic disorders and therapies
        associated with, VIII:20.2*t*
Listeria monocytogenes
    in fever of unknown origin, VIII:4.3*t*
    in meningitis, VIII:12.7*t*
        treatment, VIII:12.6*t*; 12.7
    in neutropenic patient, VIII:20.3*t*
    in organ transplant recipients, VIII:21.6
Livedo reticularis, with leg ulcers, V:12.5; 12.5*t*
Liver spots, V:1.5*f*
Local anesthetics, VII:11.8*t*
    allergic reactions to, VII:11.7–11.8
    topical, adverse effects, V:17.7

Phototoxicity (*continued*)
  photopatch testing contraindicated in, V:13.5
  photo tests for, V:13.3*t*
  treatment, V:13.5
Phthalic anhydride, and hypersensitivity pneumonitis, VII:4.2*t*
Phthirus pubis, in sexually transmitted diseases, VIII:10.1*t*
Physical therapy
  for hemochromatosis, VI:13.5
  for osteoarthritis, VI:15.3
  for shoulder pain, VI:16.2
Pigeon breeders, hypersensitivity pneumonitis in, VII:4.4
Pigmentation, abnormal. *See also* Hyperpigmentation; Hypopigmentation
  in systemic sclerosis, V:14.11; 14.11*f*
Pigmented villonodular synovitis, VI:18.4
Piperacillin
  and amikacin, for soft-tissue infections, VIII:8.8*t*
  and aminoglycoside, for secondary peritonitis, VIII:14.5*t*
  and gentamicin
    for nosocomial pneumonia, VIII:7.4*t*
    for soft-tissue infections, VIII:8.8*t*
  for neutropenia, VIII:20.5
  for osteomyelitis, VIII:15.6*t*
  pharmacokinetics, VIII:3.6*t*
  for primary peritonitis, VIII:14.2*t*
  and tazobactam
    pharmacokinetics, VIII:3.6*t*
    for soft-tissue infections, VIII:8.8*t*
    spectrum of *in vitro* activity, VIII:3.5*t*
  and tobramycin
    for sepsis, VIII:1.5*t*
    for soft-tissue infections, VIII:8.8*t*
  use with β-lactamase inhibitors, VIII:3.4
Piperazines
  characteristics, VII:5.6*t*
  dosage and administration, VII:8.8*t*
Piperidines
  characteristics, VII:5.6*t*
  dosage and administration, VII:8.8*t*
Pirbuterol, for asthma, VII:1.4
Piroxicam
  adverse effects, V:17.2; 17.4; 17.5
  cross-reactivity, VII:11.9*t*
  for palindromic rheumatism, VI:18.2
Pituitary disorders
  cutaneous manifestations, V:21.9*t*
  musculoskeletal manifestations, VI:13.4
Pituitary surgery, for Cushing's disease, V:21.8
Pityriasis, V:4.7; 4.7*f*
Pityriasis rosea, clinical features, V:8.3*t*
Pityriasis rotunda
  associated malignancies, V:19.8*t*
  clinical characteristics, V:19.8*t*
Pityriasis rubra pilaris, clinical features, V:8.3*t*
Pityrosporum ovale, V:9.6
Plaque, definition, V:1.3*t*
Plasma cell dyscrasias, rheumatic manifestations, VI:17.3
Plasma exchange, VII:17.4
Plasmapheresis, VII:17.3–17.4
  for digital ulcers in Raynaud's phenomenon, VI:5.3
  for idiopathic inflammatory myopathies, VI:6.8
  for maintenance therapy in renal disease with SLE, VI:4.5
  for scleroderma, VI:5.8*t*
Plasmodium spp., in fever of unknown origin, VIII:4.3*t*
Plasmodium falciparum, drug-resistant, VIII:23.4

Plesiomonas shigelloides
  in diarrhea, VIII:13.3*t*
  in traveler's diarrhea, VIII:13.5
Pneumococcal bacteremia, incidence, VIII:2.3; 2.3*f*
Pneumococcal disease, mortality from, VIII:2.1; 2.2*t*
Pneumococcal vaccine, VIII:2.1–2.3
  administration in HIV, VII:16.8
  adverse reactions to, VIII:2.2
  aggressive use, VIII:2.2–2.3
  dosage and administration, VIII:2.2
  future, VIII:2.8*t*
  for HIV-infected (AIDS) patient, VIII:2.6*t*
  indications for, VIII:2.2*t*
    prevalence, VIII:2.2; 2.3*f*
  routine immunization of adults with, VIII:2.2*t*
Pneumoconiosis, differential diagnosis, VII:4.6
Pneumocystis spp., neoplastic disorders and therapies associated with, VIII:20.2*t*
Pneumocystis carinii
  in neutropenic patient, VIII:20.3*t*
  in organ transplant recipients, VIII:21.6
  pneumonia
    and fever of unknown origin in HIV-infected (AIDS) patient, VIII:4.6
    in HIV-infected (AIDS) patient, VIII:22.3–22.4
      diagnosis, VIII:22.4
      prevention, VIII:22.3*t*; 22.3–22.4
      treatment, VIII:22.4
    nosocomial, VIII:7.3
    prophylaxis for, VII:16.7
Pneumonia. *See also Pneumocystis carinii*, pneumonia
  aspiration, causes, VIII:5.5
  atypical
    causes, VIII:5.5
    characteristics, VIII:5.2*t*
  bacterial, characteristics, VIII:5.2*t*
  community-acquired, etiologic agents, VIII:5.3*t*
  etiologic agents, VIII:5.3–5.6
  evaluation in, VIII:5.1–5.3
    epidemiologic issues in, VIII:5.2*t*
  hospitalization for, VIII:5.1
    indications for, VIII:5.3
  increased mortality from, risk factors for, VIII:5.3*t*
  mixed bacterial, VIII:5.4*f*
  nosocomial, VIII:7.1–7.6
    bacteriologic classification, VIII:7.3*t*
    bacteriology, VIII:7.2–7.3
    clinical features, VIII:7.3
    diagnosis, VIII:7.3
    diagnostic criteria for, VIII:7.3*t*
    mortality from, VIII:7.1
    pathogenesis, VIII:7.1; 7.2*t*
    prevalence, VIII:7.1
    prevention, VIII:7.4–7.5; 7.5*t*
    treatment, VIII:7.4; 7.4*t*
  outpatient treatment, VIII:5.6–5.7
    with antibiotics, VIII:5.6*t*
    patient follow-up for, VIII:5.7
  prevalence, VIII:5.1
  prevention, VIII:5.7
  radiographic findings in, VIII:5.2
  sputum studies in, VIII:5.2–5.3
  symptoms, VIII:5.1–5.2
  underlying conditions in, VIII:5.2
Pocket erosion, natural radiographic history, VI:2.7*f*
POEMS syndrome, in plasma cell dyscrasias, VI:17.3; 17.3*t*
Poikiloderma, in dermatomyositis, V:14.6; 14.7*f*

Poliomyelitis vaccine, VIII:23.4
Polio vaccine, VII:17.8*t*
  oral, for HIV-infected (AIDS) patient, VIII:2.6*t*
  for travelers, VIII:2.7*t*
Pollen immunotherapy, VII:17.7
Polyarteritis nodosa, VII:14.4
  cutaneous, VI:7.6; 10.12
  diagnostic criteria for, VII:14.2*t*
  differential diagnosis, VII:14.4
  prevalence, VII:14.4
  symptoms, VII:14.4
  treatment, VII:14.3*t*
Polyarteritis overlap syndrome, VII:14.4–14.5
Polyarthritis
  chronic, classification, VI:2.2*t*
  early, differential diagnosis, VI:12.6
  poststreptococcal, characteristics, VI:9.2*t*
Polyclonal antibody, for antirejection prophylaxis, VIII:21.2
Polyclonal sera, for cancer patient host defenses, VIII:20.6
Polycystic ovary disease
  differential diagnosis, V:21.8
  treatment, V:21.8
Polycythemia vera, pruritus in, V:11.3
Poly-Histine-D, VII:5.7
Polymorphous light eruption, V:13.2–13.3; 13.3*f*
  photo tests for, V:13.3*t*
  treatment, V:13.2–13.3
Polymyalgia rheumatica, VII:14.6
  erythrocyte sedimentation rate in, VI:1.5
Polymyositis, VI:6.1–6.8. *See also* Idiopathic inflammatory myopathy(ies); Myositis
  in adults, VI:6.1–6.2
    clinical features, VI:6.2
  clinical features, VI:6.1–6.4
  vs. dermatomyositis, V:14.6
  prognosis, V:14.9
Polymyositis/dermatomyositis. *See also* Collagen vascular disease
  clinical manifestations, VI:3.2; 3.2*t*
  pathophysiology, VI:3.2
  serologic manifestations, VI:3.3*t*
Polymyxin B, pharmacokinetics, VIII:3.7*t*
Polymyxins, VIII:3.2*t*
  spectrum of *in vitro* activity, VIII:3.5*t*
Polyserositis, recurrent. *See* Familial Mediterranean fever
Polysporin, topical, for infected diabetic leg and foot ulcers, V:21.4
Polyunsaturated ethyl ester lipids, for psoriatic arthritis, VI:10.4*t*
Porcine protein, and hypersensitivity pneumonitis, VII:4.2*t*
Porphyria cutanea tarda, V:21.8
  bullae and erosion in, V:21.9*f*
  diagnosis, V:21.9
  hypertrichosis form, V:21.9*f*
Porphyrias, cutaneous manifestations, V:21.8–21.9
Positive end-expiratory pressure, for sepsis, VIII:1.6*f*
Postantibiotic effect, VIII:3.8
Posterior uveitis, in Behçet's disease, V:16.4
Post-herpetic neuralgia, V:3.7
Posttransplant lymphoproliferative disorder, EBV-associated, VIII:21.5
  clinical manifestations, VIII:21.5
  management, VIII:21.5
Potassium channel blockers, for asthma, VII:1.7
Potassium hydroxide, in diagnosis of dermatophytoses, V:4.4

Strongyloides stercoralis
  in neutropenic patient, VIII:20.3*t*
  in organ transplant recipients, VIII:21.2
Subconjunctival hemorrhages, VII:7.3*t*
Subperiosteal bone resorption, in hyperparathy-
    roidism, VI:13.3; 13.3*f*
Sucralfate, for scleroderma gastrointestinal disease,
    VI:5.8*t*
Sulbactam. *See* Ampicillin
Sulconazole, spectrum of activity, V:4.5*t*
Sulfadiazine, for toxoplasmosis, VIII:22.5
Sulfapyridine, for pyoderma gangrenosum, V:16.6
Sulfasalazine
  adverse effects, V:17.7
  for enteropathic or reactive arthritis, VI:8.9
  for peripheral arthritis in ankylosing spondylitis,
    VI:8.7
  for psoriatic arthritis, VI:10.4*t*
Sulfites, adverse effects, VII:1.5
Sulfonamide, adverse effects, V:17.4
Sulfonamides
  adverse effects, V:17.2; 17.3; 17.5; 17.7,
    VII:11.2*t*; 11.8–11.9
  contraindications to, V:18.6
  in prevention of *Pneumocystis carinii* infection in
    organ transplant recipients, VIII:21.6
  reactions to, VII:4.5
  for soft-tissue infections, VIII:8.8*t*
  topical, adverse effects, V:17.7
Sulindac
  for ankylosing spondylitis, VI:8.7
  cross-reactivity, VII:11.9*t*
Sunlight
  electromagnetic radiation from, classification,
    V:13.1; 13.2*t*
  skin exposure to, effects, V:13.1; 13.2*t*
Sunscreen, V:13.3
  for chronic actinic dermatitis, V:13.6
  for cutaneous disease in myositis, V:14.8
  for cutaneous lupus erythematosus, V:14.5;
    14.5*t*
  for herpes labialis-associated erythema multi-
    forme, V:15.6
  for photosensitivity drug eruption prophylaxis,
    V:17.5
Superficial pustular perifolliculitis, V:2.4*t*; 2.4–2.5
Suppurative pelvic thrombophlebitis, VIII:14.10
Supraglottic structures, VIII:6.8*f*
Surgery
  for chronic sinusitis, VIII:6.5
  and immune system, VII:17.2*t*
Sweet's syndrome, V:16.3; 16.3*f*, VI:10.9; 10.10*f*
  associated malignancies, V:19.8*t*
  clinical features, V:16.3; 19.8*t*
  differential diagnosis, V:16.3
  histopathology, V:16.3
  patient evaluation in, V:16.3
  prognosis, V:16.3
  treatment, V:16.3
Symmetric synovitis of wrists and carpal joints,
    diagnosis, VI:2.2
Sympathectomy
  microsurgical digital, for digital ulcers in
    Raynaud's phenomenon, VI:5.3
  pharmacologic cervical, for digital ulcers in
    Raynaud's phenomenon, VI:5.3
Syndesmophytes, VI:8.4; 8.5*f*
Synechia, VII:5.4*f*
Synovial biopsy, VI:1.3
  in diagnosis of tubercular arthritis, VIII:16.9
Synovial chondromatosis, VI:18.4
Synovial fluid
  analysis, in evaluation of monarthritis,
    VI:12.4–12.6

appearance, VI:12.4; 12.5*f*
  in gout, VI:12.4; 12.5*f*
  in traumatized joints, VI:12.4; 12.5*f*
cell counts, VI:1.2; 12.5
characteristics
  in arthritis, VI:12.5*t*
  in infectious arthritis, VIII:16.3; 16.4*t*
crystal identification in, VI:12.5–12.6
crystals in, VI:1.2–1.3; 1.3*f*
culture, VI:1.2
gross characteristics, VI:1.2
Synovial sarcoma, VI:18.4
Synovial soft-tissue swelling, VI:2.3*f*
Synovitis, crystal-induced, differential diagnosis,
    VI:18.2
Syphilis, VIII:10.1*t*; 10.7
  arthritis from, VI:14.3–14.4
  diagnosis, VIII:10.7
  early, treatment, VIII:10.5*t*
  in HIV-infected (AIDS) patient, VIII:10.7;
    22.6
    treatment, VIII:22.6
  in laryngitis, VIII:6.9*t*
  nontreponemal serologic tests for, VIII:10.5*t*
  secondary, cutaneous involvement in, clinical
    features, V:8.3*t*
  treatment, VIII:10.7
  treponemal serologic tests for, VIII:10.5*t*
Syringomas, V:7.7; 7.7*f*
Systemic disorders, with prominent cutaneous
    manifestations, V:18.4–18.6; 18.6*t*
Systemic inflammatory response syndrome,
    VIII:1.1–1.7
  definition, VIII:1.2*t*
  iatrogenic, VIII:1.1
Systemic lupus erythematosus, V:14.1–14.6,
    VI:1.5; 4.1–4.7. *See also* Collagen
    vascular disease
  butterfly facial rash in, VI:4.2*f*
  chronic arthritis in, drug therapy for, VI:4.3*t*
  clinical manifestations, VI:3.2; 3.2*t*
  cutaneous, V:14.1–14.6
    chronic, differential diagnosis, V:14.2
    evaluation, V:14.5*t*
    laboratory abnormalities in, V:14.4
    subacute, V:14.3, VI:4.4*f*
      annular lesions in, V:14.3; 14.3*f*
      differential diagnosis, V:14.2
      disease associations, V:14.3
      papulosquamous lesions in, V:14.3; 14.3*f*;
        14.4*f*
    treatment, V:14.4–14.6; 14.5*t*
  diagnostic criteria for, V:14.2*t*, VI:4.2*t*
  drug-induced, V:17.6, VI:1.5; 1.5*t*
  malar eruption in, V:10.4
  mucocutaneous lesions in, classification, V:14.2*t*
  musculoskeletal features, VI:4.3
  neuropsychiatric manifestations, VI:4.5–4.6;
    4.6*t*
    diagnostic measures in, VI:4.6*t*
  new therapies for, VI:4.6–4.7
  pathophysiology, VI:3.1
  in pharyngitis, VIII:6.6*t*
  photosensitivity in, V:13.6
  serologic manifestations, VI:3.3*t*
  treatment
    for constitutional symptoms, VI:4.3–4.4
    for rash, VI:4.3–4.4
    for serositis, VI:4.3–4.4
Systemic necrotizing vasculitis, VII:14.3–14.6;
    14.5*t*
  complications, VII:14.3
  polyarteritis nodosa group, VII:14.4*t*; 14.4–14.5
  diagnosis, VII:14.5

Systemic sclerosis, V:14.10–14.11, VI:5.4–5.9. *See
    also* Collagen vascular disease
  clinical manifestations, VI:3.2; 3.2*t*, 5.4–5.6
  diffuse vs. limited, V:14.10
  serologic manifestations, VI:3.3*t*
  systemic disease in, V:14.11

T

Tachycardia, in sepsis, VIII:1.3
Tachyphylaxis, VII:1.5
Tachypnea, in sepsis, VIII:1.3
Takayasu's arteritis, VI:7.3–7.4, VII:14.7
  angiographic findings in, VI:7.4; 7.4*f*
Tar, for psoriasis, VI:10.3*t*
Target lesions, in bullous erythema multiforme,
    V:17.4; 17.4*f*
Tattoo, clinical features, V:6.5*t*
Technetium diphosphonate scanning, in diagnosis
    of infectious arthritis, VI:14.2
Telangiectasia, in systemic sclerosis, V:14.11; 14.11*f*
Temporal arteritis. *See also* Giant cell vasculitis
  erythrocyte sedimentation rate in, VI:1.5
Temporal artery, enlarged, in large vessel vasculitis,
    VI:7.3; 7.3*f*
Tendon infections, VI:14.5
Tendon xanthomas, in hyperlipidemia, VI:17.6; 17.6*f*
Tenosynovitis, VI:14.5
  in disseminated gonococcal infection, VIII:10.8
Terbinafine
  dosage and administration, V:4.6
  spectrum of activity, V:4.5*t*
Terbutaline, for asthma, VII:1.4
Terconazole, for candidiasis, VIII:10.5*t*
Terfenadine
  actions, VII:5.6–5.7
  adverse effects, VII:5.6; 8.8
  for angioedema and urticaria, VII:8.8
  contraindications to, VII:11.4*t*
  dosage and administration, VII:8.8*t*
  drug interactions, V:15.3
  drugs that retard metabolism, VII:5.6
  for rhinitis, VII:5.5
  for urticaria, V:15.3
Test dosing, for adverse reactions to local anesthet-
    ics, VII:11.9*t*
Tetanus
  incidence
    by age group, VIII:2.6*t*
    in U.S., 1955-1991, VIII:2.6*t*
  toxoid, in patient with history of adverse reac-
    tion attributed to tetanus, VII:11.8*t*
  vaccine, VII:17.8*t*
Tetanus/diphtheria, mortality from, VIII:2.2*t*
Tetanus-diphtheria vaccine
  administration in HIV, VII:16.8
  routine immunization of adults with, VIII:2.2*t*
  toxoid, VIII:2.5
  schedule for, VIII:2.5
Tetracycline(s), VIII:3.2*t*
  for acne fulminans, VI:10.5*t*
  adverse effects, V:17.5, VII:11.2*t*
  for bowel-associated dermatosis-arthritis
    syndrome, V:16.6
  for chlamydia-induced reactive arthritis, VI:8.9
  pharmacokinetics, VIII:3.7*t*
  for pharyngitis, VIII:6.8*t*
  for pneumonia, VIII:5.6*t*
  for Rocky Mountain spotted fever, V:18.6
  for soft-tissue infections, VIII:8.8*t*
  spectrum of *in vitro* activity, VIII:3.5*t*
  for stomatitis from antineoplastic therapy,
    V:19.10

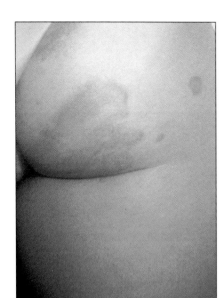

Chapter 8, Figure 2,
p. VII:8.2

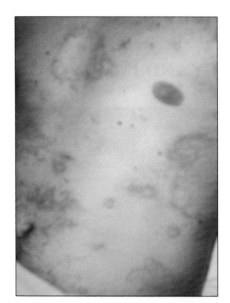

Chapter 8, Figure 3,
p. VII:8.2

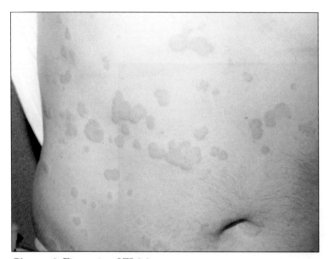

Chapter 8, Figure 4, p. VII:8.2

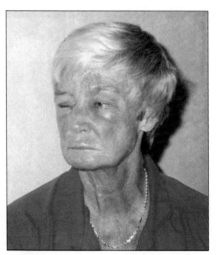

Chapter 8, Figure 5, p. VII:8.2

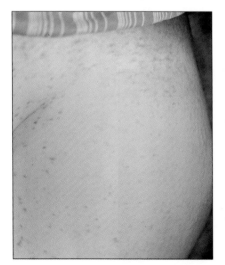

Chapter 8, Figure 9, p. VII:8.5

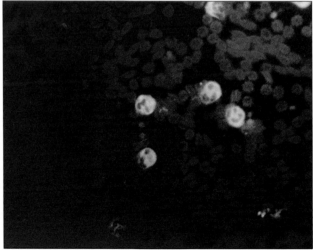

Chapter 14, Figure 4, p. VII:14.6

VIII. INFECTIOUS DISEASES

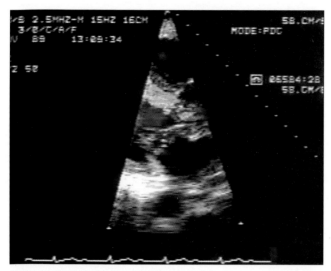

Chapter 11, Figure 3B, p. VIII:11.6

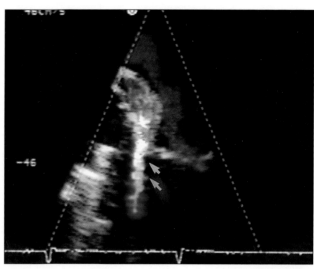

Chapter 11, Figure 4B, p. VIII:11.7

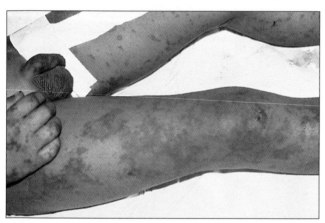

Chapter 12, Figure 2, p. VIII:12.3

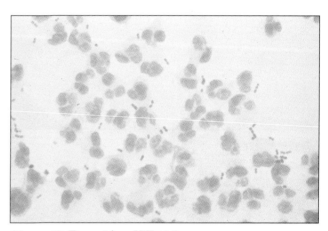

Chapter 12, Figure 3A, p. VIII:12.5

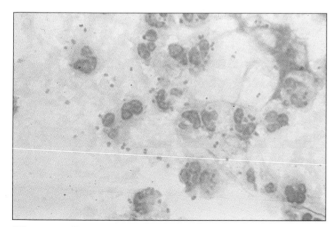

Chapter 12, Figure 3B, p. VIII:12.5

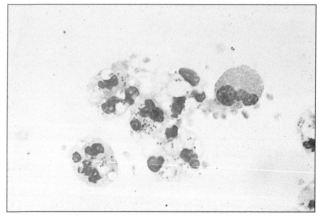

Chapter 12, Figure 3C, p. VIII:12.5